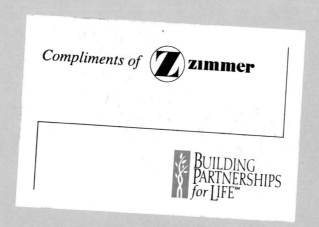

THE ADULT HIP

THE ADULT HIP

Volume II

Editors

John J. Callaghan, M.D.
Department of Orthopaedics
University of Iowa
Iowa City, Iowa 52242

Aaron G. Rosenberg, M.D.
Department of Orthopaedic Surgery
Arthritis and Orthopaedic Institute
Rush Medical College
Chicago, Illinois 60612

Harry E. Rubash, M.D.
Department of Orthopaedic Surgery
University of Pittsburgh Medical Center
Pittsburgh, Pennsylvania 15213

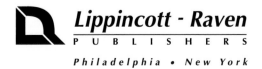

Lippincott - Raven
PUBLISHERS

Philadelphia • New York

Acquisitions Editor: Kathey Alexander
Developmental Editor: Rhoda Dunn
Manufacturing Manager: Dennis Teston
Production Manager: Maxine Langweil
Production Editor: Loretta Cummings
Cover Designer: Karen Quigley
Indexer: Maria L. Coughlin
Compositor: Lippincott–Raven Electronic Production
Printer: Kingsport Press

Printed in the United States of America

9 8 7 6 5 4 3 2 1

The adult hip / editors, John J. Callaghan, Aaron G. Rosenberg, Harry E. Rubash.
   p. cm.
   Includes bibliographical references and index.
   ISBN 0–397–51704–1 (2 v. set) — ISBN 0–7817–1429–X (2 v. set with CD)
   1. Hip joint—Surgery.   2. Hip joint—Diseases.   3. Artificial hip joint.   I. Callaghan, John J.
   II. Rosenberg, Aaron G.   III. Rubash, Harry E.
   [DNLM: 1. Hip joint—surgery.   2. Hip Prosthesis.   3. Joint Diseases—surgery.   4. Hip.
   5. Bone Diseases—surgery.   6. Biocompatible Materials.   WE 860 A2435 1998]
   RD549.A36   1998
   617.5′81—dc21
   DNLM/DLC
   for Library of Congress   97–28141
                                            CIP

To my wife, Kim,
and our children, Patrick and Katie,
for their love, friendship, and never-ending support

J.J.C.

To my wife, Iris,
whose love, support, and example fill my life and world,
and to our wonderful children, AJ, Jess, Becca, and Cody,
who put everything into perspective

A.G.R.

To my wife, Kimberly,
for her love, support, and friendship throughout the years,
and to my children, Bradley, Steven, and Kristin,
for their youth, enthusiasm, vigor, and complexities

H.E.R.

Contents

VOLUME I

SECTION I: HISTORY OF HIP SURGERY

SECTION II: BASIC SCIENCE

Anatomy

Biomaterials

VOLUME II

SECTION V: TOTAL HIP ARTHROPLASTY

Economics and Utilization of Hip Arthroplasty

Primary Total Hip Arthroplasty

Sepsis

SECTION VII: REVISION OF TOTAL HIP ARTHROPLASTY

Revision of the Acetabular Component

Revision of the Femoral Component

Contributing Authors

Roy K. Aaron, M.D.
Clinical Associate Professor
Department of Orthopaedics
Brown University School of Medicine
154 Waterman Street
Providence, Rhode Island 02906

Thomas P. Andriacchi, Ph.D.
Professor
Department of Orthopaedic Surgery
Rush-Presbyterian-St. Luke's Medical Center
1653 West Congress Parkway
Chicago, Illinois 60612

Miguel A. Ayerza, M.D.
Instructor
Department of Orthopaedic Surgery
Italian Hospital of Buenos Aires
Potosí 4125
1199 Buenos Aires
Argentina

W. Timothy Ballard, M.D.
Chattanooga Orthopaedic Group
2415 McCallie Avenue
Chattanooga, Tennessee 37404

William L. Bargar, M.D.
Assistant Clinical Professor
Department of Orthopaedics
University of California Davis School of Medicine
1020 29th Street
Sacramento, California 95816

Robert L. Barrack, M.D.
Professor
Department of Orthopaedic Surgery
Tulane University Medical Center
1430 Tulane Avenue
New Orleans, Louisiana 70112

Arnold T. Berman, M.D.
Department of Orthopaedic Surgery
Allegheny University Hospitals
230 North Broad Street
Philadelphia, Pennsylvania 19102

Daniel J. Berry, M.D.
Consultant in Orthopaedic Surgery
Mayo Clinic;
Assistant Professor of Orthopaedics
Mayo Medical School; and
Department of Orthopaedics
Mayo Foundation
200 First Street SW
Rochester, Minnesota 55905

Jonathan Black, Ph.D.
Principal
IMN Biomaterials
409 Dorothy Drive
King of Prussia, Pennsylvania 19406-2004

J. David Blaha, M.D.
Professor and Chairman
Department of Orthopaedics
West Virginia University
Morgantown, West Virginia 26506-9196

Patrick J. Boland, M.D., F.R.C.S., F.R.C.S.I.
Department of Orthopaedic Surgery
Memorial Sloan-Kettering Cancer Center
1275 York Avenue
New York, New York 10021

Mathias P. G. Bostrom, M.D.
Assistant Attending Orthopaedic Surgeon
Department of Orthopaedics
The Hospital for Special Surgery
Cornell University Medical College
535 East 70th Street
New York, New York 10021

Robert B. Bourne, M.D., F.R.C.S.C.
Professor of Surgery
Department of Orthopaedic Surgery
London Health Sciences Centre
The University of Western Ontario
339 Windermere Road
London, Ontario N6A 5A5
Canada

Barry D. Brause, M.D.
215 East 68th Street
New York, New York 10021

Calvin R. Brown, Jr., M.D.
Assistant Professor
Section of Rheumatology
Department of Internal Medicine
Rush-Presbyterian-St. Luke's Medical Center
1725 West Harrison Street
Chicago, Illinois 60612

Thomas D. Brown, Ph.D.
Richard C. Johnston Professor of Orthopaedic
  Biomechanics
Department of Orthopaedic Surgery
The University of Iowa Hospitals and Clinics
2430 Steindler Building
Iowa City, Iowa 52242-1008

William D. Bugbee, M.D.
Assistant Clinical Professor
Department of Orthopaedics
University of California at San Diego
200 West Arbor Drive
San Diego, California 92103

Pieter Buma, Ph.D.
Department of Orthopaedics
University Hospital Nijmegen
P.O. Box 9101
6500 HB Nijmegen
The Netherlands

John J. Callaghan, M.D.
Professor
Department of Orthopaedics
University of Iowa
200 Hawkins Drive
Iowa City, Iowa 52242

Hugh U. Cameron, M.D., Ch.B.,
  F.R.C.S.(C.)
Associate Professor
Departments of Surgery, Pathology, and
  Engineering
Orthopaedic and Arthritic Hospital
43 Wellesley Street E
Toronto, Ontario M4Y 1H1
Canada

William N. Capello, M.D.
Professor
Department of Orthopaedic Surgery
Indiana University Medical Center
541 Clinical Drive
Indianapolis, Indiana 46202-5111

Robert J. Carangelo, M.D.
Department of Orthopaedics
University of Connecticut
10 Talcott Notch
Farmington, Connecticut 06034

John J. Carbone, M.D.
Department of Orthopaedic Surgery
Johns Hopkins Bayview Medical Center
4940 Eastern Avenue
Baltimore, Maryland 21224-2780

Michael A. Catino, M.D.
Department of Orthopaedic Surgery
University of Pittsburgh
  Medical Center
3471 Fifth Avenue
Pittsburgh, Pennsylvania 15213-3221

Hugh P. Chandler, M.D.
Department of Orthopaedic Surgery
Massachusetts General Hospital
15 Parkman Street
Boston, Massachusetts 02114

Michael J. Chmell, M.D.
Clinical Instructor
Department of Orthopaedic Surgery
University of Illinois, Rockford
5668 East State Street
Rockford, Illinois 61108

Michael J. Christie, M.D.
Arthritis and Joint Replacement Center
Vanderbilt University Medical Center
1500 21st Avenue South
Nashville, Tennessee 37212

Ian C. Clarke, Ph.D.
Harbor–UCLA Medical Center
University of California, Los Angeles
1000 West Carson Street
Torrance, California 90509

Dennis K. Collis, M.D.
Orthopaedic and Fracture Clinic
Sacred Heart Medical Center
1200 Hilyard Street
Eugene, Oregon 97401

Christopher P. Comstock, M.D.
Attending Staff Pediatric
  Orthopaedic Surgeon
Department of Orthopaedic Surgery
Driscoll Children s Hospital
3533 South Alameda
Corpus Christi, Texas 78466-6530

Tim K. Conlan
Division of Adult Reconstructive Surgery
Department of Orthopaedic Surgery
University of Pittsburgh Medical Center
3471 Fifth Avenue
Pittsburgh, Pennsylvania 15213-3221

Lawrence S. Crossett, M.D.
Assistant Professor
Department of Orthopaedic Surgery
University of Pittsburgh Medical Center
3471 Fifth Avenue
Pittsburgh, Pennsylvania 15213-3221

John M. Cuckler, M.D.
Professor
Department of Orthopaedic Surgery
University Hospital
University of Alabama at Birmingham
1813 Sixth Avenue South
Birmingham, Alabama 35294-3295

Lawrence P. Davis, M.D.
Associate Professor
Department of Radiology
Wayne State University
Detroit, Michigan 48202

David K. DeBoer, M.D.
Arthritis and Joint Replacement Center
Vanderbilt University Medical Center
1500 21st Avenue South
Nashville, Tennessee 37212

Paul E. DiCesare
Department of Orthopaedic Surgery
Hospital for Joint Diseases
301 East 17th Street
New York, New York 10003

William J. Donnelly, M.B.B.S., B.Med.Sc.,
F.R.A.C.S. (Orth.)
Director
Department of Orthopaedics
Princess Alexandria Hospital
100 Heather Street
Wilston
Brisbane, Queensland
Australia

Lawrence D. Dorr, M.D.
Department of Orthopaedics
University of Southern California Hospital
1510 San Pablo Street
Los Angeles, California 90033-4634

Clive P. Duncan, M.B., M.Sc., F.R.C.S.C.
Professor and Chairman
Department of Orthopaedics
Vancouver Hospital and Health Sciences Center
University of British Columbia
910 West 10th Avenue
Vancouver, British Columbia V5Z 4E1
Canada

Harold K. Dunn, M.D.
Professor and Chairman
Department of Orthopaedics
University of Utah School of Medicine
50 North Medical Drive
Salt Lake City, Utah 84132

Jeffrey J. Eckardt, M.D.
Professor
Department of Orthopaedic Surgery
UCLA Center for Health Sciences
University of California, Los Angeles
10833 LeConte Avenue
Los Angeles, California 90095

Thomas A. Einhorn, M.D.
Professor and Chairman
Department of Orthopaedic Surgery
Boston University School of Medicine
One Boston Medical Center Place
Boston, Massachusetts 02118-2393

Reginald A. Elson, F.R.C.S.
Department of Orthopaedics
Northern General Hospital
Sheffield S5 7AU
United Kingdom

Roger H. Emerson, M.D.
Clinical Associate Professor
Department of Orthopaedics
University of Texas Southwestern Medical School
6300 West Parker Road
Plano, Texas 75093-7916

Charles A. Engh, M.D.
Associate Clinical Professor
Department of Orthopaedics
Anderson Orthopaedic Clinic
National Hospital Medical Center
2445 Army-Navy Drive
Arlington, Virginia 22206-2905

Brian G. Evans, M.D.
Assistant Professor
Department of Orthopaedic Surgery
Georgetown University Medical Center
3800 Reservoir Road NW
Washington, D.C. 20007-2197

Robin L. Evans, R.N., M.S.N., ONC, CCRC
Clinical Research Coordinator/Instructor
Departments of Orthopaedic Surgery and
    Acute/Tertiary Care
University of Pittsburgh Medical Center
3471 Fifth Avenue
Pittsburgh, Pennsylvania 15213-3221

Thomas K. Fehring, M.D.
Charlotte Orthopaedic Specialists
1915 Randolph Road
Charlotte, North Carolina 28207

Judy R. Feinberg, Ph.D.
Assistant Professor
Department of Orthopaedic Surgery
Indiana University Medical Center
541 Clinical Drive
Indianapolis, Indiana 46202-5111

Anthony B. Fiorillo, M.D.
Clinical Instructor in Medicine
Department of Medicine
University of Pittsburgh Medical Center
580 South Aiken Avenue
Pittsburgh, Pennsylvania 15232-1531

Robert H. Fitzgerald, Jr., M.S., M.D.
Professor and Chairman
Department of Orthopaedic Surgery
Hospital of the University of Pennsylvania
3400 Spruce Street
Philadelphia, Pennsylvania 19104-4283

Patrick G. Flynn, P.T.
Staff Physical Therapist
Department of Physical Therapy
University of Pittsburgh Medical Center
3471 Fifth Avenue
Pittsburgh, Pennsylvania 15213-3221

Robert J. Foster, Sc.D.
Associate Research Scientist
Department of Orthopaedic Surgery
Columbia University
630 West 168th Street
New York, New York 10032

Michael A. R. Freeman, M.D., F.R.C.S.
Department of Orthopaedic Surgery
Royal London Hospital–University of London
Whitechapel Road
London WIN 2DE
England

Jorge O. Galante, M.D., D.Med.Sci.
Professor
Department of Orthopaedic Surgery
Rush-Presbyterian–St. Luke's Medical Center
1725 West Harrison Street
Chicago, Illinois 60612-3833

Timothy M. Ganey, Ph.D.
Orthopaedic Research Director
Georgia Baptist Medical Center
303 Parkway Drive NE
Atlanta, Georgia 30312

Reinhold Ganz, M.D.
Professor and Chairman
Department of Orthopaedics
University of Berne, Inselspital
Freiburgstrasse
CH-3010, Berne
Switzerland

Jean W. M. Gardeniers, M.D., Ph.D.
Department of Orthopaedics
University Hospital Nijmegen
P.O. Box 9101
6500 HB Nijmegen
The Netherlands

Kevin L. Garvin, M.D.
Professor
Department of Orthopaedic Surgery
University of Nebraska Medical Center
600 South 42nd Street
Omaha, Nebraska 68198-1080

Rudolph G. T. Geesink, M.D., Ph.D.
Department of Orthopaedic Surgery
University Hospital Maastricht
Peter Debyelaan 25, Postbus 5800
6202 AZ Maastricht
The Netherlands

Graham A. Gie, M.D.
Consultant Orthopaedic Surgeon
The Princess Elizabeth Orthopaedic Hospital
2 The Quadrant
Wonford Road
Exeter, Devon EX2 4LE
England

Jeremy L. Gilbert, Ph.D.
Associate Professor
Division of Biomaterials
Northwestern University
311 East Chicago Avenue
Chicago, Illinois 60611

Andrew H. Glassman, M.S., M.D.
Director, Joint Replacement Program
National Hospital Medical Center
2445 Army-Navy Drive
Arlington, Virginia 22206-2905

Victor M. Goldberg, M.D.
Charles M. Mendon Professor and Chairman
Department of Orthopaedics
Case Western Reserve University Hospital
11100 Euclid Avenue
Cleveland, Ohio 44106

Peter Griss, M.D., Ph.D.
Klinikum der Philipps Universitat
Hausanschrift Baldingerstrasse
35043 Marburg
Germany

Jason E. Guevara
Division of Adult Reconstructive Surgery
Department of Orthopaedic Surgery
University of Pittsburgh Medical Center
3471 Fifth Avenue
Pittsburgh, Pennsylvania 15213-3221

John E. Hall, M.D.
Professor
Department of Orthopaedic Surgery
Boston Children's Hospital
Harvard Medical School
300 Longwood Avenue
Boston, Massachusetts 02115

William H. Harris, M.D.
Chief, Hip and Implant Unit
Director, Orthopaedic Biomechanics
  Laboratory
Clinical Professor
Department of Orthopaedic Surgery
Massachusetts General Hospital
Harvard Medical School
55 Fruit Street
Boston, Massachusetts 02114

James M. Hartford, M.D.
Division of Orthopaedic Surgery
University of Kentucky
800 Rose Street
Lexington, Kentucky 40536-0084

Carl T. Hasselman, M.D.
Department of Orthopaedic Surgery
Musculoskeletal Research Center
University of Pittsburgh
E 1641 Bioscience Tower
Pittsburgh, Pennsylvania 15213

John H. Healey, M.D.
Associate Professor of Orthopaedic Surgery
Cornell University Medical College; and
Chief of Orthopaedic Surgery
Memorial Sloan-Kettering Cancer Center
1275 York Avenue
New York, New York 10021

William L. Healy, M.D.
Chairman
Department of Orthopaedic Surgery
Lahey Hitchcock Medical Center
41 Mall Road
Burlington, Massachusetts 01805

Edward J. Hellman, M.D.
Assistant Professor
Department of Orthopaedic Surgery
Indiana University Medical Center
541 Clinical Drive
Indianapolis, Indiana 46202-5111

Peggy S. Hockenberry, P.T.
Coordinator
Department of Physical Therapy
University of Pittsburgh Medical Center
200 Lothrop Street
Pittsburgh, Pennsylvania 15213-3221

Nicolette H. M. Hoefnagels, M.S.C.
Department of Orthopaedic Surgery
University Hospital Maastricht
Peter Debyelaan 25, Postbus 5800
6202 AZ Maastricht
The Netherlands

James G. Howe, M.D.
Professor and Chairman
Departments of Orthopaedics and Rehabilitation
University of Vermont, Fletcher Allen Health Care
440 Stafford Hall
Burlington, Vermont 05405

William J. Hozack, M.D.
Associate Professor
Department of Orthopaedic Surgery
The Rothman Institute
Thomas Jefferson University Hospital
800 Spruce Street
Philadelphia, Pennsylvania 19107

Rik Huiskes, Ph.D.
Professor of Biomechanics
Department of Orthopaedics
University Hospital Nijmegen
Th. Craanenlaan 7, P.O. Box 9101
6500 HB Nijmegen
The Netherlands

David S. Hungerford, M.D.
Professor
Department of Orthopaedic Surgery
Johns Hopkins University at Good
  Samaritan Hospital
5601 Loch Raven Boulevard
Baltimore, Maryland 21239

Michael H. Huo, M.D.
Department of Orthopaedic Surgery
Johns Hopkins Bayview Medical Center
4940 Eastern Avenue
Baltimore, Maryland 21224-2780

Debra E. Hurwitz, Ph.D.
Assistant Professor
Department of Orthopaedic Surgery
Rush-Presbyterian–St. Luke's
  Medical Center
1653 West Congress Parkway
Chicago, Illinois 60612

Joshua J. Jacobs, M.D.
Associate Professor
Director of the Section of Biomaterials
Department of Orthopaedic Surgery
Rush University
1725 West Harrison Street
Chicago, Illinois 60612

Murali Jasty, M.D.
Clinical Associate Professor
Department of Orthopaedic Surgery
Massachusetts General Hospital
Harvard Medical School
55 Fruit Street
Boston, Massachusetts 02114

Norman A. Johanson, M.D.
Associate Professor
Department of Orthopaedic Surgery
Temple University School of Medicine
3401 North Broad Street
Philadelphia, Pennsylvania 19140

Richard C. Johnston, M.D.
Department of Orthopaedics
University of Iowa
200 Hawkins Drive
Iowa City, Iowa 52242

Ravindra P. Joshi, M.D.
Department of Orthopaedic Surgery
New York Orthopaedic Hospital Associates; and
Department of Joint Replacement/Revision Surgery
Columbia-Presbyterian Medical Center
161 Fort Washington Avenue
New York, New York 10032

Scott S. Kelley, M.D.
Assistant Professor
Department of Orthopaedics
University of North Carolina
  School of Medicine
242 Burnett-Womack Building
Chapel Hill, North Carolina 27599-7055

Heino Kienapfel, M.D., Ph.D.
Klinikum der Philipps Universitat
Hausanschrift Baldingerstrasse
35043 Marburg
Germany

Hui-Taek Kim, M.D.
Assistant Professor
Department of Orthopaedic Surgery
Pusan National University Hospital
1 Ga-10, Ami-Dong, Seo-Gu
Pusan, 602-739
Korea

Paul R. Kim, M.D., F.R.C.S.C.
Department of Orthopaedic Surgery
London Health Sciences Centre
The University of Western Ontario
339 Windermere Road
London, Ontario N6A 5A5
Canada

Seneki Kobayashi, M.D., Ph.D.
Assistant Professor
Department of Orthopaedic Surgery
Shinshu University School of Medicine
Asahi 3-1-1
Matsumoto 390
Japan

Anil B. Krishnamurthy, M.D.
Assistant Professor
Department of Orthopaedic Surgery
Wright State University
30 Apple Street
Dayton, Ohio 45409

Ken N. Kuo, M.D.
Professor of Orthopaedic Surgery
Associate Chairman of Education
Department of Orthopaedic Surgery
Rush-Presbyterian–St. Luke's
* Medical Center*
1725 West Harrison Street
Chicago, Illinois 60612

Paul F. Lachiewicz, M.D.
Associate Professor of Orthopaedics
Department of Orthopaedics
University of North Carolina School of Medicine
242 Burnett-Womack Building
Chapel Hill, North Carolina 27599-7055

Bobbie Lambert, R.N.
Departments of Orthopaedics and Rehabilitation
University of Vermont, Fletcher Allen Health Care
440 Stafford Hall
Burlington, Vermont 05405

Joseph M. Lane, M.D.
Department of Orthopaedic Surgery
Hospital for Special Surgery
535 East 70th Street
New York, New York 10021

Eugene P. Lautenschlager, Ph.D.
Professor of Biological Materials
Department of Dental Basic and Behavioral
* Sciences*
Northwestern University
313 East Chicago Avenue
Chicago, Illinois 60611

Jack E. Lemons, Ph.D.
Professor
Division of Orthopaedic Surgery
Departments of Biomaterials and Surgery
Schools of Medicine and Dentistry
University of Alabama, Birmingham
1919 Seventh Avenue South
Birmingham, Alabama 35294-3295

Steven Li, M.D.
The Hospital for Special Surgery
535 East 70th Street
New York, New York 10021

Jay R. Lieberman, M.D.
Department of Orthopaedic Surgery
UCLA Medical Center
University of California, Los Angeles
10833 LeConte Avenue
Los Angeles, California 90095

Robin S. M. Ling, M.D., F.A.C.S.
Honorary Professor of Orthopaedic
* Biomechanical Engineering*
The University of Exeter
2 The Quadrant
Wonford Road
Exeter EX2 4LE
Devon, England

John P. Lubicky, M.D.
Professor
Department of Orthopaedic Surgery
Rush Medical College; and
Shriners Hospital for Children
2211 North Oak Park Avenue
Chicago, Illinois 60707

William J. Maloney, M.D.
Associate Professor
Department of Orthopaedic Surgery
Barnes-Jewish Hospital
Washington University School of Medicine
One Barnes Hospital Plaza
St. Louis, Missouri 63110

J. Bohannon Mason, M.D.
Otto E. Aufranc Fellow in Adult
* Reconstructive Surgery*
Tufts University School of Medicine
Medford, Massachusetts 02155

Bassam A. Masri, M.D., F.R.C.S.C.
Clinical Assistant Professor and Head
Division of Reconstructive Orthopaedics
Department of Orthopaedics
Vancouver Hospital and Health Sciences Center
University of British Columbia
930-943 West Broadway
Vancouver, British Columbia V5Z 4E1
Canada

Kevin R. Math, M.D.
Assistant Professor
Department of Radiology
Albert Einstein College of Medicine
Bronx, New York; and
Attending Radiologist and Physician-in-Charge
Department of Musculoskeletal Imaging
Beth Israel Medical Center
170 East End Avenue
New York, New York 10128

Tadami Matsumoto, M.D.
Associate Professor
Department of Orthopaedic Surgery
University of Kanazawa School of Medicine
Takara-machi, 13-1
Kanazawa, Ishikawa 920
Japan

James P. McAuley, M.D., F.R.C.S.(C.)
Associate Professor
Division of Orthopaedic Surgery
Department of Surgery
Ottawa General Hospital
University of Ottawa
501 Smyth Road
Ottawa, Ontario, K1H 8L6
Canada

Andrew A. McBeath, M.D.
Frederick J. Gaenslen Professor and Chairman
Division of Orthopaedic Surgery
Department of Surgery
University of Wisconsin Hospital and Clinics
600 Highland Avenue
Madison, Wisconsin 53792-3228

Joseph C. McCarthy, M.D.
Associate Clinical Professor
Department of Orthopaedic Surgery
New England Baptist Hospital
125 Parker Hill Avenue
Boston, Massachusetts 02120

Donald E. McCollum, M.D.
Professor
Department of Orthopaedic Surgery
Duke University Medical Center
Durham, North Carolina 27710

William A. McGann, M.D.
1 Shrader Street
San Francisco, California 94117

Harry A. McKellop, Ph.D.
Associate Professor
Department of Orthopaedics and Biomedical
* Engineering*
The J. Vernon Luck Orthopaedic Research Center
University of Southern California
2400 South Flower Street
Los Angeles, California 90007

Theresa M. McKillip, P.A.C.
Department of Orthopaedic Surgery
University of Nebraska Medical Center
600 South 42 Street
Omaha, Nebraska 68198-1080

Patrick A. Meere, M.D.
Department of Orthopaedic Surgery
Hospital for Joint Diseases
301 East 17th Street
New York, New York 10003

W. E. Michael Mikhail, M.D.
Professor of Orthopaedic
* Bioengineering Research*
Clinical Professor of Orthopaedic Surgery
Medical College
University of Ohio
Regency Orthopaedics
2000 Regency Court
Toledo, Ohio 43623

Eric C. Mirsky, M.D.
Department of Orthopaedic Surgery
The Mount Sinai School of Medicine
5 East 98th Street
New York, New York 10029

Craig G. Mohler, M.D.
Orthopaedic and Fracture Clinic
Sacred Heart Medical Center
1200 Hilyard Street
Eugene, Oregon 97401

Michael A. Mont, M.D.
Associate Professor
Department of Orthopaedic Surgery
Johns Hopkins University at
* The Good Samaritan Hospital*
5601 Loch Raven Boulevard
Baltimore, Maryland 21239

Gue Moreau, M.D.
Division of Orthopaedic Surgery
Department of Surgery
Ottawa General Hospital
University of Ottawa
501 Smyth Road
Ottawa, Ontario, K1H 8L6
Canada

Van C. Mow, Ph.D.
Professor of Mechanical Engineering and
* Orthopaedic Bioengineering*
Department of Orthopaedic Surgery
Columbia University
630 West 168th Street
New York, New York 10032

Michael C. Munin, M.D.
Assistant Professor
Division of Physical Medicine and
 Rehabilitation
Department of Orthopaedic Surgery
University of Pittsburgh Medical Center
3471 Fifth Avenue
Pittsburgh, Pennsylvania 15213-3221

D. Luis Muscolo, M.D.
Director, Research Laboratory
Vice-Chairman, Department of
 Orthopaedic Surgery
Italian Hospital of Buenos Aires
Potosí 4215
1199 Buenos Aires
Argentina

Ohannes A. Nercessian, M.D.
Assistant Professor
Department of Orthopaedic Surgery
Columbia-Presbyterian Medical Center
161 Fort Washington Avenue
New York, New York 10032

John A. Ogden, M.D.
Clinical Professor
Director of Orthopaedics
Georgia Baptist Medical Center
303 Parkway Drive Northeast
Atlanta, Georgia 30312

Douglas E. Padgett, M.D.
Assistant Professor
Department of Orthopaedic Surgery
The Hospital for Special Surgery
535 East 70th Street
New York, New York 10021

Wayne G. Paprosky, M.D.
Associate Professor
Department of Orthopaedic Surgery
Rush-Presbyterian–St. Luke's Medical Center
25 North Winfield Road
Chicago, Illinois 60190

Leonard F. Peltier, M.D., Ph.D.
Professor Emeritus
Section of Orthopaedics
The University of Arizona College of Medicine
Tucson, Arizona 85724-5064

Brad L. Penenberg, M.D.
8635 West Third Street
Los Angeles, California 90048

Christopher L. Peters, M.D.
Assistant Professor
Department of Orthopaedic Surgery
University of Utah School of Medicine
50 North Medical Drive
Salt Lake City, Utah 84132

William Petty, M.D.
Professor
Department of Orthopaedics
University of Florida College of Medicine
1600 SW Archer Road
Gainesville, Florida 32610-0246

Robert Poss, M.D.
Department of Orthopaedic Surgery
Brigham and Women's Hospital
75 Francis Street
Boston, Massachusetts 02115

Hollis G. Potter, M.D.
Chief, Division of Magnetic Resonance Imaging
Department of Radiology
The Hospital for Special Surgery
535 East 70th Street
New York, New York 10021

Louis Quartararo, M.D.
Department of Orthopaedic Surgery
Allegheny University Hospitals
230 North Broad Street
Philadelphia, Pennsylvania 19102

Dheeraj K. Rajan, M.D.
Department of Radiology
Wayne State University
Detroit, Michigan 48202

Chitranjan S. Ranawat, M.D.
Department of Orthopaedic Surgery
Lenox Hill Hospital
William Black Hall
130 East 77th Street
New York, New York 10021

José A. Rodriguez, M.D.
Clinical Instructor
Cornell University Medical College; and
Department of Orthopaedic Surgery
Lenox Hill Hospital
William Black Hall
130 East 77th Street
New York, New York 10021

Leon Root, M.D.
Professor of Clinical Surgery (Orthopaedics)
Department of Orthopaedics
The Hospital for Special Surgery
535 East 70th Street
New York, New York 10021

Aaron G. Rosenberg, M.D.
Professor
Department of Orthopaedic Surgery
Arthritis and Orthopaedic Institute
Rush Medical College
1725 West Harrison Street
Chicago, Illinois 60612

Richard H. Rothman, M.D., Ph.D.
James Edwards Professor and Chairman
Department of Orthopaedic Surgery
The Rothman Institute
Thomas Jefferson University
800 Spruce Street
Philadelphia, Pennsylvania 19107

Harry E. Rubash, M.D.
Professor
Clinical Vice Chairman
Department of Orthopaedic Surgery
University of Pittsburgh Medical Center
3471 Fifth Avenue
Pittsburgh, Pennsylvania 15213-3221

Mazen Said, M.D.
Department of Orthopaedics
Center for Implant Surgery
BNAI-ZION Medical Center
47 Golomb Street, P.O. Box 4940
Haifa 31048
Israel

Susumu Saito, M.D.
Chief, Department of Orthopaedic Surgery
Sumitomo Hospital
5-2-2 Nakanoshima, Kita-ku
Osaka 530
Japan

Toyonori Sakamaki, M.D.
Department of Orthopaedic Surgery
Keio University School of Medicine
Tokyo
Japan

Eduardo A. Salvati, M.D.
Professor of Orthopaedic Surgery
The Hospital for Special Surgery
535 East 70th Street
New York, New York 10021

Jan W. Schimmel, M.D., Ph.D.
Department of Orthopaedics
University Hospital Nijmegen
P.O. Box 9101
6500 HB Nijmegen
The Netherlands

Thomas P. Schmalzried, M.D.
Joint Replacement Institute
Orthopaedic Hospital
2400 South Flower Street
Los Angeles, California 90007

B. Willem Schreurs, M.D., Ph.D.
Department of Orthopaedics
University Hospital Nijmegen
P.O. Box 9101
6500 HB Nijmegen
The Netherlands

Steven F. Schutzer, M.D.
Orthopaedic Associates of Hartford
85 Seymour Street
Hartford, Connecticut 06106

Gareth Scott
Department of Orthopaedic Surgery
Royal London Hospital–University of London
Whitechapel Road
London W1N 2DE
England

Arun S. Shanbhag, Ph.D.
Assistant Professor of Orthopaedic Surgery,
   Mechanical Engineering, and Bioengineering
Department of Orthopaedic Surgery
University of Pittsburgh
E-1641 Biomedical Science Tower
Pittsburgh, Pennsylvania 15213

Peter F. Sharkey, M.D.
Assistant Professor
Department of Orthopaedic Surgery
The Rothman Institute
Thomas Jefferson University Hospital
850 Walnut Street
Philadelphia, Pennsylvania 19107

Nigel E. Sharrock, M.B., Ch.B.
Senior Scientist
Department of Anesthesiology
The Hospital for Special Surgery
535 East 70th Street
New York, New York 10021

Craig D. Silverton, D.O.
Assistant Professor
Department of Orthopaedic Surgery
Rush-Presbyterian–St. Luke s Medical Center
1725 West Harrison Street
Chicago, Illinois 60614

Raj K. Sinha
Department of Orthopaedic Surgery
University of Pittsburgh Medical Center
Kauffman Building
3471 Fifth Avenue
Pittsburgh, Pennsylvania 15213-3221

Tom J. J. H. Slooff, M.D., Ph.D.
Professor
Department of Orthopaedics
University Hospital Nijmegen
P.O. Box 9101
6500 HB Nijmegen
The Netherlands

Francis X. Solano, Jr., M.D.
Clinical Associate Professor of Medicine, and
 Obstetrics and Gynecology
Department of Medicine
University of Pittsburgh Medical Center
580 South Aiken Avenue
Pittsburgh, Pennsylvania 15232-1531

Nicholas G. Sotereanos, M.D.
Department of Orthopaedic Surgery
University of Pittsburgh Medical Center
3471 Fifth Avenue
Pittsburgh, Pennsylvania 15213-3221

Sharon Stevenson, D.V.M., Ph.D.
Department of Orthopaedics
Case Western Reserve University Hospital
11100 Euclid Avenue
Cleveland, Ohio 44106

Nobuhiko Sugano, M.D., Ph.D.
Assistant Professor
Department of Orthopaedic Surgery
Osaka University School of Medicine
2-2 Yamadaoka
Suita 565
Japan

Dale R. Sumner, Ph.D.
Professor and Chairman, Department of Anatomy
Director, Section of Bone Biology
Department of Orthopaedic Surgery
Rush-Presbyterian–St. Luke's Medical Center
1653 West Congress Parkway
Chicago, Illinois 60612

Kunio Takaoka, M.D., Ph.D.
Professor
Department of Orthopaedic Surgery
Shinshu University School of Medicine
Asahi 3-1-1
Matsumoto 390
Japan

Russell G. Tigges, M.D.
Department of Orthopaedics
Massachusetts General Hospital
15 Parkman Street
Boston, Massachusetts 02114

Wendy Toplak, O.T.R.
Head of Occupational Therapy
University of Pittsburgh Medical Center
3471 Fifth Avenue
Pittsburgh, Pennsylvania 15213-3221

Jeffrey D. Towers, M.D.
Assistant Professor of Radiology and
 Orthopaedics
Department of Radiology
University of Pittsburgh Medical Center
200 Lothrop Street
Pittsburgh, Pennsylvania 15213

Robert T. Trousdale, M.D.
Assistant Professor
Mayo Graduate School of Medicine;
Department of Orthopaedic Surgery
The Mayo Clinic and Foundation
200 First Street SW
Rochester, Minnesota 55905

Thomas P. Vail, M.D.
Assistant Professor
Department of Orthopaedic Surgery
Duke University Medical Center
Duke South Orange Zone
Durham, North Carolina 27710

Nico Verdonschot
Department of Orthopaedics
University Hospital Nijmegen
Th. Craanenlaan 7, P.O. Box 9101
6500 HB Nijmegen
The Netherlands

Steven R. Wardell, M.D.
Otto E. Aufranc Fellow in Adult
 Reconstructive Surgery
New England Baptist Hospital
125 Parker Hill Avenue
Boston, Massachusetts 02120

Ray C. Wasielewski, M.D.
Division of Orthopaedic Surgery
Ohio State University
Doan Hall
410 West Tenth Avenue
Columbus, Ohio 43210-1282

Lars R. A. Weidenhielm, M.D., Ph.D.
Associate Professor, Karolinska Institute
Senior Consultant
Department of Orthopaedics
St. Goran Hospital
St. Goransplan 1
5-11281 Stockholm
Sweden

Stuart L. Weinstein, M.D.
Ignacio V. Ponseti Professor of
  Orthopaedic Surgery
Department of Orthopaedic Surgery
University of Iowa Hospital
Iowa City, Iowa 52242

Dennis R. Wenger, M.D.
Clinical Professor of Orthopaedic Surgery
University of California at San Diego; and
Director, Department of Pediatric Orthopaedics
Children's Hospital
3030 Children's Way
San Diego, California 92123-4228

Janet E. Whirlow, M.D.
Arizona Center for Joint Replacement
3333 East Camelback Road
Phoenix, Arizona 85018-3424

Richard E. White, Jr., M.D.
Clinical Assistant Professor
Department of Orthopaedic Surgery and
  Rehabilitation
University of New Mexico School of Medicine
1122 Lomas Boulevard NE
Albuquerque, New Mexico 87131

Philip Z. Wirganowicz, M.D.
Assistant Professor
Department of Orthopaedic Surgery
University of Pennsylvania
3400 Spruce Street
Philadelphia, Pennsylvania 19104

Richard L. Wixson, M.D.
Professor of Clinical Orthopaedic Surgery
Department of Orthopaedic Surgery
Northwestern University Medical School
676 St. Clair Street
Chicago, Illinois 60611

Steven T. Woolson, M.D.
Clinical Professor
Division of Orthopaedic Surgery
Stanford University Medical School
300 Pasteur Drive
Stanford, California 94305

Shigeru Yanagimoto, M.D.
Department of Orthopaedic Surgery
Keio University School of Medicine
35 Shinanomachi Shinjuku-ku
Tokyo 160
Japan

George W. Zimmerman
Division of Adult Reconstructive Surgery
Department of Orthopaedic Surgery
University of Pittsburgh Medical Center
3471 Fifth Avenue
Pittsburgh, Pennsylvania 15213-3221

Joseph D. Zuckerman, M.D.
Chairman
Department of Orthopaedic Surgery
Hospital for Joint Diseases
301 East 17th Street
New York, New York 10003

Foreword

Advances in the field of total hip replacement surgery are occurring at an accelerating rate. Simply consider the recent remarkable advances in the concepts, techniques, and materials of total hip replacement. For example, the number one problem in total hip replacement is periprosthetic osteolysis. Our present understanding of this problem is dramatically better than it was just a short time ago. With the improvement in the conceptual features of periprosthetic osteolysis have come improvements in implant design, materials, and surgical techniques. *The Adult Hip* consolidates and integrates this rapidly increasing information.

This two-volume set is much more than just a text on total hip surgery; it provides succinct presentations of hip surgery, development, anatomy, and biomechanics, as well as an especially strong section on biomechanics and wear. In addition to a detailed presentation of perioperative considerations, the text provides important information on the alternatives to total hip arthroplasty.

It is a substantial achievement to bring all of these advances into one beautifully integrated text that comprehensively assesses the current state-of-the-art advances in adult hip surgery. The editors are vigorous, thoughtful, and critical. They have selected outstanding contributors and have ensured that the presentations are balanced, inclusive, and lucid. The authors draw deeply from the wellsprings of creative innovation and evaluation of all aspects of total hip replacement, enabling the reader to benefit from their skills and knowledge.

Finally, this text deals admirably with the three important "hows" of adult hip surgery: how to assess problems, how to interpret concepts, and how to manage patients.

The editors and contributors to this text are to be congratulated. We, as surgeons, gain immeasurably from this compilation of timely advances, enabling us to better serve our patients.

William H. Harris, M.D.

Preface

As students of surgery, and hip surgery in particular, we are acutely aware of the giants in our field who have paved the way for our contemporary ability to diagnose and treat hip diseases. We are fortunate to live in a time when access to information is more readily obtained than it was during their time. This book represents our contribution to this reality.

An enormous amount of investigative work has been performed and reported on the normal hip, the disease processes affecting it, and treatment of these diseases, but until now this material has not been available in one complete and convenient source. We developed *The Adult Hip* to provide a comprehensive, organized text on adult hip pathology and treatment. We were fortunate to attract the most respected world authorities in this field, and the book reflects the depth of their various knowledge and expertise.

The 101 chapters in *The Adult Hip* are organized as two volumes with seven major sections. The "Basic Science" section provides the necessary underpinnings for sound clinical judgement. It includes pertinent information concerning anatomy, biomaterial, and wear, as well as the biology of grafts and osteolysis. Distinctive features of the clinical sections include a beautifully illustrated chapter on surgical anatomy and approaches, as well as in-depth coverage of alternatives to arthroplasty. In addition, eminent authorities provide detailed analyses on evaluation and imaging of the hip, the various disorders that affect the adult hip, and important details of perioperative management from anesthesia and nursing standpoints. Because it remains the most performed hip operation, total hip arthroplasty receives exhaustive attention, including indications, contraindications, technical details, complications, and outcomes, as well as the economic impact of both primary and revision procedures. The inclusion of multiple authors, representing varying and sometimes opposing points of view, accurately represents the profusion of surgical techniques and approaches to the problem of contemporary hip arthroplasty. Some of these approaches are so new that their utility is not yet clear; but they represent potential solutions to problems that have not yet been adequately addressed.

This text can serve as a comprehensive review for medical students, researchers and students in the basic sciences related to hip reconstruction, orthopaedic residents, and fellows in adult reconstructive hip surgery. At the same time, it is a valuable resource for those seeking practical advice and expertise concerning the details of hip reconstruction, including general orthopaedic surgeons, experienced hip surgeons, and others who care for patients with hip problems. All of these groups will find information to broaden their scope of knowledge and clinical performance.

To take advantage of modern communications techniques, an interactive CD-ROM version of the book is available, providing 30 minutes of video clips, Medline abstracts linked to key references in each chapter, and additional artwork not included in the text. The CD-ROM also features quick searches by topic, keyword, and author; hypertext links; help menus; windowing features; and print capabilities.

Our goal for this edition of *The Adult Hip* is to set a new standard for a text on adult hip surgery. We hope that we have captured the extensive advances in the field of hip surgery, especially since the development of total hip arthroplasty, and that all readers will better understand the disorders of the adult hip and their treatments.

Acknowledgments

I have many people to acknowledge for helping make this book possible: my parents, who promoted intellectual curiosity and the search for truth; my teachers, from whose inspiration came my devotion to the profession; Emil T. Hofman and the faculty at the University of Notre Dame; Wilton H. Bunch and the faculty at Loyola Stritch School of Medicine; Richard C. Johnston, my father in hip surgery, and the faculty at the University of Iowa; Eduardo A. Salvati, my mentor in hip surgery, and the faculty at the Hospital for Special Surgery; my friends and colleagues in the Hip Society; my students who have endured my passion for the understanding of the hip and the dissemination of that understanding; Lori Yoder, my secretary, who handled all of the coordination of faxes, messages, and manuscripts crucial to the timely completion of this book; Rhoda Dunn and Kathey Alexander at Lippincott–Raven Publishers, who handled every detail of the editing process and assured the timely submission of manuscripts, which is indeed a huge task for such a production as this book; and finally, and most importantly, to the authors, who have sacrificed their time and energy in the preparation of this text.

J. J. C.

This work would not be possible without the examples, guidance, and teaching of my mentors: Henry J. Mankin, who taught me more about what it means to be a physician and a surgeon in one year than I have ever learned; Jorge O. Galante, who trained me, supported me, and guided my development as an educator and investigator; Regina Barden, the nurse clinician whose example of professionalism, attention to detail, comprehensive patient care, and search for truth and excellence in research have been an inspiration both for me and for my patients; and Natalie Slopecki, whose concern for making sure things do not fall through the cracks has kept me afloat for the last dozen years.

A. G. R.

The Adult Hip has been a dream of mine for the past decade. Many people have been instrumental in the development of this concept and in seeing it to fruition: my mother and late father, who instilled in me the importance of my family and a dedication to my profession; Albert B. Ferguson, Jr., from whose inspiration and guidance came my devotion to a career in academic orthopaedic surgery; Dana C. Mears, whose creativity and innovations in the complexities of reconstructive surgery kindled my desire to study the adult hip; William H. Harris, my mentor in hip surgery whose compassion and genius have guided the field of arthroplasty for more than two decades, and who continues to teach me what it means to be an educator, investigator, and gentleman; Edward N. Hanley, Jr., my friend, surrogate brother, and visionary in many aspects of life; James H. Herndon, whose wisdom, insight, and leadership have contributed greatly to the field of orthopaedic surgery and have guided my development as an academic orthopaedist; Savio L-Y Woo, who has taught me the importance of simplicity and cooperation in the pursuit of science; my students, residents, and fellows, who have tolerantly endured my determination to pursue studies of the adult hip; and Robin Evans, my research nurse, whose professionalism, hard work, and dedication to orthopaedic research have been an inspiration to us all—the many authors and co-authors who contributed to the success of this text.

H. E. R.

SECTION V

Total Hip Arthroplasty

The Adult Hip, edited by J. J. Callaghan,
A. G. Rosenberg, and H. E. Rubash.
Lippincott–Raven Publishers, Philadelphia © 1998.

CHAPTER 51

Overview of Total Hip Arthroplasty

Jorge O. Galante

Over the last 30 years, we have seen drastic changes in our ability to manage patients with joint disabilities. The development of total hip replacement in the sixties by Sir John Charnley represents a milestone in orthopedic surgery (11). At the Consensus Development Conference (49) sponsored by the National Institute of Health in September 1994, on the subject of total hip replacement, the following conclusions, among others, were reached: "Total hip replacement is an option for nearly all patients with disease of the hip that causes chronic discomfort and functional impairment." "Most patient have an excellent prognosis for long-term improvement in symptoms and physical functions."

Although the preceding statements are correct, they do not provide a complete reflection of the current state of total joint replacement. In the past two decades, a number of innovations and technological improvements have been introduced. Many of these changes have had an important effect and have resulted in significant improvements with drastic reductions in failure rates. On the other hand, many innovations in technology have failed to live up to their promise. In many instances, practices and techniques of the past were superior to those used more recently. These issues will be discussed under a number of headings, including indications, fixation, remodeling, and wear and osteolysis.

INDICATIONS

The indications for total hip replacement have evolved since the introduction of the procedure. Total hip replace-

ment is indicated in patients exhibiting hip joint deterioration from a number of causes, including degenerative arthritis, rheumatoid arthritis, ankylosing spondylitis, primary and secondary avascular necrosis, arthritis, ankylosis secondary to previous infections, spontaneous ankylosis, postsurgical ankylosis, benign and malignant bone tumors around the hip joint, and hip fractures.

Pain and the ensuing disability in the face of failure of conservative measures constitute the main reasons for performing the procedure and the basis for the most satisfactory postoperative outcomes. Limitation of motion and deformity in the absence of pain are reasonable justifications for the procedure, provided that they result in significant disability. For example, bony ankylosis, with disability secondary to deformity, associated spinal problems, or deterioration of the ipsilateral or contralateral knee joint, is an excellent indication for a total hip replacement of the ankylosed joint.

In the decade of the seventies, age was an overwhelming consideration. Because of the uncertainty surrounding long-term efficacy of the procedure and the potential for late failure, only the elderly were considered reasonable candidates. The procedure was thought to be contraindicated in young patients, particularly those below the fourth or fifth decades of life. As data on long-term survivorship has become available, age limits have been extended. Total hip replacement can be considered, given the appropriate conditions, in any age group after skeletal maturity.

However, the surgeon and the patient must be aware of the shortcoming of the procedure. Joint replacement cannot be successfully used in the young and active individual without a change in activity levels leading to a more sedentary lifestyle. Manual labor, heavy lifting, high-intensity sport activities are all capable of leading to pre-

J. O. Galante: Department of Orthopaedic Surgery, Rush-Presbyterian–St. Luke's Medical Center, Chicago, Illinois 60612-3833.

mature failure, the need for revision surgery, and consequently to a potentially severe degree of physical handicap in the future.

We must understand that there are limitations inherent to the materials used. Polyethylene socket wear and the resulting granulomatous reaction (with potential bone destruction) plays a critical role in the long-term survival of a total joint replacement. Thus, although it is very reasonable to think in terms of 15-year lifetimes, it becomes more difficult to predict survivorship for longer periods, particularly if the patient is young and active. The surgeon and the patient should discuss these issues at length so that an informed decision can be made about whether to proceed with the operation and whether an appropriate lifestyle can be maintained thereafter. It is important that the patient's expectations be realistic, particularly in the younger age group.

An area of some controversy is that of femoral neck fractures in the elderly (37,70). In most algorithms for treatment, reduction and internal fixation is recommended for the patient who is less than 65 years old and has no chronic illnesses and good femoral bone stock. Prosthetic replacement is used in the older age group. Three types of replacements are feasible: a unipolar, a bipolar, and a total hip replacement. I use a unipolar cemented prosthesis in the elderly patients with a low level of activity and a limited life expectancy. Otherwise, I believe that a total hip replacement is the procedure of choice and a better alternative to a bipolar prosthesis, which is frequently recommended. Although functional outcomes in the short term may not be all together different between these three different procedures, the potential for failure and revision surgery due to acetabular protrusion, wear, loosening, or other factors, may be lower with a total hip replacement. There is support for this viewpoint in the orthopedic literature (21), but there is a lack of well-designed, prospective, adequately controlled clinical trials that provide an objective scientific rationale for this decision.

The presence of active local or systemic infection remains a significant contraindication to a total hip replacement. Common sense and good surgical judgment are important tools that the orthopedic surgeon should use in defining indications for total hip replacement in patients with other medical problems, including advanced stage obesity and other comorbidities.

FIXATION

Fixation of the prosthetic components was initially thought to be the Achilles heel of joint replacement and the most likely mechanism of failure. Aseptic loosening and the development of paraprosthetic osteolysis were attributed to the use of acrylic cement and the reaction to its degradation products. Considerable research efforts were invested in the late 1970s and 1980s towards both the improvement of cement techniques and the development of technologies that avoided the use of acrylic cement altogether.

Aseptic loosening represents, still today, the most common indication for revision surgery. Data from the Swedish Hip Registry, indicates that among 4858 revision arthroplasties performed between 1979 and 1990, 3836 (or 79%) were performed for aseptic loosening (39). In our institution, aseptic loosening represents the reason for 78% of all the revisions performed.

To some degree, these numbers pose a paradox. At a time when very low failure rates due to aseptic loosening are reported, it still remains the most frequent cause of failure, although the total number of revisions remains constant. Certainly, many of these failures may be the product of surgeries performed before modern cement techniques and contemporary prosthetic designs were introduced. Some of these failures may be the product of design principles and techniques that were introduced as improvements but resulted in disastrous consequences. An additional reason to explain the persisting high number of revisions due to aseptic loosening might be that the results reported by clinical investigators at major clinical centers are not representative of the outcomes seen in the orthopedic community at large, where failure rates might be higher. Technical expertise with either cemented or cementless techniques is closely related to experience and, thus, surgery performed by surgeons who perform a limited number of such operations might possibly explain a higher rate of failure.

The mechanism of loosening can be seen as secondary to mechanical or biological factors (60,80,81). From a mechanical viewpoint, the repetitive nature of the external loads generates stresses at the prostheses and the interfaces that may eventually lead to failure of the cement and its bonds to the prosthetic device and to the bone. In the case of cementless stems, mechanical failure can occur if the areas available for osseointegration and ingrowth are limited by design, or if the extent of ingrowth was small to begin with.

The biologic mechanism involves degradation of the cement–bone or of the cementless interface resulting from the migration of wear particles. These particles may originate from wear of the polyethylene at the joint articular surface, from corrosion products generated at the Morse taper cone junction of the femoral head, and from abraded cement or metal debris from the implant. These particles have been clearly linked to a granulomatous reaction leading to membrane formation, osteolysis, and eventual implant loosening. In practice, although both mechanical and biologic effects operate in the loosening process, the dominating factor may be one or the other, depending on a number of circumstances, including implant design, fixation mode, and technique, as well as biologic factors unique to the individual.

Fixation is best discussed under two separate headings, cement and cementless. Although some of the basic mechanical and biologic considerations are similar for these two technologies, there are fundamental differences and there is still a great deal of controversy over the relative merits of one approach versus the other.

Regarding femoral fixation, long-term results of cemented total hip replacement using early designs and conventional techniques have shown variable results (1,5, 11,35,56,61,64,69). Although the decade of the 1980s saw the introduction of a number of changes in cementing technologies and implant design, and a number of these developments have drastically reduced the short- and intermediate-term femoral failure rate (27–29,46,54, 55), because of the simultaneous introduction of high-strength metal alloys, design changes, and new cement techniques, it is not always possible to evaluate the relative merits of one development over the other.

Femoral stem fractures were not uncommon in the late 1970s and early 1980s (9,10,19). Failure mechanisms included the use of cast cobalt–chrome and stainless steel (two alloys with relatively low fatigue strength) and the presence of metallic defects, which, when coupled with stem loosening, varus position, or loss or proximal support, led to the mechanical conditions that favored the occurrence of fatigue fractures of the stem. The introduction of high-strength metal alloys including forged cobalt–chrome alloy, titanium-6-aluminum-4-vanadium, and high-strength stainless steel has resulted in a drastic decrease in the incidence of stem fractures.

Their occurrence, however, has not been totally eliminated. Undetectable metallic defects can still occur and, given the appropriate set of circumstances, can lead to a fatigue failure. Sporadically, such fractures occur and can be traced back to a change in manufacturing techniques or other production events.

The surgeon should also remember that porous-coated metal stems do not truly incorporate high-strength metal alloys. The process of sintering a porous surface to the underlying substrate leads to a substantial decrease in fatigue strength for both cobalt–chrome and titanium alloys. Through appropriate design, implants with adequate strength characteristics can be manufactured. The surgeon should be careful and use appropriate informed judgment when choosing a cementless implant if the anatomy requires the use of a very small femoral stem in a patient who is otherwise of normal body build and activity level.

Regarding the specific choice of metallic alloys for cemented femoral stems, I believe that forged cobalt–chrome alloy is the material of choice. We have observed a high incidence of loosening with cemented titanium stems. This might be from a number of causes. In some instances, the use of titanium femoral heads resulted in increased wear and resultant particulate production leading to eventual loosening and osteolysis.

Titanium has a lower elastic modulus and thus a titanium alloy stem will be less rigid than a comparable stem made from cobalt–chrome alloy (57). This may lead to increased cement stresses and eventual mechanical failure. In addition, micromotion between the implant and the surrounding cement envelope would be more likely to produce abrasion and increased particulate production in a titanium stem given its poor surface abrasion resistance.

A number of improvements in stem design have also contributed to a decrease in the incidence of loosening. The main effect of these design features has been the reduction of cement stresses, decreasing the possibility of fracture of the cement mantle. Desirable stem characteristics include the elimination of sharp corners to reduce cement-stress concentrations. Proximal cross sections should preferably be trapezoidal. The stem should be straight and tapered to adapt to the anatomy of the femur. It should be available in multiple sizes to allow for the maintenance of a uniform thickness in the mantle of cement, regardless of the size of the femur in which it is implanted. It should not reach past the isthmus. It should provide a variety of offsets to allow for proper reconstruction of the anatomy of the hip joint. It should allow for appropriate centralization within the cement mantle. There is some controversy and conflicting evidence regarding the ideal surface characteristics of the stem and, hence, of the cement–stem interface.

One of the scenarios proposed for the failure process of a cemented total hip arthroplasty is initiation by debonding at the cement–stem interface (80,81). This promotes cement failure as a result of increased cement stresses, and it also leads to the generation of cement wear particles. Eventually, for both mechanical and biologic reasons, failure occurs at the cement–bone interface as well. Efforts were then directed to strengthening the cement–stem interface to prevent debonding. Thus, precoating with acrylic cement or roughened surfaces was introduced to fulfill that goal.

A different philosophy proposes the use of a smooth or polished stem surface that does not bond to the cement, to allow it to subside within the cement mantle. It was shown using analytical methods that this approach did produce an elevation of cement stresses, but that the stress patterns at the cement–bone interface were less detrimental than those introduced with a bonded stem (81). This was probably because of an increase in interface compression that might reduce the possibility of cement–bone interface failure.

A stem that does not bond to the cement mantle should be smooth or polished and should be collarless to allow for stem subsidence. There are some practical additional advantages to the use of a polished or smooth surface stem: for example, revision is a much easier undertaking than with a bonded precoated prosthesis.

From a practical viewpoint, excellent and equivalent intermediate and long-term results have been reported with both precoated and smooth-surface stems in spite of their drastically different design principles (3,39,48,61). This indicates that the quality of the cement mantle plays a most critical role in the long-term prevention of failure, overshadowing to some extent some of the stem design considerations discussed previously.

Contemporary cement techniques have been introduced for the purpose of optimizing the strength of the cement and improving its distribution (28,29,47). These include vacuum mixing or centrifugation, canal lavage, plugging the canal, retrograde injection of cement, and cement pressurization. In addition, the use of appropriate rasps and centralizers allows the surgeon to produce a cement mantle that is complete, free of defects, circumferential, and of nearly uniform thickness. These are important elements in avoiding both failure of the cement and the potential presence of tracks for particle migration.

Using these principles, failure rates of 1% to 3% at 10 and 15 years have been reported (25,48,50,58). Thus, a well-cemented femoral stem, using contemporary materials, designs, and cementing techniques, has the potential for excellent survivorship and represents the best alternative for the vast majority of patients who are candidates for a total hip arthroplasty today.

In contrast to the excellent intermediate and long-term results reported with cemented femoral fixation, the use of cement in the acetabulum has not universally met the same level of success. Loosening rates of 7% to 40% at 10 years have been reported even with the use of modern cement techniques (11,30,47,48,52,69).

From a technical viewpoint, it is more difficult to obtain satisfactory conditions for cementing in the acetabulum than in the femur; it is more difficult to obtain an enclosed cavity that allows pressurization of the cement in a reproducible manner, and it is more difficult to create a dry field without seepage of blood, particularly if the surgeon uses a posterolateral approach. There may also be biologic differences when compared with the femur: the characteristics of the periacetabular trabecular bone may allow easier progression of reactive membranes at the cement–bone interface. Thus, many surgeons today, including myself, prefer to use cementless techniques in the acetabulum.

Cementless techniques were introduced in the 1970s and early 1980s as a potential solution for what was then perceived to be a failure of acrylic cement. They are generally based on the use of a porous material that allows bone ingrowth. Roughened surfaces and bioactive ceramic coatings are also in use clinically to promote bone ongrowth as a method of fixation.

Prerequisites for bone ingrowth include the use of a biocompatible material, a pore size ideally in the 100- to 400-μm range, intimate contact between the pore surface and the surrounding bone, and minimal initial micromotion. Given those conditions, a process akin to primary bone formation, without an enchondral phase, will take place. Within days after implantation, blood cellular elements can be seen within the pore structure. After a week, mature bony trabeculae are found. Eventually, haversian remodeling will lead to a mature bone structure.

Successful bone ingrowth can be accomplished with a number of pore structures manufactured with different technologies. From a clinical viewpoint, both titanium and cobalt–chrome alloys have been used successfully (15,18,46). However, it is my perception that titanium offers a better biologic potential for reproducible successful osseointegration.

My own experience has been with the use of a porous titanium fiber–metal composite (20,38). The material is made by molding and sintering unalloyed titanium fibers. This results in a porous structure with an average pore diameter of 250 μm at about 50% density compaction. The material is compliant, a feature that favors impaction by press-fitting techniques. It can be bonded by a sintering process to a metallic surface, or bonded directly to polyethylene or other polymers by a molding process. It can also be manufactured with wrought cobalt–chrome alloy wires.

A material used extensively in Europe is the so-called corundum blasted titanium alloy surface (63). This surface, with irregularities within a prescribed range (5 to 10 μm) in depth, is capable of producing bone ongrowth and excellent osseointegration. The microgeometry of the surface plays a critical role in creating a favorable biologic environment. Excellent results have been reported clinically with cementless femoral stems manufactured in this manner. The radiologic appearances are characteristic of osseointegrated stems without radiolucencies or reactive linear densities.

Highly crystalline hydroxyapatite applied as a thin coating has been successfully used in the past 5 to 10 years (4,17,22). Intermediate-term results are excellent, but there is some concern about the possibility of slow resorption of the ceramic and late debonding.

Our initial experience with a first-generation cementless stem was not successful. We reported a high incidence of loosening and osteolysis (44). One of the fundamental reasons for failure was the use of noncircumferential porous coatings. We have shown, both experimentally and in autopsy specimens, that in the nonporous coated areas of the stem, a connective tissue membrane forms (6,78). This membrane serves as a pathway that allows polyethylene and other particulates produced at the joint level to reach the most distal areas of the stem–bone interface. Histiocytes containing multiple polyethylene-like particles can be identified in the membrane histologically. Thus, distal femoral osteolysis, and in some instances secondary loosening, became in the long-term, the dominant mechanism of failure. It is essential that a porous-coated cementless stem incorporate a circumferential coating to seal the medullary cavity and thus prevent the distal migration of particles.

The porous coating should cover a sufficiently large surface of the stem to provide an adequate area for fixation. In our first-generation design, about 10% of the surface was porous coated, an area probably insufficient, as we have seen evidence of secondary loosening in autopsy specimens (78).

Femoral stems can be extensively coated through their whole length, or proximally partially coated. I believe that in primary surgery it is desirable to use proximally coated stems. This principle will promote proximal stress transfer and in theory decrease the extent and severity of proximal bone resorption. Their potential removal is facilitated by the limitation of the porous coating to the proximal region. Extensively coated stems, which provide stability by fixation in the distal portion of the prosthesis, should be used only in revision surgery. The presence of proximally deficient femurs requires, in those circumstances, extensive coating to obtain stability by distal fixation.

Patient selection criteria play an important role in the prevention of failure. The quality of the bone stock is an important variable. The presence of osteoporosis requires the use of large-diameter stems which, in conjunction with thin porotic cortices, can lead to severe stress shielding. In addition, initial stabilization of the prosthesis becomes more difficult or inadequate. Age, because of its relation to osteoporosis, becomes a significant factor.

Given all of the above qualifications, adequate design and materials, proper technique, and appropriate patient selection criteria, excellent intermediate-term results can be obtained. Our own experience with a second-generation cementless stem showed a rate of loosening of 2% at an average 7-year follow-up and no distal osteolysis, an experience that compares favorably with our use of the hybrid prosthesis. Furthermore, these excellent intermediate-term follow-up results were obtained in a patient population with an average age of 50 years, a group of patients that are at notorious risk for failure.

My indications for the use of cementless stems include younger patients (less than 65 years old) with normal life expectancy and adequate bone stock. The choice of a cementless stem for the younger patient is not based on the premise that the stem will function without failure for a longer time than a cemented stem; it is rather because a potential revision may be easier with a proximally coated cementless stem than with a stem implanted with contemporary cement techniques.

Regarding the acetabulum, in the past decade, biologic fixation of porous-coated implants has challenged the use of acrylic cement as the preferred method of fixation. Experience with cemented acetabular components has shown that the rate of aseptic loosening increases with time, especially after the first 8 to 10 postoperative years (11,30,47,52,69). The mechanism of loosening has been proposed to be mainly biologic in nature, with particulate debris migrating along the host bone–cement interface as the initiating event (60). This is followed by an inflammatory tissue response, periprosthetic bone loss, and eventual implant loosening. To provide a successful alternative to cement, cementless components must demonstrate a lower rate of loosening and a lower incidence of osteolysis, the major causes of long-term failure.

Our own experience with a cementless hemispherical porous-coated prosthesis at an average 9-year follow-up was very satisfactory (72). There were 204 total hip arthroplasties in 184 patients with an average age of 51 years. The acetabula were inserted line to line, without press-fit impaction, and were fixed with three to five cancellous bone screws. There were no revisions performed for aseptic loosening. Only one acetabular component (0.6%) had migrated and the incidence of osteolysis was 5%.

Using the Kaplan-Meier technique, with a definition of failure that included revision or reoperation for any cause that related to the acetabular component, there was a 97% chance of survival at 10 years. Most of the problems and complications were seen in the younger patients. If only the group of patients over 70 years of age was considered, there were no complications, revisions, or reoperations.

This experience leads me to conclude that cementless hemispherical porous-coated acetabular prostheses can provide clinical results at up to 10 years that are as good or better than those reported with the use of cement.

There are some issues of concern that affect potential longer-term survivorship. The histologic appearance of the prosthesis–bone interface was studied in uncomplicated, retrieved autopsy specimens (51). Bone ingrowth was a common feature. This would indicate that stable fixation can be accomplished in a reproducible manner. Of concern in the longer-term implants were the presence of membrane and small granuloma containing particulate wear debris in screw holes with or without screws. In some instances, these membranes invaded the screw tracks or the interface adjacent to the screw holes. Particulate wear debris and granuloma were also seen at the rim of the components, but penetration of the bone–implant interface by this route was limited. Thus, screw holes with or without screws may serve as pathways for migration of particulate debris to the bone–porous coating interface and thus may be a factor leading to eventual failure.

The long-term problem affecting survivorship of the implant is wear and the resultant biologic response to the wear debris. Furthermore, it is the young patient that is at risk, both because of the time factor involved and their potential level of activity. It stands to reason that efforts should not only be directed to minimize particulate production, but also to limit their potential migration. That is the basis for a number of improvements that have been incorporated into many contemporary cementless acetabular components. This includes better locking mechanisms, improved manufacturing tolerances, and smooth inner metallic surfaces to decrease the possibility of wear at the convex surface of the polyethylene, absence of holes to eliminate internal pathways for particle migration, and full hemispheres to facilitate impaction of the implant without screws.

Appropriately designed cementless hemispherical porous-coated implants can provide excellent acetabular reconstruction for the vast majority of patients. There are some exceptions. Cementless implants should not be used in conjunction with a massive auto- or allograft, particularly if the prosthesis depends on the graft for support. Bone ingrowth cannot be expected at the graft–porous surface interface, and possible graft resorption may lead to late migration.

Patients who have received large doses of radiation to treat pelvic malignancies are at increased risk of loosening and failure with both cemented and cementless acetabula (31). The surgeon and the patient must be aware of these risks and make an appropriate decision as to the best technique to be used. At this time, I believe that cement with an adjuvant metallic support device may be the best alternative.

With the above exceptions, in primary surgery I use cementless acetabular reconstruction for all of my patients. The acetabulum is reamed to obtain a concentric surface of subchondral bleeding bone. A cup without holes that is 2 mm larger than the last reamer used is then impacted in place. Screws are not needed for most patients. Screws or some other form of immediate fixation may be used in instances of severe osteoporosis or deficient bone stock, or in the elderly patient where a concern for late development of osteolysis is not an issue.

In my own practice, a hybrid total hip arthroplasty, with a cementless acetabulum and a cemented femur, constitutes the best choice for all patients over the age of 65. In the younger patient with normal life expectancy and good femoral bone stock, a cementless total hip arthroplasty is a good alternative.

What does the future hold in the area of fixation? I believe that cementless fixation will continue to be used in the femur and in the acetabulum, particularly as we extend our indications to the younger patients. Furthermore, the reproducibility and extent of fixation may be substantially improved through enhancement by a variety of techniques. Tricalcium phosphates applied over the porous coating have been shown to significantly increase the strength of fixation and the occurrence of ingrowth in the experimental animal (53). This material has the desirable property of being resorbed within weeks after implantation. It has been used in clinical studies as well and it appears to improve the radiologic and clinical status of patients with cementless femoral stems.

A very promising avenue is that offered by the use of the so-called growth factors (66). The transforming growth factor-beta (TGF-β) family of proteins are polypeptide growth factors that have diverse effects on cell growth, differentiation, and function and are receiving considerable attention for potential clinical uses. They have been shown both *in vitro* and *in vivo* to have an effect on bone metabolism and repair. They have also been shown to significantly increase the amount of bone ingrowth in porous coatings. The potential future application of these factors is interesting in terms of increasing the reproducibility and the extent of ingrowth in primary surgery. This may have secondary long-term effects as well in preventing the progression of particle migration. They may be, though, of particular importance as a method of bone regeneration and ingrowth in the bone-deficient revision femur or acetabulum, a very difficult problem encountered in reconstructive surgery.

BONE REMODELING

Bone remodeling is a potential cause of long-term failure, particularly in cementless implants (32). Although bone loss secondary to cortical remodeling has not been shown to be a wide-spread clinical problem at the present time, it is an issue of concern in some specific patient populations.

Significant bone resorption has been reported with very large, very stiff metallic stems. Stem diameter, the extent of porous coating, the presence of bone ingrowth, the age and sex of the patient, and the presence of preexisting osteopenia have all been shown to be potential risk factors (13,14,16,71). Certainly, the use of large rigid stems in combination with preexisting osteopenia can lead to a nearly total loss of the cortex, with dramatic radiologic appearances and serious clinical consequences.

There are a number of design features of the stem that can affect the bone's mechanical environment and thus induce bone remodeling. These include the presence and absence of a porous coating, the type of porous coating, the location of the porous coating, and the stiffness of the stem (7,65,67,68,74). Experimental models have shown that the presence of a porous coating affects the rate of the bone loss process rather than its severity. Furthermore, the porous coating type does not influence either the amount or the pattern of bone remodeling in the long term. The data from experimental studies suggest that the rate of bone loss can be slowed by reducing the amount of porous coating but, ultimately, the magnitude is not substantially altered. Stiffness of the stem, on the other hand, has been shown to be an important variable affecting the overall extent of the bone-remodeling process.

We have used the dog as an experimental model, performing a unilateral total hip arthroplasty and using the opposite side as the control. After implantation of a cementless metallic stem, a pattern of bone remodeling and secondary bone loss occurs, characterized by proximal atrophy and distal cortical hypertrophy. In this model, a reduction in stem stiffness was effective in reducing proximal bone loss (73).

A number of design strategies can be utilized to decrease the bending stiffness of the stem, a variable critical to the process of bone resorption. One is a change in cross section, the second is the use of a prosthetic device made from a composite material or a low-modulus material. Changes in cross section are only moderately effective because the shape and dimensions of canal filling stems are imposed by the shape and dimensions of the host femur. Some reduction in stiffness is feasible by the incorporation of flutes and other similar geometrical changes, but these affect mostly the mid and distal stem areas and not the most proximal region.

The use of a low-modulus device is an attractive option. A cemented prosthesis is a lower-modulus device because the cross section is reduced as an intervening layer of cement is interposed between the cortex and the metallic stem. However, given the appropriate set of circumstances, such as the use of a large cemented stem, bone loss after cemented total hip replacement can be of the same order of magnitude as that following cementless total hip replacement (12,45).

Low-stiffness composite stems have been found to be effective in the experimental animal and they provide the basis for future developments in cementless femoral design (73). Further analytical and experimental work is needed to provide the structural framework that will allow us to accurately predict and prevent bone loss caused by stress shielding in total hip arthroplasty.

WEAR AND OSTEOLYSIS

During the first decade of extensive use of joint replacement devices, mechanical factors appeared, for the most part, to be responsible for the failures observed. Accordingly, much of the research in the field was engineering in nature. As design and materials improved, we have come to realize that biologic factors (that is, the response of the organism) play a critical role in the failure process.

Wear, the generation of debris, and the subsequent tissue reactions have emerged as the central problem limiting long-term longevity of total joint replacements. In addition, focal osteolysis is a major clinical problem (32).

Charnley may have been the first to recognize the phenomenon of osteolysis in total hip replacement, initially describing it as an "alteration in the texture of the cortex" (11). It has since been recognized by a number of authors in both loose and stable cemented components (18). It was at one time called cement disease, before the true pathogenesis of the problem was recognized.

Osteolysis is common in loose cemented components. It can occur in stable cemented implants where a defi-

ciency in the cement mantle and a communication between the joint and the focal lesion have been recognized and thought to be critical for its appearance (2,41).

The process has also been described in both loose and well-fixed uncemented implants, indicating that the absence of acrylic cement does not preclude the occurrence of osteolysis (40). In a review of total hip arthroplasty performed with the uncemented HGP (Harris-Galante) titanium-based alloy stem (44), 8% of 110 radiographically stable hips showed focal femoral osteolysis at an average 5.5-year follow-up. When we looked at the same patient population with a minimum follow-up of 10 years, the incidence was 27%, demonstrating that the incidence of femoral osteolysis in this patient population increased with time. These patients tend to be younger and more active, and they are essentially asymptomatic. Long-term radiographic follow-up of all patients after total hip arthroplasty, especially those with uncemented implants, is thus mandatory to identify the process prior to the occurrence of major complications resulting from progressive bone loss.

Other authors have described a 10% to 20% incidence of osteolysis with other uncemented implants fabricated either from cobalt–chrome or titanium alloy (18). The lesions tend to be proximal in designs with circumferential coatings, as contrasted with systems without circumferential porous coatings, where the lesions tend to be located more distally along the femoral stem.

Acetabular osteolysis occurs in association with both cemented and uncemented acetabular components as well (42,60,72,83). In uncemented components, the incidence is related to the type of prosthesis and length of follow-up. The differences in reported frequency are thought to be related to differences in either the thickness of the polyethylene insert, the relative stability of the insert, the congruity between the insert and the concave surface of the metal shell, the diameter of the femoral head, the quality of the polyethylene, or a combination of these factors.

The histopathology of the lytic lesion is well defined (2,82). It is characterized by granuloma formation with foci of intense histiocytic infiltration and foreign-body giant cells in association with dense fibrous tissue. Fine, opaque black granules can be seen within the histiocytes and under polarized light, and minute, strongly birefringent particles (characteristic of polyethylene) can be observed within the cytoplasm of the histiocytes. In the case of cemented implants, a large number of polymethylmethacrylate particles can also be seen.

One of the pertinent questions relates to the composition and characteristics of the wear debris. A study of material recovered from osteolytic areas revealed that 70% to 90% of the particles were ultra-high-molecular-weight polyethylene (62). The mean size was approximately 0.5 μm, and 92% of the particles were below 1 μm in size. In addition, corrosion products, titanium alloy, unalloyed titanium, cobalt–chrome, stainless steel, and silicates have also been identified. Volumetrically, though, submicron ultra-high-molecular-weight polyethylene particles constitute the dominant wear product (8,43).

It is hypothesized that the generation of wear particles and their migration into the joint cavity and periprosthetic spaces may stimulate macrophage recruitment and phagocytosis (26,59,82). This, in turn, stimulates secretions of various cellular mediators that interact and modify the activities of one another, resulting in either histiocytic or osteoclastic bone resorption (24,34).

This process is under intense scrutiny and further research is needed to clarify the role of the various bone-resorbing agents and the relative importance of the various types of particulate materials. Techniques that are being applied today include immunohistochemistry and *in situ* hybridization, powerful tools that will help us understand the basic cellular mechanisms involved.

What is the origin of the particles and how do they access the areas of the lesion?

Polyethylene particles represent mostly, although not exclusively, wear debris from the articular surfaces. They have easy access to the proximal medial cortex and the trochanteric regions of the hip. Lytic lesions in these areas are common, but they acquire clinical significance only if large granulomas develop. The distal femoral canal is accessible through defects in the cement mantle in the case of cemented implants. As mentioned previously, noncircumferentially coated porous implants or press-fit stems without a coating can provide a direct pathway to the distal stem (6,78).

The convex surface of the polyethylene insert in modular acetabula can also be a source of wear debris, particularly with earlier prosthetic designs. Access to the peri-acetabular trabecular bone structure is generally provided through holes in the metallic shell.

Fretting and corrosion at modular junctions have recently been recognized as important potential sources of particulate debris (23,33,75–77,79). The phenomena can occur both in mixed tapers (cobalt-based alloy-titanium alloy) and in tapers and heads made from the same alloy. The process involves a number of variables including metallurgical state, taper geometry, and manufacturing tolerances. It is thought to be the product of both fretting and crevice corrosion mechanisms.

The corrosion products have been identified to be primarily chromium phosphates. They have been identified at the taper junction, in the joint capsule, at the lytic lesion, and in the articular surface of the polyethylene. They are seen in the tissues as green plates, but they are also seen as submicron particles within histiocytes and, in certain cases, they can be the dominant particulate species. In some clinical cases of osteolysis, corrosion can be identified as the basis for the mechanism of failure.

Modularity was introduced in the 1980s as an important advance in prosthetic design. Modularity has obvious advantages for both the surgeon and the manufacturer. It adds versatility to the surgical procedure and results in a substantial decrease in prosthesis inventory and costs. However, it has the obvious disadvantage of adding an additional source of particulate debris and an additional potential cause for failure. Certainly, the incorporation of increased modularity in some new implant systems is a reason for concern. For these reasons, there is a growing interest among many surgeons for a return to nonmodular monolytic stems, a design principle that was time-tested and proven in the original Charnley femoral prosthesis.

Other particulate debris that have potential clinical significance include metallic particles, most frequently seen in loose implants where gross interfacial motion may be present. Silicates can be seen and are probably remnants of the surface-processing technique used during manufacturing. Stainless steel particles are usually produced as debris from cerclage wires or cables used for trochanteric fixation. These particulate species can have biologic effects of their own or migrate to the joint and act as a third body to increase polyethylene wear.

Although all of the above types of particles may have biologic effects, there is a consensus that polyethylene particles represent the most biologically active agent, as their size and large numbers give rise to an enormous surface area for interaction with the surrounding tissues.

For that reason, methods to decrease the severity of polyethylene wear are critical to increase the longevity of total hip prosthesis. A number of factors govern the rate of polyethylene wear, and some of these, including the choice of femoral head diameter and polyethylene thickness, are under direct control of the surgeon. There is increasing evidence that smaller-diameter heads are associated with lower rates of wear (36), thus femoral heads with a 32-mm diameter should not be routinely used. Although a 22-mm head diameter represents the ideal choice from the viewpoint of wear, its use is not practical in many prosthetic systems, particularly of the cementless type, because the large diameter of their neck tapers severely restricts range of motion and increases the potential for postoperative dislocation. Certainly, with smaller, metal-backed acetabular components, less than 50 mm in diameter, the use of a 22-mm head is almost essential to maintain a reasonable thickness of polyethylene.

A great deal of progress has occurred in recent years as a better understanding has been reached of some of the factors that govern the quality and uniformity of polyethylene. This has allowed the development of improved fabrication modalities and sterilization techniques. Sterilization by radiation in inert atmospheres or using other environments and techniques such as ethylene dioxide has become current practice. There are a number of new approaches being studied to develop ultra-high-molecular-weight polyethylene with a different molecular structure, such as with increased crosslinkage. to improve wear resistance. Ceramic heads have been introduced as another method of decreasing polyethylene wear. Although wear can be decreased both in laboratory and in clinical settings, the introduction of a ceramic head may pose additional problems including fracture of the ceramic component (18). Furthermore, the clinical benefit of using ceramic heads has not been demonstrated conclusively.

The use of alternate bearing systems, such as metal–metal and ceramic–ceramic, is being considered both experimentally and clinically. Both of these types of systems have been used in Europe during the last few years. Extensive clinical application in the United States is probably several years away, because a number of regulatory issues must be resolved prior to their wide-spread introduction. It is in the younger patient population where these alternate bearing systems are of particular interest.

For the foreseeable future, joint replacement using conventional contemporary materials and designs will remain the cornerstone for restoration of joint function. At this stage in the development and use of joint replacement devices, it is incumbent upon the orthopedic surgeon to analyze in depth the reason for failures and, in particular, to avoid the widespread use of new techniques without adequate long-term evaluation. Appropriate judgment based on scientific information and common sense should be used in the choice of an implant system.

Cost is an overwhelming consideration in today's socioeconomic environment, and technologic improvement should only be applied where it is truly needed. It is the younger, more active patients who are at risk and in need for improved solutions.

Wear and its related biologic problems are at the heart of most failures seen today, and will be responsible for most of the failures that we will see in the future. It is in this area that most of the clinical and laboratory research efforts are being directed. It is not easy to predict the behavior of biologic systems. Thus, there is no substitute for ongoing close scrutiny and long-term follow-up of the different patient populations, the introduction of well-designed prospective clinical studies, and in-depth research directed to the *in vitro* and *in vivo* behavior of the materials and designs used in joint replacement surgery.

REFERENCES

1. Amstutz HC, Markolf KL, McNeice GM, Gruen TA. Loosening of total hip components: cause and prevention. In: *The hip: proceedings of the fourth open scientific meeting of the Hip Society*. St. Louis: CV Mosby, 1976:102–116.
2. Anthony PP, Gie GA, Howie CR, et al. Localized endosteal bone lysis in relation to the femoral components of cemented total hip arthroplasties. *J Bone Joint Surg* 1990;72B:971–979.
3. Barrack RL, Mulroy RD, Harris WH. Improved cementing technique and femoral component loosening in young patients with hip arthroplasty: a 12-year radiographic review. *J Bone Joint Surg* 1992;74B:385.
4. Bauer TW, Geesink RCT, Zimmerman R, McMahon JT. Hydroxyapatite-coated femoral stems: histological analysis of components retrieved at autopsy. *J Bone Joint Surg* 1991;73A:1439–1452.
5. Beckenbaugh RD, Ilstrup DM. Total hip arthroplasty. A review of 333 cases with long follow-up. *J Bone Joint Surg* 1978;60A:306–313.
6. Bobyn JD, Jacobs JJ, Tanzer M, et al. The susceptibility of smooth implant surfaces to periimplant fibrosis and migration of polyethylene wear debris. *Clin Orthop* 1995;311:21–39.
7. Bobyn JD, Pilliar RM, Binnington AG, Szivek JA. The effect of proximally and fully porous-coated canine hip stem design on bone modeling. *J Orthop Res* 1987;5:393–408.
8. Campbell P, McKellop H, Yeom B, et al. Isolation and characterization of UHMWPE particles from periprosthetic tissues. *Trans Soc Biomater* 1994;17:391.
9. Carlsson AS, Gentz CF, Stenport J. Fracture of the femoral prosthesis in total hip replacement according to Charnley. *Acta Orthop Scand* 1977;48:650.
10. Charnley J. Fracture of femoral prosthesis in total hip replacement. *Clin Orthop* 1975;111:105–120.
11. Charnley J. *Low friction arthroplasty of the hip: theory and practice*. New York: Springer-Verlag, 1979.
12. Cohen B, Rushton N. Bone remodelling in the proximal femur after Charnley total hip arthroplasty. *J Bone Joint Surg* 1995;77B:815–819.
13. Engh CA, Bobyn JD, Glassman AH. Porous-coated hip replacement: the factors governing bone ingrowth stress shielding and clinical results. *J Bone Joint Surg* 1987;69B:45–55.
14. Engh CA, Bobyn JD. The influence of stem size and extent of porous coating on femoral bone resorption after primary cementless hip arthroplasty. *Clin Orthop* 1988;231:7.
15. Engh CA, Hooten JP, Zetti-Schaffer KF, et al. Porous-coated total hip replacement. *Clin Orthop* 1994;298:89–96.
16. Engh CA, McGovern TF, Bobyn JD, Harris WH. A quantitative evaluation of periprosthetic bone-remodeling after cementless total hip arthroplasty. *J Bone Joint Surg* 1992;74A:1009–1020.
17. Friedman RJ, Bauer TW, Garg K, Jiang M, An YH, Draughn RA. Histological and mechanical comparison of hydroxyapatite-coated cobalt-chrome and titanium implants in the rabbit femur. *J Appl Biomater* 1995;6:231–235.
18. Friedman RJ, Black J, Galante JO, et al. Current concepts in orthopaedic biomaterials and implant fixation. *J Bone Joint Surg* 1993; 75A:1086–1109.
19. Galante JO, Rostoker W, Doyle JM. Failed femoral stems in total hip prostheses. *J Bone Joint Surg* 1975;57A:230–236.
20. Galante JO, Rostoker W, Lueck R, Ray RD. Sintered fiber composites as a basis for attachment of implants to bone. *J Bone Joint Surg* 1971; 53A:101–114.
21. Gebhard JS, Amstutz HC, Zinar DM, Dorey RJ. A comparison of total hip arthroplasty for treatment of acute fracture of the femoral neck. *Clin Orthop* 1992;282:123–131.
22. Geesink RG, Hoefnagels NH. Six-year results of hydroxyapatite-coated total hip replacement. *J Bone Joint Surg* 1995;77B:534–537.
23. Gilbert JL, Buckley CA, Jacobs JJ. In-vivo corrosion of modular hip prosthesis components in mixed and similar metal combinations. The effect of crevice, stress, motion, and alloy coupling. *J Biomed Mater Res* 1993;27:1533–1544.
24. Glant TT, Jacobs JJ, Molnar G, et al. Bone resorption activity of particulate-stimulated macrophages. *J Bone Mineral Res* 1993;8:1071–1079.
25. Goetz DD, Smith EJ, Harris WH. The prevalence of femoral osteolysis associated with components inserted with or without cement in total hip replacements. A retrospective matched-pair series. *J Bone Joint Surg* 1994;76A:1121–1129.
26. Goldring SR, Schiller AL, Roelke M, et al. The synovial-like membrane at the bone-cement interface in loose total hip replacements and its proposed role in bone lysis. *J Bone Joint Surg* 1983;65A:575–584.
27. Gruen TA, McNeice GM, Amstutz HC. "Mode of failure" of cemented stem-type femoral components: a radiographic analysis of loosening. *Clin Orthop* 1979;141:17–27.
28. Harris WH, Maloney WJ. Hybrid total hip arthroplasty. *Clin Orthop* 1989;249:21–29.
29. Harris WH, McGann WA. Loosening of the femoral component after use of the medullary plug cement technique. *J Bone Joint Surg* 1982;64A:1063–1067.
30. Hodgkinson JP, Maskell AP, Paul A, Wroblewski BM. Flanged acetabular components in cemented Charnley hip arthroplasty. Ten-year follow-up of 350 patients. *J Bone Joint Surg* 1993;75B:464–467.
31. Jacobs JJ, Kull LR, Frey GA, et al. Early failure of acetabular components inserted without cement after previous pelvic irradiation. *J Bone Joint Surg* 1995;77A:1829–1835.
32. Jacobs JJ, Sumner DR, Galante JO. Mechanisms of bone loss associated with total hip replacement. *Orthop Clin North Am* 1993;24:583–590.
33. Jacobs JJ, Urban RM, Gilbert JL, et al. Local and distant products of modularity. *Clin Orthop* 1995;319:94–105.

34. Jiranek WA, Machado M, Jasty M, et al. Production of cytokines around loosened cemented acetabular components: analysis with immunohistochemical techniques and in situ hybridization. *J Bone Joint Surg* 1993;75A:863–879.

35. Ling RSM. Loosening experiences at Exeter. *Orthop Trans* 1981;5:351.

36. Livermore J, Ilstrup MS, Morrey B. Effect of femoral head size on wear of the polyethylene acetabular component. *J Bone Joint Surg* 1990; 72A:518–528.

37. Lu-Yao GL, Keller RB, Littenberg B, Wennenberg JE. Outcomes after displaced fractures of the femoral neck. A meta-analysis of one hundred and six published reports. *J Bone Joint Surg* 1994;76A:15–25.

38. Lueck R, Galante JO, Rostoker W, Ray RD. Development of an open pore metallic implant to permit attachment to bone. *Surg Form* 1969; 20:456.

39. Malchau H, Herberts P, Ahnfelt C. Prognosis of total hip replacement in Sweden. Follow-up of 92,675 operations performed 1978–1990. *Acta Orthop Scand* 1993:64:497–506.

40. Maloney WJ, Jasty M, Harris WH, et al. Endosteal erosion in association with stable uncemented femoral components. *J Bone Joint Surg* 1990;72A:1025–1034.

41. Maloney WJ, Jasty M, Rosenberg A, et al. Bone lysis in well-fixed cemented femoral components. *J Bone Joint Surg* 1990;72B:966–970.

42. Maloney WJ, Peters P, Engh CA, Chandler H. Severe osteolysis of the pelvis in association with acetabular replacement without cement. *J Bone Joint Surg* 1993;75A:1627–1635.

43. Maloney WJ, Smith RL, Huene D, et al. Particulate wear debris: characterization and quantitation from membranes around failed cementless femoral replacements. *Trans Orthop Res Soc* 1993;18:294.

44. Martell JM, Pierson RH, Jacobs JJ, Rosenberg AG, Maley M, Galante JO. Primary total hip reconstruction with a titanium fiber-coated prosthesis inserted without cement. *J Bone Joint Surg* 1993;75A:554–571.

45. McCarthy CK, Steinberg GG, Agren M, Leahey D, Wyman E, Baran DT. Quantifying bone loss from the proximal femur after total hip arthroplasty. *J Bone Joint Surg* 1991;73B:774–778.

46. Mohler CG, Kull LR, Martell JM, Rosenberg AG, Galante JO. Total hip replacement with insertion of an acetabular component without cement and a femoral component with cement. Four to seven-year results. *J Bone Joint Surg* 1995;77A:86–96.

47. Mulroy RD, Harris WH. The effect of improved cementing techniques on component loosening in total hip replacement: an 11 year radiographic review. *J Bone Joint Surg* 1990;72B:757–760.

48. Mulroy W, Harris WH. Non-septic, cemented femoral revision total hip arthroplasty using so-called second generation cementing techniques: 15 year radiographic review. *J Bone Joint Surg* 1995;77A:1845–1852.

49. NIH Consensus Statement. *Total hip replacement.* 1994;12(5).

50. Oishi CS, Walker RH, Colwell CW Jr. The femoral component in total hip arthroplasty. Six to eight-year follow-up of one hundred consecutive patients after use of a third-generation cementing technique. *J Bone Joint Surg* 1994;76A:1130–1136.

51. Pidhorz LE, Urban RM, Jacobs JJ, Sumner DR, Galante JO. A quantitative study of bone and soft tissue in cementless porous-coated acetabular components retrieved at autopsy. *J Arthroplasty* 1993;8:213–225.

52. Ranawat CS, Deshmukh RG, Peters LE, Umlas ME. Prediction of the long-term durability of all-polyethylene cemented sockets. *Clin Orthop* 1985;317:89–105.

53. Rivero DP, Fox J, Skipor AK, Urban RM, Galante JO. Calcium phosphate-coated porous titanium implants for enhanced skeletal fixation. *J Biomed Mat Res* 1988;22:181–201.

54. Roberts DW, Poss R, Kelly K. Radiographic comparison of cement techniques in total hip arthroplasty. *J Arthroplasty* 1986;1:241–247.

55. Russotti GM, Coventry MB, Stauffer RN. Cemented total hip arthroplasty with contemporary techniques: a five year minimum follow-up study. *Clin Orthop* 1988;235:141.

56. Salvati EA, Wilson PD Jr, Jolley MN, Vakili F, Aglietti P, Brown GC. A ten-year follow-up study of our first one hundred consecutive Charnley total hip replacements. *J Bone Joint Surgery* 1981;63A:753–767.

57. Sarmiento A. Low modulus of elasticity prosthesis (Ti-6Al-4V) in total hip arthroplasty. *Orthop Trans* 1981;5:357.

58. Schmalzried TP, Harris WH. Hybrid total hip replacement. A 6.5 year follow-up study. *J Bone Joint Surg* 1993;75B:608–615.

59. Schmalzried TP, Jasty M, Harris WH. Periprosthetic bone loss in total hip arthroplasty: polyethylene wear debris and the concept of the effective joint space. *J Bone Joint Surg* 1992;74A:849–863.

60. Schmalzried TP, Kwong IM, Jasty M, et al. The mechanisms of loosening of cemented acetabular components in total hip arthroplasty: analysis of specimens retrieved at autopsy. *Clin Orthop* 1992;274:60–68.

61. Schulte KR, Callaghan JJ, Kelley SS, Johnston RC. The outcome of Charnley total hip arthroplasty with cement. *J Bone Joint Surg* 1993; 75A:961–975.

62. Shanbhag AS, Jacobs JJ, Glant TT, et al. Composition and morphology of wear debris in failed uncemented total hip arthroplasty. *J Bone Joint Surg* 1994;76B:60–67.

63. Spotorno L, Romangnoli S, Ivaldo N, Grappiolo G, Bibbiani E, Blaha JO, Guen TA. The CLS system. Theoretical concept and results. *Acta Orthop Belgica* 1993;59:144–148.

64. Stauffer RN. Ten year follow-up study of total hip replacement, with particular reference to roentgenographic loosening of the components. *J Bone Joint Surg* 1982;64A:970–982.

65. Sumner DR, Galante JO. Determinants of stress shielding: design vs. materials vs. interface. *Clin Orthop* 1992;274:202–212.

66. Sumner DR, Turner TM, Purchio AF, Gombotz WR, Urban RM, Galante JO. Enhancement of bone ingrowth by transforming growth factor-β. *J Bone Joint Surg* 1995;77A:1135–1147.

67. Sumner DR, Turner TM, Urban RM, Galante JO. Remodeling and ingrowth of bone at two years in a canine total hip-arthroplasty model. *J Bone Joint Surg* 1992;74A:239–250.

68. Sumner DR, Turner TM, Urban RM, Galante JO. Experimental studies of bone remodeling in total hip replacement. *Clin Orthop* 1992;275: 83–90.

69. Sutherland CJ, Wilde AH, Borden LS, Marks KE. A ten-year follow-up of one hundred consecutive Muller curved-stem total hip replacement arthroplasty. *J Bone Joint Surg* 1982;64A:970–982.

70. Swiontrowski MF. Current concepts review. Intracapsular fractures of the hip. *J Bone Joint Surg* 1994:76A:129–138.

71. Sychterz CJ, Engh CA. The influence of clinical factors on periprosthetic bone remodeling. *Clin Orthop* 1996:322:285–292.

72. Tompkins GS, Jacobs JJ, Kull LR, Rosenberg AG, Galante JO. Primary total hip reconstruction with a porous acetabular component. Seven to ten year results. *J Bone Joint Surg* 1997;79A:169–176.

73. Turner TM, Sumner DR, Raginsky B, Funk CM, Igloria R, Urban RM, Galante JO. Proximal bone loss is reduced (but not eliminated) with low modulus stems in cementless THR: a two-year canine study. *Trans Orthop Res Soc* 1996:21:235.

74. Turner TM, Sumner DR, Urban RM, Rivero DP, Galante JO. A comparative study of porous coatings in a weight-bearing total hip-arthroplasty model. *J Bone Joint Surg* 1986;68A:1396–1409.

75. Urban RM, Jacobs JJ, Gavrllovic J, Turner TM, Galante JO. Dissemination of metal-alloy particles to the liver and spleen of patients with total hip or knee replacement prostheses. *Trans Fifth World Biomat Congress* Toronto 1996;660.

76. Urban RM, Jacobs JJ, Gilbert JL, et al. Characterization of solid products of corrosion generated by modular-head femoral stems of different designs and materials. In: Marlowe DE, Parr JE, Mayor MB, eds. *Modularity of orthopedic implants, ASTM STP 1301*, American Society for Testing Materials 1997.

77. Urban RM, Jacobs JJ, Gilbert JL, Galante JO. Migration of corrosion products from modular hip prostheses: particle microanalysis and histopathological findings. *J Bone Joint Surg* 1994;76A:1346–1359.

78. Urban RM, Jacobs JJ, Sumner DR, Peters CL, Voss FR, Galante JO. The bone-implant interface in femoral stems with non-circumferential porous coating: a study of specimens retrieved at autopsy. *J Bone and Joint Surg* 1996:78A;1068–1081.

79. Urban RM, Jacobs JJ, Tomlinson MJ, Black J, Turner TM, Galante JO. Particles of metal alloys and their corrosion products in the liver, spleen, and para-aortic lymph nodes of patients with total hip replacement prostheses. *Trans Orthop Res Soc* 1995;20:241.

80. Verdonschot N, Hulskes R. Dynamic creep behavior of acrylic bone cement. *J Biomed Mater Res* 1995;29:575–581.

81. Verdonschot N, Hulskes R. Mechanical effects of stem cement interface characteristics in total hip replacement. *Clin Orthop* 1996;329: 326–336.

82. Willert HG, Semlitsch M. Reactions of the articular capsule to wear products of artificial joint prostheses. *J Biomed Mater Res* 1977;11: 157–164.

83. Zicat B, Engh C, Gokcen E. Patterns of osteolysis around total hip components inserted with and without cement. *J Bone Joint Surg* 1995; 77A:432–439.

The Adult Hip, edited by J. J. Callaghan,
A. G. Rosenberg, and H. E. Rubash.
Lippincott–Raven Publishers, Philadelphia © 1998.

CHAPTER 52

Cost Effectiveness of Total Hip Arthroplasty

Robert B. Bourne and Paul R. Kim

The editor emeritus of *The New England Journal of Medicine,* Arnold Relman, has described three eras in medicine since World War II: the era of expansion, the era of cost containment, and the contemporary era of assessment and accountability (16). The reasons for greater scrutiny of medical practice are multiple, but they seem to center around the perception that medical costs are escalating out of control and that there is a lack of quality assurance.

Many factors have led to the escalation of medical costs. Affluence, expensive new technologies, and an aging population all have contributed to cost dilemmas (5). Health-care costs currently consume anywhere from 6% to 15% of a first-world country's gross domestic product. Projections for the future are staggering, suggesting that 25% or more of a nation's gross domestic product might be consumed by health care within the next 25 years. The current upward spiral of medical costs seems unacceptable, leading both private and public health-care providers to seek greater cost efficiencies.

Coupled with the issue of cost concerns is the concept of quality assurance. Several studies have demonstrated that greater health-care expenditure per capita, more beds per capita, and longer length of stay do not equate with improved patient health (21). Indeed, some nations with the lowest health-care expenditures have the longest average life spans and the lowest perinatal mortality rates. In addition, considerable variance has been noted in surgical rates from country to country or even from region to region within the same nation. Economists point to this lack of standardization as being a major factor contributing to escalating health-care costs. Others point to these same statistics as an indication of needless intervention and have encouraged the development of practice standards.

The outcomes movement has arisen from the issues of cost and quality assurance, but it has been given considerable impetus by private health management organizations that wish to provide quality medical care in a cost-effective manner. These organizations have led the way in terms of developing practice guidelines, clinical pathways, and cost-effectiveness research. In addition, government health-care providers have entered the fray, comparing cost to quality-adjusted life-years (cost to QALY) data. More recently, health-care providers have been examining individual procedures, such as total hip arthroplasty, in terms of cost-effective practice. In our center, we have assessed total hip arthroplasty in terms of cost to QALY and have found that total hip arthroplasty is one of the most cost-effective medical interventions known (6). Healy and Barber have also conducted cost-effectiveness studies and presented these at the 1995 meeting of the American Academy of Orthopaedic Surgeons. They have demonstrated that significant cost savings might be achieved by matching patients in terms of age, medical status, activity level, and bone stock with expensive or less expensive total hip replacements.

The study of cost-effectiveness parameters by the orthopedic surgeon is somewhat new. Some fears exist that long-term results will be compromised by this approach. Nevertheless, as cost-effectiveness data gain greater importance in the field of health-care policy, it would seem appropriate that the total hip replacement surgeon is better served by being well informed in this regard.

R. B. Bourne and P. R. Kim: Department of Orthopaedic Surgery, London Health Sciences Centre, The University of Western Ontario, London, Ontario N6A 5A5, Canada.

METHODOLOGIES TO DETERMINE COST-TO-UTILITY RATIOS

Growing interest in the evaluation and comparison of differing treatment regimens in medicine is being driven by the combination of ever-increasing health-care costs and shrinking health-care resources. To evaluate the cost effectiveness of total hip arthroplasty, and particularly to compare it with other treatment modalities, it is necessary to use standardized cost and utility assessments. To understand these clinical epidemiology methodologies, it is necessary to understand the terminology used.

Evaluation of differing treatment regimens in terms of cost effectiveness involves an economic assessment. This requires a calculation of the dollar costs of the therapy or treatment being studied. Up until this point, most economic assessments have been based on charges rather than costs. Tertiary care institutions that support costly cardiac, neurosurgical, trauma, or transplant programs often have charges that are 30% greater than community hospitals without these expensive services. It is obviously of great importance to determine the actual cost rather than the charge for a particular service.

The calculation of costs includes both direct and indirect costs. Costs associated directly with the delivery of medical care include outpatient-related costs (i.e., drug costs, consultation fees), inpatient-related costs (i.e., hospital costs, surgical fees), and patient-specific costs (i.e., transportation costs, home-care service fees). Indirect costs include earnings a patient may have foregone while undergoing treatment or while affected by illness.

There are three basic forms of economic evaluation utilized, as summarized in Table 1 (8). For each type, the costs of treatment are compared with the outcomes of treatment. Cost effectiveness analysis is a comparison of two differ treatments or programs, comparing the costs as related to a common effect that may differ in magnitude (7). An example would be comparing two different hip prostheses with respect to clinical outcome, using a spe-

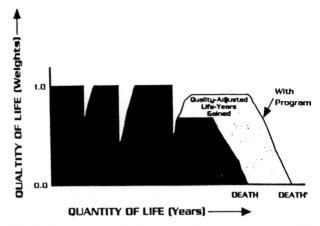

FIG. 1. The area under the curve is measured in quality-adjusted life-years (QALY). With this type of analysis, one can compare across disciplines.

cific rating scale. In a cost-effectiveness analysis, one does not assign a dollar value to the outcome: outcome measurement depends on the rating scale used. Cost-benefit analysis measures both the costs and the consequences of alternative treatments in dollar terms (7). The life of an individual consists of two major components, (a) the quantity (years) and, (b) the quality of life. This can be demonstrated graphically: Figure 1 shows a hypothetical life profile of an individual with and without a particular treatment program. The area between the two curves represents the QALY gained: increases in both the quantity and the quality of life. This provides a single comprehensive measure of health improvement, which allows one to compare various treatments across different health disciplines.

There are a wide variety of measures currently used to assess health-related quality of life. These can be divided into three main areas (Table 2) (6,7). The first group comprises disease-specific measures that assess outcome with tools developed specifically for a certain condition: health-related quality of life is assessed as it pertains to a certain disease. Examples are the Western Ontario McMaster (WOMAC) Arthritis index (2), the Harris Hip Score (9), and the d'Aubigne-Postel Hip Score (14). The WOMAC scale was developed specifically to assess patients suffering from osteoarthritis of the hip and knee. This index been shown to be both valid and reliable (1,3). The second group consists of patient-specific outcome measures. The McMaster Toronto Arthritis (MACTAR) scale represents this group. It assesses the effectiveness of a treatment in relieving patient complaints (20).

The third group consists of global outcome measures. These instruments can be applied to any number of patient populations, and they are in a sense generic. They typically cover areas such as physical function, social and emotional function, pain, and self-care. They can be subdivided into health profiles and utility measures. Health

TABLE 1. *Major study designs for economic evaluations*

Type of analysis	Compares	To
Cost	$ Value of resources used up	Clinical effects
Cost/utility	$ Value of resources used up	Quality of life produced by the clinical effects
Cost/benefit	$ Value of resources used up	$ Value of resources saved or created

Based on Feeny DH, Torrence GW, Labelle R. Integrating economic evaluations and quality of life assessments. In: Spilker B, ed. *Quality of life and pharmacoeconomics in clinical trials*, 2nd ed. Philadelphia: Lippincott-Raven 1996: 85–95.

TABLE 2. *Groupings of ways to assess health-related quality of life*

Disease-specific
  Western Ontario McMaster Arthritis index (WOMAC)
  Harris Hip Score
  D'Aubigne and Postel Score
Patient-specific
  McMaster Toronto Arthritis index (MACTAR)
Global assessment
  Health profiles
    Sickness impact profile
  Utility measures
    Time trade-off
    Standard gamble

profiles provide separate scores for a number of different categories of health-related quality-of-life issues. An example is the Sickness Impact Profile as developed by Bergner et al. (4). It was designed to provide a more sensitive measure of a patient's progress by assessing activities associated with everyday living. Utility measures are widely applicable and give general scores, usually on a scale of 0 (representing death) to 1 (representing perfect health) (18,19). They can be applied and compared to a broad range of health-care treatments or programs. Utility measures also allow the patient and researcher to assess both the positive and negative aspects of treatment. These aspects are both included in the final score, which represents all aspects of health-related quality of life. With disease-specific measures, the positive and negative aspects of treatment are measured separately, so it is not possible to determine what trade-offs the patient is willing to make for a certain treatment. This same deficiency is also found in health profile measurements.

The two types of utility measures most commonly used are the time trade-off and the standard gamble techniques (18,19). The time trade-off technique, simply stated, asks the respondent to choose between two possibilities: to live in health state A for a certain time *(x)*, or to live in health state B for a certain time *(y)*. The outcome at the end of both time periods *x* and *y* is the same (usually death). Times *x* and *y* are varied in a systematic fashion to identify a point at which the respondent is indifferent between the two possibilities. This concept has been used by McNeil et al. (15), who presented a group of individuals with two treatment options for laryngeal cancer. The first was laryngectomy, which offers survival but loss of voice, and the second was radiation, which preserves voice but has the risk of shorter survival. On average, individuals indicated that they would trade off 14% of their full life expectancy to avoid loss of speech. This demonstrates the concept of time trade-off. One can also apply this to loss of mobility or function from any disease, including arthritis of the hip. The standard gamble is a type of lottery in which the respondent is presented with two choices. Choice A involves a single outcome

with a 100% chance of occurring, whereas choice B involves two alternatives, one perfect health (the most preferred state) and the other sickness (the least preferred state). The chances of these two alternatives occurring are varied until the respondent is indifferent to choosing between choice A and choice B.

When these methodologies utilizing utility measures are coupled with costs, formulation of cost-to-utility ratios can be determined. The results are expressed in cost/QALY (19). This ratio can be calculated for the treatment of different conditions or diseases and therefore a comparison of cost effectiveness between unlike procedures can be done. Laupacis et al. have studied the issue of cost to utility ratios in depth (12). Using the cost/QALY, they found that interventions costing less than $20,000/QALY are extremely cost effective and should be utilized. Those interventions costing between $20,001 and $100,000/QALY are moderately cost effective and probably should be funded but require discussion. Interventions that cost more than $100,000/QALY might be effective but are extremely costly and require considerable analysis before being implemented. Naylor et al. have debated this approach, stating both ethical and validity concerns. The ethical concerns center around whether or not interventions with a cost/QALY ratio over $100,000 should be denied to the population. Validity concerns center around the accuracy of the clinical methodologies used and the accuracy of the costing data. Despite these potential shortcomings, cost-to-utility ratios are being utilized with greater frequency.

A COST-TO-UTILITY ANALYSIS OF TOTAL HIP REPLACEMENT

In 1987, a blinded, randomized clinical trial was initiated to compare contemporary cemented and cementless total hip replacements in terms of disease-specific, patient-specific, global, functional capacity, and cost-to-utility ratios (6,10–13,16). At 5 to 8 years of follow-up, the revision rates and clinical outcomes are similar for the two prostheses. The disease-specific (Fig. 2), patient-specific (Fig. 3), global (Fig. 4), and functional capacity (Fig. 5) outcomes were similar for the cemented and cementless implants utilized.

To perform the cost-to-utility ratios, accurate costing was performed on 100 patients in terms of inpatient (hospital and physician) and outpatient (outpatient and third-party) costs. Total hip replacement was demonstrated to be a type A intervention with a cost-to-QALY ratio of approximately $8,000 (12). The cost-to-QALY ratio for total hip replacement was then compared to that for the treatment of moderate hypertension, the treatment of osteoporosis, the treatment of coronary artery bypass, hemodialysis, liver transplantation, and universal precautions for human immune virus deficiency (Fig. 6). As

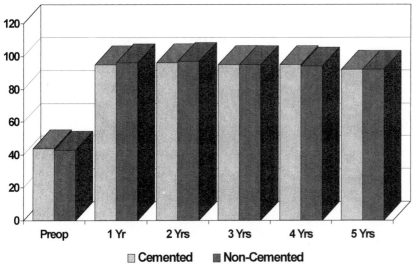

A

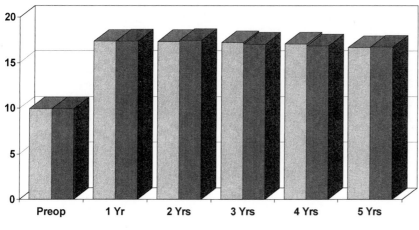

B

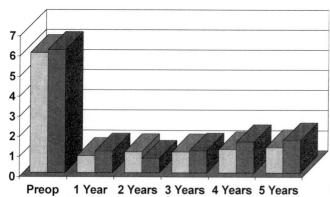

C

FIG. 2. Examples of disease-specific outcome measures comparing cemented and cementless total hip replacements. **A:** Harris Hip Score. **B:** D'Aubigne-Postel. **C:** WOMAC, MACTAR.

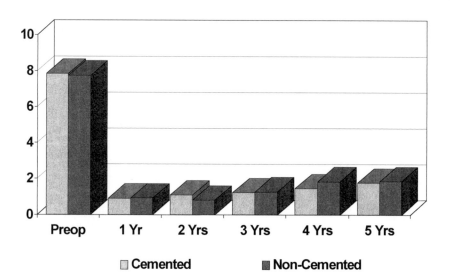

FIG. 3. Example of MACTAR patient-specific outcomes comparing cemented and cementless total hip replacements.

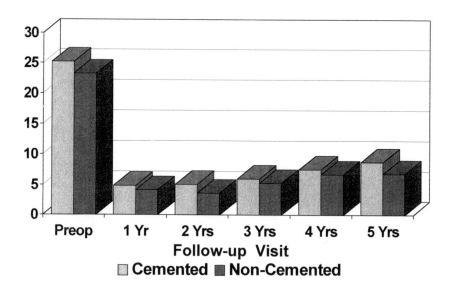

FIG. 4. Example of the Sickness Impact Profile global physical score comparing cemented and cementless total hip replacements.

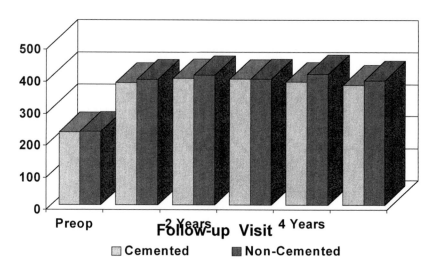

FIG. 5. Example of a functional capacity outcome (the 6-minute walk) comparing cemented and cementless total hip replacements (distance measured in meters).

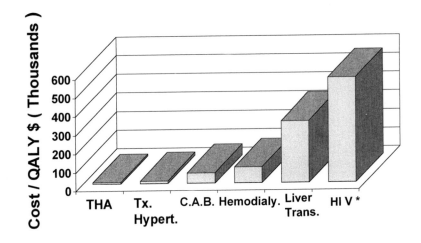

FIG. 6. Cost/utility ratios comparing cost effectiveness of treating total hip arthroplasty (THA), moderate hypertension (Tx—Hypert.), coronary artery disease (C.A.B.), hemodialysis (Hemodial.), liver transplantation (L. transp.), and universal precautions against human immunodeficiency virus (HIV).

* **Cost / Additional Life Saved**

most cost to utility ratios were, costing and utility data were utilized for 2 years. It will be of interest to repeat the costing data at 5, 10, and more years of follow-up.

DISCUSSION

Total hip arthroplasty is one of the most cost-effective medical interventions known. The detailed analysis of the quality of life and cost-effectiveness aspects of total hip replacement have other ramifications. In terms of global health, we have determined that a symptomatic patient with a severely arthritic hip is just as disabled as a patient with intractable angina or one on hemodialysis. Similar disruption of patient social interactions, ability to work, and sleep patterns occurs with osteoarthritis of the hip as with so-called life-threatening disorders. Furthermore, once total hip replacement is performed, these patients are reverted to virtually normal health, as opposed to those on hemodialysis or those treated with a coronary artery bypass. Hence, cost-to-utility data are extremely important in demonstrating the disability of a patient with osteoarthritis of the hip as well as the efficacy of total hip replacement and its cost effectiveness in comparison to other medical and surgical interventions.

REFERENCES

1. Bellamy N. Pain assessment in osteoarthritis: experience with the WOMAC osteoarthritis index. *Semin Arthritis Rheum* 1989;18:14–17.
2. Bellamy N, Buchanan WW. A preliminary evaluation of the dimensionality and clinical importance of pain and disability in osteoarthritis of the hip and knee. *Clin Rheumatol* 1986;5:231–241.
3. Bellamy N, Buchanan WW, Goldsmith CH, Campbell J, Stitt LW. Validation study of WOMAC: a health status instrument for measuring clinically important patient relevant outcomes to antirheumatic drug therapy inpatients with osteoarthritis of the hip or knee. *J Rheumatol* 1988;15:1833–1840.
4. Bergner M, Bobbitt RA, Carter WB, Gilson BS. The sickness impact profile: development and final revision of a health status measure. *Med Care* 1981;19:787–805.
5. Bourne RB. Some clinical research is not cost-effective: weaknesses of outcome studies. *Spine* 1995;20:1–4.
6. Bourne RB, Rorabeck CH, Laupacis A, Feeny D, Tugwell PS, Wong C, Bullas R. Total hip replacement. The case of noncemented femoral fixation because of age. *Can J Surg* 1995;38(1):S61.
7. Drummond MF, Stoddart GL, Torrance GW. Methods for the economic evaluation of health care programs [abstr]. 1987.
8. Feeny DH, Torrence GW, Labelle R. Integrating economic evaluations and quality of life assessments. In: Spilker B, ed. *Quality of life and pharmacoeconomics in clinical trials*, 2nd ed. Philadelphia: Lippincott-Raven 1996;85–95.
9. Harris WH. Traumatic arthritis of the hip after dislocation and acetabular fractures: treatment by mold arthroplasty. *J Bone Joint Surg* 1969;51A:737.
10. Laupacis A, Bourne RB, Rorabeck CH, Feeny D, et al. The effect of elective total hip replacement upon health-related quality of life. *J Bone Joint Surg* 1993;75A:1619.
11. Laupacis A, Bourne RB, Rorabeck CH, Wong C, Tugwell P, Leslie K, Bullas R. Costs of elective total hip arthroplasty: cemented versus noncemented. *J Arthroplasty* 1994;9:481.
12. Laupacis A, Feeny D, Detsky AS, Tugwell P. How attractive does a new technology have to be to warrant adoption and utilization? Tentative guidelines for using clinical and economic evaluations. *Can Med Assoc J* 1992;146:473–481.
13. Laupacis A, Rorabeck CH, Bourne RB, Feeny D, et al. Randomized trials in orthopaedics: why, how and when? *J Bone Joint Surg* 1989;71A:535.
14. Merle d'Aubigne R, Postel, M. Functional results of hip arthroplasty with acrylic prostheses. *J Bone Joint Surg* 1954;36A:451.
15. McNeil BJ, Weichselbaum R, Pauker SG. Speech and survival: trade-offs between quality and quantity of life in laryngeal cancer. *N Engl J Med* 1981;305:982–987.
16. Relman AS. Assessment and accountability: the third revolution in medical care. *N Engl J Med* 1988;3:21.
17. Rorabeck CH, Bourne RB, Laupacis A, Feeny D, Wong C, Tugwell P, Leslie K, Bullas R. A double-blind study of 250 cases comparing cemented with cementless total hip arthroplasty: cost-effectiveness and its impact on health-related quality of life. *Clin Orthop* 1994;198:156.
18. Torrance GW. Utility approach to measuring health-related quality of life [review]. *J Chronic Dis* 1987;40:593–603.
19. Torrance GE, Feeny D. Utilities and quality-adjusted life years. *J Technol Assess Health Care* 1989;5:559–575.
20. Tugwell P, Bombardier C, Buchanan WW, Goldsmith CH, Grace E, Hanna B. The MACTAR patient preference disability questionnaire—an individualized functional priority approach for assessing improvement in physical disability in clinical trials in rheumatoid arthritis. *J Rheum* 1987;14:446.
21. Wennberg JE. Population illness rates do not explain population hospitalization rate. *Med Care* 1987;25:354.

The Adult Hip, edited by J. J. Callaghan,
A. G. Rosenberg, and H. E. Rubash.
Lippincott–Raven Publishers, Philadelphia © 1998.

CHAPTER 53

The Economics of Total Hip Arthroplasty

William L. Healy

Total hip arthroplasty (THA) surgery is a clinically and cost-effective treatment that can predictably relieve pain and improve function for patients with painful, arthritic hips (11,13,18). The prevalence of hip replacement surgery in the United States increased to 258,300 surgical cases in 1994, which represents a 3.6% increase from 1993 (16). During 1994, 137,415 primary THAs, 93,439 partial hip replacements, and 27,446 revision THAs were performed in the United States.

Despite its widespread success, THA has been targeted for cost control because of its high cost per procedure and its increasing prevalence in an aging American population. Since the introduction of the Medicare Diagnosis-Related Group (DRG) hospital-payment system in 1984, payment to hospitals for THA has evolved to primarily a case-price reimbursement system. When hospitals deliver hip replacement operations, they receive a predetermined payment. If their expenses exceed the payment, they lose money. If they control their expenses to less than the payment, they profit. During the past 10 years, the hospital payment for THA has increased at less than the rate of inflation.

During the past few years, many hospitals have had trouble breaking even or making a profit on primary THA surgery. In 1989, Mt. Sinai Hospital in Cleveland lost $500,000 on 200 total joint-replacement operations (7). Surgeons at Lutheran General Hospital in Park Ridge, Illinois, evaluated 44 hip replacements performed during 1991 (8). Their DRG reimbursement was $11,300 per case. However, their average cost to deliver hip replacement operations was $11,790 per case, which meant a loss of $490 per hip replacement operation in 1991 (8).

When surgeons at the Hospital for Special Surgery in New York City reviewed 1020 primary hip replacements performed in 1992, they noted that the hospital lost $238 per case or 1.5% of the hospital cost to deliver those operations (6). When patients were stratified by age, they noted that the hospital lost more money on older patients. If the Medicare budget is cut, this trend at the Hospital for Special Surgery will be even more of a problem because approximately two thirds of joint-replacement operations are performed on Medicare patients (6). Despite the clinical efficacy of THA, hospitals will find it difficult to remain in the hip replacement business if they consistently lose money on THA. Thus, the cost of THA is a critical issue for surgeons and hospitals who deliver hip replacement surgery.

In 1996, Americans confront a paradox in public opinion regarding health care. Many Americans believe too much money is being spent on health care, and it should be possible to decrease the expense while increasing quality. It is not clear that these conflicting goals can be achieved. However, it is clear that in the short term, Americans want to spend less money on health care. This desire for health care cost reduction presents a problem for patients, surgeons, and hospitals who value THA.

COST OF TOTAL HIP ARTHROPLASTY

In an effort to define and understand the economics of THA, an analysis (3) was made of the hospital cost of hip replacement surgery during the 1980s at the Lahey Clinic. Forty-four patients treated with hip replacement surgery in 1981 were compared with 104 patients treated with hip replacement surgery in 1990. Hospital bills were evaluated and charges were assigned to hospital service centers.

W. L. Healy: Department of Orthopaedic Surgery, Lahey Hitchcock Medical Center, Burlington, Massachusetts 01805.

Charges on the hospital bills were converted to cost by government-mandated, hospital-specific, cost-to-charge ratios. These cost-to-charge ratios provide an accurate and reliable estimate of cost. Economic comparisons between the two groups of patients were made with actual dollars and with inflation-adjusted dollars. That study (3) noted that the hospital cost to deliver hip replacement at Lahey Clinic during the 1980s was controlled at the rate of inflation. The hospital cost for THA in 1981 was $8,428. The hospital cost for THA in 1990 was $12,348. This change represented a 46% increase in actual dollars and a 2% increase in inflation-adjusted dollars. The consumer price index increased 43.8% during this interval.

The most significant decrease in cost associated with hip replacement during the 1980s was the cost of the hospital room, which decreased from 50% of the hospital cost for hip replacement in 1981 to 37% of the hospital cost for hip replacement in 1990. In sharp contrast, the cost of the hip implant increased from 11% of the hospital cost for hip replacement in 1981 to 24% of the hospital cost for hip replacement in 1990. The cost of a hip implant increased 212% in actual dollars from 1981 to 1990 and 118% in inflation-adjusted dollars.

Success in controlling the hospital cost for hip replacement during the 1980s occurred by utilization control or volume reductions. Hip replacement operations were delivered with shorter hospital stay, less time in the operating room, fewer tests, less therapy, and fewer medications. Failure in controlling the hospital cost for hip replacement during the 1980s was the result of a universal failure to control unit costs of services and supplies required for hip replacement surgery. This study documented that further control of the hospital cost for hip replacement would require control of unit costs and that the single biggest unit cost associated with THA was the cost of the implant.

A similar study (17) of the hospital cost for THA was performed at the University of Texas at Houston using a cost-accounting system (Decision Support System, TSI, Boston, Massachusetts). Fifty primary hip replacements performed during 1992 were studied. The average hospital cost for these operations was $13,826. The hip implant consumed $4,769 or 34.4% of the total hospital cost of primary hip replacement. These authors (17) used a different cost-accounting method than that used in the Lahey Hitchcock study, but the results of their evaluation were similar.

COST OF REVISION TOTAL HIP ARTHROPLASTY

As the prevalence of primary hip replacement surgery increased during each year of the past decade, the prevalence of revision hip replacement surgery also increased. In 1994, 27,446 revision hip replacement operations were performed in the United States, which represented a 2.7% increase over 1993. In 1992, the number of revision hip replacement surgeries increased by 18%, whereas the number of primary hip replacement surgeries increased by only 9% (16). The increase in the number of revision hip replacement surgeries presents a problem for hospitals because revision hip surgery consumes more hospital resources than primary hip replacement surgery. However, the reimbursement to the hospital for revision surgery is not much higher than that for primary hip replacement surgery.

At the Lahey Hitchcock Medical Center, revision hip replacement surgery is associated with greater preoperative planning than primary hip replacement, and in 1992, the average operating-room time for revision THA was 78% longer than that for primary THA. According to 1992 Medicare statistics (15), revision THA was associated with a 15% longer length of hospital stay than primary THA, and revision THA generated 20% more hospital charges than primary THA.

Surgeons at Tulane University Medical Center in New Orleans compared two groups of patients who had primary and revision THA operations performed between 1990 and 1992 (4). In these patients, revision THA was associated with significantly increased operating-room time, increased intraoperative blood loss, increased use of bone graft procedures, increased postoperative complications, and increased length of hospital stay. They calculated that the work performed by the surgeon and the risks taken by the surgeon were significantly greater for revision THA. However, the reimbursement to the surgeon was not significantly higher for revision THA than for primary THA.

Lavernia et al. (12) performed a cost analysis of primary and revision THA at the Good Samaritan Hospital, Johns Hopkins University School of Medicine, comparing patients who received surgery within the years 1987 through 1990. In this study, the time spent in the operating room for patients undergoing revision THA was 109% longer than that of patients undergoing primary THA, and patients spent 92% more time in the hospital after revision THA. Charges for hip implants in this study were 25% higher for revision surgery, and hospital charges were 59% higher for revision surgery.

McGrory et al. (14) evaluated 36 revision THA operations performed at Massachusetts General Hospital between 1992 and 1994. The average hospital charge was $32,734, the average hospital cost was $24,494, and the average reimbursement by Medicare was $14,035. Average reimbursement was only 57.3% of the real hospital cost.

Ritter et al. (19) compared their experience with primary and revision THA in 1991. They performed 250 primary THA and 73 revision THA operations. Average length of stay in the hospital was 5.9 days for primary THA and 6.0 days for revision THA. Surgeons spent 77% more time in the operating room when performing revision THA operations than when performing primary THA operations. Despite 77% more work for revision THA operations, the Medicare payment increased only 30.8%, from $1,363 for primary THA to $1,782 for revision THA, under the reimbursement schedules for Medicare in the state of Indiana.

Revision hip replacement surgery presents a problem for hospitals because the charges and costs for revision THA are significantly higher than the charges and costs for primary THA. However, the reimbursement to the hospital is essentially the same for revision and primary THA, according to the DRG 209 Medicare reimbursement schedule. It should not be surprising to medical economists that few American hospitals specialize in revision total-hip replacement. In 1992, 2648 hospitals performed at least one revision hip replacement operation. However, 50% of the these hospitals performed five or fewer revisions, and only three hospitals in the United States performed more than 200 revision hip replacement operations in 1992 (15). At Lahey Hitchcock Medical Center, we performed 231 hip replacement operations in 1995, 189 (82%) of which were primary THA, and 42 (18%) of which were revision THA.

Revision hip replacement surgery requires more work and more surgical risk than does primary hip replacement surgery. However, the professional reimbursement for revision THA is essentially the same as for primary THA. Depending on the number of components exchanged during revision hip replacement surgery, the professional reimbursement may be less for more difficult revision hip-replacement operations. Furthermore, professional reimbursement for both primary and revision hip replacement surgery is scheduled to decrease, according to the Medicare payment schedules.

COST CONTAINMENT IN TOTAL HIP ARTHROPLASTY

The crisis regarding the cost of health care in the United States has created a need to reduce the cost of THA. The Federal Government, managed-care organizations, insurance companies, employers, and patients have demanded that health-care costs be decreased. Surgeons and hospitals must address this universal demand to control costs if they hope to continue to deliver successful hip replacement operations to their patients in the future.

Methods for controlling the costs of THA include reducing the number of operations performed, reducing utilization of services and supplies required for THA, and reducing the unit costs of services and supplies required for THA (Table 1).

In consideration of the increasing prevalence of THA surgery, the aging population in the United States, and the increasing desire of older citizens to remain active, it is unlikely that the number of THA operations performed

TABLE 1. *Methods of reducing the cost of THA*

Reduce volume of THA operations
    Disincentives for patients to seek THA
    Disincentives for surgeons to perform THA
    Disincentives for hospitals to deliver THA
Reduce utilization of services and supplies for THA
    Utilization review
    Clinical pathways
    Early hospital discharge to rehabilitation facility
Reduce unit costs of services and supplies for THA
    Reduce implant cost
        Vendor discount
        Implant standardization/demand matching
        Competitive bid purchasing

THA, total hip arthroplasty.

will decrease without social manipulation. Formalized rationing of surgical procedures could achieve this goal. Disincentives for patients to seek THA, for surgeons to perform THA, and for hospitals to deliver THA might decrease the volume of THA in this country. The managed-care revolution, with introduction of capitated payment systems, may reduce the number of THA operations performed in this country. If primary-care physicians have an economic disincentive to refer patients for hip replacement surgery, the total number of THA operations may be decreased. This author does not expect the total volume of hip replacement surgery to decrease in this country. However, if the volume of THA operations is maintained at 1994 levels, this would represent a relative decrease in THA in relation to the population and in relation to the specific population greater than 60 years of age.

The cost of THA can be successfully controlled by reducing utilization of services and supplies required for the procedure. Utilization review has successfully reduced length of stay in the hospital for general medical populations (21). Utilization review programs have successfully reduced the number of diagnostic and surgical procedures performed in a fee-for-service health insurance plan in New York City (20). Orthopedic surgeons at Stanford (22) demonstrated that a utilization review program for THA implemented from 1984 to 1986 could reduce length of stay and hospital cost for THA.

Utilization of the services and supplies required for hip replacement surgery has been reduced by clinical pathways. Clinical pathways are flow charts, or algorithms, for the total care of a patient from the time of diagnosis of a problem through treatment, until a desired outcome is achieved. Clinical pathways have been designed to improve the clinical efficiency, cost effectiveness, and quality of THA. Surgeons at Lutheran General Hospital in Parkridge, Illinois (8), used a clinical pathway for THA to reduce length of stay in the hospital from 12.3 days in 1988 to 6.2 days in 1991. The clinical pathway at Lutheran General Hospital also converted a $2,835 loss for primary THA reimbursed by Medicare in 1988 to a

$490 loss for primary THA reimbursed by Medicare in 1991 (8). Froimson (7) used a case-management program that was similar to a clinical pathway to convert a $500,000 loss on 200 joint replacements in 1989 to a profit on joint-replacement surgery in 1991 and 1992.

Surgeons at the Mayo Clinic (1) demonstrated that a utilization review program, which reduced variations among surgeons who perform THA, was associated with decreased length of hospital stay and decreased hospital charges for THA.

1995
HIP

LAHEY HITCHCOCK CLINIC
HIP IMPLANT STANDARDIZATION PROGRAM
Patient Data Sheet

NAME: _____ LC#: _____ DATE OF SURGERY: _____

SIDE: L R SURGEON: _____

THA PATIENT TYPE SCORE: (Circle appropriate level for each category)

Age: _____	**Weight:** _____	**Expected[+]Activity:**
1. > 75.	1. Less than 120.	1. Sedentary.
2. 70-75.	2. 120-149.	2. Household ambulator.
3. 65-69.	3. 150-179.	3. Community ambulator.
4. 60-64.	4. 180-200.	4. No walking limit.
5. < 60.	5. Greater than 200.	5. Sports/heavy work.
(Add 5 points for < 55 years old)		(* following T.H.A.)

Health:[**]	**Bone Stock:**[***](Femoral index)	
1. Poor.	1. $\geq$.63	
2. Fair.	2. .56-.62	inner diameter
3. Moderate.	3. .49-.55	
4. Good.	4. .42-.48	outer diameter
5. Excellent.	5. $\leq$.41	

AGE: _____   PATIENT TYPE SCORE: _____

WEIGHT: _____   DEMAND CATEGORY: _____

ACTIVITY: _____   (See Implant Selection Chart)

HEALTH: _____   ACETABULAR IMPLANT: _____

BONE STOCK: _____   FEMORAL IMPLANT: _____

TOTAL: _____

A   William L. Healy, M.D.

FIG. 1. Front **(A)** and back **(B)** of Lahey Hitchcock Medical Center Hip Implant Standardization Program: Patient Data Sheet.

1. **Poor:** (ASA 4) → Decompensated diseases/short life expectancy. A patient with an incapacitating disease that is a constant threat to life (heart failure, renal failure).

2. **Fair:** (ASA 3) → Fair control of chronic diseases. A patient with a severe systemic disease that limits activity (angina, obstructive pulmonary disease, prior myocardial infarction).

3. **Moderate:** (ASA 2-) → Medications controlling chronic diseases. A patient with a mild, systemic disease controlled with medication (mild diabetes, controlled hypertension, anemia, chronic bronchitis, morbid obesity).

4. **Good:** (ASA 2+) → No medications. History of chronic medical problems under control. A patient with an inactive, mild, systemic disease (mild diabetes, hypertension, anemia, chronic bronchitis, morbid obesity).

5. **Excellent:** (ASA 1) → No medications. No chronic diseases. A normal, healthy patient.

***
BONE STOCK

Based on Femoral Index (Healey, Vigorita, Lane: JBJS April 1985)

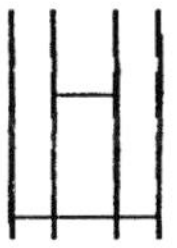

Femoral Index* = $\dfrac{\text{Inner Diameter (Canal)}}{\text{Outer Diameter (Cortical Bone)}}$

inner diameter*

outer diameter*

*Measured 8 cm. distal to the proximal aspect of the lesser trochanter

.50 ± .09 → osteoarthritis

.56 ± .08 → osteoporosis

HIP IMPLANT SELECTION:

DEMAND CATEGORY:	SCORE:	CUP:	STEM:
I (high demand)	22-25[+]	Choice	Choice
II	18-21	Choice	Cemented
III	12-17	Choice (age ≤ 75) .... Cemented (polyethylene) (age ≥ 76)	Cemented
IV (low demand)	≤ 11	Cemented (polyethylene)	Cemented

William L. Healy, M.D.

WLH/mejr/REV:9/95

B

FIG. 1. *Continued.*

Some hospitals have used early discharge to skilled nursing facilities and rehabilitation hospitals as a way of decreasing length of stay, decreasing hospital costs, and increasing profit from THA operations. Medicare DRG payment is delivered to the acute care hospital as soon as the patient is discharged. Patients in skilled nursing facilities and rehabilitation hospitals accrue new charges on a different Medicare payment schedule. This method of early discharge to reduce utilization is actually a cost-shifting methodology that will be discouraged by global payment systems that are being developed by the Health Care Financing Administration.

At a certain point after implementation of a utilization review program, a clinical pathway, and an early discharge program, the value of these programs in reducing the cost of THA is diminished. After these programs were implemented at Lahey Hitchcock Medical Center, the daily hospital cost for 302 DRG-209 discharges during 1994 was evaluated. For these 302 THA operations, the average hospital cost was $9,312, and the average length of stay in the hospital was 5.69 days. Sixty-nine percent of the hospital cost was spent on hospital days 1 and 2. The distribution of hospital costs during the first 6 days of hospitalization included day 1, $5,064; day 2, $1,068; day 3, $777; day 4, $789; day 5, $655; and day 6, $532. These data clearly demonstrate that the greatest opportunity for THA cost control at Lahey Hitchcock Medical Center is during the first 48 hours of hospitalization.

The cost of THA can be reduced by reducing the unit costs of services and supplies required for the operation. The hip implant cost is the single biggest component of the hospital cost for THA. Implant cost is a fixed cost of total joint arthroplasty, and it is appropriate to focus on implant costs when attempting to control the cost of hip replacement surgery. In their May 1992 position statement, Containing the Cost of Orthopaedic Implants, the American Academy of Orthopaedic Surgeons (2) encouraged orthopedic surgeons to work toward containing the cost of orthopedic implants. Although the Academy emphasized that the selection of the implant should remain with the surgeon, they strongly advised surgeons to collaborate with hospitals to contain the cost of implants. In an editorial in June 1994 (5), The Journal of Bone and Joint Surgery also encouraged surgeons to control the cost of implants. This editorial stated that, because surgeons are the prime consumers of orthopedic implants, it is surgeons who ultimately have the ability to control the cost of those implants.

Methods for controlling the cost of hip implants include negotiation of vendor discounts, standardization of hip implants, and purchasing of hip implants by competitive bid. Negotiating vendor discounts and the purchasing of implants by competitive bid require good business practices by hospital administrators and surgeons. When these practices are employed, hospitals can achieve appreciable savings on the costs of implants.

In an attempt to assist surgeons with the objective selection of hip implants, to decrease variability in the selection of hip implants, and to decrease the average cost of hip implants to Lahey Hitchcock Medical Center, the surgeons at that institution developed a hip implant standardization program (10). Five objective patient characteristics were used to evaluate the demand a patient might place on a hip implant: age, weight, expected activity after THA, general health (ASA score), and bone stock (femoral index). Patients were assigned to four demand categories, and implants of various designs, materials, and cost were assigned to those four demand categories. The cost of the implants typically decreased from demand category I (high) to demand category IV (low). All hip implants were approved by the Food and Drug Administration for all patients (Fig. 1).

The hip implant standardization program was retrospectively tested in 103 hip replacement operations performed during 1991. If the hip implant standardization program had been in place during 1991, the hospital would have saved 25.7% of the actual cost of hip implants spent on those 103 patients. The standardization program also showed the potential to decrease by 10% the amount of DRG-209 dollars spent on hip implants for each hip replacement operation (10). In comparing his experience with hip replacement surgery in 1989 and 1992, Froimson (7) used a standardization program or demand-matching system to reduce the cost of hip implants by $1,000 per case.

IMPACT OF COST-REDUCTION PROGRAMS ON QUALITY OF TOTAL HIP ARTHROPLASTY

Cost-reduction programs have demonstrated the ability to reduce the cost of THA. However, the impact of these cost-reduction tools on the quality of patient outcome after hip replacement surgery has not been evaluated. Although hospitals need to reduce the cost of THA to survive in difficult economic times for providers of health care, surgeons face the dilemma of advocating for the welfare of their patients and cooperating with cost-control initiatives at their hospitals.

Surgeons at the Lahey Hitchcock Medical Center evaluated the impact of a THA clinical pathway and a hip implant standardization program on the outcome of 127 patients who received hip replacement operations. The control group included 63 patients who had hip replacement surgery in 1991, who were treated *without* a clinical pathway or implant standardization. The study group included 64 patients who had hip replacement surgery in 1993 and who were treated *with* a clinical pathway and implant standardization. Median follow-up for the patients in the 1991 group was 4.0 years. Median follow-up for the patients in the 1993 group was 2.0 years (9).

Before hip replacement surgery, the two patient populations were similar in age, weight, activity, general health, occupation, preoperative Harris Hip Score, preoperative Merle, D'Aubigne, Postel Hip Score, and a preoperative visual analog pain score. The two groups of patients were dissimilar when hip implants were compared. Differences in choice of implant would be expected based on the implementation of the implant standardization program in the 1993 study group.

Hip pain was relieved successfully in both groups without any difference between groups ($p < .5$). Both groups demonstrated clinical improvement without any difference between groups, as demonstrated by Harris Hip Score ($p > .5$) and Merle, D'Aubigne, Postel Hip Score ($p < .5$). When stratified by Charnley Class, postoperative hip scores decreased with increasing Charnley Class (increasing disability).

Patient outcome after hip replacement surgery improved universally, and outcome was not different between the groups of patients in 1991 and 1993, as measured by level of activity, ability to climb stairs, amount of support needed for walking, distance walked, and occupation of the patient at the time of follow-up. Responses of the patients to the following questions were similar for both groups of patients: Hip pain interfering with sleep? Increased function/activity of daily living? Increased enjoyment of recreational activities? Decreased hip pain? Decreased amount of medication taken for hip pain? and Satisfaction with THA? (Table 2).

In general, patients in both groups reported clinical improvement and satisfaction after hip replacement surgery, and no differences were observed between groups in terms of outcome or satisfaction.

Complications during hospitalization were evaluated by looking specifically for operative complications, anesthetic complications, medical complications, thromboembolic complications, infection, problems with wound healing, and instability or dislocation. Two hospital complications occurred in both the 1991 control group and the 1993 study group. No significant difference in complication rates was observed between these two groups.

The hip replacement clinical pathway was associated with a reduced length of stay in the hospital for the 1993 group compared with the 1991 group. Length of stay decreased from 8.49 days in 1991 to 5.80 days in 1993 ($p < .001$).

The introduction of the cost-reduction programs was associated with a reduction in hospital cost for patients in the 1993 group compared with patients in the 1991 group. The mean hospital cost for THA in 1991 was $9,706. The mean hospital cost for THA in 1993 was $9,067 dollars ($p < .05$). This statistically significant difference in hospital cost was also significant when inflation-adjusted dollars were compared. These hospital costs were derived from a validated cost-accounting program (TSI, Inc., Boston, MA), which determined actual hospital costs.

The implant standardization program was associated with a change in the selection of hip implants by the surgeons and a decrease in the cost of hip implants. In 1991, 100% of acetabular cups were cementless implants; in 1993, 95% of acetabular cups were cementless implants. Selection of the acetabular cups did not change appreciably. Selection of femoral implants, however, did change considerably. In 1991, 65% of femoral implants were cemented; in 1993, 98% of femoral implants were cemented. This change in the selection of implants was associated with a reduction in the average cost of hip implant per case, from $3,856 in 1991 to $3,553 in 1993. This reduction of 8.5% is statistically significant ($p < .001$).

TABLE 2. *Impact of cost-reduction programs on THA at the Lahey Hitchcock Clinic*

	Control group (1991) No clinical pathway No implant standardization		Study group (1993) Clinical pathway Implant standardization		Postoperative comparison
	Preoperative	Postoperative	Preoperative	Postoperative	
Number/minimum follow-up	63/4.0 yr		64/2.0 yr		
Pain analog score (range, 0–10)	8.95 (7–10)	1.05 (0–6)	9.36 (6–13)	0.84 (0–5)	$p < .5$
Harris Hip Score (range, 0–100)	38.24 (18–68)	89.75 (57–100)	34.09 (13–67)	89.34 (56–100)	$p > .5$
Merle, D'Aubigne, Postel Hip Score (0–18)	9.24 (4–14)	15.90 (12–18)	9.36 (6–13)	16.16 (9–18)	$p < .5$
Decreased pain with THA	62 (98.4%)		64 (100%)		$p = .4961$
Increased function with THA	63 (100%)		63 (98.4%)		$p = .5039$
Patient satisfaction	63 (100%)		63 (98.4%)		$p = .5039$
Hospital ALOS (days)	8.49 (4–13)		5.80 (3–13)		$p < .001$
Mean hospital cost (actual dollars)	$9,706.00		$9,067.00		$p < .05$
Mean hospital cost (inflation-adjusted dollars)	$10,569.00		$9,873.00		$p < .05$

ALOS, average length of stay.
Statistical significance, $p < .05$.

CONCLUSION

It is important for surgeons and hospitals who value THA to be concerned about its cost. Health-care reform is ongoing in the health-care marketplace, with the managed care revolution reaching every corner of the United States. It was estimated that 70% of Americans would be covered by some kind of managed care in January 1996. As a way of controlling costs, some members of Congress have suggested changing Medicare from a discounted fee-for-service product to a managed-care, health-care product.

Surgeons and hospitals face a dilemma in continuing to provide quality THA in an environment that requires reduction of cost. It is appropriate to apply continuous quality-improvement programs to increase the efficiency and quality of hip replacement surgery. A limit exists as to how far the cost of hip replacement surgery can be reduced. Surgeons need to be careful to stop short of a yet-to-be-defined quality limit, if that limit is demonstrated to impact negatively on the outcome of their patients after THA.

REFERENCES

1. Amadio PC, Naessens J, Rice R, Ilstrup D. Quality improvement in an integrated group practice setting. *American Academy of Orthopaedic Surgeons Annual Meeting*, Scientific Program. Orlando, FL: February 18, 1995:175.
2. American Academy of Orthopaedic Surgeons. *Containing the cost of orthopaedic implants*. Rosemont, IL: The American Academy of Orthopaedic Surgeons, May 1992.
3. Barber TC, Healy WL. The hospital cost of total hip arthroplasty: a comparison between 1981 and 1990. *J Bone Joint Surg* 1993;75A:321–325.
4. Barrack RL, Hoffman G, Tejeiro WV, Carpenter LJ. Surgical work input and risk in primary versus revision total joint arthroplasty. *J Arthroplasty* 1995;10:281–286.
5. Clark CR. Cost containment: total joint implants. *J Bone Joint Surg* 1994;76A:799–800.
6. Evans BG, Bear BJ, Salvati EA, Reynolds JR, Malakoff S. Relationship of age to hospital cost and reimbursement for primary total hip arthroplasty. From the annual meeting of *American Academy of Orthopaedic Surgeons*, scientific program. New Orleans, LA: February 24, 1994:77.
7. Froimson AI. Rational uses of resources in total joint surgery. From the annual meeting of *American Academy of Orthopaedic Surgeons*, scientific program. New Orleans, LA: February 24, 1994;76.
8. Goldstein WM, Patek RM, Stine J, Szpila K. Cost analysis of total hip and total knee arthroplasty in the Medicare patient: a strategy in dealing with DRGs. Scientific Exhibit at the annual meeting of *American Academy of Orthopaedic Surgeons*. Washington, DC: February 20–25, 1992;308.
9. Healy WL, Ayers ME, Iorio R, Patch DA, Pfeifer BA. Impact of a clinical pathway on implant standardization of total hip arthroplasty: a clinical and economic study of patient outcome. The 1996 annual meeting of the *American Academy of Orthopaedic Surgeons*, scientific program. Atlanta, GA: February 24, 1996.
10. Healy WL, Kirven FM, Iorio R, Patch DA, Pfeifer BA. Implant standardization for total hip arthroplasty: an implant selection and cost reduction program. *J Arthroplasty* 1995;10:177–183.
11. Laupacis A, Bourne R, Rorabeck C, Feeny D, Wong C, Tugwell P, Leslie K, Bullas R. The effect of elective total hip replacement upon health-related quality of life. *J Bone Joint Surg* 1993;75A:1619–1626.
12. Lavernia CJ, Drakeford MK, Tsao AK, Gittelsohn A, Krackow KA, Hungerford DS. Revision and primary hip and knee arthroplasty: a cost analysis. *Clin Orthop* 1995;311:136–141.
13. Liang MH, Cullen KE, Larson MO, Thompson MS, Schwartz JA, Fossel AH, Roberts WN, Sledor CB. Cost effectiveness of total joint arthroplasty in osteoarthritis. *Arthritis Rheum* 1986;29:937–943.
14. McGrory BJ, Seger RF, Harris WH. Hospital charges, costs, and reimbursement for revision total hip arthroplasty in Medicare patients. From the 1996 annual meeting of the *American Academy of Orthopaedic Surgeons*, scientific program. Atlanta, GA: February 24, 1996:200.
15. Mendenhall S. A closer look at revisions. *Orthopaedic Network News* 1993;4:6.
16. Mendenhall S. 1995 Hip and knee implant review. *Orthopaedic Network News* 1995;6:1.
17. Meyers SJ, Reuben JD, Moye LA, Zong J. The actual inpatient costs of primary and revision total joint replacements. Read at the 65th annual meeting of the *American Academy of Orthopaedic Surgeons*. New Orleans, LA: February 1994.
18. Rissanen P, Aro S, Slatis P, Sintonen H, Paavolainen P. Health and quality of life before and after hip or knee arthroplasty. *J Arthroplasty* 1995;10:169–175.
19. Ritter MA, Carr KD, Keating EM, Faris PM, Bankoff DL, Ireland PH. Revision total joint arthroplasty: Does Medicare reimbursement justify time spent? *(abstr)*. *J Arthroplasty* 1994;9:115.
20. Rosenberg SN, Allen DR, Handte JS, Jackson TC, Leto L, Rodstein BM, Stratton SD, Westfall G, Yasser R. Effective utilization review in a fee-for-service health insurance plan. *N Engl J Med* 1995;333:1326–1330.
21. Schwartz WB, Mendelson DN. Hospital cost containment in the 1980s. Hard lessons learned and prospects for the 1990s. *N Engl J Med* 1991; 324:1037–1042; *erratum*, 1991;325:71.
22. Sommers LS, Schurman DJ, Jamison JQ, Woolson ST, Robison BL, Silverman JF. Clinician-directed hospital cost management for total hip arthroplasty patients. *Clin Orthop* 1990;258:168–175.

The Adult Hip, edited by J. J. Callaghan,
A. G. Rosenberg, and H. E. Rubash.
Lippincott–Raven Publishers, Philadelphia © 1998.

CHAPTER 54

Outcomes Assessment

Norman A. Johanson

The increasing cost of health care, and a near obsession with obtaining rapid access to any potentially promising medical or surgical treatment, no matter how costly, are two major strands in the Gordian knot that symbolizes the U.S. economy. Add the increasing public demand for a legal right to quality health care, and this mixture synergistically applies dangerous internal stresses to our economic and ethical infrastructure. Serious illnesses without a cure, treatments that no third party is willing to pay for, and patients suffering because the supposed "right" treatment was not selected, strengthen the case for serious consideration of the outcomes approach. *Outcomes* has become a hot topic—a buzzword. More than the term *result*, *outcome* has an official sound, an air of finality, and seems to be somehow connected to better science. The discussion in this chapter will focus on the multifaceted nature of outcomes assessment and how its meaning is highly dependent on who the observer is and what the incentives and expected benefits of outcomes assessment are.

Outcomes may mean the fulfillment of long-awaited expectations of pain relief and restoration of function to the hopeful orthopedic patient. In addition to these desirable outcomes, range of motion, radiographic findings, or a laboratory test may be of particular interest to the operating surgeon. The researcher may see outcomes as a con-

stellation of proxy measures for the health of populations. A governmental approach to outcomes might be concerned with the volume and intensity of services for a condition, and their relationship with morbidity, mortality, and rehospitalization. Likewise, private insurers may be primarily interested in outcomes as they determine economic risk and, ultimately, corporate viability.

This chapter summarizes outcomes assessment development, beginning with its infancy at the turn of the century, and reaching maturity in the 1990s. From Codman's "Idea" (9) to Relman's era of assessment and accountability (54), the incentives for measuring outcomes have changed and the technology of measurement instruments has evolved to a high level of sophistication. But the fundamental concepts that drove the early movement have persisted. The challenge to find the best ways to evaluate and document the change (for better or worse) in patient health status brought about by medical or surgical treatment, and then to compare it to that which would occur with no treatment at all, remains. Detailed analyses of the various processes of care, quality improvement of health care organizations, and cost analysis are meaningless unless the patient's actual health status is factored into the equation. Outcomes assessment is a patient-centered process. What follows is an account of the forces that have helped to place the measurement of actual health outcomes and the patient side by side at the center of the health care debate.

N. A. Johanson: Department of Orthopaedic Surgery, Temple University School of Medicine, Philadelphia, Pennsylvania 19140.

HISTORY OF THE OUTCOMES MOVEMENT: CODMAN'S "END RESULT IDEA"

At the turn of the century, E. A. Codman and his senior partner F. B. Harrington implemented the "End Result System" into their surgical practice (9,48). This system was designed to routinely follow-up and document the outcomes of various treatments for the stated purpose of improving the "efficiency" of patient care. They believed that this type of evaluation should be performed systematically and without bias to provide as accurate a picture of the patient's clinical status as was possible. Codman later went on to advocate the use of his system in hospitals, a concept which was met with some resistance in Boston, but which has recently been vindicated by a late twentieth century effort by health-care providers to better understand the outcomes of their treatments. Codman was unsuccessful in convincing the Board of Trustees of the Massachusetts General Hospital of the merits of his system. Because of this, he left that hospital in 1911 to start his own. The following passage from the autobiographical preface to his book, *The Shoulder*, published using his own money in 1934, describes his reasons for venturing out on his own:

> I determined that, as any increased opportunity at the M.G.H. [the Massachusetts General Hospital] was most unlikely since the tradition of a seniority system was so firmly fixed, I would start a small hospital where I would be my own master and could work out my own ideas. I especially wished to make it an example of the End Result Idea. There would be no trustees to consult or other members of the staff to placate, if I wished to state publicly the actual results of the treatment which the patients received. In other words, I would make this small hospital an example of the advantage of an organization based on actual efficiency analysis of the results of treatment. (9)

This strikingly contemporary-sounding statement has echoed throughout the remainder of the century. The importance of the idea was missed by most of Codman's peers, primarily because there was little incentive driving them toward a more sophisticated methodological approach to evaluating their clinical outcomes and to using the results to drive the improvement of efficiency and quality. Codman, in fact, saw substantial negative incentives that governed their behavior. His frustration with the general resistance to his ideas came to a climax at a meeting of the Suffolk District Medical Society at the Boston Medical Library in January, 1915. The topic of discussion was hospital efficiency, and at the conclusion of the meeting Codman unveiled a giant cartoon depicting what he perceived to be the economic, political, and academic obstacles to realizing progress toward his goal. His description of the cartoon was as follows:

> It depicts President Lowell standing on the Cambridge Bridge, wondering whether it would be possible for the professors of the Medical School to support themselves on their salaries, if they had no opportunity to practice among the rich people of the Back Bay. The Back Bay is represented as an ostrich with her head in a pile of sand devouring humbugs and kicking out her golden eggs blindly to the professors, who show more interest in the golden eggs than they do in medical science. On the right is the Massachusetts General Hospital with its board of trustees deliberating as to whether, if they really used the End Result System, and let the Back Bay know how many mistakes were made on the hospital patients, she would still be willing to give her golden eggs to support the hospital, and would still employ the members of their staff and thus save the expense of their salaries. (9)

Many of those present at the meetings were outraged, but undaunted by this, Codman continued to advocate outcomes assessment by physicians and hospitals:

> Am I a victim of a dominant idea because I am willing to make the main object of my life the demonstration of the importance of the simple plan that hospitals should constantly inquire into the results of the treatment of their patients, and modify their organizations when necessary to obtain better results? (9)

In 1914, Codman was instrumental in forming the Committee on the Standardization of Hospitals. The American College of Surgeons, which was formed in 1913, absorbed Codman's committee in 1917. The committee became the driving force behind the standardization of hospital care in the United States. The process was later refined in the birth of the Joint Commission on Accreditation of Hospitals (48). Later in his career, Codman was reinstated at Harvard for the purpose of running the Registry of Bone Sarcoma, which he had originally created for the standardization of treatment of this difficult group of tumors.

VOLUME, COST, AND QUALITY: CONTEMPORARY CHALLENGES

Rapid Expansion of Health Care in the United States

The legacy of E. A. Codman was temporarily obscured by the spectacular expansion and specialization of health care during the middle portion of this century (54). Scientific breakthroughs, technological advancements, and the political and economic climate in this country synergistically supported the rapid growth of biomedical research and the resulting plethora of health-care services. Virtually unlimited economic resources were made available for the treatment and cure of various diseases, and, in the rush toward the new and the interesting, there was little incentive to carefully study their cost and their actual effectiveness. In addition, the rapid changes in diagnostic and treatment modalities during this revolutionary period complicated the comparisons of treatments and outcomes for a given condition over several years.

This factor has had particular relevance to orthopedic surgery, where the short-term benefits of newer and, theoretically, better implantable devices were not always weighed against the higher cost and long-term liabilities that may not have characterized more time-tested designs which they replaced. Implant wear, particulate debris, and osteolysis are problems that are rarely seen within 5 years of implantation, and therefore only the long-term results are pertinent for comparing this type of implant performance (40,49,58).

As the volume of health-care services rapidly grew in the United States during the 1950s and 1960s, variation in the distribution of providers and treatments among populations became more evident. What was seen as an undersupply of providers and care provided the rationale for a building boom of hospitals and medical schools. It was not clear, however, how much of the apparent undersupply resulted from problems of the distribution of physicians and health services. The advent of large regional or national computerized databases containing hospital discharge abstracts has facilitated investigation into the variations in utilization rates of various services (8,15,31,32,39,44,51,64). Hip fracture, and hip and knee arthritis are three conditions that have received considerable attention, primarily because the treatment alternatives involve the utilization of costly surgical technology as well as in-patient care in elderly patients who are insured by the federal government. In 1989, total knee replacement (TKR) and total hip replacement (THR) rated fourth and fifth, respectively, among all Part B allowed Medicare charges (52). In aggregate, TKR and THR accounted for 4% of all Part B allowed charges, a total of 327 million dollars. The estimated total cost of TKR and THR in 1985 was 4 billion dollars. In the last decade, the cost has nearly doubled. Therefore, it is not surprising that, after recognizing significant variations in the rate of TKR and THR utilization among small areas, states, and regions of the United States, health policy makers would ask the inevitable question, "Which rate is right?" (65). Why is the performance rate of surgical repair of hip fracture relatively constant throughout the country, whereas in 1982 someone living in Boston was 1.75 times more likely to receive a TKR and 1.5 times more likely to receive a THR than someone living in New Haven, Connecticut? (66). Why are the highest rates of Medicare TKR and THR in the less-populated western states? (51). And why, in the mid 1980s, was the annual per capita in-patient expenditure 889 dollars in Boston and 451 dollars in New Haven? (66). The answers to these important questions are not yet clear. They await the development of testable hypotheses and the generation of large databases with appropriate data reliably collected from a wide variety of (orthopedic) settings. This is more likely to occur now than in Codman's time because of the recent advent of powerful incentives to do so, as well as the increased technologic ability to collect and analyze data.

Cost Containment

Arnold Relman has described the decade of the 1980s as the era of cost containment (54). The issue of cost containment has proven to be the alarm that has reawakened Codman's dormant ideas. The competition for diminishing resources has established outcomes assessment as an essential feature of any rational system that purports to have the patient at the focal point of health-services delivery, while attempting to flex under the economic strain. The process of adopting an outcomes approach has intensified as health-care providers are moving to accept part or all of the financial risk in the care of populations through capitated agreements (28). The emphasis is shifting rapidly from the proliferation of treatments that have been shown to be efficacious under well-prescribed and narrowly defined conditions, to the wholesale elimination of treatments that have not been shown to be generally effective when utilized by the larger community of providers in a representative population. The proven efficacy of a treatment is no longer enough to justify its general use. A commonly used treatment should be shown to be among the most cost effective in its class (36). In the current health-care environment, it is more common to ask which treatment alternatives work and how much they cost than to ask what's new and interesting. Implant "demand matching," although it is not necessarily data driven, is an example of such a development (24). This process, among others, has gained considerable popularity among cost-conscious hospitals and orthopedic surgeons.

Assessment and Accountability: The Definition of Quality

Codman's end result idea has reached full flower in what Relman has called the present era of assessment and accountability (54). Interestingly, this idea has been fully incorporated into modern industry prior to arriving in the health-care environment. Concepts such as total quality management as the foundation for the corporate approach to assessment and accountability issues are now commonplace. As the house of medicine has evolved from being a cottage industry into the broader competitive marketplace, a similar transformation is taking place (33). The fundamental problem for health-care professionals, however, is to arrive at a definition of the "product" being produced, and then to formulate meaningful quality standards. The Wall Street Journal summarized "medicine's industrial revolution" in stating:

The industry is quickly moving to rationalize health care delivery, measure the costs and benefits of treatments, and compare the outcomes of different providers." (33)

The article continued with a rather optimistic assessment of the ease with which the product of medicine will be defined, and the efficiency with which quality of care will be measured:

A healthy patient is a unit of production, and for all units of production there is an optimal production function. For the first time in the history of medicine, thanks to numerous, concurrent, interdependent breakthroughs in health care information technology and statistics, such functions can now be calculated." (33)

The details of defining a healthy patient, in light of all the costly health services currently available to the consumer, have made devilish work for all who are truly interested in maintaining the traditional patient advocacy role of the medical profession, in distinction to the emerging business image of the health-care provider, casting him or her as either an entrepreneur or a trade unionist (14,28). Relman has underscored the crucial question that is now being addressed to the medical profession:

The key question is: Will medicine bow and become essentially a business or will it remain a profession? . . . Will we act as businessmen in a system that is becoming increasingly entrepreneurial or will we choose to remain a profession, with all the obligations for self-regulation and protection of the public interest that this commitment implies? (53)

It is clear that the work of defining quality in orthopedic surgery must proceed with a concerted and generalized effort to collect data at the delivery level that accurately and reliably describe the patient's clinical status, and that document the changes brought about by various treatments. Chassin (7) has suggested three essential criteria for characterizing a good measure of quality: (a) It must have high sensitivity and specificity; (b) There should be a proven or well-accepted relationship between the measure and a health-care outcome that patients and physicians care about; and (c) The health-care outcome that is measured should have a proven or well-accepted relationship to a specific process of care, so that the physician can do something to improve the outcome. Important outcomes data for most orthopedic procedures extend far beyond that which can be gleaned from administrative data or retrospectively gleaned chart data (43,45). Therefore, prospective data collection instruments that are sensitive, specific, and related to patient symptoms and expectations are needed to define quality (16). Greenfield (19) supported this concept in his evaluation of the state of outcomes research in 1989:

Careful attention must first be paid to the nature of the outcomes chosen to evaluate care. Death, for example, would be expected to be an important but relatively unusual consequence of most medical and surgical care. Therefore, to eval-

uate the effectiveness of care for the majority of patients, other outcome measures must be used, such as the reduction of symptoms, improvement in daily functioning, or improvement in the sense of well-being and the health-related quality of life. (19)

Managed Care and Quality

Outcomes assessment is currently thought of by many practitioners today as a mechanism for automatically enhancing one's ability to negotiate successfully with powerful managed-care insurers (60). The line of reasoning for this is that if superior outcomes can be documented, a provider will be rewarded with more patient referrals. From the insurers point of view, however, the ultimate goal may be to reduce the number of providers and limit access to certain types of costly treatment. The actual measurement of the quality of an individual's outcome may be less important than achieving the primary goal of cost reduction. The current practice of economic credentialing, which bases the assessment of quality on administrative data derived from billing and utilization records, is an example of low-cost, high-efficiency outcome assessment. Many health maintenance organizations (HMOs) are devising or have devised performance measures that define efficiency, effectiveness, and patient satisfaction (60). The current issue is not *whether* outcomes will be used in selecting or deselecting physicians and surgeons from a plan or network, but *which* patient outcomes will be judged to be most representative of the quality of a practitioners care.

The managed-care sector is currently unimpressed with the contribution that the medical outcomes literature has made toward developing measures of quality that directly relate to the actual clinical status of the patient before and after treatment. One important reason for this may be that the clinical data required to document these changes are much more costly to obtain than are administrative data (45). In addition, the legal ramifications of the health insurance industry gaining access to sensitive patient-derived data, and facilitating the sharing of these data with enlarging networks, have barely been explored (62,68). But these considerations are peripheral to a more fundamental reason that has allowed insurers to behave in such a cavalier fashion. Until recently, the medical community has not adequately set forth uniform data elements that should be collected before and after treatment on patients with commonly occurring conditions. Consequently, there is not a well-defined spectrum of validated and risk-adjusted outcomes for most medical and surgical treatments (19). Until the appropriate outcomes are defined, the quality measures that are used will appear strikingly superficial, arbitrary, and self-serving. Nonetheless, insurer-defined quality measures will become increasingly more powerful in determining practice patterns and financial reimbursement, unless credible and feasible alternatives are demonstrated by the medical profession. In 1993, the National Committee for Quality Assurance (NCQA), a Washington-based coalition of managed-care organizations and employers, issued The Health Plan Employer Data and Information Set (HEDIS) (60). This is an instrument that has been used to compare the global quality of various health plans. As the pressure for quality emanates from the health plans to the individual providers, more specific measures will be needed to define the quality of any particular practice.

Greenfield has said, "Outcomes are dangerous, treacherous, and not friends of providers" (61). This is because of the difficulties encountered with adapting what was once the domain of health-care researchers to the application orientation of the practitioner who will be evaluated by the emerging quality measures. Greenfield has underscored the necessity of retaining a sound fundamental methodological framework as outcomes assessment moves into the clinical environment. The following factors have been underscored for assuring sound "research-oriented" clinical assessment: (a) Conclusions should be hypothesis driven; (b) Relevant outcomes must be measured; (c) Case mix must be controlled to determine the relative importance of coexistent conditions versus the index condition; (d) Nondisease factors such as socioeconomic status must be considered; (e) Optimal time intervals for assessment should be defined; and (f) Adequate statistical power should be provided (61). The task of bringing these rigorous criteria into the area of clinical assessment appears at first glance to be daunting. On closer inspection, however, the real issue is not the simplification of an overly complicated and irrelevant research methodology. The primary problem is the establishment of an accepted uniform condition-specific or region-specific data set to be used in conjunction with a global health status measure. As data are collected and analyzed, a progressive streamlining or condensing of instruments would occur by the elimination of highly correlated or redundant elements. The ultimate goal is the integration of a highly efficient outcome assessment process into the actual delivery of care. This goal is close to being reached in several areas of orthopedic practice.

The American Medical Association (AMA) has recently taken steps to fill the "quality void" by developing the Physician Performance Assessment Program (13). Although it is unclear how such a centralized program can impact subspecialty care, the stated emphasis demonstrates a commitment to forming a potential buffer between managed-care plans and individual providers:

The emphasis will be on developing quality measures that make sense—based, for example, on outcomes, not over-reliance on raw economics. (13)

What the AMA intends to do is serve as an agent to promote professionally based quality standards and to "be a force to ensure that quality, fairness and accountability are made part of the system" (13). Its ability to do so will in large part be determined by the cooperation among the diverse specialties of medicine to define particular outcomes and generate the necessary data in a timely fashion.

Practice Guidelines

Practice guidelines have been espoused by those who wish to contain costs by reducing variations in practice (10,12,23,50,55). Many approach practice guidelines with the assumption that, by implementing them, proportionately more high-cost practice patterns would be eliminated than would be established, and that the overall volume of services for a given condition could somehow be controlled in the process. But from a global perspective, practice guidelines are only one step in what has come to be called the Best Practice Cycle (1). Practice guidelines describe an array of appropriate and inappropriate treatments for well defined conditions (26,27). Initially the guidelines arise from a consensus of experts or a state-of-the-art practice that can be gleaned from the literature. The guidelines, however, must be modified utilizing outcomes data gathered from many different practice environments involving a variety of populations to ensure generalizability, and to allow the necessary flexibility for patient preference (25,69). Comparisons must be made utilizing the methodological criteria mentioned in the preceding section. Series of cycles are needed for a thorough refinement of practice guidelines into a "best practice" that can be disseminated and used as a reliable guide to clinical behavior (1). The gradual evolution of practice guidelines, therefore, should be brought about by iterative reporting back to the providers the results of analysis of amalgamated data that they themselves have supplied. The obvious necessity of agreement and cooperation by clinicians in this process cannot be understated. The process must be driven by actual outcomes data that accurately document the conditions, treatments, and outcomes precisely enough so that the conclusions and recommendations will facilitate noticeable implementation (change in practice), and produce significant measurable effects of the changes that are made. Only with outcomes data will the Best Practice Cycle avoid "begging the question" regarding the appropriate care in cases where there is no uniform agreement on the best diagnostic and/or treatment alternatives. Whereas practice guidelines may have a beneficial effect on minimizing variations in practice, outcomes assessment should primarily be viewed as a vehicle to point the direction toward better, higher quality practice. Powerful justification for utilizing or withholding certain costly procedures or treatments would undoubtedly emerge as a valuable byproduct of the cycle. In addition, as risk is accepted by providers in an environment of high-level scrutiny by consumers and the media, the strength of both positive and negative arguments for costly or conservative treatment will be increasingly crucial (14).

MODERN SOLUTIONS TO OUTCOMES ASSESSMENT

The Environment of Outcomes Assessment

The best outcomes assessment is performed utilizing data that most closely describe the patient's demography, comorbidity, general health status, disease-specific symptoms, quality of life, and satisfaction with care before the initiation of any treatment, and after treatment at an interval defined to detect the maximum benefit (16, 61). The location best suited for the performance of outcomes assessment is the outpatient setting. The hospital environment is a progressively shrinking window of care in orthopedic patients, whereas the bulk of patient care has shifted to the home and various outpatient care facilities that are now sites for outcome assessment and documentation. Therefore, any strategy to enhance the quality of orthopedic outcomes assessment must address the feasibility of integrating data collection and reporting into the routines of office practice. The advent of inexpensive computing has opened a door of opportunity for efficiently performing office-based outcomes assessment, and for enhancing the quality of the medical record (62, 68). The recent development of validated patient-administered questionnaire instruments for assessment of many common orthopedic conditions has provided the tools for the full implementation of an outcomes approach to clinical decision making.

Outcome Assessment Instruments: An Overview

It is widely believed that the most reliable instruments for measuring clinical outcomes are either validated patient-administered questionnaires or questionnaires administered by a highly skilled observer other than the treating physician (16). For reasons pertaining to cost, the self-administered questionnaire has emerged as the gold standard for outcomes assessment. It is important that the patient's own view of the severity and importance of his or her symptoms should be considered when selecting items for a scale to measure clinical outcomes (25,69). The symptoms or functions that are most severely affected by the disease, and most important to the patient, should be addressed. The scale's sensitivity to change after treatment is dependent on the appropriateness of question selection. For example, a scale that addresses a patient's tolerance for strenuous physical activity and ability to engage in competitive sports is not as likely to reflect improvement after a total hip replacement as one that measures the difficulty with walking ten blocks and

performing light housework. Wright et al. showed, in a study of 72 patients who were preparing to undergo total hip replacement, that there was considerable variation in the severity and importance of the patients' symptoms (69). In addition, issues such as pain specifically occurring at night, during recreation, and during sexual activity were found to be frequent complaints not included in traditionally used hip rating scales.

The issue of questionnaire-based outcomes assessment is naturally met by physicians with some degree of ambivalence (41). Its methodology represents a fundamental departure from traditional clinical data collection that emphasizes a physician-performed history and physical examination. The history and physical, along with ancillary laboratory and radiographic tests, are necessary for establishing a diagnosis and for formulating treatment alternatives. However, a crucial problem is the intra- and interobserver variation in the actual data collection (3,4, 6,29). Moreover, important questions regarding the validity of physician versus patient-based outcome assessment have recently been raised. Lieberman et al. (38) have reported significant differences between the physician's assessment and the patient's responses to a questionnaire after total hip replacement. The physician's evaluation was regularly more favorable than the patient's. The discrepancy increased in patients with inferior surgical results. Compounding these problems is the wide array of language that is used to describe the patient's general health status and disease-specific symptoms (30). Settings in which physicians do not customarily perform systematic collection of clinical data for research purposes are more likely to demonstrate these variations. It is also necessary to gather data from a diversity of orthopedic practices to maximize the ability to generalize any conclusions regarding the appropriateness and effectiveness of care. Outcomes assessment should be performed both at academic centers and in nonacademic settings.

The first hip scales were developed to objectively measure the patient's clinical status before and after hip surgery (3–5,11,22,34,67). In a recent report, Bryant et al. analyzed 19 published hip scores (5). In this study, ten of the most popular scoring systems were compared when they were used to measure the long-term outcome of hip arthroplasty in 47 procedures (41 patients). It was noted that among the scoring systems, pain was most frequently rated and was the most heavily weighted variable. Pain measurement is most frequently measured using response categories that contain anchoring adjectives such as *severe*, *moderate*, *mild*, or *none*, with a corresponding point value assigned to each category. This strategy was frequently modified by mixing descriptors of pain such as *none* or *ignores* in the Harris Hip Score (22), or severity of pain with medication utilization and functional limitation as in the HSS Hip Rating System (67). In all traditional scores, the physician was given the responsibility of assigning the patient to one category. In the case of mixed or ambiguous descriptors, it was the physician's judgment that determined which of them applied or was most important in any given case. Therefore, the likelihood of both inter- and intraobserver variation was significantly increased, potentially compromising the validity of the scores. This problem is not unique to hip evaluation. Similar observations regarding pain assessment in traditional global knee rating systems have been made (11).

Functional evaluations among hip scores vary in the factors chosen and the point values assigned to each factor. Among the 19 hip scoring systems that Bryant evaluated, walking distance, walking aids, and limp were assessed with a frequency of more than 50% (5). Other frequently utilized variables were tying shoelaces (8 of 19), stair climbing (7 of 19), and work (7 of 19). Sitting, bathing, foot care, public transportation, car driving, dressing, and sports were addressed in only five or fewer scoring systems. The striking feature of this summary of hip scoring systems is the variation of inclusion or exclusion of particular functional abilities. For example, the Harris Hip Score addresses walking distance, support, limp, stairs, footwear, public transportation, and sitting (22). The Iowa hip score includes several additional functions such as dressing, housework, squatting, riding in a car, and carrying objects (34). In comparison, the modified d'Aubigne HSS Hip Rating System is relatively cursory in its functional assessment, combining walking distance, support, and limp to form a single variable, and similarly combining shopping, housework, desk work, and working (67). The irregularity with which functional assessment is handled is not unique to hip scoring systems. Drake et al. (11) reported a nearly identical situation in a report on 34 knee rating systems.

Hip rating scores report hip range of motion in a variety of ways: (a) summing the arcs of motion in the three cardinal planes (flexion, abduction, rotation) (5), (b) utilizing the Gade index modified by Harris (22), or (c) utilizing functional activities as proxy measures of range of motion (41). The first two strategies require a detailed physical examination to complete. This may be a significant problem when an actual follow-up visit is not possible. Bryant et al. (5) observed that both the Gade index and the summation of arcs of movement are highly correlated with the measurement of flexion arc alone. This finding supports the concept of hip range of motion being most conveniently inferred from functional performance data.

The high level of variability among traditional hip scores has resulted in a diverse group of instruments using different language and definitions, scaling factors, and weighting of the various domains. Some scales create an aggregate global score and others do not. Some scales define excellent, good, fair, and poor results, and others specify results as acceptable and unacceptable. What has resulted is an array of disparate descriptive terms and numerical scores that cannot be compared with each other. Moreover, the scales have not been validated by a scientifically rigorous process. Hence, the majority of the published long-term studies on the result of total hip replacements have been noted to have significant methodological deficiencies (18,20).

At the National Institutes of Health (NIH) Consensus Conference on Total Hip-Joint Replacement in the United States, held in 1982, the need for improved methodology in the approach to patient evaluations was noted:

> Improved quantitative methods for the functional evaluation of hip replacement patients should be utilized and developed further. (46)

In an editorial by J. O. Galante in the 1985 *Journal of Bone and Joint Surgery*, the following observation was made:

> A system for evaluating the results of hip surgery should ideally provide objective parameters that can be measured in a reproducible manner by independent observers. All of the systems that are used today have common flaws, in that much of the information is of a subjective nature. (17)

In response to Galante's call for orthopedic surgeons to "agree to a uniform method of evaluating and reporting the results of hip-replacement surgery," the Hip Society, Society International Congress of Orthopaedics and Traumatology (SICOT), and the American Association of Orthopaedic Surgeons (AAOS) convened a task force that arrived at an agreement on a system of clinical and radiographic terminology, referred to as CART (30). Published in 1990 by Johnston et al., CART was described as "building-blocks of information" that could be combined to form a common language for the reporting of total hip replacement results. This was a significant step toward defining a core minimal data set of items to be used in the evaluation of patients being treated for hip arthritis (37). The next challenge was to adapt the concepts and terminology embodied in this consensus into the methodological framework of outcomes assessment that has evolved during the 1980s. This approach has been supported by the NIH consensus panel on total hip replacement that convened in 1994 (47).

Instrument Validation

The requirements for a clinical outcome assessment instrument are similar to those for a laboratory instrument. It must be valid or accurate in its description of a real clinical state. It must be reliable or precise when used on a stable patient, and responsive in demonstrating a quantitative change that is appropriate to the observed clinical change (6,16,29).

The face validity of an outcome assessment instrument is the least complex and least expensive way to ensure that the instrument will in fact measure what it purports to measure. This entails knowledgeable observers, or a panel of experts, deciding that the instrument contains the essential elements, questions, or probes for defining the indications and expected outcomes of a given treatment. Each question should have an array of responses that are clearly defined, mutually exclusive, and ordered in a hierarchical progression (6). This is accomplished using terms that denote severity, frequency, distance, time, or functional impairment on either a visual analog scale with anchors under the scale, or a Likert scale with multiple response options.

The criterion validity of an instrument is checked by comparing the responses with gold standards that have measurable characteristics and a known relationship with a particular outcome. In the hip rating questionnaire (HRQ) developed and validated at the Hospital for Special Surgery, the authors correlated the patient's self-reported walking score with the results of a 6-minute walking distance test (29). The Pearson correlation coefficient (r) was .6, suggesting that patients who actually could walk farther tended to have higher estimates of their own walking ability.

The construct validity of an instrument is evaluated utilizing a more highly technical and theoretical process, analyzing how the various responses correlate with each other in describing a particular health concept. For example, in validating a hip questionnaire, one might hypothesize that pain severity and limitation of walking distance would have a moderate correlation. In the HRQ, this was in fact found to be the case, with $r = .43$. Limitation of walking distance was also found to be moderately correlated with the need and frequency of walking assistance ($r = .39$), difficulty with stairs ($r = .41$), and difficulty using public transportation ($r = .39$) (29).

Reliability is a measure of reproducibility or precision of the instrument. It has been defined as the extent to which the same assessment will be made on a particular phenomenon in the absence of any true interval change. This feature of an instrument is very important because it defines the variability or background noise that is inherent in the instrument itself. The reliability is tested by administering the instrument twice to a stable patient. The responses from the first and second administration may be evaluated using the Kappa statistic for ordinal data and either the Pearson correlation coefficient or an intraclass correlation coefficient for dimensional data (29,59). It is important to check the reproducibility of each individual question, no matter how simple or straightforward it may appear. For example, in the pretesting phase of the HRQ, the question, Do you have stairs at home?, was not reproducible. Eight out of 52 stable patients responded differently the second time to this apparently simple yes-or-no question. The Kappa statistic, which measures the degree of agreement that exceeds chance alone, was .57. A Kappa of 1 represents perfect agreement, and .6 is regarded as the minimum acceptable

agreement. On this basis, the stairs-at-home question was eliminated from the questionnaire.

An instrument's responsiveness describes its ability to detect clinically important change. It represents the signal intensity that is measured to determine the effectiveness of a treatment (29). Classically, the response to total hip replacement has been measured by the extent to which the hip score changes. It must be remembered, however, that the noise level, or variation, caused by less-than-perfect reliability needs to be accounted for in defining the clinically important difference. When planning a prospective study, the sample size required to detect a qualitative advantage of one form of treatment over another will be directly proportional to the magnitude of difference that is considered clinically important, and inversely proportional to the reliability (Kappa value) of the instrument. Guyatt et al. (21) described a technique for determining the "responsiveness index" for an outcome assessment instrument (29). This was calculated by dividing the minimum clinically important change by the square root of twice the mean square error. The mean square error is an alternative numerical representation of the reliability. Using this index, the sample size for a hypothetical prospective study comparing two different treatments for hip arthritis can be calculated. If the 100-point HRQ scale were used as the primary outcome measure, to detect with 90% power at an alpha level of .05 (one-tailed), the total score difference of 12 points between the results of two treatments, only 19 patients would be required in each treatment group. This example has significant implications regarding the economy of conducting clinical research with instruments that have excellent responsiveness and reliability.

The SF-36 and the WOMAC

Two validated instruments, the SF-36 (63) used for general health status assessment, and the WOMAC (2), which is used to assess disease-specific hip and knee symptoms, have gained general acceptance for outcomes assessment in hip and knee arthritis. General health status measures are useful for evaluating the health of patients with a variety of medical conditions. Unlike disease-specific measures, general health status instruments facilitate the comparison of treatments across disease boundaries. The SF-36 was developed during the Medical Outcomes Study, an observational study conducted between 1986 and 1990 on adult patients in Boston, Chicago, and Los Angeles. At 6-month intervals over a 2-year period, 2546 patients were surveyed. The short form, containing 36 questions, evolved out of this process. The SF-36 measures three major health attributes that include eight health concepts. Functional status as an attribute takes into account the concepts of physical function, social function, and role limitations caused by either physical or emotional problems. Well-being encompasses mental health, energy/fatigue, and pain. The attribute of overall health includes the patients' perceptions of their current health, expectations of the future, and the changes in their health over the past year.

In two separate prospective studies, Ritter et ql. (57) and McGuigan et al. (42) demonstrated statistically significant improvement in most subscales of the SF-36 when preoperative scores are compared with 2-year postoperative scores after total hip replacement. The preoperative scores, however, did not predict postoperative improvement, casting some doubt on the utility of the SF-36 for evaluating the indications for surgery. Nevertheless, the SF-36 clearly demonstrated the dramatic impact that hip replacement has on quality of life. Other analyses of both hip and knee replacement using different instruments have come to similar conclusions (56).

The WOMAC, or Western Ontario and McMaster University Osteoarthritis Index, is a disease-specific measure that was developed and validated for patients who have osteoarthritis of the hip or knee (2). The WOMAC contains three domains: pain (five questions), stiffness (two questions), and physical function (17 questions). The issues addressed by the WOMAC have much in common with many of the traditionally used hip scales, and therefore it has already gained wide acceptance among orthopedic surgeons. In a prospective study of 188 patients, Laupacis et al. (35) have shown that total hip replacement resulted in improvement in all three WOMAC domains. Ninety of these patients were followed for 2 years. Improvement was also noted in general health status and global health-related quality of life.

AAOS Lower Extremity Instrument

In 1994, the AAOS, in conjunction with the Council on Musculoskeletal Subspecialty Societies (COMSS), convened a meeting in Tarpon Springs, Florida. Task forces were formed to complete questionnaire-based outcome assessment instruments that would cover the spine, upper extremity, lower extremity, and pediatrics. The lower extremity instrument was tested for reproducibility in 1995 and is scheduled for sensitivity testing in 1996. The guiding concept was to develop a core group of questions that would apply to all lower extremity problems, and a series of modules that would more specifically apply to specialties such as arthritis, sports, foot and ankle, and tumor. The AAOS has fully supported the development of these instruments and plans to further implement their testing under the auspices of the Committee on Outcomes Research and the Task Force on Data Management. During a pilot test in the fall of 1995, the Task Force on Data Management demonstrated the feasibility of electronically transmitting outcomes data to a central site. A permanent central repository for further data collection is planned. Taken together with the recent statement by the AMA regarding the Physician Performance Assessment Program (13), it appears that the AAOS is well positioned to interface with this effort at the subspecialty level.

CONCLUSION

The outcomes movement nears the end of the twentieth century as a rapidly generalized and multifaceted process. Unlike Codman's private efforts to implement his End Result System, the call for outcomes assessment today is issued within health plans, hospitals, and medical societies on a daily basis. The technology of outcomes assessment has matured to the point where it is ready for integration into clinical practice. Computing technology is now available at reasonable cost and with adequate power to facilitate the construction of databases that form the foundation of the electronic medical record. Most importantly, the medical community has the incentive to define quality in a methodologically rigorous fashion, utilizing outcomes data and practice guidelines. Althouggh the term *outcome* has varying meanings for the patient, physician, researcher, government, insurer, and society at large, its foundational concepts have become a dominant force in the debates that continue on health-care reform. Codman's idea has survived and, in fact, prevailed. Orthopedics has a long tradition of outcomes assessment, and for that reason the orthopedic community has a unique opportunity to take a leadership role in the job of demonstrating effectiveness of medical and surgical treatments for musculoskeletal disease. If this needed leadership emerges successfully, it will provide many with hope for a more rational, patient-centered, and cost-effective health-care system.

REFERENCES

1. Beed, G. Implementing outcomes research: When theory meets reality. *Manag Care Med* 1995;April:27–31.
2. Bellamy N, Buchanan WW, Goldsmith CH, Campbell J, Stitt LW. Validation study of WOMAC: a health status instrument for measuring clinically important patient relevant outcomes to antirheumatic drug therapy in patients with osteoarthritis of the hip or knee. *J Rheumatol* 1988;15:1833–1840.
3. Bellamy N, Campbell J. Hip and knee rating scales for total joint arthroplasty: a critical but constructive review. Part 1. *J Orthop Rheum* 1989;3:3–21.
4. Bellamy N, Campbell J. Hip and knee rating scales for total joint arthroplasty: a critical but constructive review. Part 2. *J Orthop Rheum* 1989;2:63–76.
5. Bryant MJ, Kernohan WG, Nixon JR, Mollan RAB. A statistical analysis of hip scores. *J Bone Joint Surg* 1993;75B:705–709.
6. Charlson M, Johanson N, Williams P. Scaling, staging and scoring. In: Troidl H, Spitzer W, McPeek B, et al., eds. *Principles and practice of research: strategies for surgical investigators.* New York: Springer-Verlag, 1991;192–200.
7. Chassin MR. Quality of care: time to act. *JAMA* 1991;266(24):3472–3473.
8. Chassin MR, Brook RH, Park RE, Keesey J, Fink A, Kosecoff J, Kahn K, Merrick N, Solomon DH. Variations in the use of medical and sur-

gical services by the medicare population. *N Engl J Med* 1986;314: 285–290.

9. Codman EA. *The shoulder*. Boston: 1934;v–xl.

10. Culhane C. Streamlining for managed care. *Am Med News* 1994;April 11:25–28.

11. Drake BG, Callahan CM, Dittus RS, Wright JG. Global rating systems used in assessing knee arthroplasty outcomes. *J Arthroplasty* 1994;9 (4):409–417.

12. Dubois RW. Practice guidelines: Why, how, and who? *Bull Rheum Dis* 1994;43(3):7–8.

13. Editorial: Seal of approval. *Am Med News* 1996;39(9):19.

14. Emanuel EJ, Brett AS. Managed competition and the patient-physician relationship. *N Engl J Med* 1993;329(12):879–882.

15. Friedman B, Elixhauser A. Increased use of an expensive, elective procedure: total hip replacements in the 1980s. *Med Care* 1993;31(7): 581–596.

16. Fries JF. Toward an understanding of patient outcome measurement. *Arthritis Rheum* 1983;26(6):697–704.

17. Galante J. The need for a standardized system for evaluating results of total hip surgery *[editorial]*. *J Bone Joint Surg* 1985;67A:511–512.

18. Gartland JJ. Orthopaedic clinical research: deficiencies in experimental design and determinations of outcome. *J Bone Joint Surg* 1988;70A: 1357–1364.

19. Greenfield S. The state of outcome research: are we on target? *N Engl J Med* 1989;320:1142–1143.

20. Gross M. A critique of the methodologies used in clinical studies of hip-joint arthroplasty published in the English-language orthopaedic literature. *J Bone Joint Surg* 1988;70A:1364–1371.

21. Guyatt G, Walter S, Norman G. Measuring change over time: assessing the usefulness of evaluative instruments. *J Chronic Dis* 1987;40: 171–178.

22. Harris WH. Traumatic arthritis of the hip after dislocation and acetabular fractures: treatment by mold arthroplasty. *J Bone Joint Surg* 1969; 51A:737–755.

23. Hayward RS, Wilson MC, Tunis SR, Bass EB, Guyatt G. User's guides to the medical literature: VIII. How to use clinical practice guidelines. A. Are the recommendations valid? *JAMA* 1995;274(7):570–574.

24. Healy WL, Kirven FM, Iorio R, Patch DA, Pfeifer BA. Implant standardization for total hip arthroplasty: an implant selection and a cost reduction program. *J Arthroplasty* 1995;10(2):177–183.

25. Hlatky M. Patient preferences and clinical guidelines. *JAMA* 1995;273 (15):1219–1230.

26. Hochberg MC, Altman RD, Brandt KD, Clark BM, Dieppe PA, Griffin MR, Moskowitz RW, Schnitzer TJ. Guidelines for the medical management of osteoarthritis: Part 1. Osteoarthritis of the hip. *Arthritis Rheum* 1995;38(11):1535–1540.

27. Hochberg MC, Altman RD, Brandt KD, Clark BM, Dieppe PA, Griffin MR, Moskowitz RW, Schnitzer TJ. Guidelines for the medical management of osteoarthritis: Part 2. Osteoarthritis of the knee. *Arthritis Rheum* 1995;38(11):1541–1546.

28. Inglehart JK. Physicians and the growth of managed care. *N Engl J Med* 1994;331(17):1167–1171.

29. Johanson NA, Charlson M, Sztrowski T, Ranawat CS. A self-administered hip-rating questionnaire for the assessment of outcome after total hip replacement. *J Bone Joint Surg* 1992;75A:1619–1626.

30. Johnston RC, Fitzgerald RH, Harris WH, Poss R, Muller ME, Sledge CB. Clinical and radiographic evaluation of total hip replacement: a standard system of terminology for reporting results. *J Bone Joint Surg* 1990;72A:161–168.

31. Keller RB, Soule DN, Wennberg JE, Hanley DF. Dealing with geographic variations in the use of hospitals. *J Bone Joint Surg* 1990;72A: 1286–1293.

32. Keller RB, Rudicel SA, Liang MH. Outcomes research in orthopaedics. *J Bone Joint Surg* 1993;75A:1562–1574.

33. Kleinke JD. Medicine's industrial revolution. *Wall Street J* 1995;Aug 21.

34. Larson CB. Rating scale for hip disabilities. *Clin Orthop* 1963;31:85–93.

35. Laupacis A, Bourne R, Rorabeck C, Feeny D, Wong C, Tugwell P, Leslie K, Bullas R. The effect of elective total hip replacement on health-related quality of life. *J Bone Joint Surg* 1993;75A:1619–1626.

36. Liang MH, Cullen K, Larson M, Thompson MS, Schwartz JA, Fossel AH, Roberts WN, Sledge CB. Cost-effectiveness of total joint arthroplasty in osteoarthritis. *Arthritis Rheum* 1986;29(8):937–943.

37. Liang MH, Katz JN, Phillips C, Sledge C, Cats-Baril W, AAOS Task Force on Outcome Studies. The total hip arthroplasty outcome evalua-

tion form of the American Academy of Orthopaedic Surgeons: results of a nominal group process. *J Bone Joint Surg* 1991;73A:639–646.

38. Lieberman JR, Dorey F, Shekelle P, Schumacher L, Thomas B, Kilgus DJ, Finerman GA. Differences between patients and physicians evaluations of outcome after total hip arthroplasty. *J Bone Joint Surg* 1996; 78A:835–838.

39. Madhok R, Lewallen DG, Wallrichs SL, Ilstrup DM, Kurland RL, Melton LJ. Trends in the utilization of primary total hip arthroplasty, 1969 through 1990: a population-based study in Olmsted County, Minnesota. *Mayo Clin Proc* 1993;68:11–18.

40. Maloney W, Peters P, Engh CA, Chandler H. Severe osteolysis of the pelvis in association with acetabular replacement without cement. *J Bone Joint Surg* 1993;75A:1627–1635.

41. McGrory BJ, Morrey BF, Rand JA, Ilstrup DM. Correlation of patient questionnaire responses and physician history in grading clinical outcome following hip and knee arthroplasty: a prospective study of 201 joint arthroplasties. *J Arthroplasty* 1996;11(1):47–57.

42. McGuigan FX, Hozack WJ, Moriarty L, Eng K, Rothman RH. Predicting quality-of-life outcomes following total joint arthroplasty: limitations of the SF-36 health status questionnaire. *J Arthroplasty* 1995; 10(6):742–747.

43. Melfi C, Holleman E, Arthur D, Katz B. Selecting a patient characteristics index for the prediction of medical outcomes using administrative claims data. *J Clin Epidemiol* 1995;48(7):917–926.

44. Melton LJ, Stauffer RN, Chao EYS, Ilstrup DM. Rates of total hip arthroplasty: a population-based study. *N Engl J Med* 1982;307: 1242–1245.

45. Mitchell JB, Bubolz T, Paul JE, Pashos CL, Escarce JJ, Muhlbaier LH, Weisman JM, Young WW, Epstein RS, Javitt JC. Using Medicare claims for outcomes research. *Med Care* 1994;32(7):JS38–JS51.

46. NIH Consensus Conference. Total hip-joint replacement in the United States. *JAMA* 1982;248:1817.

47. NIH Consensus Conference. Total hip replacement. *JAMA* 1995;273 (24):1950–1956.

48. O'Leary DS. Measurement and accountability: taking careful aim. *The Joint Commission Journal on Quality Improvement*. 1995;21(7): 354–357.

49. Owen TD, Moran CG, Smith SR, Pinder IM. Results of uncemented porous-coated anatomic total hip replacement. *J Bone Joint Surg* 1994; 76B:258–262.

50. Pauly MV. Practice guidelines: Can they save money? Should they? *J Law Med Ethics* 1995;325:65–74.

51. Peterson M, Hollenberg J, Szatrowski T, Johanson NA, Mancuso CA, Charlson ME. Geographic variations in the rates of elective total hip and knee arthroplasties among Medicare beneficiaries in the United States. *J Bone Joint Surg* 1992;74A:1530–1539.

52. Praemer A, Furner S, Rice DP. *Musculoskeletal conditions in the United States*. Park Ridge, IL: American Academy of Orthopaedic Surgeons, 1992;135–136.

53. Relman AS. Shattuck lecture—The health care industry: Where is it taking us? *N Engl J Med* 1991;854–859.

54. Relman AS. Assessment and accountability: the third revolution in medical care. *N Engl J Med* 1988;319:1220–1222.

55. Richardson WS, Detsky AS. User's guide to the medical literature: VII. How to use a clinical decision analysis. A. Are the results of the study valid? *JAMA* 1995;273(16):1292–1295.

56. Rissanen P, Aro S, Slatis P, Sintonen H, Paavolainen P. Health and quality of life before and after hip or knee arthroplasty. *J. Arthroplasty* 1995;10(2):169–175.

57. Ritter MA, Albohm MJ, Keating EM, Faris PM, Meding JB. Comparative outcomes of total joint arthroplasty. *J Arthroplasty* 1995;10(6): 737–741.

58. Schmalzried TP, Guttmann D, Grecula M, Amstutz HC. The relationship between the design, position, and articular wear of acetabular components inserted without cement and the development of pelvic osteolysis. *J Bone Joint Surg* 1994;76A:677–688.

59. Spitzer RL, Cohen J, Fleiss JL, et al. Quantification of agreement in psychiatric diagnosis: a new approach. *Arch Gen Psychiatr* 1967;17: 83–87.

60. USQA quality monitor. *J Health Performance Improvement* 1994;1(1): 1–15.

61. Voelker R. Medical news and perspectives: creating a basis for good outcomes. *JAMA* 1995;273(18):1401.

62. Wallace S. The computerized patient record. *Byte* 1994;May:67–75.

63. Ware JE, Sherbourne CD. The MOS 36-item short-form health survey (SF-36). *Med Care* 1992;30:473.

64. Wennberg J, Gittelsohn A. Variations in medical care among small areas. *Sci Am* 1982;246(4)120–134.

65. Wennberg J. Which rate is right? *N Engl J Med* 1986;314(5):310–311.

66. Wennberg J, Freeeeman J, Culp WJ. Are hospital services rationed in New Haven or over-utilized in Boston? *Lancet* 1987;1:1185–1189.

67. Wilson PD Jr, Amstutz HC, Czerniecki A, Salvati EA, Mendes DG. Total hip replacement with fixation by acrylic cement: a preliminary study of 100 consecutive McKee-Farrar prosthetic replacements. *J Bone Joint Surg* 1972;54A:207–236.

68. Woodward B. The computer-based patient record and confidentiality. *N Engl J Med* 1995;333(21):1419–1422.

69. Wright JG, Rudicel S, Feinstein AR. Ask patients what they want: evaluation of individual complaints before total hip replacement. *J Bone Joint Surg* 1994;76B:229–234.

The Adult Hip, edited by J. J. Callaghan,
A. G. Rosenberg, and H. E. Rubash.
Lippincott–Raven Publishers, Philadelphia © 1998.

CHAPTER 55

Critical Pathways in Total Hip Arthroplasty

James G. Howe and Bobbie Lambert

Coordinated, multidisciplinary planning for the care of the total hip arthroplasty (THA) patient can ensure maximal benefits to the patient and the health-care system. This chapter will describe a 10-year experience coordinating the care of patients undergoing THA, including the initial development of a clinical path, the expansion of that concept to include case management of the entire episode of care (a patient-care program), and the revision or development of clinical paths that cover specific phases of the experience.

Total hip arthroplasty has revolutionized the care of the arthritic patient. The procedures are associated with low complication rates and significant improvements in comfort and functional status (14). Laupacis et al. (13) have demonstrated that THA is a cost-effective medical treatment. As the demands for THA increase and the relative health care dollars decrease, society will focus on value, as defined by the relationship between quality and cost (V = Q/C), with both service and outcome quality being measured. It is hypothesized that a well-developed coordinated care program will maximize value by ensuring quality while reducing costs.

There are many terms that describe coordination of care. Case management or care management is generally defined as a system that focuses on the accountability of an identified individual or group for coordinating the care for a patient (or a group of patients) across a continuum of care; ensuring and facilitating the achievement of qual-

ity, clinical, and cost outcomes; negotiating, procuring, and coordinating services and resources needed by the patient and family; intervening at key points (and/or at significant variances) for individual patients; addressing and resolving patterns in aggregate variances that have a negative quality-to-cost impact; and creating opportunities and systems to enhance outcomes (3).

The term *patient care program* has been used to describe coordination of care. A patient care program is defined as a program that coordinates the health care activities of all involved care sites for a specific patient program or diagnostic category throughout the full continuum of care. A clinical path is a shorthand version used by care givers: it outlines a series of expected events that occur in the care of a patient. For a specific group of patients, the events are standardized with respect to a very clear description of the event, timing of the event, expected goals, and ability to measure the event. Other similar terms that refer to organizing care include *care maps*, *protocols*, *algorithms*, *guidelines*, *practice parameters*, and *care continuum*. Although there is overlap, each defines a specific process or intent. An algorithm, for example, is a step-by-step decision process. Many algorithms can be associated with one patient care program.

Clinical pathways have been utilized by many institutions to maintain quality and standardize or decrease utilization of services and supplies (1,6,7,15). A recent national poll of 188 health-care providers by Anderson Consulting found that four-fifths of health-care organizations currently use clinical paths. Of the remaining one-fifth, most plan to begin to use paths in the near future (5). Implementation results in a decreased length of stay

J. G. Howe and B. Lambert: Departments of Orthopaedics and Rehabilitation, University of Vermont, Fletcher Allen Health Care, Burlington, Vermont 05405.

and thus a significant reduction in cost. The clinical pathway may document every step in the journey from diagnosis, through treatment, to follow-up. Once the steps are documented, they are more readily available for analysis, evaluation, and modification. The use of a pathway fosters the approach of total quality management. One of the major benefits of the use of pathways is that they provide a forum for physicians and the entire health-care team to work together in a multidisciplinary process.

DEVELOPMENT AND IMPLEMENTATION OF THE CLINICAL PATHWAY

After some experience with diagnostic-related group (DRG) reimbursement in the late 1980s, it became apparent that hospitals would incur a loss on DRG 209 (covering total joint replacement). This was very disturbing information, especially for the surgeons who had built their clinical practice and academic career around this procedure. Stimulated by the clinician and strongly supported by hospital administration, a process was initiated to look closely at all institutional aspects of total hip replacement. The team was multidisciplinary, including doctors, nurses, administrators, therapists, and a social worker. All areas of the institution that participated in the care, either directly or indirectly, were represented or consulted. The focus was on optimizing inpatient care and outcomes. A first draft of the critical pathway was developed based on current practice. Each hospital area and process involved in the care of the total hip patient was evaluated, with specific goals and expectations for service and care delivery. The areas or processes identified were: surgical scheduling, preoperative medical evaluation, patient education, postoperative rehabilitation, and postoperative pain. Subcommittees worked on each area and developed recommendations that were discussed, modified, and then accepted by consensus by the entire group. The result of this work was a clinical path for THR that was implemented on the inpatient unit of The University of Vermont College of Medicine in 1990.

Documentation and daily responsibilities were important issues in implementation and continued review. The clinical path form, which listed daily tests, treatments, activities, and expectations, was kept in the patient's room and all care givers were expected to follow the detailed program unless the patients condition required some modification. In that case, a variance was noted and explained. The nurse caring for the patient was responsible for monitoring the pathway and coordinating communications.

The results from the first clinical pathway were very gratifying. There was a documented decrease in length of hospitalization and cost (Table 1). DRG 209 became a source of revenue for the hospital rather than a financial drain. Along with the decrease in length of stay and cost,

TABLE 1. *Results of the implementation of the first clinical pathway*

Year	LOS	Cost	DRG reimbursement
1990	10.10		
1991	7.38	12,839	
1992	7.87	12,137	
1993	7.51	12,517	
1994	6.24	11,270	
1995			12,266
1996			12,024

LOS, length of stay; DRG, diagnosis-related group.

the quality of the experience for the patient improved. Outcomes remained unchanged as measured by complication rates and Harris Hip Scores. The pathway gave documentation to the total hip experience. It stimulated group discussion, study, and the initiation of quality improvement projects around the care of the patients undergoing total hip procedures.

In 1994, the Orthopaedic Service at The University of Vermont College of Medicine initiated a project to review the total hip clinical pathway and evaluate the care of that patient population. The length of stay decreased dramatically after introduction of the clinical pathway, and it compared favorably with the literature, which described reductions in length of stay (attributed to clinical paths) to 7 days (2), 11 days (12), or 5.9 days for low risk patients (17). The cost and length-of-stay history are described in Table 1.

Likewise, in 1994, the lengths of stay for total joint patients in our rehabilitation unit were below the national average (i.e., 13 days compared to 15 days nationally and 16 days regionally). Onset days (days the patient is in the acute-care hospital before transfer to rehabilitation), however, could be improved. The majority of our patients were discharged home (Table 2).

DEVELOPMENT OF THE PATIENT CARE PROGRAM

Although results continued to improve, it was decided to expand the inpatient clinical path to become a true case management system, including the physician's office,

TABLE 2. *Distribution of destinations after patient discharge*

Year	Discharge destination	Number of patients (%)
1994	Home	254 (82.2)
	Rehabilitation unit	37 (12)
	Nursing home	18 (5.8)
1995	Home	273 (80.3)
	Rehabilitation unit	51 (15)
	Nursing home	16 (4.7)

improving coordination among all care givers, and extending the pathway beyond the inpatient hospital to post-hospital care either at home or in a rehabilitation unit. The clinical path is a central feature of the patient care program, which also includes new systems for preoperative evaluation, patient education, demand matching of prostheses, and post-hospital referral and follow-up.

Several areas were targeted for improvement during revision:

1. Improve the transition from physician's office to inpatient unit, and from inpatient unit to post-hospital care (either home or rehabilitation unit).
2. Decrease duplication of documentation.
3. Increase patient involvement via patient and family education.
4. Build on the existing clinical paths and algorithm with a periodic assessment process, to continually modify and improve.
5. Work with the Visiting Nurse Association (VNA) locally and throughout the region to develop consistent home care plans.
6. Include education and research as part of the clinical pathways.
7. Use the value equation ($V = Q/C$) as a measure of the success of the clinical pathway.

As the rework commenced, the group expanded its representation from the original committee to include the VNA, physician outpatient office, patient education specialist, quality assurance specialist, and rehabilitation referral coordinator.

RESULTS OF REVISION AND MODIFICATIONS

The results of revision were more than a mere modification, but rather a reengineering of the total hip clinical process. The pathway began to take on the feel of an integrated system. Each team member was encouraged to extend his or her thinking beyond the care site in order to understand, appreciate, and coordinate efforts with care givers throughout the patient's entire experience from office to home. Some of the highlights of the redesign follow.

EDUCATION

Staff in all disciplines and at each site where the patients are cared for need to be well versed in the overall patient care program and to understand their specific responsibilities. To accomplish this, an extensive document describing the development, purpose, and content of the total hip clinical pathway was developed and used by members of the Total Hip Clinical Pathway Task Force who met with the different disciplines to review their

responsibilities in detail. The document was distributed widely. The role of a service coordinator was conceived during this development of the pathway. This person was responsible for ensuring that the pathway was followed throughout the patient's experience from office, preoperative assessment, hospitalization, home or rehabilitation unit, and finally a return visit to the orthopedist. Because this was the first expanded pathway across sites, oversight was important. As the staff at various sites became familiar with their responsibilities, the need for the monitoring and involvement of the service coordinator decreased.

The education of the patient begins at the initial visit to the orthopedist's office. In addition to the information that one would expect the physician to convey to the patient, a video (12 minutes) about the total hip replacement is shown. A second video, which focuses on the nursing unit and postoperative rehabilitation, is given to the patient to take home and watch.

A strong belief that patients and their families need and want to be as knowledgeable as possible about their care led to an emphasis on patient education throughout the episode of care. A patient version of the clinical path was developed, using language understandable at a sixth-grade level. All disciplines use the same patient version to give instructions, so duplication is avoided and the information is consistent. The concept of the clinical path, its purpose, and its value to the patient are explained, first in the orthopedist's office and then at each care site. The patient is given the Patient Version which has three parts: before surgery, in hospital, and at home (Appendix 1). During each phase, the staff uses the patient's version to teach and review with the patient both the current progress and the next steps to be taken. Responses from patients have been very positive when the pathways were used by staff. When the staff did not review the pathway with the patient, some patients would note that the staff had a lot of paperwork, but they were not able to identify the value of this paperwork.

PREOPERATIVE EVALUATION

The purpose of the preoperative evaluation is to ensure that the patient is ready for surgery and is entering surgery with the lowest possible risk. Ultimately, it is the anesthesiologist who must decide if the patient is completely worked up and ready for surgery. In the past, the lack of coordination among primary physicians, orthopedists, and anesthesiologists has resulted in delays in proper assessment and has been a significant reason for the cancellation or delay of surgery. After discussion with the anesthesiologists, they agreed to take responsibility for organizing and monitoring the preoperative work-up. They also developed a consensus among themselves as to the content of an adequate work-up for the common medical problems seen in total hip patients. The patient is given a packet with forms for the preoperative evaluation. This packet accompanies the patient as he or she progresses through the care site, thus eliminating the need for document duplication. A letter containing recommendations for the preoperative evaluation is included with the packet and the patient is instructed to give it to the primary care physician.

One major breakthrough in avoiding duplicate documentation resulted from having the patient fill out a medication sheet listing all medication, dose and frequency, and describing medications used for pain control. This form is reviewed for accuracy by the primary physician and kept by the patient who gives it to the staff at the preoperative visit, where it is copied and used as documentation in the patient's record. The original remains with the patient to be reviewed and copied as needed at the next care site. The patient is given the responsibility of keeping track of his or her forms, and of bringing the completed history, physical, and test results from the primary physician to their preoperative visit. We have found most patients are able to manage this responsibility well.

At the time of the initial visit, the nursing staff evaluates the patient's knowledge and capability for postoperative care at home. If they feel the patient would benefit from a preoperative home assessment, the VNA is contacted. A VNA physical therapist then visits the home to evaluate the patient and home, and to suggest modifications as required. During the home visit, the physical therapist assesses the potential need for transfer to the inpatient rehabilitation unit at the time of discharge. If the patient meets criteria, the rehabilitation unit is notified and a tentative reservation made for 4 days after surgery. This preoperative notification has saved several days' delay in transfer for each patient, resulting in significant cost savings for the acute-care hospital.

As a final step, the patient with the completed packet is evaluated by anesthesia approximately 1 week before the surgery in the ambulatory service center. At this time, the nursing and medical staff review with the patient the clinical path for the next phase (in the hospital).

REDUCING DUPLICATION

An attempt to eliminate duplication of records occurred at every step. The inpatient pathway (Appendix 2) is kept by the patient's room. The printed pathway contains all expected occurrences in a manner that can be easily read or reviewed. The nurses take primary responsibility for the form, although all providers make notations and sign off each day. Most of the charting for the nurses and physicians is done on the pathway form and no notes are written in the clinical record, unless there is a variance from the pathway.

ANTICOAGULATION

Over the last 25 years, many different medications have been used at our institution to prevent deep venous thrombosis and pulmonary embolism. With the introduction of the initial hospital pathway in 1990, the resident staff worked with the pharmacists to develop a warfarin dosing algorithm. The decision algorithm allowed the pharmacist to adjust the dose of warfarin based on the protime. The residents provided only oversight. This program freed up the residents and markedly improved the quality of anticoagulation.

As the length of hospitalization decreased from 11 to 5 days, it became apparent that anticoagulation would need to continue after discharge. An anticoagulation service was established with overall supervision from the medicine department. The pharmacists, using a dosing algorithm, are responsible for adjusting the patient's warfarin doses. The target INR is 1.8 to 3.0. The warfarin is started the night prior to surgery and continued for 4 weeks. The pharmacist gives the patient instructions prior to discharge and coordinates all the postdischarge blood drawing (reviewing the protimes) and phone calls to the patient. This program has been a success as measured by outcome and service quality and cost.

OPERATING ROOM

At least 70% of the routine costs for total hip arthroplasty are incurred in the first 24 hours of hospitalization. Supplies used in the operating room afford an opportunity for cost saving. The use of standardized surgical packs and demand matching to guide prosthetic choice, for instance, are two programs that can be instituted to decrease cost. Custom surgical packs refer to presterilized packs containing many of the standardized items used for a specific procedure, such as drapes, suction hoses, knife blades, suture, light handles, cautery, dressings, and other items. Total joint arthroplasty lends itself to the use of custom packs. Purchasing these packs resulted in an initial annual savings of approximately $60,000 for the hospital. The surgical custom packs also increased efficiency, thereby decreasing the operating room turn-over time, and approximately 22,560 items were removed from inventory. The surgical pack system eliminated approximately 110,000 process steps from the organization, resulting in both space and personnel savings.

Prosthetic implant costs increased as a percent of total hospital charges from 11% in 1981 to 24% in 1990 (10,11). Instituting a program of demand matching can significantly lower prosthetic cost. The goal of demand matching is to match the patient with the most appropriate prosthesis. This will maintain quality to the patient while decreasing cost. Patients are classified into demand categories by several criteria. The criteria, well established in the literature, include age, weight, activity level, life expectancy, and bone quality. We use four demand categories from demand to low demand. Similarly, prostheses are classified by their capacity to accept demand. This classification is less than scientific and is primarily based on clinical results, actual and theoretical scientific advantage, and personal philosophy. Demand matching can be computerized.

To demonstrate the impact of demand matching, 51 consecutive primary total hip patients were analyzed. The total actual prosthetic cost for these patients was $207,525. Applying the above criteria via the computer demand matching program, the 51 patients fell into four groups: 12 high demand, 17 mid/high demand, 8 mid/low demand, and 14 low demand. Comparing prices of the prosthesis in use at the time showed that high-demand components average $5,535, whereas low-demand averaged $3,365, a difference of $2,170. The demand-matching prosthetic cost for the 51 patients was $175,009. This represents a per case savings of $637.53 on prosthesis costs. Demand matching also facilitates a cost-and-outcomes comparison from surgeon to surgeon. A demand-matching program can be flexible, allowing each surgeon to have both a personalized demand profile and a personalized prosthetic demand classification. This will aid in program implementation.

TABLE 3. *Categories evaluated as measures of success*

Outcomes
Harris Hip Score or knee score (measured pre-op, 6 months post-op, and yearly
SF 36 (or other measure of functional health when developed by FAHC)
Unplanned readmits within 10 days
Unplanned office visits
FIM (rehab patients only, admission, discharge, follow-up)
Complications (see follow-up questionnaire later)

Process
Variances from clinical path
Canceled surgery (not at patient request)
Pre-op warfarin and antibiotic
Patient scheduled for rehab moved on day 4
Patients moved to rehab who were not prescheduled

Cost
Length of stay
Cost per case/reimbursement/margin

Patient satisfaction
Press-Ganey and/or rehab inpatient survey
UH outpatient survey
Questionnaire re prep video (ABC, B3)
Postdischarge telephone call from service coordinator

FAHC, Fletcher Allen Health Care; pre-op, preoperatively; post-op, postoperatively; rehab, rehabilitation.

MEASURES OF SUCCESS

One of the first tasks of such a process is to define measures of success and how they would be reported. Four categories were evaluated: outcomes, process, cost, and patient satisfaction (Table 3).

Data are collected on an ongoing basis and coordinated by the quality assurance group. Data are analyzed and a written quarterly report submitted to the Total Hip Clinical Pathway Program Committee. Analysis includes trending, identification of opportunities for improvement, areas for further investigation, and areas in need of modification. A written summary is presented.

PATHWAYS: A FORM OF CLINICAL REENGINEERING

Reengineering as described by Michael Hammer (4,8,9) has dramatically affected all of corporate America. Medicine is an industry that can benefit from reengineering. The medical environment mandates change, and the development of patient care programs and clinical pathways is an obvious answer. Seven principles emerged from the recent University of California, San Francisco (UCSF) Reengineering Projects (16). They bear noting:

1. All projects must be physician initiated.
2. All projects have their aim in cost containment.
3. All reengineering projects must adhere to the 80/20 rules.
4. Each reengineering project includes the development of specific outcomes measures.
5. Reengineering teams are composed of decision makers who represent all major departments that provide care to the involved patients.
6. Reengineering projects are incremental and proceed at their own paces.
7. No meetings are held unless the clinical champions are present.

The description of the development of the total hip patient care program represents a beginning step in clinical reengineering. It can be used as a model for continuing refinement of the care processes, as the centerpiece of the patient care program, and its impact on outcomes for the patient and organization depends on the continuing disciplined and consistent use of the pathway by all disciplines. It is essential to monitor important aspects of the pathway on an ongoing basis, responding to trends identified by this process, and to see the pathway as a work in progress, with the potential for ongoing continuous improvement in the management of patients undergoing total hip arthroplasty.

REFERENCES

1. Amadio PC, Naessens J, Rice R, Ilstrup D. Quality improvement in an integrated group practice setting. *Annual meeting of the American Academy of Orthopedic Surgeons*, scientific program. Orlando, FL. Feb. 18, 1995;175.
2. American Health Consultants. Back on their feet: education readies orthopedic patients for fast discharge. *Hospital Benchmarks* 1995;2(4): 41–43.
3. Center for Case Management. *Concurrent and retrospective uses of variances from clinical pathways, first national conference.* Boston, MA, 1995;A-5.
4. Champy J. *Reengineering management: the mandate for new leadership.* New York: HarperBusiness, 1995.
5. *Clinical Path Survey*, Anderson Consulting for Decision Support Systems, December 1995.
6. Fromson AI. Rational uses of resources in total joint surgery. *Annual meeting of the American Academy of Orthopedic Surgeons*, scientific program. Feb. 24, New Orleans, LA, 1994;76.
7. Goldstein WM, Patek RM, Stine J, Szpila K. Cost analysis of total knee and total hip arthroplasty in the Medicare patient. a strategy in dealing with DRGs. *Annual meeting of the American Academy of Orthopedic Surgeons*, scientific program. Washington, DC, Feb. 20–25, 1992;308.
8. Hammer M, Champy J. *Reengineering the corporation: a manifesto for business revolution.* New York: HarperBusiness, 1993.
9. Hammer M, Stanton, S. *The reengineering revolution: a handbook.* New York: HarperBusiness, 1995.
10. Healy WL, Finn D. The hospital cost and the cost of the implant for total knee arthroplasty: a comparison between 1983 and 1991 for one hospital. *J Bone Joint Surg* 1994;76A:801–806.
11. Healy WL, Kirven FM, Iorio R, Patch DA. Implant standardization for total hip arthroplasty: an implant selection and cost reduction program. *J Arthroplasty* 1995;10:177–183.
12. Holle ML, Rick C, Sliefert MK, Stephens K. Integrating patient care delivery. *J Nursing Admin* 1995;25(7,8):32–37.
13. Laupacis A, Feeny D, Detsky AS, Tugwell AX. How attractive does a new technology have to be to warrant adoption and utilization? Tentative guidelines for using clinical and economical evaluation. *Can Med Assoc J* 1992;146:473.
14. Rorabeck CH, Bourne RB, Laupacis A, Feeny D, Wong C, Tugwell P, Leslie K, Bullas R. A double-blind study of 250 cases comparing cemented with cementless total hip arthroplasty. Cost-effectiveness and its impact on health-related quality of life. *Clin Orthop* 1994;298: 156.
15. Sommers LS, Schurman DJ, Jamison JQ, Woolson ST, Robison BL, Silverman JF. Clinical-directed hospital cost management for total hip arthroplasty patients. *Clin Orthop* 1990;258:168–175.
16. Weber DO. Aggressive physician-led clinical reengineering helps University of California-San Francisco Medical Center stay competitive. *Strateg Health Excell* 1996;9(5).
17. Weingarten S, Reidninger M, Conner L, Siebens H, Varis G, Alter A, Ellrodt G. Hip replacement and hip semiarthroplasty surgery: potential opportunities to shorten lengths of hospital stay. *Am J Med* 1994;97: 208–213.

APPENDIX 1

TOTAL HIP

CLINICAL PATHWAY
Patient Version

Your Ambulatory Services Center (ASC) appointment is on
_____ at _____

Your Surgery is scheduled for
_____ at _____

On the day of surgery, you need to arrive at ASC at _____

Your first office post-operative appointment is on
_____ at _____

BEFORE SURGERY

In order to provide you the best possible care the many people involved in your care are guided by clinical pathways. This is your copy of the pathway to **Total Hip Replacement**. Please bring it with you to your preoperative visit so that you can review it with the nurse there.

Date			
Day	**Orthopaedic Office Visit**	**Home visit by VNA Physical Therapist**	**Ambulatory Services Center Visit**
Who You See	- You will see the surgeon & the nurse or medical office assistant - You will be asked to make an appointment to see your family doctor to have a history, physical & any necessary tests	- If you do not have a home visit the information in this column will be given to you at the Ambulatory Services Center visit. - A physical therapist will meet with you and your family.	- You will meet with your health team, which includes nurses, an anesthesiologist, & your orthopaedic doctor's resident.
Information You Give	- The information you give & the results of exams & tests will be given to your health team (doctors, nurses, therapists, social workers). - The consent for surgery may be signed at this time.	- You will have a chance to identify any problems & discuss home set-up, equipment, Rehab, insurance, advance directives & whether extra help is needed at home.	- The consent form for surgery & anesthesia must be complete. - You will be asked if you have any advance directives. - You will meet with the different members of your health team to be checked & to discuss surgery. - Bring x-rays, test results & any other reports done by your family doctor.
Treatments			- You will be given & shown how to use an inspirometer, to help with breathing. Bring it with you on the day of your surgery. - You will be given betadine sponges & shown how to use them.
Tests			- You will have blood drawn & urine tested if not already done. - You may need to have other tests or see other specialists.
Medications	- You will be given a medication/allergy sheet to fill out. Bring this with you to all appointments.		- You will be given one dose of a blood thinner to take the night before surgery.
Patient Education	- You will see a video about surgery. - Your doctor will discuss test results, the need for surgery-its risks & complications, recovery & going back to work. - You will be mailed a video to watch at home on exercising and recovery. You will also get a handout explaining how to prepare for surgery & what to expect at your visit to Ambulatory Services Center. If you want, we can arrange for you to talk with a patient who has had the surgery.	- The physical therapist will discuss & answer your questions. - You will be told who to call if you have any questions or problems.	- You will learn what to expect the day of surgery & during your recovery. You will also get a handout that explains this. - You will go over what to do the night before surgery.
Discharge Planning	- You and your health team will discuss how to take care of any special needs you have. A discharge plan will be set up. - Your primary care doctor will be notified about your plans for surgery.	- You will plan with the physical therapist how to set up your home & help during recovery.	

Advance Directives

Many people have asked us the meaning of the term "Advance Directive." It means telling your medical team ahead of time what you would, or would not, want done if you were unable to speak for yourself in an emergency situation. This could happen if you were unconscious, physically unable to talk, or mentally unable to make decisions for yourself.

A Living Will is one kind of advance directive. A Living Will usually concerns what you would want to be done if there were little hope of recovery. For example, would you want artificial means to be used to support your breathing, circulation, liver, kidneys or feeding? Living Wills sometimes contain other instructions, such as organ donation information.

A Durable Power of Attorney means that you can legally choose someone else who will speak for you and make decisions for you if you are unable to do so yourself. You, yourself, can write out the specific instructions that they will follow.

You do not need to have an Advance Directive. However, if you do have one, you should tell us about it.

If you do not have an Advance Directive, but would like more information about them, including Living Wills, please ask for an information booklet about them at Ambulatory Care.

Lifeline

Lifeline is a service which can be purchased by you. There is a low, one time sign-on fee plus a monthly fee (not covered by insurance). This service can be installed in a day or two once you call 1-800-286-5463 or 1-802-654-1212.

For people living alone, Lifeline is a way to quickly and easily get help if you need it. Just press the help button that you will be given to wear. This sends a signal for help to the Lifeline Response Center. They will immediately send someone to assist you.

They also have an inactivity alarm - if you don't check in with them after a period of time, the Response Center will call for immediate help to be sent to you.

Things to Do Before Surgery

Blood Transfusions
Daily Medications
Insurance
Family Doctor Exam
Appointments

Blood Transfusions: Blood transfusions are common in total joint replacement surgery. Units of blood come from one of two sources: the Red Cross's blood bank or yourself. Patients can donate their own blood up to 35-40 days before surgery through the Autologous Blood Program. This blood can be transfused back to you as needed during or after surgery. This option is encouraged whenever medically possible. If you do this, you will need to take iron supplements before donating the first unit of blood. If you and your surgeon decide that you will use autologous blood, the office will send a prescription to the Red Cross. The Red Cross will contact you for an appointment.

Daily Medications: You should stop taking any non-steroidal anti-inflammatory medications (such as Advil, Motrin, Naprosyn, Relafen, Day-Pro, Oruval) or any medications containing aspirin three weeks before your surgery. These medications act as anti-coagulants or blood thinners. They increase the length of time it takes to stop bleeding. If you need relief, take Extra-Strength Tylenol as a substitute.

You will be taking a blood thinner starting the day before surgery & continuing for four weeks after discharge. This is done to prevent blood clots.

Insurance: We want to help prevent problems with insurance paying for this surgery. Please check with your insurance company to be sure that there are no special forms or requirements to fill out. They are becoming more common.

Family Doctor Exam: Once we know the date of your surgery, you should make an appointment to see your family doctor within 30 days of your surgery. You will give your doctor a history & physical form to fill out (it's in the colored folder). After they are filled out you should take this and any other test results and hand carry them to your pre-operative Ambulatory Service Center appointment.

Appointments: You will be mailed the date & time to visit the Ambulatory Service Center. This is usually a week before your surgery. Please plan on taking 3-4 hours. Your surgery will be done at the Medical Center campus of Fletcher Allen Health Care. On the day of surgery, please report to the Ambulatory Service Center at the time given you. This time is usually 1½ hours before the start of surgery.

Specific Instructions:

_____

_____

_____

<u>Ambulatory Service Center</u>

Pre-Operative Visit

The Ambulatory Service Center (ASC) at the Medical Center Campus of the Fletcher Allen Health Care (FAHC) provides care to patients requiring outpatient procedures as well as those requiring surgery.

- Please make sure that you bring your history and physical form with you to your appointment.

- Your pre-operative visit could last two to four hours. This is because of the number of tests and people you will need to meet.

- Several tests are done to discover any health problem that might interfere with surgery. Eat as you normally would, unless otherwise instructed by your doctor.

- The nurses in the ASC will collect information to help them take better care of you and will coordinate your visit. Occasionally, you will be given special instructions. This may be a special diet, medications, and/or bowel laxatives. These will be ordered if necessary and will be fully explained to you during this visit.

- Since this is a teaching hospital, residents (doctors in specialty training programs) will meet with you to answer questions about the surgery. They will continue to care for you and see you each day in the hospital (someone is on call 24 hours a day) and will work closely with your attending orthopaedic surgeon.

- You will also meet with an anesthesiologist who will explain the various types of anesthesia and discuss the best one for you. If you are a smoker, you should try to stop smoking for as long as possible before your surgery or to at least cut down. This will keep your lungs clearer and reduce the risk of developing a cold or pneumonia after surgery. Also, the hospital is now smoke-free.

TOTAL HIP

CLINICAL PATHWAY
Patient Version

AT HOME

Hip Replacement

Date		
Day	**At Home**	**You Can Expect at 6 weeks**
Who You See	You will meet with a physical therapist within the first forty-eight hours after discharge.	You will be seen at the Orthopedic Surgeon's Office at 6 weeks, 3 months, 6 months, and one year after surgery, and then every 2 years.
Treatments	- Staples are removed in the office or by VNA 10-14 days after surgery. - Once steri-strips begin to fall off they can be removed. - Continue to wear TEDS for six weeks after surgery. - Continue to elevate leg when sitting. - Continue to sleep or lie down with pillow between legs. - Continue to do CSMT checks daily	
Tests	- You will have x-rays taken at some of your office visits. - If you are taking blood thinners, you will have blood drawn at least once a week.	
Mobility/Activity	- Continue exercise program set up by Physical Therapy. - Limit riding in a car to necessary appointments - Do not take a shower until 24 hours after sutures/staples have been removed.	- Everyone differs. Usually, you will now be using a cane. - Precautions will be lifted by your doctor. Once lifted, would expect you would be able to bend 90° at the hip in 2-3 weeks. - Continue with exercise work-outs 2-3 times each day.
Diet	- Regular	
Medications	- Continue to take medications for pain control, if needed. - Take medications as prescribed before going to the dentist for cleaning or any work done on the teeth or gums. - Take blood thinners as directed.	- The need for medication should be greatly decreased or gone. - There may still be some incisional discomfort off and on. - Take medications as prescribed, for visits to the dentist. - Discontinue taking blood thinners, as directed.
Patient Education	- Check daily for signs or symptoms of complications. Call the office if you notice any.	- Continue to use cane if walking on uneven, slippery or unfamiliar ground.

EXERCISES

You should have 2-3 exercise work-outs every day. Do each exercise a minimum of 10 times, gradually increasing as you work with your therapist. These exercises will help you gain strength and mobility.

1. Ankle pumps: Bend your ankles up and down.

2. Quad Sets: Tighten your thigh muscle and push the back of your knee into the bed. Hold for 6 seconds.

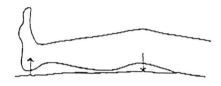

3. Gluteal Sets: Squeeze your buttocks together. Hold for 6 seconds.

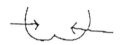

4. Hip Rotation: Keep leg straight and roll out so kneecaps point to side. Return to starting position - kneecaps point to ceiling.

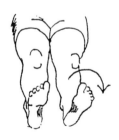

5. Hip Abduction: Keep leg straight and kneecap pointed towards ceiling, slide your leg out to side, then back to center.

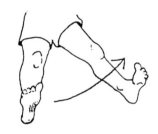

6. Hip Flexion: Slide your heel toward buttock, bending your knee. DO NOT bend more than 70°.

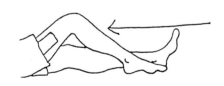

STANDING UP, holding on to a counter.

7. Knee Flexion: While standing with your hip straight, bend your knee behind you.

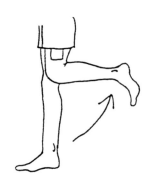

8. Hip Extension: Keep your knee straight, and lift your leg behind you without bending forward.

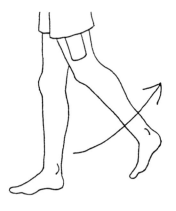

9. Hip Flexion: Lift your knee up, but NOT beyond a 70° angle.

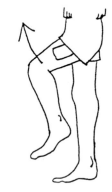

10. Hip Abduction: Keep your leg straight, toes pointed forward and lift your leg out to the side, then back to center. DO NOT cross legs.

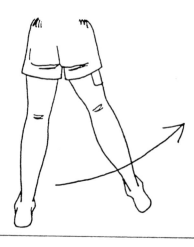

Going Home

Precautions:

1. NO hip bending beyond 70 degrees

2. NO crossing of legs

3. NO rolling kneecap in

4. Limit riding in a car for six weeks, except for necessary appointments.

5. DENTAL WORK:

    After total joint surgery, you need to take antibiotics any time you have dental work done. This is to prevent infection of your new total joint. You will be given 2 dental cards telling you what to take and when. Please, give one of the cards to your dentist, who can prescribe these antibiotics for you.

6. SITTING:

    - Choose a firm chair with arms. Avoid low or overstuffed chairs.
    - Keep your knees apart.
    - DO NOT bend forward (DO slouch so hips kept forward).
    - DO NOT sit for longer than 45 minutes at a time.
    - Use elevated toilet seat until told otherwise.

7. SLEEPING:

    - Use either your abductor pillow or 2 bed pillows between your legs.
    - DO NOT sleep on your operated side.
    - If you sleep on non-operated side, keep your pillows between your legs.

8. WALKING:

    - Continue to use your walker/crutches for balance while standing or walking.
    - Check the tips of your walker or crutches. Tighten the screws on your crutches daily.
    - Remember to remove scatter rugs.

9. STAIRS:

    - Going up, lead with non-operated leg.
    - Going down, lead with operated leg and crutches/walker.

Daily Checks

SIGNS AND SYMPTOMS OF COMPLICATIONS:

Call your doctor if you notice:

> Increase in pain or redness
> Increase in swelling
> Any drainage
> Fever
> Unexplained calf tenderness, redness, increased warmth
> Chest pain or shortness of breath.

Check the circulation of the operated leg by doing CSMT checks twice a day. CSMT stands for Color, Sensation, Motion and Temperature. Here's how to do it.

COLOR: Check the color of the toes/foot of the operated side. Is the color normal? Is it the same as your normal side? Call your doctor if it has become more pale or the color is fading compared to your normal side.

SENSATION: Check the feeling of the toes of your operated side. Are you able to move them when you want? Call your doctor if your feeling has decreased or now you cannot feel anything.

MOTION: Check the toes of your operated side. Are you able to move them when you want? Call your doctor if this movement has decreased or you are now unable to move your toes.

TEMPERATURE: Check the degree of warmth of the toes on your operated side. Is it the same as your normal side? Call your doctor if the skin of your operated side has become cooler or cold compared to your normal side.

REMEMBER: If you have ANY problems, call your doctor's office. A physician is ALWAYS on call. The best time to reach the office nurse is between 8 am and 4:30 pm, Monday through Friday.

TOTAL HIP

CLINICAL PATHWAY
Patient Version

IN HOSPITAL

Date		
Day	Day of Surgery	Day 1 After Surgery
Who You See	- Respiratory, Physical Therapy & Occupational Therapy (if needed)	- Pharmacy
Information You Give	- You will be asked if you have any advance directives.	
Treatments	BEFORE SURGERY: - You will change into a gown. - You will have an IV started. AFTER SURGERY: - You will have a venodyne & TEDs (elastic stockings) placed on your leg to help with circulation. - You will have a tube to drain urine. - You may have oxygen. - The nurse will closely watch your vital signs (blood pressure, temperature, pulse & breathing), check your circulation (CSMT), bowel sounds & incision. - You will use an inspirometer & cough every 2 hrs.	- Continue vital signs, CSMT, TEDs, venodynes, inspirometer, bowel sounds & incision check. (It is not unusual to run a temperature the first few days). - Oxygen will be discontinued as soon as you are breathing well on your own. - IV tubing will be removed.
Tests	Blood drawn	Blood Drawn
Mobility/ Activity	You will: - stay in bed & the nurse will turn you often to help circulation & breathing. - you will have a special pillow placed between your legs. This is called an abductor pillow. - you will need to do ankle pumps every hour.	You will: - have a nurse with you when you first sit up, since you may feel dizzy. - start PT: stand at the bedside with a walker & take a few steps. Start leg exercises. - use a trapeze to help you move around in bed. - sit in a hip chair 1 hr, 2 times. - learn how to get in & out of bed & hip chair. - continue with pillow.
Diet	You will be limited to ice chips & sips of clear liquids.	If no problems with clear liquids, you will start taking full liquids & later start a regular diet.
Medications	- You may be given Duramorph (a pain medication) with your spinal anesthesia during surgery. This should control pain for about 16-18 hours. - Let the nurse know if you are having pain. - Antibiotics started before surgery will be continued.	- Duramorph will start to wear off & you will be given other pain meds either IV or orally. - ASK for pain meds when you need them. - You will start taking daily medications.
Patient Education	- Your family may wait in the Surgical Waiting Room & will be told of your progress. They will be able to visit you briefly in the recovery room & for longer periods later when you move from the Recovery Room to the nursing floor.	- Your nurse & physical therapist will explain the equipment & the do's & don't for total hips. - They will also explain what they are doing & signs & symptoms they are watching for. - The pharmacist will talk with you about the blood thinner you are taking.
Discharge Planning		- The Health Team will discuss with you & your family needs for care & equipment at home.

Common Questions After Hip Surgery

How much pain will I have after surgery?
Everyone differs. You may feel some pulling and soreness around your incision for the first few days. Usually, the hip and leg pain you experienced before surgery will be much less, or gone.

What about pain medication?
Duramorph is a pain medication that is given to you during the operation. It usually keeps you free from pain for the first 24 hours, but often causes itching. Be sure to let the nurse know if you have any itching, so you can be given something to relieve it. Once the effects of the Duramorph wear off, you may have some pain. Medication has been ordered by your doctor to relieve pain, but YOU MUST ASK for it. The doctor will specify that it should be given *when needed.*

What if the medication makes me sick or dizzy?
Let your nurse or doctor know and they will find another drug for you to take as a substitute.

Should I try to get through the pain without taking pain medication?
Pain can slow down your activity. Taking pain medication will make it easier for you to move about and do your exercises. ASK for pain medication when needed.

How much swelling is normal?
Extra fluids given during surgery and trauma from the surgery itself cause swelling, which you may see for the first few days after your surgery. It most often appears in the legs, genitals, and around the incision. Some swelling--especially in the operated leg-- is common. It will tend to be greater, though, if you stand too long, let your legs hang down while sitting, or fail to keep your muscles active.

How long do I need to wear TED stockings?
Wear the stockings until you go back for your six-week follow-up visit with your doctor. You can take them off a couple of hours during the day, but you should wear them at night. They help keep swelling down and prevent blood clots from forming in your veins.

How should I care for my incision?
Have someone check it every day and watch for increased redness, draining, swelling or warmth. If the incision is dry, you do not need to keep it covered, unless your clothes irritate it.

Who will take the stitches, or staples, out?
Either your physician will remove the stitches in the office or the physical therapist will do this at your home, usually between the 10th and 14th day after surgery. Do not shower until they have been removed.

How long will I need an abductor pillow between my legs?
Usually the pillow is used for the first few days in the hospital to make sure you don't cross your legs or roll them inward. After that, you can usually switch to regular pillows.

How often should I elevate my leg?
Keep your leg elevated when sitting. Be sure to take several breaks every hour. Get up and walk or put the leg down.

What activities can I do during the first two weeks at home?
Exercises, walking and light work like preparing a simple meal are okay. But don't stand too long or get overtired. Don't try to do lifting or heavy housework, like vacuuming or yard work. Don't sit in a chair all day. Moving around will help your circulation as well as your joints.

If I do twice as many exercises each day, will I recover twice as fast?
No. You should exercise two to three times a day. If you do more, you might irritate the tissues around the joint.

How soon will I be able to use a cane?
There is not one answer for everyone. The physical therapist will help you decide when the time is right.

Why do I have to wait six weeks before riding in a car?
Most important is that you might damage your hip, in the case of an accident or even with sudden, forceful impact. (You should be aware that some insurance companies will not cover home health services if you are not really "house-bound"). It is all right to drive to medical appointments.

Will I need special equipment at home?
Yes, you will need a raised toilet seat and a walker or crutches, as well as a tub seat. If the bathroom is on the second floor, a commode would be a good idea.

Should I make any change to my home?
Yes. Remove scatter rugs and other safety hazards on the floor. Rearrange furniture, if necessary, to be sure you have enough room to move around with a walker. If both hips are done at the same time, it is better not to use the stairs, so you may need to arrange a bed downstairs. If you must use the stairs, try to go up and down only once a day.

When will I be discharged?
Discharge is usually in 5 to 7 days after surgery, or 12 to 14 days if both hips are done. Your health-care team will talk with you soon after your surgery, so that you have time to make arrangements for equipment and help you may need at home.

When are my follow-up appointments?
These are usually six weeks, three months, six months and one year after surgery.

Day 2 after Surgery	Day 3–4 after Surgery	Discharge (Days 4 or 5)
- Social Service if needed		
- Continue: vital signs, CSMT, venodynes, TEDs, inspirometer, bowel sounds & incision check. - The tube in your bladder will be taken out. - If tests show you need a blood transfusion, it will be given.	- Continue: vital signs, TEDs, inspirometer, CSMT, bowel sounds & incision checks. - Discontinue Venodynes. - Your dressing will be removed on Day 4.	On the day of discharge we expect: - pain is taken care of with oral meds - bodily functions are normal for you & lungs are clear - the wound is healing
Blood drawn & urine tested	Blood drawn	- You will know when to make an appointment to check your blood.
You will: - continue with hip pillow & trapeze - PT: do some walking in hallways & to the bathroom. You will be shown how to get on & off a raised toilet seat. - sit in a hip chair 1½ hrs, 2-3 times.	You will: - continue with pillow. - start moving in bed without trapeze. - Be shown how to go up & down stairs, in & out of car by P T before discharge. - walk longer distances with less help. - sit in hip chair for 1½ 2-3 times - Day 4 & 5 sit for 2 hrs 2-3 times	On the day of discharge you will: - understand total joint do's & don'ts - walk safely with walker or crutches. - be able to get in & out of bed & chair, on & off toilet, up & down stairs, & in & out of car with walker or crutches - be able to follow your exercise program at home
Regular diet if bowel sounds heard	Regular	Regular (you will understand a special diet if you need one)
- Ask for pain meds when you need them - You will be given laxatives if needed. - You will watch a video about blood thinners. - Continue daily medications.	- Ask for pain meds when you need them. - You will be given laxatives if needed. - A pharmacist will discuss blood thinners. - Continue daily medications.	- Your doctor will give you medication prescriptions. - You will understand your medications & how to control pain. - You understand the reason you may want to take pain meds 1hr before exercising.
- Nurses will continue answer any questions about your care & go over do's & don't for total hips. - The video on exercising & recovery can be watched on the TV hospital channel.	- PT will discuss with you & your family safety in your home. - PT will discuss your home exercise program with you. - Nurses will discuss signs & symptoms of infection, blood clots, & CSMT with you.	- You will understand the signs & symptoms of infection & blood clots & when to call the doctor. - You will know who to call if you have any questions or problems. - You will know where & when your follow-up care is to take place.
- PT & doctors will discuss your progress & where your follow-up therapy will take place.	- Your health team will discuss discharge plans to make sure needed equipment & care has been arranged in your home on Day 3. - Occupational Therapy (OT) will see you if needed on Day 3. - If you are going to Rehab you may go on Day 4. This is usually a 12-14 day program.	- All your home care needs will have been arranged with equipment in place. - You will be given instructions on: showering, care of wound, medications, equipment, activity, therapy visits, and follow-up visits with your doctor. - Your primary care doctor will be told about your stay in the hospital & discharge.

APPENDIX 2

Hospital Areas

Parking

Follow the signs around to the Emergency Department. There is a parking lot for temporary parking for your family to use until you go to surgery. Then they will need to use the main lot in the front. The entrance to the Ambulatory Service Center is next to the Emergency Room.

Family Waiting Area

The family waiting room is in the main lobby. Your family will be notified when your operation is over and you are in the recovery room. A cafeteria is located next to the lobby for their use.

Operating Room

The operating room is a bright, cool room where you will be attended by nurses, surgeons and the anesthesiologist. In the operating room, the staff wears surgical gowns, caps and masks to keep the area as sterile as possible.

Recovery Room

When your operation is complete, you will be taken to the recovery room or to one of the Intensive Care Rooms. These are bright and busy places equipped with monitors and machines used for your care.

It is normal to feel some confusion as you awaken. Often you feel cold, but warm blankets are available if you need them. The nurses will check your blood pressure often and will also check the area of surgery. Often oxygen is used until you are fully awake. If you had general anesthesia, your throat may feel dry and a little sore from the breathing tube used during the operation. The area of your surgery may hurt and burn. Ask the nurse for medication to relieve the pain.

You will be brought to your regular room as soon as you are fully over the acute recovery period. Your family will be able to visit with you once you are in your regular room.

Regular Room

Private rooms are not usually available. Friends and family can visit with you throughout the day, but it is expected that they will not stay overnight. (Pediatrics is an exception). Each room has a phone for your use and individual TV controls. For a daily fee, your TV control will be hooked up. Someone comes each day to see if you want to sign up for the TV or you can call directly.

Acute Hospital Phase
Total Hip Replacement   Clinical Pathway
Fletcher Allen Health Care

Addressograph

Expected LOS: 5 days

Category	DOS (once arrived on B3) On Target / Variance	D E N	POSTOP DAY 1 On Target / Variance	D E N	POSTOP DAY 2 On Target / Variance	D E N
Date / Day						
Consults	• Respiratory • Physical Therapy • Occupational Therapy prn		• Pharmacy		• Rehab (if needed) • Patient/Family Service if needed	
Measurements / Treatments	• Vital signs with CSMT checks as ordered • I+O q2hr • IV • Check bowel sounds • Foley • O2 – SAT prn O2 prn • Inspirometry q1hr while awake • Check breath sounds • Check dressing q2hr • TEDS/Venodynes		• Vital signs q4hr with CSMT checks • I+O qshift • IV to saline lock • ————————> • ————————> • O2 discontinued • ————————> • ————————> • Check dressing for drainage		• Vital signs bid with CSMT checks qshift • ————————> • D/C saline lock • BM (assess need for laxatives) • Discontinue foley/ I+O cath vs PVR cath • ————————> • Change dressing (by physician) • ————————>	
Tests	• Pro Time • Hemagram		• ————————> • ————————> • Lytes, BUN, Creatinine		• ————————> • ————————> • Urine Screen	
Mobility/Activity	• Bedrest with turning • Abductor pillow • THR protocol		• Physical Therapy • Hip chair 2 X 1hr with 2 assist • ————————> • ————————> • ————————> • Bed exercises with PT		• ————————> • Hip chair 2-3 X 1 1/2 hr with 1 assist • ————————> • ————————> • ————————> • BRP using RTS with 1 assist	
Diet/Nutrition	• Sips of clear liquids ————> full liquids • Ice chips		• Regular		• ————————>	
Medications	• Review current medications/ allergies • Duramorph protocol • Warfarin (Coumadin) • Toradol • Analgesics as ordered • Kefzol X 3 doses		• Tylenol #3 • Percocet • ————————> • ————————>		• ————————> • ————————> • ————————> • MOM • Senekot • Pericolace • Dulcolax • Fleets enema	
Patient/Family Education	• Family visit • Orient to unit on admission • Orient to C + DB and inspirometer • Review clinical pathway		• Review clinical pathway • THR precautions • S/S infection S/S DVT • CSMT checks • Homans signs • Pharmacist introduces Coumadin protocol		• ————————> • ————————> • ————————> • ————————> • Coumadin video (or verbal instruction by pharmacist)	
Discharge Planning	• Review data base for discharge needs & plans		• VNA		• PT notify Rehab & PT regarding transfer to Rehab PRN	
Team Variance Identification (write focus note if variance)						
Team Signatures						
Physician Evaluation	• Alert & oriented • Lungs clear • Calves non tender		• Alert & oriented • Lungs clear • Calves non tender • Dressing changed – wound benign		• Alert & oriented • Lungs clear • Calves non tender • Wound benign	
Physician Variance Identificaton (write focus note if variance)						
Physician Signatures						

5/02/94   Revised: 01/16/96 jeh HTHRCP.SAM Orthopaedic Unit 656-2430

Form# 015392 (2/96)

Acute Hospital Phase
Total Hip Replacement   Clinical Pathway
Fletcher Allen Health Care

Addressograph

	POSTOP DAY 3	D	E	N	DAY 4	D	E	N	DAY 5	D	E	N	EXPECTED OUTCOMES	D	E	N
Date	On Target				On Target				On Target				On Target			
Day	Variance				Variance				Variance				Variance			
Consults																
Measurements / Treatments	• VS BID with CSMT q8hr				• VS and CSMT checks at discharge								• Patient's VS to baseline normal			
	• Inspirometer				• ————————>								• Lungs are clear			
	• Voiding				• ————————>								• Patient has normal voiding pattern			
	• Dressing change/ open to air				Check incision line								• Incision area is healing as expected			
	• BM (follow up if no BM Day #2)				• ————————>								• Bowel function is normal			
	• TEDS												• No UTI			
	• Discontinue venodyne															
Tests	• Protime				• ————————>											
	• Hemagram															
Mobility /Activity	• Physical Therapy				• ————————>								• Patient verbalizes activity restrictions and rationale			
	• Hip chair 2-3 X 1 1/2 hr - 1 assist with family				• Hip chair 2-3 X 2hr – 1 assist with family								• Patient can demonstrate exercises			
	• Abductor pillow				• ————————>								• Safe with walker			
	• THR protocol				• ————————>								• Safe with transfer			
	• BRP with RTS with 1 assist				• BRP – 1 assist with walker using RTS											
Diet	• Regular (PTA diet)				• ————————>								• Tolerates regular diet			
Medications	• Percocet				• ————————>								• Patient verbalizes correct use of medications			
	• Tylenol #3				• ————————>								• Pain controlled with oral medications			
	• Warfarin (Coumadin)				• ————————>								• Patient understands follow-up regarding Coumadin			
	• Pericolace				• ————————>											
	• Fleets enema				• ————————>											
	• Dulcolax				• ————————>											
	• MOM				• ————————>											
	• Senekot				• ————————>											
Patient/Family Education	• THR precautions				• Drug instruction sheets reviewed								• Patient knows who to call with questions			
	• S/S infection / SS DVT				• CSMT instructions								• Patient verbalizes signs & symptoms of blood clots and infection			
	• CSMT checks				• MD instructions											
	• Pharmacy will review home Coumadin				• RN review Coumadin knowledge											
	• PT discusses safety in home, exercises & equipment															
Discharge Planning	• Final arrangements for equipment and home care				• Nursing discharge form								• Pt/family states that home care needs have been arranged			
					• VNA referral (PT if needed)								• Equipment in place			
					• Day 4: transfer to Rehab if appropriate											
Team Variance Identification (Write focus note if variance)																
Team Signatures																
Physician Evaluation	• Alert & oriented				• Alert & oriented				• Alert & oriented				• Alert & oriented			
	• Lungs clear				• Lungs clear				• Lungs clear				• Lungs clear			
	• Calves non tender				• Calves non tender				• Calves non tender				• Calves non tender			
	• Wound benign				• Wound benign				• Wound benign				• Wound benign			
Physician Variance Identification (Write focus note if variance)																
Physician Signature																

5/03/1994 Revised: 12/11/95 jeh HTHRCP2.SAM

Acute Hospital Phase
Total Knee Replacement Clinical Pathway
Fletcher Allen Health Care

Addressograph

Expected LOS: 4 - 5 days

		D	E	N			D	E	N			D	E	N
Date	On Target					On Target					On Target			
Day	DOS (once arrived on B3) Variance				POSTOP DAY 1 Variance					POSTOP DAY 2 Variance				
Consults	• Respiratory				• Pharmacy					• Rehab (if needed)				
	• Physical Therapy									• Patient/Family Service if needed				
	• Occupational Therapy prn													
Measurements / Treatments	• Vital signs with CSMT checks as ordered				• Vital signs q4hr with CSMT checks					• Vital signs bid with CSMT checks qshift				
	• I+O q2hr				• I+O qshift					• ——————>				
	• IV				• IV to saline lock					• D/C saline lock				
	• Check bowel sounds				• ——————>					• BM (assess need for laxatives)				
	• Foley				• ——————>					• Discontinue foley/ I+O cath vs PVR cath				
	• O2 – SAT prn O2 prn				• O2 discontinued									
	• Inspirometry q 1hr while awake				• ——————>					• ——————>				
	• Check breath sounds													
	• Check dressing q2hr				• Check dressing for drainage					• Change dressing (by physician)				
	• TEDS/Venodynes				• ——————>					• ——————>				
Tests	• Pro Time				• ——————>					• ——————>				
	• Hemagram				• ——————>					• ——————>				
					• Lytes, BUN, Creatinine					• Urine Screen				
Mobility/Activity					• Physical Therapy					• Walk in hall with Physical Therapy				
	• Bedrest with turning				• Chair 1 hour X 2					• Chair 2-3 X 1 1/2 hr with 1 assist				
	• TKR protocol				• ——————>					• ——————>				
					• CPM started					• ——————>				
	• Ankle pumps every hour				• Bed exercises with PT					• ——————>				
										• BRP using RTS with 1 assist				
Diet/Nutrition	• Sips of clear liquids ————> full liquids				• Regular					• ——————>				
	• Ice chips													
Medications	• Review current medications/ allergies													
	• Duramorph protocol													
					• Tylenol #3					• ——————>				
					• Percocet					• ——————>				
	• Warfarin (Coumadin)				• ——————>					• ——————>				
	• Toradol				• ——————>									
	• Analgesics as ordered									• MOM				
	• Kefzol X 3 doses									• Senekot				
										• Pericolace				
										• Dulcolax				
										• Fleets enema				
Patient/Family Education	• Family visit				• Review clinical pathway					• ——————>				
	• Orient to unit on admission				• TKR precautions					• ——————>				
	• Orient to C + DB and inspirometer				• S/S infection S/S DVT					• ——————>				
	• Review clinical pathway				• CSMT checks					• ——————>				
					• Homans signs					• Coumadin video (or verbal instruction by pharmacist)				
					• Pharmacist introduces Coumadin protocol									
Discharge Planning	• Review data base for discharge needs & plans				• VNA					• PT notify Rehab & PT regarding transfer to Rehab PRN				
Team Variance Identificaton (write focus note if variance)														
Team Signatures														
Physician Evaluation	• Alert & oriented				• Alert & oriented					• Alert & oriented				
	• Lungs clear				• Lungs clear					• Lungs clear				
	• Calves non tender				• Calves non tender					• Calves non tender				
					• Dressing changed — wound benign					• Wound benign				
Physician Variance Identificiaton (write focus note if variance)														
Physician Signatures														

5/02/94   Revised: 1/16/96 jeh HTHRCP.SAM Orthopaedic Unit 656-2430

Form# 015393 (2/96)

Acute Hospital Phase
Total Knee Replacement Clinical Pathway
Fletcher Allen Health Care

Addressograph

	POSTOP DAY 3	D	E	N	DAY 4	D	E	N	DAY 5	D	E	N	EXPECTED OUTCOMES	D	E	N
Date	On Target				On Target				On Target				On Target			
Day	Variance				Variance				Variance				Variance			
Consults																
Measurements / Treatments	• VS BID with CSMT q8hr				• VS and CSMT checks at discharge								• Patient's VS to baseline normal			
	• Inspirometer				• ------------>								• Lungs are clear			
	• Voiding				• ------------>								• Patient has normal voiding pattern			
	• Dressing change				Check incision line - remove dressing								• Incision area is healing as expected			
	• BM (follow up if no BM Day #2)				• ------------>								• Bowel function is normal			
	• TEDS												• No UTI			
	• Discontinue venodyne															
Tests	• Protime				• ------------>											
	• Hemagram															
Mobility /Activity	• Physical Therapy walk in hall				• Up and down stairs, in and out of car								• Patient verbalizes activity restrictions and rationale			
	• Chair 2-3 X 1 1/2 hr with 1 assist				• Chair 2-3 X 2hr — with 1 assist								• Patient can demonstrate exercises			
	• CPM increase knee bend				• ------------>								• Safe with walker or crutches			
	• TKR protocol				• ------------>								• Safe with transfer			
	• BRP with RTS with 1 assist				• BRP — 1 assist with walker using RTS											
Diet	• Regular (PTA diet)				• ------------>								• Tolerates regular diet			
Medications	• Percocet				• ------------>								• Patient verbalizes correct use of medications			
	• Tylenol #3				• ------------>								• Pain controlled with oral medications			
	• Warfarin (Coumadin)				• ------------>								• Patient understands follow-up regarding Coumadin			
	• Pericolace				• ------------>											
	• Fleets enema				• ------------>											
	• Dulcolax				• ------------>											
	• MOM				• ------------>											
	• Senekot				• ------------>											
Patient/Family Education	• TKR precautions				• Drug instruction sheets reviewed								• Patient knows who to call with questions			
	• S/S infection / SS DVT				• CSMT instructions								• Patient verbalizes signs & symptoms of blood clots and infection			
	• CSMT checks				• MD instructions											
	• Pharmacy will review home Coumadin				• RN review Coumadin knowledge											
	• PT discusses safety in home, exercises & equipment															
Discharge Planning	• Final arrangements for equipment and home care				• Nursing discharge form								• Pt/family states that home care needs have been arranged			
					• VNA referral (PT if needed)								• Equipment in place			
					• Day 4: transfer to Rehab if appropriate											
Team Variance Identification (Write focus note if variance)																
Team Signatures																
Physician Evaluation	• Alert & oriented				• Alert & oriented				• Alert & oriented				• Alert & oriented			
	• Lungs clear				• Lungs clear				• Lungs clear				• Lungs clear			
	• Calves non tender				• Calves non tender				• Calves non tender				• Calves non tender			
	• Wound benign				• Wound benign				• Wound benign				• Wound benign			
Physician Variance Identification (Write focus note if variance)																
Physician Signature																

5/03/1994 Revised: 1/09/96 jeh HTHRCP2.SAM
Form #718-003

The Adult Hip, edited by J. J. Callaghan,
A. G. Rosenberg, and H. E. Rubash.
Lippincott–Raven Publishers, Philadelphia © 1998.

CHAPTER 56

Primary Total Hip Arthroplasty: Indications and Contraindications

Thomas K. Fehring and Aaron G. Rosenberg

Total hip arthroplasty (THA) is one of the true triumphs of modern medical science. For centuries, people with disabling hip conditions were faced with living out their years in pain. The relentless progression of hip disease usually led to a downward spiral of limited function and ultimate immobility for most patients unfortunate enough to be afflicted.

With the advent of THA, this outlook changed dramatically. Many debilitating hip processes that in the past had required crutch ambulation or wheelchair use became treatable. With pain relief, these patients could go on to a useful existence without burdening their family or society. This procedure has allowed those patients with hip disease to continue to live independently. Few operations can claim such a benefit to both the patient and society as a whole.

Today, over 100,000 THAs are performed annually in the United States, a testament to the ability of this procedure to relieve pain and improve function. The goal of this chapter is to define the indications and contraindications for THA and to define for whom this procedure is most appropriate.

T. K. Fehring: Charlotte Orthopaedic Specialists, Charlotte, North Carolina 28207.

A. G. Rosenberg: Department of Orthopaedic Surgery, Arthritis and Orthopaedic Institute, Rush Medical College, Chicago, Illinois 60612.

INDICATIONS

To try to enunciate golden rules to guide the choice of patients for total hip arthroplasty is an impossible task. (John Charnley, 1979)

The terms *indications* and *contraindications*, while carrying the ring of specificity, actually represent the end points of a complex decision-making process that must be carried out by the medical practitioner in conjunction with the patient. Any medical decision making requires consideration of the potential risks and benefits of a particular intervention. This type of risk-to-benefit calculation is relatively uncomplicated for many diagnostic interventions, but there is clearly more at stake in most therapeutic interventions, particularly surgical ones.

Although there is a burgeoning literature devoted to the thought processes and rationale involved in medical decision making, there is no consensus on the specific methods that are most appropriately used to determine when a particular intervention is indicated (7,9,10,14,15). Surgical decision making represents a fascinating, complex subset of these processes, undertaken to determine whether or not active intervention is in the best interest of the patient. Wide variations noted in the rate of regional performance of multiple surgical techniques (including total joint replacement) demonstrate that indications are far from universally agreed upon (12,13,16). Clearly, the consequences of surgical intervention must be carefully evaluated by both the patient and the surgeon. In more complex cases, this may require the full range of the surgeon's analytical skills, as well as the ability to effectively communicate with the patient.

Indications can be defined as those situations where an individual patient will benefit from the intervention, with sufficient likelihood of success to warrant the risks involved in the intervention. Contraindications would connote the opposite; the risks involved, or the likelihood of interventions to fail to achieve the desired results, outweigh the expected benefit. Determining whether or not a given procedure is indicated or contraindicated involves the careful evaluation of the patient's complaints, pathology, and overall health status. The surgeon must also perform the complex task of weighing the multiple probabilities associated with both positive and adverse outcomes, many of which are based on less than adequate data.

Important considerations in the performance of any elective surgical procedure are the relative risks of perioperative events, which may carry significant morbidity or mortality. Total hip arthroplasty as initially practiced, and before the risk of thromboembolic disease was well understood, carried with it a mortality risk from pulmonary embolism alone of up to 3%. Although the incidence of this and other serious complications has been substantially reduced, the surgeon contemplating elective surgical intervention must compare the potential long-term benefits of pain reduction and improved function with complications that may occur.

A simple example of the tradeoffs that must be evaluated is in the setting of pharmacologic intervention for prophylaxis of deep venous thrombosis. The benefits of thrombosis and embolism reduction may be accompanied by an increased risk of serious bleeding complications (5,8). This weighing of risks and expected benefits, common in reconstructive surgical practice, keeps much of surgical decision making in the realm of heuristic rather than algorithmic problem solving.

Various models of decision making have been evaluated to determine whether they represent a reasonable approximation of the way clinicians actually make clinical decisions. Although none of these models have been found to completely represent the way in which clinicians think, a widely accepted and useful method of decision making is the theory of expected utility. Its use in decision making is called expected utility analysis. This technique requires the surgeon to list the potential benefits of any intervention and assign to each benefit both a probability for its occurrence and a numerical ranking of its expected utility or benefit. Expected utility theory posits that the decision maker reaches a decision by finding the product of each expected outcome's worth (utility) and the probability of that particular outcome's occurrence, and then summing these products. The product of the various positive utilities (otherwise known as benefits: pain relief, independence in activities of daily living, return to employment) is compared to the product of the negative utilities (risks: death, pain, nerve injury), and an expected-utility figure is

obtained. This figure then may be compared to the utility figures generated by other therapeutic choices. Rational decision making would lead the clinician to choose the therapy with the greatest overall utility. The calculations might be expressed in an equation as follows:

Expected utility =
    (benefit of utility A × probability of utility A)
    − (benefit of utility B × probability of utility B)
    − (further products of benefits and their probabilities)
        − (risk of utility A × probability of risk A)
        − (risk of utility B × probability of risk B)
        − (further products of risks and their probabilities)

This risk-to-benefit analysis is rarely accomplished for many orthopedic utilities. In business decision making, such utilities are mainly economic factors and can be compared in terms such as dollars. But medical decision making, where factors such as pain, various functional parameters, and quality-of-life issues must be taken into account, is potentially more complex, and direct conversion to a standard utility rating is much more difficult. Furthermore, most of the risks and benefit utilities are subjective, not associated with well-described or accurate probabilities; clinicians are unlikely to use statistical analytic methods to make specific decisions for individual patients. Nonetheless, an approximation of this technique may be quite useful.

Because of the lack of known probabilities, the term *subjective utilities analysis* should be employed. Such analysis, even on an informal basis, can assist the surgeon in the complex decision-making process. To make such complex decisions, the surgeon must not only accurately assess multiple patient-related factors but also his or her own skills, experiences, and resources. It may be helpful to communicate with the patient all of the potential risks and benefits involved in the specific interventions.

The number of factors to be considered when contemplating a THA is relatively large. The remainder of this chapter will review those factors that determine when hip arthroplasty surgery is or is not indicated.

One factor that should be kept in mind when evaluating a patient for hip arthroplasty is that the surgery has time-limited results. In general, the service life of arthroplasty is related to complications of fixation, wear, or material failure. Although many researchers have demonstrated relatively high component survival with a variety of fixation methods and component designs, it is difficult to imagine a young adult with a normal life span outliving a total hip implant. Thus age is an important factor in the decision to proceed with THA (1–4). Assuming no excessive co-morbidities or other hip joint pathology, the older patient is generally a better candidate for arthroplasty: the implant will most likely outlive the patient. The younger individual, on the other hand, may well require multiple surgeries over his or her lifetime, with deteriorating function.

Other factors that influence the success of the THA include weight and expected activity levels. The 18-year-old patient with severe multiarticular inflammatory arthritis and a persistent adduction contracture interfering with hygiene and impeding any attempts at ambulation would be expected to stress a THA significantly less than a 30-year-old former professional football player who is over 6 feet tall, weighs 270 pounds, and suffers from isolated posttraumatic arthritis of the hip.

The pediatric or young adult patient clearly deserves an attempt at alternative treatments, such as arthrodesis or osteotomy. It is important that such treatment alternatives relieve symptoms for an adequate length of time to justify major intervention. It is also important that such intervention does not make subsequent treatment exceedingly complex.

Conservative treatment should be attempted prior to proceeding with THA. This may include the use of assistive devices for ambulation, weight loss, systemic or local medications, physiotherapy, and activity modification. A concerted effort at nonsurgical therapy may be more reasonable in the younger patient than in the elderly, where prolonged attempts are time consuming and rarely as effective in relieving symptoms and improving function as THA. Based on the studies relating age and hip arthroplasty, these modalities should be attempted more aggressively in the younger patient than in the elderly. In some settings, the symptoms, physical findings, and radiographic changes are severe enough to warrant consideration of THA even if the patient has had no prior conservative treatment. However, in most cases, particularly in younger patients, it may be wiser to demonstrate to the patient that conservative or nonsurgical treatment will not relieve symptoms or improve function, prior to recommending more aggressive treatment with more substantial potential risks and complications.

Symptom severity is another important factor to consider in determining whether arthroplasty is indicated. Pain is the most common complaint prior to surgical intervention, and it is often activity related. In the patient whose symptoms are clearly amenable to activity modification, and in whom THA is not an ideal operation because of age, co-morbidities, or other factors, the surgeon should opt for conservative treatment. An obvious example would be a young athletic man whose hip pain limits only his athletic activity. THA would not be expected to hold up to the rigors of athletic competition, so such activity would be contraindicated after THA. If the individual has little or no symptoms with activity modification, then this is a more reasonable course than proceeding with THA. The potential serious long-term consequences of THA outweighs the relatively small benefit obtained, as the patient must abandon competitive athletic competition in either case.

Thus, behavior modification plays a role in the treatment of hip disease. In attempting to understand a patient's pain pattern, the clinician must decide whether a patient has realistically modified activity to accommodate the damaged joint. If the patient is unwilling to make lifestyle changes to accommodate the degenerative joint, then he or she will probably not make lifestyle changes to extend the life of a prosthetic joint. The patient unwilling to give up sports or other joint-stressful avocations that cause substantial discomfort, is probably not having enough pain to warrant intervention. On the other hand, it seems unreasonable to ask patients to modify their lifestyle to the point of extreme inactivity.

Limitation in functional ability is another important factor in determining the appropriateness of THA. Understanding the patient's requirements for the activities of daily living is essential. The ability to perform a job, to do household tasks, and to maintain personal hygiene is a measure of the effect of hip function on lifestyle. Walking tolerance (the length of time or distance one can walk without rest) can be an important benchmark. In general, if a patient cannot perform activities of daily living despite conservative treatment, hip function has decreased to the point where intervention may be indicated.

THE GOALS OF THA

The goals of THA are to relieve pain and improve function. If these goals are kept in the forefront of a clinician's mind, the task of deciding who would benefit from this procedure is not difficult. However, as Charnley intimated, there are no golden rules. The primary indication for THA is disabling pain. Hip pain is usually characterized by groin or anterior thigh pain. It generally worsens with activity and is relieved by rest. This pain rarely extends below the knee. Buttock pain is occasionally seen and must be distinguished from radicular or referred low back pain.

Patients have variable pain tolerances. An understanding of this concept is important in deciding the appropriateness of THA. It is not the clinician's role to argue with the patient's perception of his or her pain pattern. It is the clinician's role, however, to determine if pain is sufficient to warrant intervention in each case.

Occasionally, one may encounter a patient who has severe limitation of function, yet has little or no pain referable to the hip joint. For example, an ankylosed or arthrodesed hip may be relatively asymptomatic but responsible for substantial back or ipsilateral knee problems. Although the patient has no complaints referable to the hip joint, conversion of the ankylosed joint would be expected to ameliorate the contiguous joint problems. Good data support the contention that fusion take-down results in a greater need for assistive devices for ambulation than existed prior to take-down (11). Thus, attempts to ameliorate symptoms in contiguous joints may result in an increase in symptoms at the operated joint. Excellent communication between surgeon and patient is necessary before establishing the need for surgery.

Sometimes, overall function is so limited that hip symptoms are minimized as a result, or the disease process continues to limit function but is no longer associated with severe or even mild pain. Examples are end-stage juvenile rheumatoid arthritis and longstanding hip dysplasia. Any intervention in these situations must be carefully considered. Understanding the patient's activity requirements, functional limitations, and expectations of life after surgery are mandatory. Only modest gains in function may be achieved secondary to longstanding hip contractures, so the clinician and patient must decide whether the gains anticipated from prosthetic replacement outweigh the risks associated with surgical intervention.

Radiographs are extremely helpful in deciding for whom THA is appropriate. However, the mere existence of moderate to severe degenerative changes radiographically is not an indication for surgery. John Charnley stated, "The x-ray does not influence the surgeon's decision whether or not to operate." It is important to remember the goals of THA—to decrease pain and increase function. Radiographs are but one component of the decision-making equation. Patients may function very well with severe radiographic changes. Likewise, patients with only moderate changes can be significantly disabled. Therefore the decision to operate must be a clinical one, not a radiographic one, even if it is felt that the radiographic picture is sure to deteriorate. However, one must be wary of the patient with only mild radiographic changes, reasonable range of motion, and non-characteristic hip pain. Chances of relieving this type of pain are remote. The patient who complains of severe pain but has only moderate radiographic changes is most difficult to deal with. Only through repeated interview and examination can the clinician understand this patient's pain pattern. The clinician must develop an understanding of what it is like to walk in this patient's shoes. He must understand this patient's lifestyle to determine if the patient is putting unrealistic demands on that particular joint. Such demands may prevent the usual conservative measures from providing tolerable relief. Occasionally, the response to an intra-articular injection of local anesthetic may help in the decision-making process.

In those patients with severe pain and severe x-ray changes, this conflict does not exist. And in patients with severe pain and normal radiographs, further evaluative studies of the hip may be indicated and the search for a diagnosis focused elsewhere.

Failure of conservative measures, on the other hand, is a prime indicator for surgical intervention. There are usually three modes of conservative treatment—cane or crutch ambulation, nonsteroidal anti-inflammatory drugs (NSAIDs), and behavior modification. These can be used alone or in combination to prolong the life of a patient's natural hip. Behavior modification to avoid impact-loading exercise may be all that is necessary to treat a patient successfully.

Cane ambulation can significantly off-load stress from a degenerative hip. However, in some societies, patients are reluctant to try this as it appears to be an admission of general infirmity.

Nonsteroidal anti-inflammatory drugs are widely used to treat arthritis of the hip. Experimenting with different forms of these agents until an effective one is found is common management. Once an adequate agent is found, liver, renal, and hematopoietic functions must be monitored routinely to ensure no adverse effect occurs. Prolonged use of various NSAIDs in an elderly person with severe disease must be weighed against the possible side effects. Recent guidelines on the conservative treatment of osteoarthritis of the hip have been published by the American College of Rheumatology (6).

Even in patients with severe disease on initial presentation, a trial of conservative treatment has merit. This allows the patient and surgeon a chance to become familiar with each other. It also gives the clinician the chance to understand the patient's lifestyle, pain tolerance, and expectations regarding intervention. It is extremely rare to recommend arthroplasty to a patient on the first encounter.

CONTRAINDICATIONS

There are few absolute contraindications to THA. Most clinicians would agree that active infection, local or systemic, is a contraindication.

Relative contraindications include morbid obesity, neurologic dysfunction, and remote infection. Although these conditions may result in a higher failure rate, substantial reduction in pain and improvement in function may overshadow the potential risks.

The presence of substantial co-morbidities may preclude the use of surgical intervention in all but the most incapacitated of patients. The risks of perioperative mortality after surgical intervention must be carefully weighed against the functional improvement and pain relief that can be expected.

There may be anatomic abnormalities of soft tissue or bone that would place the patient at increased risk from the surgical procedure. For example, an elderly patient with an ancient femoral neck fracture with substantial shortening and rotational deformity, and with concomitant severely atherosclerotic femoral vessels, may be at substantially increased risk, after lengthening and rotational release, of femoral artery thrombosis.

PATIENT SELECTION

> When total hip becomes a true science, there ought to be no need for a chapter on how to select patients, because then all hip disorders will be treated by total hip replacements. (John Charnley)

The science of THA probably has progressed to this point in patients over 60 years old, in whom activity level has usually diminished and expectations tend to be reasonable. There have been outstanding results in this group. The revision rate in this population is acceptable, and, for the vast majority, the initial surgery will be the only one.

In the 40- to 60-year-old age group however, activity levels remain high and patients' expectations regarding longevity of their implant often exceed the life of the implant. For most disorders, THA may be the most appropriate surgical intervention in this age group, but the timing of this intervention must be made carefully. Many of these patients have heard about the clinical success of their older friends and acquaintances. They frequently demand similar intervention without understanding that in their age group, early surgical intervention may lead to subsequent revision.

> The surgeon should turn a deaf ear to the exaggerated adjectives used to describe pain....Physical signs must take precedence over subjective sensation in this age group.... X-ray findings are of great importance in this group. (John Charnley)

In those patients less than 40 years old, the stakes regarding surgical intervention go up dramatically. Life expectancy now stretches into the seventh and eighth decades, but a prosthetic hip placed in one of these patients cannot, in most cases, be expected to last 40 years. Even in the best of circumstances, these patients can count on at least one revision during their lifetime.

Therefore, in this age group, the science of hip arthroplasty probably has not progressed to the point where prosthetic replacement should be offered to all patients. Behavior modifications and other conservative modalities must be maximized. Unfortunately, the success of THA has colored the patient's perception of nonprosthetic options in treating hip disease. Although hip fusion may be the most appropriate treatment, this option is frequently not accepted by the patient. If an appropriate osteotomy can extend the life of the natural hip, it should be given serious consideration. The surgeon who is contemplating THA in the younger patient should be familiar with the indications for alternative hip salvage procedures, so that THA is not the only option. Although it is not necessary for all surgeons who treat arthritis of the hip to be familiar with the operative techniques involved in hip salvage, they should be able to suggest to those younger patients alternative treatments that will reduce pain and improve functional capability and still allow for THA at a later date.

It is important to discuss candidly with young patients the possibility of multiple revisions during their lifetime. They must understand that, even though they have pain relief, they may need to decrease their activity level after the THA in order to extend the life of their implant. The possibility of an eventual resection arthroplasty should be mentioned along with other age-related complications.

Finally, Charnley's "pseudarthrosis test" can be used to determining the wisdom of proceeding with arthroplasty in a young patient: if a patient with severe hip disease would be no worse off with a pseudarthrosis of the hip than they are currently, then prosthetic intervention is probably indicated.

TIMING OF SURGICAL INTERVENTION

The timing of surgical intervention is a critical part of the decision making in THA. The patient who has exhausted all conservative measures (and who meets appropriate radiographic and clinical criteria to warrant intervention) must decide whether the symptoms are severe enough to proceed with arthroplasty.

It must be stressed that this is most often a *patient decision*, not a radiographic decision. The clinician's job is to educate the patient about the disease, not to make the decision to intervene. The decision to have a hip replaced should be made by an informed patient. Even when the alternatives are limited, patients often want the clinician to make the decision for them. To do so is not wise.

To help a patient with this decision, two questions can be asked: Is your hip keeping you from performing *reasonable* activities of daily living? Does it keep you from doing the things that are important to you? If the answers are Yes, and the patient is medically stable and meets objective criteria, then hip replacement is probably in their best interest.

PATIENT EXPECTATIONS

A patient occasionally enters into this process with unrealistic expectations, which must be tempered by the experience of the surgeon, who must have communications skills and an understanding of the patient's psychological make-up.

The patient must understand that hip arthroplasty is not a panacea for multiple physical problems: it affects but one joint. An improved gait pattern may help an aching back to some degree, but it may have little effect on other musculoskeletal disorders. In fact, occasionally with hip pain no longer limiting function, some patients find other joints painful as their activity level now exceeds their preoperative function.

The patient must also understand the functional limitations that may still exist after hip arthroplasty. After years of contracture, normal range of motion may not be restored. Positions may have to be avoided to prevent instability. These concepts should be discussed preoperatively with the patient.

Finally, it is important to explain that the patient must assume responsibility for the prosthetic hip. This implant is a walking device designed to relieve pain, not a device for impact-loading sports or heavy manual labor. If the hip is abused, the consequences include diminished longevity of the hip and the need for subsequent revision surgery.

CONCLUSIONS

Surgical decision making varies from simple to complex. It is the job of the surgeon to assess all the patient-related factors involved in the surgical decision and to communicate the information to the patient, keeping in mind the patient's psychological make-up and intellectual capacity. This may be time consuming and difficult. When the surgeon does not have good data on outcomes and risks for specific conditions or anatomic variations, it may be difficult to assess the real benefits and risks of surgery. Nonetheless, time spent in this exercise will reward the surgeon with patients who fully understand the goals of surgery and are better able to cooperate with their own recovery. This results in a happier patient population and a more satisfying surgical practice—perhaps the ultimate goals of the hip arthroplasty surgeon.

REFERENCES

1. Charnley J. *Low friction arthroplasty of the hip: theory and practice.* New York: Springer-Verlag, 1979.
2. Collis DK. Cemented total hip replacement in patients that are less than fifty years old. *J Bone Joint Surg* 1984;66A:353–359.
3. Dorr LD, Luckett M, Conaty JP. Total hip arthroplasties in patients younger than 45 years: a nine to ten year follow-up study. *Clin Orthop* 1990;260:215–221.
4. Halley DK, Wroblewski BM. Long term results of low friction arthroplasty in patients 30 years of age or younger. *Clin Orthop* 1986;211: 43–50.
5. Harris WH, Salzman EW, Athanasoulis CA, et al. Aspirin prophylaxis of venous thromboembolism following total hip replacement: warfarin vs. dextran 40. *JAMA* 1972;220:1319–1322.
6. Hochberg MC, Altman RD, Brandt KD, Clark BM, Sieppe PA, Griffin MR, Moskowitz RW, Schnitzer TJ. Guidelines for the medical management of osteoarthritis. Part 1. Osteoarthritis of the hip. *Arthritis Rheum* 1995;38(11):1535–1540.
7. Kassirer JP, Kopelman RI. *Learning clinical reasoning.* Baltimore: Williams & Wilkins, 1991.
8. Paiment GD, Beisaw NE, Harris WH, et al. Advances in prevention of venous thromboembolic disease after elective hip surgery. *Instruct Course Lect* 1990;39:413–421.
9. Riegelman RK. *Minimizing medical mistakes—the art of medical decision making.* Boston: Little, Brown, 1991.
10. Riegelman RK. *The measures of medicine—benefits, harms, and costs.* Cambridge: Blackwell Science, 1995.
11. Reikera O, Bjerkreim I, Gunderson R. Total hip arthroplasty for arthrodesed Hips—5–13 year results. *J Arthroplasty* 10:529–531.
12. Rutkow I, Gittelsohn A, Zuidema G. Surgical decision making: the reliability of clinical judgment. *Ann Surg* 1979;190:409–415.
13. Rutkow I. Surgical decision making: the reproducibility of clinical judgment. *Ann Surg* 1982;117:337–342.
14. Schwartz S, Griffin T. Medical thinking—the psychology of medical judgment and decision making. New York: Springer-Verlag, 1986.
15. Sox HC, Blatt MA, Higgins MC, Marton KI. Medical decision making. Boston: Butterworth-Heinemann, 1988.
16. Wennberg J. Dealing with medical practice variation: a proposal for action. *Health Affairs* 1984;3:6–9.

The Adult Hip, edited by J. J. Callaghan,
A. G. Rosenberg, and H. E. Rubash.
Lippincott–Raven Publishers, Philadelphia © 1998.

CHAPTER 57

Classification of Acetabular and Femoral Deficiencies

Tim K. Conlan, Jason E. Guevara, George W. Zimmerman, and Harry E. Rubash

As both primary and revision total hip arthroplasty operations have become more common, so have the bone deficiencies encountered in revision surgery. The presence of host bone affects the success in achieving the primary goal in revision arthroplasty, which is a stable implant with anatomic restoration. If the bone is substantially deficient, anatomic restoration may have to be sacrificed to obtain a stable implant. If the implant cannot be stabilized, either a custom implant or a structural allograft must be used.

Various classification systems have been proposed for assessing bone stock when femoral and acetabular deficiencies exist prior to revision surgery. The purpose of a good classification system is to help the surgeon choose an appropriate method of treatment with a reasonably expected outcome. It also provides a uniform nomenclature and allows comparisons of data among different studies. The hallmark of a useful orthopedic classification is easy-to-remember terms that are practical as a guideline for treatment options.

ACETABULAR DEFICIENCIES IN TOTAL HIP ARTHROPLASTY

Revision surgery of the acetabular component in total hip implants is not consistently successful. Cemented acetabular revision procedures using improved cementing techniques have had suboptimal results, with a high rate of component loosening and migration (4). Alternative methods of reconstruction, including the use of a bipolar component with morselized bone allograft as well as a threaded screw ring acetabular component, have been abandoned because of unsatisfactory results. Porous-coated cementless acetabular components have produced good intermediate-term results when used in revisions (26,30,32,41,42). They are the most commonly used components in both primary and revision reconstructions.

Bone deficiency in the acetabulum can be encountered in primary and revision acetabular reconstruction. Primary deficiencies result from either an abnormality of growth or a condition that alters the shape of the acetabulum. Both types of deficiencies can be divided into those contained within the acetabulum and those that affect its peripheral rim. Contained deficiencies are associated with inflammatory disorders, metabolic disorders, tumors, infection, trauma, osteoarthritis, previous surgery, and iatrogenic causes (3). Bone deficiencies

T. K. Conlan, J. E. Guevara, G. W. Zimmerman, H. E. Rubash: Division of Adult Reconstructive Surgery, Department of Orthopaedic Surgery, University of Pittsburgh Medical Center, Pittsburgh, Pennsylvania 15213-3221.

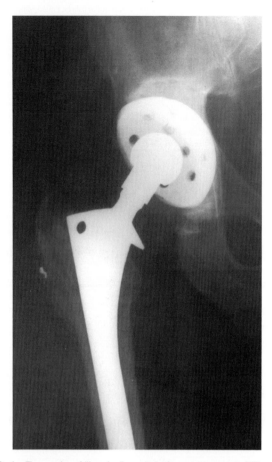

FIG. 1. Example of "jumbo" acetabular component. Fifty-one-year-old male with acetabular reconstruction using a 76 mm cup secondary to significant bone loss status post THA with a cemented acetabular cup.

maximized using peripheral fixation while the patient's own structures can be used as a basis for cementless reconstruction. Such a large component lowers the center of hip rotation to a more anatomic location. Care must be taken to avoid lateralization. The success of this technique has been largely attributed to integrity of the posterior column (32,41).

A high hip center can be achieved by placing a small cementless component into the remaining bone stock of the superior iliac wing. Proximal displacement without lateralization of the acetabulum is recommended (25,39,43). Superolateral relocation of the hip center causes a significant increase in hip joint force and redirects the total joint force medially along the femoral neck. Superior relocation, on the other hand, does not change the joint force (12). In addition, significantly higher rates of femoral loosening have occurred with superolateral positioning of cemented acetabular components compared with near-anatomic positioning. A high hip center is associated with a significantly higher rate of aseptic loosening of the femoral component than of the acetabular component (24). Schutzer and Harris found no acetabular loosening or need for revision associated with a high hip center using a cementless acetabular component (40).

encountered during revision arthroplasty continue to be the most common and are seen with multiple revisions, aseptic loosening and component migration, infection, osteolysis, and iatrogenic causes.

The goals of acetabular reconstruction as put forth by the American Academy of Orthopaedic Surgeons (AAOS) Committee on the Hip are to restore the hip to its center of rotation, obtain implant stability, restore acetabular integrity, and restore continuity of the acetabulum (10). In most cases, these goals can be accomplished using cementless technique and a porous-coated hemispherical component fixed with screws (16,26,32,41,42). If severe bone deficiency or the inability to restore the center of hip rotation preclude stability of the acetabular component, several other reconstruction methods are available. These options include the use of an oversized ("jumbo") acetabular component (Fig. 1); a high hip center (Fig. 2); a metal reinforcement ring support with bone graft (Fig. 3); a bi-lobed, oblong, double component; or a structural allograft with a standard or revision component.

With the jumbo acetabular component (greater than 70-mm outer diameter), support of the component can be

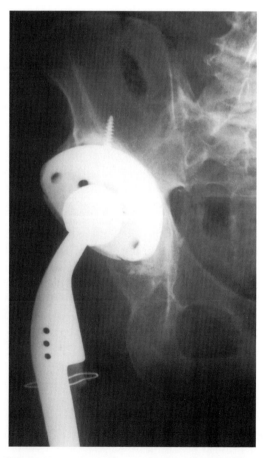

FIG. 2. High hip center acetabular reconstruction.

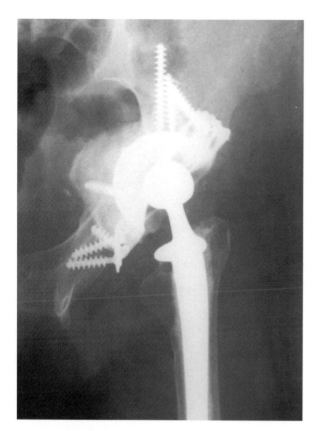

FIG. 3. Acetabular reconstruction using metal reinforcement and bone graft. This 72-year-old woman had acetabular reconstruction using a metal cage and bone graft secondary to pelvic discontinuity.

The use of metal reinforcing rings in conjunction with bone grafting has been recommended only for elderly patients with limited expectations and poor host bone quality, for whom more extensive reconstruction procedures are not thought to be reasonable options (38). This technique has resulted in higher rates of migration among patients with good host bone, and the type of deficiency reconstructed is an important factor in the success of the implant (44). Berry and Mueller reported a high failure rate for the reconstruction of major defects with metal reinforcement rings (12% with a mean follow-up of 5 years) (2). These devices currently are used where cementless porous-coated sockets will have little host bone contact and thus a high likelihood of failure. The rings may be used in the reconstruction of massive bone loss associated with acetabular discontinuity, but follow-up reports for this application are limited.

The use of the bi-lobed, oblong, coated acetabular component is a new cementless technique that appears promising but has only short-term follow-up data. This method restores the normal hip center of rotation, avoids late graft collapse, and may facilitate bone ingrowth. It does not restore bone stock and is technically more difficult to perform than a hemispherical socket. According to

Berry, the Mayo Clinic experience with 15 components followed for 6 to 39 months produced no radiographic loosening or need for revision of the acetabulum (personal communication, 1996).

The use of structural allograft to reconstruct acetabular bone stock has become controversial. Although early reports demonstrated excellent results, the long-term performance for cemented acetabular bulk allograft has been poor (22,31). Mulroy and Harris reported a failure rate of 47% at 11 years (31). Gross and associates reported good long-term results for the use of large bulk allograft to treat major defects (19).

A variety of components and techniques have been used to treat many of the acetabular deficiencies encountered in revision surgery, making long-term follow-up and comparison of these results difficult. There have been numerous reports of acetabular reconstruction using a variety of terms to describe the bone deficiency. Some of the terms used include *protrusio, intra-acetabular, minor column,* and *global deficiencies.*

A clear understanding of the surgical anatomy and radiographic presentation of the acetabulum is necessary to understand acetabular reconstruction. The bone supporting the acetabulum needs to be addressed to ensure adequate support of the component when a deficiency is encountered. The acetabulum is a hemisphere contained within the posterior and anterior columns. The acetabulum is better described as being contained within the open arms of an inverted Y formed by the posterior column (the ilioischial component) and an anterior column that extends from the anterior iliac crest to the symphysis (27). Both columns unite above the midpoint of the anterior column. This junction constitutes the roof of the acetabulum. These structures are referred to in all classification systems describing reconstruction of the acetabulum with bone deficiencies.

Radiographically, the posterior column is best visualized using the iliac oblique pelvic view. The anterior column is best visualized using the obturator oblique pelvic view. The anterior wall is best seen on the iliac oblique view. The medial wall of the acetabulum is formed by the quadrilateral plate medially and the cotyloid fossa laterally. The acetabular teardrop comprises this inferomedial portion of the acetabulum in anteroposterior (AP) pelvic roentgenograms and defines the interior (medial lip) and the exterior (lateral lip) of the acetabular wall. This well-defined shadow is a more suitable landmark than Kohler's line (the ilioischial line), which varies with the obliquity of the AP roentgenogram (Fig. 4) (18).

AAOS Committee on the Hip

The AAOS Committee on the Hip published a classification for acetabular bone deficiency in June 1989 (10). The goals of this committee were to provide a simple, standard nomenclature for accurately describing the bone

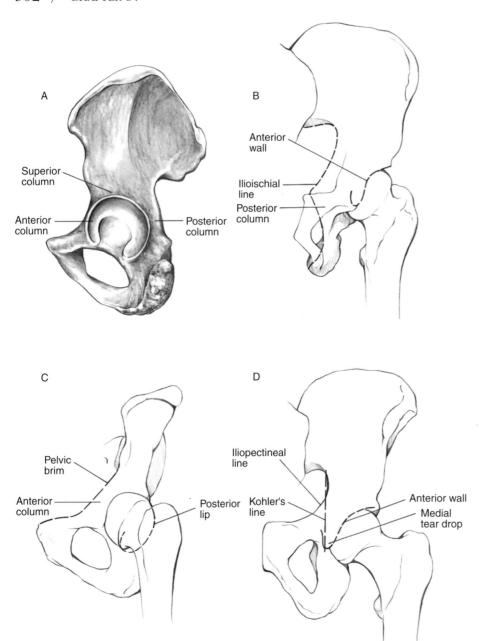

FIG. 4. A: Lateral view of hemipelvis and acetabulum. The anterior column extends from the iliac crest to the symphysis pubis. The posterior column begins at the sciatic notch and extends posteriorly and inferiorly to the pubic ramus. The superior dome is the weight-bearing roof of the acetabulum. **B:** Iliac oblique view of the pelvis and acetabulum. This is the best view to visualize the posterior column outlined by the ilioischial line. The anterior lip of the acetabulum is also well seen. **C:** Obturator oblique view of the pelvis and acetabulum. This is the best view to visualize the anterior column denoted by the pelvic brim and the iliopectineal line. The posterior acetabular lip can also be identified best on this view. **D:** Anterior view of the pelvis. The cotyloid fossa and the quadrilateral plate of the acetabulum correspond to the medial tear drop. The integrity of the ilioischial line (Kohler's line) is used to determine the severity of acetabular medialization.

deficiency in both primary and revision reconstruction of the acetabulum. The classification was intended to be generic in terms of the treatment modality used (Table 1).

This system divides bone deficiencies into two categories: those located in the cavitary area of the hemisphere, leaving the rim of the acetabulum intact, and those that erode the rim. In this classification, the rim includes the medial wall.

A loss of the supporting bone rim around the acetabulum is called a segmental defect (type I) (Fig. 5). Segmental defects are not contained defects. They can be located superiorly, anteriorly, posteriorly, or centrally (a medial defect). A medial segmental defect is present if there is a violation of the medial wall.

TABLE 1. *American Academy of Orthopaedic Surgeons acetabular deficiency classification*

Type I	Segmental deficiencies
	Peripheral
	Superior, anterior, posterior
	Central (medial wall absent)
Type II	Cavitary deficiencies
	Peripheral
	Superior, anterior, posterior
	Central (medial wall intact)
Type III	Combined deficiencies
Type IV	Pelvic discontinuity
Type V	Arthrodesis

With permission, from D'Antonio JA, Capello WN, Borden LS, et al. Classification and management of acetabular abnormalities in total hip arthroplasty. *Clin Orthop* 1989;243:127.

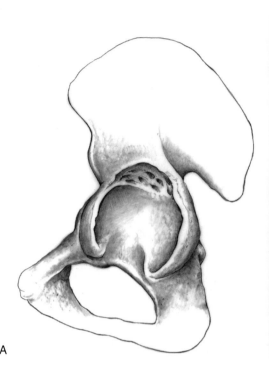

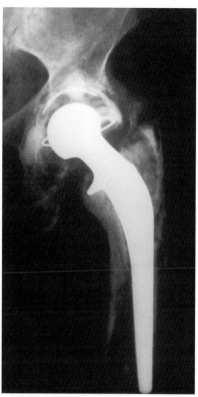

FIG. 5. A: Type I acetabular segmental defect. (With permission, from D'Antonio JA, Capello WN, Borden LS, et al. Classification and management of acetabular abnormalities in total hip arthroplasty. *Clin Orthop* 1989;243:127.) **B:** This 68-year-old man had a segmental type I defect to the superior peripheral acetabular rim after total hip arthroplasty.

A loss of volume in the sphere of the acetabulum with an intact rim is called a cavitary defect (type II) (Fig. 6). These are contained bone defects with a supportive intact rim consistently present. Cavitary defects can be located superiorly, anteriorly, posteriorly, or medially. A medial cavitary deficiency previously was called a protrusio defect, in which, in a revision setting, osteolysis causes the medial wall to expand into the pelvis. The particulate debris generated by wear particles may cause large cavitary lesions, and their location can vary depending on the type of acetabular component used.

Many deficiencies encountered in revision surgery are a combination of these two types and are classified separately (type III) (Fig. 7). It is not uncommon to see a failed cemented acetabulum that has migrated superiorly as well as medially, but periprosthetic bone deficiencies can be located in any quadrant of the acetabulum.

The remainder of the AAOS classification system consists of pelvic discontinuity and arthrodesis of the hip. Pelvic discontinuity (type IV) (Fig. 8), is defined as a defect across the anterior and posterior columns with total separation of the superior from the inferior portion of the acetabulum. Hip arthrodesis (type V) (Fig. 9) is not a bone deficiency, but it is included in the classification because the hemisphere is entirely consolidated.

The AAOS classification system is very inclusive but generalizes the type of acetabular deficiency. It can be used in both primary and revision reconstruction, it has the highest consensus among adult reconstructive sur-

geons, and it is becoming more prevalent in the literature. It does not help with selection of prosthesis type or reconstruction technique for a particular defect. Many published reports use this classification but are not specific in noting locations of the defects and do not correlate the system with the treatment used.

Other classification systems have been described in the literature. All of them encompass peripheral uncontained defects around the acetabular rim and contained cavitary defects with an intact acetabular rim.

Chandler and Penenberg

Chandler and Penenberg eloquently described their system, which is based on the review of 76 acetabular grafts performed for acetabular revisions (5) (Table 2). They divided the acetabulum into three anatomic zones: the rim, the medial wall, and the intra-acetabular area, which lies between the rim and the medial wall. They found four types of deficiencies, alone and in various combinations.

This classification is similar to that of the AAOS in that rim defects are equivalent to segmental defects (type I, AAOS), and intra-acetabular defects are equivalent to cavitary defects (type II, AAOS). Rim defects were the most common deficiency in Chandler and Penenberg's series. Most of the isolated cases were associated with congenital hip dysplasia, whereas the combination defects involving the rim occurred after previous recon-

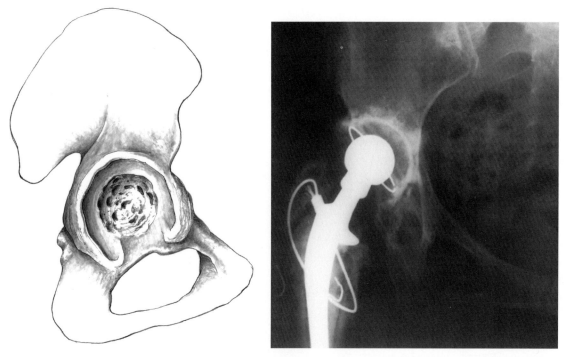

FIG. 6. A: Type II acetabular cavitary defect. (With permission, from D'Antonio JA, Capello WN, Borden LS, et al. Classification and management of acetabular abnormalities in total hip arthroplasty. *Clin Orthop* 1989;243:127.) **B:** This 62-year-old woman had superior and medial migration of the cemented acetabular component creating type II cavitary defects with maintained intact rim support.

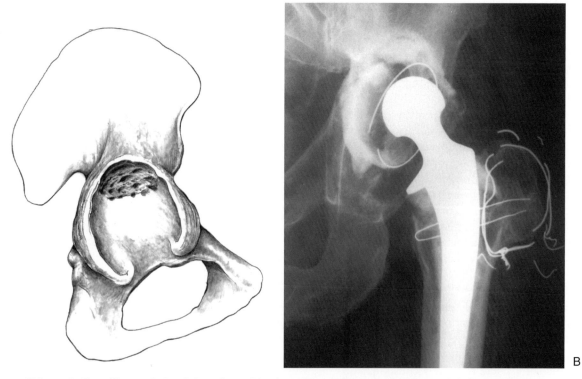

FIG. 7. A: Type III acetabular defect. A combination of the cavitary and segmental defects. (With permission, from D'Antonio JA, Capello WN, Borden LS, et al. Classification and management of acetabular abnormalities in total hip arthroplasty. *Clin Orthop* 1989;243:127.) **B:** This 51-year-old man had both cavitary and segmental acetabular defects. Type III defect with significant circumferential bone loss and component loosening.

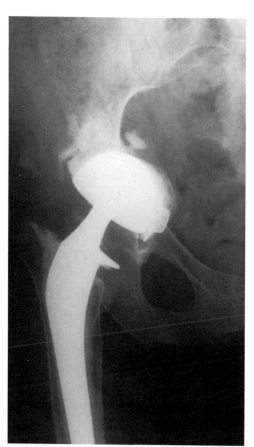

FIG. 8. Type IV acetabular defect. Pelvic discontinuity where the anterior and the posterior columns are disrupted creating an unstable condition in this 72-year-old woman.

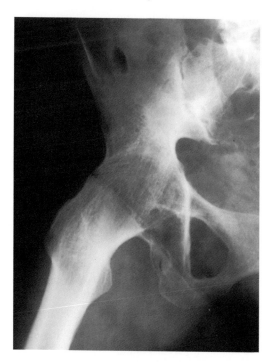

FIG. 9. Type V acetabular defect. Acetabulofemoral arthrodesis with complete consolidation and filling of the acetabular cavity with an abundance of bone.

structive failures. This system includes two separate categories of medial-wall defects: those with a segmental defect (perforation) and those with a cavitary defect (protrusio). In addition, the combination defect (type III, AAOS) is subdivided, although the authors had found few cases in each subdivision. A reconstructive method has been developed for each type of defect, but no generalized treatment method recommended. This system's specificity may be a drawback although it more clearly defines the involved bone deficiency. Chandler and Penenberg's book on reconstruction of the acetabulum and the femur is an excellent reference for specific examples and treatment methods (5).

Gross and Associates

The simple classification devised by Gross and associates (19) was based on the type of bone grafting used to reconstitute acetabular bone stock (Table 3).

The type of allograft used was based on whether the defect was contained or uncontained. Over half of the large defects reviewed were the protrusio type. Gross et al. classified large pelvic defects as either a contained cavitary defect (protrusio), or as a structural rim defect, the latter being subdivided as minor or major column involvement. A minor column defect, referred to as a shelf defect, was described as a loss of part of the rim but with less than 50% of the corresponding acetabular wall deficient. A major column defect, referred to as an acetabular defect, was defined as a loss of one or both columns with a corresponding acetabular wall deficiency greater than 50%.

This classification emphasizes cases in which bulk allograft is used, and 40% of the authors' reconstructions required structural allograft. It can be used with some primary deficiencies, such as congenital hip dysplasia, with a characteristic superolateral deficiency, and with classic protrusio-type defects. However, this system does not specify defect location, classifying defects is based on size and graft type, and the reconstruction method is weighted toward structural allografts.

Engh and Glassman

The AAOS classification system was modified by Engh and Glassman (15,16). Their method of grading acetabular bone stock damage was considered simpler, consisting of only three categories (Table 4).

With the intact acetabular rim and cavity of a minimal defect, rim fixation is possible and bone ingrowth likely. For a moderate defect, fixation of the intact acetabular rim is possible, but cavitary damage means that bone ingrowth is unlikely. Because a severe defect includes damage of both the rim (out-of-round, weak, or broken) and cavity, successful rim fixation and bone ingrowth are

TABLE 2. *Chandler and Penenberg acetabular bone deficiency classification*

1. Rim defects
2. Intra-acetabular defect
3. Protrusio of the medial wall of the acetabulum
4. Perforation of the medial wall of the acetabulum
5. Combined acetabular defects
    A. Protrusio and perforation of the medial wall of the acetabulum
    B. Superior rim and intra-acetabular defects
    C. Superior rim and intra-acetabular defects with medial-wall perforation
    D. Superior acetabular defects and perforation of the medial wall
    E. Global deficiency (complex anterior, superior, and intra-acetabular area deficient)
    F. Column defects (anterior or posterior rim and intra-acetabular defect with medial-wall perforation or pelvic discontinuity)

Modified and with permission, from Chandler HP, Penenberg BL. Acetabular reconstruction. In: Chandler HP, Penenberg BL, eds. *Bone stock deficiency in total hip replacement: classification and management.* Thorofare, NJ: Slack, 1989;49.

unlikely. This classification system fails to describe the amount of bone loss and offers no algorithm for treatment. The purported advantages of this limited number of categories were depiction of the type of defect facilitating communication, while avoiding the creation of multiple subgroups that provide few cases for statistical analysis. Among the 152 acetabular revisions they reviewed, 67 were considered minimal defects, 56 moderate, and 29 severe. They had a high failure rate in this series, which was attributed to poor implant choice and extensive bone loss.

Paprosky and Colleagues

Paprosky and co-workers have written extensively on acetabular bone deficiencies. They developed a classification system based on recurrent patterns of acetabular bone loss and defined specific radiographic criteria to assess each defect preoperatively (36,37). This system classifies the degree to which the acetabular rim is intact and able to provide initial support to allow osseointegration of the acetabular component (Table 5). Preoperative assessment of component migration indicates which structures are present to support the acetabular component. The authors found that the type of reconstruction necessary can thus be determined preoperatively, and they proposed a treatment method for each type of defect.

The preoperative radiographic criteria used are the amount of acetabular cup migration, the amount of ischial lysis, the degree of teardrop lysis, and the integrity of Kohler's line. Together, these criteria characterize the

host bone available for component fixation. The authors derived these criteria by comparing preoperative roentgenograms with intraoperative findings of bone deficiency. They found that component migration of less than 2 cm correlated with an intact superior dome and osteolysis of the ischium (a posterior wall deficiency); osteolysis of the teardrop (a medial wall deficiency); and violation of Kohler's line (an anterior column deficiency). They then classified defects based on whether the remaining bone could support a cementless component (type 1), partially support it (type 2), or not support it at all (type 3).

A type 1 defect has an intact acetabular rim with no component migration and only local osteolysis (Fig. 10). A type 2 defect has a distorted rim with superior or medial bone loss, intact anterior and posterior columns, and minimal ischial lysis. Type 2 defects are further divided based on the direction of migration of the failed acetabular component. There is less than 2 cm of migration of the prosthesis with this defect. A type 2A defect involves superomedial migration, resulting in a distorted superior rim without superior prosthesis contact (Fig. 11). In a type 2B defect, superolateral migration of the component leads to loss of the superior rim and dome, but the anterior and posterior column provide support (Fig. 12). A type 2C defect is characterized by medial migration, which results in a loss of the medial wall (Fig. 13).

In a type 3 defect, the rim is inadequate for component stability, and either the anterior or the posterior column is not supportive of component fixation. These defects pro-

TABLE 3. *Classification of pelvic defects by Gross et al.*

Small defect
  Autograft
  Modified implant
Large defect (allograft)
  Contained cavitary defect (protrusio)
  Structural defect
    Minor column (shelf grafts)
    Major column (acetabular allografts)

TABLE 4. *Engh and Glassman classification of acetabular bone stock damage*

Type	Bone loss (rim)	Bone loss (cavity)
Minimal	Intact	Intact
Moderate	Deficient	Intact
Severe	Deficient	Deficient

Modified from Engh CA, Glassman AH, Griffin WL, Mayer JG. Results of cementless revision for failed cemented total hip arthroplasty. *Clin Orthop* 1988;235:93.

TABLE 5. *Paprosky classification of acetabular defects*

Defect	Rim	Walls/dome	Columns	Migration	Teardrop lysis
Type 1	Intact	Intact	Intact/supportive	None	None
Type 2	Distorted	Distorted	Intact/supportive	Less than 2 cm	
2A	Distorted	Intact	Intact/supportive	Superomedial	Minimal
2B	Missing	Distorted	Intact/supportive	Superolateral	Minimal
2C	Distorted	Intact	Intact/supportive	Medial	Severe
Type 3	Missing	Compromised	Nonsupportive	Greater than 2 cm	
3A	Missing	Compromised	Nonsupportive	Superolateral	Moderate
3B	Missing	Compromised	Nonsupportive	Superomedial	Severe

Modified and with permission, from Paprosky WG, Perona PG, Lawrence JM. Acetabular defect classification and surgical reconstruction in revision arthroplasty. A six year followup evaluation. *J Arthroplasty* 1994;9:34.

hibit support of a cementless component alone because of extensive migration of the component (more than 2 cm above the normal hip center). They are subdivided based on the degree to which the integrity of the medial wall can support a prosthesis and the amount of host bone available for fixation. In type 3A, the medial wall is present, as confirmed by an intact medial teardrop border, intact or expanded Kohler's line, and 50% to 70% of the host bone is available for component fixation (Fig. 14). A type 3B defect has no medial wall, confirmed by an obliterated teardrop, severe ischial lysis, Kohler's line violated, and less than 50% of the host bone available for component fixation (Fig. 15).

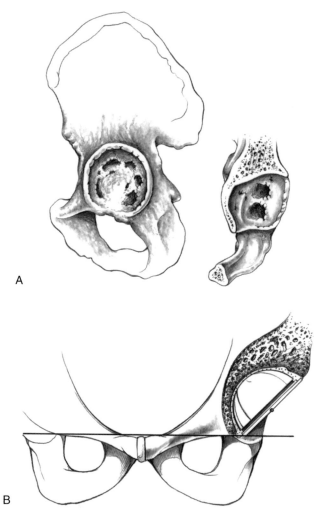

FIG. 10. A,B: Type 1 acetabular defect with intact rim and supportive columns. The defect is minimal and is secondary to localized lysis. (With permission, from Paprosky WG, Perona PG, Lawrence JM. Acetabular defect classification and surgical reconstruction in revision arthroplasty. A six year followup evaluation. *J Arthroplasty* 1994;9:34.)

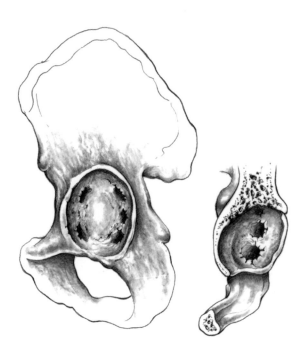

FIG. 11. Type 2A acetabular defect with superior bone lysis, but the rim remains intact. The deformity is generalized oval enlargement of the acetabulum. (With permission, from Paprosky WG, Perona PG, Lawrence JM. Acetabular defect classification and surgical reconstruction in revision arthroplasty. A six year followup evaluation. *J Arthroplasty* 1994; 9:35.)

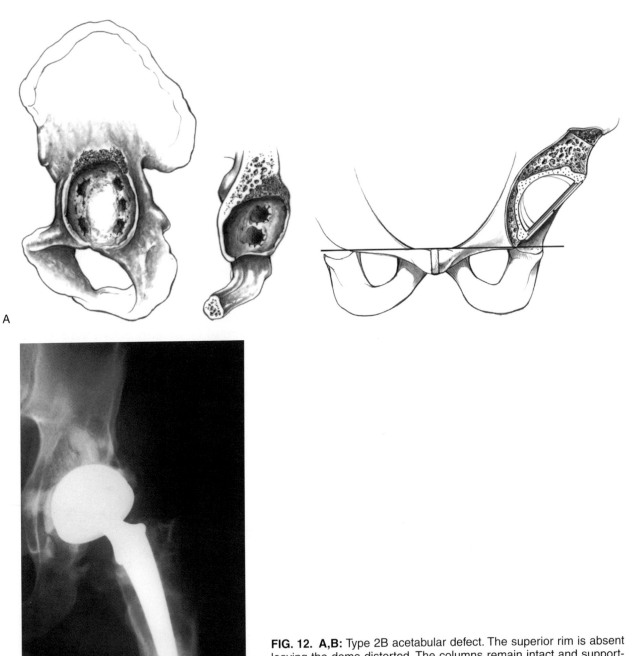

FIG. 12. A,B: Type 2B acetabular defect. The superior rim is absent leaving the dome distorted. The columns remain intact and supportive. (With permission, from Paprosky WG, Perona PG, Lawrence JM. Acetabular defect classification and surgical reconstruction in revision arthroplasty. A six year followup evaluation. *J Arthroplasty* 1994; 9:36.) **C:** This 72-year-old male had a type 2B acetabular defect with loss of the superior rim and superolateral migration of the acetabular component.

Other Acetabular Classifications

In addition to the in-depth work of Paprosky et al. on cementless revisions, others have advocated the classification of defects based on the intraoperative stability of the porous-coated cementless acetabular component. Hungerford classified defects in cementless reconstruc-

tions by the amount of graft used and the stability the graft provided (23). Borden described a "press fit" classification system because he found it difficult to correlate the AAOS classification system with his results (personal communication). In a press fit type I reconstruction, the acetabulum provides complete component stability with no graft requirement. A press fit type II reconstruction

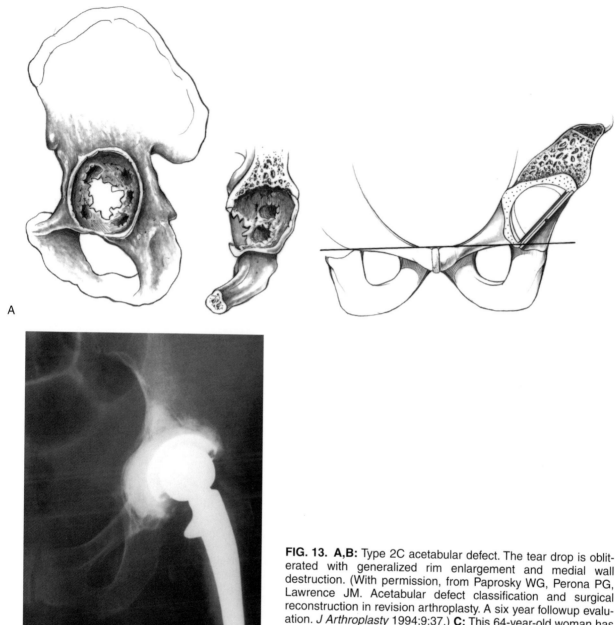

FIG. 13. A,B: Type 2C acetabular defect. The tear drop is obliterated with generalized rim enlargement and medial wall destruction. (With permission, from Paprosky WG, Perona PG, Lawrence JM. Acetabular defect classification and surgical reconstruction in revision arthroplasty. A six year followup evaluation. *J Arthroplasty* 1994;9:37.) **C:** This 64-year-old woman has a type 2C acetabular defect. The acetabular component has migrated medially and superiorly to compromise the medial tear drop.

requires bone grafting for the defects, but the acetabulum still provides component stability. A press fit type III reconstruction requires the use of structural bone grafting for component stability. Tanzer et al. also described staging the severity of the bone loss observed at the time of revision (42). D'Antonio contended the AAOS classification did not adequately address the quantity of bone loss when using cementless components. He also proposed grading the severity of bone loss in relation to the type of reconstruction after classifying the deficiency (Table 6) (7,8). For example, if a defect exists but the acetabular component is stabilized by the remaining bone, restora-

tion of bone integrity is performed without bone graft instead of a structural restoration.

The grading systems of Tanzer et al. and of D'Antonio are similar to Hungerford's and Borden's and based on the same concepts used by Engh and Paprosky.

Each of these classification systems that have been described has certain benefits. Most are based on the integrity of the acetabular supportive structures, which are necessary for cementless reconstruction, as well as the acetabular volume, which is necessary for containment of the prosthesis. The availability of a wide range of components has helped solve many of the problems of

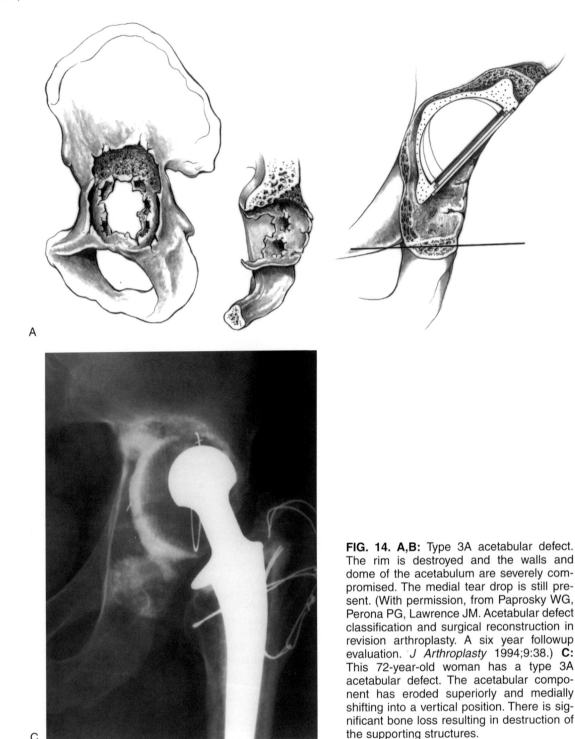

A

B

C

FIG. 14. A,B: Type 3A acetabular defect. The rim is destroyed and the walls and dome of the acetabulum are severely compromised. The medial tear drop is still present. (With permission, from Paprosky WG, Perona PG, Lawrence JM. Acetabular defect classification and surgical reconstruction in revision arthroplasty. A six year followup evaluation. *J Arthroplasty* 1994;9:38.) **C:** This 72-year-old woman has a type 3A acetabular defect. The acetabular component has eroded superiorly and medially shifting into a vertical position. There is significant bone loss resulting in destruction of the supporting structures.

reconstructing acetabular bone deficiencies and has reduced the need for structural allografts. The choice of bone graft depends on the type of deficiency and the choice of acetabular component. Most acetabular deficiencies are structurally supportive. There is little controversy regarding their treatment, with intermediate results being good. However, the severity of defects has not been quantified adequately. Two recent reviews of cementless revision surgery found that more than 80% of cases required some form of bone graft, but few required bulk allograft (26,32,41). The majority of the deficiencies were cavitary. When structural support is not present, the appropriate type of reconstruction remains a subject of debate. Paprosky has provided guidelines for preoperatively assessing acetabular defects that may require structural support. The AAOS classification of bone deficiencies is very general but does not specifically relate a treatment method to a type of defect. Addressing the

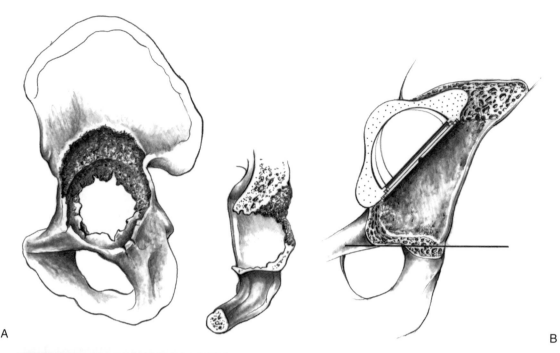

A   B

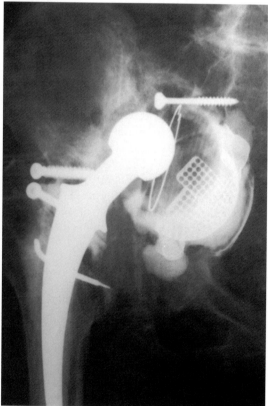

C

FIG. 15. A,B: Type 3B acetabular defect. There is complete obliteration of the medial tear drop and severe lysis. The columns are extremely nonsupportive and the walls and dome of the acetabulum are severely compromised. (With permission, from Paprosky WG, Perona PG, Lawrence JM. Acetabular defect classification and surgical reconstruction in revision arthroplasty. A six year followup evaluation. *J Arthroplasty* 1994;9:39.) **C:** This 89-year-old woman has a type 3B acetabular defect. The medial wall is destroyed and the acetabular component has migrated intrapelvicly. There are no supportive structures with severe bone loss.

TABLE 6. *Grading system of severity of acetabular bone loss (D'Antonio)*

Grade I	Complete prosthetic host bone contact
	No bone graft required
Grade II	Incomplete prosthetic host bone contact
	Prosthesis stable in host bone
	Filler graft may be added
Grade III	Incomplete prosthetic host bone contact
	Prosthesis is not stable in host bone
	Structural bone graft required to stabilize the prosthesis

With permission, from D'Antonio JA. Classification of acetabular bone defects. In: Galante JO, Rosenberg AG, Callaghan JJ, eds. *Total hip revision surgery.* New York: Raven Press, 1995;305–310.

severity of bone loss related to the stability of a cementless acetabular component in conjunction with the AAOS classification and the location of this defect may facilitate better comparison of the treatment methods used.

FEMORAL BONE DEFICIENCIES IN TOTAL HIP ARTHROPLASTY

Primary total hip arthroplasties rarely are complicated by femoral bone defects. In occasional cases of developmental dysplasia of the hip, the femur has excessive anteversion, and with some congenital abnormalities, the femoral canal may be too small for conventional femoral stems. The quality of bone deteriorates with various disorders, for example Gaucher's disease, osteopetrosis, tumors, Paget's disease, and metabolic bone diseases. Prior fractures and osteotomies or previously placed hardware also can complicate a primary procedure.

In contrast, an underlying femoral bone defect typically is present in a femoral hip revision. The classification of femoral bone deficiencies has evolved from very simple systems to many elaborate forms that usually describe and support a treatment algorithm. Their profusion and variety has led to confusion in trying to compare the results of treatments for a particular deficiency reported in the literature. Many of the more recently proposed classification systems were developed to help provide a basis for a femoral hip revision. The seven major classifications in use today are discussed below.

Chandler and Penenberg

In 1989, Chandler and Penenberg classified six main categories of femoral bone deficiencies encountered in their series of femoral reconstructions in revised total hip arthroplasties (Table 7) (6). The classification was based on femoral anatomy, and they discussed how each defect led to their treatment of 43 hips in 37 patients with a clinical follow-up of 19 months.

Chandler and Penenberg described two types of calcar bone loss, which is a common defect in revision total hip arthroplasty. Seven hips (16%) had a calcar intramedullary deficiency, usually associated with a failed femoral stem that had subsided and was in varus alignment. The nonsupportive calcar rim was treated with an iliac crest bone graft or a napkin-ring allograft. Four hips (9%) had a total calcar deficiency in a loose, cemented, varus femoral component with associated thinning of the lateral cortex at the distal stem tip. They treated this defect with an allograft calcar and distal strut allograft.

Trochanteric Deficiency

Because the greater trochanter is important in hip stability and abductor strength, defects here were considered as a separate category. The authors found 11 hips (26%) with defects in the greater trochanter. They treated this deficiency with a femoral head/neck split allograft.

Cortical Thinning

Cortical thinning without complete violation of cortical stability was an isolated defect in two hips (5%) and was combined with other femoral defects in 10 hips (23%). All 12 of these (28%) were associated with a failed cemented femoral component, and most involved the lateral cortex. The authors treated the defects using onlay cortical strut allografts extending 8 cm proximal and distal to the thinned cortical area. They used an uncemented femoral component of standard length and did not necessarily bypass the thinned cortical region.

Cortical Perforation

The complete loss of a segment of femoral cortex can result from osteolysis, infection, or penetration of a loose

---

TABLE 7. *Chandler-Penenberg classification of femoral bone deficiencies*

Calcar deficiency
   Intramedullary
   Total
Trochanteric deficiency
Cortical thinning
Cortical perforation
Femoral fractures about or below the stem of a femoral component
   Fractures of the patient's femur
   Fatigue fracture of an allograft
Circumferential deficiency of the metaphysis and proximal diaphysis
   Loss of the trochanter and metaphysis with a thin shell of the diaphysis remaining
   Total loss of the proximal femur

With permission, from Chandler HP, Penenberg BL. Femoral reconstruction. In: Chandler HP, Penenberg BL, eds. *Bone stock deficiency in total hip replacement: classification and management.* Thorofare, NJ: Slack, 1989;104.

femoral component. It may also be iatrogenic, having been caused during revision surgery either inadvertently or intentionally (e.g., cortical windows used to facilitate cement extraction). Chandler and Penenberg found isolated cortical defects in five hips (12%) and cortical perforation as part of a combined defect in nine hips (21%). They treated this defect by filling the window with iliac crest autograft and overlay strut allograft. The believed that a standard-length uncemented femoral component could be used even if they did not bypass the perforated segment.

Femoral Fractures About or Below the Stem of a Femoral Component

Periprosthetic fractures can occur about or below the femoral component. The authors noted four hips (11%) with periprosthetic fractures of the native femur and two hips (5%) with a fracture at a proximal allograft to native host bone junction. They treated the femoral fractures with medial/lateral strut allografts, spanning 12 cm, proximally and distally and supplemented with iliac crest autograft. For failure at the junction of a proximal femoral allograft and host bone, they used a medial strut allograft with a tension band lateral 12-hole supracondylar dynamic compression blade plate and a standard-length femoral prosthesis.

Circumferential Deficiency of the Metaphysis and Proximal Diaphysis

One of the most challenging problems in the revision of a total hip arthroplasty arises with complete loss of the proximal femur. This may occur in severe cases of osteolysis, stress shielding, or failure of a custom proximal femoral replacement. The authors found 11 hips (26%) with a circumferential proximal femoral deficiency. Their treatment consisted of a proximal femoral allograft with an uncemented standard or long-stem prosthesis onlay strut allograft and a standard-length stem with a supplemental tension band dynamic compression blade plate.

The Chandler-Penenberg classification provides a treatment option for each category of femoral bone deficiency. Unfortunately, this classification does not adequately quantitate the lesions (e.g., cortical thinning).

Additionally, several of the proposed allograft reconstructions are no longer favored for reconstructive hip replacements. Instead of small napkin allografts for defects in the calcar region, a calcar replacement femoral component now typically is used. Similarly, a cortical defect now is often bypassed by two cortical diameters with a long-stem prosthesis.

Endo-Klinik

In 1987, Engelbrecht and Heinert presented a femoral bone loss classification based primarily on radiographic assessment of a loose cemented femoral component (14). Termed the Endo-Klinik classification, it comprises four basic grades of femoral bone loss (Table 8) (13,14,17).

In grade 1, the cemented femoral component is loose with a few radiolucent lines in the upper half of the cement mantle. These signs may result from an early debonding of the prosthesis–cement interface, osteolysis, or a poor cementing technique. Very little bone loss can be expected in these cases.

In grade 2, a more pronounced radiolucent zone about the cement mantle portends subsequent endosteal erosion of the proximal femur. This erosion produces a large deficiency in the proximal metaphysis, but adequate bone stock remains in the diaphysis. Subsidence also can be seen in grade 2.

Grade 3 is characterized by a widened medullary cavity, a subsided loose femoral component in varus alignment, and expansion of the upper femur. A cortical defect may be present if the prosthesis has perforated the lateral cortex.

Grade 4 is the most severe femoral bone defect in the Endo-Klinik classification. The failed total hip arthroplasty has a large, proximal femoral deficiency that extends into the diaphysis, making reconstruction a challenging endeavor.

This classification frequently has been used in reporting the results of the Ling technique. Gie et al. reported on 56 cases of impaction allografting in cemented revisions, followed for 18 to 49 months (17). Most of the bone loss deficits in this series [40 patients (71%)] were grade 2. Thirteen patients (23%) had a grade 3 deficit, and only three (5%) had a grade 1 femoral defect. The authors noted, however, that several of the grade 3 cases

---

TABLE 8. *The Endo-Klinik classification of loss of femoral bone stock*

Grade 1	Radiolucent lines confined to the upper half of the cement mantle; clinical signs of loosening
Grade 2	Generalized radiolucent zones and endosteal erosion of the upper femur leading to widening of the medullary cavity
Grade 3	Widening of the medullary cavity by expansion of the upper femur
Grade 4	Gross destruction of the upper third of the femur with involvement of the middle third, precluding the insertion of even a long-stemmed prosthesis

With permission, from Gie GA, Linder L, Ling RSM, Simon J-P, Slooff TJJH, Timperley AJ. Impacted cancellous allografts and cement for revision total hip arthroplasty. *J Bone Joint Surg* 1993;75B:15.

were very close to grade 4. In this small sample, the loss of bone stock did not correlate with postoperative pain.

Elting et al. reported on 27 patients who underwent the Ling technique of impaction allograft cemented revisions and were followed for 2 to 5 years (13). Eleven patients (41%) had an Endo-Klinik grade 1 defect; ten patients (37%), grade 2; five patients (18%), grade 3; and one patient (4%), grade 4. They found that, with their reconstructive method, the amount of preoperative bone stock loss did not correlate with the postoperative Harris Hip Score.

The Endo-Klinik system is easy to use when the preoperative radiographic signs are typical. It also promotes a better understanding of the progression of a loose cemented prosthesis. However, this classification is not specific for the location of bone loss, it lacks a subdivision, and it usually is used only with the Ling technique of total hip revision.

Engh and Associates

In 1988, Engh and associates described a simple classification of femoral bone deficiencies with only three categories (Table 9) (1,16,29). Their goal was to enable the direct comparison of results after a total hip arthroplasty revision according to the amount of femoral bone loss at the time of the revision.

With mild bone stock damage, removal of the primary implant leaves an intact femoral neck and calcar, and the quality and quantity of bone in the metaphyseal region is sufficient to allow treatment similar to that with a primary total hip arthroplasty. Immediate implant stability is easily achieved in this situation during a cementless revision. With moderate bone stock damage, the metaphyseal region demonstrates enough bone loss to prevent revision total hip arthroplasty using a proximally coated prosthesis. Engh and associates believe that such deficiency compromises the osteogenic potential proximally, necessitating distal fixation with a fully coated prosthesis. Severe bone stock damage refers to revision cases in which a standard-length prosthesis cannot be used because of bone loss in the isthmus and shaft. Immediate

TABLE 9. *Engh classification of bone stock damage*

Bone	Damage
Minimal	Minimal or no damage
Moderate	Proximal damage only (neck and intertrochanteric)
Severe	Damage to both the proximal femur and the femoral shaft

With permission, from Engh CA, Glassman AH, Griffin WL, Mayer JG. Results of cementless revision for failed cemented total hip arthroplasty. *Clin Orthop* 1988;235:93.

stability cannot be achieved and a long-stem prosthesis is needed.

Engh and co-workers evaluated the fixation of 127 revised femoral components to determine if moderate or severe bone stock deficiency at the time of revision led to a change in radiographic findings (15). This group included 105 (83%) cases involving moderate bone loss and 22 (17%) with severe bone stock damage, and it excluded the minimal bone damage category (e.g., cementless endoprosthesis and surface replacement revisions). The authors found no correlation between the two groups; the implants were stable in 96% of moderate cases and 95% of the severe cases.

The classification proposed by Engh and associates is easy to remember, with simple terms. Unfortunately, it fails to consider specific regions and does not provide a treatment algorithm for complex cases in which structural bone grafting is needed. Additional conditions are not included, such as a distal diaphyseal defect with no or minimal bone stock loss proximal in the metaphyseal region.

Gross and Associates

In 1993, Gross et al. noted that all femoral bone defects could be generalized into two basic categories: intraluminal and cortical (20,29). Intraluminal bone loss was defined as the loss of cancellous bone, with the cortex remaining sufficiently strong to support an implant without supplemental allografting. Cortical bone loss was subdivided into noncircumferential (type I) and circumferential (type II) damage. In type I, the cortical defect can be repaired using a strut allograft. Type II was further classified as either type IIA, a calcar defect less than 3 cm long, or type IIB, a proximal femoral defect longer than 3 cm. A type IIA defect requires extensive bone grafting to achieve implant stability.

This classification is easy to conceptualize and is very basic in its applications. However, it considers only whether the femoral cortex is intact and if the remaining cortex can support an implant without the need for a strut allograft. The simple categories are too limited because they do not address combined defects or indicate whether a cemented or uncemented revision is preferable.

Hahnemann University

In 1990, Berman and associates presented the classification used at the Hahnemann University Hospital for revision total hip arthroplasties (1). Femoral bone stock deficiency is broken down into five categories on the basis of the need for bone grafting, primarily in cementless revisions (Table 10).

Although this classification includes treatment options for each subgroup, a system that relies on a 3-inch zone

TABLE 10. *Hahnemann University: femoral bone stock loss*

F1	Represents a loose component with adequate bone stock in which a cemented or uncemented component can be placed without concern about cortical support
F2	Indicates moderate bone loss with intrinsic host bone stability which may require cancellous grafting
F3	Represents severe proximal bone loss of less than 3 inches where proximal femoral replacement or strut grafting is indicated
F4	Describes severe proximal and distal bone loss of more than 3 inches, which would typically require allograft replacement
F5	Represents fracture of the femoral stem or shaft in which case defects must be spanned by twice the diameter of the shaft, and onlay graft may be indicated

From Amstutz HC, Luetzow WF, Moreland JR. Revision of femoral component: cemented and cementless. In: Amstutz HC, ed. *Hip arthroplasty.* New York: Churchill Livingstone, 1991;829–853.

measurement fails to account for variation in the size of the femur. This classification also suffers from the use of vague terms such as *moderate bone loss* without quantitating the regional bone loss sufficiently for treatment planning.

Mallory

In 1988, Mallory described a simple classification of proximal femoral defects that he had identified during revisions of failed cemented total hip arthroplasties (1,21,28,29). It includes three main types based on the viability of the cortex and the medullary contents in terms of supporting the reimplantation of a femoral prosthesis (Table 11).

Type I femoral bone defects occur when the medullary contents and the cortex are intact after removal of a failed femoral component. This condition can occur with a poorly cemented primary hip prosthesis in which a thin cement mantle has loosened but not damaged the surrounding bone. A cup arthroplasty revision or a loose press-fit endoprosthesis also may leave a type I femoral bone defect. These defects leave sufficient bone to allow either a cemented or an uncemented revision.

Type II defects occur when the femur lacks medullary contents secondary to a failed loose prosthesis, migration of the stem, and/or osteolysis. The femoral cortex is still intact in these cases, allowing several revision options. Although the loss of metaphyseal cancellous bone precludes proximal fixation during revision, the intact cortical bone distally enables uncemented implantation of a prosthesis with distal fixation.

Type III deformities involve destruction of both the medullary contents and the femoral cortex. Damage to the structural cortex is divided by location into three subgroups: type IIIA, above the lesser trochanter; type IIIB, from the lesser trochanter to the isthmus region; and type IIIC, a severe femoral cortex bone deficiency extending below the isthmus level. A femur with a type III defect may require a proximal femoral allograft and a long-stem prosthesis.

Among 160 patients followed for 2 to 6 years, Mallory grouped 48 patients (30%) in type I, 96 patients (60%) in type II, and 16 patients (10%) in type III (27). Postoperatively, the Harris Hip Score improved by 40 points or more for 90% of the patients. All patients with a type I or II defect had good to excellent results, and only 10% with a type III defect had postoperative pain, a limp, or a progressive radiolucency about the femoral component.

The Mallory classification is useful for assessing proximal bone quality. The principle of dividing bone defects into cancellous and cortical categories is valuable in determining the available reconstructive options. However, this classification is not specific enough for treatment options because it uses distance subdivisions that include the lesser trochanter to the isthmus in a single subtype. Type IIIB is too general and does not allow direct comparisons between a small lesser trochanter defect and a large diaphyseal defect or the combination.

Paprosky

In 1990, Paprosky described a new classification of femoral bone deficiencies in total hip arthroplasty. It was based on the degree of bone loss and the quality of the remaining diaphyseal bone support for a cementless femoral component (Table 12) (29,33–35).

A revision involving a type 1 defect is very similar to a primary total hip arthroplasty in that metaphyseal and diaphyseal bone loss are minimal. There is only partial damage of the calcar and the anteroposterior proximal bone stock. Revision arthroplasty can be performed without supplemental bone grafting.

TABLE 11. *Mallory classification of bony deformities (28)*

Type	Femoral deficits
Type I	Intact cortex and medullary content
Type II	Intact cortex but deficient medullary content
Type III	Deficits of both the cortex and medullary canal
A	Proximal to lesser trochanter
B	Lesser trochanter to isthmus
C	Isthmus and distally

TABLE 12. *Paprosky femoral defect classification*

Type	Femoral defect
1	Minimal metaphyseal and diaphyseal bone loss
2A	Absent calcar extending just below the intertrochanteric level
2B	Anterolateral metaphyseal bone loss
2C	Absent calcar with posteromedial metaphyseal bone loss
3A	2A plus diaphyseal bone loss
3B	2B plus diaphyseal bone loss
3C	2C plus diaphyseal bone loss

With permission, from Pak JH, Paprosky WG, Jablonsky WS, Lawrence JM. Femoral strut allografts in cementless revision total hip arthroplasty. *Clin Orthop* 1993;295:173.

Type 2 femoral defects have more extensive metaphyseal bone loss proximally, with complete loss of the calcar and a major anteroposterior deficiency. Despite the extensive loss of bone, the diaphyseal region remains intact and able to support a femoral component. There are three subgroups in this category: type 2A represents a nonsupportive calcar but an intact diaphysis. In type 2B, the anterolateral metaphyseal region is deficient with an intact diaphysis, and in type 2C, the calcar is absent with a deficient posteromedial section of the proximal metaphysis.

Type 3 lesions are the most severe, with complete circumferential bone loss in the metaphysis that extends to, and involves, the diaphysis. All three subgroups require a diaphyseal strut allograft. Each corresponding subgroup in this category has the same defect as in type 2A, 2B, and 2C, but with the additional involvement of the diaphysis.

Among 297 patients who underwent revision arthroplasty using an extensively coated, cementless femoral component, Paprosky classified the femoral defects as type 1 or 2A in 45 patients (15%), as type 2B or 2C in 156 patients (53%), and as type 3 in 96 patients (32%) (34). Preoperative and postoperative Postel and D'Aubigne scores were obtained for each group, and those with types 1 or 2A improved from 5.2 to 10.5; those with types 2B or 2C improved from 4.9 to 10.2; and those with type 3 improved from 4.3 to 9.6. With a follow-up of 5 to 14 years, good to excellent results were obtained even in patients with severe bone loss using a long-stem extensively coated cementless revision femoral component supplemented with strut allografts.

A valuable advantage of the Paprosky classification is that it provides excellent guidelines for the type of strut graft needed in an uncemented femoral revision. Additionally, the ability of the remaining bone stock to support a revision prosthesis is well detailed. Unfortunately, this classification is complex and is difficult to apply to cemented revisions. Moreover, it does not address greater trochanteric deficiencies, which are a unique problem encountered in total hip arthroplasty revisions.

AAOS Classification of Femoral Abnormalities

The AAOS Committee on the Hip developed a comprehensive classification that is based on anatomic location and can be used in both primary and revision hip arthroplasty (9,11,29). To clarify the system, the developers classified defects that occur in the cancellous bone as well as the cortical bone, and they used nomenclature identical to that used in their classification of acetabular bone deficiencies (10). The two basic categories of bone loss are a segmental and cavitary defect in the femur. The AAOS Committee on the Hip Femoral Abnormality Classification (9,11,29) was also designed to address problems unique to primary or revision hip reconstructions which include combined defects, malalignment, femoral stenosis, and femoral discontinuity (Table 13).

Segmental

A segmental femoral defect is a loss of supportive cortical bone (Fig. 16). A segmental defect can be located proximally, intercalary, or within the greater trochanter. In the proximal region, a partial segmental defect can be located anteriorly, medially, or posteriorly in any of the three main levels (see Fig. 16). An intercalary defect is a single perforation with normal femoral cortex proximal and distal to it, similar to a cortical window. Greater trochanter segmental defects were classified separately to address the specific difficulties often encountered in a total hip femoral revision.

Cavitary

A cavitary defect is a cancellous bone deficiency causing excavation of the endosteal cortical bone that is contained intermedullary with no extension out through the cortical bone (Fig. 17). This type of defect is usually present in most total hip arthroplasty revisions. Ectasia refers to a cavitary defect that has expanded the periosteal

TABLE 13. *AAOS classification of femoral abnormalities*

Segmental
Proximal
Partial
Complete
Intercalary
Greater trochanter
Cavitary
Combined segmental and cavitary
Malalignment
Rotational
Angular
Stenosis
Discontinuity

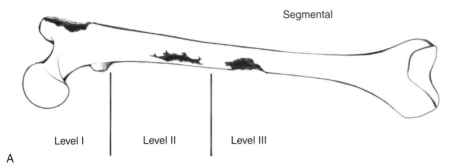

Segmental

Level I   Level II   Level III

A

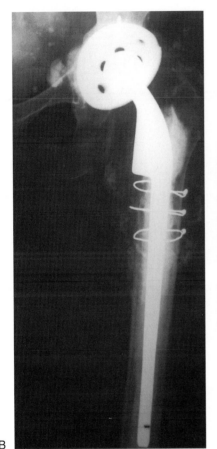

B

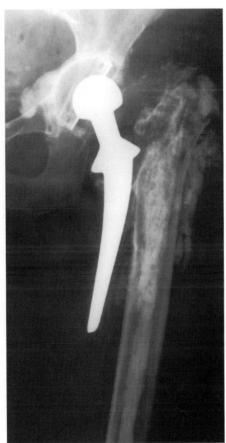

C

FIG. 16. A: Segmental defect. (With permission, from D'Antonio J, McCarthy JC, Bargar WL, et al. Classification of femoral abnormalities in total hip arthroplasty. *Clin Orthop* 1993;296:134.) **B:** This patient has a failed THA where the femoral component has eroded out of the femur leaving a segmental calcar deficiency. **C:** A cemented long stem calcar replacement prosthesis was used in this revision.

region of the bone deforming the cortex to a thin ballooned appearance (see Fig. 17A,D).

Combined Segmental and Cavitary

Combined defects can be caused by osteolysis, a fracture of the stem, iatrogenic perforation, overzealous extraction of a femoral component, or prolonged aseptic loosening of the femoral component, which typically has moved into varus alignment and/or has subsided (Fig. 18). Combined femoral bone defects make preoperative planning important when determining the surgical technique of revision total hip arthroplasty (see Fig. 18B).

Malalignment

The AAOS Committee on the Hip added this category to address both primary and revision settings. There are two types of malalignments: rotational and angular (Fig. 19A). Rotational deformities are frequently encountered in cases of developmental dysplasia of the hip in which excessive femoral anteversion may be seen. Angular deformities may occur with a large bowed femur or in cases of Paget's (Figs. 19B,C; 20).

Stenosis

Femoral stenosis is the narrowing of the femoral canal to a diameter less than that of the isthmus (Fig. 21). This

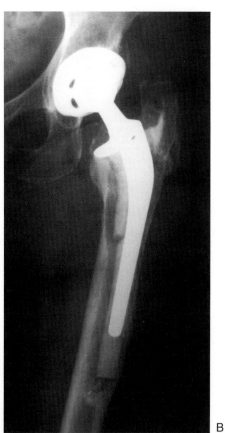

II. Cavitary

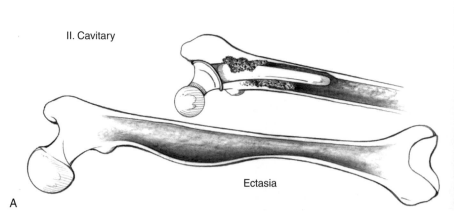

Ectasia

A

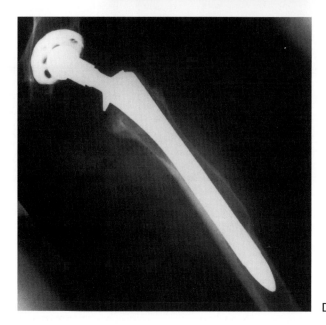

B

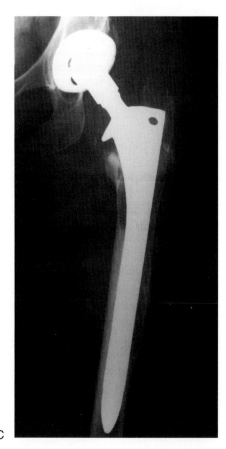

C

D

FIG. 17. A: Cavitary defect. (With permission, from D'Antonio J, McCarthy JC, Bargar WL, et al. Classification of femoral abnormalities in total hip arthroplasty. *Clin Orthop* 1993; 296:134.) **B:** This patient has a failed cemented femoral component with a broken cement column and a large cavitary defect. **C:** A long-stem cementless revision stem was used in the revision. **D:** This follow-up lateral radiograph demonstrates the ectatic femoral cortex.

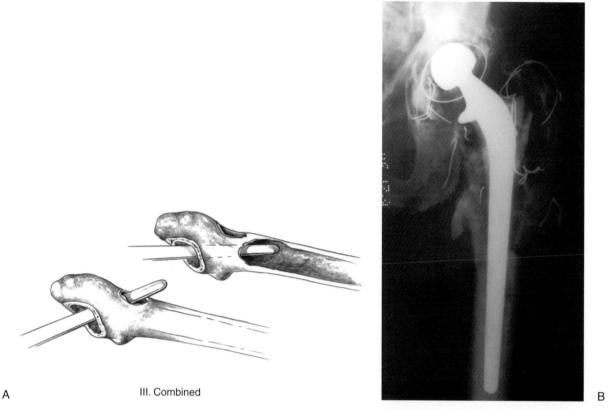

A   III. Combined   B

FIG. 18. A: Combined segmental and cavitary defect. (With permission, from D'Antonio J, McCarthy JC, Bargar WL, et al. Classification of femoral abnormalities in total hip arthroplasty. *Clin Orthop* 1993;296:135.) **B:** This patient demonstrates a large segmental and cavitary defect present in the proximal third of the femur. A proximal femoral allograft or a proximal femoral replacement prosthesis will be used in the near future revision.

condition can arise after a femur fracture, open reduction and internal fixation (see Fig. 21B,C), bony hypertrophy, malunion, or a large pedestal at the tip of a loose cementless femoral prosthesis.

Discontinuity

Femoral discontinuity is either a new or old femur fracture (Fig. 22A). In a primary total hip arthroplasty, a femoral nonunion may be present from an old fracture site. Periprosthetic femoral fractures are the most common cause of discontinuity (see Fig. 22B,C).

Levels

This classification system also uses three levels when describing the location of the femoral abnormality defects (see Fig. 16A). Level I is defined as bone proximal to the inferior portion of the lesser trochanter. Level

II is from the inferior lesser trochanter to 10 cm distal, and level III involves the femoral bone distal to level II. The inferior border of the lesser trochanter was chosen as a simple guide for special reconstructive situations that arise when the lesser trochanter is completely absent. Finally, a grading system for reporting the results of femoral implants was devised (Table 14). The strengths of the AAOS Committee on the Hip Femoral Abnormality Classification are that it is comprehensive, applicable to both primary and revision procedures. It is based on anatomic lesions of the femur that include rotational, stenotic, and discontinuous lesions, and it uses the nomenclature that is currently accepted for reporting acetabular bone deficiencies.

The weakness of this system is that it is difficult to remember. The classification comprises femoral abnormalities, rather than femoral bone deficiencies such as the preceding acetabular classification. This classification does discuss the different levels, but a cavitary defect may be a small portion laterally in the diaphyseal region of an uncemented prosthesis that has fallen into varus

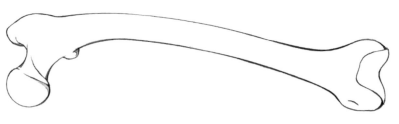

A

IV. Malalignment

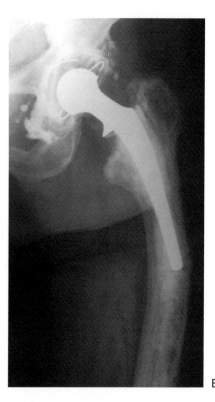

B

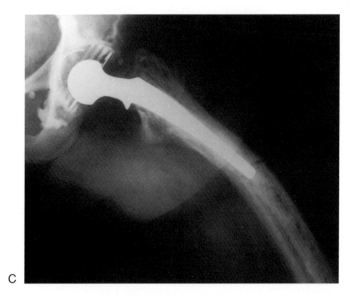

C

FIG. 19. A: Malalignment. (With permission, from D'Antonio J, McCarthy JC, Bargar WL, et al. Classi-fication of femoral abnormalities in total hip arthro-plasty. *Clin Orthop* 1993;296:135.) **B,C:** This patient with Paget's disease demonstrates a revision situa-tion with a marked bowing of the femur. Looser's lines are easily visible laterally.

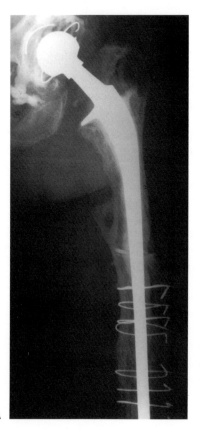

A

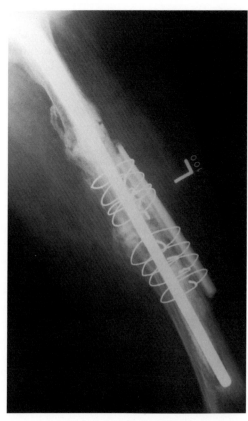

B

FIG. 20. A,B: Malalignment. A long-stem cemented femoral component with a two-level femoral osteotomy and a lateral onlay strut allograft was used in this malalignment revision.

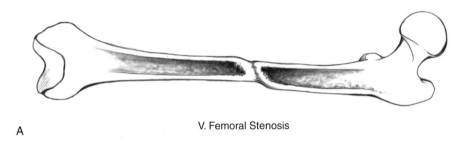

V. Femoral Stenosis

A

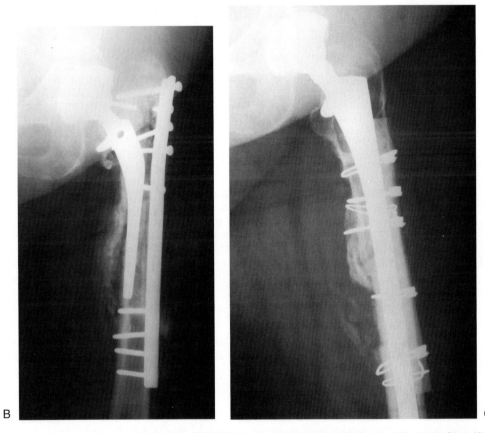

B

C

FIG. 21. A: Stenosis. (With permission, from D'Antonio J, McCarthy JC, Bargar WL, et al. Classification of femoral abnormalities in total hip arthroplasty. *Clin Orthop* 1993;296:136.) **B:** A periprosthetic fracture was unsuccessfully managed by an open reduction and internal fixation. The proximal fixation has failed with a segmental defect present. On careful inspection, the femoral canal has a complete stenosis at the most proximal of the distal screws. **C:** A cementless long-stem revision component was used after drilling/reaming past the stenotic femoral canal. A supplemental onlay allograft was applied laterally.

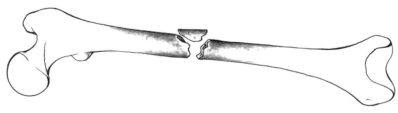

A   VI. Femoral Discontinuity

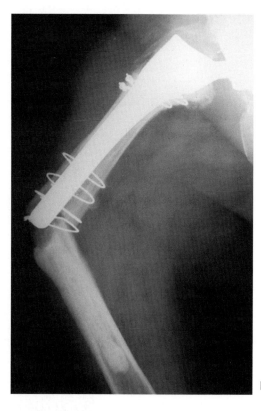

B

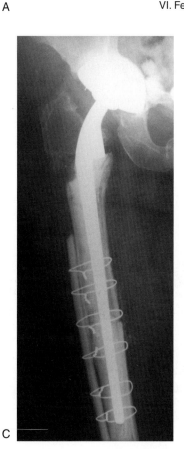

C

FIG. 22. A: Discontinuity. (With permission, from D'Antonio J, McCarthy JC, Bargar WL, et al. Classification of femoral abnormalities in total hip arthroplasty. *Clin Orthop* 1993;296:136.) **B:** This failed revision demonstrates a periprosthetic femur fracture. **C:** A long-stem short-body calcar replacement prosthesis was used in the revision supplemented by an onlay strut allograft laterally. The previous greater trochanteric fibrous stable union was managed conservatively.

alignment or a large ectatic osteolytic lesion in Gruen zones 2, 3, 4, 5, or 6 from a failed uncemented implant. Both will be classified simply as level II cavitary defects.

It is imperative to use a comprehensive bone deficiency classification to help provide a treatment algorithm, and to allow a direct comparison of results used in different surgical techniques in total hip reconstructions. The current

gold standard classification system is that proposed by the AAOS Committee on the Hip (9,11,29). This system takes into account almost all situations encountered during a primary or a revision total hip arthroplasty. Total hip arthroplasty is becoming more complex and this system is currently the best one available.

TABLE 14. *A grading system for the results of femoral implants*

Grade I	Complete prosthetic host bone contact No bone graft required
Grade II	Incomplete prosthetic host bone contact Prosthesis stable in host bone Filler graft may be added
Grade III	Incomplete prosthetic host bone contact Prosthesis is not stable in host bone Structural bone graft required to stabilize the prosthesis

REFERENCES

1. Amstutz HC, Luetzow WF, Moreland JR. Revision of femoral component: cemented and cementless. In: Amstutz HC, ed. *Hip arthroplasty*. New York: Churchill Livingstone, 1991;829–853.
2. Berry DJ, Muller ME. Revision arthroplasty using an anti-protrusio cage for massive acetabular bone deficiency. *J Bone Joint Surg* 1992;74B:711–715.
3. Borden LS, Greenky SS. The difficult primary total hip replacement: acetabular problems. In: Steinberg ME, ed. *The hip and its disorders*. Philadelphia: WB Saunders, 1991;1007–1019.
4. Callaghan JJ, Salvati EA, Pellici PM, et al. Results of revision for mechanical failure after cemented total hip replacement 1979-1982. A two to five-year followup. *J Bone Joint Surg* 1988;67A:1074–1085.
5. Chandler HP, Penenberg BL. Acetabular reconstruction. In: Chandler

HP, Penenberg BL, eds. *Bone stock deficiency in total hip replacement: classification and management*. Thorofare, NJ: Slack, 1989;47–102.

6. Chandler HP, Penenberg BL. Femoral reconstruction. In: Chandler HP, Penenberg BL, eds. *Bone stock deficiency in total hip replacement: classification and management*. Thorofare, NJ: Slack, 1989;103–164.

7. D'Antonio JA. Prosthetic bone loss of the acetabulum. Classification and management. *Orthop Clin North Am* 1992;23:279–290.

8. D'Antonio JA. Classification of acetabular bone defects. In: Galante JO, Rosenberg AG, Callaghan JJ, eds. *Total hip revision surgery*. New York: Raven Press, 1995;305–310.

9. D'Antonio JA. Classification of femoral bony abnormalities. In: Galante JO, Rosenberg AG, Callaghan JJ, eds. *Total hip revision surgery*. New York: Raven Press, 1995;351–358.

10. D'Antonio JA, Capello WN, Borden LS, et al. Classification and management of acetabular abnormalities in total hip arthroplasty. *Clin Orthop* 1989;243:126–137.

11. D'Antonio J, McCarthy JC, Bargar WL, et al. Classification of femoral abnormalities in total hip arthroplasty. *Clin Orthop* 1993;296:133–139.

12. Doehring TC, Rubash HE, Shelley FJ, Schwendeman LJ, Donaldson TK, Navalgund YA. Effect of superior and superolateral relocation of the hip center on hip joint forces: an experimental and analytical analysis. *J Arthroplasty* 1996;11:693–703.

13. Elting JJ, Zicat BA, Mikhail WEM, Hubbell JC, House BS. Impaction grafting: preliminary report of a new method for exchange femoral arthroplasty. *Orthopedics* 1995;18:107–112.

14. Engelbrecht E, Heinert K. *Klassifikation und Behandlungsrichtlinien von Knochensubstanzverlusten bei Revisionsoperationen am Huftgelenk-mittelfristige Ergebnisse. Primare und Revisionsalloarthroplastik Hrsg—Endo-Klinik, Hamburg*. Berlin: Springer-Verlag, 1987;189–201.

15. Engh CA, Glassman AH. Cementless revision of failed total hip replacement: an update. *Instr Course Lect* 1991;40:189–197.

16. Engh EA, Glassman AH, Griffin WL, Mayer JL. Results of cementless revision for failed cemented total hip arthroplasty. *Clin Orthop* 1988;235:91–110.

17. Gie GA, Linder L, Ling RSM, Simon J-P, Slooff TJJH, Timperley AJ. Impacted cancellous allografts and cement for revision total hip arthroplasty. *J Bone Joint Surg* 1993;75B:14–21.

18. Goodman SB, Adler SJ, Fyhrie DP, Schurman DJ. The acetabular teardrop and its relevance to acetabular migration. *Clin Orthop* 1988;236:199–204.

19. Gross AE, Allan DG, Catre M, et al. Bone grafts in hip replacement surgery: the pelvic side. *Orthop Clin North Am* 1993;24:679–695.

20. Gross AE, Allen DG, Lavoie GJ, Oakeshott RD. Revision arthroplasty of the proximal femur using allograft bone. *Orthop Clin North Am* 1993;24:705–715.

21. Head WC, Wagner RA, Emerson RH, Malinin TI. Restoration of femoral bone stock in revision total hip arthroplasty. *Orthop Clin North Am* 1993;24:697–703.

22. Hooten JP, Engh CA Jr, Engh CA. Failure of structural acetabular allografts in cementless revision arthroplasty. *J Bone Joint Surg* 1994;76B:419–422.

23. Hungerford DS, Krakow KA, Lennox DW. The PCA primary and revision hip systems. In: Fitzgerald R, ed. *Noncemented total hip arthroplasty*. New York, Raven Press, 1988.

24. Kelly SS. High hip center in revision arthroplasty. *J Arthroplasty* 1994;9:503–510.

25. Kwong LM, Jasty M, Harris WH. Proximal placement of acetabular component in total hip arthroplasty: a long term followup study. *J Arthroplasty* 1993;8:341–346.

26. Lachiewicz PF, Hussamy OD. Revision of the acetabulum without cement with use of the Harris-Galante porous-coated implant. Two to eight-year results. *J Bone Joint Surg* 1994;76A:1834–1839.

27. Letournel E, Judet R. Anatomy of acetabulum. In: Elson RU, ed. *Fractures of the acetabulum*, 2nd ed. Berlin: Springer-Verlag, 1997;17–22.

28. Mallory TH. Preparation of the proximal femur in cementless total hip revision. *Clin Orthop* 1988;235:47–60.

29. Masri BA, Duncan CP. Classification of bone loss in total hip arthroplasty. In: Pritchard DJ ed. *Instr Course Lect* 1996;45:199–208.

30. McGann WA, Welch RB, Picetti III GD. Acetabular preparation in cementless revision total hip arthroplasty. *Clin Orthop* 1988;235:35–46.

31. Mulroy RD Jr, Harris WH. Failure of acetabular autogenous grafts in total hip arthroplasty. *J Bone Joint Surg* 1990;72A:1536–1540.

32. Padgett DE, Kull LR, Rosenberg AG, Sumner DR, Galante JO. Revision of the acetabular component without cement after total hip arthroplasty. Three to six-year followup. *J Bone Joint Surg* 1993;75A:663–673.

33. Pak JH, Paprosky WG, Jablonsky WS, Lawrence JM. Femoral strut allografts in cementless revision total hip arthroplasty. *Clin Orthop* 1993;295:172–178.

34. Paprosky WG, Krishnamurthy A, MacDonald SJ. Five to fourteen year follow-up of 300 cementless femoral revision arthroplasties with extensively coated components. *Scientific exhibit at the 63rd annual meeting of the American Academy of Orthopaedic Surgeons*, Atlanta, GA, 1996.

35. Paprosky WG, Lawrence J, Cameron H. Femoral defect classification. Clinical application. *Orthop Rev* 1990;19(suppl 9):9–15.

36. Paprosky WG, Magnus RE. Principles of bone grafting in revision total hip arthroplasty. Acetabular technique. *Clin Orthop* 1994;298:147–155.

37. Paprosky WG, Perona PG, Lawrence JM. Acetabular defect classification and surgical reconstruction in revision arthroplasty. A six year followup evaluation. *J Arthroplasty* 1994;9:33–44.

38. Possai KW, Dorr LD, McPherson EJ. Metal ring support for deficient acetabular bone in total hip replacement. In: Pritchard DJ, ed. *Instr Course Lect* 1996;45:161–169.

39. Russotti GM, Harris WH. Proximal placement of the acetabular component in total hip arthroplasty: a long term followup study. *J Bone Joint Surg* 1991;73A:587–592.

40. Schutzer SF, Harris WH. High placement of porous-coated acetabular component in complex total hip arthroplasty. *J Arthroplasty* 1994;9:359–367.

41. Silverton CD, Rosenberg AG, Sheinkop MB, Kull LR, Galante JO. Revision total hip arthroplasty using a cementless acetabular component. Technique and results. *Clin Orthop* 1995;319:201–208.

42. Tanzer M, Drucker D, Jasty M, McDonald M, Harris WH. Revision of the acetabular component with an uncemented Harris-Galante porous-coated prosthesis. *J Bone Joint Surg* 1992;74A:987–994.

43. Yoder SA, Brand RA, Pedersen DR, O'Gorman TW. Total hip acetabular component position affects component loosening rates. *Clin Orthop* 1988;228:79–87.

44. Zehntner MK, Ganz R. Midterm results of acetabular allograft reconstruction with the acetabular reinforcement ring during total hip revision. *J Arthroplasty* 1994;9:469–479.

The Adult Hip, edited by J. J. Callaghan,
A. G. Rosenberg, and H. E. Rubash.
Lippincott–Raven Publishers, Philadelphia © 1998.

CHAPTER 58

Preoperative Planning

Robert L. Barrack

Total hip replacement is one of the most dramatically successful procedures performed in medicine (35). Relief of pain and restoration of function are predictably achieved in a very high percentage of cases. In a sense, however, hip replacement has fallen victim to its own success. Not only is a good or excellent result expected in virtually all cases, but cost-effective utilization of resources has also become a priority (62). Financial constraints make it necessary to achieve good results while conserving resources. These resources include operating room time, blood loss, implants, and instruments. Perhaps the overriding factor in achieving savings is the avoidance of complications (41). In order to achieve efficient utilization of resources, minimize complication rates, and achieve consistent, reproducible results, thoughtful preoperative planning is essential. Preoperative planning allows surgeons to shorten their learning curve when performing new procedures or when initially utilizing certain implant systems. It allows formulation of alternative plans and anticipation of intraoperative challenges in cases that are unusual in any way. Appropriate implants can be selected, and the need for special equipment or implants can be predicted preoperatively. An appropriate operative approach can also be chosen.

In the past, discussions of preoperative planning have focused almost entirely on the radiographic exercise of templating (17,22,24). Although templating is a crucial step in the planning process, facts obtained from the history, review of systems, physical examination, and gen-

eral review of radiographs provide equally valuable information in planning the procedure. By combining this data with careful templating, the surgeon has the best chance of achieving successful, reproducible results while efficiently utilizing resources and minimizing perioperative complications.

HISTORICAL FACTORS

Preoperative planning begins with a careful history and review of systems. Much of this is reviewed in previous chapters; however, it is appropriate to revisit some important items here. Once again, the nature and location of symptoms should be reviewed. If the symptoms are not classic for pathology originating in the hip joint, other extrinsic sources of symptoms and referred pain should be considered. Tests to help localize the symptoms to the hip joint may be an appropriate part of the preoperative assessment. If the pain is gluteal and has a radicular component, physical and radiographic examination of the lumbar spine is appropriate. Degenerative arthritis of the spine and hip often coexist, and differentiating the origin of symptoms may be a challenge. Local injections can be useful in problematic cases. If the pain pattern is suggestive of a significant element of nerve root symptoms, an epidural steroid injection may be considered. If a significant portion of the symptoms are relieved, the diagnosis of pain originating in the hip joints should be reassessed. If the pain is well localized laterally, a trochanteric injection may be considered, and if dramatic relief is obtained, further conservative treatment is probably warranted. If

R. L. Barrack: Department of Orthopaedic Surgery, Tulane University Medical Center, New Orleans, Louisiana 70112.

the nature of the pain is unusual and the origin remains in doubt, an anesthetic arthrogram may yield useful information (23). Medial thigh or knee pain, for instance, may be referred from the hip as in the adolescent. In such cases, relief of symptoms by an injection helps assure the diagnosis. If symptoms of activity-related muscle aching or cramping are present, vascular claudication should be considered. Peripheral vascular disease is particularly common in older men who are diabetic or smokers.

Certain items from the history have a significant impact on preoperative planning. It is appropriate to start with enquiries about childhood hip pathology, although in many instances, if treatment occurred early in childhood, patients are not cognizant of the specific diagnosis. It is helpful to determine if there is any recollection of treatment in braces or casts or any surgery on the hip. A history of brace or cast treatment points to the possibility of developmental dysplasia of the hip (DDH) or Perthes disease, which should be further evaluated with radiographs. Torsional deformities of the lower extremities are even more common and should be confirmed on physical exam. A history of sepsis is perhaps the most

important in terms of the impact on preoperative planning. Most often, sepsis will have occurred early in childhood and may not be volunteered by patients without specific questioning. Although active infection is a contraindication, infection in the distant past is not (42,45). It does, however, require further evaluation. In studies from the Mayo Clinic, a history of septic arthritis of the knee was associated with a risk of subsequent total knee infection of 5% to 10%, and 15% if there had been associated osteomyelitis (40). Although similar rates of subsequent infection are not available for hip replacement after previous infection, an increased level of risk would be expected. Evaluation for quiescent infection is therefore advisable. Sedimentation rate and aspiration should be considered. If there is a suggestion of osteomyelitis based on history or radiographic review, nuclear medicine scans, such as indium, may be helpful. Whereas increased uptake in the joint is expected with any degenerative arthritis of the hip, a focus of uptake in the metaphyseal region is a cause for concern. In this case, either open biopsy, or fluoroscopic or computed tomography (CT)-directed biopsy may be considered, depending on the lesion location.

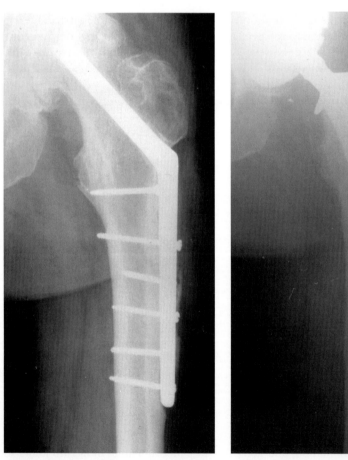

A   B

FIG. 1. A: Preoperative radiograph demonstrating previous internal fixation device requiring special extraction equipment. **B:** A long cementless stem was elected to bypass screw holes and the area of cortical thinning beneath the plate.

If surgery is undertaken in cases of previous sepsis, it is probably prudent to plan to do intraoperative frozen sections of any abnormal tissue encountered. If acute inflammatory cells are encountered, deferring hip replacement with debridement and a possible resection arthroplasty is probably advisable. Intraoperative cultures and Gram stains should also be considered when there is a history of sepsis. This requires that intravenous antibiotics be withheld until cultures are obtained. If preoperative and intraoperative assessment does not indicate indolent infection, as is often the case, and cemented components are implanted, the use of antibiotic-impregnated cement may be advisable as in any case of hip replacement considered at higher risk for infection.

The history of any prior hip surgery is relevant for planning purposes. Prior incisions must be considered in planning the operative approach. Longitudinal incisions should be incorporated when possible. If it is necessary to cross a prior incision, it is probably best to do so at a 90-degree angle to minimize the risk of skin slough at the apex (19). In general, the incidence of wound problems is low with incisions placed about the hip. Problems have been reported, however, with longitudinal parallel incisions placed anterior to a previous incision (60). This seems to compromise circulation to the intervening skin bridge, and skin slough has been reported in this scenario.

The presence of previous implants from prior hip surgery is of obvious relevance in preoperative planning. It is helpful to know the type and manufacturer of any internal fixation device that was previously placed in order to plan its removal. In some cases, extraction devices that are unique to the component requiring removal are available. Generic screw removal systems are also available. The presence of channels, screw holes, and bone remodeling, resulting from previous implants, may alter the planned component selection for hip replacement. Longer stems may be indicated to bypass stress risers from screw holes or a thinned cortex from previously applied plates (Fig. 1).

A history of other previous surgical intervention may also be relevant. Many older total hip candidates may have coexisting vascular diseases. The presence of a previous ipsilateral vascular bypass graft is a concern (Fig. 2). In such cases, preoperative vascular consultation is probably advisable to determine the status of the graft preoperatively and to assist in monitoring the vascular status postoperatively. The lower extremity is placed in extreme positions during total hip replacement, particularly during femoral canal preparation. These positions are known to kink the femoral vessels (8) and to place grafts at risk for thrombosis. The length of time the extremity is maintained in extreme positions should be kept to a minimum in such cases, and it is probably advisable to replace the limb in a more physiologic position every few minutes to lower the risk of thrombosis. At the

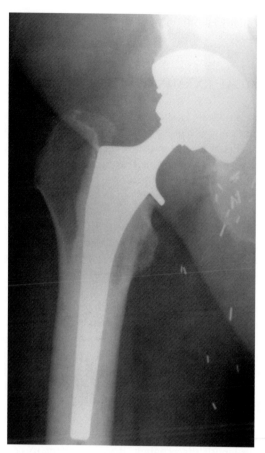

FIG. 2. Postoperative radiograph demonstrating multiple vascular clips from previous vascular bypass procedure. Vascular surgery consultation was obtained preoperatively.

end of the procedure, evaluation of the vascular status of the limb in the operating room is probably advisable. Cameron has described an operative approach to minimize the risk of graft occlusion in this clinical scenario (15). Trochanteric osteotomy and wide exposure are described to avoid placing the limb in extreme positions. Although this clinical situation is relatively uncommon, the consequences are potentially devastating, so that awareness of the vascular status, particularly the presence of previous vascular grafts, is important.

The history of previous medical conditions and/or treatment is also of potential importance. Patients who have had previous pelvic radiation may not fare as well with uncemented acetabular components (39,49). A number of drugs, including steroids and cytotoxic agents, are thought to inhibit bone ingrowth (12,69). The effect of these drugs on the clinical results of uncemented components has not yet been well established. If patients have been on such drugs chronically and continued use is anticipated, the use of cemented components may be more appropriate.

Although total hip replacement is a very commonly performed procedure, a careful history and review of systems remains an important part of the preoperative planning process.

PHYSICAL EXAMINATION

The physical examination also contributes crucial information to the preoperative plan. The exam traditionally begins with observation. The skin and soft tissue about the hip are examined, with particular attention to the planning of possible incisions. The implication of previous incisions has been discussed previously. The patient's standing posture should be noted. Patients with excessive lumbar lordosis have a different orientation of the acetabulum in the erect posture that may impact component stability. When the acetabular component is inserted, the lordosis may be corrected, particularly when surgery is performed in the lateral decubitus position. To compensate for this, it has been suggested that the component be placed in more anteversion (or flexion) in order to be more stable when the patient assumes an upright posture (3). Observation of the iliac crests from behind is important in assessing the presence of pelvic obliquity. This frequently signifies a limb-length discrepancy. The obliquity is corrected by placing blocks under the short limb until the pelvis is even. The block thickness necessary to achieve a level pelvis is recorded as one measure of limb-length discrepancy. It is important to correlate this with the patient's own feeling of leg length, tape-measure distances from the anterior inferior iliac spine to the medial malleolus, and radiographic measurements. The block test is generally considered the most accurate clinical measurement (28,36). If there is wide discrepancy between various clinical measurements, or between clinical and radiographic measurements, a scanogram may be helpful in determining the true relative limb length. Computed tomography is also accurate for measuring limb length. A study comparing orthoroentgenography with CT found that the cost and time were equivalent, but CT was more accurate in the presence of a flexion deformity and had far less radiation exposure (1). The amount of clinical discrepancy should be recorded and correlated with radiographic measures. There are a number of instruments available for estimating length changes intraoperatively (53,76), and these are particularly useful when significant length changes are planned. If lengthening of more than 2 cm is anticipated, somatosensory evoked potential (SSEP) may be advisable (73). This degree of lengthening is rare, however, in primary hip arthroplasty, unless significant DDH is present.

After performing the block test, the Trendelenburg test can be done as a clinical test of abductor muscle weakness (36). This should be correlated with observation of gait for the Trendelenburg or gluteus medius lurch as a sign of functional muscle weakness as well as the results of manual muscle testing (resisted side-lying abduction).

If a patient has significant muscle weakness (three out of five or less with manual testing) an underlying cause should be sought. Some degree of weakness can be expected secondary to chronic hip pain and inflammation. The presence of significant abductor weakness may alter the operative plan. It may be more advantageous to increase the femoral offset by component selection and placement and/or by lateralizing the trochanter. It is also advisable to place the components in a very stable position to help compensate for the absence of strong abductors. In the absence of functional abductors, the use of a constrained acetabular liner has also been suggested (48). This is certainly much more common in the revision situation than in primary total hip replacement.

Observation of gait can also reveal rotational deformities of the lower extremities. Intoeing, for example, may be indicative of internal femoral torsion or excessive femoral anteversion. This can be confirmed on physical exam by the presence of excessive internal rotation of the femur (greater than 70°) and limited external rotation (36). If excessive femoral anteversion is suspected on the basis of gait, physical exam, history, or radiographs suggestive of moderate or severe DDH, CT can be performed to quantify the degree of the anteversion. A plain radiograph technique has been described (63) but is not as accurate. The condition is often bilateral and the patient should be advised that limb rotation may be somewhat asymmetric postoperatively. The presence of excessive anteversion can significantly alter the preoperative plan, particularly if an uncemented stem is planned, which is often the case because these patients tend to be on the younger side of the general total hip population.

After observation of gait, the active and passive ranges of motion are typically tested and recorded. Severe restriction in range of motion can be a significant factor in selection of the operative approach, which will be discussed later. The presence of contractures is also a significant factor in preoperative planning. The Thomas test is classically used to test for the presence of flexion contracture (36). Significant degrees of flexion contracture are most common in patients who are wheelchair bound and/or have inflammatory joint disease. Preoperative physical therapy may be advisable to lessen the degree of contracture. The presence of other contractures, such as an adduction contracture, should be noted on physical exam, and, here too, preoperative therapy may be considered to reduce the amount of correction required at surgery. The degree of contracture also can affect the choice of operative approach. If abduction is limited to the point of limiting ability to prep and drape the extremity, or to rotate or maneuver the hip in order to perform a standard approach, a preoperative adductor tenotomy is an option (Fig. 3). This can be performed as a separate procedure with the patient supine. The adductor longus can be released directly from the pubis through a percutaneous incision. The presence of contracture makes length-

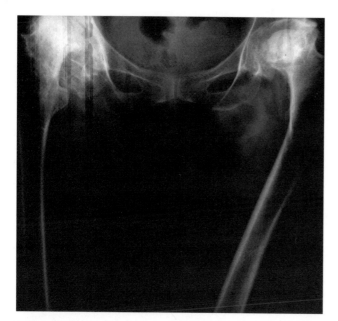

FIG. 3. Patient with severe adduction contracture of left hip underwent adductor tenotomy to facilitate hip replacement.

would preclude postoperative ambulation, than they should be addressed first. Patients with multiple joint involvement will invariably require ambulatory aides such as a walker, crutches, or at least a cane, and they must have adequate upper extremity function to utilize these devices. The joints of the lower extremity also have a logical sequence. A plantigrade foot is essential for effective gait. If foot or ankle pathology precludes plantigrade gait and is the source of significant symptoms, this should be corrected prior to hip replacement. Knee replacement, on the other hand, is most often deferred until after ipsilateral hip replacement for a number of reasons (3). It is difficult to perform knee replacement with an ankylosed hip, and rehabilitation is likewise more difficult with a stiff or painful hip. Several muscle groups cross both the hip and knee joint, so hip replacement may change the tension or direction of pull of muscles crossing the knee. Hip replacement can also change the rotation of the extremity, which could have significant impact on the alignment and stability of a knee replacement. Internal rotation of the femur could adversely effect patellar tracking and stability, for instance.

ening of the extremity more difficult. If the extremity is short preoperatively, the patient should be advised that some or all of the limb length discrepancy may remain.

The review of systems and physical exam should also include the contralateral hip and other involved joints, as their status may impact the overall preoperative plan. If the other hip is severely involved to the point of limiting the patient's ability to ambulate postoperatively, bilateral hip replacement may be considered (58,65). This is often the case in patients who have significant flexion and adduction contractures of both hips, and in patients who are wheelchair dependent (Fig. 4). In such cases, the degree of contracture and range of motion are particularly important to note bilaterally. When bilateral hip replacements are performed, it may be prudent to obtain radiographs in the operating room at the conclusion of the case to ensure that both hips are reduced. This is particularly an issue when patients are positioned in the lateral decubitus position, because there is considerable movement of the patient while in an anesthetized state and the hips are vulnerable to dislocation.

The status of other joints is also a factor in planning the surgical procedures. This is particularly the case with rheumatoid patients. A detailed discussion of the appropriate sequence of surgical procedures in rheumatoid patients is beyond the scope of this discussion, but some general principles are worth mentioning. In most cases, there is one joint that is the source of the vast majority of the patient's symptoms and functional disability, and this is the focus of immediate attention. When several joints contribute significant symptoms and disability, an overall plan for staging procedures is appropriate (50,72). If upper extremity joints are involved to an extent that

A

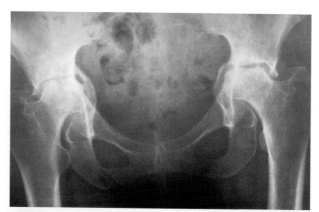

B

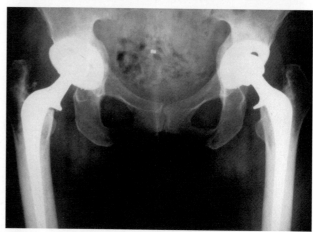

FIG. 4. A: Preoperative radiograph demonstrating severe bilateral hip disease in wheelchair-dependent patient. **B:** Bilateral hip replacement was performed under a single anesthesia because of the presence of contractures and the anticipated difficulty in ambulation after a single hip replacement.

CHOICE OF OPERATIVE APPROACH

Choosing the surgical approach is an important aspect of preoperative planning. In reality, most surgeons utilize the same operative approach for the vast majority of cases based on their training, experience, and level of comfort. Most primary cases can be done through the same approach without difficulty. There are, however, instances where certain surgical approaches may be advantageous, based on information derived from the history, physical examination, and radiographic review. A history of prior surgery is an important consideration in planning the incision. As noted previously, a longitudinal incision placed anterior and parallel to a previous posterior incision seem to be more prone to wound necrosis. In such a case, it is safer to incorporate the previous skin incision with longer incisions proximally and distally to allow a fascial incision at a more routine midline location (61). The history of a prior posterior approach has been suggested as a relative contraindication to a second posterior approach because of concerns of instability (25). This is not a universally accepted principle, however.

Obese or very muscular patients require some modification of operative approach. Longer incisions are often advisable and the availability of deeper retractors that can reach the depth of the wound and the rim of the acetabulum are necessary. It is also advisable to arrange for an adequate number of assistants in surgery. Whereas routine primary hip surgery may be performed with a single assistant, a second assistant is advisable with a very large patient. Availability of the wide array of self-retaining hip retractors now available may also be of benefit in such cases. If a standard posterior approach is selected in a large patient, certain additional measures may be necessary to obtain adequate exposure. The entire quadratus femoris and gluteal sling can be released from the femur, and the reflected head of the rectus femoris and the anterior capsule can be released as well to mobilize the femur to provide adequate exposure to ream the acetabulum and insert the acetabular component in the proper orientation. If the femur is not mobilized and retracted anteriorly to an adequate extent, there is a great tendency to insert the components in neutral or retroversion rather than the 20° to 30° of anteversion that is desirable. This probably contributes to the higher incidence of dislocation for total hips performed through a posterior approach. This is particularly true when the patient is positioned in the lateral decubitus position. In this position, the orientation of the pelvis changes with relative forward flexion and caudal tilt of the pelvis, which must be compensated for by

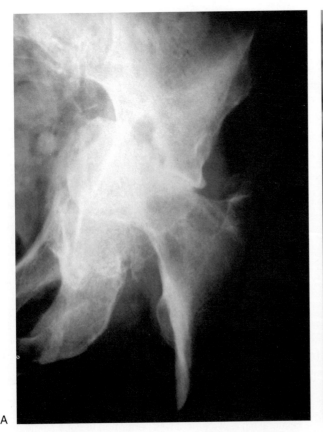

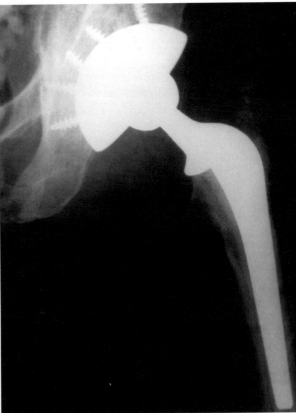

A

B

FIG. 5. A: Preoperative radiograph showing severe posttraumatic protrusio acetabuli. **B:** Total hip was performed through a posterior approach by cutting the head *in situ.*

adding an additional degree of anteversion and less abduction or inclination (51).

Other options to consider for surgical approach include trochanteric osteotomy. The use of a triradiate approach has also been described in the obese patient (46).

The presence of contractures as determined on physical exam may influence the choice of surgical approach. Patients with flexion and/or adduction contractures, particularly those who spend a lot of time in a wheelchair, are prone to recurrence of contracture postoperatively. This is particularly true of patients with spasticity, such as the older patient who has had a cerebrovascular accident or the occasional patient with cerebral palsy who is considered for hip replacement (10). In such cases, a standard posterior approach is probably associated with higher risk of dislocation, and an anterolateral or direct lateral approach may have some advantages in terms of stability.

The presence of a stiff or ankylosed hip may also have impact on the choice of operative approach. If a posterior approach is selected, than the same modifications for exposure as described in the obese patient may be applicable. Trochanteric osteotomy may also be considered. The cause of the ankylosis should be considered, however. If there is heterotopic ossification present, or if the patient is at high risk for heterotopic ossification, and perioperative radiation therapy is planned, the option of the trochanteric osteotomy is less attractive because of the possible deleterious effects of radiation on trochanteric union. There is some evidence that the direct lateral approach may predispose to heterotopic ossification, especially when uncemented implants are utilized (9). This may also be a factor to consider in such patients.

The presence of protrusio acetabuli may have a bearing on the choice of operative approach. In most cases, the femoral head can be cut *in situ* and removed, allowing the use of a standard operative approach (Fig. 5). This is preferable to forcibly dislocating the head by rotating the femur, which risks fracture of the femur or less frequently the acetabulum or pelvis. In the presence of a stiff hip or a large patient, a more extensile approach such as trochanteric osteotomy may be planned. (Fig. 6) When trochanteric osteotomy is anticipated as a significant possibility based on preoperative planning, it is probably prudent not to begin with a direct lateral approach. Although a standard posterior or anterolateral approach can be combined with trochanteric osteotomy, combining a direct lateral approach with trochanteric osteotomy has been discouraged (19).

In cases where trochanteric osteotomy is considered, a modification that has been popularized in recent years is the trochanteric slide (31). This provides a degree of exposure similar to that of a trochanteric osteotomy, but it has the advantage of maintaining soft-tissue attachment both proximally and distally, which should improve vascularity and trochanteric healing as well as lowering the

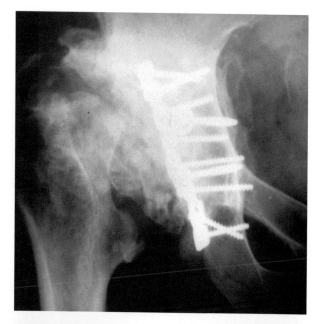

A

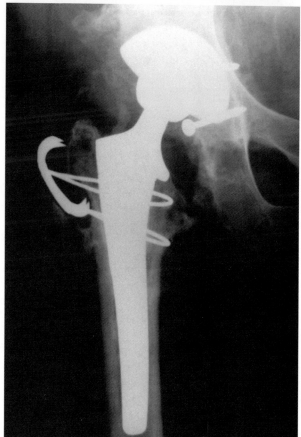

B

FIG. 6. A: Severe posttraumatic arthritis after posterior column plating. **B:** Because of the combination of obesity, extensive heterotopic ossification, and ankylosis of the hip, a transtrochanteric approach was utilized.

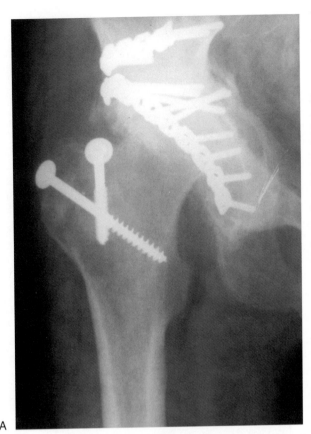 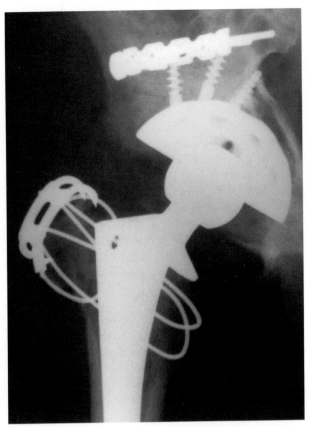

FIG. 7. Because of the presence of a posterior column plate **(A)**, a combined posterior and trochanteric approach was utilized **(B)**.

risk of proximal migration. If significant leg lengthening is anticipated, however, this approach may be more difficult to utilize.

A final factor in planning the operative approach is the need for access to a particular anatomic region. If there is a bony deficiency of the acetabulum or hardware from previous surgery present, the surgical approach must allow direct access to that region. If a posterior column plate is present, for example, a posterior approach is necessary (Fig. 7). Posterior column plates are often in direct proximity to the sciatic nerve, which may actually be encased in scar tissue adherent to the plate. Plate removal may be necessary to ream the acetabulum, in which case SSEP monitoring may be considered to warn of potential nerve damage. If there is an anterior acetabular deficiency, on the other hand, an anterolateral or direct lateral approach may be more appropriate.

RADIOGRAPHIC TECHNIQUE

The first step in preoperative radiographic analysis involves obtaining consistent, appropriate radiographs for review. As in virtually all aspects of orthopedics, a minimum of two views required, one in the anteroposterior

(AP) projection and one lateral view. In practice, three views are preferable. An AP view of the pelvis is necessary to estimate relative limb length. The beam is centered over the pubis in the midline. A more accurate assessment of the dimensions of the proximal femur is obtained from an AP view centered over the hip. The standard distance from the x-ray tube to the table top is 40 inches. If a grid cassette is placed directly beneath the hip, magnification of the bones of approximately 10% is seen in an average-size patient. Placing a cassette directly beneath the extremity is common in the operating room, but in most radiology departments a bucky tray is placed in a compartment approximately 2 inches below the table top, resulting in magnification of 15% to 20% (29,30). The degree of magnification is directly related to the distance from the bone to the cassette. In an obese patient, therefore, the magnification can be over 25%, whereas in a thin patient it can be less than 15% (18). This represents a wide range for templating purposes, and therefore the use of a magnification marker is useful, particularly with patients of above- or below-average size. A typical magnification marker consists of a Plexiglas bar within which two spherical metal balls are embedded exactly 100 mm apart (17). The distance between the two resulting circular radiographic images is measured and the number of

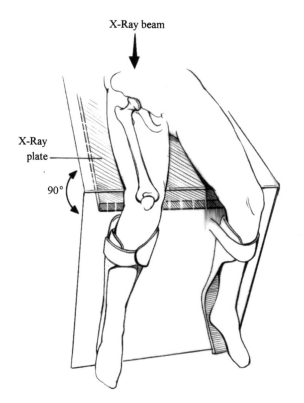

FIG. 8. Positioning of the patient with flexion contracture of the hip or knee.

millimeters measured above 100 represents the degree of magnification. This is still an estimate, however, because the marker must be taped to the skin or elevated with an accompanying stand to a level estimating the level of the center of the femur.

The AP pelvis and hip radiograph should be obtained with the patient lying flat on the table and the lower

extremities internally rotated 15° to 20°. One technique for improving consistency of positioning that has been suggested is to flex the knees over the end of the table (13,30). If a flexion contracture has been noted on physical examination, the radiographic technique should be modified. If a standard AP radiograph is obtained in the presence of a flexion contracture, typically the femur will be off of the table top with the patient supine or there will be increased lumbar lordosis. If the hip is flexed for an AP radiograph, it will result in a greater degree of magnification, foreshortening the image, and often rotation of the femur as well. These inaccuracies can be minimized by obtaining the AP radiographs in a semi-sitting position (Fig. 8). It is also desirable to obtain the AP radiographs in 15° to 20° of internal rotation to bring the femoral neck into a parallel orientation relative to the cassette and thus perpendicular to the x-ray tube in the average patient. This gives a more accurate depiction of the proximal femoral geometry and true femoral offset. Patients tend to naturally assume a posture of external rotation of the hips when lying supine. In addition, patients with degenerative disease tend to lose internal rotation early and later develop external rotation contractures, accentuating the tendency for AP radiographs to be taken with the hip externally rotated. Radiographs in external rotation make the intertrochanteric area appear more narrow, the femoral offset less, and the lesser trochanter more prominent. Internal rotation has the opposite effect: increasing the offset, making the intertrochanteric area larger, and making the lesser trochanter much less prominent (Fig. 9). A recent study demonstrated that rotation of the femur has a significant effect on the measurement of both the neck–shaft angle and femoral offset (32). As a result of all of these factors, preoperative planning based on malrotated radiographs is inaccurate and will provide subop-

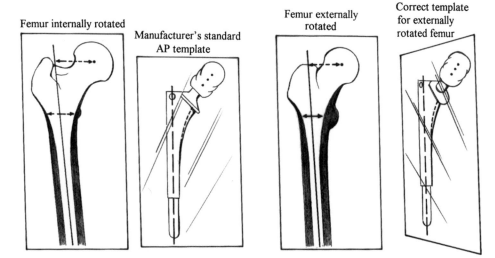

FIG. 9. Internal rotation of the femur brings the hip into the plane of the acetabulum, which changes the apparent offset, metaphyseal dimensions and neck–shaft angle.

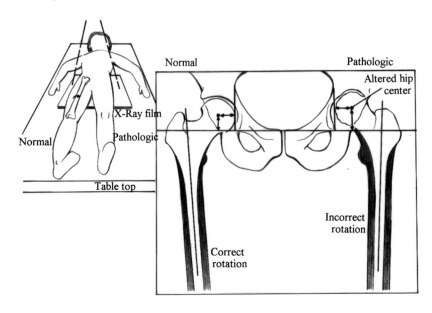

FIG. 10. If patient is unable to internally rotate pathologic hip, femoral templating can be performed on contralateral normal hip.

timal information for the preoperative plan. If the pathologic hip cannot be internally rotated 15°, templating can be done on the contralateral normal or less involved side (Fig. 10). This assumes that the internal geometry of the contralateral hip is an accurate representation of that of the pathologic hip, a supposition that has been supported by a number of authors (22,24,30). In many cases, however, both hips have external rotation contractures. In such cases, a posteroanterior radiograph can be obtained with the patient placed prone, with the affected limb in 15° to 20° of external rotation and the hip directly against the table top (Fig. 11).

If there has been a previous fracture or osteotomy, long films of the entire femur are advisable. A standing film that includes the hip, knee, and ankle will give a more accurate assessment of the effect of the angular deformity on the overall limb alignment. In patients with posttraumatic arthritis subsequent to acetabular fractures, further radiographic evaluation is advisable. Judet views can help assess the acetabular margins, but a CT scan can be invaluable in such cases. This is particular concern in avascular necrosis (AVN) or posttraumatic arthritis after hip dislocations. In such cases, there is often an associated fracture of the posterior wall, whose presence or magnitude may not have been appreciated at the time of the injury. Computed tomography gives an accurate assessment of the presence and extent of such deficiencies (Fig. 12).

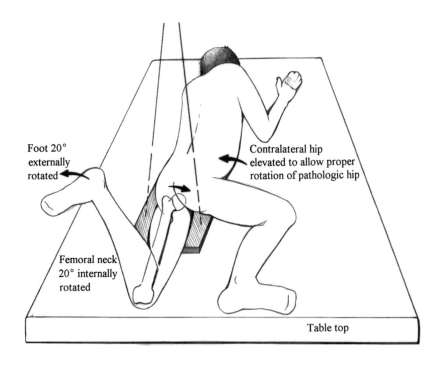

FIG. 11. Positioning of the patient with external rotation contracture of both hips.

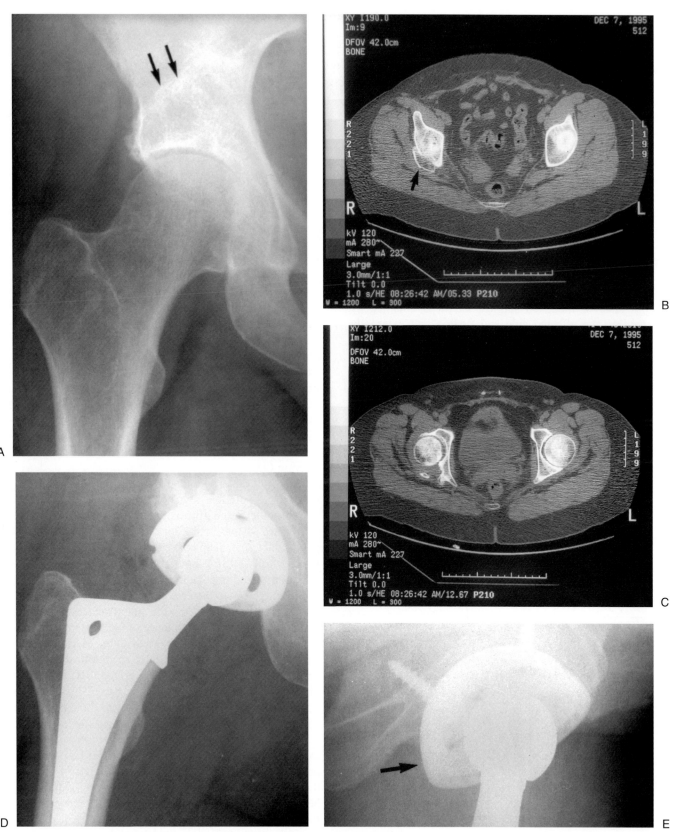

FIG. 12. Preoperative radiograph **(A)** of a patient with posttraumatic arthritis secondary to fracture dislocation of the hip. Subtle density indicates a significant posterior wall fragment *(arrow)*. A CT scan demonstrated a large posterior wall fragment that migrated superiorly **(B)** and a significant posterior wall defect **(C)**. Screw fixation of the acetabular component was utilized **(D)** because of partial uncoverage of the component posteriorly as a result of the defect **(E)**.

The preferred lateral projection of the hip advocated by most authors for preoperative planning is a modification of the frog-leg lateral, the table-down or Lowenstein lateral x-ray. This is obtained with the patient supine and the hip externally rotated so that the hip, knee, and ankle are contacting the table top (Fig. 13A). The femur is usually closer to the table in this position than in the standard AP radiograph, because the distance to the femur is less and results in less magnification. Again, a magnification marker is useful in estimating the degree of magnification. This projection is best for determining the maximum bow of the femur and estimating the true degree of anteversion of the femoral neck. To obtain an orthogonal view to the AP projection with the limb internally rotated, the knee can be lifted at an angle of 15° to 20° from the table top (see Fig. 13B).

Other lateral radiographic views have been described for the hip, both before and after hip arthroplasty. The cross table or modified surgical lateral is obtained by extending the affected side and flexing and externally rotating the contralateral side. This is a more useful lateral projection of the acetabulum than of the femur. This

femur is magnified and foreshortened because of the distance from the cassette (13). The frog-leg lateral is obtained with the hip flexed and externally rotated, the knee flexed, and the foot typically braced against the contralateral knee. Again, the femur is magnified a variable amount because of the distance from the cassette, and this does not yield as consistent an image as the Lowenstein lateral for preoperative lateral templating of the femur.

Radiographic Review

Once standard radiographic views are obtained, it is appropriate to review the films in a general way to confirm the original or working diagnosis prior to embarking on preoperative planning. If the trabecular pattern is coarsened and irregular, for instance, Paget's disease should be considered. Laboratory values from serum and urine may be appropriate to determine if the patient is in the active, lytic phase of the disease, in which case medical treatment with deferral of surgery may be appropriate (11,43,52). This would also alert the surgeon to carefully review long films of the femur in the AP and lateral projections for bowing, which could make stem insertion difficult. It may be difficult to distinguish bone pain from Paget's disease from the accompanying degenerative joint disease. Intra-articular injection of a local anesthetic has been suggested as a method of making this distinction (43).

Other relevant systemic diseases may be discovered by general radiographic review. If the patient is male with hypertrophic osteoarthritis, and prominent syndesmophytes are visible in the lower lumbar spine on the AP pelvis view, the diagnosis of diffuse idiopathic skeletal hyperostosis (DISH) should be entertained. Perioperative radiation or indomethacin may be elected in such cases for prophylaxis of heterotopic ossification. In patients with sickle cell disease, the intertrochanteric region should be examined for evidence of bone infarcts or obliteration of the intramedullary canal (Fig. 14A). The bone can be very sclerotic and require special drills to penetrate and reestablish the canal (see Fig. 14B). There is a high risk of perforation in such cases (21), and fluoroscopy may even be advisable to lower the risk. Similar concerns exist in osteopetrosis and Paget's disease (14).

After confirming the diagnosis, radiographs should be examined for bone quality. This is an important factor for prosthesis selection for many surgeons (22). In the past, the Singh index was commonly utilized (68), and it has been modified for purposes of classifying bone density for preoperative component selection (30). More recently, Dossick et al. (27) described a method of classifying proximal femoral geometry based on the calcar-to-canal ratio. The outer diameter of the femur at the midportion of the lesser trochanter is divided by the diameter at a point 10 cm distal (Fig. 15). A ratio of less than 0.5 is

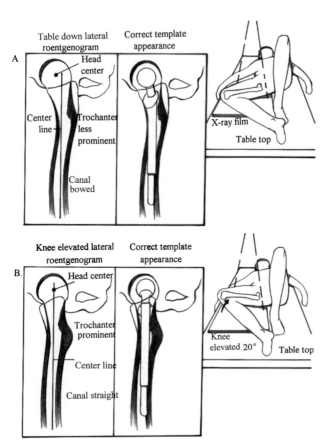

FIG. 13. Patient positioning for modified frog-leg lateral (Lowenstein lateral) view. With the knee flat on the table, the maximum anterior bow of the femur is visualized **(A)**. With the knee 20° elevated, the view is rotated 90° (orthogonal) from the AP view **(B)**.

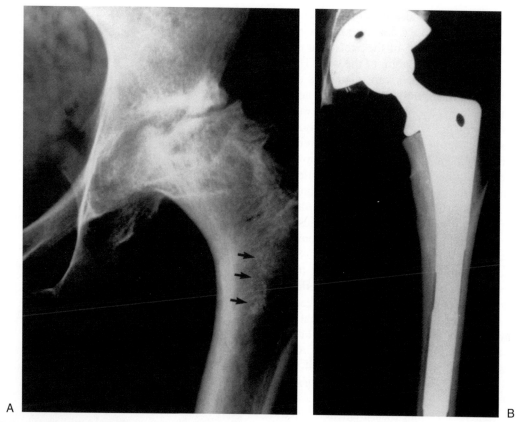

FIG. 14. A: A patient with sickle cell anemia has subtle calcification and density changes in the inter-trochanteric area *(arrows)*. B: Drills and high-speed burrs were necessary to reestablish the canal prior to insertion of a cementless femoral stem.

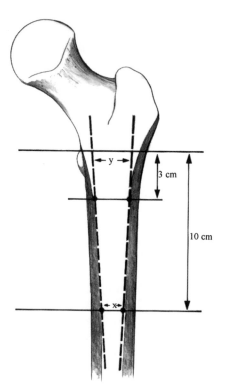

FIG. 15. Measurement of the calcar-to-canal ratio.

classified as type A, between 0.5 and 0.75 is type B, and more than 0.75 is type C. Type A bone has also been described qualitatively as demonstrating cortices on both the AP and lateral radiographs, whereas type B bone has thinning of the posterior cortex on the lateral view, and type C has thinning of cortices on both views, typical of a "stovepipe" femur (27). Type A bone is generally believed to be most amenable to an uncemented femoral component (26). Type C bone favors the use of a cemented stem, and type B bone is intermediate.

Radiographic Landmarks

Prior to actual templating, it is useful to mark anatomic landmarks and record certain measurements. In the past, the ilioischial line (Kohler's line) has been used to estimate the degree of protrusio acetabuli radiographically. This line extends from the sciatic notch to the lateral edge of the obturator foramen. A study by Goodman et al. demonstrated that estimates of protrusion based on this landmark were variable depending on the degree of pelvic rotation (33). Kohler's line is actually posterior to the medial wall of the pelvis and only overlies it on a true AP view. The acetabular teardrop is an anatomic landmark present in the inferomedial aspect of the acetabulum just superior and lateral to the obturator foramen. Its lateral lip represents the exterior of the acetabular wall and the medial lip the interior margin of the wall. These relationships do not vary as much with rotation as does Kohler's line, and the teardrop represents an actual anatomic landmark of the inferomedial acetabulum rather than a radiographic image. The teardrop has become a pivotal landmark for preoperative planning as well as postoperative measurement of component migration. A horizontal line can be constructed connecting the inferior margins of both teardrops on the AP pelvis radiographs. Vertical lines are constructed bisecting the teardrops extending superiorly. The center of the femoral heads are located, and the horizontal and vertical distance from the teardrop to the center of the head can be determined. Special templates devised by Müller facilitate taking these measurements (Müller Foundation, Bern, Switzerland) (75). Templates of concentric circles can be utilized to locate the center of the head (Fig. 16). The horizontal and vertical coordinates give an accurate recording of the center of rotation of the normal and pathologic hip. Average coordinates reported in normal adults are 14 mm vertical and 37 mm horizontal from the acetabular teardrop (64,67).

Another important radiographic measurement is that of limb length. This is commonly estimated by drawing a horizontal line along the inferior margin of both ischial tuberosities (interischial line) (34). The vertical distance from this line to either the top or the bottom of the lesser trochanter of each hip is measured. The distance between the two is recorded as the limb length discrepancy (Fig. 17). This should be correlated with clinical measurements and any significant difference should be evaluated and resolved prior to surgery. The presence of flexion contracture may result in a clinical measurement of shortening, whereas adduction contracture may give the appearance of lengthening. The amount of desired lengthening should be well established preoperatively and incorporated into the plan. If the operative limb appears long preoperatively, the patient should be advised that it may well remain long postoperatively, because shortening may increase the risk of instability. Change in limb length is a major cause of litigation in total hip replacement, the most common problem being lengthening of the operative limb. This risk can be minimized by careful preoperative planning, and if lengthening appears to be a potential problem, this should be emphasized in preoperative counseling and informed consent.

The neck–shaft angle, defined as the angle between the central axis of the femur and the axis of the femoral neck, is a useful measurement. There is wide variation of this angle, with a reported mean of 124.7 ± 7.4 (56). If the neck–shaft angle of the component utilized varies significantly from the anatomic angle, the level of the neck resection will be affected.

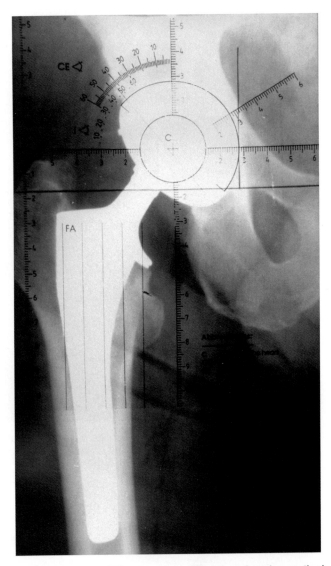

FIG. 16. Use of Müller templates to determine the vertical and horizontal distances from the teardrop to the center of rotation. These can be used preoperatively as well as postoperatively.

The femoral offset is defined as the perpendicular distance from the neutral long axis of the femur and the center of rotation of the hip. (see Fig. 17). Restoring the normal degree of offset is a primary goal of hip replacement, thus making this measurement valuable. Because the amount of offset is affected by the degenerative process, it is useful to measure the offset on the contralateral normal hip.

The degree of acetabular dysplasia can be measured as described by Ranawat (57). A line is drawn from the inferior edge of the teardrop to the superolateral edge of the acetabulum (see Fig. 17). The angle between this line and the line connecting the teardrops should be 45°, which indicates that some degree of dysplasia is present.

A measurement of academic interest is the abductor moment arm. This is estimated by drawing a line between

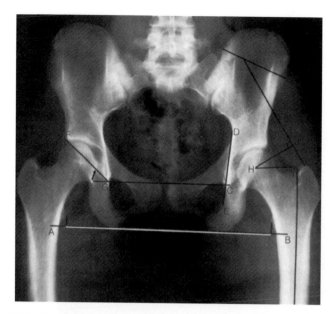

FIG. 17. Preoperative measurements include interischial line (AB), Kohler's line (DE), interteardrop line (CG), offset (HI), and abductor moment arm (HJ).

the anterior superior and posterior superior iliac spines. A line is drawn from a point one third of the way from the posterior to the anterior superior spine, to the tip of the trochanter (see Fig. 17). This approximates the line of the pull of the gluteus medius (23). A perpendicular is then constructed from the center of rotation of the head to this line, and its length represents the abductor moment arm.

TEMPLATING

Restoring proper hip biomechanics was a primary objective of total hip replacement as described by Charnley (20). Preoperative measurement of x-rays was emphasized in his original text. With the use of cement on both the acetabular and the femoral side, the surgeon has the ability to vary the placement of either component within the cement envelope. With the widespread use of cementless implants in the 1980s, the placement of components became largely determined by the patient's anatomy. Surgeons therefore lost the ability to customize component placement, and preoperative templating became even more crucial in planning the cementless total hip replacement. Dr. Charles Engh can be credited with refining the radiographic techniques and templating principles required for the more demanding challenge presented in preoperative planning for the cementless total hip replacement (29,30). This can best be accomplished by careful preoperative templating of appropriate radiographs. The general goals are to restore as nearly as possible the anatomic or premorbid center of rotation and femoral offset, while equalizing limb length.

Acetabular Side

Templating appropriately begins with the acetabular side, because this is the sequence that is followed in surgery. The acetabular template is placed just lateral to the lateral edge of the teardrop at a 45-degree angle. Ideally, the cup should be completely covered by bone and should span the distance between the teardrop and the superolateral margin of the acetabulum. The component size that best accomplishes this with minimal removal of subchondral bone is selected. For cemented sockets, a uniform 2- to 3-mm space must be left for cement. This is often indicated on templates by a dashed line. The center of rotation is marked through the template. If the component's medial edge is just lateral to the teardrop, the horizontal and vertical distances from the teardrop should closely approximate those of the contralateral normal hip. Müller templates facilitate comparison of the proposed center of rotation to that of the normal side (75).

Protrusio Acetabuli Cases

Protrusio acetabuli is present in a number of primary hip replacements, particularly in cases of rheumatoid arthritis, ankylosing spondylitis, Paget's disease, and any metabolic bone disease that weakens the subchondral bone. Leaving the hip center in the medialized location is not advisable, because there is often not optimal structural support for the component in that position, and the opportunity to restore medial bone should be utilized. The femoral head can be morselized and used as a medial graft to lateralize the component to a more normal anatomic position. It should be noted that a large volume of morselized bone may be necessary to achieve component lateralization, and it may be necessary to utilize additional allograft material in addition to the autograft from the femoral head (Fig. 18).

Lateralizing the component in cases of protrusio acetabuli has the additional advantage of increasing femoral offset and decreasing the tendency for impingement. Because the cup is contacting bone graft medially rather than structurally supportive subchondral bone, a large component is needed to achieve peripheral rim contact. Failure to achieve initial stability through a tight rim fit risks fracture of the medial wall during insertion or medial migration and recurrence of protrusio acetabuli over time.

Significant lengthening occurs through the acetabulum in protrusio acetabuli cases. It is therefore common to lengthen the involved extremity during reconstruction. This is often desirable, since the limb is often short in these cases. Protrusio acetabuli is often bilateral and, when it is, both hips are often involved with the pathologic process. In such cases, the patient should be advised that there may be a significant degree of lengthening of

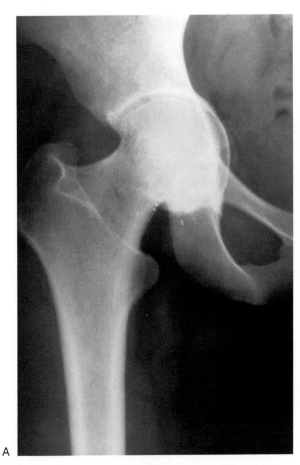 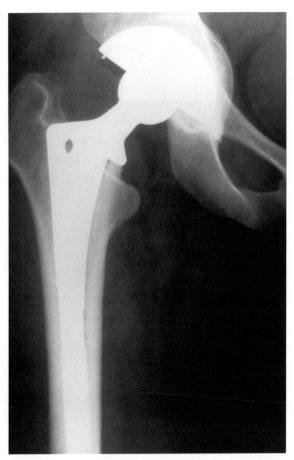

FIG. 18. A: Preoperative radiograph of patient with primary protrusio. **B:** Morselizing femoral head plus additional allograft was necessary to densely pack bone medially. Low neck cut was necessary to avoid overlengthening.

the first hip, but that there will be the opportunity to equalize the limb length when the other hip replacement is performed.

In cases of longstanding protrusio acetabuli, there is often ankylosis of the hip with contracture of the capsule and surrounding soft tissue. When lengthening occurs through lateralizing the socket, the amount of further lengthening that can reasonably be obtained may be limited. As a result, a lower neck cut and shorter prosthetic neck segment may be utilized in these cases (see Fig. 18B).

In cases where protrusio acetabuli is associated with severe osteoporosis, as in juvenile rheumatoid arthritis, it is occasionally prudent to consider a protrusio ring or cage. Insertion of an uncemented press-fit component in such cases can risk acetabular or pelvic fracture.

Lateralized Acetabulum

In many cases of degenerative osteoarthritis, the presence of hypertrophic osteophytes in the acetabulum causes lateralization of the hip's center of rotation. This occurs most often in men with hypertrophic osteoarthritis. This becomes apparent during templating when 1 or 2 cm of reaming is noted to be necessary to place the component in the vicinity of the teardrop. Failure to recognize this will result in placement of the acetabular component in a lateralized position with incomplete bony coverage and suboptimal stability, particularly when a press-fit cementless acetabular component is implanted without screws (Fig. 19). Complete peripheral rim contact is desirable to obtain immediate stability with press-fit acetabular components. Complete bony coverage is also desirable for cemented sockets. Higher degrees of cemented acetabular component coverage have been associated with lower loosening rates (66). A recent study has also shown that increased horizontal distance from the teardrop (lack of adequate medialization of a lateralized acetabulum) was the most significant factor predictive of an unfavorable radiographic appearance of a cemented acetabular component (44).

Identifying the anatomic location of the hip joint in such cases can be difficult. The most reliable structural

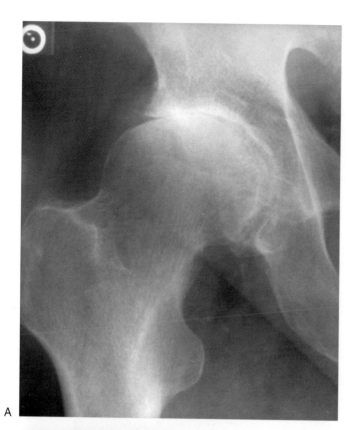

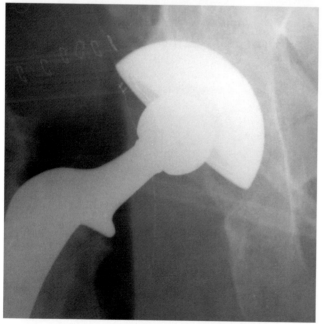

FIG. 19. A: Preoperative radiograph with lateralized acetabulum. **B:** Inadequate reaming of medial osteophyte left the acetabular component laterally displaced and incompletely covered.

landmark is the transverse acetabular ligament that marks the inferior border of the true acetabulum and the location of the teardrop (24). Often, the cotyloid notch or "horseshoe" is completely overgrown with cartilage and not visually discernible. If reaming is initiated above the transverse acetabular ligament in a straight medial direction for several millimeters, the location of the notch becomes apparent and it can be curetted of bone, cartilage, and soft tissue, and the unicortical inner plate of the acetabulum can be visualized at its base. Straight medial reaming to within a few millimeters of the planned depth of reaming is advisable to avoid superior placement of the component. If reaming is initiated at the 45-degree angle in such a scenario, the reamers will cut a path that is equally superior and medial resulting in higher cup placement. This can be avoiding by straight medial reaming with smaller reamers to close to the desired depth initially, followed by progressively larger reamers to enlarge the periphery in the desired orientation (Fig. 20).

It is not necessary or desirable to ream the entire way to the unicortical plate in all such cases. If the acetabular component is completely contained within bone, further reaming may be counterproductive. It is probably better to maintain bone stock and leave the component somewhat lateralized. Charnley (20) emphasized the risk of impingement, instability, and restricted motion, which could result from overreaming in such cases. Leaving the cup in this position relatively increases offset and the abductor moment arm, which is generally advantageous.

Superolateral Migration

In addition to medial and lateral displacement, many degenerative hips migrate in a superolateral direction. This is most common in women with some degree of dysplasia. Because of the shallowness of the acetabulum and the incomplete coverage of the femoral head, forces are concentrated on the superolateral joint margin, which initially becomes flattened and eventually erodes away with subsequent superior migration of the hip and shortening of the extremity (Fig. 21). This becomes apparent when the template is placed adjacent to the teardrop and a significant portion of the lateral margin remains uncovered (see Fig. 21B). A number of options exist in such cases. If there is a well-established pseudoacetabulum, a smaller component can be placed at a high hip center (64,67). There are a number of potential disadvantages to this approach. The supporting bone available in this location is small in dimension and may not provide adequate coverage. Small components are often required, necessitating the use of a 22-mm head to allow for adequate polyethylene thickness. This exacerbates the tendency for instability resulting from impingement on the anterior column and anterior inferior iliac spine with flexion and internal rotation, and on the ischium in extension and external

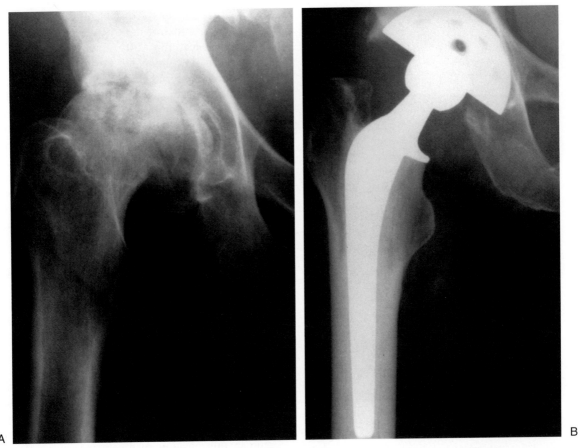

FIG. 20. A: Lateralized acetabulum with extensive medial osteophyte. **B:** Medial reaming allowed complete coverage and placement of component at level of teardrop.

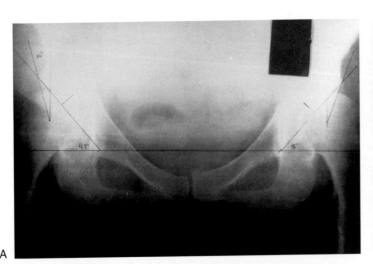
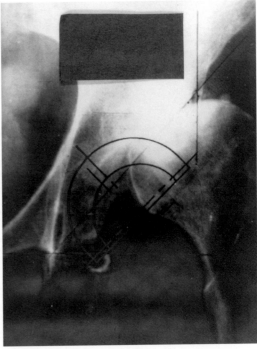

FIG. 21. A: Radiograph showing incomplete coverage of the femoral head and early degenerative arthritis. **B:** Three years later, there is superolateral migration with erosion and flattening.

rotation. There is also substantial evidence that superior and lateral placement increases forces across the hip, thereby increasing the risks of accelerated polyethylene wear and acetabular loosening. A well-defined pseudoacetabulum is more common in severe degrees of dysplasia or complete dislocations (whose management is discussed elsewhere). In the more subtle degrees of dysplasia and accompanying migration, there is often inadequate bone to ream in the superolateral margin, and anatomic cup placement is preferred (6,7).

When the template is placed adjacent to the teardrop and the lateral margin is uncovered, a number of options exist. Medial reaming to the subchondral plate and use of a low-profile cup will minimize the degree of uncoverage. Ten percent to 20% uncoverage can be accepted, and screws can be used to augment fixation of cementless components because there will not be circumferential peripheral contact. In cemented components, cement augmentation of the superolateral deficiency has been described without deleterious effects on component fixation in the 5- to 10-year time frame (55). The acetabular component can be positioned somewhat vertically, and an offset liner can be placed in the superior position to compensate for this. If the cup remains more than 10% to 20% uncovered in spite of all of these maneuvers, a structural graft fixed to the pelvis can be considered (Fig. 22). This possibility should be recognized during templating, because a significant amount of additional equipment may be required. Surgical techniques for implanting cementless components with structural femoral head autograft have been described (6,7). Equipment utilized typically includes drills, taps, screws, and washers from a typical fracture fixation set. Titanium or cobalt chrome screws and washers have a the-

oretical advantage over stainless steel, because the screws will be in close proximity and in the same aqueous environment as the acetabular and femoral head components. A high-speed burr and cup arthroplasty reamers have been found to be useful in shaping the graft.

When structural grafting is performed, significant lengthening will occur through the acetabular component. This may necessitate a lower neck cut and shorter prosthetic neck length to avoid overlengthening. In cases where significant length changes are anticipated, it is particularly appropriate to use one of a number of intraoperative devices to measure length (74,77). Most such devices utilize a pin fixed superiorly in the ilium and a fixed point laterally on the femur, and the distance between the two points is measured with the extremity in the same position before hip dislocation and after trial reduction. If lengthening of more than 2 cm is anticipated, the use of SSEP is an option to consider to minimize the risk of nerve palsy (73).

The presence of hip dysplasia should also alert the surgeon to the possibility of excessive femoral anteversion, which is a common coexisting condition. If a cemented stem is selected, a smaller, straighter stem, such as a congenital-hip-dysplasia (CDH) stem, may be necessary. The stem can simply be rotated within the cement column to compensate for the excessive anteversion. In these cases, however, the greater trochanter is often posteriorly rotated, and during trial reduction the direction of pull of the abductors should be observed and the hip should be carefully checked for impingement of the trochanter in extension and external rotation. It may be necessary to osteotomize the trochanter and reattach it further anteriorly and laterally.

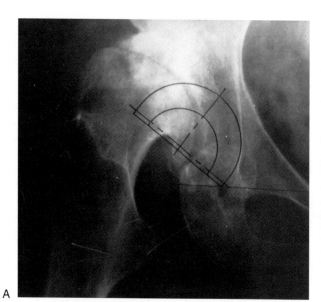
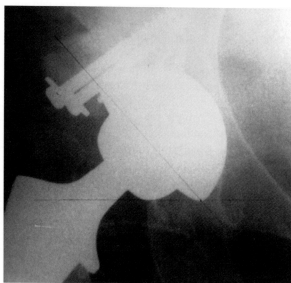

A

B

FIG. 22. A: Significant superior deficit remains with cup placed in anatomic position. **B:** Structural graft allows restoration of normal center of rotation.

If an uncemented, press-fit stem is selected, excessive anteversion presents a challenge for which there are a number of potential solutions. A custom prosthesis can be generated with a CT scan that allows fit and fill of the distorted anatomy along with appropriate adjustment in the version of the prosthetic neck relative to the shaft. This has the disadvantage of the additional expense of the scan and the prosthesis, as well as the commitment to a single component geometry than may not be stable when implanted in the anatomic environment of that particular patient. A modular stem can be utilized with a metaphyseal portion oriented to the degree of anteversion of the patient's anatomy (16). The stem can then be rotated within the metaphyseal portion in a variety of positions until maximal stability is achieved. If an off-the-shelf cementless stem is utilized, there are at least two options. If the stem is straight and parallel-sided and the neck is anteverted 10°, implanting a left stem in a right hip (or vice versa) will provide relative retroversion of 20°, which may be adequate for mild or moderate degrees of excessive anteversion. Another option includes performing a subtrochanteric osteotomy of the femur to derotate the proximal fragment prior to inserting the cementless stem (37,38,70).

Because of all of the surgical implications of increased femoral anteversion, it is important to recognize this entity preoperatively. With careful attention to the details of the physical examination and radiographic review, this should not be difficult in the majority of cases.

Identifying the Center of Rotation

The ideal position for the acetabular template (and component) is achieved by placing the inferomedial edge adjacent to the lateral margin of the teardrop. In most patients, this will restore the center of rotation very close to an anatomic and desirable location. This can be checked by measuring the horizontal and vertical distances from the teardrop to the templated center of rotation, and comparing them to the coordinates from the teardrop to the center of the normal or unaffected contralateral hip. If the distances are equal and there is no difference in limb length, than this point can be utilized as the point about which the reconstruction can be planned. If a limb-length discrepancy is present with the affected side short, which is most often the case, the center of rotation planning point is moved superiorly above the templating point the number of millimeters of the planned correction, and this point is utilized for subsequent templating.

Femoral Templating

After the planned center of rotation of the reconstruction is marked on the radiograph, the femur is templated, referencing from this point. The goals and emphasis of femoral templating vary depending on whether a cementless proximally coated, cementless extensively coated, or cemented stem is planned. It also varies somewhat depending on whether the stem is straight or anatomic. Although in practice most surgeons have a strong tendency to implant the same type of stem for most of their cases, it is prudent to template for both a cemented and cementless stem, particularly in cases where any anatomic abnormality is identified. Cementless components require immediate stable fixation at the time of implantation. If difficulty is encountered in reaming and broaching, or immediate stability is not achieved, it is probably best to implant a cemented stem.

Component size is judged from the AP radiograph of the hip. For proximally coated components, proximal fit and fill are generally emphasized. For extensively coated cementless stems, fixation is obtained distally, so a tight fit in the isthmus is sought. Contact of the stem medially and laterally with the endosteal sidewalls over several centimeters is recommended (29,30). For cemented stems, it is important to leave adequate room for a cement mantle. A 2- to 3-mm circumferential cement mantle is optimal. It is crucial to perform femoral templating on radiographs with the correct degree of rotation (15° to 20° of internal rotation) to most accurately predict stem size, neck length, offset, and neck resection level. If the affected side has an external rotation contracture and the contralateral side is normal, then templating begins with acetabular templating on the affected side. The center of rotation is marked on the x-ray, and the horizontal and vertical distances from the teardrops are measured. These coordinates are used to transpose the center of rotation to the unaffected side where femoral templating can be performed (29).

The femoral template is moved vertically until the center of the femoral head template is at the same vertical height as the planned acetabular center of rotation. Regardless of the stem type utilized, the templates should be kept centered along the neutral axis of the femur, rather than in any varus or valgus inclination. Ideally, femoral bone stock should be maintained and neck cuts should be planned between 1 and 2 cm above the lesser trochanter. If the center of rotation of the femur overlies the planned center of rotation of the hip, then length and offset will be restored. The neck resection level is marked though the template and the distance above the lesser trochanter can be measured with a ruler with the appropriate level of magnification, so the appropriate neck resection level can be reproduced during surgery. If the center of the femoral head template lies medial to the planned center of hip rotation when the template is at the appropriate height, stem insertion to this level will increase femoral offset, which is generally an advantage, particularly if it is a matter of a few millimeters. Excessive increase in offset may cause prominence of the trochanter with a tendency towards bursitis and should be avoided.

If the center of the femoral head template lies lateral to the planned center of hip rotation, then the reconstruction will decrease femoral offset, and this is particularly to be avoided. Charnley (20) was among the first to emphasize restoring normal hip biomechanics as a goal of hip replacement, and one of the cornerstones of this philosophy was restoring or increasing abductor moment arm. He accomplished this by utilizing a component of appropriate offset, making the neck cut at the appropriate level, and lateralizing the trochanter. Now that trochanteric osteotomy is rarely performed in primary total hip arthroplasty, the major tool at the disposal of the surgeon for increasing the abductor moment arm is restoring or increasing the femoral offset (71).

Decreasing offset has a number of negative effects. The decrease in abductor moment arm decreases abductor strength. A study from McGrory et al. (54) showed less strength in isokinetic testing in hips with lesser offset. Another study by Rothman et al. (61) showed a higher incidence of limp with low-offset hip replacements. Lowering the abductor moment arm increases joint reaction forces, which could lead either to higher rates of acetabular loosening or increased rates of polyethylene wear. Robinson et al. (59) were able to demonstrate a correlation between low offset and higher rate of polyethylene wear. Finally, decreasing offset leads to laxity in the abductor musculature, which could lead to a higher incidence of instability. Increasing evidence of the advantage of restoring offset has led to a resurgence of interest in this concept (71).

A number of options exist to avoid performing a reconstruction that decreases offset. Seating the component lower, using a long neck cut, and utilizing a longer head will compensate for small decreases in offset (Fig. 23). This sacrifices bone, however, and it changes the fit of the proximal femoral component, which is a particular concern in proximally coated cementless stems. Anatomic stems in particular must have the neck cut made at a predetermined height to avoid anterior impingement of

the tip of the stem distally. A larger-size component may be considered if going to the next size increases the base offset. The anatomy of the femur may preclude this, however. If a cemented stem is utilized, adequate room for the cement mantle must be assured if a large stem is considered. This might entail drilling of the femur to ensure a 2-mm mantle. Another option is switching to a different stem design that has a higher base offset. Offset can be increased in a number of ways, including changing the neck–shaft angle, changing the proximal geometry, and medializing the take-off point of the neck from the stem. Because of the complexity of going from one stem to another, it is important to plan the strategy for restoring offset preoperatively. In recent years, a popular solution has been the dual offset total hip. This allows the same stem and the same neck resection level to be utilized with two different base offsets (Fig. 24).

The neck resection should be planned so as to utilize a neck length without a "skirt," or thickened extension of the head, as this tends to impinge at extremes of motion (47). Such impingement will result in restricted motion, polyethylene wear, and/or instability. Most implant systems offer four or five head choices, of which the first two or three do not have a skirt or extension. Generally, reconstructions are planned around a short neck length (high neck cut), because calcar planers are often utilized and the broach can always be countersunk and further planing done. Alternatively, the neck can be re-cut. This is preferable to too low a resection level, resulting in the necessity of utilizing a long or extra-long neck, which typically comes with a skirt.

After planning the size and neck resection level, the lateral radiographs must be templated to assure fit can be achieved with the planned stem diameter and length. If stem impingement is predicted, options include varying the entry point in the AP plane, switching to an anatomic (bowed) stem, or implanting a cemented stem (Fig. 25).

The AP radiograph is also useful for planning an entry point. By drawing the neutral axis of the femur and

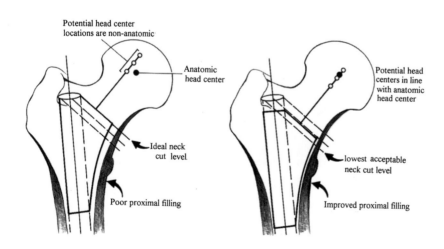

FIG. 23. Seating component lower and using longer neck affects offset as well as proximal fill.

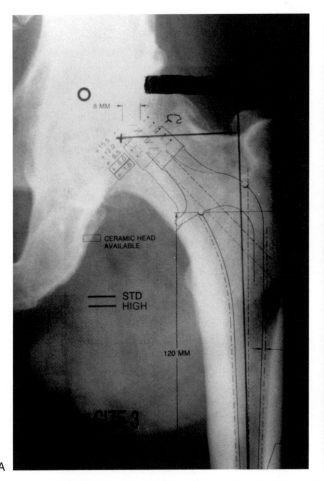

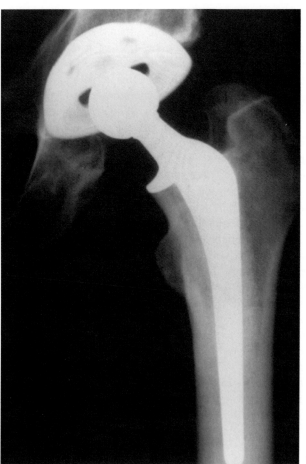

A

B

FIG. 24. A: Preoperative radiograph of patient with a high-offset total hip, requiring the extra offset option to reproduce the anatomic offset. **B:** High-offset component restored anatomic offset.

extending it proximally, the appropriate entry point can be located. This is more crucial in a cementless stem. Typically, this involves a lateral entry site near the pyriformis fossa and requires removal of any remnants of the lateral aspect of the femoral neck.

The planned component size and distal canal diameter should be measured on the AP radiograph and used as a reference during surgery. If difficulty is encountered seating reamers and broaches below the planned size, often the entry point is incorrect, usually medial, and reaming and broaching is often being done in a varus orientation. If difficulties persist, an intraoperative x-ray with a broach in place will often confirm the problem (Fig. 26). If reaming of the femur is proceeding above the planned size, it may also be prudent to obtain an intraoperative radiograph with a reamer or broach in place. Reamers can ream away cortical bone, particularly in osteoporotic patients, leading to potential complications. If cortical bone is being reamed without significant resistance, the choice of a cementless stem should probably be reconsidered. Isthmus diameter is also helpful to know for selecting the appropriate-size canal plug for cemented stems.

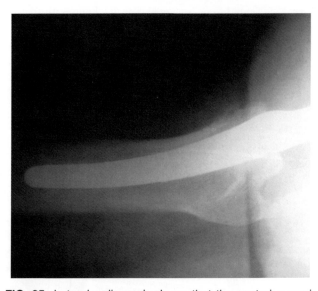

FIG. 25. Lateral radiograph shows that the posterior proximal femur was well accommodated by an anatomic stem. The use of a straight stem would have required a more posterolateral entry point to center the component in the lateral plane.

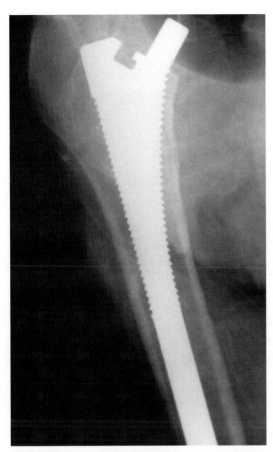

FIG. 26. Intraoperative radiograph with broach well below the anticipated size shows the relative varus and medial entry points.

Neck–Shaft Angle

If the neck–shaft angle is measured preoperatively, it can be compared to the neck–shaft angle of the implant to be utilized. If there is a difference of more than a few degrees, a predictable pattern of intraoperative adjustments can be made. The average neck–shaft angle is approximately 125°, whereas most implant systems have a neck–shaft angle of 130° to 135°. Values significantly lower than this represent coxa vara, and values above this represent coxa valga.

Coxa Vara

Patients with coxa vara have higher than usual femoral offset. This can be compensated for by utilizing a component with a lower neck–shaft angle, or by making a lower neck cut and utilizing a longer neck. Making a standard-length neck cut can significantly lengthen the leg without restoring offset. The use of high-offset components or components with a lower neck–shaft angle help preserve bone by minimizing the necessity of the low neck cut (Fig. 27).

Coxa Valga

The opposite situation exists when the patient's neck–shaft angle significantly exceeds that of the prosthesis. There is a relatively low offset and more length. To compensate for this with a component with less valgus, it is necessary to make a higher neck cut and use a shorter neck to maintain length and offset (see Fig. 27).

Coxa Breva

When avascular necrosis of the capital femoral epiphysis occurs early in life, as in Perthes disease, a short femoral neck (coxa breva) can result. In these cases, length and offset are usually increased when using a standard acetabular component. If a standard neck cut and neck length are employed, overlengthening may occur. Often a low neck cut and short head may be necessary to avoid this (Fig. 28).

Accuracy of Templating

A recent study demonstrated that an experienced surgeon can preoperatively predict component size in 95%

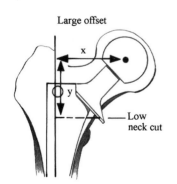
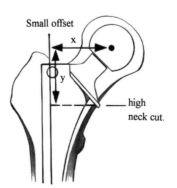

FIG. 27. Variations in component positioning depend on the patient's anatomy. Using a fixed neck–shaft angle prosthesis and coxa vara, a low neck cut combined with a longer neck prosthesis is necessary to reproduce anatomy. In coxa valga, a high neck cut and a shorter neck prosthesis are necessary to reproduce, length and offset.

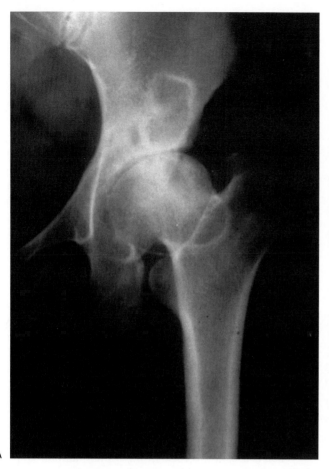

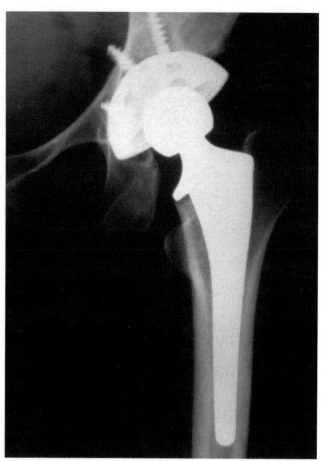

A   B

FIG. 28. A: Preoperative radiograph demonstrates coxa breva secondary to Perthes disease. **B:** Postoperative radiograph demonstrates that a standard cup resulted in lengthening that restored equal lengths, but a low neck cut and short neck were necessary to avoid overlengthening.

of cases (18). When preoperative planning was combined with intraoperative limb-length measurement, lengthening of more than 6.0 mm was seen in only 25% of patients, the lowest report by far (76,2). Clearly, the best chance of restoring hip center of rotation, leg length, and femoral offset is through careful preoperative planning.

CONCLUSION

Preoperative planning is crucial to the success of primary total hip arthroplasty. Data gathered from the history, review of systems, physical examination, review of radiographs, and templating are synthesized into an organized plan of attack for each case. Based on this information, the operative approach is selected as well as the type of components to be utilized. If cementless components are planned, it is often prudent to have an alternative plan for the use of a cemented component. The sizes of components anticipated are recorded, and if significant deviation from the plan occurs intraoperatively, an explanation should be sought. Intraoperative x-rays can often resolve

the discrepancy. With such an organized approach, the need for adequate implants, instruments, and graft material can be anticipated, and intraoperative surprises can be minimized. This shifts the learning curve in favor of the surgeons, shortens operative time, and minimizes complications. Such an approach is also more likely to lead to consistent, reproducible results, while making the most efficient use of available resources.

ACKNOWLEDGMENTS

The author wishes to thank Mrs. Gerrie Savage for her tireless efforts in compiling and editing material for this chapter.

REFERENCES

1. Aaron A, Weinstein D, Thickman D, Eilert R. Comparison of orthoroentgenography and computed tomography in the measurement of limb-length discrepancy. *J Bone Joint Surg Am* 1992;74(6):897–902.
2. Abraham WD, Dimon JH III. Leg length discrepancy in total hip arthroplasty. *Orthop Clin North Am* 1992;23(2):201–209.

3. Aufranc OE, Aufranc ST. Evaluation of the patient with an arthritic hip. In: Stillwell WT, ed. *The art of total hip arthroplasty*. Florida: Grune & Stratton, 1987;123–132.

4. Balderston RA. Surgical approaches. In: Balderston RA, Rothman RH, Booth RE, Hozack WJ, eds. *The hip*. Philadelphia: Lea & Febiger, 1992;70–91.

5. Balderston RA, Hillard WDB, Iannotti JP, et al. Treatment of the septic hip with total hip arthroplasty. *Clin Orthop* 1987;221:231–237.

6. Barrack RL, Newland CC. Uncemented total hip arthroplasty with superior acetabular deficiency. *J Arthroplasty* 1990;5(2):159–167.

7. Barrack RL, Newland CC. A technique of acetabular reconstruction for uncemented total hip replacement. *Orthop Rev* 1990;19(10):807–816.

8. Binns M, Pho R. Femoral vein occlusion during hip arthroplasty. *Clin Orthop* 1990;255:168–172.

9. Bischoff R, Dunlap J, Carpenter L, DeMouy E, Barrack RL. Heterotopic ossification following uncemented total hip arthroplasty. Effect of the operative approach. *J Arthroplasty* 1994;9(6):641–644.

10. Buly RL, Huo M, Root L, Binzer T, Wilson PD Jr. Total hip arthroplasty in cerebral palsy. Long-term follow-up results. *Clin Orthop* 1993;296:148–153.

11. Cafflin FS, Singer FR. Paget's disease of bone: path of physiology, diagnosis, and management. *J Am Acad Orthop Surg* 1995;3(6):336–344.

12. Callaghan JJ. The clinical results and basic science of total hip arthroplasty with porous-coated prosthesis. *J Bone Joint Surg Am* 1993;75(2):299–310.

13. Cameron HU, ed. *The technique of total hip arthroplasty*. St. Louis: Mosby, 1992.

14. Cameron HU. Hip replacement in the absence of a medullary canal. *Contemp Orthop* 1991;22(6):669–672.

15. Cameron HU. Hip surgery in aortofemoral bypass patient. *Orthop Rev* 1988;17:195–197.

16. Cameron HU. The use of a distally fluted long stem hip prosthesis in correction of angular deformities of the femur. *Contemp Orthop* 1990;20:159–162.

17. Capello WN. Preoperative planning of the total hip arthroplasty. *Inst Course Lect* 1986;35:249–257.

18. Carter LW, Stovall DO, Young TR. Determination of accuracy of preoperative templating of noncemented femoral prostheses. *J Arthroplasty* 1995;10(4):507–513.

19. Chandler HP, Penenberg BL. Surgical approaches. In: Chandler HP, Penenberg BL, eds. *Bone stock deficiency in total hip replacement. Classification and management*. New Jersey: SLACK, 1989;41–46.

20. Charnley J. *Low friction arthroplasty of the hip*. New York: Springer-Verlag, 1979.

21. Clarke HJ, Jinnah RH, Brooker AF, Michaelson JD. Total replacement of the hip for avascular necrosis in sickle cell disease. *J Bone Joint Surg Br* 1989;71(3):465–470.

22. D'Antonio JA. Preoperative templating and choosing the implant for primary THA in the young patient. *Inst Course Lect* 1994;43:339–346.

23. DeOrio JK, Blasser KE. Indications and patient selection. In: Morrey BF, ed. *Joint replacement arthroplasty*. New York: Churchill Livingstone, 1991;547–559.

24. Dore DD, Rubash H. Primary total hip arthroplasty in the older patient: optimizing the results. *Instr Course Lect* 1994;43:347–357.

25. Dorr LD. Optimizing results of total joint arthroplasty. *Inst Course Lect* 1985;34:401–404.

26. Dorr LD. Total hip replacement using the APR system. *Techniques Orthop* 1986;1(3):22–34.

27. Dossick PH, Dorr LD, Gruen T, Saberi MT. Techniques for preoperative planning and postoperative evaluation of noncemented hip arthroplasty. *Techniques Orthop* 1991;6(3):1–6.

28. Edeen J, Sharkey PF, Alexander AH. Clinical significance of leg-length inequality after total hip arthroplasty. *Am J Orthop* 1995;24(4):347–351.

29. Engh CA. Recent advances in cementless total hip arthroplasty using the AML prosthesis. *Techniques Orthop* 1991;6(3):59–72.

30. Engh CA, Bobyn JD, eds. *Biological fixation in total hip arthroplasty*. New Jersey: SLACK, 1985.

31. Glassman AH, Engh CA, Bobyn JD. A technique of extensile exposure for total hip arthroplasty. *J Arthroplasty* 1987;2(1):11–21.

32. Goldberg BA, Joshi AB, Patel M, Kamaric E. Effect of axial rotation on the measurement of the physiologic valgus angle, neck–shaft angle, and the medial head offset of the femur. Presented at the *62nd annual meeting of the American Academy of Orthopaedic Surgeons*, Orlando, FL, 1995.

33. Goodman SB, Adler SJ, Fyhrie DP, Schurman DJ. The acetabular teardrop and its relevance to acetabular migration. *Clin Orthop* 1988;236:199–204.

34. Gore DR, Murray MP, Gardner GM, Sepic SB. Roentgenographic measurements after Müller total hip replacement. *J Bone Joint Surg Am* 1977;59:948–953.

35. Harris WH, Sledge CB. Total hip and total knee replacement (1). *N Engl J Med* 1990;323(11):725–731.

36. Hoppenfeld S. *Physical examination of the spine and extremities*. New York: Appleton-Century-Crofts, 1976.

37. Holtgrewe JL, Hungerford DS. Primary and revision total hip replacement without cement and with associated femoral osteotomy. *J Bone Joint Surg Am* 1989;71(10):1487–1495.

38. Huo MH, Zatorski LE, Keggi KJ. Oblique femoral osteotomy in cementless total hip arthroplasty. Prospective consecutive series with a 3-year minimum follow-up period. *J Arthroplasty* 1995;10(3):319–327.

39. Jacobs JJ, Kull LR, Frey GA, Gitelis S, Sheinkop MB, Kramer TS, Rosenberg AG. Early failure of acetabular components inserted without cement after previous pelvic irradiation. *J Bone Joint Surg Am* 1995;77(12):1829–1835.

40. Jerry GJ, Rand JA, Ilstrup D. Old sepsis prior to total knee arthroplasty. *Clin Orthop* 1988;236:135–140.

41. Johnston RC. Cost effectiveness of total hip replacement. Presented at the *22nd annual meeting of the Harvard Hip Course*, Boston, MA, 1992.

42. Jupiter JB, Archmurray W, Lowell JD, Harris WH. Total hip arthroplasty in the treatment of adult hips with current or quiescent sepsis. *J Bone Joint Surg Am* 1981;63:194–200.

43. Kaplan FS, Singer FR. Paget's disease of bone: pathophysiology, diagnosis, and management. *J Am Acad Orthop Surg* 1995;3(6):336–344.

44. Karachalios T, Hartofilakidis G, Zacharakis N, Tsekoura M. A 12 to 18 year radiographic follow-up study of Charnley low-friction arthroplasty. The role of the center of rotation. *Clin Orthop* 1993;296:140–147.

45. Kim YH. Total arthroplasty of the hip after childhood sepsis. *J Bone Joint Surg Br* 1991;73(5):783–786.

46. Krackow KA, Steinman H, Cohn BT, Jones LC. Clinical experience with a triradiate exposure of the hip for difficult total hip arthroplasty. *J Arthroplasty* 1988;3(3):267–278.

47. Krushell RJ, Burke DW, Harris WH. Range of motion in contemporary total hip arthroplasty. The impact of modular head–neck components. *J Arthroplasty* 1991;6(2):97–101.

48. Lombardi AV, Mallory TH, Kraus TJ, Vaughn BK. Preliminary report on the S-ROM constraining acetabular insert: a retrospective clinical experience. *Orthopedics* 1991;14(3):297–303.

49. Massin P, Duparc J. Total hip replacement in irradiated hips. A retrospective study of 71 cases. *J Bone Joint Surg Br* 1995;77(6):847–852.

50. Maynard MJ, Ranawat CS, Flynn WF Jr, Umlas ME. Total hip replacement arthroplasty in patients with inflammatory arthritis. *Semin Arthroplasty* 1995;6(3):145–166.

51. McCollum DE, Gray WJ. Dislocation after total hip arthroplasty. Causes and prevention. *Clin Orthop* 1990;(261):159–170.

52. McDonald DJ, Sim FH. Paget's disease. In: Morrey BF, ed. *Joint replacement arthroplasty*. New York: Churchill Livingstone, 1991;725–730.

53. McGee HM, Scott JH. A simple method of obtaining equal leg length in total hip arthroplasty. *Clin Orthop* 1985;194:269–270.

54. McGrory BJ, Morrey BF, Cahalan TD, An KN, Cabanela ME. Effect of femoral offset on range of motion and abductor muscle strength after total hip arthroplasty. *J Bone Joint Surg Br* 1995;77(6):865–869.

55. McQueary FG, Johnston RC. Coxarthrosis after congenital dysplasia: treatment by total hip arthroplasty without acetabular bone grafting. *J Bone Joint Surg Am* 1988;70:1190–1144.

56. Noble PC, Alexander JW, Lindahl LJ, Yew DT, Granberry WM, Tullos HS. The anatomic basis of femoral component design. *Clin Orthop* 1988;235:148–164.

57. Ranawat CS. Preoperative planning for total hip arthroplasty. In: Dorr LD, ed. *Techniques in orthopaedics: revision of total hip and knee*. Baltimore: University Park Press, 1984;1–7.

58. Ritter MA, Stringer EA. Bilateral total hip arthroplasty: a single procedure. *Clin Orthop* 1980;149:185–190.

59. Robinson EJ, Devane PA, Bourne RB, Rorabeck CH, Hardie R. Effect of implant position on polyethylene wear in total hip arthroplasty. Pre-

sented at the *62nd annual meeting of the American Academy of Orthopaedic Surgeons*, Orlando, FL, 1995.

60. Rothman RH, Hozack WJ, eds. *Complications of total hip arthroplasty.* Philadelphia: WB Saunders, 1988.

61. Rothman RH, Hearn SL, Eng KO, Hozack WJ. The effect of varying femoral offset on component fixation in cemented total hip arthroplasty. Presented at the *60th annual meeting of the American Academy of Orthopaedic Surgeons*, San Francisco, CA, 1993.

62. Rorabeck CH, Bourne RB, Laupacis A, Feeny D, Wong C, Tugwell P, Leslie K, Bullas R. A double-blind study of 250 cases comparing cemented with cementless total hip arthroplasty. Cost-effectiveness and its impact on health-related quality of life. *Clin Orthop* 1994;298:156–164.

63. Ruby L, Mital MA, O'Connor J, Patel U. Anteversion of the femoral neck. *J Bone Joint Surg Am* 1979;61(1):46–51.

64. Russotti GM, Harris WH. Proximal placement of the acetabular component in THA: a long-term study. *J Bone Joint Surg Am* 1991;73:587–592.

65. Salvati EA, Hughes P, Lacichiewicz P. Bilateral total hip replacement arthroplasty in one stage. *J Bone Joint Surg Am* 1978;60:640–644.

66. Sarmiento A, Ebramzadeh E, Gogan WJ, McKellop H. Cup containment and orientation in cemented total hip arthroplasties. *J Bone Joint Surg Br* 1990;72:996–1002.

67. Schutzer SF, Harris WH. High placement of porous-coated acetabular components in complex total hip arthroplasty. *J Arthroplasty* 1994;9(4):359–367.

68. Singh M, Nagrath AR, Maini PS. Changes in trabecular pattern of the upper end of the femur as an index of osteoporosis. *J Bone Joint Surg Am* 1970;52(3):457–467.

69. Specter M. Factors augmenting or inhibiting biological fixation. *The hip.* 1987;213–224.

70. Sponseller PD, McBeath AA. Subtrochanteric osteotomy with intramedullary fixation for arthroplasty of the dysplastic hip. A case report. *J Arthroplasty* 1988;3(4):351–354.

71. Steinberg B, Harris WH. The "offset" problem in total hip arthroplasty. *Contemp Orthop* 1922;24:556–562.

72. Tsahakis PJ, Brick GW, Poss R. Surgery of the hip. In: Sledge CB, Ruddy S, Harris ED Jr, Kelley WN, eds. *Arthrtitis surgery*. Philadelphia: WB Saunders, 1994;780–793.

73. Wasielewski RC, Crossett LS, Rubash HE. Neural and vascular injury in total hip arthroplasty. *Orthop Clin North Am* 1992;23(2):219–235.

74. Williamson JA, Reckling FW. Limb-length discrepancy and related problems following total hip joint replacement. *Clin Orthop* 1978;134:135–138.

75. Wilson MG, Nikpoor N, Aliabadi P, Poss R, Weissman BN. The fate of acetabular allografts after bipolar revision arthroplasty of the hip. A radiographic review. *J Bone Joint Surg Am* 1989;71(10):1469–1479.

76. Woolson ST. Leg length equalization during THR. *Orthopedics* 1990;13(1):17–21.

77. Woolson ST, Harris WH. A method of intraoperative limb length measurement in total hip arthroplasty. *Clin Orthop* 1985;194:207–210.

The Adult Hip, edited by J. J. Callaghan,
A. G. Rosenberg, and H. E. Rubash.
Lippincott–Raven Publishers, Philadelphia © 1998.

CHAPTER 59

General Principles of Surgical Technique

Ohannes A. Nercessian and Ravindra P. Joshi

In no other musculoskeletal surgical procedures, and in very few surgical procedures in general, are the basic principles of surgical technique as essential for a favorable outcome as in the total hip arthroplasty procedure. This chapter will outline the operating room environment, the patient positioning, the skin preparation and draping, the use of assistants, and the wound closure necessary to optimize the results of total hip arthroplasty.

THE OPERATING ROOM ENVIRONMENT

To achieve a successful outcome of any surgical procedure, all efforts must be made to prevent or decrease the risk of postoperative complications, including the prevention of surgical infection. Operating room personnel must practice aseptic techniques with respect to the patient, to the operating room instruments, and to themselves. Discipline and efficiency during the procedure will reduce operative times, one factor demonstrated to reduce infection. Optimally, a designated surgical team should become proficient in the procedure.

In 1867, Lister (24) introduced the use of carbolic acid compresses in open fractures and reported a decrease in the infection rate. He then introduced the concept of antiseptic preparation of the skin before elective incisions, and he subsequently popularized use of carbolic acid in all fields of surgery. The classic listerism involved spraying the surgical instrument, the wound, and the surgeons

performing the procedures with carbolic acid. Lister's aseptic technique had significant clinical benefit in abolishing the fulminating and often epidemic hospital sepsis such as infection caused by *Clostridium* organisms. However, infection caused by skin organisms such as *Staphylococcus* and *Streptococcus* species have remained common.

The orthopedic and other surgical literature are replete with reports addressing wound infection and preventive operating room techniques. Similarly, progress in bacteriology and the use of antibiotics over the past few decades has considerably reduced the incidence of postoperative infections and the morbidity and morality associated with such infection. Nevertheless, infection following total hip arthroplasty is a major complication associated with considerable morbidity and mortality as well as cost of the treatment. The introduction of massive amounts of foreign body during the operation makes the total hip arthroplasty procedure more susceptible to the development of infection, and it makes the postoperative treatment of infection more difficult. Prevention of this complication is essential for successful short- and long-term outcome.

Factors critical to the development of infection are the disease-producing dose of organisms, the virulence of the organism, and the ability of the host to fight or resist the infection. In 1957, Elek et al. (15) reported that more than 1 million viable staphylococci were necessary to produce infection by intradermal injection in human volunteers. When foreign material such as silk was inserted at the same time, infection could be caused by as few as 100 viable organisms. Charnley (3–6) reported that in total hip arthroplasty, the wound could be infected with a far lower dose of infecting organism. Hence a cause-and-

O. A. Nercessian and R. P. Joshi: Department Orthopaedic Surgery, Columbia-Presbyterian Medical Center, New York, New York 10032.

effect relationship between the foreign material in the surgical wound and increased risk or extent of infection exists.

The first line of defense in preventing infection is to control the site of entry of the organism (the surgical wound and the operating room environment). Some particles, such as epithelial scales, are shed from the operating room personnel. These particles come from exposed parts of the body, such as the face and upper neck and chest, the perineum, and the nasopharynx. Bathing or showering of the personnel prior to the surgical procedure reduces the shedding for short intervals (minutes) but has no long-term effect on shedding. The larger the number of operating room personnel, the larger the number of shed particles. Therefore, the number of persons must be kept to a minimum. Only personnel required for successful completion of the operation should be in the operating room. Traffic in and out of the operating room should be minimized, and eliminated if possible.

The microorganisms associated with wound colonization are predominantly the same as those found in the skin and in the infected postoperative total hip replacement. They include *Staphylococcus epidermidis, Staphylococcus aureus,* and *Streptococcus viridans.* A high correlation between the presence of wound colonization and the development of deep wound sepsis has been reported by Fitzgerald (17,18).

The conventional ventilation system does not control the infecting dust particles generated by the personnel in the operating room as does a high-flow ventilatory system. The conventional or the standard operating room has a low air exchange rate (25 to 30 times per hour). In contrast, the clean air operating room has a positive pressure zone of unidirectional airflow that generates an exchange rate of 300 to 400 time per hour, as well as high-efficiency filtration of particles 2 μm or less. In 1982, Salvati et al. (31) investigated the effect of horizontal laminar airflow ventilation systems on the infection rate in more than 3000 total hip and total knee arthroplasties. They found the infection rate decreased from 1.4% to 0.9% in total hip arthroplasty when performed in horizontal laminar airflow, whereas the incidence of infection increased from 1.4% to 3.9% in total knee arthroplasty. These differences were statistically significant in both groups. Salvati et al. (31) attributed the discrepancy to the position of the patient and the operating team in the operating room in relation to the airflow. The vertical airflow with an enclosure system, which Charnley advocated, creates a positive pressure inside the enclosure that forces air out through the bottom of the enclosure. A controlled study (3,6) confirmed the favorable outcomes resulting from the improved air circulation provided by the enclosure.

Statistical data (12,13) obtained retrospectively from 17 major teaching institutions on 21,903 total hip arthroplasties revealed inconclusive results for the advantage of the clean air over antibiotics. However, the results indicated low infection rates when both were used. The authors concluded that the clean air room was considered essential if the surgeon did not use prophylactic antibiotics, especially in institutions where it was difficult to control traffic in the operating room.

Lidwell et al. (23) reported a multicenter prospective study in Britain on over 8000 total hip replacements. Their results demonstrated that the use of an ultraclean air room during total joint arthroplasty reduced postoperative wound infection. The use of whole body exhaust systems also increased protection against infection. Their result suggested that ultraclean air and antibiotic prophylactics had independent and cumulative effects in preventing postoperative joint infection.

Ultraviolet (UV) light has been shown to decrease the bacterial count in the operating room. A report by the National Research Council study (20,21) indicated significant reduction in postoperative wound infection rates. Although UV lighting is relatively inexpensive and easy to install, there are hazards to its use. Conjunctivitis occurs when the eyes are directly exposed to UV radiation for 2 to 3 minutes at a time. Skin burning and dryness of the surgical wound have been noted. The operating room personnel must use special eye shields to protect against UV radiation, and sun screening solution to protect the exposed parts of the body. Lowell et al. (25,26) at the Peter Bent Brigham Hospital reported a significant decrease in infection rates with the use of UV radiation. For primary total hip surgery, the infection rate dropped from 2.1% to 0.4%, and for all total hip surgery, from 3.00% to 0.53%.

The surgical mask is intended to prevent bacteria and particles from the nasopharynx from spreading to the operating room environment. It has become an absolute requirement in operating rooms throughout the world. Sompolinsky and co-workers (34) demonstrated that the nasopharynx can occasionally serve as a source of wound infection. Masks may decrease contamination of the wound by as much as 90%. Ritter et al. (30) have shown that the filtration efficiency of most disposable masks is greater than 95%. Cloth masks are inefficient and thin masks allow bacteria to escape easily (11). Improper application of the mask increases the number of bacteria that escape and enter the wound. With the use of body exhaust systems and the space suits, the use of the masks can be safely eliminated.

In a study (7) conducted with conventional cloth surgical gowns, light microscopy demonstrated pores of 1 to 50 μm in size, large enough for bacteria to pass through. This route of infection may be significant in procedures such as total hip replacement, where the surgeon's hands and surgical equipment often come in contact with the surgeon's gown. Disposable synthetic fiber gowns are impermeable to most particles. These gowns are resistant to water and impervious to bacterial penetration. The use of gowns and hoods with an exhaust system provides a complete barrier between the surgical personnel and the wound. All surgical personnel should remember the basic surgical concepts of remaining sterile throughout the surgery by avoiding contact with the backs of the gowns of other surgical team members, avoiding the wiping of debris on the front of one's own gown, and avoiding the placement of hands in the axilla (all high-bacterial-count areas).

SURGICAL SCRUB AND GLOVING

Surgical scrub is a routine practice fundamental to prophylaxis against infection. The added protection of a high quality surgical glove is essential in handling surgical wounds involving instrumentation, soft tissue, and bone. The 10-minute hand scrub is an unnecessary ritual, although in comparing several cleansing agents, Dineen (10) demonstrated differences between 5- and 10-minute scrubs. Some have suggested that a 1-minute scrub may be adequate because of the slight difference in bacterial count of fingertips examined after 1 minute of scrubbing and up to 2 hours of scrubbing. Bernard (1) has also shown no difference in reducing bacterial counts with 3-, 5-, or 10-minute scrubs.

Most gloves have been punctured during long operations that require the use of much equipment. Gloves should be continually checked for holes. The practice of changing gloves frequently is a good and rational discipline. Butterfield (2) demonstrated glove perforations in 70% of cases. Bacterial counts of *S. aureus* reaching 18,000 have been reported when gloves have been punctured (8). All surgical team members should wear two pairs of high-quality gloves. However, no scientific report has proved that the punctured glove is the source of postsurgical infection.

The outer gloves are the pair most often punctured and contaminated after performing a draping procedure. In one study, the greatest number of colonies (44%) grew from gloves used for draping (27). This finding confirms the need to change gloves after draping. In that study, the surgeons who used their hands most strenuously developed more holes in their gloves.

Soiling of the wound by contamination during postoperative recovery can also be a source of exogenous infection. The first 24 hours after surgery appears to be the most important period for direct contamination (22). Natural epithelial formation has begun at the end of this period and provides a barrier to contamination.

PATIENT POSITIONING

Although the approach used in total hip arthroplasty is the choice of the surgeon based on his experience, patient positioning must be carefully performed. The position of the acetabular component is dependent on the position of the patient's pelvis, despite careful reliance on bony landmarks. To avoid vascular and neurologic complications in the contralateral leg, care must be exercised in padding the pressure points. Similarly, in anesthetized patients the movement and positioning of the upper extremities must be done carefully. All extremities must be adequately protected with padding.

After the patient is brought to the operating room, the right or left hip to be operated on should be clearly marked. The radiograph confirming the pathology must be available on the operating room radiographic view box. The side to be operated on should be verified.

The choice of anesthesia involves the anesthesiologist, the patient, and the surgeon, and it is based on the preoperative evaluation, the length of the procedure, and the general health of the patient (28). The anesthesiologist makes the final recommendation. After induction of anesthesia, an indwelling Foley catheter is inserted using sterile technique. The indwelling catheter can be used by the anesthesiologist to monitor the hemodynamic status of the patient and control fluid administration intraoperatively. It also is helpful to the patient and staff postoperatively to avoid the need for intermittent catheterization. The Foley catheter is securely taped to the opposite (nonoperative) inner thigh, leaving enough slack to avoid tugging or pulling of the catheter during positioning.

Once the Foley catheter is inserted, the patient is placed in the desired position (i.e., supine for the transtrochanteric approach or lateral decubitus for the posterolateral approach). The turning of the patient must be done gently in an organized fashion. The anesthesiologist controls the head and neck of the patient, holding the endotracheal tube securely in place to avoid dislodgement of the tube or overstretching of the cervical spine. One surgical team member controls the hands and shoulders of the patient and another controls the patient's hips. The ipsilateral arm is positioned in no more than 90-degree forward flexion and slight adduction. An axillary pad is placed by lifting the patient's chest and positioning the pad distal to the contralateral axilla. The contralateral arm must be kept in no greater than 90-degree forward flexion, and all extremities are padded over their bony protuberances (29).

The operating room table must be kept in absolute horizontal position parallel to the floor. Any position such as Trendelenburg or reverse Trendelenburg, which is often chosen by the anesthesiologist during induction of anesthesia, must be corrected back to the horizontal position. This is done to avoid malposition of the acetabulum component during the procedure.

Although a number of holders have been devised to place the patient in the lateral decubitus position, several principles are relevant to all types. The pubis and sacrum must be secured. The placement of the pubic clamp must be done cautiously with the pad directed against the pubic symphysis. Placement of the pad more inferiorly could

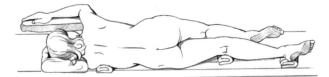

FIG. 1. Patient in the true lateral position with the head, arms, axilla, and contralateral leg well padded.

cause occlusion or compromise of the femoral vessels of the opposite limb, which may remain unrecognized and lead to severe and often disastrous complication (33). Placement of the pad superiorly may compromise the ipsilateral femoral vessels, and it may often prevent adequate flexion and adduction of the operated hip, a requirement for assessment of hip stability. A direct check of the area and the distal pulses of the contralateral extremity is essential prior to draping of the patient.

The sacral pad is applied over the mid sacrum. The upper edge of the sacral pad should be at least 3 to 5 inches away from the most posterior end of the skin incision. When the patient is securely positioned in the lateral decubitus position (Fig. 1), the position of the pelvis is checked so that the patient is not tilted in the anterior or posterior direction (Fig. 2). Chest positioners and pillows between the arms are helpful in preventing anterior displacement of the torso. Inadequate fixation of the pelvis can lead to anterior pelvis tilt during the procedure, which can in turn cause unrecognized retroversion of the acetabular component.

The perineum is isolated using an adhesive U-shaped plastic drape.

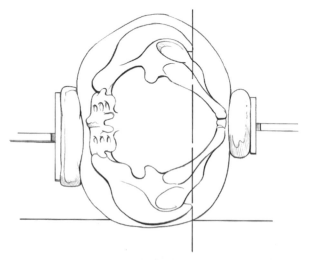

FIG. 2. Pelvis must be well secured in the lateral position, keeping the pelvis vertical. If the pelvis is tilted forward, the surgeon will perceive more anteversion of the acetabular component than is actually present.

SKIN PREPARATION AND DRAPING

After positioning of the patient, the skin preparation and draping is performed. The skin preparation and hair removal is done in the operating room or induction room. The method of hair removal and the time elapsed before surgery can affect the rate of bacterial colonization of the site. In one study (8), razor shaving of the skin at the operative site was found to cause a high incidence of skin contamination. The use of chemical agents for hair removal was demonstrated to reduce the infection rate to 1.6% compared to 5.6% using razor shaving as a control (32).

Cruse (9), in a series of 20,105 operations, found that clipping the hair at the surgical site reduced wound infection. The rate when the site had been shaved was 2.3%, when clipped it was 1.9%, and when no attempt had been made to remove the hair it was 0.9%. The author attributed the increased rate to the razor-induced trauma that created a port of entry for the skin bacteria. However, hair at the site of the operation has been incriminated as an important source of surgical contamination. Traumatization or nicking of the skin at the site of the surgical incision must be avoided.

After hair removal from the site of the operation is complete, the surgical site along with the entire leg, buttock, and trunk is washed with bactericidal soap (Betadine soap) for approximately 5 minutes. This soap is then rinsed with alcohol, and the dried skin is then painted with Betadine or an iodine solution. Fitzgerald and Washington (19) demonstrated better efficacy using a soap that leaves an antibacteria barrier than using ordinary soap. He recommended defatting the skin with alcohol and Freon and painting it with tincture of iodine. Freon, an environmental hazard, has been eliminated and instead only alcohol is used. Other authors (14) have demonstrated the bactericidal and bacteriostatic effectiveness of hexachlorophane compound. This latter compound can be used in patients with an allergy to iodine and iodine-containing solutions.

Once skin preparation is completed, the draping is started. The purpose of the draping is to provide a sterile operative field while leaving a minimal area of the skin exposed. The draping is done once the surgeon and the assistant have put on their gowns, gloves, and the vacuum body exhaust system. Care must be taken to avoid contamination of the surgical site, the surgeon's sterile gown, and the drapes themselves. The drapes should be impervious to bacteria and fluid and should be abrasion resistant. They should filter bacteria and allow breathing of the skin. Disposable drapes made of microporous textiles are preferred.

The operated limb must be draped freely to avoid contamination of the wound. Four towels are applied anterior, posterior, superior, and inferior (at the groin) to the hip and buttock, leaving adequate room for the final incision. The draping closes in on the wound with each layer of draping.

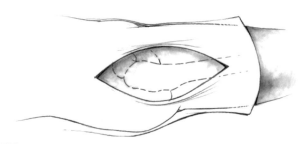

FIG. 3. When the leg has been draped, the leg must be free, and the groin and buttock must be sealed from the wound.

The patient's foot and leg are placed in a sterile impermeable bag. The bag is rolled up to the level of the knee and a sterile elastic wrapping is gently applied over the bag to prevent venous stasis. A long leg stockinette is then applied over the leg and brought all the way up to the trunk of the patient. This stockinette is secured in place with a U-shaped drape extending to the posterior and anterior aspects of the surgical site. Two split drapes are then applied from the inferior and superior aspects of the wound. A fenestrated drape is applied putting the operated limb through the fenestrated site. The upper part of the patient's leg has two layers of draping, the lower part three layers of sterile draping. The stockinette is cut to expose the surgical site on the lateral thigh and posterior lateral buttock. An iodoform-impregnated plastic adhesive drape is then applied covering the site of the incision and the edges of the stockinette.

The bacteria from the surface of the skin can migrate during the surgery and infect the wound. Applications of the iodoform-impregnated adhesive drape (Steri-drapes) reduces this contamination. In some studies (16,30), bacterial sampling of the wound after application of iodoform-impregnated drapes showed that wound contamination was reduced from 15% to 1.6%. The skin must be dry for the application of the Steri-drape to ensure full adherence. Whatever method of draping is utilized, the incision should be well exposed, the groin should be well sealed from the operative sight, and the leg should be draped so as to allow full hip, knee, and ankle motion without contamination (Fig. 3).

USE OF ASSISTANTS

The total hip arthroplasty procedure is a major surgical undertaking that cannot be done without assistance. A team of personnel (surgeons, assistants, and surgical scrub nurse) is necessary to ensure the execution of the surgical procedure under optimal conditions in a safe and functional operating room environment. One assistant is an absolute necessity for completion of a total hip arthroplasty procedure, but two or three assistants are optimal for efficiency. The surgical team must rehearse all the technical steps of the procedure together, and the

surgical assistants must be well versed with the technique of surgery. In difficult or technically demanding procedures or circumstances, the team must also rehearse one or more alternative technical plans for a successful outcome of the surgery. In more complex procedures, numerous pieces of complex equipment are introduced, and the surgical staff must be familiar with the use of this equipment. Lack of familiarity with procedures and equipment can result in suboptimal performance, unnecessary repetitions of some technical steps, prolongation of the time of the surgery, and suboptimal results. This is especially prudent in assigning the operating room staff. Although the operating room staff is expected to be familiar with all areas of surgery, in the technically demanding total hip arthroplasty it is beneficial to assign a selected number of staff with in-depth knowledge and experience in this procedure. Arbitrary staff assignment results in uncertainty, apprehension, and hesitation during surgery. A specialized team approach is most beneficial because it allows staff to develop a professional rapport with other surgical team members. Working with the team, each staff member becomes aware of the style of each surgeon and thereby can anticipate needs and assist accurately and efficiently. The specialized team members develop greater awareness of the inventory and equipment required for a specific procedure. With an experienced team, the procedure is carried out and completed with ease and efficiency, reducing operating room time.

In a teaching hospital environment, new residents are assigned to each service for a given interval of time (usually a senior or a junior resident for 6-week intervals). Because of this uncontrolled change, it is a priority that the surgical team rehearse the technical steps of the procedure. The team must familiarize themselves with the procedure by reviewing and reading available information in textbooks or published articles. In a teaching environment, the resident staff will be more experienced and specialized at the end of the rotation than at the start of the rotation. Having one member of the team (the hip fellow) in all scheduled total hip procedures during the year will make the transition from the end of the rotation of the first group of residents to the beginning of the next group uneventful. In institutions where a hip fellowship is unavailable, a physician's assistant with thorough technical experience in total hip arthroplasty can be substantially beneficial to the surgical team.

In most instances, the surgical team performing the total hip arthroplasty consists of the surgeon, the first assistant, and the second assistant. In the posterolateral approach to the hip, the surgeon's position will be posterior to the patient's buttock, the first assistant directly opposite to the surgeon, anterior to the patient, and the second assistant next to the first assistant close to the patient's foot. The operating room technician will stand at the foot of the operating table.

The function of the surgeon is to perform or to supervise the performance of every step of the surgical procedure. The function of the first assistant is to provide adequate exposure by retraction and maintaining a clear and bloodless field for proper visualization. The function of the second assistant is to provide retraction and steady position of the patient's limb. Proper limb positioning is a skill that sometimes is not adequately appreciated.

SKIN INCISION AND OLD INCISION

The incision should be adequate in length for access and visualization of the hip anatomy. In obese or muscular patients with difficult anatomic pathologies, additional lengthening of the incision may be necessary. Remember, incisions heal side to side, not end to end. Faulty draping may cover a portion of the incision area requiring a short proximal limb of the incision. This may make the acetabular exposure difficult during surgery.

In a patient who has undergone previous hip surgery and presents with one or more than one old surgical scar, placement of the skin incision must be carefully planned. If only a single scar is present and its position is adequate, it should be used. This skin incision is carefully marked and excised. The excision of the old scar improves the blood supply and healing of the skin. Old surgical incisions that are not along the planned incision site should be ignored. Inclusion of part of the old surgical scar with the new incision can be attempted. As a rule, new incisions should not cross old surgical scars and skin islands between the old and the new incision should be avoided to prevent skin necrosis. In complex cases, a sham incision can be made and closed. The surgeon can come back later through the same incision. If necrosis occurs at the sham incision site, the surgeon should consider plastic surgery consultation for closure of the reconstructed wound. Cases with previous procedures, where all of the skin around the greater trochanter has been scarred and no underlying adipose tissue remains, should be considered for vastus lateralis greater trochanteric flap coverage at the time of reconstruction. After the skin incision is made, the subcutaneous tissue is incised to expose the fascia lata. Up to 1 inch of the fascia is freed of adipose tissue on each side of the proposed fascia incision to allow closure of the fascia without adipose interposition (Fig. 4). Sewing or clamping towels to this fascia during the operation will also protect the skin and adipose tissue from excessive retraction.

WOUND CLOSURE

After the approach to the hip and preparation and insertion of the total hip arthroplasty components are performed, meticulous wound closure is important to prevent hematoma formation and to prevent postoperative wound drainage. Wound hemostasis is important. Branches of the lateral femoral circumflex vessels anteriorly, the medial femoral circumflex vessels posteriorly, the obturator vessels (along the inferior acetabular rim and transverse acetabular ligament), and the perforating vessels from the profundus femoris (in the area of gluteus maximus tendon insertion) need to be ligated or cauterized. Use of drains is controversial, but many surgeons still place a drain deep to the fascia lata.

The fascia lata requires reapproximation. If the patient is obese, some form of tissue retention sutures should be applied in the adipose layer. Remnants of Scarpi's and Camper's fascia (remnants of the abdominal fascia, which continue into the adipose tissue of the thigh) provide layers for reapproximation of the adipose tissue. Charnley originally used retention wire sutures, which were crimped over foam bolsters and removed at 1 to 2 weeks postoperatively (Fig. 5). If retention sutures are not used, a compressive dressing that circumferentially covers the thigh and pelvis should be utilized. If the patient is in the lateral decubitus position during surgery, care must be taken to keep the hip located when positioning the patient supine. The senior person in the room should keep one hand on the lateral pelvis and cradle the thigh and knee in abduction and external rotation (with the other arm, forearm, and hand) during the entire move to the supine position. Pillows or splints should be placed between the legs and the patient should be transferred to a hospital bed rather than to a cart: the latter may cause adduction of the legs and would require a second transfer to the hospital bed.

DISCUSSION

The total hip arthroplasty procedure requires large amounts of technical equipment and the introduction of large foreign material loads to the body, and it therefore requires the optimization of general surgical principles. Efficiency and proficiency with this operation requires a

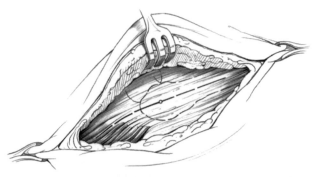

FIG. 4. Adipose tissue must be freed from the underlying fascia lata on both sides of the incision into the fascia to allow closure of the fascia without strangulation of the adipose tissue.

A

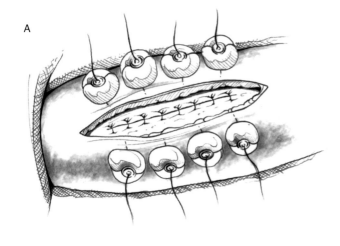

B

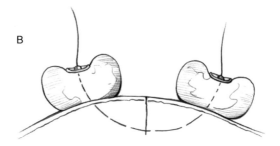

C

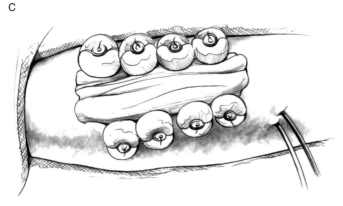

FIG. 5. Original Charnley technique for superficial wound closure. **A:** Open wound with wires placed in subcutaneous tissue and foam pads in position. **B:** Cross section of suture technique. **C:** Final dressing after tightening of the wires and application of pressure dressing that is secured by foam.

skilled surgical team that works together on a regular basis. Aseptic surgical technique is paramount throughout the procedure. From the study of this operation, much has been learned about the prevention of surgical infections in general. The procedure should be performed in a routine manner for the straightforward primary hip replacement. The operating environment should assure aseptic technique. Patient positioning, skin preparation and draping, use of assistants, incisions and closures should all be precise and reproducible.

REFERENCES

1. Bernard HR. The effect of scrub time on hand antisepsis using povidone-iodine surgical scrub for 3-, 5-, 10-minute scrubs. In: Polk HC, Ehrenkranz NJ, eds. *Therapeutic advances and new clinical implications: medical and surgical antisepsis with Betadine microbicides.* Norwalk, Conn: Purdue Frederick, 1972.
2. Butterfield WC. Puncture wounds in surgical gloves. *Conn Med J* 1970;34:180.
3. Charnley J, Eftekhar N. Postoperative infection in total prosthetic replacement arthroplasty of the hip joint with special reference to the bacterial contact on the air in the operating room. *Br J Surg* 1969; 56:641.
4. Charnley J. Low friction arthroplasty of the hip. In: Charnley J, ed. *Theory and Practice.* New York: Springer-Verlag, 1979.
5. Charnley J. Postoperative infection after total hip replacement with special reference to air contamination in the operating room. *Clin Orthop* 1972;87:167.
6. Charnley J. A sterile air operating theatre enclosure. *Br J Surg* 1965;51:195.
7. Charnley J, Eftekhar NS. Penetration of gown material by organism from surgeon's body. *Lancet* 1969;1:172.
8. Cole WR, Bernard HR. Inadequacies of present methods of surgical skin preparation. *Arch Surg* 1964;89:215.
9. Cruse PJR. Postoperative study of 20105 surgical wounds with emphasis on use of topical antibiotics and prophylactic antibiotics. Presented at the *4th symposium on Control of Surgical Infection,* Washington, DC, Nov. 1972.
10. Dineen P. An evaluation of the duration of the surgical scrub. *Surg Gynecol Obstet* 1969;129:1181.
11. Dineen P. Microbial filtration by surgical masks. *Surg Gynecol Obstet* 1971;133:812.
12. Eftekhar NS. *Total hip arthroplasty,* vol. 1. St. Louis: Mosby Yearbook, 1993;870.
13. Eftekhar NS. Controversy of the clean air and total hip replacement. In: the Hip Society. *The hip: proceedings of the second open scientific meeting of the Hip Society.* St. Louis: Mosby Yearbook, 1974.
14. Eitzen HE, Ritter MA, French MV, et al. A microbiological in-use

comparison of surgical hand washing agents. *J Bone Joint Surg* 1979; 61A:403.

15. Elek SD, Cohen PE. The virulence of *Staphylococcus pyogenes* of man: a study of the problems of wound infections. *Br J Exp Pathol* 1957;38:573.

16. Fairclough JA, Johnson D, Mackie I. The prevention of wound contamination by skin organism by the preoperative application of an iodophor impregnated plastic adhesive drape. *J Int Med Res* 1986;14:105.

17. Fitzgerald RH Jr, Peterson LF, et al. Bacterial colonization of wound and sepsis in total hip arthroplasty. *J Bone Joint Surg* 1973;55:1242.

18. Fitzgerald RH Jr, Peterson LF. Wound colonization in deep wound sepsis. In: Eftekhar NS, ed. *Infection in total joint replacement surgery: Prevention and management.* St. Louis: Mosby Yearbook, 1984.

19. Fitzgerald RH Jr, Washington JA II. Contamination of operative wound. *Orthop Clin North Am* 1975;6:1105.

20. Goldner JL, Allen BL Jr. Ultraviolet light in orthopaedic operating room at Duke University: 35 year experience 1937 to 1973. *Clin Orthop* 1973;96:195.

21. Hart D, Nicks J. Ultraviolet radiation in the operating room intensities used and bactericidal effect. *Arch Surg* 1961;82:449.

22. Heifetz CJ, Richards FO, Lawrence MS. Comparison of wound healing with and without dressings; experimental study. *Arch Surg* 1952; 65:746.

23. Lidwell OM, Lowbury EJ, White W, et al. Effect of ultra-clean air in operating room on deep sepsis in the total knee replacement: a randomized study. *Br Med J* 1982;285:10.

24. Lister J. A new method of treatment of compound fracture, abscess, etc. with observation on the condition of suppuration. *Lancet* 1967;1:326.

25. Lowell JD. Use of ultraviolet radiation in total hip replacement surgery. In: Eftekhar NS, ed. *Infection in joint replacement surgery. Prevention and management.* St. Louis: Mosby Yearbook, 1984.

26. Lowell JD, Kundsin RB. Ultraviolet radiation. Its beneficial effect on the operating room environment and the incidence of deep wound infection after total hip and total knee arthroplasty. *Instr Course Lect* 1977;26:58–65.

27. McCue SF, Berg EW, Saunders EA. Efficacy of double-gloving as a barrier to microbial contamination during total joint arthroplasty. *J Bone Joint Surg* 1981;3:811.

28. Modig J. Regional anesthesia and blood loss. *Acta Anesthesiol Scand* 1988;2(suppl 89)44.

29. Nercessian OA, O'Connor D, Allen A, Posta A. Neurological injury in the upper extremity following total hip arthroplasty. *Orthop Trans* 1994;18(1):1086.

30. Ritter MA, Campbell ED. Retrospective evaluation of an iodophor-incorporated antimicrobial plastic adhesive wound drape. *Clin Orthop* 1975;111:147.

31. Salvati EA, Robinson RP, Zeno SM, et al. Infection rates after 3175 total hip and total knee replacements performed with and without a horizontal unidirectional filtered air flow system. *J Bone Joint Surg* 1982;64:525.

32. Seropian R, Reynolds BM. Wound infection after preoperative depilatory vs. razor preparation. *Am J Surg* 1971;121:251.

33. Smith JW, Pellici PM, Shrrock N, et al. Complications after total hip replacement. The contralateral limb. *J Bone Joint Surg* 1989;71A (4):528.

34. Sompolinsky D, Hermann Z, Ording P, et al. A series of postoperative infections. *J Infect Dis* 1957;100:1.

The Adult Hip, edited by J. J. Callaghan,
A. G. Rosenberg, and H. E. Rubash.
Lippincott–Raven Publishers, Philadelphia © 1998.

CHAPTER 60

The Cemented Femoral Component

William J. Maloney and James M. Hartford

Cemented total hip arthroplasty was first introduced by Sir John Charnley in 1961. At that time, he published an article entitled *Arthroplasty of the Hip: A New Operation* (19). Since this report, the surgical technique and implants have been modified in an attempt to improve the reliability and reproducibility of the procedure. Some of these changes have resulted in improved longevity and some have not. The focus of this chapter will be to discuss the clinical results and surgical technique as it relates to primary cemented femoral component replacement.

The reported success of primary cemented femoral components has varied in the literature (2,9,114,116). To understand the reasons for this variability, one must be familiar with the evolution of current cement techniques and the concept of generations in cement technique. *First-generation cementing technique* refers to finger-packing doughy cement into the unplugged femoral canal. The femoral components often had sharp

corners with a narrow medial border and were made of stainless steel. Although some surgeons were able to achieve a satisfactory cement mantle using this method, for most surgeons it resulted in incomplete (inadequate) cement mantles. Second-generation cementing technique involved plugging the medullary canal, cleaning the canal with pulsatile lavage, and inserting the cement in a retrograde fashion using a cement gun. The implants of this generation were made of super alloys. Implant designs had been modified to remove sharp corners on the implants. In addition, most of these implants had a broad medial border. Third-generation cementing included all second-generation techniques plus porosity reduction of the cement, pressurization of the cement mantle, and surface modifications on the implants. Surface modifications on the implants included micro- and macro-texturing as well as industrial application of polymethylmethacrylate (PMMA) to the implant in an attempt to improve the bond between implant and cement. Recent application of the term *fourth-generation cement technique* has been made in the literature. Fourth-generation cementing refers to all the elements of third-generation technique plus stem centralization proximally and distally to ensure adequate and symmetric cement mantles.

W. J. Maloney: Department of Orthopaedic Surgery, Barnes-Jewish Hospital, Washington University School of Medicine, St. Louis, Missouri 63110.

J. M. Hartford: Division of Orthopaedic Surgery, University of Kentucky, Lexington, Kentucky 40536-0084.

In reviewing the published results of cemented total hip arthroplasty, it is also important to be aware of the reported criteria of failure. Endpoints commonly used to define a failed total hip replacement include the need for revision surgery, clinical failure (a painful arthroplasty), and radiographic failure (loose implant). The reported failure rate depends on the author's definition of failure and may vary considerably from one report to the next. It is useful when reviewing reports to assess the mechanical failure rate for a given device. The mechanical failure rate for a particular implant can be defined by the percentage of cases in a given series requiring revision surgery, plus the percentage of cases determined to be radiographically loose.

RADIOGRAPHIC ASSESSMENT

Evaluation of femoral component stability is usually reported using a zonal analysis as described by Gruen et al. (50). This system divides the femur into seven zones on the anteroposterior (AP) radiograph (Fig. 1) and has subsequently been modified to include seven additional zones on the lateral radiograph. However, the definition of what constitutes a radiographically loose implant is not universally agreed upon. One system defines definite loosening of a cemented femoral component when one of the following criteria is met: (a) implant subsidence or change in implant position on serial radiographs; (b) new metal–cement radiolucency (not present on the initial

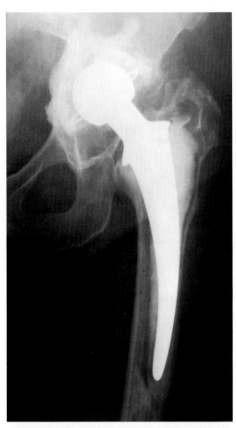

FIG. 2. Extensive radiolucency at the cement–bone interface of this cemented femoral component, with a cement fracture at the tip of the stem indicative of loosening.

postoperative radiograph); (c) cement mantle fracture; and (d) implant fracture (Fig. 2).

Radiographic criteria of cemented femoral component stability as described by Harris also defines categories of probably and possibly loose components. Radiographs that demonstrate a continuous radiolucent line at the cement–bone interface are graded "probably loose" (56). If there is an incomplete radiolucent line occupying between 50% and 99% of the cement–bone interface, the implant is graded as "possibly loose." However, recent autopsy studies in which the remodeling at the cement–bone interface has been evaluated have pointed out the problem of making sweeping generalizations concerning the significance of radiolucencies between cement and bone on the femoral side (65,73,79). In these autopsy studies, radiolucencies were most commonly related to skeletal remodeling and not to the formation of a soft-tissue membrane between cement and bone. An inner cortex commonly formed immediately adjacent to the cement mantle, and it is not distinguishable from the cement on clinical radiographs. Between the inner and outer cortex, a second medullary canal formed that appeared as a radiolucency on clinical radiographs (Fig. 3). In contrast to the typical cement–bone radiolucency that is associated with fibrous tissue formation, the radi-

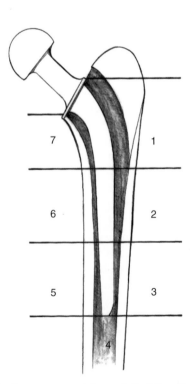

FIG. 1. Gruen zones 1 through 7, AP radiograph.

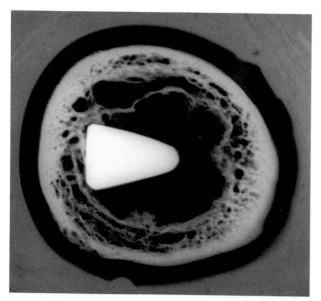

FIG. 3. Radiograph of a cross section through the diaphysis from a patient who had undergone a cemented total hip arthroplasty 17 years prior to death. The cement is radiolucent because of a lack of barium. Note the inner cortex around the cement mantle and the formation of a second medullary canal between the inner and outer cortex. A clinical radiograph tangential to the second medullary canal will demonstrate a radiolucency. (From Morrey BF. *Biological Material and Mechanical Considerations of Joint Replacement.* New York: Raven Press, with permission.)

olucency that forms as a result of bone remodeling is nonprogressive and is not associated with the formation of sclerotic lines. As a result, the criteria for loosening as well as the definition of a radiolucent line as it pertains to fibrous tissue formation needs to be reevaluated.

The amount of subsidence of the femoral component that can be reproducibly measured on clinical radiographs is not well defined. Many authors use 2 mm on the femoral component side as the criterion for loosening (12). Roentgen stereophotogrammetric analysis (RSA), used predominantly as a research tool, has been able to identify femoral migration as small as 0.02 mm. This modality can identify early migration of components, helping to predict later loosening and clinical failure. Early subsidence of a cemented femoral stem of 1.2 mm within the first 2 years of follow-up has been associated with the need for early revision of the component (70,104). When compared to evaluation of serial radiographs, arthrography and radionuclide studies have not provided any significant additional information on cemented femoral component stability.

CLINICAL RESULTS: FIRST-GENERATION CEMENTING

Cemented total hip replacement using first-generation cementing techniques in North America were disappoint-

ing. Failure rates on the femoral side of up to 20% to 24% at 5 years, which increased to 30% to 40% at 10 years, were reported (2,116). In one study of 100 consecutive Mueller total hip replacements followed for 10 years, 20 patients with 22 arthroplasties had died without having revision surgery (114). Twenty arthroplasties had been revised. Nineteen revision surgeries were performed for aseptic loosening of one or both components. Overall, the mechanical failure rate on the femoral side was 40%. Aseptic loosening was often associated with osteolysis. In another study, Stauffer reported that the mechanical failure rate of cemented Charnley low-friction arthroplasties went from 24% at 5 years to almost 30% at 10 years (116).

Not all studies using first-generation cementing techniques have reported poor results. For example, Schulte et al. (110) reported the 20-year results of 330 Charnley cemented prostheses inserted from 1970 to 1972. At the 20-year follow-up evaluation, 83 patients with 98 hips were still living. In this series, the mechanical failure rate (revised, and radiographically loose but not revised) was 6% for all 322 femoral components. For the patients surviving 20 years, the mechanical failure rate was 7% for 98 femoral components. The excellent long-term clinical results presented in this study can be attributed to the expert handling of bone cement resulting in satisfactory cement mantles despite using first-generation techniques.

CONTEMPORARY CEMENT TECHNIQUE

The goal in femoral cementing is to optimize the cement–bone interface. To obtain this goal reproducibly, attention to technical detail is important. Careful attention to technical factors helps to create a cement mantle free of mantle defects with a minimum 2-mm thickness, and a femoral component that it is centered in the cement mantle in neutral alignment. The steps outlined below detail how to achieve this goal, and their rational is explained.

Canal Preparation

To optimize the cement–bone interface, proper preparation of the femoral canal is important. The femoral canal is first prepared with a series of broaches that create an envelope for the implant. The broaches should be designed so that they are larger than the component that is to be implanted, allowing adequate room for cement. Once the largest broach that can be placed into the femoral canal has been inserted, collar cone provisionals can be used to perform a trial reduction, checking hip stability and leg length. The broach is then removed and loose cancellous bone can be taken away with a curette. This helps improve cement intrusion into the remaining cancellous bone. Reamers should not be used to prepare the femoral canal when cement is being used. By removing stable cancellous bone, reaming creates a smooth endosteal surface, which in turns decreases the interfacial shear strength between cement and bone.

Next, the femoral canal must be plugged. Plugging allows for greater intrusion pressure and better filling. The femoral canal can be plugged with bone cement, bone, or commercially available plastic plugs. The plug should be placed 2 to 3 cm distal to the level of the tip of the femoral component (Fig. 4). This placement allows the cement mantle distance an equal distance below the tip of the stem. It is important to remember that pressurization of the cement is dependent on a secure distal plug. Maltry et al. have shown that commercial plugs vary in their ability to maintain their position without being dislodged during cement pressurization (82).

The femoral canal should then be cleaned using a pressurized lavage system. This serves two purposes: By removing marrow, fat, and blood, the risk of embolism is reduced. This in turn improves cement intrusion into the bone. A study by Majkowski et al. compared interfacial

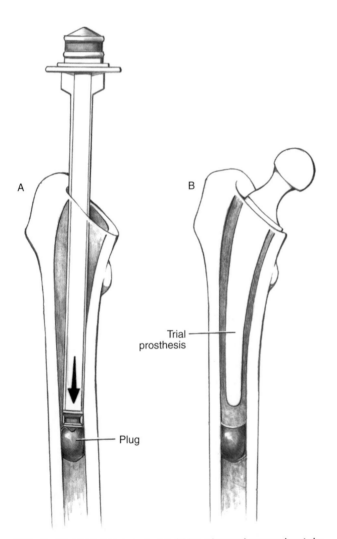

FIG. 4. The femoral canal should be plugged approximately 2 cm distal to the anticipated length of the femoral stem.

shear strength and cement intrusion into unprepared trabecular bone, bone prepared with irrigation, and bone prepared with pressurized lavage (78). Pressurized lavage led to a significant increase in the depth of cement penetration and interfacial shear strength when compared to unprepared bone. The canal can then be dried using suction, and dry and adrenaline-soaked sponges. Several other factors, including the use of spinal anesthesia and the use of hydrogen peroxide and iced saline, have also been shown to decrease bleeding from the cancellous bone of the femoral canal (7). A dry femoral canal at the time of cement insertion further helps to optimize this interface.

Cement Preparation

Controversy continues to exist concerning the benefit of porosity reduction in cemented total hip arthroplasty. It is clear, however, that cement fails in fatigue, and it has been estimated that the hip is loaded approximately 1 million times a year during gait. Laboratory testing has demonstrated that centrifugation decreases the pore size in cement to 200 to 400 µm in diameter (Fig. 5) (15). For any given specimen, this results in an increase in cross-sectional area. Fatigue data from this study demonstrated a 24% increase in ultimate tensile strain of standard test specimens, and a 136% increase in tension-compression fatigue strength as a result of centrifugation. Davies et al. showed that porosity reduction improved the fatigue life of bone cement by a factor of 5 (33). Similar benefits have been demonstrated with vacuum mixing (124).

Several *in vitro* models have been used to study the effects of porosity reduction in the face of surface imperfections (33). In general, these studies have demonstrated a beneficial effect of porosity reduction (30,33,124). Davies et al. showed that centrifuged Simplex-P bone cement (Howmedica, Rutherford, New Jersey) was able to withstand significantly more cycles before failure at all strain levels tested, when compared to uncentrifuged test specimens, despite notching of the test specimens (30). Examination of the fracture surfaces demonstrated multiple pores (Fig. 6). Vacuum mixing also reduces porosity and improves the mechanical properties of cement (123). These studies suggest that the increase in strength demonstrated with porosity reduction is independent of surface conditions.

One study undertaken to evaluate the effect of specimen notching did not show a beneficial effect in terms of increased strength (99). The results of this study showed that in the presence of a notch, there was no difference between specimens with or without porosity reduction. It should be noted that specimens used in this study were 26 by 90 mm. The exothermic reaction in a specimen of this size would be expected to increase the material temperature to the boiling point of the monomer.

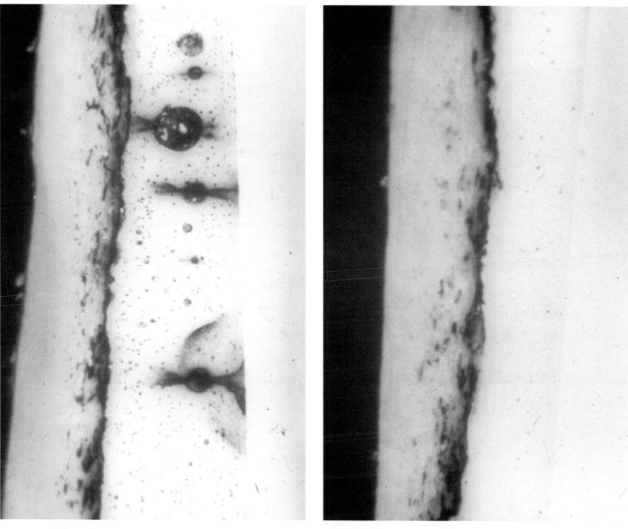

FIG. 5. Bone–cement–prosthesis composite (left to right). **A:** In the absence of porosity reduction, note the multiple voids in the cement mantle. **B:** The cement has been centrifuged prior to insertion. Note the marked reduction in the number and size of the voids.

Cement viscosity may also play a role in the success of cemented femoral components. *In vitro* tests have revealed the structural superiority of high viscosity over low viscosity cement (45). Clinically, a statistically significant survival rate has been reported with the use of high-viscosity cement for femoral components as compared to low-viscosity cement (58).

Cement Insertion and Pressurization

Bone cement is most reliably injected into the femoral canal using a cement gun. Cement should be injected in a retrograde fashion to avoid trapping air between the plug and cement and to ensure a more uniform distribution of cement in the femoral canal (Fig. 7). Care should be taken to avoid leaving the tip of the nozzle in the cement mantle as cement is being injected, as this can also intro-duce voids in the cement column. Once the femoral canal has been filled with bone cement, the cement mantle should be pressurized (Fig. 8). It has been shown that the strength of the cement–bone interface is directly related to the depth of penetration of cement into bone. Data suggest that a penetration depth of 4 mm provides the optimal strength for the cement–bone interface (5). It is obviously not possible to achieve this depth of penetration in the diaphysis where the bone is primarily dense cortical bone. However, in the metaphysis where there is more cancellous bone, this can be achieved in some regions. To obtain this type of cement penetration, it is necessary to use some type or pressurization system, as pressurization of the cement will increase penetration into the bone (83).

It is technically relatively easy to obtain high intrusion pressures in the diaphysis, but it is more difficult to obtain similar pressure in the proximal femur (metaphyseal region). Three commercially available cement pres-

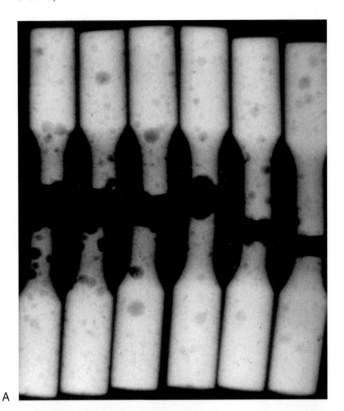

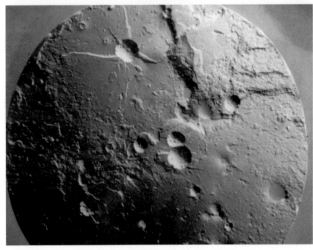

FIG. 6. A: Radiograph of multiple test specimens using non-centrifuged cement after fatigue testing. Note the voids present throughout the test specimens. **B:** Scanning electron micrograph of the fracture surface.

surization systems were recently evaluated to test their effectiveness at generating high intrusion pressures (31). The use of all three systems resulted in average peak cement pressures at the cement–bone interface, including the proximal region of the femur, of over 30 pounds per square inch (psi) with *in vitro* testing. After the *in vitro* study, one of the systems was evaluated intraoperatively. In ten primary cases, the average peak intrusion pressure in the proximal femur was 32 psi (±10). In revision cases, the average peak intrusion pressure was significantly less

(19 ± 9 psi). In a previous study, Rey et al. showed that a cement pressure of 20 psi produced a cement intrusion depth of 8 mm for LVC cement, 2.2 mm for Simplex-P cement, and 1.4 mm for Palacos cement in bovine trabecular bone, which is more dense than human cancellous bone (Fig. 9) (97).

Concerns have been raised in the past about PMMA pressurization and necrosis of cortical bone. One study showed that there was slightly increased bone resorption and decreased bone formation with pressurization (90). However this has not been proven to be of clinical significance.

Stem Centralization and Cement Mantle Thickness

Most contemporary cemented stems are designed to be used with stem centralizers. Some centralization devices are applied to the stem at the time of manufacturing, and others require assembly in the operating room (Fig. 10). These devices are designed to aid in centering the stem within the canal to ensure a more uniform cement man-

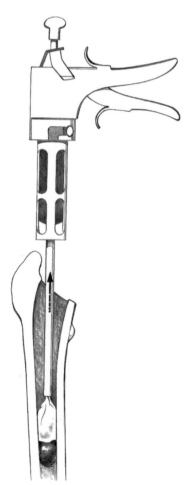

FIG. 7. The cement should be inserted in a retrograde fashion using a reliable cement gun.

undergoing unilateral total hip arthroplasty employing third-generation cement techniques followed for an average of 6 to 8 years (93). Eighty-nine patients survived. The rate of mechanical failure was 1%. In a study by Goldberg et al. using modern cement techniques as well as proximal and distal centralizers, at an average follow-up of 5.7 years, there were no radiographic cases of possible, probable, or definite loosening (48). Using the proximal and distal centralizers, 73% of the stems were in neutral position, 20% were within 1° to 2° of neutral, and only 7% were malaligned by greater than 2°.

CEMENTED TOTAL HIP REPLACEMENT IN THE YOUNGER PATIENT

Early reports on the results of total hip replacement in the young adult using first-generation cementing techniques were poor. Chandler et al. reported on a series of 29 patients who were less than 30 years of age at the time of their primary procedure (18). At an average follow-up of 5.5 years, five patients had undergone revision for loosening of the femoral component. In addition, one patient had an identified loose component on radiograph. Reporting similar results, Dorr followed a series of 108 cemented primary hips in patients under 45 years of age (35–37). At 4.5 years after surgery, three femoral components had been revised. Seventy-two percent of the patients were graded as having a satisfactory result. But by 9 years, 14 stems were revised and only 58% of the patients had a satisfactory result. At 15 years, 24 of the 49 patients in whom follow-up could be attained had undergone revision of the femoral component. Patients who were less than 30 years old had a worse outcome than patients between 30 and 45 years of age.

More recent studies have reported somewhat better results in the younger patient. Collis, in a series of 51 patients under the age of 50 followed from 12 to 18 years, reported ten femoral components revisions and three radiographically loose stems (24). Sullivan et al. reviewed a series of patients under 50 who were followed from 16 to 22 years (118). They found an 8% failure rate of the cemented stems. Solomon et al., after reviewing 156 stems implanted in patients under 50 years of age followed for 3 to 16 years, identified a femoral revision rate of 5.4% and a radiographic loosening rate of 4.3% (113).

As in older patients, modern cementing technique has led to improvements in long-term results for cemented femoral stems in the young patient. Ballard et al., reviewing 42 hips in patients under 50 years old with a follow-up of 10 years, identified two femoral components revised for aseptic loosening (6). Five components were identified as definitely loose by radiographic criteria. The overall loosening rate was 16%. Barrack et al. reviewed 44 patients under 50 years of age undergoing total hip arthroplasty using second-generation cementing techniques (8).

The follow-up was 10 to 14.8 years. They identified one definitely loose component by radiographic criteria. No femoral components had been revised. The mechanical failure rate was 2%. It is clear from these studies that surgical technique is an important determinant of long-term outcome with cemented femoral components.

FACTORS RELATED TO FAILURE

Technical factors in terms of cementing technique have proven important for long-term survival. Tapadiya et al. compared matched sets of failed and successful femoral components (119). On initial postoperative radiographs, they identified a statistically significant greater incidence of cement–bone radiolucencies in the failed group. These radiolucencies, or gaps, were indicative of incomplete cement filling. When femoral cement–bone radiolucency, collar–calcar contact, femoral metal–cement radiolucency, femoral cement mantle adequacy, cement distal to the stem tip, and femoral component stem position were analyzed together, the failed group showed a statistically significant higher percentage of adverse radiographic findings ($p < .006$), again emphasizing the importance of technique on outcome.

Several studies have suggested that varus orientation of the femoral stem has been associated with a higher percentage of aseptic loosening (9,26,27,39,72,94,107,114, 116). Varus positioning of the stem results in a thin or nonexistent cement mantle in the proximal medial and distal lateral zones. Callaghan et al. reviewed a series of patients who had revision hip surgery for aseptic loosening of the femoral component. Stem loosening correlated with varus position in 50% and an inadequate cement mantle in 34% (16). Embranzadeh et al., in evaluating cement mantles, identified increased evidence of loosening in stems placed in more than 5° of varus (39). They identified improved outcomes in femurs with less than 2 mm of proximal medial cancellous bone, and stems with a cement mantle between 2 and 5 mm in thickness. These studies demonstrate the importance of technique for long-term survival of cemented femoral components.

More recently, Barrack et al. proposed a grading system for cement technique (8). They rated cementing technique on a scale of A to D. "A" cementing refers to complete filling of the proximal portion of the diaphysis so that it is difficult to distinguish cortex from cement. This is commonly referred to as white-out. "B" cement technique refers to near complete filling of the diaphysis however one can distinguish cortex from cement in some areas. "C" cement technique is divided into C1 and C2 technique. "C1" refers to an incomplete cement mantle in the proximal portion of the diaphysis in which greater than 50% of the cement–bone interface demonstrates radiolucencies. "C2" refers to a case where the mantle is less than 1 mm thick, or metal is up against bone. For example, a component placed in varus with the tip of the stem up against the lateral cortex would be rated C2. Finally, "D" cementing refers to a cement mantle with gross deficiencies such as no cement below the stem, major defects in the mantle, or multiple large voids in the mantle. It has been shown that aseptic loosening correlates with cement technique, with C and D mantles performing worst. Cement technique should be graded on the first postoperative radiographs. Radiolucencies secondary to remodeling changes and membrane formation make grading cement technique on follow-up radiographs less accurate.

Clinical variables have also been evaluated as risk factors associated with mechanical failure of cemented total hip replacements. Schurman et al. reported that the type of prosthesis, the preoperative Harris Hip Score, and the surgeon did not correlate with the need for revision (111). Increased weight, however, was associated with an increased risk of failure; only 8% of patients less than 68 kilograms required revision 12 years after the index operation. In contrast, 15% of patients weighing more than 68 kilograms required revision at the same time point. Many of the failures in the under-68-kg group occurred in the first 2 years. These early failures could be attributed to technical errors. Excluding the early failures, only 3.4% of the under-68-kg group required revision. Older patients did better than younger patients, and women did better than men. Patients with a diagnosis of posttraumatic arthritis did worse than a comparable osteoarthritic population. Regression tree analysis demonstrated that patients who weighed less than 75 kg had the best outcome. In this group, the chance of survival at 12 years was 90%.

MECHANISMS OF FAILURE

With regard to failure of the cemented femoral component, much attention has been paid to the soft-tissue membrane that forms at the cement–bone interface. This membrane has been implicated in bone resorption, and the process was once incorrectly referred to a as cement disease. On the femoral side, this membrane occurs late in the loosening process and does not appear to be responsible for the initiation of aseptic loosening. In contrast, mechanical factors appear responsible for the initiation of femoral loosening in most cases. Autopsy studies have shown that

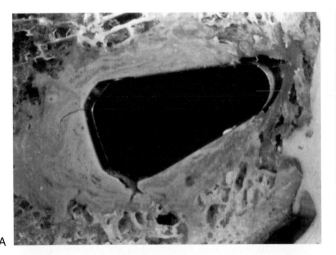

A

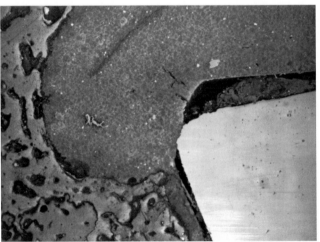

B

C

FIG. 11. **A:** Cross section through the metaphysis demonstrating a debonded implant. Note the gap between the metal and cement with fracture of the cement mantle. **B:** Scanning electron micrograph demonstrating a debonded implant. The implant has rotated into retroversion. Note the fibrous tissue that has migrated into the gap between metal and cement. **C:** Scanning electron micrograph of a cement mantle after the implant has been removed. Note the fracture of the cement mantle, which extends down the metal–cement interface. (Parts A and B reprinted from Morrey BF. *Biological Material and Mechanical Considerations of Joint Replacement.* New York: Raven Press, with permission.)

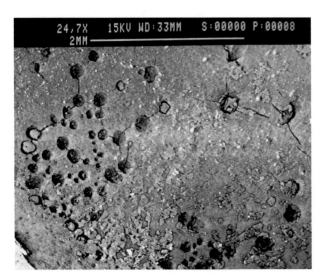

FIG. 12. Multiple pores in a cement mantle; fracture is associated with the pores. (From *British Journal of Bone and Joint Surgery* 1991;73B:556, with permission.)

debonding between the stem and cement initially occurs at the cement–metal interface (Fig. 11) (64,79). Finite element studies have shown that when debonding occurs at the cement–metal interface, high peak stresses in the cement mantle are produced (53,54). Out-of-plane forces involved with stair climbing produce peak stresses in the cement mantle proximally and near the distal tip of the stem. These stresses are high enough to initiate cement cracks. Cracks are more prone to form in areas of thin cement, or adjacent to cement mantle defects. In addition, pores in the cement were sites for crack initiation and crack propagation (Fig. 12). Once these mechanical events have occurred, biologic processes become more important. As a result of debonding and cement fracture, stability of the stem is compromised and particulate polymeric debris can gain access to the endosteal bone. Debris stimulates a foreign-body reaction, which causes bone resorption and results in the fibrous tissue membrane commonly seen at revision surgery (49,66).

It has been suggested in the past that the fibrous layer that develops at the cement–bone interface will eventually lead to loosening of the implant (14,42). The particulate-induced soft-tissue membrane that invades the cement–bone interface begins at the pseudocapsule and extends along the cement–bone interface. This has different implications for the acetabular and femoral components. In the proximal femur, the interdigitation between trabecular bone and cement probably acts as a barrier for migration of debris along this interface. In contrast, the same degree of cement–bone interdigitation is not seen in the subchondral bone around the periphery of the acetabulum. Therefore, the acetabular cement–bone interface is probably a lower-resistance pathway for particle-laden joint fluid compared to the femoral cement–bone interface. There are also some geometric differences between

the acetabulum and femur. The mouth of the acetabular component, which is accessible to soft-tissue membrane invasion, is relatively large compared to the cement–bone interface of the acetabulum. In contrast, the mouth of the femur is relatively small compared to the overall surface area at the cement–bone interface of the femoral component. A granuloma that extends 2 to 3 cm from the periphery of the acetabulum towards the acetabular dome is going to have a significant effect on cemented acetabular stability compared to a granuloma extending 2 to 3 cm distally from the proximal end of the femur. Finally the cemented femoral and acetabular components function in a different mechanical environment. High shear and torsion forces are present on the femoral side, whereas the acetabulum is primarily loaded under compression. These factors explain in part the differences in the mechanism and rates of cemented femoral and acetabular component loosening.

SKELETAL REMODELING

The skeletal changes that occur in the proximal femur after total hip replacement surgery are a good example of mechanically induced bone remodeling that can occur in an otherwise normal skeleton. It is clear that mechanical loading environment influences the balance between bone formation and resorption (23,68,120,125). Wolff's Law describes the relationship between mechanical load and adaptive bone remodeling. In the normal lower extremity, load is transmitted from the femoral head through the femoral neck to the cortical bone of the proximal femur. Load transmission to the proximal femur is markedly altered after total hip arthroplasty. Load normally carried by proximal femur alone is now shared by the implant and bone. *In vitro* testing has shown that insertion of a cemented stem results in a marked decrease in the cortical strain in the proximal femur (79,92). On average, the strain measured in the proximal medial femoral cortex (the calcar region) after insertion of a cemented femoral component is only 15% of that measured in the intact femur prior to implantation. Similar results have been reported after insertion of extensively porous-coated implants. These findings confirm predictions made by finite element studies (63).

Adaptive remodeling theory predicts that the reduction in stress and strain results in resorptive remodeling (63). Radiographically, this phenomenon is best illustrated by the osteopenia that occurs in the calcar region. This phenomenon has been widely referred as stress shielding (Fig. 13). As a result of load sharing, adaptive bone remodeling theory predicts that resorptive remodeling would continue until there is normalization of cortical strain patterns. Analysis of autopsy specimens has not confirmed this prediction. In a study of cadaveric femurs in patients who had previously undergone cemented femoral replacement, the strain patterns along the medial femoral cortex were analyzed (79). With adaptive remodeling that occurs *in vivo*,

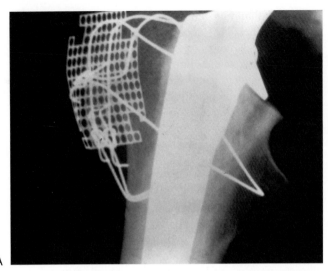 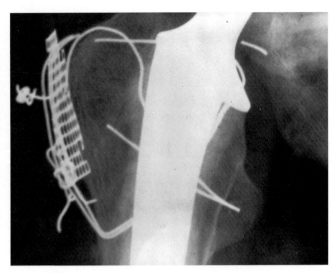

A   B

FIG. 13. A: Early postoperative radiograph after a cemented total hip arthroplasty. Note the thickness of bone in the calcar region. **B:** Radiograph from the same patient approximately 10 years after surgery. Note the bone atrophy in the calcar region compared to the early postoperative radiograph. (From Schurman, Maloney, Smith. *Osteoporosis.* Academic Press, Inc., with permission.)

the strain in the calcar region increases to approximately 30% to 40% of that measured distally. This process occurs relatively rapidly in the first 1 to 2 years after surgery. Although a new "strain equilibrium" appeared to be reached, the strain patterns did not normalize even 17 years after surgery. Despite the fact that the calcar strains did not normalize *in vivo,* the bone in the calcar region did not completely disappear. It appears, at least in the human femur, that there is a point beyond which mechanical factors will not lead to further bone loss.

In examining the bony remodeling that occurs clinically after total hip arthroplasty, it is important to understand the normal age-related changes that occur in the proximal femur in the absence of a hip replacement, particularly the enlargement of the femoral canal diameter that tends to occur after age 45 (103,112). Smith and Walker reported that the diameter of the femoral diaphysis increased an average of 4.4 mm in women between the ages of 45 and 90 (112). In addition to canal widening, cortical bone tends to become thinner and more porotic with advancing age.

Based on radiographic studies, several authors have suggested that the skeletal remodeling that occurs after total hip replacement may be associated with aseptic loosening of the implants. It has been suggested that with aging, the cortex will grow away from the cement and lead to loosening. In a study comparing 30 patients with aseptic loosening of a cemented femoral component with a group of matched controls, Hoffman et al. reported that in those patients with aseptic loosening, the femoral canal expanded at a rate 4 times that of the control group (60). They suggested that medullary enlargement may play a role in failure. Morsher and Ittenson also found that canal expansion occurs at an accelerated rated for the first 2 years after cemented total hip arthroplasty and felt this may play a role in the loosening process (88). In another radiographic study, Comadoll et al. examined the radiographs of 26 cemented total hip arthroplasties an average of 10.4 years after surgery (25). This study found a significant decrease in the cortical thickness and an increase in canal diameter for both men and women. The

FIG. 14. A: Autopsy specimens from a patient who had a unilateral cemented total hip arthroplasty 15 years prior to death. **B:** Radiographs of the same specimens. (From *American Journal of Bone and Joint Surgery* 1990;72A:1222, with permission.) **C:** Radiographs of cross sections from the metaphyseal region of the right (left side) and left (right side) femurs from the same patient. The left femur had a cemented femoral component implanted 15 years prior to death. The right femur had a similar implant placed in the laboratory for comparison. Note the atrophy of the cortical bone circumferentially, as well as the trabecularization of the cortical bone in the calcar region of the right femur. (From *American Journal of Bone and Joint Surgery,* 1990;72A:1222, with permission.) **D:** Radiographs of cross sections from the metaphyseal region of the right (left side) and the left (right side) femurs from the same patient. Note the densification of bone around the cement mantle of the left femur. **E:** Scanning electron micrograph of the cement–bone interface. Note the densification of bone at this interface and the lack of gaps between and bone, consistent with osseointegration. (From *Journal Arthroplasty* 1993;8:81, with permission.) **F:** Higher-power scanning electron micrograph of the cement–bone interface, demonstrating osseointegration between cement and bone. (From *AAOS Orthopaedic Knowledge Update*: Hip and Knee Reconstruction, by Maloney.)

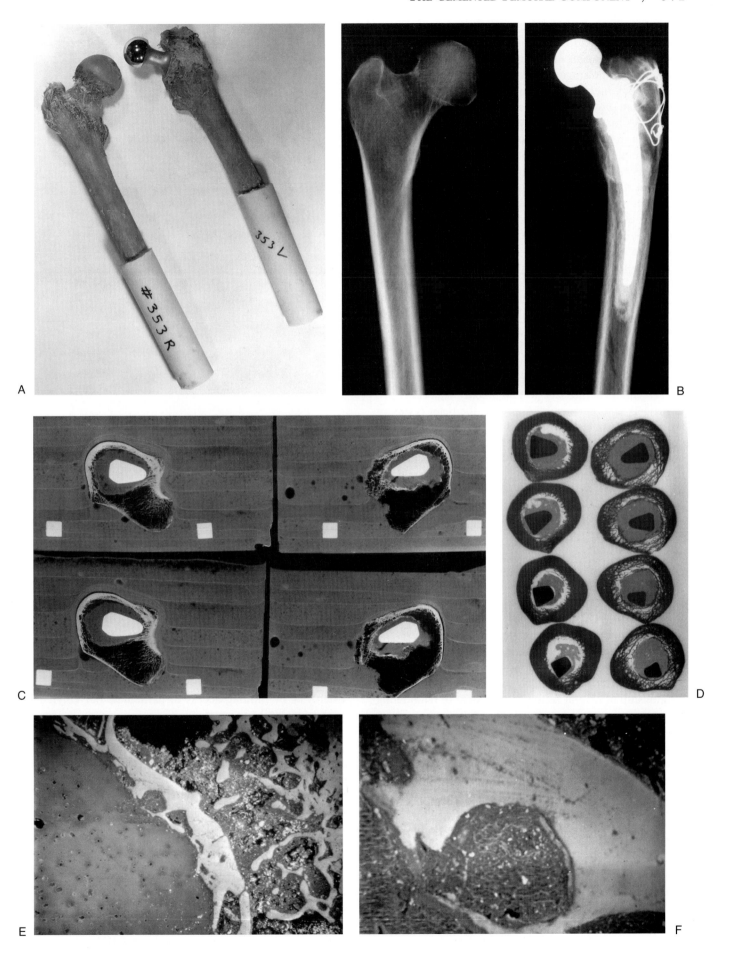

authors concluded that this may cause a separation between cement and bone over time. In contrast, Poss et al. measured a mean rate of cortical expansion of 0.33 mm/year and average loss of cortical bone of 0.15 mm/year at a mean of 11.5 years after cemented total hip replacement (96), values similar to those observed in normal aging. In addition, they were unable to identify any consistent patterns when comparing the implanted to the contralateral intact femur.

Autopsy studies have not supported the hypothesis that mechanically induced osteoporosis and canal widening associated with normal age-related bone remodeling play a role in aseptic loosening of cemented femoral components (65,73,79). Biomechanical studies of autopsy specimens up to 17 years after surgery showed that the femoral components remain mechanically well fixed over time (79). Osseointegration occurs at the bone–cement interface. Maloney et al. and Jasty et al. have performed serial sections of the proximal portion of the femur and femoral component in clinically well-fixed total hip stems retrieved at autopsy (65,79). The histology shows host bone directly against cement. Only rare areas of intervening fibrous tissue were noted. Densification of bone at the cement–bone interface was commonly seen (Fig. 14). In patients with unilateral hip disease, the outer cortex of the operated femur was often thinned and relatively osteoporotic compared to the contralateral intact femur. The inner cortex was not distinguishable from the cement mantle on clinical radiographs. A second medullary canal formed between the inner and outer cortex. The second medullary canal is seen as a radiolucency between the outer cortex and cement on clinical radiographs. This may be misinterpreted as representing fibrous tissue formation (65,73,79). These studies show that age-related remodeling does not play a role in aseptic loosening.

Direct examination of autopsy specimens is also a valuable tool for quantification of the extent of resorptive remodeling (81). Transverse sectioning permits evaluation of the remodeling process by level (metaphyseal and diaphyseal) and quadrant (anterior, posterior, medial, and lateral). Maloney et al. performed a multivariate analysis in patients with unilateral hip disease to determine the relationship of several factors to the extent of remodeling (81). Bone-mineral density of the contralateral femur strongly correlated with the percent decrease of bone-mineral density of the remodeled femur. Based on these data, it appears that patients with poor bone to begin with are at risk for the greatest bone loss on a percentage basis.

OSTEOLYSIS

Osteolysis, once refered to as cement disease, commonly occurs in association with aseptic loosening (Fig. 15). Histologic studies of interface tissue recovered at the time of revision surgery has demonstrated a classic foreign body granuloma with an abundance of macrophages

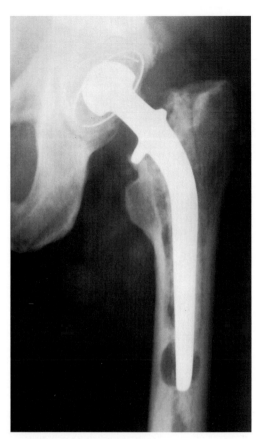

FIG. 15. Osteolysis around a cemented femoral component once referred to as cement disease.

(42,49,57). Particulate debris, whether PMMA, polyethylene, titanium, or cobalt–chrome, is thought to initiate the osteolytic process. Cementless technology was introduced in part to avoid osteolysis associated with loosening of cemented components. Unfortunately, this was not realized. In a study where both cemented and noncemented components were assessed for osteolysis in a matched pair fashion, the authors concluded that the access of particulate debris to the periprosthetic interface was essential for the initiation of osteolysis (46). They also felt that current third-generation cementing techniques helped provide protection against the femoral osteolysis by limiting access of particulate polyethylene to the cement–bone interface.

Fragmentation of the cement mantle has been identified as a source for PMMA particles and focal osteolysis. In a study examining autopsy specimens with cemented femoral components. areas of focal femoral osteolysis were identified (Fig. 16). Examination of the areas of lysis revealed fractures in the cement mantle with generation of particulate debris (Fig. 17) (80). Review of the tissue at the cement–bone interface revealed macrophage and giant-cell foreign-body granulomatous reaction (66). Anthony et al. reported four cases of focal osteolysis with stable cemented femoral components (3). At revision surgery, cement mantle defects were identified at the site

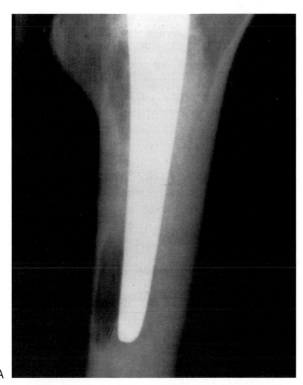
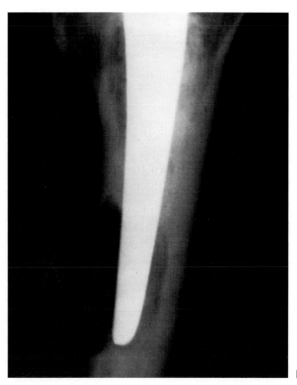

A   B

FIG. 16. A: Localized osteolysis around a radiographically stable cemented femoral component. **B:** Radiograph demonstrated progression of the lesion.

of the osteolytic defects. The authors hypothesized that these defects provided access of joint fluid contents into the endosteal surface.

Animal studies support the postulate that bulk methylmethacrylate is well tolerated biologically. A report by Miller et al. evaluated the biologic response of PMMA implants in canine femoral diaphysis (86). At 1 to 42 weeks, there was no evidence of inflammation or cell death. Data from a rabbit model study also demonstrated that new bone could be deposited directly on bone cement, and that bone could fill gaps that initially were present between cement and bone (38).

On a cellular level, arachidonic acid mediators have been shown to be released from macrophages after exposure to particulate PMMA. The exposure to PMMA was also associated with cellular injury (61). Cell culture studies have shown that particulate PMMA stimulates release of a variety of bone-resorbing factors including interleukin-1, tumor necrosis factor, and prostaglandin E_2 from mononuclear cells (59). Conditioned media from these cultures results in bone resorption when added to limb bone assay models.

The precise role of the immune system in the biologic response to particulate debris is controversial. Jasty et al. demonstrated that a typical foreign-body response results when immunodeficient mice are challenged with PMMA particles (66). Subcutaneous injections of PMMA in immunodeficient mice produced granulomas consisting of macrophages and giant cells, suggesting that lympho-

cytes were not a necessary component in the biologic response to particulate debris. Similarly, when Santavirta et al. added PMMA particles to lymphocytes in culture no significant reaction was noted (106). Results of these studies suggest that the immune system does not play a significant role in the response to wear debris. In immunohistochemical studies, however, lymphocytes have been identified in the soft-tissue membrane around failed implants (up to 10% of the cells present) (67).

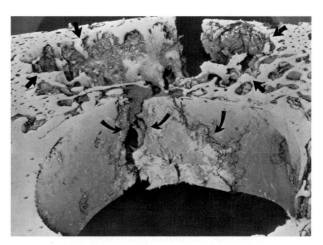

FIG. 17. Scanning electron micrograph of a cross section through the diaphysis of a femur, demonstrating fragmentation of a thin cement mantle *(arrows)* with an osteolytic defect in the adjacent cortex.

These cells may be important in modulating the biologic response to wear debris.

DESIGN ISSUES

Collar

Controversy exists over the use of a collared prosthesis in cemented total hip arthroplasty. Finite element as well as *in vitro* studies have shown that a collar results in increased load transfer from to the proximal femur compared to collarless implants. This may reduce stress shielding of the proximal femur and reduce strain in the proximal medial cement mantle (28,55,84,92). Data from clinical studies show that, with modern instrumentation, collar–medial neck contact can be achieved initially in 90% of cases and maintained in 88% of these cases (108). In a prospective randomized study of collared versus collarless prostheses, Fitzgerald et al. showed a higher incidence of loose femoral components among hips inserted without collars (41). In contrast, Meding et al. reported on a randomized series with 5-year follow-up, finding that the presence of the collar had no effect on fixation, osteopenia, or clinical scores (85).

Proponents of the collarless femoral component may agree on the reduction of the proximal femoral strain in *in vitro* studies with the use of the collar, but *in vivo* such reductions do not appear clinically significant, as seen by the absence of osteopenia on radiographs. The proponents of a collarless stems point to the difficulty of obtaining and maintaining adequate calcar–collar contact. There have been several early reports on the resorption of the medial femoral neck under a collar (11,20,26). Proponents of the collarless stem also point to the problems of proximal medial neck resorption under the collar and the possible generation of wear debris secondary to the micromotion between the collar and cement as well as the collar and the calcar (77). A prospective study by Rickards and Duncan examined the results of 98 HD2 prostheses (Howmedica, Rutherford, New Jersey) (98). In 26% of the initial cases, unsatisfactory collar–calcar contact was obtained. Of the remaining patients, 76% lost the collar–calcar contact over the course of 2 years. However, as noted above, collar–calcar contact can be achieved and maintained in a much higher percentage of patients using modern instrumentation.

Metal–Cement Interface

Failure of the cement–metal interface has been identified as an initiating factor in the failure of cemented femoral stems (64). *In vitro* studies have supported this postulate, showing increased strains of the cement mantle when debonding of the cement–metal interface occurs (29,51,54). To improve the longevity of cemented femoral stems, the cement–metal interface has been enhanced through surface texture modifications of the femoral component including micro- and macro-texturing and component pre-coating with PMMA. *In vitro* experiments comparing pre-coating with smooth and porous-coated femoral implants have shown that precoating strengthens the metal–cement interface even in the presence of contaminants such as blood (32,34).

The concept of surface texture modifications is not universally accepted. Gardiner and Hozack reported 17 femoral prosthesis that had undergone surface modifications and failed at a mean of 37 months after surgery (43). These authors as well as others have postulated that the improved cement–prostheses bond transferred increased stresses to the cement–bone interface, leading to early failure at this interface (43,77). However, increased load transfer is unlikely to represent a mechanism for loosening in these failures. Considering the experience with cementless implants where all load is transferred at the metal–bone interface, it is unlikely there would be an adverse biologic response as a result of increase load transfer at the cement–bone interface. Analysis of autopsy specimens with pre-coated femoral components has shown no evidence of failure at the cement–bone interface. In addition, the published results with the Harris pre-coat prosthesis (Zimmer, Warsaw, IN) have been good (87,93,108). It is more likely these failures were associated with poor cementing, including thin cement mantles or mantle defects.

SPECIAL PROBLEMS

Most long-term reports on cemented total hip replacement have study groups that include patients with a variety of diagnoses. Osteoarthritic patients usually make up the majority of these study groups, but patients with other diagnoses such as rheumatoid arthritis, avascular necrosis, and developmental dysplasia are often included. Some diagnoses, such as developmental dysplasia or juvenile rheumatoid arthritis, represent special problems and are worth evaluating independently.

Congenital Dislocation of the Hip

Total hip replacement for neglected congenital dislocation of the hip and severe dysplasia present several technical challenges. On the femoral side, the issues of leg length and offset are of key concern. The preservation of proximal bone stock is also important. Deformity of the proximal femur and small intramedullary canal may result in the need for special or custom femoral components. Careful preoperative planning is important to ensure an adequate selection of implants at surgery.

Limb lengthening is often required in an attempt to equalize limb lengths. A greater incidence of trochanteric nonunion is identified with lengthening of the leg more than 2 cm. With limb lengthening, the incidence of nerve palsy in patients with developmental dysplasia or dislocation increases and has been reported to be approximately 5% (4).

Anwar et al. reported on 34 cemented total hip replacements in 28 patients for neglected congenital dislocation of the hip with a follow-up of 5.6 to 14 years (mean, 9.4 years) (4). Radiographic loosening occurred in three femoral components and was attributed to poor cementing technique. In another long-term study by Garvin et al. (8 to 16.5 years), five revisions of the femoral component were performed out of 29 cemented hip arthroplasties (44). Four of the five failures, however, were fractured Trapezoidal-28 (Zimmer, Warsaw, IN) stems. The remaining case was for femoral loosening.

Custom-designed femoral components have been evaluated with good results for severe dysplasia of the hip. In a series of 19 dysplastic hips, custom components were used with design features including a varus neck to reduce impingement and improve the effective lever arm of the abductors (62). With a mean follow-up of 57 months, (range, 27 to 108), the survival rate for the femoral component was 93%. The authors felt that the clinical results justified the use of a custom prostheses in the situation in which a standard prostheses could not provide an anatomic restoration of the hip.

Juvenile Rheumatoid Arthritis

Patients requiring total hip replacement for juvenile rheumatoid arthritis often have polyarticular involvement and are severely disabled. The local anatomy in these patients is often abnormal secondary to soft-tissue contractures and bony deformity. Hypoplasia of the femur is common, sometimes requiring special or custom implants.

The short-term results of cemented total hip arthroplasty in this patient population were encouraging. Longer-term studies, though, have reported high failure rates. In one report of 96 primary cemented total hip arthroplasties in 54 patients at a minimum of 5 years after surgery (mean, 11.5 years), revision surgery was performed in 25% of patients, and 17 patients had radiographically loose stems (123). The factors thought to be responsible for the high failure rate were the high vascularity of the bone as well as the high degree of osteoporosis. All the stems in this series were inserted with first-generation cementing technique. In another report (74), 62 cemented hip replacements in 34 patients were followed up for 2 to 11 years (mean, 6 years). Although only two patients required revision (one loose acetabular component and one broken femoral stem), 8% of the femoral components demonstrated progressive radiolucencies or migration. A recent radiologic review of 57

total hip arthroplasties in 34 adolescents with chronic juvenile rheumatoid arthritis was performed by Williams and McCullough (122). One femoral component had been revised and six showed evidence of radiologic loosening. A factor suggested for the loosening was the dynamic state of the immature skeleton with frequent cortical remodeling.

In general, these reports include surgeries performed over many years, so the cement technique may have changed during the course of the study. Although patients with juvenile rheumatoid arthritis are young, the relatively high failure rates are higher than might be expected considering their low body weight and activity level. Factors such as poor bone quality and highly vascular bone, which may compromise cement technique, have been cited as possible causes of the high failure rate in this patient population. Although long-term follow-up studies of patients with juvenile rheumatoid arthritis show increased rates of loosening. The significant benefits of pain relief and improved range of motion should not be overlooked.

Fracture of the Acetabulum

The prevalence of posttraumatic arthritis after acetabular fracture ranges from 12% to 57% (17,76,95,102). The risk of developing posttraumatic arthritis increases with increased comminution and displacement, and with involvement of the weight-bearing surface (75). Avascular necrosis of the femoral head is another potential problem after trauma. The frequency of avascular necrosis of the femoral head after acetabular fracture ranges from 2% to 40% (75,117,121).

In general, the results of primary cemented hip replacement after pelvic trauma are not as good as the results reported for primary osteoarthritis. This may be in part because these patients tend to be younger and more active. Additionally, the distorted or compromised bony anatomy may play a role in implant fixation. Romness and Lewallen reviewed 55 primary total hip arthroplasties in 53 patients with a history of previous acetabular fracture (101). At the time of primary arthroplasty, the average age was 56 years. The patients were followed for an average of 7.5 years. In this study, the revision rate was 7.8%. Almost 16% of the patients had symptomatic loosening. Radiographic loosening was demonstrated in 29.4%. The authors concluded that their loosening and failure rates were much higher than the current reported rates of routine primary arthroplasty, but that they were similar to the early reports of routine total hip arthroplasty using first-generation techniques.

Sickle-Cell Hemoglobinopathy

Sickle-cell hemoglobinopathies have been associated with femoral head osteonecrosis. Sickling can result in occlusion of the small vessels in the femoral head, which may produce infarction. Collapse of the femoral head and secondary degenerative joint disease result (22). Complication rates in these patients undergoing total hip replacement are high. A study reviewing 28 arthroplasties in 25 patients with sickle-cell anemia and osteonecrosis of the femoral head found a 49% complication rate within the 7.5-year follow-up (1). The infection rate was close to 20%. Seventeen of the femoral stems were cemented. Ten of these had been revised. The high complication rate included seven infections, two intraoperative fractures, three urinary tract infections, three sickle-cell crises, and two episodes of excessive blood loss.

The authors concluded that the risk-to-benefit ratio in patients with sickle-cell hemoglobinopathy is high. They recommended a preoperative hematology consultation, preoperative transfusion to achieve a hemoglobin A level of greater than 50%, perioperative antibiotics, hydration and oxygenation to prevent crisis, and caution in the use of bone cement because of high failure rates.

The high loosening rates of total hip arthroplasties for osteonecrosis resulting from sickle cell hemoglobinopathy may be related to bone remodeling and bone quality. The chronic anemia in these patients results in marrow proliferation. In the proximal femur, this proliferation results in canal widening. In addition, these patients often have associated cortical thinning. The high infection rates may be related to a deficiency in the immune system in these patients. Patients with sickle-cell disease also are functionally asplenic as a result of autoinfarction of the spleen.

Ankylosing Spondylitis

Ankylosing spondylitis has been traditionally felt to be a risk factor for the development of heterotopic bone after total hip arthroplasty. The reported rates of ectopic bone formation vary from 4% to 61.7%. In one recent large study, clinically important heterotopic bone developed in 11% of cases (71). All of these patients had either previous hip surgery, a postoperative infection, or complete ankylosis preoperatively. The authors concluded that routine prophylaxis for uncomplicated total hip arthroplasty was not necessary.

Renal Transplant

Osteonecrosis is a recognized complication of renal transplantation. Chronic immunosuppression with corticosteroids has been implicated as the major factor in the etiology of the osteonecrosis. Despite several different approaches to early osteonecrosis, collapse of the femoral head ultimately occurs. Treatment with total hip arthroplasty has been advocated. A review of 50 patients with osteonecrosis of the femoral head after renal transplant was performed by Cheng et al. (21). The femoral components had a survival rate of 97% at 5 years and 87% at 10 years. Cemented femoral prostheses appear to have satisfactory results after transplantation. The results are analogous to those in older patients without renal transplant.

REFERENCES

1. Acurio MT, Friedman RJ. Hip arthroplasty in patients with sickle-cell hemoglobinopathy. *J Bone Joint Surg* 1992;74B:367–371.
2. Amstutz HC, Markolf KL, McNeice GM, et al. Loosening of total hip components: cause and prevention. In: Evarts CM, ed. *The hip. Proceedings of the fourth open scientific meeting of The Hip Society.* St. Louis: CV Mosby, 1976:102–116.
3. Anthony PP, Gie GA, Howie CR, Ling RSM. Localised endosteal bone lysis in relation to the femoral components of cemented total hip arthroplasties. *J Bone Joint Surg* 1990;72B:971–979.
4. Anwar MM, Sugano N, Mashura K, Kadoweki T, Takaoka K, Ono K. Total hip arthroplasty in the neglected congenital dislocation of the hip. A five to 14-year follow-up study. *Clin Orthop* 1993;295:127–134.
5. Askew MJ, SteegeJW, Lewis JL, et al. Effect of cement pressure and bone strength on polymethylmethacrylate fixation. *J Orthop Res* 1984;1:412–420.
6. Ballard WT, Callaghan JJ, Sullivan PM, Johnston RC. The results of improved cementing techniques for total hip arthroplasty in patients less than fifty years old. A ten year follow-up study. *J Bone Joint Surg* 1994;76A:959–964.
7. Bannister GC, Young SK, Baker AS, Mackinnon JG, Magnusson PA. Control of bleeding in cemented arthroplasty. *J Bone Joint Surg* 1990;72B:444–446.
8. Barrack RL, Mulroy RD, Harris WH. Improved cementing techniques and femoral component loosening in young patients with hip arthroplasty. A 12 year radiographic review. *J Bone Joint Surg* 1992;74B:385–389.
9. Beckenbaugh RD, Ilstrup D. Total hip arthroplasty. A review of 333 cases with long follow-up. *J Bone Joint Surg* 1978;60A:306–313.
10. Berger RA, Seel MJ, Wood K, D'Antonio J, Rubash HE. The effect of centralizing device on cement mantle deficiencies and initial prosthetic alignment in total hip arthroplasty. *Journal of Arthroplasty* 1977;12:434.
11. Blacker GJ, Charnley J. Changes in the upper femur after low friction arthroplasty of the hip. *Clin Orthop* 1978;137:15–23.
12. Brand RA, Pedersen DR, Yoder SA. How definition of loosening affects the incidence of loose total hip reconstructions. *Clin Orthop* 1986;210:185–191.
13. Brien WW, Salvati EA, Klein R, Brause B, Stern S. Antibiotic impregnated bone cement in total hip arthroplasty. An in vivo comparison of the elution properties of Tobramycin and Vancomycin. *Clin Orthop* 1993;296:242–248.
14. Bullough RG, Dicarlo EF, Hansraj KK, Neves MC. Pathologic studies of total joint replacement. *Orthop Clin North Am* 1988;19:611–625.
15. Burke DW, Gates EI, Harris WH. Centrifugation as a method of improving tensile and fatigue properties of acrylic bone cement. *J Bone Joint Surg* 1984;66A:1265–1273.
16. Callaghan JJ, Salvati EA, Pellicci PM, Wilson PD, Ranawat CS. Results of revision for mechanical failure after cemented total hip replacement, 1979 to 1982. *J Bone Joint Surg* 1985;67A:1074–1085.
17. Carnesale PG, Stewart MJ, Barnes SN. Acetabular disruption and central fracture-dislocation of the hip. a long term study. *J Bone Joint Surg* 1975;57A:1054–1059.
18. Chandler HP, Reineck FT, Wixson RL, McCarthy JC. Total hip replacement in patients younger than thirty years old. *J Bone Joint Surg* 1981;63A:1426–1434.
19. Charnley J. Arthroplasty of the hip: a new operation. *Lancet* 1961;i:1129–1132.
20. Charnley J, Cupic Z. The nine and ten year results of low-friction arthroplasty of the hip. *Clin Orthop* 1973;95:9–25.
21. Cheng EY, Klibanoff JE, Robinson HJ, Bradford DS. Total hip arthroplasty with cement after renal transplantation. *J Bone Joint Surg* 1995;77A:1535–1541.

22. Chung SM, Ralston EL. Necrosis of the femoral head associated with sickle cell anemia and its genetic variants. *J Bone Joint Surg* 1969; 51A:33–58.

23. Churches AE, Howlett CR, Waldron KJ, Ward GW. The response of living bone to controlled time varying loading: method and preliminary results. *J Biomech* 1979;12:35–45.

24. Collis DK. Long term follow-up of cemented total hip replacements in patients who were less than fifty years old. *J Bone Joint Surg* 1991;73A:593–597.

25. Comadoll JL, Sherman RE, Gustilo RB, Bechtold JE. Radiographic changes in bone dimensions in asymptomatic cemented total hip arthroplasties. Results of nine to thirteen-year follow-up. *J Bone Joint Surg* 1988;70A:433–438.

26. Cotterill PB, Hunter GA, Tile M. A radiographic analysis of 166 Charnley-Müller total hip arthroplasties. *Clin Orthop* 1982;163: 120–126.

27. Coudane H, Fery A, Sommelet J, Lacoste J, Leduc P, Gaucher A. Aseptic loosening o f cemented total arthroplasties of the hip in relation to position of the prosthesis. New utilization of the Tschaprow-Cramer statistical test. *Acta Orthop Scand* 1981;52:201–205.

28. Crowninshield RD, Brand RA, Johnston RC, Pedersen DR. An analyses of collar function and the use of titanium in femoral prostheses. *Clin Orthop* 1981;158:270–277.

29. Crowninshield RD, Tolbert JR. Cement strain measurement surrounding loose and well fixed femoral component stems. *J Biomed Mater Res* 1983;17:819–825.

30. Davies JP, Burke DW, O'Connor DO, Harris WH. Comparison of the fatigue characteristics of centrifuge and uncentrifuged Simplex P bone cement. *J Orthop Res* 1987;5:366–371.

31. Davies JP, Harris WH. In vitro and in vivo studies of pressurization of femoral cement in total hip arthroplasty. *J Arthroplasty* 1993;8: 585–591.

32. Davies JP, Harris WH. Strength of cement-metal interface in fatigue. Comparison of smooth, porous, and precoated specimens. *Clin Mater* 1993;12:121–126.

33. Davies JP, O'Connor DO, Burke DW, Jasty M, Harris WH. The effect of centrifugation on the fatigue life of bone cement in the presence of surface irregularities. *Clin Orthop* 1988;229:156–161.

34. Davies JP, Singer G, Harris WH. The effect of a thin coating of polymethylmethacrylate on the torsional fatigue strength of the cement-metal interface. *J Applied Biomaterials* 1992;3:45–49.

35. Dorr LD, Kane TJ III, Conaty JP. Long term results of cemented total hip arthroplasty in patients forty-five years old or younger. A 16 year follow-up study. *J Arthroplasty* 1994;9:453–456.

36. Dorr LD, Luckett M, Conaty JP. Total hip arthroplasties in patients younger than forty-five years. A nine- to ten-year follow-up study. *Clin Orthop* 1990;260:215–219.

37. Dorr LD, Takei GK, Conaty JP. Total hip arthroplasties in patients less than forty-five years old. *J Bone Joint Surg* 1983;65A:474–479.

38. Draenert K. Histomorphology of the bone-to-cement interface. Remodeling of the cortex and revascularization of the medullary canal in animal experiments. In: *The hip. Proceedings of the ninth open scientific meeting of the Hip Society*. St. Louis: CV Mosby, 1981;71–110.

39. Ebramzadah E, Sarmiento A, Mckellop HA, Llinas A, Gogan W. The cement mantle in total hip arthroplasty. *J Bone Joint Surg* 1994;76A: 77–87.

40. Estok DM, Harrigan TP, Harris WH. Finite element analysis of cement strains at the tip of an idealized cemented femoral component. *Trans Orthop Res Soc* 1991;16:504.

41. Fitzgerald RH, Rand JA, Ilstrup D, Kelley SS. A prospective randomized study of collared versus a collarless femoral component. *Orthop Trans* 1990;14:639.

42. Freeman MAR, Bradley GW, Revell PA. Observations upon the interface between bone and polymethylmethacrylate cement. *J Bone Joint Surg* 1982;64B:489–493.

43. Gardiner RC, Hozack WJ. Failure of the cement-bone interface. A consequence of strengthening the cement-prosthesis interface? *J Bone Joint Surg* 1994;76B:49–52.

44. Garvin KC, Bowen MK, Salvati EA, Ranawat CS. Long term results of total hip arthroplasty in congenital dislocation and dysplasia of the hip. *J Bone Joint Surg* 1991;73A:1348–1354.

45. Gates EI, Carter DR, Harris WH. Comparative fatigue behavior of different bone cements. *Clin Orthop* 1984;189:294–299.

46. Goetz DD, Smith EJ, Harris WH. The prevalence of osteolysis associated with components inserted with or without cement in total hip replacements. *J Bone Joint Surg* 1994;76A:1121–1127.

47. Goldberg BA, Al-Habbel G, Noble PC, Paravic M, Tullos HS. A fourth generation cemented femoral prosthesis: clinical and radiographic results. *Orthop Trans* 1995;19:546.

48. Goldberg BA, Noble PC, Tullos HS. The performance of modular femoral stem centralizers in cemented total hip arthroplasty. *Orthop Trans* 1995;19:522.

49. Goldring SR, Schiller AL, Roelke M, Roelke CM, O'Neil DA, Harris WH. The synovial-like membrane at the bone-cement interface in loose total hip replacements and its proposed role in bone lysis. *J Bone Joint Surg* 1983;65A:575–584.

50. Gruen TA, McNiece G, Amstutz HC. Modes of failure of cemented stem-type femoral components. A radiographic analysis of loosening. *Clin Orthop* 1979;141:17–27.

51. Hampton SJ, Andriacchi TP, Dragnitch LF, Galante JO. Stresses following stem-cement bond failure in femoral total hip implants. *Trans Orthop Res Soc* 1981;6:144.

52. Hanson PB, Walker RH. Total hip arthroplasty cemented femoral component distal stem centralizer: effect on stem alignment and cement mantle. *Journal of Arthroplasty* 1995;10:683.

53. Harrigan TP, Kareh JA, O'Connor DO, Burke DW. A finite element study of the initiation of failure of fixation in cemented total hip components. *J Orthop Res* 1992;10:134–144.

54. Harrigan TP, Harris WH. A three dimensional non-linear finite element study of the effect of cement-prosthesis debonding in cemented femoral total hip components. *J Biomech* 1991;24:1047–1058.

55. Harris WH. Is it advantageous to strengthen the cement-metal interface and use a collar for cemented femoral components of total hip replacements? *Clin Orthop* 1992;285:67–71.

56. Harris WH, McGann WA. Loosening of the femoral component after use of the medullary-plug cementing technique. *J Bone Joint Surg* 1986;68A:1064–1066.

57. Harris WH, Schiller AL, Schouller JM, Freiberg RA, Scott R. Extensive localized bone resorption in the femur following total hip replacement. *J Bone Joint Surg* 1976;58A:612–618.

58. Havelin LI, Espehaug B, Vollset SE, Engesaeter, LB. The effect of the type of cement on early revision of Charnley total hip prosthesis. *J Bone Joint Surg* 1995;77A:1543–1550.

59. Herman JH, Sowder WG, Anderson D, Appel AM, Hopson CN. Polymethyl-methacrylate induced release of bone resorbing factors. *J Bone Joint Surg* 1989;71A:1530–1541.

60. Hoffman AA, Wyatt RWB, France EP, Bigler GT, Daniels AU, Hess WE. Endosteal bone loss after total hip arthroplasty. *Clin Orthop* 1989;245:138–144.

61. Horowitz SM, Gautsch TC, Frondoza CG, Riley L. Macrophage exposure to polymethyl-methacrylate leads to mediator release and injury. *J Orthop Res* 1991;9:406–413.

62. Huo MH, Salvati EA, Lieberman JR, Burstein AH, Wilson PD. Custom-designed femoral prostheses in total hip arthroplasty done with cement for severe dysplasia of the hip. *J Bone Joint Surg* 1993;75A:1497–1504.

63. Huskies R. The various stress patterns of press-fit, ingrown, and cemented femoral stems. *Clin Orthop* 1990;261:27–38.

64. Jasty M, Maloney WJ, Bragdon CR, et al. The initiation of failure in cemented femoral components of hip arthroplasty. *J Bone Joint Surg* 1991;73B:551–558.

65. Jasty M, Maloney WJ, Bragdon CR, Haire T, Harris WH. Histomorphological studies of the long-term skeletal responses to well fixed cemented femoral components. *J Bone Joint Surg* 1990;72A: 1220–1229.

66. Jasty M, Jiranek W, Harris WH. Acrylic fragmentation in total hip replacements and its biologic consequences. *Clin Orthop* 1992;285: 116–128.

67. Jiranek WA, Machado M, Jasty M, et al. Production of cytokines around loosened cemented acetabular components. Analysis with immunohistochemical techniques and in situ hybridization. *J Bone Joint Surg* 1993;75A:863–879.

68. Jones HH, Priest JD, Hayes WC, Tichenor CC, Nagel DA. Humeral Hypertrophy in response to exercise. *J Bone Joint Surg* 1977;59A: 204–208.

69. Josefsson G, Kolmert L. Prophylaxis with systemic antibiotics versus gentamicin bone cement in total hip arthroplasty. A ten year survey of 1,688 hips. *Clin Orthop* 1993;292:210–214.

70. Karrholm J, Borssen B, Gudmund L, Snorrsason F. Does early micromotion of femoral prosthesis matter? *J Bone Joint Surg* 1994;76B: 912–917.

71. Kilgus DJ, Namba RS, Gorek JE, et al. Total hip replacement for patients who have ankylosing spondylitis: the importance of formation of heterotopic bone and the durability of fixation of cemented components. *J Bone Joint Surg* 1990;72A:834–839.

72. Kristionsen B, Jensen JS. Biomechanical factors in loosening of the Stanmore hip. *Acta Orthop Scand* 1985;56:21–24.

73. Kwong LM, Jasty M, Mulroy RD, Maloney WJ, Bragdon C, Harris WH. Histology of the radiolucent line. *J Bone Joint Surg* 1992;74B: 67–73.

74. Lachiewicz PF, McCaskill B, Inglis A, Ranawat CS. Total hip arthroplasty in juvenile rheumatoid arthritis. Two to eleven-year results. *J Bone Joint Surg* 1986;68A:502–508.

75. Larson CB. Fracture dislocation of the hip. *Clin Orthop* 1973;92: 147–154.

76. Letournel E. Acetabular fractures. Classification and management. *Clin Orthop* 1980;151:81–106.

77. Ling RSM. The use of a collar and precoating on cemented femoral stems is unnecessary and detrimental. *Clin Orthop* 1992;285:73–83.

78. Majkowski RS, Miles AW, Bannister GC, Perkins J, Taylor GJS. Bone surface preparation in cemented joint replacement. *J Bone Joint Surg* 1993;75B:459–463.

79. Maloney WJ, Jasty M, Burke DW, O'Connor DO, Zalenski EB, Bragdon C, Harris WH. Biomechanical and histologic investigation of cemented total hip arthroplasties. *Clin Orthop* 1989;249:129–140.

80. Maloney WJ, Jasty M, Rosenberg A, Harris WH. Bone lysis in well fixed cemented femoral components. *J Bone Joint Surg* 1990;72B: 966–970.

81. Maloney WJ, Sychterz C, Bragdon C, McGovern T, Jasty M, Engh CA, Harris WH. Femoral bone remodeling after total hip arthroplasty: the skeletal response to well-fixed femoral components inserted with and without cement. *Clin Orthop* 1996;333:15.

82. Maltry JA, Noble PC, Kamaric E, Tullos HS. Factors influencing pressurization of the femoral canal during cemented total hip arthroplasty. *J Arthroplasty* 1995;10:492–497.

83. Markolf KC, Amstutz HC. Penetration and flow of acrylic bone cement. *Clin Orthop* 1976;121:99–102.

84. Markolf KC, Amstutz HC, Hischowitz DL. The effect of calcar contact on femoral micromovement. *J Bone Joint Surg* 1980;62A: 1315–1323.

85. Meding JB, Faris PM, Keeting EM. The comparison of collared and collarless femoral components in primary and cemented total hip arthroplasty. *Orthop Trans* 1995;19:402.

86. Miller J, Burke DC, Stachiewicz JW, Amed AM, Kelebay LC. Pathophysiology of loosening of femoral components in total hip arthroplasty. Clinical and experimental study of cement fracture and loosening of the cement-bone interface. In: *The hip. Proceedings of the sixth open scientific meeting of the Hip Society*. St. Louis: CV Mosby, 1978;64–86.

87. Mohler CG, Kull LR, Martell JM, Rosenberg AG, Galante JO. Total hip replacement with insertion of an acetabular component without cement and a femoral component with cement. Four to seven-year results. *J Bone Joint Surg* 1995;77A:86–96.

88. Morscher E, Ittenson F. Knochen-remodelling und lockerung des protheseenschaftes bei huftporthesen. Symposium des Argeitskreises fur Ostelologie Davos 12/13, 4 1984. *Acta Med Aust* 1984;32:16.

89. Mulroy WF, Estok DM, Harris WH. Total hip arthroplasty with use of so-called second-generation cementing techniques. *J Bone Joint Surg* 1995;77A:1845–1852.

90. Oates KM, Barrera DL, Tucker WN, Chau CCH, Bugbee WO, Convey FR. In vivo effect of pressurization of polymethylmethacrylate bone-cement. Biomechanical and histologic analysis. *J Arthroplasty* 1995; 10:373–381.

91. O'Connor D, Burke DW, Sedlacek RC, Harris WH. Peak cement strains in cemented femoral total hip. *Trans Orthop Res Soc* 1991;16:220.

92. Oh I, Harris WH. Proximal strain distribution in the loaded femur. An in vitro comparison of the distributions in the intact femur and after insertion of different hip replacement femoral components. *J Bone Joint Surg* 1978;60A:75–85.

93. Oishi CS, Walker RH, Colwell CW. The femoral component in total hip arthroplasty. Six to eight year follow-up after use of third generation cementing technique. *J Bone Joint Surg* 1994;76A:1130–1136.

94. Olsson SS, Jernberger A, Tryggo D. Clinical and radiological long term results after Charnley-Müller total hip replacement. A 5 to 10 year follow-up study with special reference to aseptic loosening. *Acta Orthop Scand* 1981;52:531–542.

95. Pennal GF, Davidson J, Garside H, et al. Results of treatment of acetabular fractures. *Clin Orthop* 1980;151:115–123.

96. Poss R, Staehlin P, Larson M. Femoral expansion in total hip arthroplasty. *J Arthroplasty* 1987;2:259–264.

97. Rey RM Jr, Paiement GD, McGann WM, et al. A study of intrusion characteristics of low viscosity cement Simplex-P and Palacos cements in a bovine cancellous model. *Clin Orthop* 1987;215: 272–278.

98. Rickards R, Duncan CP. The collar-calcar contact controversy. *J Bone Joint Surg* 1986;68B:851.

99. Rimnac CM, Wright, TM, McGill DL. The effect of centrifugation on the fracture properties of acrylic bone cements. *J Bone Joint Surg* 1986;68A:281–287.

100. Rockborn P, Olsson SS. Loosening and bone resorption in Exeter hip arthroplasties. Review of a minimum of five years. *J Bone Joint Surg* 1993;75B:865–868.

101. Romness DW, LeWallen DG. Total hip arthroplasty after fracture of the acetabulum. Long term results. *J Bone Joint Surg* 1990;72B: 761–764.

102. Rowe CR, Lowell JD. Prognosis of fractures of the acetabulum. *J Bone Joint Surg* 1961;43A:30–59.

103. Ruff CB, Hayes WC. Subperiosteal expansion and cortical remodeling of the human femur and tibia with aging. *Science* 1982;217: 945–948.

104. Ryd L. Roentgen stereophotogrammetric analysis of prosthetic fixation in the hip and knee joint. *Clin Orthop* 1992;276:56–65.

105. Russotti GM, Coventry MB, Stauffer RN. Cemented total hip arthroplasty with contemporary techniques. A five year minimum follow-up study. *Clin Orthop* 1988;235:141–147.

106. Santavirta S, Nordstrom D, Metsarinne K, Konttinen YT. Biocompatibility of poly-ethylene and host response to loosening of cementless total hip replacement. *Clin Orthop* 1993;297:100–110.

107. Sarmiento A, Turner TM, Latta LL, Tarr RR. Factors contributing to lysis of the femoral neck in total hip arthroplasty. *Clin Orthop* 1979; 145:208–212.

108. Schmalzried TP, Harris WH. Hybrid total hip replacement: a six and one-half year follow-up. *J Bone Joint Surg* 1993;75B:608–615.

109. Schmalzried TP, Maloney WJ, Jasty M, Kwong LM, Harris WH. Autopsy studies of the bone-cement interface in well-fixed cemented total hip arthroplasties. *J Arthroplasty* 1993;8:179–188.

110. Schulte KR, Callaghan JJ, Kelley SS, Johnston RC. The outcome of Charnley total hip arthroplasty with cement after a minimum twenty-year follow-up. *J Bone Joint Surg* 1993;75A:961–975.

111. Schurman DJ, Bloch DA, Tanner CM. Conventional cemented total hip arthroplasty. Assessment of clinical factors associated with revision for mechanical failure. *Clin Orthop* 1989;240:173–180.

112. Smith RW, Walker RR. Femoral expansion in aging women: implication for osteoporosis and fracture. *Science* 1964;145–156.

113. Solomon MI, Dall DM, Learmonth ID, Davenport JM. Survivorship of cemented total hip arthroplasty in patients fifty years of age or younger. *J Arthroplasty* 1992;7S:347–352.

114. Sutherland CJ, Wilde AH, Borden LS, Marks KE. A ten year follow-up of one hundred consecutive Müller curved stem total hip-replacement arthroplasties. *J Bone Joint Surg* 1982;64A:970–982.

115. Star MJ, Colwell CW, Kelman GJ, Ballock RT, Walker RH. Suboptimal (thin) distal cement mantle thickness as a contributory factor in total hip arthroplasty femoral component failure. A retrospective radiographic analysis favoring distal stem centralization. *J Arthroplasty* 1994;9:143–149.

116. Stauffer RN. A ten year follow-up study of total hip replacements with particular reference to roentgenographic loosening of the components. *J Bone Joint Surg* 1982;64A:983–990.

117. Stewart MJ, Milford LW. Fracture-dislocation of the hip: an end result study. *J Bone Joint Surg* 1954;36A:315–342.

118. Sullivan PM, Mackenzie JR, Callaghan JJ, Johnston RC. Total hip arthroplasty with cement in patients who are less than fifty years old. A sixteen to twenty-two year follow-up study. *J Bone Joint Surg* 1994;76A:863–869.

119. Tapadiya D, Walker RH, Schurman DJ. Prediction of outcome of total hip arthroplasty based on initial postoperative radiographic analysis.

Matched paired comparisons of failed versus successful femoral components. *Clin Orthop* 1984;186:5–15.

120. Tonino AJ, Davidson CL, Klopper PJ, Linclau LA. Protection from stress in bone and its effects. *J Bone Joint Surg* 1976;58B:107–112.

121. Urist MR. Fracture dislocation of the hip joint. The nature of the traumatic lesion, treatment, late complications and end result. *J Bone Joint Surg* 1948;30A:699–727.

122. Williams WW, McCullough CJ. Results of cemented total hip replacement in juvenile chronic arthritis. A radiologic review. *J Bone Joint Surg* 1993;75B:872–874.

123. Witt JD, Swann M, Ansell BM. Total hip replacement for juvenile chronic arthritis. *J Bone Joint Surg* 1991;73B:770–773.

124. Wixon RL, Lautenschlager EP, Novak MA. Vacuum mixing of acrylic bone cement. *J Arthroplasty* 1987;2:141–149.

125. Woo AL-Y, Kuei SS, Amiel D, et al. The effect of prolonged physical training on the properties of lone bone: a study of Wolff's law. *J Bone Joint Surg* 1981;63A:780–787.

126. Wright TM, Sullivan DJ, Arnoczky SP. The effect of antibiotic addition on the fracture properties of bone cement. *Acta Orthop Scand* 1984;55:414.

The Adult Hip, edited by J. J. Callaghan,
A. G. Rosenberg, and H. E. Rubash.
Lippincott–Raven Publishers, Philadelphia © 1998.

CHAPTER 61

The Cemented Acetabular Component

Chitranjan S. Ranawat and José A. Rodriguez

Although the use of methylmethacrylate cement for prosthetic fixation had been reported previously in the orthopedic literature (26,67), Charnley is credited with pioneering the study and use of bone cement for the fixation of prosthetic hip implants (67). Working with a dental materials chemist, D. C. Smith, Charnley experimented with self-curing acrylic cement in the laboratory during 1956 and 1957. He performed his first human operation using cement in 1958, and he reported the first six cases in 1960 (14). Thereafter, the use of bone cement proliferated in Europe, and in 1967 three centers were reporting their results with cemented total hip arthroplasty (13,43,45). Until 1971, the use of methylmethacrylate bone cement in the United States was restricted by the Food and Drug Administration to a few licensed centers.

As the understanding of the variables of cement fixation improved, the technique of cemented acetabular replacement was modified to improve the depth of penetration of the cement. This included fixation holes (43,45), extension of the lateral wall of the polyethylene to allow the implant to compress the cement (15), cleaning of the bony surface to remove marrow elements (68), and the use of a water-filled balloon to pressurize the cement (38,67).

Charnley's original experiments with total hip replacement used polytetrafluoroethylene (Teflon) as the bearing surface of the acetabular component because of its low coefficient of friction. Although the early clinical results with this technique were positive, the wear of the Teflon surface was much higher than anticipated, resulting in large areas of caseous reactive tissue around the implant and surrounding bone, with subsequent fixation failure (15). In 1962, high-density polyethylene was chosen as the preferred bearing surface. Although the coefficient of friction was 5 times higher than that of Teflon, the wear resistance was noted to be 500 to 1000 times better. Since that time, ultra-high-molecular-weight polyethylene has remained the standard in bearing surfaces for total joint replacement.

RADIOGRAPHIC EVALUATION

Radiographic evaluation of the cemented socket has as its primary goal an assessment of the position and fixation quality of the implant. The position of the socket is evaluated as previously described with respect to the acetabular teardrop (8). A line is drawn that joins the inferior margins of the two acetabular teardrops. The intersection of this line with the line marking the plane of opening of the socket determines the angle of abduction. The horizontal distance between this intersection point and the inferior margin of the acetabular component is noted. The vertical distance from the inferior margin of the acetabular component to the inter-teardrop line is also noted. These two measurements are compared in postoperative and follow-up radiographs to assess for changes in socket position. Our goal in positioning the socket is

C. S. Ranawat and J. A. Rodriguez: Department of Orthopaedic Surgery, Lenox Hill Hospital, William Black Hall, New York, New York 10021.

approximately 40° of abduction and 15° of anteversion. At least 80% of the cemented socket should be covered with acetabular bone.

There are different opinions as to which radiographic findings are indicative of loosening of the acetabular component. This assessment is made by observing the quality of the cement–bone interface in each of the three zones defined by DeLee and Charnley (22). Obvious migration of the socket (with respect to previous studies) or cement mantle fracture can be considered evidence of loosening of the socket. In addition, a progressive radiolucency of greater that 2 mm throughout the interface would be highly suggestive of loosening. However, standard radiographic assessment is less sensitive than computed tomography scans or oblique views of the pelvis in ascertaining the presence of radiolucent lines (61). There is evidence that the presence of any continuous lucency is highly correlated with loosening of the socket when tested at revision surgery (29). On the other hand, a continuous radiolucency at the cement–bone interface is perfectly consistent with an excellent clinical result in elderly or low-demand patients (15,47).

Our goal in radiographic evaluation is to critically assess the quality of fixation of the cemented socket. We use a modified point system, evaluating the appearance of the cement–bone interface in each of the three zones (22), with the lateral-most zone subdivided into 1A and 1B (54,70) (Table 1). A grade 1 interface has a homogeneous merge of cement interdigitating with the cancellous bone, without rounding off or radiolucency (Fig. 1). A grade 2 interface has rounding off of the cement, or a thin (<1 mm) radiolucency. A grade 3 interface has an obvious lucent line of at least 1 mm (Fig. 2). Grade 4 is reserved for evidence of migration of the socket. The numerical grade for zones 1A and 1B are averaged, and the sum of the grades is used as a numerical score.

In this way, a perfect interface in three zones would score a 3. So-called bottoming out of the socket (a zone 2 cement mantle of less than 1 mm) and protrusio deformity are assigned to grade 2 (Fig. 3). A socket with a score above 4 points is considered not well fixed. Using this classification allows a prediction of the longevity of the implant based on the early postoperative radiograph (Fig. 4) (54).

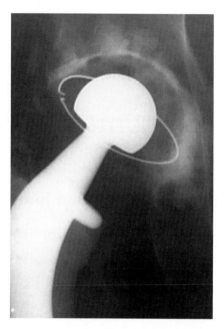

FIG. 1. One month postoperative and 13-year follow-up radiographs of a 56-year-old man with an index diagnosis of idiopathic osteonecrosis.

DESIGN FEATURES

The rigidity of fixation of the cemented acetabular components is at its greatest at the time of initial implantation. For this reason, the polyethylene socket design must seek to optimize the initial fixation of the implant to the cement, as well as fixation of the cement to the bone.

Oh has demonstrated in a laboratory study that design features that increase the surface area of polyethylene in contact with the cement will significantly increase the resistance to torsional loads (49). This was accomplished with peripheral pegs on the polyethylene, as well as grooves within the polyethylene. In this way the cement–implant interface is strengthened.

Strengthening of the cement–bone interface was studied by Oh using a circumferential flange of polyethylene at the periphery of the implant and measuring the effect it has on the cement during implantation (49). This modifi-

TABLE 1. *Examples of the acetabular scoring system*

Description of the bone–cement interface	Grade in zone I	Grade in zone II	Grade in zone III	Acetabular score (sum of grades in the three zones)
Perfect interface in all zones	1	1	1	3
Thin lateral radiolucency	1.5	1	1	3.5
Thin radiolucency in zone I	2	1	1	4
Thin radiolucency in zones I and II	2	2	1	5
Wide radiolucency in zone I	3	1	1	5
Thin global radiolucency	2	2	2	6
Wide global radiolucency	3	3	3	9
Migration (>3 mm)	4	4	4	12

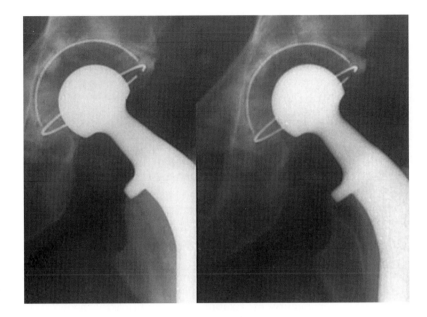

FIG. 2. Radiographs of a 64-year-old woman at 1 month and 15 years after surgery. A 1-mm cement–bone interface radiolucency is evident in zone 1a in the 1-month radiograph, for a score of 3.5. At 15 years follow-up, the lucency has progressed to encompass most of zone 1 and has become wider laterally for a score of 4.0. The remainder of the interface is well preserved.

cation was noted to significantly improve the cement intrusion pressures and the final depth of cement intrusion into the cancellous bone of a cadaveric acetabulum.

Oh also examined the strain present within the cement, and how it changes with respect to socket placement

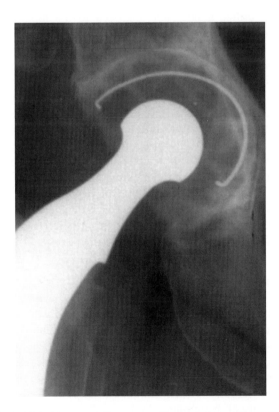

FIG. 3. The 15-year follow-up radiograph in a 50-year-old woman with rheumatoid arthritis and protrusio deformity. A circumferential 1-mm radiolucency is evident for a radiographic score of 6.0. The limited activity that her arthritis dictates has minimized the wear of the polyethylene and thereby maintained the integrity of the construct.

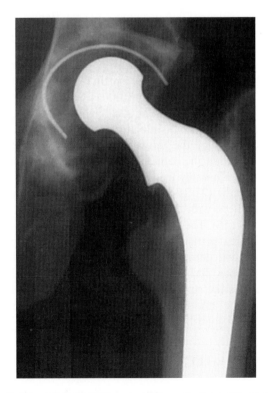

FIG. 4. The 15-year follow-up radiograph for a 26-year-old woman with pauciarticular rheumatoid arthritis. A large area of balloon-like osteolysis is present in zone 1, and the remainder of the cement–bone interface is preserved.

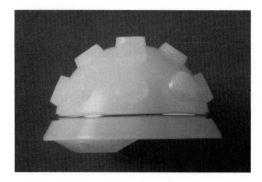

FIG. 5. Lateral view of a size 46 polyethylene socket for use with cement, demonstrating the peripheral polyethylene pegs and circumferential flange on the mouth of the implant to maintain a proper cement mantle.

within a prepared acetabulum (49). Eccentric placement of the socket within the acetabulum, and bottoming out of the socket, each increased the measured strain within the cement. This study demonstrated the importance of maintaining a concentric cement mantle of 3 to 4 mm within the prepared bed. This goal can also be achieved with the combination of polyethylene pegs with a circumferential flange at the periphery of the implant (Fig. 5).

The preparation of polyethylene has also been shown to affect the longevity of the cemented socket. In a retrospective review of 236 cemented sockets, Bankston et al. (3) have shown that sockets machined from extruded polyethylene bar stock had a significantly higher wear rate compared to sockets that were compression molded directly from the polyethylene resin (0.05 mm/year compared with 0.11 mm/year; $p = .0001$). Similar results have been reported based on surgically retrieved specimens (57) as well as on hip simulator data.

The effect of the thickness of polyethylene on the stresses within the cement–bone interface were demonstrated by Charnley using a photoelastic model comparing a small- (22.25-mm) and large- (50-mm) diameter femoral head with the same outer diameter as the socket (56 mm) (15). The thinner polyethylene model had 50% higher stresses transmitted to the surrounding tissues, and this was concentrated over a smaller arc. Finite element analysis has further shown that thicker polyethylene diminishes the stresses in the subchondral bone (18), as well as the stresses within the polyethylene itself (5), which may contribute to an accelerated wear rate.

SURGICAL TECHNIQUE

The technique of cementing the acetabular component has been previously described (17,53,55,56). The following describes the technical details that assist in achieving good quality cement fixation in a reproducible fashion.

Anesthesia

The use of epidural anesthesia with hypotension has the dual benefit of providing a dry surgical field with improved cement penetration into the cancellous bone (4), as well as an improvement in blood loss and hemodynamic factors, which results in a diminished rate of thromboembolic complications (37,63). A mean arterial blood pressure of 60 to 70 mm Hg can be safely achieved in most patients, using arterial lines and Swan-Ganz catheters to monitor the blood pressures and epinephrine infusion to support the blood pressure as needed.

A retrospective study of 20 patient pairs matched for age, sex, diagnosis, and body weight was performed comparing normotensive general anesthesia maintaining a systolic blood pressure of 110 mm Hg with hypotensive epidural anesthesia and a mean arterial blood pressure of 60 mm Hg (53). In these patients, the radiographic score for quality of fixation was significantly better with hypotensive epidural anesthesia. Clinical studies have had similar findings of improved fixation and longevity with hypotensive epidural anesthesia (54,56).

Exposure

We utilize a posterior approach to the hip in most cases. Wide exposure of the acetabulum is required and can be achieved by releasing the restraints to anterior retraction of the proximal femur. The gluteus maximus tendinous insertion on the proximal femur is completely released, and the posterior third of the insertion of the gluteus minimus is released from the superior femoral neck and capsule. With inferior capsulotomy and release of the tendinous origin of the reflected head of the rectus femoris from the supra-acetabular region, an adequate anterior translation of the proximal femur will result. The bony margins of the acetabulum are exposed by resecting the labrum circumferentially. The pulvinar is resected, and the transverse acetabular ligament is left in place to assist in the pressurization of the cement.

Preparation of the Acetabular Bed

The goal in preparing the acetabular bed is to achieve an adequate cancellous surface area for implant fixation while preserving the strong subchondral bone for support. Studies have demonstrated the negative effect of removing the subchondral bone of the acetabulum on the initial stability of the implant (9,65), as well as on longevity of the implant (23,35,66). Reaming should proceed progressively until the cancellous bone of the medullary cavities of the pubis and ischium are just becoming visible, while preserving the medial wall of the acetabulum. Because the anatomy of the acetabulum is elliptical, the superior subchondral bone remains, and it

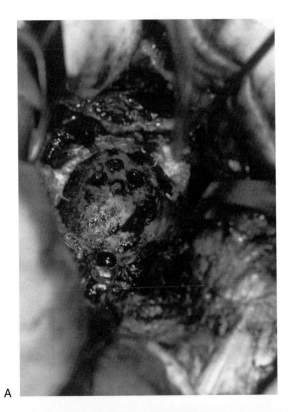

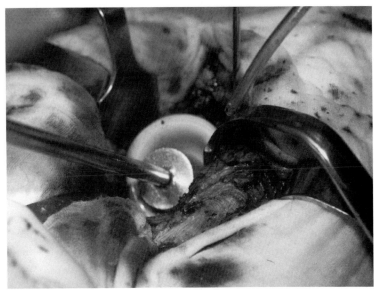

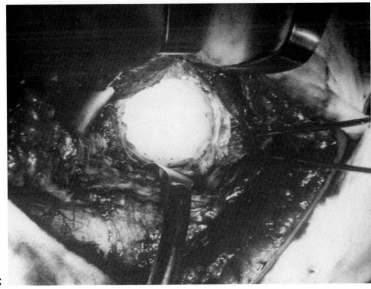

FIG. 6. Intraoperative photo of an acetabulum prepared with fixation holes **(A)**, with the pressurizing bulb in place **(B)**, and after completion of pressurization **(C)**. Note the wide exposure of the acetabulum that is achieved, along with the quality of the cement bed.

may still have a small amount of articular cartilage at its lateral edge that should be removed. The sizing of the implant should allow for a 2- to 4-mm cement mantle circumferentially; therefore, a socket outer diameter of 2 mm smaller than the last reamer used is chosen.

The strength of the macrolock achieved with the cement is related to the surface area available for cement intrusion (23,49). The surface area is maximized by fashioning multiple fixation holes with the use of a high-speed burr. Two large fixation holes (6-mm width, 10-mm depth) are created in the superior subchondral bone

of the ilium, and one each within the pubic and ischial medullary cavities (53,55). The cysts are debrided of soft tissue and the sclerotic margins are prepared with a burr. Multiple smaller holes are then created in the remaining subchondral bone. These holes are then cleaned with pulsatile irrigation, and dry sponge is packed into the large fixation holes until the cement is ready for implantation. Some type of trial implant should be used to assess for the presence of overhanging bone or soft tissue that might engage the acetabular component as it is being inserted, and these should be removed.

Cement Application

Simplex cement is utilized because of its superior intrusion properties, strength, and handling characteristics. The cement reagents are heated in a blanket warmer to accelerate the rate of polymerization. While the acetabulum is being prepared, the cement is mixed in an open bowl for 30 seconds and then allowed to sit for 1 or 2 minutes as the remaining air bubbles created during the mixing process dissipate. When the cement reaches a doughy consistency, it is applied to the back surface of the implant as the final irrigation and drying of the bony bed is performed.

The cement is placed into the acetabulum and swiftly digitally pressurized into the large fixation holes, followed by a sturdy rubber balloon (Fig. 6). This provides a uniform pressurization of the cement into the cancellous bone. *In vitro* studies using cadaveric acetabula have demonstrated that finger-packing results in the high interface pressures only within the anchoring holes (49). Sustained external pressurization (1 to 2 minutes) markedly increases the interface pressures and the depth of cement penetration into the remainder of the cancellous bone (49), while also significantly improving pushout strength of the implant (48).

The cement is cleared from the inferior margin of the acetabulum prior to placing the socket, to identify the floor of the acetabulum and the margin of the transverse acetabular ligament where the inferior margin of the socket should lie. Any blood that has pooled in the cement bed is dried with a sponge as the acetabular component is implanted. Pressure is maintained on the prosthesis until the cement polymerizes using a small pusher that sits within the socket to minimize the transmission of minor hand movement to the cement.

The position of the acetabular component is assessed with respect to the bony landmarks of the hip. Preoperative templating should allow an estimate of the desired position of the implant with respect to the anterolateral margin as well as the inferior margin of the acetabulum, and this can be reproduced intraoperatively. The location of the pubis and ischium are noted by palpating the outer margins of the rami as well as by noting the position of the prepared fixation holes. These fixation holes should be equally covered by the implant and cement in most cases. In addition, the anterior and posterior walls of the acetabulum can provide additional guidance, allowing placement of the socket in sufficient anteversion to match the anterior wall. Unfortunately, bony deformities, such as dysplasia, protrusio, and large osteophyte formation, are sufficiently common to make a single landmark inadequate for evaluation in all patients.

We utilize a trial implant to define the peripheral margin of the acetabular component, and we mark the desired position prior to mixing the cement.

MEASUREMENT OF WEAR

Wear of the articulating surface occurs with great variability of direction (32,39,64). The actual penetration of the femoral head into the socket occurs in three dimensions (32,64). The volume of particulate polyethylene that is created in this process is called the volumetric wear. However, our ability to measure wear is based on two-dimensional radiographs. The radiographic change in the thickness of the socket at the maximal point of wear is referred to as linear wear. Volumetric wear is then calculated based on a simple trigonometric formula in turn based on the measured linear wear and the square of the radius of the articulating head. A 32-mm head can be expected to generate substantially more volumetric wear than a 22-mm head with the same measured linear wear. Because calculation is based on a one-dimensional measurement, it probably represents an underestimation of the actual volume of wear particles produced (32).

Charnley recognized early the importance of measuring the apparent linear wear of the polyethylene on follow-up radiographs. To aid in this task, he added a wire marker. Charnley and Cupic first published a technique for measuring the penetration of the prosthetic femoral head into the socket using a uniradiographic technique (12). However, this technique proved to be of questionable reliability, depending on the magnification of the radiograph, the position of the film, and the placement of the wire marker (16).

In trying to address the apparent error in the uniradiographic technique of measuring linear wear, Livermore et al. developed a duoradiographic technique, comparing the minimum thickness of the socket in the most recent radiograph with the thickness in the postoperative film (39). In addition, they used the cement–bone interface as the point of measuring, rather than the wire marker. The Livermore technique was improved by digitizing the films, thereby diminishing the error of the measurement by allowing manipulation and magnification of the image (7).

Ohlin and Sevlik have described a technique of measuring the change in position of the center of the femoral head compared to the center of the socket (51). Rodriguez et al. have described a technique using digitized radiographs and commercially available software to define the center of rotation of the prosthetic femoral head and of the socket, where the computer software measures the difference between these two points (Fig. 7) (59). A similar technique used in Europe is called EBRA (30,50).

Martell et al. designed a software package that recognizes the borders of the socket and prosthetic head and measures the difference between these points (41). This technique minimizes the human error inherent in defining these points, and it improves the reproducibility of the measurement. Devane et al. (21) have created a software

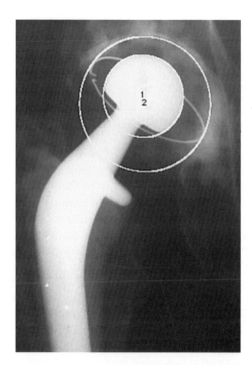

FIG. 7. This image demonstrates the use of specialized computer software to calculate the distance between the center of curvature of the socket relative to that of the femoral head as a means of measuring linear polyethylene wear.

package with an additional benefit: the exact dimensional specifications of a given implant provided by the manufacturer are included (20). These known dimensions are compared with the digitized images of orthogonal views of the socket. All magnification correction and dimensional differences are calculated by the software. In this way, they have been able to directly measure linear wear in two planes and thereby more accurately calculate the three-dimensional or volumetric wear.

Using these techniques, polyethylene wear in cemented sockets has been shown to have a great deal of variability (Table 2). The type of bearing surface (3), the size of the articulating head (39), the presence of metal backing (11,59), acetabular orientation (6,59), and the preparation of the polyethylene (3,57) have each been shown to affect the polyethylene wear rate. Clinical factors such as weight and sex have been shown by some studies to affect the wear rate (59). Using a 22-mm stainless steel head with an all-polyethylene socket, the average linear wear rate tends to vary between 0.07 and 0.15 mm/year (2,7,39,62). With a 28-mm cobalt–chrome (CoCr) head in an all-polyethylene socket, the average linear wear rate varies between 0.05 and 0.13 mm/year (3,11,28,39,59). The inherent differences in the techniques of measuring polyethylene wear make comparisons between studies difficult to interpret. However, using the same technique, measured differences are more reliable (44,59).

TABLE 2. *Polyethylene wear rates using different total hip replacement systems*

Author (ref.)	Number	Cup	Head	Ave. linear wear rate (mm/yr)	Ave. volumetric wear rate (mm³/yr)
Schulte et al. (62)	298	cem, poly (Charnley)	22 Stainless	0.074	n.a.
Livermore et al. (39)	227	cem, poly (Charnley)	22 Stainless	0.13	51.3
	98	(T-28)	28 Stainless	0.08	52.1
	60	(Müller)	32 Stainless	0.10	91.1
Jacobsen et al. (31)	70	cem, poly (Charnley)	22 Stainless	0.12	n.a.
Bankston et al. (3)	162	cem, poly (Triad)	28 CoCr	0.12	70.9
	74	cem, poly (Tr-28)	28 CoCr	0.05	33.3
Hernandez et al. (28)	65	noncem, Ti (Biomet)	28 Ti, cemented	0.22	139
	66	noncem, Ti (Biomet)	28 Ti, uncem	0.14	92
Woolsen and Murphey (69)	80	noncem Ti (HGP)	28 CoCr	0.14	n.a.
Latimer and Lachiewicz (36)	136	noncem Ti (HGP)	28 CoCr	0.10	n.a.
Martell and Berdia (41)	25	noncem Ti (HGP)	28 CoCr	0.21	n.a.
Rodriguez et al. (59)	50	cem, poly (Triad)	28 CoCr	0.11	n.a.
	50	cem, CoCr (Triad)	28 CoCr	0.18	n.a.
	50	noncem Ti (HGP)	28 CoCr	0.12	n.a.
McKenzie et al. (44)	175	cem, poly (Zimmer)	28 CoCr	0.08	n.a.
	99	cem, Ti (Ti BAC)	28 CoCr	0.12	n.a.
	144	noncem, Ti (HGP)	28 CoCr	0.14	n.a.
Callaghan, Pedersen, et al. (7)	61	cem, poly (Charnley)	22 Stainless	0.10	40.69
	20	cem, poly (Iowa)	28 CoCr	0.12	70.88
	43	cem Ti (Ti BAC)	28 CoCr	0.11	65.78
	63	noncem, Ti (HGP)	28 CoCr	0.07	40.78
Sychterz et al. (64)	8	cem, poly (mixed)	32 CoCr	0.04	23
	18	noncem Ti (mixed)	32 CoCr	0.08	47.9
Devane et al. (21)	80	noncem Ti (HGP)	32 CoCr	0.13	130

cem, cemented; HGP, Harris Gallante Prosthesis; noncem, noncemented; poly, polyethylene; Ti, titanium; Ti BAC, titanium-based acetabular component; n.a., not available.

MECHANICAL AND RETRIEVAL STUDIES OF THE INTERFACE

Although studies of total hip arthroplasty implants retrieved at revision surgery can be of value in understanding aspects of the failed implant, they provide little insight as to the mechanism of failure in the well-functioning implant. In attempting to document the natural history of the cemented socket, authors have examined autopsy retrieval specimens for mechanical and cellular details of implants in asymptomatic patients (15,24,50,61).

Charnley (15) has reported on 26 postmortem specimens of acetabular components implanted during the late 1960s and early 1970s using early cement technique that included a reaming of all subchondral bone to a cancellous bed, no bone preparation, and finger-packing of the cement. The patients were chosen because of their successful clinical outcome. In this group, all sockets appeared to have a fibrous membrane interposed between the cement and the bone, varying between 0.5 and 1.5 mm in thickness. Fornasier et al. (24) published similar findings from an autopsy retrieval study of 14 hips, noting a correlation between the extent of birefringent polyethylene particles evident by light microscopy and the thickness of the membrane. They proposed that cellular events are at work at the cement–bone interface in the absence of symptoms that may progress to loosening.

Schmalzreid et al. (61) have published a detailed study of 14 retrieved hemipelves following cemented total hip replacement. These specimens were evaluated radiographically as well as by light microscopy and scanning electron microscopy, and seven specimens were subjected to torque load-displacement testing. In the mechanical testing, the degree of measured displacement of the socket relative to the bone was directly related to the volumetric wear of the polyethylene, as well as to the extent of radiolucencies of the cement–bone interface.

Microscopy revealed that some soft-tissue interposition between the bone and cement was evident in every specimen. In those specimens that were most stable to mechanical testing, the soft-tissue interposition was found only peripherally, at the intra-articular portions of the cement–bone interface. The remainder of the interface was notable for intimate apposition of the bone to the cement, without intervening soft tissue. A transition zone was present between the regions of soft-tissue interposition and the regions of intimate bone–cement contact. This transition zone was notable for the presence of macrophages and evidence of bone resorption.

These findings would suggest that in a well-cemented acetabular component, the process of loosening may be the result of a cellular rather than a mechanical process, determined by the host reaction to polyethylene debris. In the face of continued use of polyethylene as a bearing surface, it is unclear whether the use of uncemented implants will result in a change in the natural history of this cellular mechanism of loosening.

METAL BACKING OF THE CEMENTED ACETABULAR COMPONENT

The addition of a metal base to the back surface of a cemented acetabular component was developed as an attempt to improve the longevity of socket fixation. The concept is based on finite element analysis of acetabular stresses, where compressive forces on the superior cancellous bone and medial wall of the acetabulum, and the tensile stresses of the peripheral subchondral bone were shown to be markedly increased after cemented socket replacement (10,18). These studies demonstrated that efforts to create a more rigid implant construct could more evenly distribute the stresses to the surrounding acetabular bone. In this way, the cement and subchondral bone would be protected from fatigue failure, particularly in the event of subchondral bone removal.

Although early reports suggested an improved outcome with cemented metal-backed sockets (42), the actual radiographic and clinical performance of metal-backed cemented implants has not fulfilled the theoretical promise of greater longevity in long-term reports from numerous centers (19). Ritter et al. have suggested that the cemented metal-backed sockets have had greater failure rates than control groups (58). At an average follow-up time of 5.2 years in 238 hips, 39% of metal-backed sockets had a complete cement–bone interface radiolucency, compared with 23% of the cemented all-polyethylene implants. Similarly, Harris has reported on 11-year-average follow-up data for 48 metal-backed cemented sockets with a 21% revision rate and 41% rate of radiographic loosening of the sockets (27).

The reasons for the inferior clinical outcomes in cemented metal-backed acetabular components are not well understood, but accelerated wear of the polyethylene has been suggested as a cause. Cates et al. examined 233 hips with metal-backed and all-polyethylene acetabular components for polyethylene wear, noting that mean linear wear rate was 37% higher in the metal-backed group (11). Rodriguez et al. studied the rate of polyethylene wear in three pair-matched cohorts of patients undergoing total hip replacement with cemented all-polyethylene sockets, cemented metal-backed sockets, and uncemented metal-backed sockets. They found that the cemented metal-backed sockets had a linear wear rate of 0.18 mm/year compared with the all-polyethylene cemented sockets where the rate was 0.11 mm/year (a 63% increase) (59). Similarly, McKenzie et al. demonstrated a significantly higher wear rate with cemented metal-backed sockets (0.12 mm/year) compared with all-polyethylene sockets (0.8 mm/year) (44).

TABLE 3. *Criteria used in the literature to describe clinical and radiographic loosening of the socket*

Author (ref.)	Prosthesis	Number of hips	Length of follow-up	Criteria for loosening	Rate
Cornell and Ranawat (17)	Charnley	85 (<55 yr)	>5 yr (ave. 10.5 yr)	1. Revision 2. Migration	0% 4%
DeLee and Charnley (22)	Charnley	141	ave. 10 yr	1. Revision 2. Migration 3. Demarcation (lateral ²/₃ of socket = type II) 4. Global demarcation (= type III)	9% 8% 52%
Stauffer (77)	Charnley	231	>10 yr	1. Revision 2. Migration, tilting or global radiolucency (>1 mm in all zones)	3% 11%
Hozack et al. (71)	Charnley	590	ave. 5.3 yr	1. Migration (>5 mm) 2. Three-zone demarcation	14% 13%
Kavanaugh et al. (33)	Charnley	166	>15 yr	1. Revision 2. Migration or global radiolucency wider than 1 mm in at least 1 zone (= probable) 3. Progressive radiolucent line less than 1 mm in all zones (= possible)	14% 50%
McCoy et al. (72)	Charnley	32	14.4–16.2 yr (ave. 15.3 yr)	1. Revision 2. Migration 3. Demarcation (121°–180°)	3% 6% 9%
Mulroy and Harris (46)	CAD, HD-2, CDH	105	10–12.7 yr (ave. 11.2 yr)	1. Revision 2. Migration or continuous radiolucent line	4% 40%
Older (52)	Charnley	153	ave. 11 yr	1. Revision 2. No demarcation (= grade 1) 3. Slight or moderate demarcation involving only the lateral quadrant (zone 1) (= grade 2) 4. Severe demarcation involving the whole circumference (could be < 1 mm) (= grade 3) 5. Migration (= grade 4)	2% 63% 22% 7% 8%
Poss et al. (73)		143	11.9 yr	1. Revision 2. Success%%63% 3. Failure	14%
Ranawat et al. (56)	Mixed	50 matched pairs	10 yr (old technique) 5 yr (modern technique)	Old cement technique: 1. Revision 2. Migration Modern cement technique: 1. Revision 2. Migration	37% 2% 14% 0%
Ritter et al. (75)	Charnley	100	10 yr	1. Revision Migration (> 5 mm)	0% 2%
Schulte (62)	Charnley	98	>20 yr	1. Revision 2. Migration (5 mm = definite) 3. Global radiolucency (= probable) 4. Lucency (50%–90% = possible)	3% 11% 18% 4%
Severt et al. (76)	T-28, Charnley, Dual-Lock	75 rheumatoid	ave. 7.4 yr	1. Revision 2. Progressive circumferential radiolucency > 2 mm (with or without migration)	3% 5.3% 8%
Ranawat (74)	Mixed	236	ave. 10 yr	1. Revision 2. Migration 3. Global lucency	0.8% 3% 3.4%
Neuman et al. (47)	Charnley	241	ave. 17.6 yr	1. Revision 2. Migration 3. Global lucency	2.5% 2% 4.6%

SURVIVAL STUDIES OF CEMENTED ACETABULAR COMPONENTS

The literature is replete with clinical series that can be used to support or refute the continued use of cemented acetabular sockets, depending on which series and which criteria are used (see Table 1). We will discuss those series with a greater than 10-year follow-up. To properly evaluate and compare reported series of cemented hip replacement, a standard set of criteria must be used to define failure (Table 3). Terms such as *definite*, *probable*, and *possible loosening* are used in the literature, with different authors applying different criteria (27,33).

The standard criteria that we apply to define clinical and radiographic failure are (a) revision of the socket for aseptic loosening, (b) radiographic evidence of migration greater than 3 mm, and (c) the appearance of a progressive, global radiolucency at the bone–cement interface. Revision of the socket for aseptic loosening is an obvious endpoint of clinical failure, and migration of the socket indicates a failure of fixation. Progressive global radiolucency is used as a criterion for failure based on the data of Hodgkinson et al., who demonstrated that 94% of sockets in this category were loose at the time of revision surgery (29).

Comparing different series of hip replacement should also take into account the exact surgical technique used as well as the implant used. For example, Mulroy and Harris reported on 105 hips using so-called modern cement technique at an average 11-year follow-up, noting socket revision or global radiolucency in 44% of cases (46). However, these sockets were mostly metal-backed, and the femoral stems were CAD and HD-2, with a very low offset, predisposing the acetabulum to higher joint reaction forces than with a Charnley implant.

Older (52) reported on a series of 153 Charnley prostheses followed for an average of 11 years. In this series, two sockets were revised, eight had migrated, and seven had a global radiolucency, for a failure rate of 11.1% (17/153). Sixty-three hips had no discernible demarcation, and 22 had demarcation within a single quadrant. Fowler et al. (25) published an extensive experience using the Exeter hip in 426 cases, followed for 10 to 16 years. Using revision or asymptomatic migration as an endpoint criterion, they noted failure in 23%. Neumann et al. published their findings on 103 Charnley total hip replacements at an average 17.6 years of follow-up, with 6 sockets that were revised, 5 of which had migrated, and 11 of which had a circumferential radiolucency (for a failure rate of 20.8%) (47).

Kavanaugh reported on an early multisurgeon series of 333 hips using Charnley implants at a mean follow-up of 15 years (33). Of these hips, 14% had been revised or migrated, and 50% had a global radiolucency. Schulte et al. (62) published the results of 98 Charnley hips at a minimum 20-year follow-up from a single surgeon series.

TABLE 4. *Preoperative diagnosis and failure rate of 236 hips*

Preoperative diagnosis	Number of hips	Percent failed
Overall	236	7.2
Juvenile rheumatoid arthritis	3	100
Ankylosing spondylitis	1	100
Legg-Calvé-Perthes disease	4	25
Rheumatoid arthritis	42	14.3
Acetabular dysplasia	15	13.3
Fracture	22	4.5
Osteoarthrosis	129	2.3
Osteonecrosis	12	0
Systemic lupus erythematosus	5	0
Paget's disease	3	0

Follow-ups averaged 10 years.

In this series, there were 11 sockets that were revised, 18 that had migrated, and 4 with a global radiolucency at the cement–bone interface, for a failure rate of 33.7% at 20 years (31).

Our experience with cemented sockets suggests that the longevity of the implant is directly related to the quality of the cement penetration into the acetabulum (54). We reported on a series of 236 hips using various implants, along with so-called modern cement technique and hypotensive epidural anesthesia, followed for an average of 10 years. Two sockets have been revised for aseptic loosening, 7 sockets have migrated, and 8 sockets have a global radiolucency, for an overall failure rate of 7%. However, in those cases where a satisfactory bone–cement interface was evident on the initial postoperative radiograph, a 2.2% failure rate was seen. The hips that did not achieve a satisfactory bone–cement interface initially, had a failure rate of 14.4%. Failure rate correlated with the preoperative diagnosis, with a higher rate of failure in patients with inflammatory arthritis, protrusio deformity, and dysplasia (Table 4). Kobayashi et al. (34) have also described risk factors.

Young age at index surgery has also been shown to diminish the longevity of implantation even with so-called modern cement technique Ballard et al. have published a series of 42 hips in patients of 50 years or younger and followed for an average of 11 years (2). In these cases, 10 sockets were revised, and 5 sockets were considered definitely loose, with none graded as probably loose, resulting in a failure rate of 36% at 10 years.

CONCLUSION

In summary, the function and longevity of the cemented all-polyethylene acetabular components in total hip replacement is dependent on many factors, including the underlying diagnosis, bone quality, prosthetic design, and the technical quality of the operation. Refinement in the prosthetic design and in the surgical environment and technique have led to an improvement in the initial fixation of the cement, with concomitant improvements in clinical survival. Autopsy retrieval studies have shown that excellent osseointegration of bone and cement can be maintained in the long term and that the mechanism of loosening of a well-fixed socket is biologic in nature. In addition, the polyethylene wear that drives this process tends to be less marked in cemented sockets than in non-cemented sockets in several studies (44,64) .

In spite of these improvements, aseptic loosening does occur. Specific diagnoses that predispose to a less favorable result with cemented sockets have been outlined and can be avoided (see Table 4). In those cases, we use uncemented porous ingrowth sockets, though it is unclear whether this will result in an improved long-term outcome compared to well-cemented sockets (36,40,69). We remain confident in our ability to achieve an adequate cement–bone bond that will last 10 to 20 years, and so we use cemented sockets in most patients of 60 years or greater.

REFERENCES

1. Askew MJ, Steege JW, Lewis JL, et al. Effect of cement pressure and bone strength on polymethylmethacrylate fixation. *J Orthop Res* 1984: 1:412–416.
2. Ballard WT, Callaghan JJ, Sullivan PM, Johnston RC. The results of improved cementing technique for total hip arthroplasty in patients less than fifty years old. A ten-year follow-up study. *J Bone Joint Surg* 1994;76A:959–966.
3. Bankston AB, Keating EM, Ranawat CS, Faris PM, Ritter MA. Comparison of polyethylene wear in machined versus molded polyethylene. *Clin Orthop* 1995;317:37–43.
4. Bannister CG, Young SK, Baker AS, Mackinnon JG, Magnusson PA. Control of bleeding in cemented arthroplasty. *J Bone Joint Surg* 1990; 72B:444–446.
5. Bartel DL, Bicknell MS, Wright TM. The effect of conformity, thickness, and material on stress in ultra high molecular weight components for total joint replacement. *J Bone Joint Surg* 1986;68A:1041–1049.
6. Bono JV, Sanford L, Toussaint JT. Severe polyethylene wear in total hip arthroplasty. Observations from retrieved AML PLUS hip implants with an ACS polyethylene liner. *J Arthoplasty* 1994;9:119–125.
7. Callaghan JJ, Pedersen DR, Olejniczak JP, Johnston RC. Radiographic measurement of wear in 5 cohorts of patients observed for 5 to 22 years. *Clin Orthop* 1995;317:14–18.
8. Callaghan JJ, Salvati EA, Pellicci PM, Wilson PD Jr, Ranawat CS. Results of revision for mechanical failure after cemented total hip replacement, 1979–1982. A two to five-year follow-up. *J Bone Joint Surg* 1985;67A:1074–1085.
9. Carter DR, Vasu R, Harris WH. Periacetabular stress distribution after joint replacement with subchondral bone retention. *Acta Orthop Scand* 1983;54:29–32.
10. Carter DR. Finite element analysis of a metal-backed acetabular component. In: Hungerford DS, ed. *The hip. Proceedings of the 11th open scientific meeting of The Hip Society.* St. Louis: CV Mosby, 1983; 216–239.
11. Cates HE, Faris PM, Keating EM, Ritter MA. Polyethylene wear in cemented metal backed acetabular cups. *J Bone Joint Surg* 1993; 75B:249–252.
12. Charnley J, Cupic Z. The nine and ten year results of low friction arthroplasty of the hip. *Clin Orthop* 1973;95:9–25.
13. Charnley J. Total prosthetic replacement for advanced coxarthrosis of the hip: introduction. Tenth international congress of orthopaedic surgery and traumatology, *Proceedings of the SICOT meeting,* Paris, 1967.
14. Charnley J. Anchorage of the femoral head prosthesis to the shaft of the femur. *J Bone Jont Surg* 1964;42B:28–30.
15. Charnley J. *Low-friction arthroplasty of the hip.* New York: Springer-Verlag, 1979.
16. Clark IC, Black K, Rennie C, Amstutz HC. Can wear from total hip arthroplasties be assessed from radiographs? *Clin Orthop* 1976;121: 126–142.
17. Cornell CN, Ranawat CS. The impact of modern cement techniques on acetabular fixation in cemented total hip replacement. *J Arthroplasty* 1986;1:197–202.
18. Crowninshield RD, Pedersen DR, Brand RA, Johnston RC. Analytical support for acetabular component metal backing. In: Hungerford DS, ed. *Proceedings of the 11th meeting of The Hip Society.* St. Louis: CV Mosby, 1983.
19. Dalstra M, Huiskies R. The influence of metal backing in cemented cups. *Proceedings of the 37th annual meeting of the Orthopaedic Research Society.* 1991;272.
20. Devane PA, Bourne RB, Rorabeck CH, Hardie RM, Horne JG. Measurement of polyethylene wear in metal-backed acetabular cups. I. Three-dimensional technique. *Clin Orthop* 1995;319:303–316.
21. Devane PA, Horne JG, Martin K, Coldham G, Krause BC. Three-dimensional polyethylene wear from a press-fit titanium total hip prosthesis: which factors influence the rate of polyethylene debris produced? *Orthop Trans* 1996;20:108.
22. DeLee JG, Charnley J. Radiological demarcation of cemented sockets in total hip replacement. *Clin Orthop* 1976;20–32.
23. Eftekar NS, Pawluk RJ. Role of surgical preparation in acetabular cup fixation. In: Hungerford DS, ed. *Proceedings of the 11th meeting of The Hip Society.* St. Louis, MO: CV Mosby, 1983;308.
24. Fornasier V, Wright J, Seligman J. The histomorphologic and morphometric study of asymptomatic hip arthroplasty. A postmortem study. *Clin Orthop* 1991;271:272–282.
25. Fowler JL, Gie GA, Lee AJC, Ling RSM. Experience with the Exeter total hip replacement since 1970. *Orthop Clin North Am* 1988;19: 477–489.
26. Haboush EJ. Arthroplasty of the hip based on biomechanics, photoelasticity, fast-setting dental acrylic, and other considerations. *Bull Hosp Joint Dis* 1953;14:242–277.
27. Harris WH, Penenberg BL. Further follow-up on socket fixation using a metal backed acetabular component for total hip replacement. *J Bone Joint Surg* 1987;69A:1140–1148.
28. Hernandez JR, Keting AM, Faris PM, Meding JB, Ritter MA. Polyethylene weaar in uncemented acetabular components. *J Bone Joint Surg* 1994;76B:263–266.
29. Hodgkinson JP, Shelley P, Wroblewski MB. The correlation between the roentgenographic appearance and operative findings at the cement-bone junction of the socket in Charnley low-friction arthroplasties. *Clin Orthop* 1988;228:105–109.
30. Ilchman T, Mjöberg B, Wingstrand H. Measurement accuracy in acetabular cup wear. *J Arthroplasty* 1995;10:636–642,
31. Jacobsson SA, Djerf K, Wahlstrom O. Twenty-year results of McKee-Farrar versus Charnley prosthesis. *Clin Orthop* 1996;329(suppl):S60–68.
32. Kabo JM, Gebhard JS, Loren G, Amstutz HC. In vivo wear of polyethylene acetabular components. *J Bone Joint Surg* 1993;75B:245–248.
33. Kavanaugh BF, Dewitz MA, Ilstrup DM, Coventry MB. Charnley total hip arthroplasty with cement. *J Bone Joint Surg* 1989;71:1496–1503.
34. Kobayashi S, Eftekar NS, Terayama K, Iorio R. Risk factors affecting radiological failure of the socket in primary Charnley low friction arthroplasty. A 10- to 20-year follow-up study. *Clin Orthop* 1994;306: 84–96.
35. Krause W, Krug W, Miller J. Strength of the cement-bone interface. *Clin Orthop* 1982;163:290–295.
36. Latimer HA, Lachiewicz PF. Porous coated acetabular components with screw fixation. *J Bone Joint Surg* 1996;78A:975–981.
37. Lieberman JR, Huo MM, Salvati EA, Sculco TP, Sharrock NE. The prevalence of deep venous thrombosis after total hip arthroplasty with hypotensive epidural anesthesia. *J Bone Joint Surg* 1994;76A: 341–348.
38. Ling RSM, Halawa M, Lee AJC, Vangala SS. Total hip replacement with the Exeter prosthesis. *J Bone Joint Surg* 1981;63B:283.
39. Livermore J, Ilstrup D, Morrey B. Effect of femoral head size on wear of the polyethylene acetabular component. *J Bone Joint Surg* 1990; 72A:518–528.
40. Malcolm AJ. Cemented and hydroxyapatite-coated hip implants. An autopsy retrieval study. In: Morrey BF, ed. *Biological, material and mechanical considerations of joint replacement.* New York: Raven Press, 1993;39–50.

41. Martell JM, Berdia S. The determination of polyethylene wear in total hip arthroplasty using computerized analysis based on digitized radiographs. Scientific exhibit. *Orthop Trans* 1995;19:476.

42. Mattingly DA, Hopson CN, Kahn A, Giannestras NJ. Aseptic loosening in metal-backed acetabular components for total hip replacement. A minimum five-year follow-up. *J Bone Joint Surg* 1985;67A:387–390.

43. McKee GK. Total prosthetic replacement for advanced coxarthrosis, Tenth international congress of orthopaedic surgery and traumatology, *Proceedings of the SICOT meeting*, Paris, 1967.

44. McKenzie MJ, Harmsen WS, Sheetz K, Berry DJ. Comparison of polyethylene wear in cemented and uncemented total hip replacements. *Orthop Trans* 1996;20:107.

45. Müller ME. Prothèses totales de hanche. Tenth international congress of orthopaedic surgery and traumatology, *Proceedings of the SICOT meeting*, Paris, 1967.

46. Mulroy RD, Harris WH. The effect of improved cementing techniques on component loosening in total hip replacement: An 11-year radiographic review. *J Bone Joint Surg* 1990;72B:757–760.

47. Neumann L, Freund KG, Sorenson KH. Long-term results of Charnley total hip replacement. Review of 92 patients at 15 to 20 years. *J Bone Joint Surg* 1994;76B:245–251.

48. Ober NS, Lavernia CJ, Reindel ES, Woo SL, Convery FR. Sustained pressurization of PMMA—a biomechanical study of the bone-cement interface. An in-vitro and in-vivo comparison. *Proc Orthop Res Soc* 1989;14:395.

49. Oh I. A comprehensive analysis of the factors affecting acetabular cup fixation and design in total hip replacement arthroplasty: a series of experimental and clinical studies. In: Hungerford DS, ed. *The hip. Proceedings of the 11th open scientific meeting of The Hip Society*. St. Louis: CV Mosby, 1983;129–177.

50. Ohlin A, Balkfors B. Stability of cemented sockets after 3-14 years. *J Arthroplasty* 1992;7:87–92.

51. Ohlin A, Sevlik G. Socket wear assessment. A comparison of three different radiographic methods. *J Arthoplasty* 1993;8:427–431.

52. Older J. Low-friction arthroplasty of the hip. *Clin Orthop* 1986;211:36–42.

53. Ranawat CS, Beaver WB, Sharrock NE, et al. Effect of hypotensive epidural anaesthesia on acetabular cement-bone fixation in total hip arthroplasty. *J Bone Joint Surg* 1991;62A:779–782.

54. Ranawat CS, Deshmuk RG, Peters LE, Umlas ME. Prediction of the long-term durability of all-polyethylene cemented sockets. *Clin Orthop* 1995;317:89–105.

55. Ranawat CS, Maynard MJ. Modern technique of cemented total hip arthroplasty. *Techniques Orthop* 1991;6:17–25.

56. Ranawat CS, Rawlins BA, Harju VT. Effect of modern cement technique on acetabular fixation in total hip arthroplasty: a retrospective study in matched pairs. *Orthop Clin North Am* 1988;19:599–603.

57. Rentfrow ED, James SP, Beauregard GP, Lee KR, McLaughlin JR. Comparison of the in vivo wear rates of 43 surgically retrieved direct compression molded and ram extruded ultra high molecular weight polyethylene acetabular components. *Biomed Sci Instrum* 1996;32:135–141.

58. Ritter MA, Keating M, Faris PM, Brugo G. Metal backed acetabular cups in total hip arthroplasty. *J Bone Joint Surg* 1990;72A:672–675.

59. Rodriguez JA, Salvati EA, Ranawat CS. Polyethylene wear in total hip arthroplasty: a radiographic study of cemented polyethylene sockets, cemented metal-backed sockets, and uncemented metal-backed sockets in matched patients. *Orthop Trans* 1996;20:107.

60. Russe W. Röntgenphotogrammetrie der kunstlichen Hüftgelenkspfanne. *Aktuelle Probl Chir Orthop* 1988;32:1–7.

61. Schmalzreid TP, Kwong LM, Jasty M, et al. The mechanism of loosening of cemented acetabular components in total hip arthroplasty. *Clin Orthop* 1992;274:60–78.

62. Schulte KR, Callaghan JJ, Kelley SS, Johnston RC. The outcome of Charnley total hip arthroplasty with cement after a minimum twenty-year follow-up. The results of one surgeon. *J Bone Joint Surg* 1993;75A:961–975.

63. Sharrock NE, Mineo R, Urquhart B. Is hypotensive anaesthesia safe in treated hypertensive patients? Experience with epidural anaesthesia. *Anesth Analg* 1989;68(suppl):S256–258.

64. Sychterz CJ, Moon KH, Terefenko KM, Engh CA Jr, Bauer TW. Wear of polyethylene cups in total hip arthroplasty. A study of specimens retrieved post mortem. *J Bone Joint Surg* 1996;78:1193–1200.

65. Vasu R, Carter DR, Harris WH. Stress distributions in the acetabular region. Before and after total hip replacement. *J Biomech* 1982;15:155–158.

66. Volz RG, Wilson RJ. Factors affecting the mechanical stability of the cemented component in total hip replacement. *J Bone Joint Surg* 1977;59A:501–507.

67. Waugh W. *John Charnley, the man and the hip.* New York: Springer-Verlag, 1990.

68. Weber BG. Pressurized cement fixation in total hip arthroplasty. *Clin Orthop* 1988;232:87–93.

69. Woolsen ST, Murphy MG. Wear of the polyethylene of Harris-Galante acetabular components inserted without cement. *J Bone Joint Surg* 1995;77A:1311–1314.

70. Wroblewski BM. Wear and loosening of the socket in the Charnley low-friction arthroplasty. *Orthop Clin North Am* 1988;19:627–630.

71. Hozack WJ, Rothman RH, Booth RE Jr, et al. Survivorship analysis of 1,041 Charnley total hip arthroplasties. *J Arthroplasty* 1990;5:41–47.

72. McCoy TH, Salvati EA, Ranawat CS, Wilson PD Jr. A fifteen-year follow-up study of one hundred Charnley low-friction arthroplasties. *Orthop Clin North Am* 1988;19:467–476.

73. Poss R, Brick GW, Wright RJ, Roberts DW, Sledge CB. *Orthop Clin North Am* 1988;19:591–598.

74. Ranawat CS, Deshmukh RG, Peters LE, Umlas ME. Prediction of the long-term durability of all-polyethylene cemented sockets based on the early radiological appearance of the bone-cement interface: a five to fifteen-year follow-up of cemented total hip replacement. *Clin Orthop* 1994;309:131–135.

75. Ritter MA, Faris PM, Keating EM, Brugo G. Influential factors in cemented acetabular cup loosening. *J Arthroplasty* 1992;7 Suppl:365–367.

76. Severt R, Wood R, Cracchiolo A, Amstutz HC. Long-term follow-up of cement total hip arthroplasty in rheumatoid arthritis. *Clin Orthop* 1991;265:137–145.

77. Stauffer RN. Ten-year follow-up study of total hip replacement. *J Bone Joint Surg* 1982;64A:989–990.

The Adult Hip, edited by J. J. Callaghan,
A. G. Rosenberg, and H. E. Rubash.
Lippincott–Raven Publishers, Philadelphia © 1998.

CHAPTER 62

The Cementless Acetabular Component

Christopher L. Peters and Harold K. Dunn

Replacement of the acetabulum with high-molecular-weight polyethylene (HMWP) using cement fixation was introduced by Sir John Charnley in November 1962. In the first 5 years after its introduction, the cemented polyethylene socket was highly successful, with a radiographic loosening rate of 4.5% (14). With longer-term follow-up, however, it became apparent that the rate of loosening of cemented acetabular components increased with time, especially after 10 to 12 years (14,46,94,112). The magnitude of the problem was evident in the fact that cemented acetabular loosening rates increased exponentially after the first 5 years, reaching 24% to 60% in multiple series with long-term follow-up (11,14,46, 94,112). Coincident with the observations of a high rate of late aseptic loosening of cemented acetabular components was the notion that methylmethacrylate was toxic to the host bone. Particulate methylmethacrylate was postulated to cause "cement disease" characterized by localized lysis of bone and acceleration of the loosening process (45).

It was this background, together with the relatively low mechanical loosening rates noted with cemented femoral components, that led numerous investigators to begin searching for an alternative method for fixation of the acetabular component to the pelvis that would improve upon previous cemented results, preserve host bone,

allow for ease of revision when necessary, and, most of all, provide lasting fixation without cement (35).

HISTORICAL DEVELOPMENT OF CEMENTLESS ACETABULAR COMPONENTS

Mechanical Fixation Devices

It is useful to divide the evolution of cementless acetabular components into (a) those devices that were designed to achieve mechanical fixation in the pelvis, generally via the geometric shape of the implant, large pegs, or threaded rings, and (b) the more current designs that were intended to achieve biologic fixation via bone ingrowth into a porous-coated surface.

Morscher (70) has described the five main types of cementless acetabular components that have been utilized to date: (a) a cylindrical socket, (b) a square socket, (c) various types of cone, (d) an ilipsoid threaded ring, and (e) a hemispheric cup (Fig. 1). Morscher further stated that the implant that interferes least with the physiologic stress patterns of the acetabulum and pelvis would likely be most successful (68–70,72). In practice, all but the hemispherical design have proven to have unacceptably high failure rates.

For example, Ring introduced a cementless metal-on-metal arthroplasty with a cone-shaped acetabular component with a long threaded rod for fixation into the poste-

C. L. Peters and H. K. Dunn: Department of Orthopedic Surgery, University of Utah School of Medicine, Salt Lake City, Utah 84132.

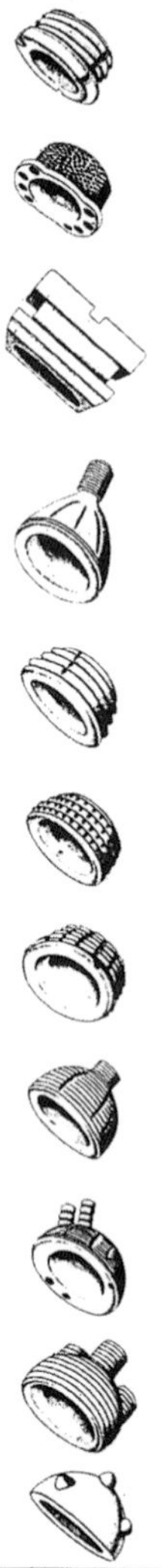

Shape	Literature		Trademark, Material, Remarks (date of first use)
Cylinder	Griss and Heimke (1981)[18]		Lindenhof, Ceramic (1974)
	R. Judet (1975)[30,31]		Judet, Porometal, Cr–Cr–Mo
Square	Griss et al. (1978)[19]		Friedrichsfeld, Ceramic (for dysplastic hip joints) (1975)
Conus	Ring (1982)[60]		Polyethylene (1979)
Obtuse cone with external thread	Mittelmeier (1974)[42]		Ceramic
Cone with external thread	Endler and Endler (1982)[14]		Endler-cup, Polyethylene (1978)
Cone with threaded screw	Parhofer and Mönch[54] (1982)		PM-prosthesis—outer cup, Ti–Al–V; inner cup, polyethylene
Truncated ellipsoid, threaded ring	Lord and Bancel (1983)[34]		Lord prosthesis—outer cup, Co–Cr; inner cup, polyethylene
Hemisphere	Boutin (1981)[5] Morscher et al. (1982)[50]		Ceramic (1971) RM-isoelastic hip endoprosthesis, polyethylene (1977) (polyacetal, 1973, abandoned)
	Knahr et al. (1983)[32]		Polyethylene
	Engelhardt (1983)[15]		Engelhardt prosthesis, ceramic (1976)

FIG. 1. Five types of cementless acetabular components as described by Morscher. (Reproduced with permission, from Morscher EW. Cementless total hip arthroplasty. *Clin Orthop* 1983;181:76–91.)

rior column of the pelvis (83). Although short-term results were good with this device, at 5 to 12 year of follow-up, 101 of 154 (66%) of these cementless acetabular components were radiographically loose in one study (2). Subsequently, Freeman et al. (30) and Ring (83) independently utilized a cone-shaped design of an all-polyethylene socket designed to achieve fixation via polyethylene pegs (Fig. 2). Although both designs were associated with good early results, high failure rates were reported after 5 years, caused by insufficient fixation, progressive socket migration, polyethylene wear, and severe bone resorption (6,54,72,73,106,110).

Similarly, three early threaded-ring designs, those of Lord and Bancel (58) (cobalt chromium alloy), Mittelmeier (66) (ceramic), and Lindenhof (107) (ceramic), generated early enthusiasm, but longer-term follow-up exhibited migration rates as high as 46% (41,43,60,88,107). One cadaver study investigating the primary fit of Lord ceramic cementless acetabular components found that the

threads of the screw-in rings were only marginally in contact with the acetabular bone (88). A factor common to the early designs described above was that mechanical fixation of the acetabular component was sufficient in the short term but insufficient in the long term, as evidenced by progressive migration of these components.

Early success with threaded or screw-in acetabular component designs in Europe led to their application in the United States in the late 1970s and early 1980s. Design changes coincident with increased usage in the United States included a shift to threaded metal-backed components made of titanium alloy, as well as a more hemispherical design with narrower thread spacing. Despite these design changes, experience with titanium alloy threaded components remained unsatisfactory. For example, Engh et al. (26) reported 21% radiographic instability at mean follow-up of only 3.9 years in 130 threaded acetabular components. Most recently Bruijn et al. (9) reported that 25% of 378 mecring threaded acetab-

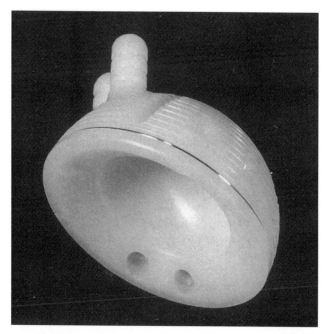

FIG. 2. Ring all-polyethylene cementless acetabular component. (Reproduced with permission, from Wilson-MacDonald J, Morscher E, Masar Z. Cementless uncoated polyethylene acetabular components in total hip replacement. *J Bone Joint Surg* 1990;72B:423.)

ular components had progressive radiographic migration. Other authors, including Apel et al. (3), Capello et al. (13), and Kennedy (48) have reported 15% to 25% radiographic failure with these devices at short- to intermediate-term follow-up. Moreover, laboratory, animal, and

retrieval studies have demonstrated the quality of threaded acetabular component fixation to be inferior to that achieved in porous-coated acetabular components with as little as 9% of the threaded component surface area in contact with bone (7,53,88,100) (Fig. 3).

Several authors have offered explanations for the inferior fixation of threaded acetabular components, especially over time. Huiskes (39), using a finite element analysis model, postulated that the relatively high rigidity of the mecring threaded acetabular component caused high local stress concentration at the site of bone–thread contact, leading to increased bone density in this area, followed sequentially by remodeling, replacement of bone by fibrous tissue, and eventual failure of the screw–bone interface. Similarly, Bruijn (9) postulated that in an attempt to achieve maximum fixation by screwing the implant in as tight as possible, the already high stresses at the bone–thread interface were raised, causing pressure necrosis, resorption of bone, and the eventual replacement of bone with fibrous tissue (53). Consistent with these data is the fact that the lack of a true micro-interlock between the acetabular component and the skeleton resulted in insufficient long-term fixation.

Biologic Fixation with Porous-Coated Components

In an effort to improve the long-term fixation of cementless acetabular components, the concept of biologic fixation, via bone ingrowth, into porous-coated acetabular components was introduced in clinical practice in 1983 and 1984 (10,25,27,31,32,96,102). Previous

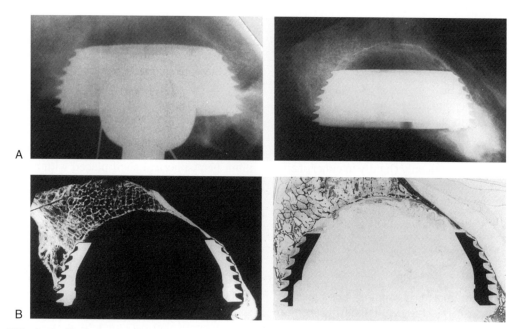

FIG. 3. A: Radiograph of screw-in acetabular component demonstrating no discernible bone–implant radiolucency. **B:** Radiograph of 2-mm-thick section of implant demonstrating minimal bone–implant contact. Reproduced with permission.

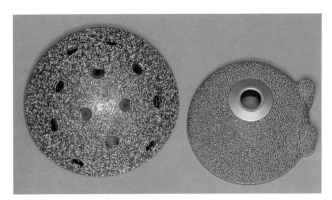

FIG. 4. The Harris-Galante porous and porous-coated anatomic acetabular components.

animal studies had demonstrated encouraging early results with both porous-coated femoral and acetabular components, and this generated enthusiasm for the ability of porous-coated acetabular components to form an enduring biologic bond to the skeleton (44,96,102). In addition, porous-coated acetabular components offered the theoretical advantages of ease of insertion because of their hemispherical shape, and possible exchange of the bearing surface via modular polyethylene liners. Thus, almost simultaneously, the Porous-Coated Anatomic (Howmedica, Rutherford, New Jersey) and the Harris-Galante (Zimmer, Warsaw, Indiana) porous acetabular components were introduced. The Porous-Coated Anatomic acetabular component was composed of chromium–cobalt alloy with a double layer of sintered chromium–cobalt beads and two peripheral pegs for rotational stability. In contrast, the Harris-Galante porous acetabular component was composed of a titanium shell with titanium fiber metal diffusion bonded to the acetabular shell. Fixation in this device was achieved with multiple 5.1-mm cancellous screws through holes in the component itself (Fig. 4).

As would be expected, the 2 to 3-year clinical and radiographic results of acetabuli reconstructed with these devices were good, with loosening rates generally less than 5% (10,23,34,63,90). Based on the excellent early results with these devices, numerous similar implants have been developed, differing only slightly in either shell geometry, metallurgy, or mechanism of fixation. Implants with this basic design continue to be used today.

CURRENT DESIGNS AND INSERTION TECHNIQUES

Virtually all porous-coated acetabular components available today have a hemispherical or modified hemispherical shape, and are made of either chromium–cobalt alloy, commercially pure titanium, or titanium-based alloy. The most common types of porous coatings in use

today continue to be sintered cobalt–chromium beads, titanium fiber metal, cancellous structured titanium, and plasma-sprayed titanium particles. Although, in the past, the site of attachment of the various porous-coated surfaces to the underlying acetabular shell has been an area of concern because of bead or particle detachment, modern-day manufacturing processes have virtually eliminated the problem of porous-coating detachment, at least at intermediate-term follow-up (10,12,37,61,63). Virtually all modern-day manufacturers make available such porous-coated acetabular components in sizes ranging from approximately 40 mm in outer diameter to as large as 80 mm, with individual sizes being available generally in 2-mm increments. The availability of numerous sizes ensures that a broad range of acetabuli, for example from extremely small diameter acetabuli typically found in patients with congenital dislocation of the hip, to extremely large acetabuli typically found in large osteoarthritic men, can be managed with a single line of cementless acetabular components.

Controversy continues to exist, however, regarding the most effective method of fixation of these components to the underlying acetabulum. Three major means of fixation were utilized in the earliest designs of porous-coated acetabular components: cancellous bone screws, antirotation pegs or lugs attached to the periphery of the metallic shell, and fixation spikes attached to the backside or periphery of the metallic shell. The second factor that must be considered, as Engh and co-workers have pointed out, is that the surface area of porous coating available for bone ingrowth varies depending on the area utilized for fixation sites such as screw holes, apical holes, or spikes (95). Therefore, the surgeon must realize that there may be a compromise between the ability to obtain initial fixation with porous-coated acetabular components and the ability to maintain this fixation over time as biologic ingrowth occurs into a limited amount of available pore space.

With this in mind, several authors have investigated the initial implant stability and surface apposition characteristics in porous-coated acetabular components utilizing spikes and screws for fixation. Perona et al. (76) compared the initial implant stability between a titanium hemispherical shell placed with a 2-mm press-fit (that is, a 2-mm oversized component) with no screws, and a 2-mm press-fit hemispherical cup with one or two dome screws, and a titanium hemispherical cup with three spikes. Their results indicated that a press-fit hemispherical component with two dome screws placed into the ilium demonstrated less motion at the ilium than a tri-spike hemispherical component, but significantly more motion at the pubis and ischium than the corresponding tri-spike component. Both the tri-spike cup and the hemispherical cup with screws had significantly less motion than the press-fit hemispherical cup without screws at all three sites on the ilium, pubis, and ischium.

In the former two cases, the amount of implant motion was compatible with bone ingrowth into porous-coated surfaces (76,77).

Schwartz et al. (95) were unable to determine a true difference in the initial surface apposition of porous-coated acetabular components of three different designs: a hemispherical titanium cup with spikes, a hemispherical cup without spikes, and a threaded hemispherical design. Of interest in this study is the fact that, although the porous-coated acetabular components were implanted by experienced surgeons in an idealized *in vitro* setting, less than complete surface contact was observed in all 12 specimens tested. Investigators observed that surface contact was limited by five factors, including the bony anatomy of the acetabulum, asymmetric reaming of the acetabulum, retention of the subchondral plate, acetabular component design, and incorrect version of the acetabular component.

The practical lessons from the studies of Perona et al. and Schwartz et al. are the following:

1. At least *in vitro*, initial fixation with spikes or screws is compatible with biologic ingrowth into porous-coated surfaces.

2. There appears to be little difference in the initial surface apposition in porous-coated acetabular components that utilize screws and those that utilize spikes for initial fixation.

3. Given the constraints of a metallic hemispherical acetabular component and a bony acetabulum that must be machined into a matching hemispherical shape, the surgeon should utilize instrumentation that would allow accurate and reproducible preparation of a hemispherically shaped acetabular bone bed.

In cementless porous-coated acetabular designs that utilized screw fixation through holes in the cup, such as the Harris-Galante porous acetabular component, the original surgical technique called for so-called line-to-line reaming of the acetabulum. This implied implantation of an acetabular component equal in diameter to the size of the last reamer utilized, followed by screw fixation to ensure initial implant stability. This technique worked well and was associated with nearly universally excellent results. For example, Martell et al. (63) reported on 121 Harris-Galante porous acetabular components with no loosening of any acetabular component at mean follow-up of 57 months. Similarly, Schmalzried and Harris reported a 0% incidence of loosening at average 68-month follow-up in a review of 83 Harris-Galante porous-coated acetabular components. Despite the excellent intermediate-term results, three areas of concern regarding the line-to-line fit with screw fixation technique became apparent.

The first of these concerns regarded the use of fixation screws into the innominate bone and the risk of damage to neighboring neurovascular structures. Although direct trauma to intra- and extrapelvic, neural, and vascular structures was extremely rare, the potential for such a devastating complication led Wasielewski et al. (103) and Keating et al. (47) to undertake two separate anatomic and radiographic studies to determine the safest zones in the acetabulum for transacetabular placement of screws. Wasielewski et al. proposed an acetabular quadrant system formed by a line extending from the anterior superior iliac spine extending through the center of the acetabulum and intersecting a perpendicular line at the center of the acetabulum (Fig. 5). Thus, the posterior-superior, posterior-inferior, anterior-superior, and anterior-inferior quadrants of the acetabulum are formed. In cadaveric anatomic specimens, it was shown that screws placed into the anterior-superior and anterior-inferior quadrants endangered the external iliac artery and vein, and the obturator neurovascular structures, respectively. It was further suggested that placement of screws in these quadrants should be avoided whenever possible. In contrast, screws placed in the posterior quadrants, perpendicular to the acetabular surface, were generally safe, especially in the posterior-superior quadrant, where screws 25 mm or longer could be safely placed in the posterior column of the acetabulum (Fig. 6). Although screws placed in the posterior-inferior quadrant were found to lie near the inferior gluteal and internal pudendal neural and vascular structures, these structures were not endangered if screws less than 25 mm in length were used (47,103).

The second concern regarding the use of acetabular transfixation screws was early evidence that both screws and screw holes could serve as pathways for the migration of wear debris and thereby possibly compromise the bone–implant interface. The fundamental concept of particulate wear debris accessibility to the bone–implant, and therefore to the screw–implant, interface was first described by Willert et al. (105) and later expanded upon by Schmalzried et al. (91), who coined the term *the concept of the effective joint space*. Based on clinical and retrieval data, these authors demonstrated that all periprosthetic regions may be accessible to joint fluid, and, therefore, also to particulate debris. This idea was further supported by clinical observations of osteolytic lesions surrounding porous-coated acetabular components, presumably caused by the presence of particulate wear debris (62,86).

For example, Maloney et al. (62) reviewed the cases of 14 patients who had osteolysis in the periacetabular region after the replacement of the acetabulum without cement at a mean follow-up of 65 months. Of note in this study was the fact that 11 of the 15 acetabular components had holes in the porous-coated acetabular shell that may have acted as conduits through which wear debris could gain access to the implant–bone interface. Similarly, Santavirta et al. (86) described six patients with osteolytic lesions in the pelvis surrounding cementless

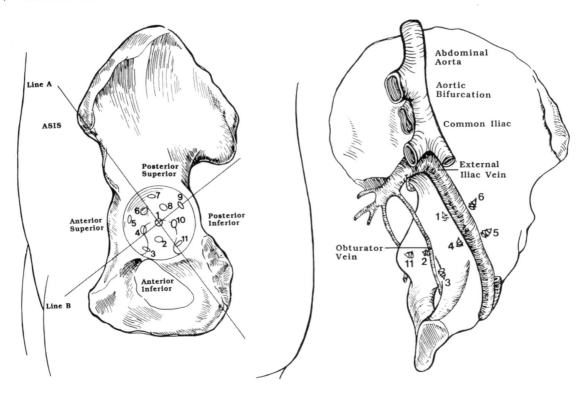

FIG. 5. Quadrant system for acetabular screw placement with cementless acetabular components. Four quadrants (anterosuperior, anteroinferior, posterosuperior, and posteroinferior) are created by a line drawn through the anterior-superior iliac spine extending through the center of the acetabulum, and a perpendicular line. (Reproduced with permission, from Wasielewski RC, Cooperstein LA, Kruger MP, Rubash HE. Acetabular anatomy and the transacetabular fixation of screws in total hip arthroplasty. *J Bone Joint Surg* 1990;72A:501–508.)

acetabular components, all of which required eventual revision of the socket. The acetabular components in this study did not contain screw holes [five Lord prostheses, one porous-coated anatomic (PCA) (Howmedica, Rutherford, New Jersey)], and thus particulate debris presumably gained access to the bone largely via the periphery of the component (86,87).

In our own series of PCA total hip replacements, 21 of 77 cementless acetabular components had failed at mean follow-up of 95 months (21). All of the failed acetabular components had evidence of eccentric polyethylene wear and were associated with major osteolytic lesions in the periacetabular bone, indicating that particulate wear debris had gained access to the bone–implant interface, presumably from a central apical hole in the metallic shell (Fig. 7). All of the acetabular implants had been radiographically stable prior to the development of the large osteolytic lesions. In a recent review (89) of a large series of resurfacing total hip arthroplasties using a press-fit titanium porous-coated acetabular component, it was again demonstrated that particulate wear debris could access the bone–implant interface. The authors sited a 70% incidence of balloon-like osteolysis in the pelvic bone sur-

rounding the acetabular implant. These clinical observations have been at least partially supported by retrieval studies that have identified metallic and polyethylene wear debris within empty screw holes of cementless acetabular components, as well as along the screw–bone interface of cups fixed with screws (79).

The final concern regarding the technique at line-to-line fit with adjunctive screw fixation for cementless acetabular components was the clinical observation of a relatively high frequency of peripheral [i.e., Delee and Charnley zones I and III (22)] radiolucent lines at short-to-intermediate-term follow-up (21,57,63,90,93). In reviewing the Harris-Galante porous-coated acetabular component at 2-to 7-year follow-up, three separate investigative groups in independent reports observed a prevalence of these radiolucent lines, ranging from 12% to 60% (21,57,63,90,93). One of these groups (90,92) was able to correlate the development of a progressive radiolucent line (a known predictor of acetabular loosening) in cemented implants, with the presence of an initial peripheral radiolucency. Because experience with cemented acetabular components had demonstrated that extensive radiolucencies were frequently associated with resorption of periacetabular bone, leading to subsequent

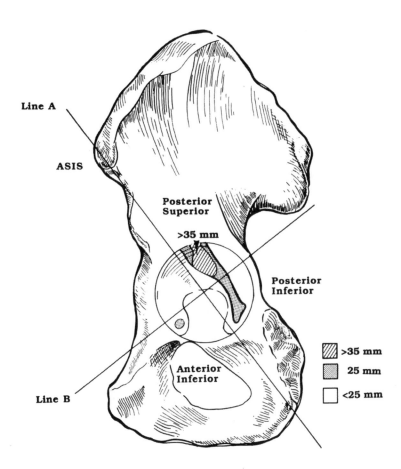

FIG. 6. Screws less than 35 mm in length that are placed into the posterosuperior quadrant, and screws less than 25 mm in length that are placed into the posteroinferior quadrant, are generally safe. (Reproduced with permission, from Wasielewski RC, Cooperstein LA, Kruger MP, Rubash HE. Acetabular anatomy and the transacetabular fixation of screws in total hip arthroplasty. *J Bone Joint Surg* 1990;72A:501–508.)

loosening, it seemed prudent to attempt to reduce the relatively high prevalence of peripheral radiolucencies that were observed when porous-coated acetabular components were implanted with the line-to-line and screw fixation technique.

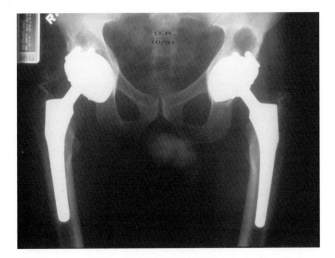

FIG. 7. Radiograph of PCA acetabular component with large osteolytic lesions in the supra-acetabular bone.

Press-Fit Fixation Technique

The method that subsequently became popular was implantation of oversized acetabular components, the so-called press-fit fixation technique. With this method, a hemispherical porous-coated acetabular component, typically 2 to 4 mm larger than the last reamer used to prepare the acetabulum, is forcefully impacted by the surgeon into the acetabulum. The objective of the technique is to press-fit the acetabular component into the host bone, obviating the need for supplemental fixation with screws or spikes. Credit is given to Gordon E. Hill, M.D., for initiation and development of this technique beginning in approximately 1985. In a review of 122 Harris-Galante porous ingrowth acetabular components implanted with this technique at average follow-up of 56 months, Schmalzried et al. (93) concluded that the press-fit technique was effective in reducing both the incidence and extent of radiolucencies at the bone–implant interface. Of note, however, was the fact that initial dome gaps (Delee and Charnley zone II) were more frequent than a comparable group of cups fixed with screws and inserted with a line-to-line fit. However, the majority of initial gaps in the polar region were not visible on 2-year follow-up radiographs, indicating that press-fit cups may undergo subtle superior migration with the early weight bearing and/or bone formation that occurs over time in the polar region.

Kwong et al. (56) investigated the optimal conditions of fit and mechanical stability of porous-coated acetabular components inserted with varying degrees of press-fit and with varying numbers of screws for adjunctive fixation. The conclusion of this study was that a 1-mm press-fit, with or without screws, provided the optimal combination of fit and stability of the acetabular component in a cadaveric model. The authors further observed that with a 2-mm press-fit incomplete seating of the implant was common, resulting in polar or zone II gaps. In addition, the use of supplemental screws did not significantly enhance stability of the implant under any press-fit conditions. In a separate cadaver study of press-fit acetabular components, MacKenzie et al. (59) demonstrated that over-sizing the acetabular component in relation to the reamed acetabular surface resulted in minimal or nonexistent polar area contact, although excellent peripheral contact was obtained. Polar gaps were significantly larger with a 4-mm oversized acetabular component than with a 2-mm oversized component or an exact-fit acetabular component.

An additional concern regarding the press-fit technique is the risk of fracture of the acetabulum. In another cadaveric study, Kim et al. (52) demonstrated that an acetabular fracture was produced in 18 of 30 (60%) acetabular specimens implanted with the press-fit technique, independent of the size of the acetabular component that was used. Fracture was significantly more common when acetabular components oversized by 4 mm were inserted with the press-fit technique, compared to cups inserted with a 2-mm press-fit (52). Thus, it appears that implantation of a grossly oversized component, for example 4 mm larger than the prepared acetabulum, is associated with a significantly higher risk of acetabular fracture.

To summarize the available data regarding the method of insertion of porous-coated acetabular components and its effect on fit and stability of the implant, it appears that the optimal technique produces a tight peripheral rim fit and minimizes the extent of polar gaps. At least with the Harris-Galante porous-coated acetabular component, this result is most likely achieved with a 1- to 2-mm oversized acetabular implant, with care being taken to ensure that the component is fully seated within the prepared acetabulum. If a tight press-fit is obtained, supplemental screws do not appear to be necessary to enhance mechanical stability. If screws are utilized, the risk of neurovascular injury and the risk of these screws serving as pathways for the migration of particulate debris to the periacetabular bone must be weighed against their capacity to provide additional fixation. The use of an excessively oversized hemispherical acetabular component, for example one that is more than 2 mm oversized, may be associated with a significant risk of acetabular fracture.

A final word of caution is that most of the available data are from cadaveric testing and are applicable to the Harris-Galante porous-coated acetabular component. This acetabular component is slightly less than a full hemisphere and contains a relatively elastic titanium fiber–metal porous-coating. Fully hemispherical cementless acetabular components, or designs with a variety of other porous coatings, may behave differently when implanted into living acetabular bone with this technique.

SURGICAL TECHNIQUE OF CEMENTLESS POROUS-COATED ACETABULAR COMPONENT INSERTION

Currently, we attempt to implant virtually all primary total hip acetabular components with a press-fit technique, and we utilize screw fixation only when initial mechanical stability is not achieved with the press-fit technique. What follows is a step-by-step summary of the method of insertion of such a porous-coated acetabular component with this technique:

1. The hip is exposed with either a posterolateral or a direct lateral approach (the surgeon's choice). After exposure of the acetabulum with anterior, posterior, and inferior retractors, the labrum is completely excised from the acetabular rim.

2. The floor of the cotyloid fossa is then exposed. Most commonly, this is performed by using a long-handled curette to remove fat and soft tissue from the horseshoe-shaped fossa. Very often, the fossa is completely obliterated by inferior medial osteophytes, and these can be removed with a 3/4-inch osteotome, which exposes the floor of the fossa.

3. An acetabular reamer approximately 6 to 10 mm smaller than the anticipated size of the acetabular component (based on preoperative templating) is then utilized to initiate reaming. The first and most important step in the reaming process is to utilize the smallest reamer to ream directly medial to the base of the cotyloid fossa (Fig. 8A). With the patient in the lateral position, this means that the surgeon places the reamer nearly perpendicular to the floor and reams centrally until the anterior and posterior margins of the lateral-most aspect of the cotyloid fossa are removed and the medial wall of the cotyloid fossa is completely exposed. Reaming then proceeds in the direction of the anticipated final cup position. Generally, this is a position of 35° to 40° of lateral opening or abduction, and 15° to 25° of forward flexion or anteversion, depending on the surgical approach that is utilized. If a direct lateral or anterolateral approach to the hip is performed, the acetabular component is usually placed in 15° to 20° of anteversion, and if a posterolateral approach is utilized, 20° to 25° is most appropriate. The acetabulum is then

expanded, using sequentially larger reamers in either 1-mm or 2-mm increments, again holding the acetabular reamer in the desired position of final cup implantation (see Fig. 8B).

4. Once an acetabular reamer makes excellent contact with the anterior and posterior walls of the acetabulum as well as the dome and lateral rim, acetabular reaming proceeds cautiously. The surgeon must determine whether sufficient subchondral or cancellous bone has been exposed to ensure bone ingrowth into a porous-coated component. If sclerotic nonbleeding bone or cartilage remains, the surgeon should continue to increase the size of the reamer until bleeding subchondral or cancellous bone is exposed throughout the majority of the acetabular bed. Care must be taken to ensure that adequate thickness of the anterior and posterior columns is available prior to increasing the size of the acetabular reamer.

5. Once an extremely tight fit with an acetabular reamer is encountered and excellent bleeding bony surfaces have been prepared, the surgeon should be able to essentially rock the entire pelvis anteriorly and posteriorly, with the reamer in place, with minimal motion visible between the rim of the acetabulum and the reamer.

6. If there is uncertainty at this point as to the hemisphericity of the prepared surface, a trial component should be inserted to ensure that there is adequate dome as well as rim contact.

7. Assuming the above requirements have been met, an acetabular component 2 mm larger than the last reamer utilized is placed onto the cup insertion device and the final implant is placed into the acetabular opening in the desired position of final implantation (see Fig. 8C).

8. The acetabular component is then firmly impacted into position utilizing several moderately sized blows to the insertion device. Care should be taken to avoid excessive impaction force in order to avoid fracture of the acetabulum at this point. Care should also be taken to ensure that the position of the acetabular component does not change during impaction.

9. Once the component has been tightly impacted into position, the insertion device is removed and the component is manually tested for stability. If there is any evidence of motion of the component in either the anteroposterior or superoinferior directions, supplemental screws should be placed into the posterior superior quadrant of the acetabulum. If no motion of the acetabular implant is visible, the component is thoroughly cleansed of debris and dried, and a modular polyethylene liner is inserted into the metal backing, with care being taken to ensure adequate seating and locking of the polyethylene (see Fig. 8D). Figure 9 outlines the clinical decision-making process for the use of supplemental screw fixation of the acetabular component in primary total hip arthroplasty.

MODULARITY ISSUES

As biologic fixation of porous-coated acetabular components became a reality in the early to mid 1980s, the advantage of a modular acetabular construct consisting of a removable polyethylene liner and a metal-backed porous-coated shell also became apparent. Chief among the advantages was the ability to exchange the polyethylene component without disturbing the biologic bone–implant interface, for example in situations where there is wear or damage of the polyethylene liner. Despite these attributes, with increased clinical use, several disadvantages of the modular construct also became apparent. These included the possibility of increased polyethylene wear, both from the articulating surface and the back-side surface, problems with conformity of the polyethylene within the metal backing of the acetabular shell, and problems with the mechanism by which the modular polyethylene liner was attached to the metal acetabular shell. The discussion below expounds upon each of these perceived or real disadvantages of modular porous-coated acetabular components.

Probably the most disconcerting observation of modular metal-backed cementless acetabular components has been the increased polyethylene wear rates compared to cemented all polyethylene sockets. The average long-term wear rate of cemented all-polyethylene acetabular components has been reported to be between 0.07 and 0.15 mm/year (15,19,33,65,82,111,112). In contrast, wear rates for cementless acetabular components have been reported to be as high as 0.77 mm/year (8,81,84). In an excellent double-blind randomized clinical trial comparing cemented and cementless total hip arthroplasties in patients with greater than 48-month follow-up, polyethylene wear and osteolysis were shown to be significantly greater in the cementless arthroplasties. Moreover, the increased linear and volumetric polyethylene wear in the cementless total hip arthroplasty group was directly related to the reduced thickness of modular, metal-backed polyethylene liners (84). Other factors thought to contribute to the increased polyethylene wear rate in cementless implants include the stiffness of the metal shell, accelerated third-body wear (chiefly from metallic particles from cementless implants), and thin unsupported modular polyethylene liners, compared to all polyethylene cemented sockets (8,81,84,85).

A related concern was the potential for polyethylene wear from the metallic-substrate-facing surface of the polyethylene, or so-called back-sided polyethylene wear. In retrieval specimens, several investigators have noted that polyethylene frequently cold-flowed into unsupported areas, such as screw holes. Consequently, even minimal micromotion at this interface offers the potential for backsided polyethylene wear (40,78,79,81,85,97). Especially alarming, if this mechanism of polyethylene

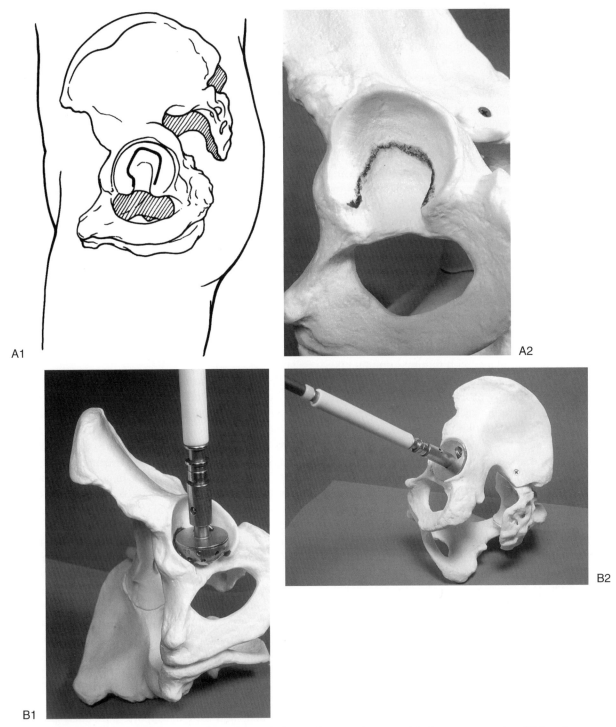

FIG. 8. The preparation and insertion technique of cementless acetabular components utilizing the press-fit technique. **A:** Complete exposure of the horseshoe shape of the cotyloid fossa after complete removal of acetabular labrum ligamentum teres and pulvinar. **B:** The acetabulum is reamed to the base of the cotyloid fossa by reaming perpendicular to the floor. This is followed by reaming the acetabulum in the anticipated final cup position: normally, 35° to 40° of abduction and 15° to 25° of anteversion.

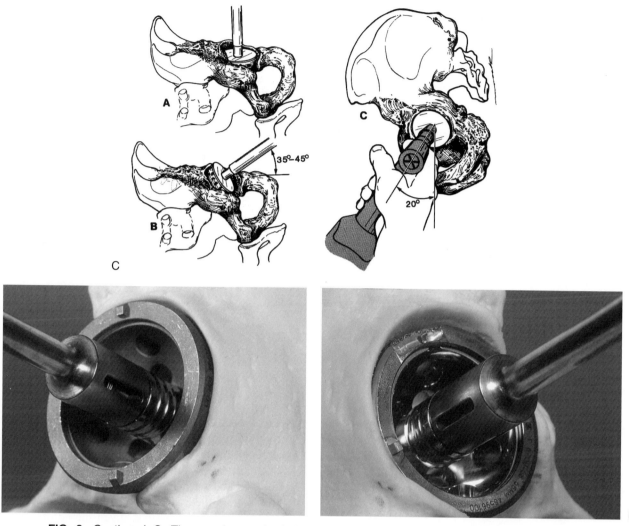

FIG. 8. *Continued.* **C:** The reaming method described in (B). Position *A* represents perpendicular reaming to the base of the cotyloid fossa. Positions *B* and *C* represent reaming of the acetabulum in the anticipated final cup position. **D:** A cup oversized by approximately 2 mm is placed into the acetabular opening, and, with multiple moderate blows, the cup is seated in the acetabulum, with care being taken to ensure complete seating of the implant. **E:** Final position of the implant press-fit between the anterior and posterior columns.

wear exists, is the proximity of wear particles to the bone–implant interface when unfilled screw holes are present.

Several recent reports regarding large osteolytic lesions surrounding modular porous-coated acetabular components have heightened concerns about polyethylene wear in these components (8,21,62,86,87). For example, Maloney et al. (62) reported 15 cases of expansile destructive lesions ballooning into the supra-acetabular portion of the pelvis. The lytic lesions were associated with radiographic evidence of asymmetric polyethylene wear in 80% of cases. The authors contributed the high rate of polyethylene wear to a number of factors, including the patients being young and active, the thin polyethylene, and the poor fixation of the liners to the metal shell.

Similarly, Bono et al. (8) reported a 78% incidence of acetabular osteolysis in 94 hip replacements performed with the Anatomic Modular Locking plus acetabular component and the Acetabular Cup System Liner (Depuy, Warsaw, Indiana). In this series, there were 15 catastrophic failures (21%) caused by wear of a thin modular polyethylene component. The acetabular component proved to be a poor design because of asymmetrical and cylindrical geometry of the polyethylene liner, predisposing the liner to increased stress at the superior rim (Fig. 10). Because the vast majority of patients with these types of acetabular osteolytic lesions are asymptomatic, many authors have emphasized the need for regular periodic radiographic follow-up of patients with cementless hip implants (8,24,81,85).

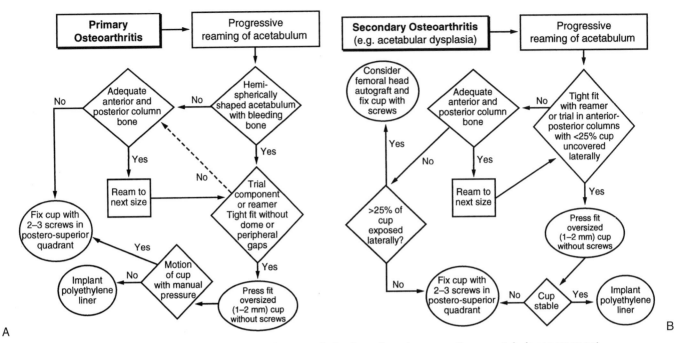

FIG. 9. Clinical algorithms for the use of screws during insertion of a cementless acetabular component utilizing the press-fit technique. **A:** Algorithm for primary osteoarthritis. **B:** Algorithm for secondary osteoarthritis.

Other areas of concern with modular polyethylene liners are the thickness of the polyethylene, the conformity between the metallic shell and the polyethylene, and the mechanism by which the polyethylene is secured to the metallic shell. Bartel et al. (5) used elasticity and finite

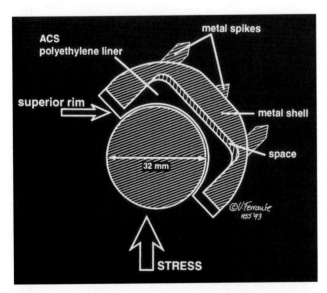

FIG. 10. The anatomic medullary locking acetabular component, and the acetabular cup system polyethylene liner that has been associated with catastrophic polyethylene wear and acetabular osteolysis. (Reproduced with permission, from Bono JV, Sanford L, Toussaint JT. Severe polyethylene wear in total hip arthroplasty. *J Arthroplasty* 1994;9:119–125.)

element models to demonstrate that a minimum polyethylene thickness, at least for the tibial component in a total knee replacement, should be 8 to 10 mm to minimize the stresses associated with surface damage. Assuming that a similar thickness would be optimal for hip replacements, manufacturers have attempted to keep acetabular polyethylene as thick as possible, given the constraints of a metal-backed shell. However, as the shell size decreases, particularly in the range of 48- to 52-mm for the outer diameter, and as femoral head size increases, the thickness of the polyethylene liner must decrease.

Also important in reducing stress, and therefore surface damage of polyethylene, is adequate congruency between the modular polyethylene and the metallic shell. If the polyethylene liner is not completely seated within the shell, and instead relies on peripheral rim contact, stress within the polyethylene should increase. Fehring et al. (29) have investigated the congruency of five modular cementless acetabular components *in vitro*. Interestingly, only 3 of 5 modular acetabular components tested were congruent under physiologic loads. It is plausible, therefore, that rim loading of polyethylene liners could contribute to increased polyethylene wear and possibly to fatigue fracture of the polyethylene at the rim.

Because at least five cases of disassembly of modular polyethylene liners from their underlying metal-backed shell have been reported, concern has been generated regarding the integrity of several locking mechanisms currently in use. *In vitro* push-out and lever-out testing has been performed on several commercially available

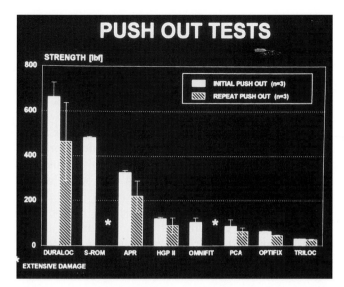

FIG. 11. Polyethylene liner push-out data. (Reproduced with permission, from Tradonsky S, Postak PD, Froimson AI, Greenwald AS. A comparison of the disassociation strength of modular acetabular components. *Clin Orthop* 1993;296: 154–160.)

systems, and the force necessary to push the liner from its shell has ranged from 663–29 lb (29,101) (Fig. 11). The force necessary to lever the polyethylene from the underlying shell has ranged from 43 to 684 lb (29,101) (Fig. 12). These results indicate that, at least *in vitro*, the quality of locking mechanisms varies tremendously. Also, as Tradonsky et al. (101) noted, it is reasonable to assume that those designs with stronger locking mecha-

nisms, if appropriately assembled, are less likely to dissociate. Also concerning in these *in vitro* tests is that repeat-liner-separation testing demonstrated approximately a 30% decrease in locking mechanism integrity and, in repeat testing, several designs demonstrated failure of the retention structures, possibly compromising the ability to replace a modular polyethylene liner.

Although it is clear that modular cementless sockets offer distinct advantages in the form of the ability to exchange a damaged articulating surface without disturbing the bone–implant interface, and in their ability to allow independent fixation of the metallic shell to the underlying bone, there are distinct and real disadvantages to modular systems. These disadvantages include a relatively high rate of polyethylene wear compared to cemented sockets, the development of osteolysis in the surrounding periacetabular bone, two possible surfaces for the origination of particulate wear debris, and dissociation or catastrophic failure of the modular polyethylene insert. Recent improvements in cementless acetabular component design have focused on eliminating many of these inherent weaknesses. For example, attempts have been made to improve not only the quality of modular polyethylene inserts, but also to improve the mechanism by which these inserts are anchored to the underlying metal shell. In addition, newer designs have focused on reducing the surface roughness and number of screw holes, and on improving the congruency between the back side of the polyethylene and the inner surface of the metal shell.

RADIOGRAPHIC EVALUATION OF CEMENTLESS ACETABULAR COMPONENTS

Because particulate-debris-induced bone resorption has been shown to frequently be a silent process, and because experience with cemented acetabular components has demonstrated a significant correlation between a complete bone–implant interface radiolucency and subsequent implant loosening, the need for regular periodic radiographic evaluation of cementless acetabular components has been emphasized (21,26,38,62). Radiographic evaluation of such implants should, at the very least, include the following: (a) the position of the acetabular component, (b) migration of the acetabular component, and (c) characterization of the bone–implant interface in the form of radiolucencies and osteolytic lesions.

The position of the acetabular component can be defined in relation to various radiographic landmarks on the pelvis. Although several different measurement systems have been used, most have utilized a system modified only slightly from that shown in Figure 13 (10,37, 64). The *x* and *y* axes can be created by a horizontal line drawn through the base of each teardrop (the *x* axis) and a vertical reference line perpendicular to the inter-tear-

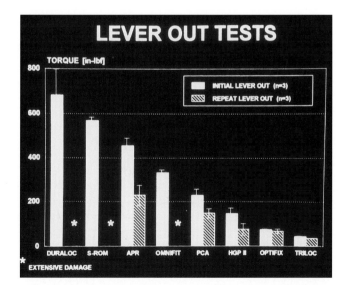

FIG. 12. Polyethylene liner lever-out data. (Reproduced with permission, from Tradonsky S, Postak PD, Froimson AI, Greenwald AS. A comparison of the disassociation strength of modular acetabular components. *Clin Orthop* 1993;296: 154–160.)

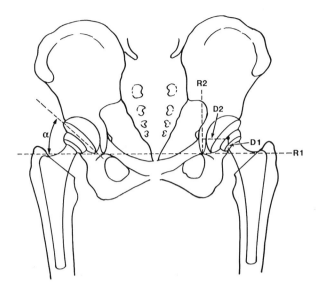

FIG. 13. Acetabular grid system for radiographic evaluation of cementless acetabular components. Alpha represents the opening angle of the acetabular implant. Reference *line 1* is the inter-teardrop line. Reference *line 2* is perpendicular to reference line 1, drawn through the middle of the teardrop. D1 is the vertical distance of the center of the acetabular component or femoral head to the inter-teardrop line (R1). D2 is the horizontal distance from the center of the femoral head or acetabular component to reference line 2.

drop line that intersects the teardrop (the y axis). Finally, a line drawn through the most lateral and most medial aspects of the metal acetabular shell intersecting the inter-teardrop line allows calculation of the opening angle of the acetabular component. The vertical position of the acetabular component can be defined by the distance between the center of the acetabular component (or femoral head) and the inter-teardrop line; the horizontal position can be defined by the difference between the hip center and the vertical reference line.

The migration of the acetabular component can then be determined by the change in these parameters measured on two successive radiographs. It is important to note that meaningful measurements can be made only from successive radiographs that are comparable. Thus, rotation, flexion, and extension of the pelvis must be considered, and magnification should be controlled either by use of an external magnification marker or by using the known diameter of the femoral head as a marker. Generally, the most useful initial anteroposterior pelvis radiograph is one obtained at the first clinical follow-up evaluation, rather than one obtained during the immediate postoperative period. Because of the inherent limitations in measuring changes in position of the acetabular component on two successive radiographs, definite acetabular component migration has been considered to be horizontal or vertical migration greater than 2 to 3 mm, or a change in the opening angle of the acetabular component of greater than 5 (10,37,57,63,64,74).

Examination of the bone–implant interface for radiolucencies or osteolytic lesions has been facilitated by a system in which the acetabular component is divided into defined zones. The most commonly utilized system is that attributed to Delee and Charnley (22), who divided the acetabulum into three equal zones, with zone I being the most lateral and zone III the medial. Recently, Martell et al. (63) have modified this system to include five zones formed by subdividing Delee and Charnley's original zone I and zone II (Fig. 14). The location of various radiolucencies and osteolytic lesions can then be defined in relation to these zones.

Because the porous-coated acetabular component–bone interface is a continuous biologic interface, development of partial radiolucencies in one or two zones has been quite common. There is some debate regarding the significance of a continuous radiolucency encompassing all zones of the acetabular component. Although it seems clear that the development of a progressive, complete radiolucency at an interface that previously had no such radiolucency would indicate loosening of the acetabular component, no data have yet correlated a nonprogressive complete bone–implant interface radiolucency with subsequent loosening of the acetabular component. A possible explanation is that because two plain radiographs do not necessarily visualize the entire bone–implant interface, it is conceivable that small areas of spot welds of bone ingrowth exist in spite of a visible complete radiolucency. Therefore, it is probably appropriate to consider a complete radiolucency of 2 mm in width around a porous-coated acetabular component to indicate possible, rather than definite, loosening of such an implant.

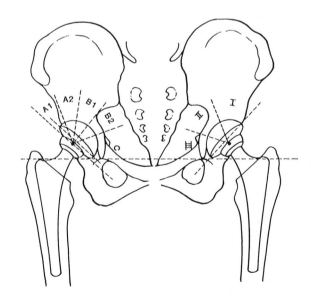

FIG. 14. Acetabular zone systems. The system of Delee and Charnley (22) is shown on the *right*, and that of Martell et al. (63) is shown on the *left*.

CLINICAL AND RADIOGRAPHIC RESULTS OF POROUS-COATED ACETABULAR COMPONENTS

There is little doubt that the most valuable scientific information is obtained from well-designed, prospective, and preferably randomized clinical trials that compare emerging techniques and designs with those for which there is reliable scientific information. Unfortunately, within the orthopedic literature there is a paucity of these types of studies, and most of the available information regarding cementless porous-coated acetabular implants is retrospective, or at best prospective, in nature. Nevertheless, a review of the literature on cementless acetabular sockets provides information regarding the clinical and radiographic performance of these sockets at short- to medium-term follow-up. It is worth noting that the longest published follow-up of a series of porous-coated acetabular components is 104 months (55). In contrast, we now have information on cemented acetabular components at a follow-up of more than 20 years (112). Thus, even 10-year cementless socket data must be considered preliminary, and final judgment of their ultimate value must wait for another decade of experience.

One randomized controlled study investigating the clinical performance and fixation of acetabular components inserted with and without cement during one-stage bilateral total hip arthroplasty exists (74). In 21 patients undergoing bilateral total hip arthroplasty, one hip was randomly allocated to have a Harris-Galante porous acetabular component inserted without cement, and the contralateral hip was treated with an all-polyethylene Charnley acetabular component with cement fixation. At a mean 27-month follow-up, there was no significant difference in the clinical performance of the hips nor was there significant difference in migration between the two designs of acetabular components using roetgenstereo-photogrammetric analysis (74). In another prospective but nonrandomized study, cemented acetabular components were compared with porous ingrowth sockets at 2- to 4-year follow-ups. Again there was no significant difference in the clinical performance of the hips. However, there was a higher rate of migration and a higher incidence of radiolucent line formation in cemented sockets (108). Based on this information, at short-term follow-up, cementless sockets are comparable to cemented sockets in terms of fixation and clinical performance.

The implantation of porous-coated acetabular components without cement began in earnest in 1983 and 1984. Since then, a large volume of data has been published by individual surgeons or centers on implants from various manufacturers. The most useful method to determine which porous-coated acetabular implant designs have fared best and which have been associated with clinical or radiographic problems is to examine the body of literature that has been germane to each individual implant.

Most of the available scientific information pertains to three porous-coated acetabular component designs, these being the Harris-Galante porous component (Zimmer, Warsaw, Indiana), the PCA (Howmedica, Rutherford, New Jersey), and the AML (anatomic medullary locking) prosthesis (Depuy, Warsaw, Indiana). Unfortunately, there is a paucity of information regarding cementless cups of other designs (Table 1).

The Harris-Galante porous acetabular component has been the most extensively studied cementless socket in the orthopedic literature (Table 2). It is made of commercially pure titanium and utilizes titanium fiber metal porous coating for bone ingrowth. Table 2 summarizes the results of nine separate series utilizing this device. Overall, experience with this implant has been excellent at short- to medium-term follow-up. The most recent series, reported by Kull et al. (55) and White et al. (104), have shown no deterioration of the results with this implant at 6- to 10-year follow-up. In total, 916 acetabular implants have been reported in the cumulative series with a revision rate of 1.3%, a loosening rate of 0.1%, and a rate of periacetabular osteolysis of 0.9% (see Table 2). Of note is that the vast majority of revision operations with this implant were performed for reasons other than loosening or loss of fixation. For example, in the separate series reported by Kull et al. (55) (180 patients) and Schmalzried and Harris (90), there were six total revision operations: two of these were for dislocation, two for failure of the polyethylene locking mechanism, and two for periacetabular lysis. It is interesting that Tradonsky et al. (101) demonstrated in *in vitro* testing that the locking mechanism of the Harris-Galante porous acetabular component was relatively weak, and 4 of 12 revision operations reported in the cumulative series of Harris-Galante porous acetabular components were performed for failure of the polyethylene locking mechanism.

The PCA acetabular component is composed of a cobalt–chromium alloy shell with sintered cobalt–chromium alloy beads for biologic fixation. Initial fixation is via peripheral pegs without supplemental screw augmentation. The early experience with the PCA acetabular component was also encouraging, with extremely low rates of acetabular loosening or revision. For example, data from Callaghan et al. (10), Hedley et al. (36), and Dodge et al. (23) at short-term follow-up (less than 3 years) showed an extremely low rate of acetabular component revision (0%) and virtually no reports of osteolysis surrounding the acetabular component. With longer-term follow-up of this socket, however, problems have become evident. In reports with longer-term follow-up, such as those reported by Davitt and Dunn (21), Owen et al. (75), and Kim and Kim (50), acetabular revision rates and the prevalence of osteolysis in the periacetabular region have risen sharply to approximately 10 to 20% (Table 3). Most alarmingly the periacetabular osteolysis has, in the vast majority of cases,

TABLE 1. *Cumulative experience with porous-coated cementless acetabular components*

Type of cup	Authors (ref.)	HHS at f/u	Age (yr)	Length of f/u (mo)	Cups (N)	Definitely loose (N)	Possibly loose (N)	Revised (N)	Reoperations (N)	Acetabular osteolysis (N)
HGP	Kull et al. (55)		51	104	180	0	3	*3	3	7
HGP (w/ screws)	Schmalzried and Harris (90)	93	59	68	83	0	0	*3	3	1
HGP (press-fit)	Schmalzried et al. (93)	92	67	56	122	0	0	1	0	0
HGP	Laschiewz et al. (57)	94	43	37	100	0	0	0	1	
HGP	Martell et al. (63)	93	49	67	121	0	0	1	0	0
HGP	Woolson and Maloney (109)	94	50	42	69	0	0	0	0	0
HGP	White et al. (104)			90	135	0	0	2	4	0
HGP	Kienapfel et al. (49)		55	39	40	0	1	0	0	
HGP	Incavo et al. (42)		63	37	66	1	5	2	0	
PCA	Dodge et al. (23)	91	58	37	44	6	0	0	0	
PCA	Heekin et al. (37)	93	58	72	91	6		2		
PCA	Davitt and Dunn (21)		56	96	77	20		17		14
PCA	Owen et al. (75)				241			26		36
PCA	Kim and Kim (50)	91	48	76	116	3		4		10
PCA	Alexander et al. (1)		55	68	89			5		
PCA	Mont et al. (67)	92	35	54	44	1		1		
AML	Kim and Kim (51)	91	48	84	51	0	0	0	0	16
AML	Engh et al. (26)		55	58	285	0	0	0	0	
AML	Piston et al. (80)		32	90	35	0	0	2		
Optifix	Incavo et al. (42)		61	29	40		2	0		
APR	Dorr (24)			67	75	0	0	0		2
LSF	Barrack et al. (4)	85		72	137	2	1	4		15
Morscher	Morscher (71)		64	17	330			2		
Total					2,571	38 (1.4%)	12 (0.5%)	75 (2.9%)		107 (4.2%)

HHS, Harris Hip Score; f/u, follow-up; HGP, Harris-Galante porous-coated component; PCA, porous-coated anatomic component; AML, anatomic medullary locking component.

TABLE 2. *Harris-Galante porous acetabular component (HGP), cumulative data*

Type of cup	Authors (ref.)	HHS at f/u	Age (yr)	Length of f/u (mo)	Cups (N)	Definitely loose (N)	Possibly loose (N)	Revised (N)	Reoper- ations (N)	Acetabular osteolysis (N)
HGP	Kull et al. (55)		51	104	180	0	3	*3	3	7
HGP (w/ screws)	Schmalzried and Harris (90)	93	59	68	83	0	0	*3	3	1
HGP (press-fit)	Schmalzried et al. (93)	92	67	56	122	0	0	1	0	0
HGP	Laschiewz et al. (57)	94	43	37	100	0	0	0	1	
HGP	Martell et al. (63)	93	49	67	121	0	0	1	0	0
HGP	Woolson and Maloney (109)	94	50	42	69	0	0	0	0	0
HGP	White et al. (104)			90	135	0	0	2	4	0
HGP	Kienapfel et al. (49)		55	39	40	0	1	0	0	
HGP	Incavo et al. (42)		63	37	66	1	5	2	2	
Total					916	1 (0.1%)	9 (1%)	12 (1.3%)	11 (11.2%)	8 (0.9%)

HHS, Harris Hip Score; f/u, follow-up.

1009

eventually required revision of the acetabular component.

The osteolysis in the PCA design has been associated with a number of factors, all leading to increased polyethylene wear. These factors have included the use of a 32-mm cobalt–chromium alloy head, progressive bead shedding leading to increased polyethylene wear by a third-body mechanism, thin unsupported polyethylene, vertical cup position, and finally, dissociation of the non-modular one-piece polyethylene articulating surface from the metal-backed shell by shearing of the central fixation peg, leading to freely mobile polyethylene and massive catastrophic wear (10,21,37,50,75).

In a cumulative series of PCA acetabular components totaling 702 cups, including series with both short- and intermediate-term follow-up, the revision rate is 7.7%, whereas the rate of acetabular osteolysis is 8.6% (see Table 3). Clearly, the increasing rate of polyethylene wear and osteolysis is of concern, and the need for regular radiographic follow-up of the patients with this implant must be emphasized.

Although less data is available, experience with the AML porous-coated acetabular component has, for the most part, paralleled that of the PCA device. The AML porous-coated acetabular component is made of cobalt–chromium alloy with cobalt–chromium alloy beads for biologic fixation. At least three separate reports totaling 371 AML sockets have been published with only two (0.5%) reported cases of revision and 22 cases (6%) of periacetabular osteolysis (Table 4) (26,51,80). Follow-up in these reports has averaged 77 months. As in the PCA series, the acetabular components reviewed at shorter-term follow-up had generally less osteolysis than hips followed for more than 7 years. With longer-term follow-up, the osteolysis rate has approached 31% in one series (51). These data do not include AML plus acetabular components, which have been shown to be associated with catastrophic polyethylene failure and acetabular osteolysis, as has been described previously.

There are a handful of reports describing the results of other commercially available porous-coated acetabular components (Table 5). For example, Dorr (24) has reported excellent results with the APR (Intermedics Orthopedics, Austin, Texas) titanium acetabular component, which utilizes cancellous structured titanium for bone ingrowth. At a mean 67-month follow-up of cups that were press-fit without screw fixation, there were no revisions and only two cups with acetabular lysis. Incavo et al. (42) also reported excellent results at 29-month follow-up with the Optifix (Richards, Memphis, Tennessee) porous-coated acetabular component in 40 hips. Barrack et al. (4) reported disappointing results with the LSF modular porous-coated acetabular component (Depuy, Warsaw, Indiana) at 72-month follow-up. In 137 cups, there was an 11% incidence of significant pelvic osteolysis, and significant radiographic evidence of polyethylene

wear was noted in over 50% of cases. Paralleling the findings of other studies with the PCA and AML acetabular components, the incidence of pelvic lysis was nonexistent at 2- to 4-year follow-up but had risen to 11% (15 cases) at a mean 72-month follow-up (4). The LSF implant is made of cobalt–chromium alloy and is coated with cobalt–chromium alloy sintered beads and utilizes screws for supplemental fixation.

A nonmodular porous-coated device designed to be press-fit into the acetabulum has been designed and extensively utilized by Morscher (68,69,71). This device has several fundamental differences from the commonly used porous-coated acetabular components. The overall design is a flattened hemisphere, designed to be 1.5 mm larger than the corresponding reaming of the acetabulum. The press-fit cup is therefore fixed to the acetabulum by the so-called snap fastener mechanism (Fig. 15) (71). In addition, the one-piece design has four layers of criss-crossed commercially pure titanium wire, which are embedded in the polyethylene, and an anchoring barrel that protrudes from the upper surface of the cup in the direction of loading of the acetabulum. Morscher has emphasized that preservation of the subchondral bone of the acetabulum in conjunction with the relatively elastic acetabular component allows optimum stress transmission from the implant itself to the acetabulum (71). Morscher has reported excellent results (two revisions and two definitely loose acetabular components) in 330 cups at only 17-month follow-up (see Table 5). Although the theoretical appeal of many of these design modifications is apparent, longer-term follow-up is necessary before definitive conclusions can be made.

Cementless porous-coated acetabular components have been used in clinical practice for over 10 years. In general, the clinical and radiographic results of these types of implants have been excellent. The Harris-Galante porous acetabular component has been the most extensively studied, and the results with this implant have been universally excellent, especially with respect to fixation of the component to the underlying host bone. The vast majority of problems related to this device have been associated with the mechanism by which the modular polyethylene component is fixed to the metal-backed shell. The relatively low rate of osteolysis in the periacetabular region with this device may be related to the intrinsic elasticity of the implant and its ability to approximate normal stress transmission in the intact pelvis. The PCA acetabular component has produced good short-term results, but there have been problems at longer-term follow-up with the polyethylene locking mechanism, severe polyethylene wear, and periacetabular osteolysis. Similarly, the AML acetabular component has provided good short-term results, but concern exists regarding the development of acetabular osteolysis with longer-term follow-up. The nonmodular porous-coated component designed by Morscher has several theoretical advantages

TABLE 3. *Porous-coated anatomic acetabular component (PCA), cumulative data*

Type of cup	Authors (ref.)	HHS at f/u	Age (yr)	Length of f/u (mo)	Cups (N)	Definitely loose (N)	Possibly loose (N)	Revised (N)	Reoperations (N)	Acetabular osteolysis (N)
PCA	Dodge et al. (23)	91	58	37	44	6	0	0	0	
PCA	Heekin et al. (37)	93	58	72	91	6		2		
PCA	Davitt and Dunn (21)		56	96	77	20		17		14
PCA	Owen et al. (75)				241			26		36
PCA	Kim and Kim (50)	91	48	76	116	3		4		10
PCA	Alexander et al. (1)		55	68	89			5		
PCA	Mont et al. (67)	92	35	54	44	1		1		
Total					702	36 (5.1%)	0	55 (7.8%)		60 (8.6%)

HHS, Harris Hip Score; f/u, follow-up.

TABLE 4. *Anatomic medullary locking porous-coated acetabular component (AML), cumulative data*

Type of cup	Authors (ref.)	HHS at f/u	Age (yr)	Length of f/u (mo)	Cups (N)	Definitely loose (N)	Possibly loose (N)	Revised (N)	Reoperations (N)	Acetabular osteolysis (N)
AML	Kim and Kim (51)	91	48	84	51	0	0	0	0	16
AML	Engh et al. (26)		55	58	285	0	0	0	0	
AML	Piston et al. (80)		32	90	35	0	0	2		6
Total					371	0 (0%)	0 (0%)	2 (0.5%)		22 (6.0%)

HHS, Harris Hip Score; f/u, follow-up.

TABLE 5. *Other porous-coated acetabular components, cumulative data*

Type of cup	Authors (ref.)	HHS at f/u	Age (yr)	Length of f/u (mo)	Cups (N)	Definitely loose (N)	Possibly loose (N)	Revised (N)	Reoperations (N)	Acetabular osteolysis (N)
Optifix	Incavo et al. (42)		61	29	40		2	0		
APR	Dorr (24)			67	75	0	0	0		
LSF	Barrack et al. (4)	85		72	137			4		2
Morscher	Morscher (71)		64	17	330	2	1	2		15

HHS, Harris Hip Score; f/u, follow-up.

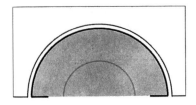

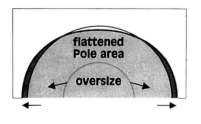

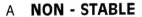

A **NON - STABLE**   B **STABLE**

FIG. 15. Photograph of the so-called snap-fastener mechanism of cup insertion with the Morscher one-piece acetabular component with flattened dome and 1- to 5-mm oversizing. (Reproduced with permission, from Morscher EW. Current status of acetabular fixation in primary total hip arthroplasty. *Clin Orthop* 1992;274:172–193.)

including an elastic one-piece construct and intrinsic press-fit stability. However, longer-term follow-up is necessary to determine the true clinical value of this device.

RETRIEVAL DATA

Although clinical and radiographic evaluations of total hip replacement implants provide useful information, only evaluation of retrieved specimens allows for microscopic characterization of the host tissue response to porous-coated devices. Moreover, it is only by careful examination of well-functioning prostheses retrieved at the time of autopsy that radiographic, clinical, and histologic correlations can be determined. The primary purpose of implant retrieval studies is three-fold: (a) to characterize the host bone–implant interface with regard to the type and geographic distribution of the host tissue response, (b) to allow histologic correlation with radiographic and clinical findings, and, more recently, (c) to determine the extent and geographic distribution of particulate wear debris.

Unfortunately, much of the early implant retrieval data were based on specimens removed at the time of revision for reasons such as dislocation, infection, or persistent pain. Furthermore, many of these specimens were in place for only a short period of time (16–18,97). Consequently, the extent and volume of bone ingrowth into porous-coated devices tended to be minimal, with much of the surface area of porous-coated acetabular implants having ingrowth of fibrous tissue only (16–18). For example, in 1988, Collier et al. (17) reported on 162 porous-coated prostheses removed by a number of surgeons at the time of revision. Fifty-eight of these implants were acetabular components. Bone ingrowth was seen in only 16% (9 of 58) of the acetabular components, which were retrieved for a variety of reasons. The retrieved acetabular specimens were in place for an average duration of only 8 months (range, 1 week to 57 months).

Similarly, Cook et al. (18) reported on 14 porous-coated acetabular components that were *in situ* for an average of only 5.5 months (range, 1 to 18 months). Most of the acetabular implants were removed for instability, dislocation, or late infection (18). Bone ingrowth was

minimal or absent in 11 of the 14 retrieved components. When ingrowth occurred, it was usually seen immediately adjacent to fixation pegs, spikes, or screws. Sumner et al. (97) reported on 25 Harris-Galante porous-coated acetabular components retrieved at the time of revision, with an average time *in situ* of only 30-weeks. Bone ingrowth was documented in 18 of the 25 cases. For the specimens with documented bone ingrowth, averages of 15% of the available surface area and 3.8% of the volume of porous-coating were occupied by bone. Thus, it became clear that the amount and distribution of bone ingrowth based on data from analysis of specimens retrieved at the time of revision was substantially less than what had been reported in animal studies and than what had been observed clinically at the time of revision (99,102). Further, these data emphasized the need for evaluation of well-functioning porous-coated implants retrieved at the time of autopsy.

Three recent studies have examined well-functioning porous-coated acetabular components retrieved at the time of autopsy (28,78,79). Specimens in these studies were generally in place for a longer period of time (average times *in situ* of 41, 45, and 50 months) and had significantly more bone ingrowth than comparable specimens retrieved at the time of revision. For example, Engh et al. (28) reported on nine porous-coated acetabular components with a mean extent of bone ingrowth of 32% and a mean area density of 48%. Interestingly, the authors did not find a correlation between radiographic evidence of bone ingrowth and histologic evidence of bone ingrowth. Areas of the bone–implant interface devoid of bone contact were generally filled with dense fibrous tissue. There was no evidence of granulomata formation or particulate-debris-induced bone resorption in these specimens.

Pidhorz et al. (79) examined 11 Harris-Galante porous acetabular components inserted with screw fixation, at an average of 41 months. The mean extent of bone ingrowth was 29.7% and, although there was no difference in the amount of bone ingrowth when the component was partitioned into nine anatomic regions, there was significantly more bone adjacent to holes containing screws than adjacent to empty screw holes (Fig. 16). Polyethylene debris was noted both in filled and empty screw holes, but no distinct granulomata

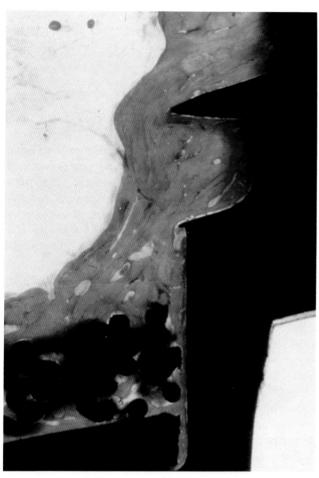

FIG. 16. Photomicrograph of the bone–implant and screw–bone interface in an autopsy-retrieved specimen at 89 months. Note abundant bone ingrowth into the porous-coating adjacent to the screw.

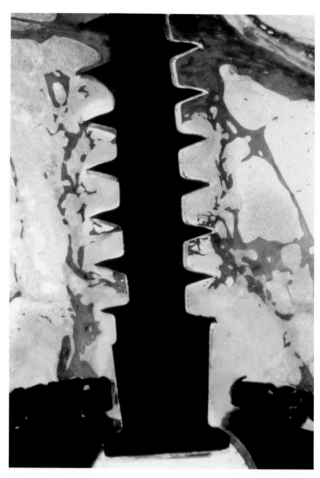

FIG. 17. Photomicrograph of autopsy-retrieved screw within a porous-coated acetabular screw component that was *in situ* for 89 months. Note the granulomatous membrane containing polyethylene debris at the screw–bone interface.

were found. This series was expanded in 1995 to include 24 Harris-Galante porous acetabular components, with several of the implants having been *in situ* for 80 to 90 months. The mean extent and volume fraction of bone ingrowth was similar to those reported previously, as was the finding of more bone ingrowth adjacent to holes filled with screws (78). In the longer-term cases, polyethylene and metal debris were noted to track along several screw–bone interfaces and in empty screw holes, although there was no evidence of screw loosening or radiographic evidence of lucency surrounding the screws (78) (Fig. 17). In both the report by Pidhorz and the expanded study of Harris-Galante porous acetabular components, there was a significant relationship between the absence of a radiolucency and the amount of bone present at the interface (78). The finding of particulate debris at the screw–bone interface probably supports the idea that screws may serve as a conduit for the migration of polyethylene and metal debris to the periacetabular bone.

To summarize the data pertaining to retrieved porous-coated acetabular components, it is important to separate the information obtained from analysis of specimens retrieved from living patients from that obtained from analysis of well-functioning specimens retrieved at the time of autopsy. Specimens retrieved from living patients for reasons such as dislocation, infection, or malposition have demonstrated little or no bone ingrowth, independent of the type of component that was retrieved. This information, together with the fact that most of the retrieved specimens were *in situ* for less than 2 years, would lead to the conclusion that the biologic and/or mechanical environment for these implants was detrimental to the ingrowth of bone into porous coating. Conversely, well-functioning acetabular components retrieved at the time of autopsy have almost uniformly demonstrated bone ingrowth into the porous coating, again independent of the type of implant. In general, approximately one third of the available surface area in these implants has been found to be in contact with bone, and significantly more bone has been observed adjacent to fixation sites such as screws or pegs. Finally, analysis of a few long-term specimens (80 to 90 months *in situ*) has indicated that particulate wear debris may access the bone–implant interface via empty holes or holes filled with screws. Continued analysis of long-term specimens is necessary to further elucidate the consequences of such debris access to the biologic interface.

FUTURE DEVELOPMENTS

Although the first decade of experience with porous-coated acetabular components has proven these devices to be at least as effective as cemented acetabular components, several possible areas of improvement have already been identified. Once such area is the enhancement of bone ingrowth into porous-coated devices. As noted, analysis of well-functioning implants has demonstrated only about one third of the available surface area of porous coating to be in contact with bone. Osteoconductive factors such as hydroxylapatite and tricalcium phosphate, and osteoinductive factors, such as transforming growth factor beta and various bone morphogenic proteins, have shown a remarkable capacity to increase the amount of bone in contact with various metallic surfaces in both human and animal studies (20,71,98).

A second area of potential improvement is that of stress transmission from the acetabular implant to the acetabulum. Morscher has emphasized the importance of reproducing "normal" stress transmission across the acetabulum with porous-coated metal implants. Important factors in this respect are a uniform optimum fit of the prosthetic acetabulum and an elastic design that provides for uniform transfer of stress while minimizing areas of stress concentration or relief (68–71). Conceivably, improvements in metal-backed acetabular component materials and design could promote more anatomic or biologic transmission of stress across the acetabulum and, thus, protect the bone–implant interface from adverse long-term sequelae.

Finally, mechanisms to prevent or at least minimize the production and possible migration of particulate wear debris will undoubtedly receive a great deal of attention in the future. Already, most manufacturers have improved the congruency between modular polyethylene liners and metal-backed shells and have improved the polyethylene liner fixation mechanism, in an effort to minimize possible production of particulate debris from nonarticulating surface sites. Also, most contemporary designs have either minimized or eliminated screw holes in the metal-backed acetabular component to eliminate potential portals of access of particulate debris. In most clinical situations of primary total hip replacement, acetabular components with three holes or less can now be utilized. Future development may include elimination of modular polyethylene liners and direct attachment of porous-coated surfaces to relatively thick all-polyethylene implants.

SUMMARY

In conclusion, experience with porous-coated acetabular components inserted without cement now extends over a 10-year period. In general, experience with these components has been excellent. For the vast majority of patients, the performance of cementless sockets has been at least equivalent to that of cemented sockets. In patients less than 50 years old, the performance of cementless sockets has surpassed that of cemented sockets. The micro-interlock obtained by bone ingrowth into porous-coated acetabular components appears to provide fixation superior to that with cemented sockets, as manifested by extremely low revision rates for migration or loss of fixation in cementless acetabular components. The press-fit technique of insertion appears to be superior to the line-to-line fit insertion technique, especially with regard to minimizing peripheral radiolucencies that may correlate with subsequent acetabular loosening. When an adequate press-fit of the acetabular component has been obtained, screws appear to add very little in the form of fixation and may potentially serve as conduits for the migration of particulate wear debris.

The vast majority of problems related to the use of cementless acetabular components have been related to the modular or nonmodular polyethylene inserts and the subsequent development of periacetabular osteolysis. Some first-generation cementless porous-coated acetabular designs have been associated with failure of the mechanism by which the polyethylene is secured to the metal-backed shell, and with development of periacetabular osteolysis in as many as 10% to 20% of reported cases. Although modern designs have attempted to minimize the problems associated with the polyethylene locking mechanism and polyethylene wear in general, the plastic portion of the socket continues to be the weak link in the system.

REFERENCES

1. Alexander N, Hungerford D, Jones L, Mont M. The correlation of acetabular failure to polyethylene manufacturing techniques in total hip arthroplasty. *American Academy of Orthopaedic Surgeons—Scientific Program.* 1995;19:316–317.
2. Andrew TA, Berridge D, Thomas A, Duke RNF. Long-term review of ring total hip arthroplasty. *Clin Orthop* 1985;201:111–122.
3. Apel DM, Smith DG, Schwartz CM, Paprosky WG. Threaded cup acetabuloplasty. *Clin Orthop* 1989;241:183–189.
4. Barrack RL, Folgueras A, Munn B, Tvedten D, Sharkey P. Pelvic lysis at 5–8 years with a porous-coated hemispherical screw fixed acetabular component. *American Academy of Orthopaedic Surgeons—Scientific Program.* 1995;19:319.
5. Bartel DL, Bicknell VL, Wright TM. The effect of conformity, thickness, and material on stresses in ultra-high-molecular weight compo-

nents for total hip replacement. *J Bone Joint Surg* 1986;68A: 1041–1051.

6. Bertin KC, Freeman MA, Morscher E, Oeri A, Ring PA. Cementless acetabular replacement using a pegged polyethylene prosthesis. *Arch Orthop Trauma Surg* 1985;104:251–261.

7. Bobyn JD, Engh CA, Glassman AH. Radiography and histology of a threaded acetabular implant. *J Bone Joint Surg* 1988;70B:302–304.

8. Bono JV, Sanford L, Toussaint JT. Severe polyethylene wear in total hip arthroplasty. *J Arthroplasty* 1994;9:119–125.

9. Bruijn JD, Seelen JL, Feenstra RM, Hansen BE, Bernoski FP. Failure of the mecring screw-ring acetabular component in total hip arthroplasty. *J Bone Joint Surg* 1995;77A:760–766.

10. Callaghan JJ, Dysart SH, Savory CG. The uncemented porous-coated anatomic total hip prosthesis. *J Bone Joint Surg* 1988;70A:337–346.

11. Callaghan JJ, Salvati EA, Pellicci PM, Wilson PD, Ranawat CS. Results of revision for mechanical failure after cemented total hip replacement, 1979 to 1982: a two- to five-year follow-up. *J Bone Joint Surg* 1985;67A:1074–1085.

12. Cameron HU. Six-year results with a microporous-coated metal hip prosthesis. *Clin Orthop* 1986;208:81–83.

13. Capello WN, Colyer RA, Kernek CB, Hile LE, Carnahan JV. Experience with non-cemented total hip replacements—Screw-in rings. *Orthop Trans* 1989;13:495.

14. Charnley J. *Low friction arthroplasty of the hip: theory and practice.* Berlin: Springer-Verlag, 1979.

15. Charnley J, Halley DK. Rate of wear in total hip replacement. *Clin Orthop* 1975;112:170–179.

16. Collier JP, Bauer TW, Bloebaum RD, Bobyn JD, Cook SD, Galante JO, Harris WH, Head WC, Jasty MJ, Mayor MB, Sumner DR, Whiteside LA. Results of implant retrieval from postmortem specimens in patients with well-functioning, long-term total hip replacement. *Clin Orthop* 1992;274:97–112.

17. Collier JP, Mayor MB, Chae JC, Surprenant VA, Surprenant HP, Dauphinais LA. Macroscopic and microscopic evidence of prosthetic fixation with porous-coated materials. *Clin Orthop* 1988;235:173–180.

18. Cook SD, Barrack RL, Thomas KA, Haddad RJ. Quantitative analysis of tissue growth into human porous total hip components. *J Arthroplasty* 1988;3:249–262.

19. Cupic Z. Long-term follow-up of Charnley arthroplasty of the hip. *Clin Orthop* 1979;141:28–43.

20. D'Antonio JA, Capello WN, Crothers OD, Jaffe WL, Manley MT. Early clinical experience with hydroxyapatite-coated femoral implants. *J Bone Joint Surg* 1992;74A:995–1008.

21. Davitt JS, Dunn HK. Porous-coated anatomic total hip arthroplasty: long term radiographic and survivorship analysis. *J Arthroplasty* 1996 (in press).

22. Delee JG, Charnley J. Radiological demarcation of cemented sockets in total hip replacement. *Clin Orthop* 1976;121:20–32.

23. Dodge BM, Fitzrandolph R, Collins DN. Noncemented porous-coated anatomic total hip arthroplasty. *Clin Orthop* 1991;269:16–24.

24. Dorr L. Five-year experience with press-fit cementless acetabular components. *13th Annual Hip and Knee Course*, Salt Lake City, Utah, Jan. 1996.

25. Engh CA, Bobyn JD, Glassman AH. Porous-coated hip replacement. *J Bone Joint Surg* 1987;69B:45–55.

26. Engh CA, Griffin WL, Marx CL. Cementless acetabular components. *J Bone Joint Surg* 1990;72B:53–59.

27. Engh CA, Massin P. Cementless total hip arthroplasty using the anatomic medullary locking stem. *Clin Orthop* 1989;249:141–158.

28. Engh CA, Zettl-Schaffer KF, Kukita Y, Sweet D, Jasty M, Bragdon C. Histological and radiographic assessment of well functioning porous-coated acetabular components. *J Bone Joint Surg* 1993;75A:814–824.

29. Fehring TK, Valadie A, Braun ER, Mobley CE, Wang P. Polyethylene liners in modular porous acetabular components: a comparative analysis. *Harris Hip Course*, given by WH Harris, Boston, MA, Sept. 1993.

30. Freeman MAR, McLeod HC, Levai J. Cementless fixation of prosthetic components in total arthroplasty of the knee and hip. *Clin Orthop* 1983;176:88–94.

31. Friedman RJ, Black J, Galante JO, Jacobs JJ, Skinner HB. Current concepts in orthopaedic biomaterials and implant fixation. *J Bone Joint Surg* 1993;75A:1086–1109.

32. Galante JO, Rostoker W, Luick R, Ray RD. Sintered fiber composites as a basis for attachment of implants to bone. *J Bone Joint Surg* 1971; 53A:101.

33. Griffith MJ. Socket wear in Charnley low friction arthroplasty of the hip. *Clin Orthop* 1978;137:37–47.

34. Haddad RJ, Cook SD, Thomas KA. Biological fixation of porous-coated implants. *J Bone Joint Surg* 1987;69A:1459–1466.

35. Harris WH, Maloney WJ. Hybrid total hip arthroplasty. *Clin Orthop* 1989;249:21–29.

36. Hedley AK, Gruen TA, Ruoff DP. Revision of failed total hip arthroplasties with uncemented porous-coated anatomic components. *Clin Orthop* 1988;235:75–90.

37. Heekin RD, Callaghan JJ, Hopkinson WJ, Savory CG, Xenos JS. The porous-coated anatomic total hip prosthesis, inserted without cement. *J Bone Joint Surg* 1993;75A:77–91.

38. Hodgkinson JP, Shelley P, Wroblewski BM. The correlation between the roentgenographic appearance and operative findings at the bone-cement junction of the socket in Charnley low friction arthroplasties. *Clin Orthop* 1988;228:105–109.

39. Huiskes R. Finite element analysis of acetabular reconstruction. *Acta Orthop Scand* 1987;58:620–625.

40. Huk OL, Bansal M, Betts F, Rimnac CM, Lieberman JR, Huo MH, Salvati EA. Polyethylene and metal debris generated by non-articulating surfaces of modular acetabular components. *J Bone Joint Surg* 1994;76B:568–574.

41. Huo MH, Martin RP, Zatorski LE, Keggi KJ. Ceramic total hip replacement done without cement. Long-term follow-up study. *American Academy of Orthopaedic Surgeons—Scientific Program.* 1995; 19:400–401.

42. Incavo SJ, DiFazio FA, Howe JG. Cementless hemispheric acetabular components: 2–4-year results. *J Arthroplasty* 1993;8:573–580.

43. Ivory JP, Kershaw CJ, Choudhry R, Parmar H, Stoyle TF. Autophor cementless total hip arthroplasty for osteoarthrosis secondary to congenital hip dysplasia. *J Arthroplasty* 1994;9:427–433.

44. Jasty M, Harris WH. Observations on factors controlling bony ingrowth into weight-bearing, porous, canine total hip replacements. In: Fitzgerald, ed. *Non-cemented total hip arthroplasty.* New York: Raven Press, 1988.

45. Jones LC, Hungerford DS. Cement disease. *Clin Orthop* 1987;225: 192–206.

46. Kavanagh BF, Dewitz MA, Ilstrup DM, Stauffer RN, Coventry MB. Charnley total hip arthroplasty with cement. *J Bone Joint Surg* 1989; 71A:1496–1503.

47. Keating EM, Ritter MA, Faris PM. Structures at risk from medially placed acetabular screws. *J Bone Joint Surg* 1990;72A:509–511.

48. Kennedy WF. Modes of failure of the threaded acetabular total hip replacement components. *Orthop Trans* 1988;1:691.

49. Kienapfel H, Pitzer W, Griss P. Three- to five-year results with the cementless Harris-Galante acetabular component used in hybrid total hip arthroplasty. *Arch Orthop Trauma Surg* 1992;111:142–147.

50. Kim Y, Kim VEM. Uncemented porous-coated anatomic total hip replacement. *J Bone Joint Surg* 1993;75B:6–13.

51. Kim Y, Kim VEM. Cementless porous-coated anatomic medullary locking total hip prosthesis. *J Arthroplasty* 1994;9:243–252.

52. Kim YS, Callaghan JJ, Ahn PB, Brown TD. Fracture of the acetabulum during insertion of an oversized hemispherical component. *J Bone Joint Surg* 1995;77A:111–117.

53. Kody MH, Kabo JM, Markolf KL, Dorey FJ, Amstutz HC. Strength of initial mechanical fixation of screw ring acetabular components. *Clin Orthop* 1990;257:146–153.

54. Krugluger J, Eyb R. Bone reaction to uncemented threaded polyethylene acetabular components. *Int Orthop* 1993;17:259–265.

55. Kull LR, Jacobs JJ, Tompkins GS, Silverton CD, Galante JO. Primary cementless acetabular reconstruction: osteolysis and interface changes at seven to ten year follow-up. *Ortho Trans* 1995;19:401.

56. Kwong LM, O'Connor DO, Sedlacek RC, Krushell RJ, Maloney WJ, Harris WH. A quantitative in vitro assessment of fit and screw fixation on the stability of a cementless hemispherical acetabular component. *J Arthroplasty* 1994;9:163–170.

57. Lachiewicz PF, Anspach WE, DeMasi R. A prospective study of 100 consecutive Harris-Galante porous total hip arthroplasties. *J Arthroplasty* 1992;7:519–526.

58. Lord G, Bancel P. The madreporic cementless total hip arthroplasty: new experimental data and a seven-year clinical follow-up study. *Clin Orthop* 1983;176:67–76.

59. MacKenzie JR, Callaghan JJ, Pedersen DR, Brown TD. Areas of contact and extent of gaps with implantation of oversized acetabular

components in total hip arthroplasty. *Clin Orthop* 1994;298:127–136.

60. Mahoney OM, Dimon JH. Unsatisfactory results with a ceramic total hip prosthesis. *J Bone Joint Surg* 1990;72A:663–671.

61. Maloney WJ, Davey JR, Harris WH. Bead loosening from a porous-coated acetabular component. *Clin Orthop* 1992;281:112–114.

62. Maloney WJ, Peters P, Engh CA, Chandler H. Severe osteolysis of the pelvis in association with acetabular replacement without cement. *J Bone Joint Surg* 1993;75A:1627–1635.

63. Martell JM, Pierson RH, Jacobs JJ, Rosenberg AG, Maley M, Galante JO. Primary total hip reconstruction with a titanium fiber-coated prosthesis inserted without cement. *J Bone Joint Surg* 1993;75A:554–571.

64. Massin P, Schmidt L, Engh CA. Evaluation of cementless acetabular component migration. *J Arthroplasty* 1989;4:245–251.

65. McCoy TH, Salvati EA, Ranawat CS, Wilson PD. A fifteen-year follow-up study of one hundred Charnley low-friction arthroplasties. *Orthop Clin North Am* 1988;19:467–476.

66. Mittelmeier H. Report on the first decennium of clinical experience with a cementless ceramic total Hip replacement. *Acta Orthop Belgica* 1985;51:367–376.

67. Mont MA, Maar DC, Krackow KA, Jacobs MA, Jones LC, Hungerford DS. Total hip replacement without cement for non-inflammatory osteoarthrosis in patients who are less than forty-five years old. *J Bone Joint Surg* 1993;75A:740–751.

68. Morscher E, Bereiter H, Lampert C. Cementless press-fit cup. *Clin Orthop* 1989;249:12–20.

69. Morscher E, Masar Z. Development and first experience with an uncemented press-fit cup. *Clin Orthop* 1988;232:96–103.

70. Morscher EW. Cementless total hip arthroplasty. *Clin Orthop* 1983;181:76–91.

71. Morscher EW. Current status of acetabular fixation in primary total hip arthroplasty. *Clin Orthop* 1992;274:172–193.

72. Morscher EW, Dick W, Kernen V. Cementless fixation of polyethylene acetabular component in total hip arthroplasty. *Arch Orthop Trauma Surg* 1982;99:223–230.

73. Nunn D. The ring uncemented plastic-on-metal total hip arthroplasty. *J Bone Joint Surg* 1988;70B:40–44.

74. Onsten I, Carlsson AS, Ohlin A, Nilsson JA. Migration of acetabular components inserted with and without cement, in one-stage bilateral hip arthroplasty. *J Bone Joint Surg* 1994;76A:185–194.

75. Owen TD, Moran CG, Smith SR, Pinder IM. Results of uncemented porous-coated anatomic total hip replacement. *J Bone Joint Surg* 1994;76B:258–262.

76. Perona PG, Lawrence J, Paprosky WG, Patwardhan AG, Sartori M. Acetabular micromotion as a measure of initial implant stability in primary hip arthroplasty. *J Arthroplasty* 1992;4:537–547.

77. Peters CL, Rosenberg AG. Bone ingrowth and total knee replacement. In: *The Knee*. New York: Elsevier Science, 1995;1:189–196.

78. Peters CL, Urban RM, Sumner DR, Koutozos C, Galante JO. Interface phenomena in well functioning porous-coated acetabular components: an autopsy retreival study. *Orthop Trans* 1995;19:401.

79. Pidhorz LE, Urban RM, Jacobs JJ, Sumner DR, Galante JO. A quantitative study of bone and soft tissues in cementless porous-coated acetabular components retrieved at autopsy. *J Arthroplasty* 1993;8:213–227.

80. Piston RW, Engh CA, De Carvalho PI, Suthers K. Osteonecrosis of the femoral head treated with total hip arthroplasty without cement. *J Bone Joint Surg* 1994;76A:202–214.

81. Poss R. Clinical aspects of modularity. *Twenty-third open scientific meeting of The Hip Society*; The first combined open meeting of the Hip Society and AAHKS, Orlando, Florida, Feb. 1995.

82. Rimnac CM, Wilson PD, Fuchs MD, Wright TM. Acetabular cup wear in total hip arthroplasty. *Orthop Clin North Am* 1988;19:631–636.

83. Ring PA. Ring UPM total hip arthroplasty. *Clin Orthop* 1983;176:115–123.

84. Robinson EJ, Devane P, Bourne RB, Rorabeck CH, Hardie R. Comparison of acetabular polyethylene wear in cemented vs cementless arthroplasty using the 3-D technique. *American Academy of Orthopaedic Surgeons—Scientific Program*. 1995;19:317.

85. Salvati EA. Acetabular and femoral observations. *Twenty-third open scientific meeting of The Hip Society*; The first combined open meeting of The Hip Society and AAHKS, Orlando, Florida, Feb. 1995.

86. Santavirta S, Hoikka V, Eskola A, Konttinen YT, Paavilainen T, Tallroth K. Aggressive granulomatous lesions in cementless total hip arthroplasty. *J Bone Joint Surg* 1990;72B:980–984.

87. Santavirta S, Konttinen YT, Hoikka V, Eskola A. Immunopathological response to loose cementless acetabular components. *J Bone Joint Surg* 1991;73B:38–42.

88. Schimmel JW, Huiskes R. Primary fit of the Lord cementless total hip. *Acta Orthop Scand* 1988;59:638–642.

89. Schmalzried TP, Guttmann D, Grecula M, Amstutz HC. The relationship between the design, position, and articular wear of acetabular components inserted without cement and the development of pelvic osteolysis. *J Bone Joint Surg* 1994;76A:677–688.

90. Schmalzried TP, Harris WH. The Harris-Galante porous-coated acetabular component with screw fixation. *J Bone Joint Surg* 1992;74A:1130–1139.

91. Schmalzried TP, Jasty M, Harris WH. Periprosthetic bone loss in total hip arthroplasty. *J Bone Joint Surg* 1992;74A:849–863.

92. Schmalzried TP, Kwong LM, Jasty M, Sedlacek RC, Harie TC, O'Connor DO, Gragdon CR, Kabo JM, Malcolm AJ, Harris WH. The mechanism of loosening of cemented acetabular components in total hip Arthroplasty. *Clin Orthop* 1992;274:60–78.

93. Schmalzried TP, Wessinger SJ, Hill GE, Harris WH. The Harris-Galante porous acetabular component press-fit without screw fixation. *J Arthroplasty* 1994;8:235–242.

94. Schulte KR, Callaghan JJ, Kelley SS, Johnston RC. The outcome of Charnley total hip arthroplasty with cement after a minimum twenty-year followup. *J Bone Joint Surg* 1993;75A:961–975.

95. Schwartz JT, Engh CA, Forte MR, Kukita Y, Grandia SK. Evaluation of initial surface apposition in porous-coated acetabular components. *Clin Orthop* 1993;293:174–187.

96. Spector M. Historical review of porous-coated implants. *J Arthroplasty* 1987;2:163–177.

97. Sumner DR, Jasty M, Jacobs JJ, Urban RM, Bragdon CR, Harris WH, Galante JO. Histology of porous-coated acetabular components: 25 cementless cups retrieved after arthroplasty. *Acta Orthop Scand* 1993;64:619–626.

98. Sumner DR, Turner TM, Gombotz WR, Urban RM, Galante JO. Transforming growth factor. *J Bone Joint Surg* 1995;77A:1135–1147.

99. Sumner DR, Turner TM, Urban RM, Galante JO. Remodeling and ingrowth of bone at two years in a canine cementless total hip-arthroplasty model. *J Bone Joint Surg* 1992;74A:239–250.

100. Tooke SM, Nugent PJ, Chotivichit A, Goodman W, Kabo JM. Comparison of in vivo cementless acetabular fixation. *Clin Orthop* 1998;235:253–260.

101. Tradonsky S, Postak PD, Froimson AI, Greenwald AS. A comparison of the disassociation strength of modular acetabular components. *Clin Orthop* 1993;296:154–160.

102. Turner TM, Sumner DR, Urban RM, Rivero DP, Galante JO. A comparative study of porous coatings in a weight-bearing total hip-arthroplasty model. *J Bone Joint Surg* 1986;68A:1396–1409.

103. Wasielewski RC, Cooperstein LA, Kruger MP, Rubash HE. Acetabular anatomy and the transacetabular fixation of screws in total hip arthroplasty. *J Bone Joint Surg* 1990;72A:501–508.

104. White RE, Devlin TC, Junick DW, Motamedi A. The Harris-Galante porous-coated acetabular component with line-to-line fit and multiple screw fixation: radiographic analysis of 135 primary hip replacements at six to ten years. *American Academy of Orthopaedic Surgeons—Scientific Program*. 1995;19:400.

105. Willert H, Buchhorn GH. Particle disease due to wear of ultrahigh molecular weight polyethylene: findings from retrieval studies. In: Morrey, ed. *Biological material, and mechanical considerations of joint replacement*. New York: Raven Press, 1993.

106. Wilson-MacDonald J, Morscher E, Masar Z. Cementless uncoated polyethylene acetabular components in total hip replacement. *J Bone Joint Surg* 1990;72B:423.

107. Winter P, Griss P, Scheller G, Moser T. Ten- to 14-year results of a ceramic hip prosthesis. *Clin Orthop* 1992;282:73–80.

108. Wixson RL, Stulberg SD, Mehlhoff M. Total hip replacement with cemented, uncemented, and hybrid prostheses. *J Bone Joint Surg* 1991;73A:257–270.

109. Woolson ST, Maloney WJ. Cementless total hip arthroplasty using a porous-coated prosthesis for bone ingrowth fixation. *J Arthroplasty* 1992;7(supplement):381–388.

110. Wroblewski BM. Wear of high-density polyethylene on bone and cartilage. *J Bone Joint Surg* 1979;61B:498–500.

111. Wroblewski BM. Direction and rate of socket wear in Charnley low-friction arthroplasty. *J Bone Joint Surg* 1985;67B:757–761.

112. Wroblewski BM. 15–21-year results of the Charnley low-friction arthroplasty. *Clin Orthop* 1986;211:30–35.

The Adult Hip, edited by J. J. Callaghan,
A. G. Rosenberg, and H. E. Rubash.
Lippincott–Raven Publishers, Philadelphia © 1998.

CHAPTER 63

Cementless Femoral Component: Modular

John M. Cuckler

Modularity in total hip arthroplasty had its inception with the advent of aluminum oxide femoral heads, initially introduced in the early 1970s in Europe as part of a hip design that used a ceramic-ceramic articular couple (9). The ability to join components of two different materials required the adaptation of a design originally intended for use in the machining industry: the Morse-type taper was adapted to fit the ceramic femoral head to the metal femoral stem, as suggested by Judet in a personal communication to Griss (21). Hip modularity was introduced in the United States in the early 1980s by the Richard's Orthopaedic Company in the form of the Auto-Phorr Hip System, based on the design of Mittelmeier (28). Although the hip system itself was unsuccessful because of thigh pain related to failure of femoral fixation, the ability to adjust neck lengths, even after implantation of the femoral stem, was soon recognized as an advantage for decreasing stem inventory requirements, and for intraoperative adjustment of neck length.

Surgeons in the era of cementless fixation of femoral stems, also initiated in the early 1980s in the United States, quickly adapted the use of the Morse taper and interchangeable femoral heads. Titanium alloy (Ti-6Al-4V) as an implant material also became popular during this time. The option of using cobalt–chrome–molybdenum (CoCrMo), aluminum oxide ceramic, or (unfortunately) titanium alloy also used the advantages of the Morse taper. Thus, the era of modularity in total hip arthroplasty began.

J. M. Cuckler: Department of Orthopaedic Surgery, University Hospital, University of Alabama at Birmingham, Birmingham, Alabama 35294-3295.

On the acetabular side, metal backing of the polyethylene insert was explored in the late 1970s as a technique of potentially enhancing the stability of the bone–cement interface. The Howmedica Corporation soon thereafter introduced an exchangeable polyethylene acetabular liner. It was hoped that this exchangeable liner would allow "simple" revision surgery when polyethylene wear occurred, similar to the concept of placing a new tread on a tire. The effects of polyethylene wear debris on loosening of the implant interface were not at that time recognized. Although the promise of exchangeable liners was not realized, modularity in acetabular design was also embraced with the advent of porous ingrowth or cementless fixation of the acetabular component. Initial cementless acetabular designs [porous-coated anatomic (PCA), anatomic medullary locking (AML)] had polyethylene inserts that were fastened in the factory and not meant to be exchangeable. However, the concept of exchangeable acetabular liners, intended to be assembled by the surgeon at the time of surgery, was introduced in the early 1980s.

For the purposes of this discussion, a modular implant will be defined as any implant that is designed for assembly by the surgeon at the time of the surgery. Other designs have used mixed material components (SIVASH) but were not designed for intraoperative assembly and will not be included in this discussion.

The latest chapter in the evolution of modularity in total hip arthroplasty began with the introduction of the SROM prosthesis in the mid 1980s by the Joint Medical Corporation. This stem design used a Morse-type taper to join a proximal metaphyseal segment to the intramedullary stem portion of the prosthesis. It was soon recognized that this design allowed more precise cementless fixation, achieving fit against the cortical bone of the femur for stability, by independently sizing the proximal and distal portions of the component. The additional advantage of unlimited adjustment of version was also immediately apparent. The particular advantages of this type of stem design in revision surgery and in the "difficult" primary case were also apparent. Other designs soon followed using a variety of modular designs, the majority of which used the Morse-type taper for assembly of the implant components.

THE RATIONALE FOR MODULARITY

The single largest advantage of modularity in total hip arthroplasty lies in the ability to adapt the component to fit the needs of both the patient and the surgeon. This is particularly critical in cementless surgery, where cortical contact of the prosthesis is necessary to achieve stability. Therefore, the surgeon may need to adjust neck length or version of the acetabular component intraoperatively to properly restore the biomechanics of the hip, and to ensure stability of the prosthesis. Femoral stem modularity allows the surgeon to fit the prosthesis to the patient, intraoperatively adapting the femoral geometry and length to the individual.

Neck length adjustment in currently available hip stems can vary as much as 35 mm, using modular femoral heads. Noble et al. have shown that relative to a given distal femoral cortical diameter, neck length in his survey of 200 cadaveric femora vary by as much as 25 mm (31). Adjustment beyond this range is particularly useful in revision surgery. However, as discussed later, it is now realized that there are limits to the ability of the Morse-type taper to safely stabilize or accommodate the long-moment arm that can exist with this type of design, leading to a reassessment of the utility of extreme adjustability of the femoral head–neck length intraoperatively.

The adaptability of acetabular liners has enabled surgeons to use liners that provide a range of additional coverage beyond the rim of the metal shell. Acetabular modularity additionally allows the surgeon to use adjunctive fixation, such as cancellous screws for fixation of the cementless socket, prior to positioning the acetabular liner. During revision surgery, it is not infrequent to encounter a worn acetabular liner, which can be easily replaced. If dislocation of a hip occurs, adjustment of the position of the extended wall portion of the liner, or replacement of a "neutral" liner with an extended wall liner, may achieve stability for the patient without further complex and risky revision. However, acetabular modularity has come at the price of liner instability, as described later. This probably results in the generation of more polyethylene wear debris, and it has even been

reported to result in disassociation of the acetabular liner from the metal shell during, for instance, closed reduction of dislocated hips (2,32,33).

Modularity of the femoral stem enables the surgeon to intraoperatively adapt the prosthesis to optimally contact cortical bone of the femur, thereby optimizing stability. In addition, stem length and stem configuration (straight versus bowed) can also be adjusted. Recently, modular proximal femoral replacement devices have been introduced to enable intraoperative adaptation to proximal bone loss during revision situations.

Noble et al., in their study of cadaveric femora, documented the wide variety of femoral anatomies that can be encountered in the human population (31). For instance, for a given medial-lateral dimension at the lesser trochanter, diaphyseal intramedullary dimensions may vary by up to 1 cm. Even greater variations are seen in the anterior-posterior dimension of the proximal femur, with variations up to 15 mm for a given distal diaphyseal diameter. Revision total hip arthroplasty, accompanied by often unpredictable degrees of femoral bone loss, further challenge the cementless reconstruction, making intraoperative adaptability of the femoral stem appealing. Particularly during revision surgery, the ability to use longer stems as required by intraoperative misadventures such as fractures, or the ability to use curved stems, is appealing. Most recently, modular revision stems have been introduced (Mallory-Head, Biomet, Incorporated; RMHS, Smith & Nephew, Inc., Memphis, TN) that allow the surgeon to intraoperatively select the extent of distal porous coating necessary to achieve distal fixation and, therefore, stability of the femoral stem (Fig. 1).

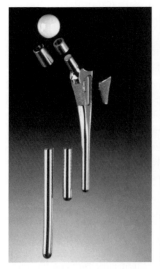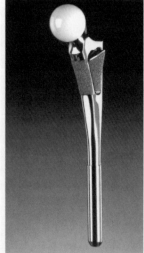

FIG. 1. An example of the Richards Modular Hip System (Smith and Nephew Richards, Inc., Memphis, Tennessee).

THE SCIENCE OF MODULARITY

The Morse Taper

The Morse taper was originally developed to allow components undergoing machining either to be fixed to a rotating system such as a lathe, or to allow the attachment of cutting tools to milling machines. The Morse taper is a truncated cone that attaches through a friction or interference fit to a similarly shaped socket. The wedge shape of the cone or taper results in a mechanical interlock, leading to stability between the components. Griss et al. are credited with the adoption of the Morse taper for attachment of an aluminum oxide ceramic head to a femoral stem, based on the suggestion of Judet (20). Boutin also began development of a ceramic–metal Morse taper junction at about the same time as the German group (5). Zweymuller et al. also adapted the Morse taper for their femoral stem to allow use of an aluminum oxide femoral head (37). Because of the brittle nature of the ceramic material, a taper angle of 5°38'22" was chosen to minimize tensile strains in the femoral head (21).

In the orthopedic industry, taper angles between 3° and 6° have been used. Unfortunately, there is a wide range of specifications among different manufacturers for Morse tapers, rendering the mixing of femoral head and stem components from different manufacturers impossible. However, there is a current trend toward the adaptation of a taper dimension and specifications promulgated by the International Standards Organization (ISO), which may eventually decrease the wide variety of taper designs and specifications that currently exist.

Because frictional forces caused by contact of the surfaces of the truncated cones are essential for stability of the implant, the effects of imprecision in machining of these surfaces has been thoroughly studied. Collier et al., in 1991, reported the observation of corrosion between mixed-metal Morse taper junctions in femoral stems retrieved at revision (11). However, Mathiesen and co-authors reported the observation of apparent corrosion at the junction of CoCr heads on CoCr stems simultaneously (27). Initially thought to be caused by galvanic corrosion, subsequent research has determined that fretting or mechanically assisted corrosion is the more probable explanation for these observations (15).

Fretting is the wear that occurs between two surfaces and is caused by micromotion. In the orthopedic environment, this is a cyclic phenomenon occurring in a biologic (i.e., electrolytic) milieu. There is evidence that the presence of biologic fluids may, in fact, reduce the propensity for fretting between two metal surfaces, much as motor oil reduces the wear in automobile engines. However, observation of fretting wear has raised concern over the potential for the wear debris generated through this process to elicit third-body wear phenomena in the articular couple of the arthroplasty, and also to induce inflammatory response to the wear debris, or even destabilization of the modular interface (4,12,26).

Corrosion is the loss of constituent ions of the metal alloy, caused by chemical interactions on the surface of a metal. This can occur in the absence of any mechanical effects on the surface of the metal, as is observed with aluminum alloy in a salt environment. Fretting corrosion is a special type of corrosion that is initiated by mechanical abrasion of the passive oxide surface of a metal, the result of micromotion between adjacent components, which can lead both to generation of particulate wear debris and to liberation of metal ions into the adjacent environment. Subsequent research has led to the consensus that fretting corrosion is the predominant mechanism resulting in the visually observable damage to the Morse taper of retrieved hip stems, and in the presence of corrosion products in the tissues surrounding failed total hip arthroplasties (6,13,15).

In the absence of micromotion, neither generation of wear debris nor corrosion products would be expected. The factors that determine the presence of micromotion have now received close attention from a variety of researchers. Probably the most critical aspect of Morse taper stability is the base diameter of the taper itself (36). Large tapers, in mechanical testing, demonstrate less bending than small tapers. The bending motion of small tapers results in more fretting wear. This explains the propensity of small tapers to demonstrate worse fretting scar at retrieval than large tapers.

Femoral neck length adjustment is achieved with modular femoral heads by varying the depth of penetration of the cone within the femoral head component. The position of the area of contact of the Morse taper components markedly affects the moment arm acting at the interface of the Morse taper. This, in turn, affects the propensity for fretting wear and fretting corrosion of the interfaces.

In addition to the length of the femoral head component, taper angle mismatch between head and neck affects the area of contact and even the position of contact between the components. Therefore, both the taper angle mismatch (the difference between the taper angles of the head and neck components) and the length of the femoral head affect the propensity for fretting wear (23). Other factors such as taper straightness, taper roundness, and quality control of the machining process are critical to the successful performance of the Morse taper modular interface. For instance, Alexander and Noble have shown that the ideal taper mismatch should be between 0 and 5 minutes larger than the taper angle of the female component (1). The precision of machining and the quality control over the machining process are critical to the stability of the taper interface. Heimke and Griss, in 1981, reported tolerances of less than 10^{-6} mm were necessary for taper stability and successful function, and they further stated, "The safety of the self-locking cone depends to a high degree on the friction between the two components. . . . The highest friction occurs between dry surfaces; any lubrication decreases the strength. . . . Since the ball has to be fixed to the stem during the operation, every possible care must be taken to clean both cones immediately before putting them together and securely fixing them, moderately pounding with a rubber, plastic, or wooden hammer" (21). Chao and his associates, based on finite element analysis, showed that the impaction force of a Morse taper interface must be sufficient to ensure stability. They also concluded that the surfaces of the Morse taper must be cleaned and dried before engagement (7).

Perhaps the most reassuring aspect of the extent of the fretting phenomenon in modular Morse taper interfaces lies in the discrepancy between observations of retrieved specimens versus those tested under laboratory simulation conditions. Dujovne and his colleagues reported, after testing SROM stems both after retrieval and in the laboratory, that "the extent of fretting observed with the *in vivo* specimens was much less than *in vitro*" (14). Similarly, despite the fact that approximately 80% of the 6 million femoral stems that have been implanted had modular head/neck junctions, fewer than 100 case reports exist in the world literature describing fretting of the Morse taper interface. To place the threat of fretting corrosion into perspective, the quantity of CoCr alloy released through wear against polyethylene has been calculated to be less than the amount of wear products from Morse taper fittings that were intentionally designed to be unstable and tested under laboratory conditions simulating 10 million cycles (23). The implication of this is that although admittedly unstable Morse tapers may liberate debris, these debris are less than the debris liberated from the normal wear of the femoral head. Well-designed Morse tapers, which liberate substantially less debris than the above experiment, can be expected to produce even less debris.

Clinical Implications

The clinical benefits of femoral head modularity are significant. The ability to intraoperatively adjust neck length is a substantial aid in adjustment of soft-tissue tension and limb length intraoperatively. Ceramic bearing surfaces are available only through the use of the Morse taper interface. During revision of the acetabular component, removal of a modular head will enhance exposure of the acetabulum. Additionally, this feature enables the surgeon to exchange heads at the time of revision in order to place a new bearing surface in contact with the revised acetabulum.

The clinical benefits of femoral head modularity appear to far outweigh the risks. Although fretting, fretting corrosion, and the potential for disassembly exists, the reports of such occurrences are few. In a survey of

experiences of American surgeons, Heck et al. found an incidence of modular femoral neck disassociation of 0.0263% (17).

The surgeon can minimize the risk of the use of the modular taper interface by always ensuring a clean, dry taper prior to the impaction of the femoral head. Impaction forces must be sufficient, within the limits provided by patient physiology and safety, to ensure complete seating of the interface. The use of larger, rather than smaller, tapers will minimize adverse contact stresses, thereby reducing the risk of fretting. Further, the use of "skirted" femoral heads to extend neck lengths should be avoided when possible to minimize contact stresses at the taper interface, and to avoid reduction in the range of motion of the prostheses (24).

Fatigue Strength

The existence of modular interfaces intuitively raises concern over the ability of the interface to withstand fatigue loading and suffer consequent fracture or breakage. Greenwald et al. have performed a comprehensive, independent assessment of fatigue performance of three modular femoral stems currently available. In this experiment, the RMHS, Impact, and SROM were tested under equivalent physiologic loads (assuming a 74-kg body weight), testing with a maximum joint force of 4 times body weight (296 kg). All stems were of equivalent size, appropriate to the hypothetical patient. Under these test conditions, both the SROM and Impact stem demonstrated failure at 2.1 times the implant service load. The RMHS demonstrated failure at 2.3 times the expected implant load. It should be noted that this test assumed no stress sharing between implant and adjacent bone. Therefore, these results represent an exceedingly severe situation not likely to be encountered *in vivo* (18). In a subsequent report of further testing in 1995, Greenwald and his colleagues found the endurance limit for the Infinity stem to be only 1.3 times the expected implant service load (19). Interestingly, fatigue failure tended to occur through the Morse-type taper when this was the modular connection interface for the stem (this includes the Impact, Infinity, and SROM).

Acetabular Modularity

The intuitive appeal of the option of exchanging acetabular liners at the time of revision surgery led to the development of modular acetabular liners in the late 1970s for metal-backed, cemented acetabular implants (16). Cementless fixation of the acetabulum emerged soon thereafter as an attractive alternative for acetabular fixation.

Initial designs of modular acetabular inserts utilized simple, bendable metal tabs for fixation of the liner at the periphery (Harris-Galante-I, Zimmer), or simple interference-fit locking mechanisms. The ability of these locking mechanisms to resist push-out or shear forces, however, was limited, as evidenced by the reports occurring soon thereafter of acetabular liner disassociation (10,35). However, disassociation of factory-assembled "one-piece" metal-backed acetabular components has also been reported (3).

Metal backing of polyethylene leads to the potential for differential motion between the polymer and the metal, which can result in the production of polyethylene wear debris. This has been confirmed in retrieval analysis of modular acetabular inserts, which have demonstrated both wear and cold flow or "creep" deformation (22,34).

Improvements in the design of the fixation of the polyethylene liner in the metal shell have focused on reduction of micromotion at the shell–liner interface. Testing of micromotion of acetabular liners has confirmed the potential contribution of this interface to accelerated wear debris production (8,25,29).

The complete elimination of motion between a low-modulus material [ultra-high-molecular-weight polyethylene (UHMWPE)] and a high-modulus material (e.g., CoCr or Ti-6Al-4V) is probably impossible, and this may represent a significant limitation of the cementless acetabular modular design. In a prospective study comparing cemented versus cementless acetabular fixation, Nayak et al. reported no statistically significant difference in the incidence of osteolysis (5% cemented, 9% cementless), but they observed different patterns of osteolysis (30). Cemented acetabular components tended to develop osteolysis in zone I, whereas cementless components demonstrated osteolysis more central in zone II.

CONCLUSIONS

Modularity in total hip arthroplasty allows intraoperative adaptability, enabling adjustment of neck length, head diameter or material, and even stem configuration. Acetabular modularity allows cementless fixation of the acetabular prosthesis, exchange of polyethylene liners, and adjunctive screw fixation of the acetabular shell.

Motion between the constituents of the implants can produce fretting wear debris and corrosion. The debris produced from unstable modular interfaces may accelerate wear of the articular couple, leading to early loosening or failure of the implant. Severe fretting or corrosion may even lead to disassembly or fracture of the implant. However, carefully designed and assembled modular prostheses appear to function satisfactorily at intermediate to long-term follow-up.

The advantages and risks of modularity must be assessed by the surgeon and balanced against the needs of the individual patient. In general, minimizing the use of modularity will maximize the benefit (i.e., avoiding the use of modular designs when clinically possible is advised). However, well-designed modular interfaces appear safe and effective, and they should be utilized when the benefit of the patient or clinical situation requires.

REFERENCES

1. Alexander JW, Noble PC. The effect of taper mismatch on the torsional properties of conical joints. *39th annual meeting, Orthopaedic Research Society*, San Francisco, CA, February 15–18, 1993;436.
2. Barrack LR, Burke DW, Cook SD, Skinner HB, Harris WH. Complications related to modularity of total hip components. *J Bone Joint Surg* 1993;75B:688–692.
3. Beaver RJ, Schemitsch EH, Gross AE. Disassembly of a one piece metal backed acetabular component. A case report. *J Bone Joint Surg* 1991;73B:908–910.
4. Bobyn JD, Tanzer M, Krygier JJ, Dujovne AR, Brooks CE. Concerns with modularity in total hip arthroplasty. *Clin Orthop* 1994;298:27–36.
5. Boutin P. Arthroplastie totale de la hanche par prosthese en alumine fritte. *Rev Chir Orthop* 1979;58:229.
6. Brown SA, Flemming CAC, Kawalec JS, Placko HE, Vassaux C, Merritt K, Payer JH, Kraay MJ. Fretting corrosion accelerates crevice corrosion of modular hip tapers. *J Appl Biomater* 1995;6:19–26.
7. Chao EYS, Suh J, Grabowski J. Mechanical strength and critical stress distribution of Morse taper lock and modular segmental prosthesis design. *38th annual meeting, Orthopaedic Research Society*, Washington, DC, February 17–20, 1992;310.
8. Chen PC, Mead EH, Pinto JG, Colwell CW Jr. Polyethylene wear debris in modular acetabular prostheses. *Clin Orthop* 1995;317:456.
9. Clarke IC. Role of ceramic implants. Design in clinical success with total hip prosthetic ceramic to ceramic bearings. *Clin Orthop* 1992;282:19–30.
10. Collier JP, Mayor MB, Jenson RV, Suprenant VA, Suprenant HP, McNamar JL, Belec L. Mechanisms of failure of modular prostheses. *Clin Orthop* 1992;285:129–139.
11. Collier JP, Surprenant VA, Jenson RE, Mayor MB. Corrosion at the interface of cobalt alloy heads on titanium alloy stems. *Clin Orthop* 1991;271:305–312.
12. Collier JP, Suprenant VA, Jenson RE, Mayor MB, Suprenant HP. Corrosion between the components of modular femoral hip prostheses. *J Bone Joint Surg* 1992;74B:511–517.
13. Cook SD, Barrack RL, Clemow AJT. Corrosion and wear at the modular interface of uncemented femoral stems. *J Bone Joint Surg* 1994;76B:68–72.
14. Dujovue AR, Bobyn JD, Krygier JJ, Wilson DR, Brooks CE. Fretting at the head neck taper of modular hip prostheses. *Proceedings of the 4th world biomaterials congress*, Berlin, Germany, April 24–28, 1992;264.
15. Gilbert JL, Buckley CA, Jacobs JJ. In vivo corrosion of modular hip prosthesis components in mixed and similar metal combinations. The effect of crevice, stress, motion, and alloy coupling. *J Biomed Mater Res* 1993;27(12):1533–1544.
16. Harris WH. A new total hip implant. *Clin Orthop* 1971;81:105–113.
17. Heck DA, Partridge CM, Ruben JD, Lanzer WL, Lewis CG, Keeting EM. Prosthetic component failures in hip arthroplasty surgery. *J Arthroplasty* 1995;10:575–580.
18. Heim CS, Postak PD, Greenwald AS. Femoral stem fatigue characteristics of modular hip designs. *Scientific exhibit, American Academy of Orthopaedic Surgeons*, San Francisco, CA, 1994.
19. Heim CS, Postak PD, Greenwald AS. Femoral stem fatigue characteristics of modular hip designs—series II. *Scientific exhibit, American Academy of Orthopaedic Surgeons*, Atlanta, GA, 1995.
20. Heimke G, Griss P, Jentshura G, Krempier B, Gugel E, Petzenhauser I, Henniche HW. Keramische und Keramikbeschichtete Knochenersatz werkstaffe. *BFMT-Forschungstiericht* 1977;T77-70:1–190.
21. Heimke G, Griss P. Five years experience with ceramic-metal composite hip endoprostheses. II. Mechanical evaluations and improvements. *Arch Orthop Traum Surg* 1981;98(3):165–171.
22. Huk OL, Bansal M, Betts F, Rimnac CM, Lieberman JR, Huo MH, Salvati EA. Polyethylene and metal debris generated by non-articulating surfaces of modular acetabular components. *J Bone Joint Surg* 1994;76B:568–574.

23. Jani SC, Sauer WA, McLean TW, Lambert RD, Covax P. Fretting corrosion mechanisms at modular implant interfaces. In: Parr JE, Mayor MB, Marlowe DE, eds. *Symposium on modularity of orthopaedic implants.* ASTM STP 1301. Philadelphia: American Society for Testing and Materials, 1996.

24. Krushell RJ, Burke DW, Harris WH. Range of motion in contemporary total hip arthoplasty. The impact of modular head-neck components. *J Arthroplasty* 1991;6:97–101.

25. Manley MT, Serekian P. Wear debris. An environmental issue in total joint replacement. *Clin Orthop* 1994;298:137–146.

26. McKellop HA, Sarmiento A, Brien W, Park SH. Interface corrosion of a modular head: total hip prosthesis. *J Arthroplasty* 1992;7:291–294.

27. Mathiesen EB, Lindgren JU, Blomgren GG, Reinholt FP. Corrosion of modular hip prostheses. *J Bone Joint Surg* 1991;73(B):569–575.

28. Mittelmeier H. Selbsthaftende Keramik-Metall-Verbund-Endoprosthese (Tragrippen Prosthese). *Med Orthop Tech* 1975;95:152–159.

29. Nashed RS, Becker DA, Gustilo RB. Are cementless acetabular components the cause of excess wear and osteolysis in total hip arthroplasty? *Clin Orthop* 1995;317:19–28.

30. Nayak N, Mulliken B, Rorabeck CH, Bourne RB, Robinson EJ. Osteolysisin cemented versus cementless acetabular components. *J Arthroplasty* 1996;11(2):1350.

31. Noble PC, Alexander JW, Lindahl W, Yew DT, Granbeny WM, Tullos HS. The anatomic basis of femoral component design. *Clin Orthop* 1988;235:148–165.

32. O'Brien RF, Chess D. Late disassembly of a modular acetabular component. A case report. *J Arthroplasty* 1992;7(suppl):453–455.

33. Retpen JB, Solgaard S. Late disassembly of modular acetabular components. A report of two cases. *Acta Orthop Scand* 1993;64:193–195.

34. Salvati EA, Lieberrnan JR, Huk OL, Evans BG. Complications of femoral and acetabular modularity. *Clin Orthop* 1995;319:85–93.

35. Tradonsky S, Postak PD, Froimson AI, Greenwald AS. A comparison of the disassociation strength of modular acetabular components. *Clin Orthop* 1993;296:154–160.

36. Young DL, Bobyn JD, Krygier JJ, Dujovne AR. Factors affecting fretting damage at the Morse taper junction of modular hip implants. Presented at the *21st meeting of the Society for Biomaterials*, San Francisco, CA, 1995;49.

37. Zweymuller K, Zhuber K, Locke H. Eine Metall-Keramik-Verbundprosthese fur den Huftgalen kersatz. *Wien Klin Wochenschr* 1977;89:548–51.

The Adult Hip, edited by J. J. Callaghan,
A. G. Rosenberg, and H. E. Rubash.
Lippincott–Raven Publishers, Philadelphia © 1998.

CHAPTER 64

Cementless Femoral Component: Extensively Coated

William D. Bugbee and Charles A. Engh

Bone ingrowth, or osseointegration, of cementless porous-coated femoral stems has proven to be a reliable and successful form of fixation. However, some features of cementless stems such as the stem geometry, the surface properties of the porous surface, and the extent of the porous surface applied to the stem continue to be the subject of debate. Clinical experience with proximally and extensively microporous-coated stems has reached nearly two decades and has led to continued enthusiasm for porous-coated stems in general and a preference for stems with more, rather than less, porous coating. The goal of this chapter is to summarize this experience. The chapter is divided into six sections: (a) historical development, (b) stem design features, (c) laboratory investigations of autopsy specimens, (d) surgical principles, (e) surgical technique, and (f) the authors' long-term clinical experience.

HISTORICAL CONTEXT

The first femoral implant to demonstrate the possibility of biologic fixation was developed by Austin-Moore in the early 1950s (17). This stem, with large fenestrations,

achieved macrointerlock with the skeleton through the placement of bone graft in these fenestrations. At the same time that John Charnley was developing the use of acrylic cement for fixation, others, such as Judet et al. (12) and Lord et al. (14), were experimenting with stems with macroporous or rough-textured surfaces. The 1970s was a time of intensive basic experimental research on surface coating and tissue ingrowth. These investigations delineated two basic criteria for bone ingrowth into porous surfaces. First, bone ingrowth could be achieved into microporous surfaces when pore size was between 50 and 500 μm (1). Second, for this bone ingrowth to be achieved, a stable implant with minimal interface motion was necessary. It was evident that the type of porous surface was not nearly as important as the interface environment that met these two criteria. On the industrial side, technology for the production of microporous surface implants was developed.

In 1977, a Food and Drug Administration (FDA)-approved clinical trial was initiated, in which primary arthroplasties were performed with a fully porous-coated femoral component with a 32-mm head size. In 1982, the results of 120 cases were presented to the FDA, and in 1983, after the FDA approved this implant, modifications were made by the manufacturer: the implant was made in a greater variety of sizes, the porous coating was removed from the distal one-eighth of the stem, and a porous-coated acetabular component was designed. In 1984, the

W. D. Bugbee: Department of Orthopaedics, University of California at San Diego, San Diego, California 92103.
C. A. Engh: Anderson Orthopaedic Clinic, Arlington, Virginia 22206.

femoral prosthesis was again modified: a Morse taper was applied to the femoral neck to make the femoral head of the prosthesis modular, and the same prosthesis was also manufactured with porous coating applied proximally to less than one-half the length of the stem. For the subsequent 3 years, prostheses with both porous coating levels were used. However, since 1988, our experience has been only with the more extensively porous-coated implant. Throughout this design evolution, patient data have been collected preoperatively, and annually postoperatively, in a computerized database. An autopsy retrieval program has allowed the study of the type of bone ingrowth into porous-coated implants, of their mechanical stability, and of the overall bone adaptation that occurs to the implant.

OPTIMUM DESIGN CHARACTERISTICS OF AN EXTENSIVELY POROUS-COATED STEM

An extensively porous-coated prosthesis can be defined as one with porous coating on more than 80% of its surface area, with a stem length that allows this porous surface to extend to the narrowest portion of the medullary canal, the femoral isthmus. The Anatomic Medullary Locking (AML) stem (Deu Puy, Warsaw, Indiana) is the only implant with this amount of porous surface that has been widely used for primary arthroplasties in the United States. The stem is made of cast cobalt–chrome. The porous surface is a powder-made beaded surface applied through a modified loose sintering process. The beads are of cobalt–chrome alloy, and their size ranges from 187 to 250 μm. The average pore size of the applied coating is 250 μm, with a range of 50 to 400 μm. On the implant itself, the porosity distribution ranges from 87% at the surface of the implant to 23% adjacent to the solid base substrate. The average porosity is 40%. The shear strength at the interface of the porous coating and the solid substrate depends on volume porosity. At 40% porosity, the substrate–coating interfacial shear strength is 21 MPa. In animal studies, when bone ingrowth occurs, the interfacial strength of the bone–implant has been shown to be up to 17 MPa for cortical bone and 5 to 6 MPa for dense cancellous bone (3). This 40% porosity has been considered the optimal balance between maximizing the strength of the porous coating–substrate interface and that of the porous coating–bone interface. Finite element studies have demonstrated that the sintering process could potentially lessen the fatigue strength of some porous-coated stems and produce stem breakage. This has been demonstrated to be of particular concern with fully porous-coated stems with a core stem diameter of less than 12 mm (13).

A critical design feature of the AML is its straight, cylindrical, nontapered distal stem geometry. Because the stem is not tapered, the implant does not wedge in place. Fixation depends instead on a so-called scratch fit between the rough external surface of the implant and a similarly shaped bone canal. The bone canal is reamed using intramedullary drills to a diameter slightly smaller in size than that of the stem. Using a straight cylindrical design makes it possible to easily prepare the inside of the femur to match the shape of the stem over a large surface area. The advantage of the extensive coating on a stem of this design is that it makes it possible to achieve biologic fixation through osseointegration over the entire length of the stem. Coating the distal part of the stem is particularly important, because it is the distal part of the stem that most consistently contacts the cortical bone. This cortical bone of the femoral diaphysis also has superior ingrowth characteristics and is of greater strength than cancellous bone. Thus, fully porous-coated stems can be equated to cemented ones in which the surgeon seeks to obtain a complete cement mantle for optimal fixation of the entire stem. Proximally coated implants function well when bone ingrowth occurs, but it is more difficult to obtain bone ingrowth with less porous coating, particularly in the revision situation and in cases with unusual anatomy. It also has been noted that in the few cases where extensively coated stems are used and osseointegration does not occur, fibrous tissue growth into the porous surface usually occurs. This alone, in the majority of cases, is adequate to provide patient satisfaction and radiographic stability. The extensive coating presumably creates a large enough area of interface bonding so that fibrous ingrowth is adequate to prevent stem subsidence. The same long-term implant stability has not been observed when bone ingrowth failure occurs with proximally porous-coated stems (19).

LABORATORY INVESTIGATION OF EXTENSIVELY COATED STEMS

Implant retrieval enables understanding of the long-term skeletal response to extensively porous-coated stems. Examining well-functioning stems and the surrounding bone makes it possible to gain valuable insight into the *in vivo* characteristics of the implant–bone system. In particular, important information has been obtained on mechanical stability, patterns of bone ingrowth, and patterns of bone remodeling.

The shear strength of the bone–porous coating interface has been evaluated in animal studies (1), which have shown that implant bonding occurs as early as 3 weeks after implantation and may reach maximum strength by 8 weeks. The maximum shear strength resulting from bone ingrowth in humans is probably slower.

Based on a determination of the percentage of the porous surface of stem containing bone ingrowth, the maximum interfacial shear strength can be calculated to reach 17 MPa in cortical bone and 5 to 6 MPa in dense cancellous bone (6). These bonds prevent micromotion between the implant and bone, but only at the areas where the two are bonded. Engh et al. (10), performing micromotion studies on autopsy-retrieved femora, have shown

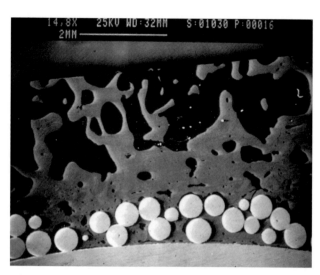

FIG. 1. Back-scatter scanning electron micrograph of bone growth into the porous surface of an Anatomic Medullary Locking (AML) implant (×15).

that when bone ingrowth occurs, the movement between the porous-coated portion of the implant and the surrounding bone is usually less than 20 μm and never exceeds 40 μm. However, with proximally porous-coated implants, the motion between the uncoated and unbonded distal smooth stem is greater. In addition, the amount of this distal (tip) micromotion is related to the extent of the implant surface that is not porous coated. Stems that were 80% coated demonstrated a maximum of 120 μm of motion at the tip, compared with 210 μm of tip micromotion for the 40% proximally coated stems. These data correlate with clinical experience. The incidence and severity of early postoperative thigh pain are greater with proximally porous-coated AML stems than with more extensively coated ones, suggesting that the increased

distal-stem tip motion occurring with the implants with less coating is a source of thigh pain (11).

After micromotion studies are complete, these specimens were embedded in plastic and sectioned for microscopic analysis. Back-scattered electron microscopy is used to study the bone ingrowth producing implant stability (6). In eight specimens studied, the percentage of the porous surface area containing bone ingrowth averaged 35%. In areas where there was bone ingrowth, 67% to 73% of the void space between the pores contained bone. Figure 1 illustrates the typical back-scattered electron microscopic appearance of bone ingrowth.

The amount of bone growth within the pores was not influenced by the anatomic location of the ingrowth. However, in concurrence with previous studies that have shown the likelihood of bone ingrowth increasing with proximity of the porous coating to cortical bone, the largest areas of bone ingrowth occurred in the areas of the femoral diaphysis with the stem fit tightest against the cortices. The greatest amount of bone ingrowth was observed to be consistently near the termination of the porous coating. At this level, compact bone directly adjacent to the porous coating showed haversian systems identical to those in the surrounding cortex.

A different pattern of bone ingrowth was observed in the more proximal areas of these specimens. The ingrowth was less predictable, but it was most frequently observed on the rounded medial and lateral corners of the implant. This bone was cancellous in nature and was usually connected to the outer cortex by hypertrophied trabeculae. This type of connecting bone was usually not visible on clinical radiographs. These patterns of cortical and cancellous bone ingrowth into porous-surfaced AML stems are shown in Figure 2. Micromotion studies performed on these same autopsy-retrieved femora prior to embedding and sectioning showed that although this con-

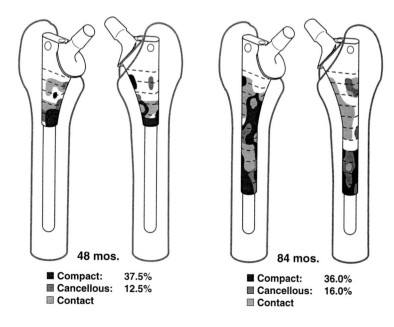

48 mos.

■ Compact: 37.5%
■ Cancellous: 12.5%
□ Contact

84 mos.

■ Compact: 36.0%
■ Cancellous: 16.0%
□ Contact

FIG. 2. Patterns of bone ingrowth into proximally and extensively porous-coated AML stems. Maps were made by scanning transverse femoral cross-sections from autopsy cases. The *dark-shaded areas* are regions of compact bone ingrowth where the porous-surfaced implant directly bonded to the femoral cortex. The *lightest-shaded areas* represent sites where the porous surface of the implant directly contacts the endosteal cortex, but bone was not visualized within the porous surface. The *intermediate shading* represents areas where there is bone ingrowth that is connected to the outer cortex by trabecular connections.

necting bone was quantitatively less proximal than distal, it was adequate to stabilize the proximal part of the implant (10).

Unfortunately, the plastic-embedded specimens used for electron microscopic analyses were valuable only for studying the areas of bone ingrowth. It was necessary to use other autopsy specimens embedded in paraffin to microscopically examine the nonbony tissue surrounding some areas of the implant. In the non-ossified marrow spaces where micromotion studies had shown minimal motion between the porous implant and the bone, fibrous tissue was frequently observed to grow within the porous surface. In other areas, there was no fibrous tissue reaction and the marrow appeared normal. In areas where mechanical testing had indicated that the micromotion between the implant exceeded 50 μm, the marrow space was filled with fibrous tissue surrounding the implant. This fibrous tissue was organized differently: it ran parallel to the implant surface. In some cases, this type of fibrous tissue was partially ossified.

In addition, histologic studies have revealed two other important bits of information. First, the ingrowth pattern did not appear related to the *in vivo* duration of the implant. Second, the relative porosity of the femoral cortex did not affect the amount of bone ingrowth. However, the specimens with the most pronounced osteoporosis tended to have predominantly cancellous or trabecular bone ingrowth rather than compact bone ingrowth (6).

One of the most compelling questions regarding porous ingrowth fixation is, How much bone ingrowth is sufficient for durable fixation? Although the percentages of ingrowth for partially and for fully porous-coated stems were similar in these studies, the total area of bone ingrowth was much greater for the fully coated stems, simply because of the larger area of porous coating. This may have clinical significance. Whereas late loosening of an extensively coated stem has never been observed, late failure of implants with limited amounts of proximal porous coating has. This suggests the possibility that insufficient quantity or quality of bone ingrowth can lead to failure, but it does not fully answer the question about how much ingrowth is enough.

Both serial clinical radiographs of the same patient and their autopsy specimens have been used to study the bone

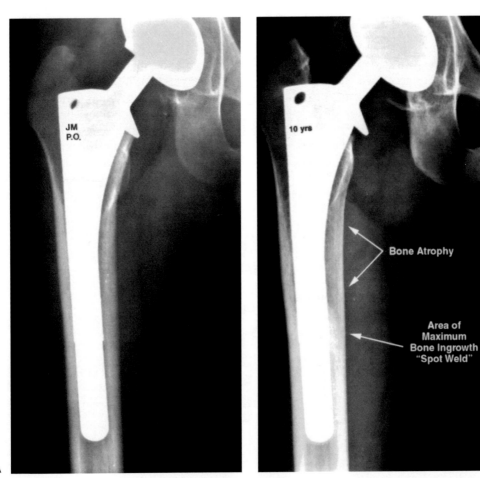

A   B

FIG. 3. A: The immediate postoperative radiographic appearance of a femur containing an osseointegrated AML prosthesis. **B:** The 10-year postoperative radiograph shows loss of bone in the cortices adjacent to the proximal two-thirds of the implant.

remodeling that occurs as the bone attempts to adapt to the implant (2,8,16,19). Three techniques have been used: subjective evaluation of serial radiographs, computer-assisted videodensitometry of the same clinical radiographs, and dual-energy x-ray absorptiometry (DEXA) analysis of autopsy-retrieved specimens. Analysis of the autopsy-retrieved specimens provides the most accurate quantitative information. There are two problems with subjective evaluation of clinical radiographs: The method is not quantitative, and it is limited by variation in radiographic technique. These two deficiencies can be partially corrected by converting these same radiographs to digital images and using a technique termed histogram-directed equalization to correct for variations in radiographic technique. A computer program can then be used to quantitate zonal changes on serial radiographs. This method has been used to evaluate 15 cementless total hip arthroplasties (9). With the AML prosthesis at 2 years postoperatively, the decrease in density in the proximal periprosthetic bone ranged from 11% to 28%. An increased density was noted adjacent to the stem tip. When serial clinical radiographs were evaluated by this method, no significant progression of periprosthetic resorptive changes was seen for the extensively porous-coated implant between the 2nd and 5th postoperative years, suggesting that some type of equilibrium was achieved at the first 2 years after the arthroplasty.

By far the most sensitive method of determining periprosthetic bone remodeling is through the use of DEXA. By using different absorptions of high- and low-radiation energies, DEXA allows direct measurement of bone mineral content. The femora of 11 patients with the well-functioning unilateral hip replacements retrieved at autopsy were analyzed (19). For this study, the contralateral femur was also retrieved and implanted with a matching prosthesis *in vitro*. This served as the control for bone mineral comparisons: an average decrease in bone mineral content of 23% in the implanted femur (range, 5% to 47%) was observed. Women experienced more bone loss than men. The average bone loss for the remodeled femur was 12% for the men, compared with 31% for the women. Zonal analysis revealed an average decrease in bone mineral content of 42% proximally, 23% in the area adjacent to the midstem, and 6% adjacent to the distal stem.

In these 11 cases, no correlation was observed between the degree of bone loss and the implant diameter of the stem that had been used, or between bone loss and the duration of implantation. The most striking finding was the strong inverse correlation between bone mineral content in the control femur and the extent of bone mineral loss in the remodeled femur ($p < .05$; $r^2 = 0.94$). This correlation suggests that the initial bone stock of the femur has the most important influence on the extent of bone remodeling. Patients with low bone mineral content in the proximal femur at the time of surgery appear prone to

more bone loss as a result of bone remodeling. Although there is a correlation between the bone mineral content and the mechanical properties of the femur, this finding suggests the intriguing possibility that the biologic state of the bone at the time of implantation has an important influence on the extent of bone remodeling.

Bone remodeling continues to be an area of intensive investigation, and the orthopedic community is beginning to understand the influence of the biologic factors, in addition to the mechanical factors, that interact to cause remodeling around cementless implants. The classic explanation of stress bypass by stiff implants does not fully explain such observations. It is increasingly recognized that all implant systems, whether cementless or cemented, elicit similar bone remodeling responses, characterized by loss of bone mineral content in the most proximal regions of the femur (15). Extensively coated stems are unique only in that they are the most well studied with respect to this phenomenon.

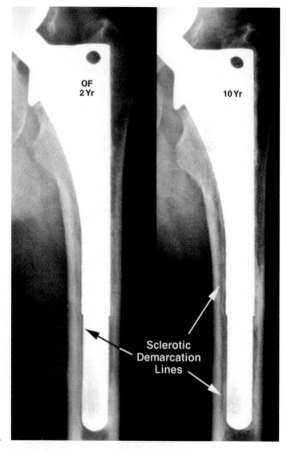

FIG. 4. The 2-year postoperative **(A)** and 10-year postoperative **(B)** radiographs of a femur containing an AML implant stabilized by fibrous tissue fixation. There was no change in the position of the implant within the femur during the 8-year interval between these two radiographs. The appearance of the bone–implant interface has also not changed, indicating implant stability.

Clinical correlation of radiographs and autopsy specimens confirms that it is possible to predict bone ingrowth into porous-coated stems based on changes in the appearance of clinical radiographs. The femur appears to respond to an extensively coated implant in a predictable fashion, in that characteristic radiographic patterns can be observed on plain radiographs (7). There are three typical responses: (a) bone ingrowth occurs; (b) bone ingrowth does not occur, but the implant is stabilized by fibrous tissue ingrowth; and (c) bone ingrowth does not occur and the stem becomes unstable. Each of these events is recognizable on plain radiographs, and recognition of these patterns is very useful in clinical practice. The typical pattern correlating with bone ingrowth is illustrated in Figure 3. The changes include densification of endosteal bone, often called spot welds, usually in the region of termination of the porous coating on the implant. Proximal to this area, femoral cortices become thinner and less radiographically dense. The extent of this proximal cortical atrophy can be variable, and this change is sometimes subtle. An additional sign of bone ingrowth is the absence of any radiodense demarcation lines next to the porous coating. These lines may occur around the smooth portion of the implant where bone ingrowth is not expected to occur, but they should not be present adjacent to the porous coating. These signs of bone ingrowth are usually clearly seen on a 1-year postoperative radiograph, and, when present, they are a reliable indicator of successful arthroplasty (4,8).

Radiographic signs of failed bone ingrowth but successful stabilization by fibrous tissue ingrowth are illustrated in Figure 4. The radiographic findings include sclerotic lines around the porous surface and less atrophy of the medial femoral neck than is observed when bone ingrowth occurs. Remodeling signs accompanied by a stem that does not show any migration on serial radiographs can be considered to be evidence that the implant is not osseointegrated but has maintained stability within the femur (i.e., stable fibrous fixation).

Signs of frank implant instability are illustrated in Figure 5. The radiographic changes include component migration, usually by subsidence and varus tilt. An additional sign of instability is progressive widening of the radiolucent space around the implant on serial radiographs.

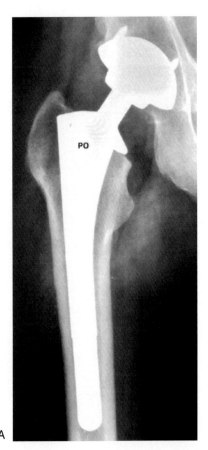
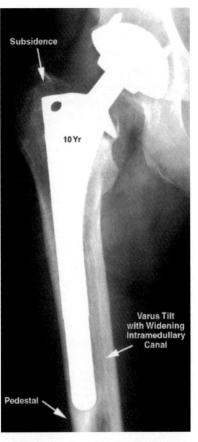

FIG. 5. The immediate postoperative **(A)** and 10-year postoperative **(B)** radiographs of a femur containing an AML implant that is not stably fixed. The positions of the implant within the femur are different on the two radiographs. The intramedullary canal has widened and new bone appears to have filled the intramedullary canal beneath the tip of the stem.

SURGICAL PRINCIPLES

Patient Selection

The development of cementless implants and the concept of osseointegration derive from clinical experience of late failures resulting from loosening of cemented implants, particularly in young, active individuals. The concept of patient matching has led many surgeons to reserve porous-coated stems for younger, active patients, particularly those characterized by good bone stock or Dorr type A or B femora. However, the nonselective use of porous-coated femoral stems for all total hip replacements over the last 20 years has demonstrated no short-term difference in clinical outcome based on age, sex, diagnosis, or bone quality (18). Patients over 65 years of age or those with osteoporosis do not have poorer clinical results or less reliable osseointegration than younger patients. The single, most important factor predicting the clinical result of extensively porous-coated stems is the quality of the initial prosthetic fit within the femur, particularly within the diaphysis (5). This finding is more a characteristic of the surgical technique than of any patient parameter.

The requirement for using an extensively coated stem therefore is simple: the presence of bone capable of providing initial mechanical support for the implant and capable of mounting an osteogenic (i.e., typical fracture healing) response sufficient for ingrowth. Exceptionally few patients do not meet these criteria.

Preoperative Planning

Careful preoperative planning using high-quality radiographs is vital to the success of porous-coated hip replacements. This templating allows for estimation of implant size, position within the bone, and location of femoral neck resection, as well as restoration of hip biomechanics (hip center, leg length, and offset). In most routine cases, preoperative templating is performed with two radiographs: an anteroposterior (AP) pelvic view and a true lateral view of the proximal one-half of the femur. The pelvic view (Fig. 6) is modified in two ways. First, the beam and the cassette are lowered to include the acetabulum and at least 8 cm of the femur. Second, the hips are internally rotated 20° to obtain a true AP view of the anteverted femoral neck. This positioning allows the radiograph to show the plane in which the implant is inserted in the femur and the plane in which the true neck–shaft angle of the femur can be measured. When the arthritic hip is stiff and cannot be rotated, either the contralateral (normal) hip is used to plan the procedure, or an AP-directed radiograph is obtained with the entire pelvis rotated to obtain the desired femoral rotation.

Templating

There are six steps in the templating process. First, the leg-length difference is calculated. This is accomplished by placing blocks beneath the feet until the pelvis is level. Second, the size and position of the acetabular component are determined. Third, the diameter of the distal, cylindrical portion of the stem is determined by placing the template in line with the center line of the femur in the femoral diaphysis. The correct size is that which fills or is slightly larger than the isthmus, so that porous coating will contact a distance of at least 5 cm of the medial and lateral endosteal cortices (Fig. 7). By placing templates of varying diameters over the isthmus, the surgeon

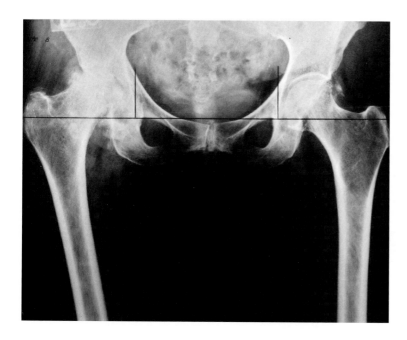

FIG. 6. An AP pelvic radiograph used for preoperative planning; both femora are rotated.

should be able to predict what caliber of drill will contact the endosteal cortices, the level at which the drill will begin cutting, and the distance over which it will cut. The fourth step is the determination of the level of the femoral neck resection and prosthetic neck length (Fig. 8). These two variables together affect the seating level of the implant and restoration of leg length and femoral offset. With the center of the acetabulum previously marked and the femoral template aligned to the diaphysis, the template is raised or lowered until one of the potential head centers directly overlays the acetabular center or lies directly above the acetabular cup center a distance equal to the desired amount of increased limb length. The level of the neck cut is then marked and the neck length chosen. The AML system contains three different proximal stem geometries: small, large, and extra large. The fifth step involves selecting the appropriate proximal implant geometry that adequately fills the proximal femur based on the level of the neck resection. The final step involves templating the lateral radiograph. With the lateral template at the desired level, the anterior and posterior sides of the straight stem should achieve three-point contact with the endosteal surface. The length should not be so

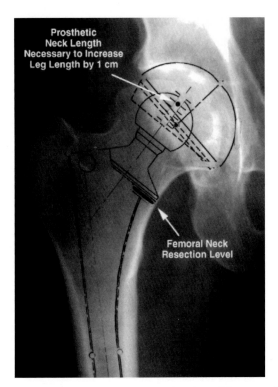

FIG. 8. Step 4 in the preoperative planning of the use of the AML femoral stem.

long as to risk perforation of the anterior femoral cortex during implantation. This is rarely a problem except in patients with distorted femoral anatomy or in revision situations where longer stem lengths are used.

SURGICAL TECHNIQUE

Aspects of the surgical technique unique and important to the successful implantation of extensively porous-coated stems include exposure, acetabular preparation and acetabular component insertion, acetabular trial positioning, femoral preparation, trial reduction, femoral component insertion, and wound closure.

Exposure

The posterior approach is used by the authors on all primary hip arthroplasties (3,5) to permit adequate exposure of both the acetabulum and the proximal femur. The patient is placed in the lateral decubitus position on the operating table, and pelvic clamps, attached to the operating table, are used to hold the patient rigidly in this position. All bony prominences and the axilla are padded. Standard draping techniques are used, with careful exclusion of the groin and perineum from the operative field. The lower (non-operated) leg is strapped to the table with the hip flexed 30° and the knee at a 90-degree flexed

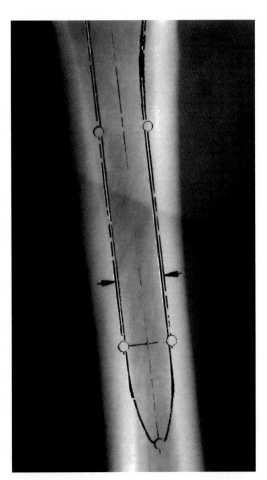

FIG. 7. Step 3 in the preoperative planning of the use of the AML femoral stem.

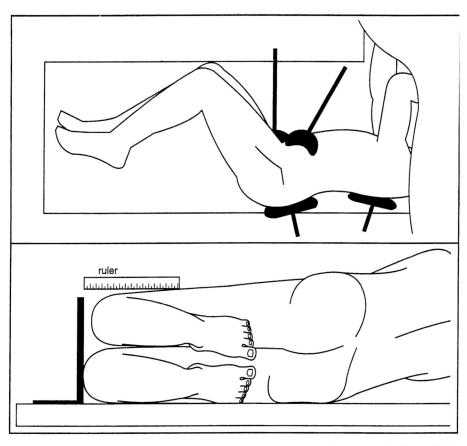

FIG. 9. Patient positioning and length measurement for surgery through a posterior lateral hip incision.

position. If the upper leg is placed directly on top of the lower leg and both knees are flexed 90°, it is possible to compare leg lengths. When the patient lies on the operating table in the lateral position, a pelvic tilt occurs. This creates an apparent leg-length discrepancy, with the upper leg appearing shorter than it actually is. The surgeon uses a right angle and a ruler to measure (at the knees) the apparent difference in femoral lengths (Fig. 9).

Once the superficial dissection is complete, the short external rotators are released from the posterolateral femur, and a posterior capsulectomy is performed. Prior to dislocation of the hip and resection of the femoral head, a ⁵⁄₃₂-inch threaded Steinmann pin is placed through the gluteus medius muscle into the ileum. The pin is then bent twice at 90-degree angles so that the exposed tip touches the greater trochanter. This point is marked with a stay stitch to monitor offset and length after placement of the trial implants. It is important to always place the upper leg back in the position it was before measurement of limb length using either of these techniques.

The hip is dislocated by flexing, adducting, and internally rotating the femur. The femur can be delivered into the surgical field with a retractor placed under the lesser trochanter. The femoral head is resected with the provisional cut. The surgeon routinely completes the capsulectomy by resecting the remaining anterior capsule (Fig.

10). With resecting of the thickened and contracted anterior capsule, patients are able to regain external rotation postoperatively. They are then able to perform routine activities such as putting on socks and shoes.

Anterior capsulectomy is accomplished by having a surgical assistant extend and internally rotate the hip

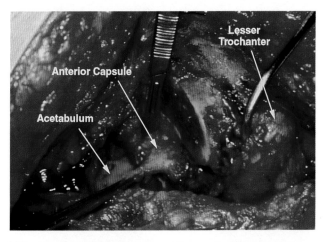

FIG. 10. The femoral head and the posterior capsule have been surgically removed. A hook beneath the lesser trochanter is used to apply traction to the femur and to tent-up the anterior capsule. The capsular attachment to the anterior neck will be cut.

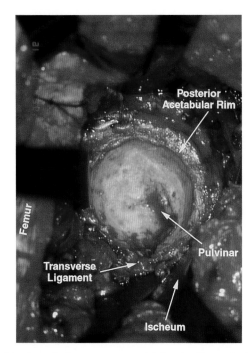

FIG. 11. Acetabular exposure obtained after anterior and posterior capsulectomy. Osteophytes have been removed from the acetabular rim. The transverse ligament has not been resected.

joint, while a second assistant applies lateral traction to the proximal femur with a bone hook (placed at the level of the lesser trochanter). This arrangement places the anterior capsule under tension so that it can be released from the anterior femur with the cautery. A curved Mayo scissors can be placed into the sheath of the psoas tendon to protect it and the underlying anterior musculature.

Once the capsule is released from the femur, a retractor can be placed over the anterior acetabular rim on the pubis, thus displacing the femur anteriorly. This anterior displacement results from detaching a portion of the gluteus maximus tendon from its insertion on the posterolateral femur. It is then easy to resect the remaining capsule, the labrum, and the transverse acetabular ligament. Next, the pulvinar (fatty tissue) is removed from the cotyloid notch (acetabular fossa), and a blunt retractor is placed into the obturator foramen. This retractor rests on the inferior edge of the acetabular fossa. This point corresponds with the lower edge of the acetabular teardrop on radiographs. The floor of the acetabular fossa corresponds with the lateral edge of the teardrop. A special posterior retractor is placed with its point in the obturator foramen. The appearance of the acetabulum with this retractor in place is shown in Figure 11. Because the entire acetabular rim must be visualized to place the cementless component, the exposure obtained using this technique is necessary.

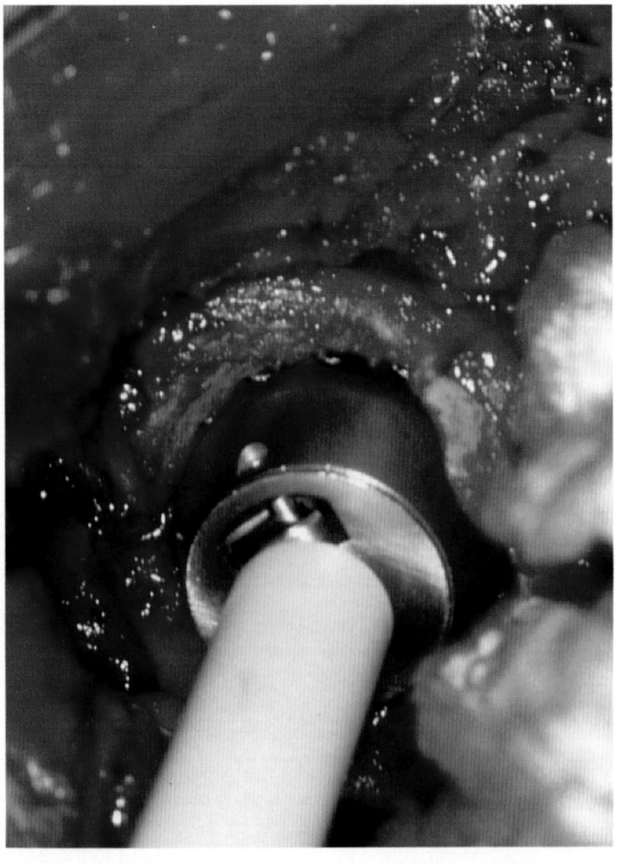

FIG. 12. The acetabular cheese-grater reamers are used with the base of the reamer parallel to the acetabular rim.

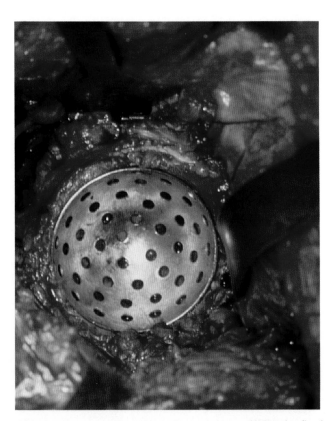

FIG. 13. An acetabular trial shell is used to estimate the fit of the porous-surfaced component.

Acetabular Preparation and Acetabular Component Insertion

The acetabulum is prepared using spherical reamers of increasing diameter. The surgical team uses cutting reamers with outside diameters measuring from 36 to 75 mm. The reamer sizes progress in 1-mm increments. The reamers should be oriented in approximately 45° of abduction and 25° of anteversion. In this orientation, the flat posterior surface of the reamer should be in the same plane as the rim of the acetabulum (Fig. 12). Reaming is continued using progressively larger reamers until all articular cartilage is removed. The subchondral plate is partially removed so that punctuate bleeding is present. However, excessive reaming of the subchondral plate and the anterior and posterior columns should be avoided. The surgical team usually does not ream to the depth of the acetabular fossa, and reaming should not proceed medially past this inner table. In general, at least two-thirds of the subchondral plate should present a healthy bleeding surface.

Acetabular Trial Positioning

Once a hemispheric acetabular bed is obtained with the debris-retaining reamers, an acetabular trial is placed to assess the coverage and optimum position of the acetabular component. Figure 13 shows the trial acetabular component in the correct position in the prepared acetabulum. The face of the trial component is also placed parallel to the acetabular opening. This usually corresponds to 45° of abduction and 20° of anteversion. The relationship between the inferior medial rim of the cup and the acetabular teardrop should be nearly identical to that recorded in the preoperative plan. This orientation defines the vertical position of the acetabular component. The horizontal position is determined by the depth to which it has been placed within the acetabular fossa. The acetabular trial should fit snugly within the acetabulum. The surgeon uses a trial that is the same diameter as the final reamer size. Surface contact between the component and the prepared acetabular cavity can be inspected through the perforations in the trial shell.

The implanted acetabulum is 1 mm larger in diameter than the final reamer used. Radius gauges are used to confirm the sizes of the acetabular trial, final reamer, and actual acetabular implant (Fig. 14). Different cup types can be used, but a cup without spikes or screw holes is preferable for most cases. The central apex hole in the cup is threaded and can be connected to an impactor. After the cup is inserted and the impactor is removed, the central

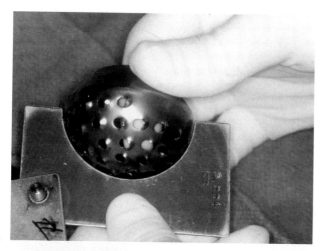

A

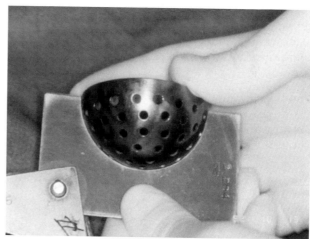

B

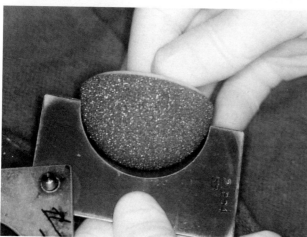

C

FIG. 14. The last acetabular reamer **(A)**, the trial cup **(B)**, and the porous-coated component **(C)** are all measured.

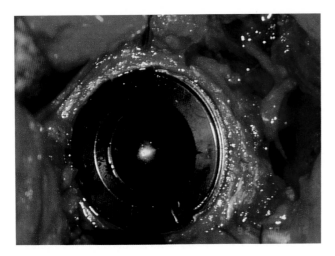

FIG. 15. A trial acetabulum polyethylene is used for the trial reduction.

hole can be filled with a threaded plug. With careful preparation of the acetabulum, excellent implant stability is obtained without the use of screw fixation. The absence of screw holes eliminates cold flow of polyethylene and the egress of polyethylene debris into the ilium. If the surgeon feels that adjunctive fixation is necessary, then a cup with spikes or holes for screw fixation can be used. After the acetabular component has been seated, a polyethylene trial liner can be inserted prior to implanting the femoral component. The porous-coated implanted shell with the trial liner inside it are illustrated in Figure 15.

Femoral Preparation

After routine acetabular preparation, the femoral neck is cut at the predetermined level. The goal of femoral preparation is to create an endosteal surface that matches the implant. This procedure involves creating a straight tube with straight rigid drills. Correct pilot hole positioning is critical for proper femoral component placement. The surgeon uses a high-speed cutting instrument to make this hole just anterior to the piriformis fossa. The pilot hole should be at least 2 mm larger than the size planned for the intramedullary canal. The position of the pilot hole can be estimated from the preoperative radiographs. Making the pilot hole larger than the anticipated distal implant size reduces the possibility of eccentric reaming of the intramedullary canal. As progressively larger drills are inserted into the medullary canal, these drills must not contact the pilot hole. If this contact does occur, the hole must be enlarged to prevent the proximally located pilot hole from influencing the direction of the drills distally. The goal is for the drills to enlarge the canal distally without proximal impingement. The location of the pilot hole and this drilling technique are illustrated in Figure 16. A small drill that fits loosely into the distal canal does not control proximal drill position. However, when larger drills are used, the tight distal diaphyseal fit will control the position of the proximal part of the drill (Fig. 17). To complete the drilling correctly, the surgeon must enlarge the pilot hole. Figure 18 is an example of a case in which an incorrectly placed pilot hole produced off-center reaming of the femoral diaphysis.

The distance drilled can be determined from the calibrations on the drill (1-cm increments). As the canal is reamed, the drill size that first begins to bite, as well as the drilling distance, should correspond relatively closely to the drill sizing from the preoperative plan. The absence of such correspondence should serve as a warning that the drilling is not being performed correctly. In this case, an intraoperative x-ray should be obtained to check the

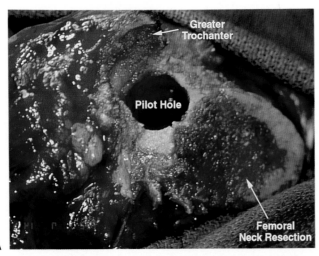
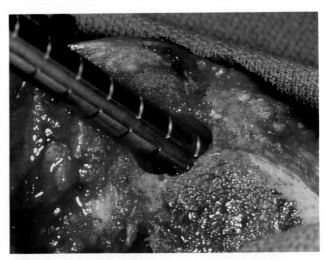

A

B

FIG. 16. The entry hole is placed as far lateral as possible in the femoral neck; this requires removal of bone from the greater trochanter **(A)**. The femoral reamers should not contact the rim of the entry/pilot hole **(B)**.

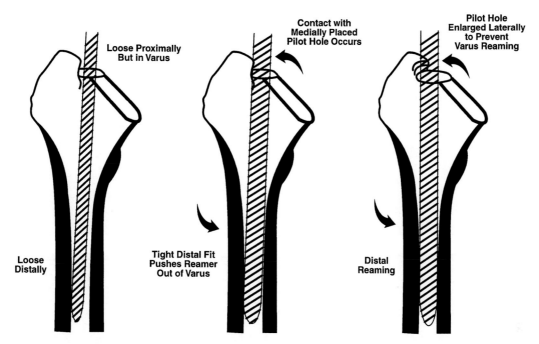

FIG. 17. These three illustrations show why it is sometimes necessary to modify the pilot hole to accommodate larger-sized reamers.

drill orientation. This problem may occur if the pilot hole is made incorrectly, thus influencing the distal path of the drill. In this scenario, a smaller-than-anticipated drill may impinge in a varus position distally. The drills should advance distally without manual pressure if reaming is concentric and centered. As larger drills are used, they will begin to bite over progressively larger distances. The surgeon prefers to have at least 3 cm of the intramedullary canal reamed in a cylindrical fashion, with this area corresponding with the circumferential porous coating of the femoral component.

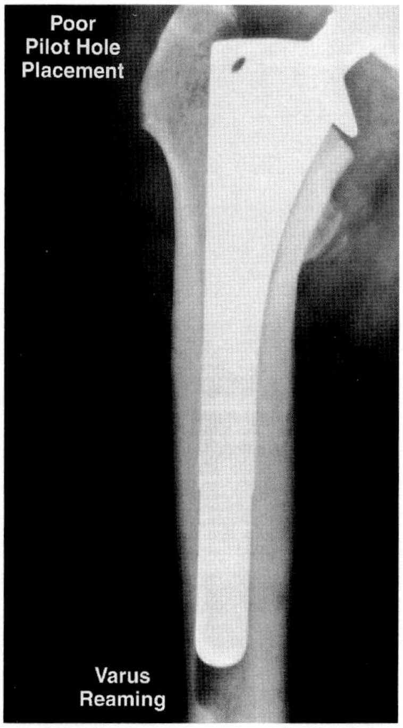

Once the distal femur has been prepared, blunt-tip proximal reamers and rasps are used to prepare the metaphyseal bone. A blunt-ended cutting reamer can be used to shape the inside of the femoral neck (Fig. 19). The rasps are driven to a point just below the level of the neck resection, and the calcar is planed flat.

Trial Reduction

With the trial rasp in place, a trial reduction can be performed using the corresponding left or right (anteverted) neck segment. Limb length and offset can both be assessed using the Steinmann pin and stitch that were placed prior to femoral head removal (Fig. 20). Leg length should also be checked with measurements at the knees (see Fig. 9). Adjustments can then be made in the femoral offset and limb length by changing the following: the neck length of the prosthesis, the implant seating level (by recutting the femoral neck and driving the implant further distally), the configuration of the neck of the prosthesis (changing from the 135-degree to the 125-degree neck–shaft angle implant), or a combination of these.

The goal is to restore equal leg length while maintaining or increasing the lateral distance between the femur and pelvis. Narrowing the lateral separation between the femur and the pelvis results in poor hip abductor tension

FIG. 18. The postoperative radiograph of a patient in whom an incorrect pilot hole caused reaming and a suboptimal position of the femoral stem.

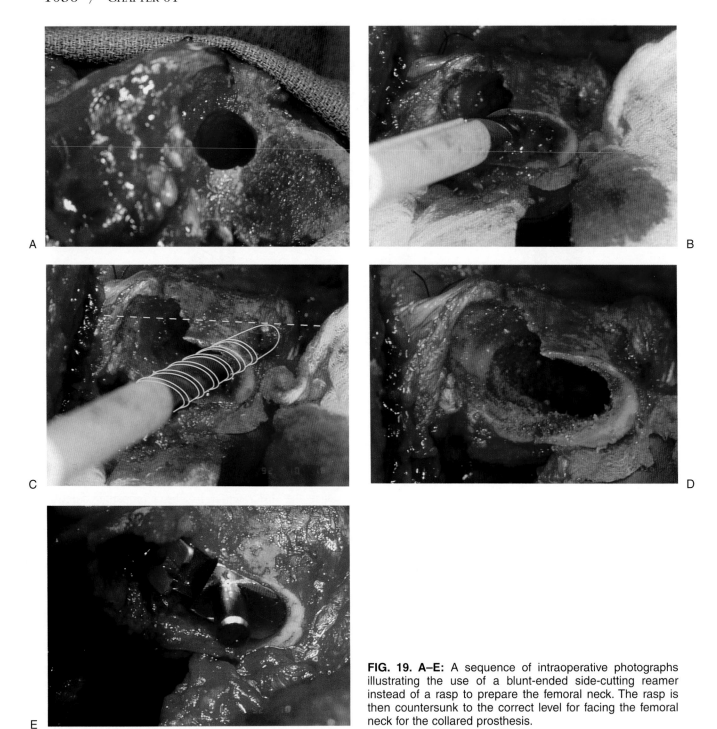

FIG. 19. A–E: A sequence of intraoperative photographs illustrating the use of a blunt-ended side-cutting reamer instead of a rasp to prepare the femoral neck. The rasp is then countersunk to the correct level for facing the femoral neck for the collared prosthesis.

and power, increased joint reactive forces, and, most important, an increased likelihood of postoperative hip dislocation.

The stability of the hip can be assessed with the trial components in place. Posterior stability is assessed with the hip in flexion, adduction, and internal rotation. In most instances, the hip should be stable when flexed 90°, when adducted 20°, and when internally rotated at least 50°. In addition to assessing posterior stability, the surgeon must

confirm anterior stability by placing the hip in full extension and external rotation. This assessment is critical when an anterior capsulectomy has been performed.

When evidence of hip instability is present, it is necessary to determine the cause. Component malalignment may be a source of instability. Once the drills and rasps have been placed, the rotation of the femoral component is essentially fixed. If excess anteversion is already present in the femur, this anteversion can be reduced 20° by using

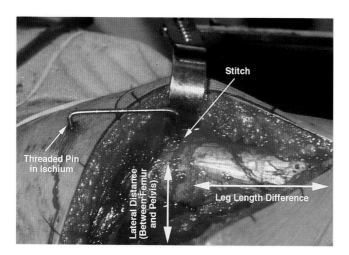

FIG. 20. The distance separating the femur from the pelvis is checked by reducing the hip and checking the relationship between the end of the iliac pin in the pelvis and a stitch previously placed in the greater trochanter.

a left femoral prosthesis neck in the right femur, or vice versa. The change in hip joint stability from this change of prosthesis should be checked with the femoral neck trial parts. Frequently, posterior instability is produced by bony impingement between an abnormally prominent anterior portion of the greater trochanter and the pelvis. This problem can be solved by resecting a portion of the anterior trochanteric prominence (Fig. 21). Impingement can also be decreased by displacing the femur a greater lateral distance away from the pelvis, lateralizing the femur. This lateralization is achieved by using a longer neck segment on the prosthesis. It is preferable that the surgeon not rely on an elevated rim on polyethylene acetabular liners to increase hip stability. An elevated rim placed posteriorly (to improve posterior stability) may actually cause anterior instability if the neck of the femoral implant impinges on the posterior elevated rim when the hip is placed in extension and external rotation.

Femoral Component Insertion

Once the surgical team is satisfied with the patient's leg length, the amount of lateralization of the femur, and the stability of the head in the cup, the trial components are removed and the identical permanent components are inserted. At this point, the surgeon must make a decision regarding the ideal amount of interference fit for the femoral component. It is best that the femoral component and final drill both be measured with a series of hole gauges (Fig. 22). In most cases, the team inserts a stem with a distal diameter 0.5 mm larger than that of the last drill. In this way, a tight initial scratch-fit is obtained in the cylindrically machined femur; however, there are exceptions. In some young patients with very hard cortical bone, the drill will bite firmly over a distance greater than 5 cm. To avoid getting the stem stuck or breaking the femur, the surgeon drills the femoral canal to the same diameter as the final implant (i.e., in a line-to-line fashion). The important point here is that the diameter of the porous-coated component be large enough so that it cannot be manually pushed down the canal farther than the level shown in Figure 23. Forceful impaction should be neces-

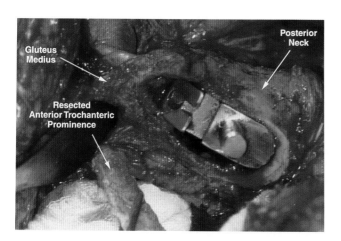

FIG. 21. Posterior hip stability can often be improved by resecting the anterior portion of the greater trochanter or part of an abnormally prominent anterior femoral neck.

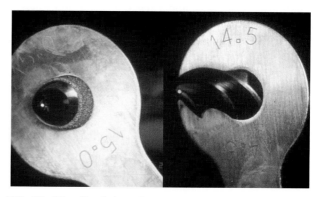

FIG. 22. The distal size of the largest reamer and the prosthesis are checked with hole gauges.

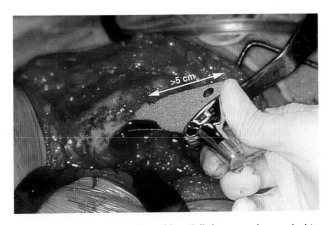

FIG. 23. Forceful impaction with a 2-lb hammer is needed to seat the implant. It should not be possible to push the implant past the point shown in the illustration.

sary to drive the prosthesis down the last 4 to 5 cm of the canal. The modular base is then placed on the trunion of the femoral neck. The selection of ball sizes includes 22, 26, 28, and 32 mm. Smaller ball sizes are preferred for younger patients and smaller patients.

Wound Closure

The wound is lavaged using pulsatile irrigation (4 liters) and closed with absorbable Vicryl suture in layers. The gluteus maximus tendon, pyriformis tendon, and short external rotators are sutured to their insertions on the posterolateral femur, and two 1/8-inch drains are inserted.

Postoperative Care

Postoperative care revolves around the concept that minimal motion at the bone–implant interface is required for successful bone ingrowth. A 3-month postoperative protective weight-bearing protocol involves the use of two crutches during the 1st month with the patient allowed touch-down weight bearing (25%), the use of one crutch and 50% weight bearing during the 2nd month, and the use of a cane during the 3rd month. This protocol is modified based on patient needs and the implant fit, particularly in revision situations. The combination of underreaming and extensive coating creates an exceptionally tight fit, and in incidences where patients are allowed early weight bearing no detrimental effects have been observed. Nonetheless, because the protective weight-bearing protocol has worked so well for so long, it is still used for postoperative care.

CLINICAL OUTCOMES OF EXTENSIVELY POROUS-COATED FEMORAL STEMS

Clinical experience with extensively porous-coated femoral stems has reached nearly two decades. Evolu-

tionary changes in stem design have affected the clinical outcome. From 1977 to 1982, only a stem with a fixed 32-mm head was available. Despite having what would presently be considered a poor initial prosthetic fit, these stems have demonstrated a 92% survival at minimum 11-year follow-up. Five stems in this group have been revised: two for instability, two for stem fracture, and one for infection.

The second evolutionary phase began in 1982 and extended to 1984. During this period, a stem was used with porous coating applied to 4.5 inches of its 6.5-inch length. The implant was manufactured in six sizes. Postoperative radiographs of slightly more than 80% of the 227 consecutive patients who underwent implantation showed the stem to adequately fill the intramedullary canal. Minimum 10-year follow-up on 174 of these patients (8) revealed that 27 have died and 21 are considered lost to follow-up. Three stems have been revised: two for symptomatic loosening, and one for sepsis (this stem was also loose). All three had failed to achieve osseointegration. One implant was removed in the 6th postoperative year, and the second in the 11th postoperative year for loosening. The infected stem was removed in the 10th postoperative year. In two of these patients, the unstable stem was replaced with another porous-coated one. In the patient with infection, the reimplantation was accomplished with antibiotic-loaded cement. In all three cases, the revisions were successful and current radiographs show the implants to appear osseointegrated. Currently, among these 174 patients with longer than 10-year follow-up, 1% (two patients) have radiographic signs of an unstable stem. Both of these patients are elderly and do not have symptoms that warrant revision. Of these stems, 92% demonstrate radiographic signs of bone ingrowth, and 7% do not appear osseointegrated, but they have maintained radiographic stability presumably by fibrous tissue ingrowth.

The third phase spanned from 1985 to 1988 and involved the use of both proximally (40%) and fully (80% to 100%) porous-coated stems of the same design. Of the 893 patients treated during this time interval, 251 received a 40% proximally porous-coated stem, and 642 received an 80% coated stem. There was no *a priori* selection for deciding which patient received which implant. At minimum 5-year follow-up, 6 of the 251 proximally coated stems required revision, whereas 3 of the 642 extensively coated stems required revision. These revisions were done for stem instability resulting from failed bone ingrowth. The conclusion was that bone ingrowth could be more predictably obtained with extensively porous-coated stems than with the proximally coated ones. Additionally, through the use of questionnaires, the authors learned that the instance of thigh pain was more prominent in patients who had received the proximally porous-coated stems (26%)

than in patients who have received the extensively coated stems (17%). When the authors limited this analysis to working-age Charnley type A patients, these differences in the clinical results were not as great. Also, in this younger-aged group, it was not possible to identify any particular patient characteristics that predisposed to greater or lesser degrees of success with each type of implant.

In 1989, a switch was made to using only the extensively porous-coated stems, and current radiographs of more than 1000 patients at follow-up of more than 2 years reveal that more than 99% have signs of osseointegration.

Clinical results mirror the radiographic experience. Satisfaction and function have been evaluated with questionnaires on all of the 174 second-generation cases with a greater than 10-year follow-up. Of these patients, 93% were totally satisfied with their arthroplasty procedure. Function improved in all but four patients in this group. In three of these four patients, the lack of a functional improvement could clearly be related to the stability of the implant (one case of a loose acetabular component and two cases with a loose femoral component).

Extensively porous-coated stems have also proved remarkably successful in revision arthroplasty. Many manufacturers now make extensively porous-coated stems specifically designed for the revision situation. These implants are typically larger in diameter and longer in length than the extensively porous-coated stems necessary for primary arthroplasty cases. The theory and technique in the revision setting are directed toward extending the porous coating distally beyond the area of diseased bone. In the United States, the long-term clinical results using this technique for revisions come from several publications. Moreland has reported seven (4.0%) revisions and three (1.7%) radiographically unstable stems in 175 cases at a mean 5-year follow-up (20). Krishnamurthy reported only five revisions in 297 cases at a 7.3-year mean follow-up. Of these 297, another two stems that had not been revised were unstable, giving a mechanical failure rate of 2.4%. In a review of 174 femoral revision procedures done by these authors between 1980 and 1986 with a minimum 5-year follow-up, ten stems have been revised (5.74%) (21). An additional two (1.1%) are radiographically unstable. Of the ten stems that have been revised, six have been revised for loosening, two for breakage, and two for infection. Survivorship analysis reveals a 90.6% survivorship of the stem at the end of the 9th year after the revision procedure.

Although clinical results of the first 10 postoperative years have been excellent, problems with the AML system at longer time intervals can be foreseen. These problems will undoubtedly result in the need for more revision procedures in the future. This will particularly be a prob-

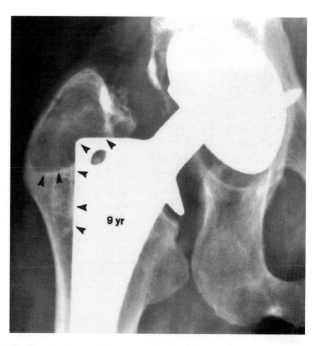

FIG. 24. Radiographic appearance of the most common large femoral osteolytic lesion observed with the AML prosthesis.

lem in those patients who were less than 65 years of age at the time of their initial arthroplasty. The anticipated problems are not related to the stem design, but to head size and the type of acetabular components used. The patterns of osteolysis observed around extensively coated stems differ from those seen around cemented and noncircumferentially porous-coated uncemented prostheses. In a review of 192 patients with extensively coated stems with fixed 32-mm heads and porous-coated cups implanted between 1982 and 1984, femoral osteolytic lesions were observed in 38 patients (20%). High-quality radiographs allow visualization of even the smallest lesions. These osteolytic lesions appear only in the periprosthetic joint space between the greater and lesser trochanters. They appear most frequently as small scalloped-out areas in the medial cortex of the femoral neck or in the greater trochanter. In most cases (29 of 38), these lesions have remained less than 1.5 cm² in size. Larger lesions most frequently occur within the greater trochanter and in some cases have resulted in late pathologic fracture. A typical large osteolytic lesion within the greater trochanter is illustrated in Figure 24. No osteolysis has been observed below the level of the lesser trochanter, suggesting that the circumferential porous coating limits the effective joint space and prevents debris access to more distal regions of the stem. Also, no distal osteolysis has been observed in cases in which the stems appear fixed by fibrous tissue ingrowth. These radiographic findings have been supported by the authors' autopsy retrieval studies that have also shown no histologic evidence of debris or granuloma formation below the level of the medial cortex of the femoral neck.

CONCLUSION

Extensively porous-coated stems were originally developed as an alternative to cemented stems in younger active patients. Although some have doubted that bone ingrowth could be consistently achieved and have expected late loosening to result when ingrowth did not occur, or they felt that the proximal bone atrophy produced by stress shielding could result in late failure, clinical experience spanning 18 years has proven that these stems perform well in all patients for primary hip arthroplasty, and even for revision hip arthroplasty. In cases with greater than 10-year follow-up, revisions for stem loosening occur in less than 2%. Proximal bone atrophy resulting from stress shielding occurs and is undesirable, but to date it has not resulted in any clinical problems. Stem fractures have not occurred in the large reported primary arthroplasty series, but they did occur in two of the earliest revision cases. Improvement in the metallurgy of these stems and changes in the sintering process for the porous surface should prevent most stem fractures in the future.

Between the basic scientific investigation of the physical and mechanical characteristics of these stems, the studies of the well-fixed retrieved implants, and the well-described prospective clinical and radiographic follow-up of patients, extensively coated stems are perhaps the most well studied of any femoral implant. The goal with extensively coated stems is to achieve as much bone ingrowth as possible, accepting the fact that when the entire stem is porous coated, the greatest amount of bone ingrowth will occur in the femoral diaphysis. Femoral implants that have extensive porous coating into the diaphysis will remain popular for several reasons: the surgical technique is easy to perform correctly, and when done correctly, the likelihood of achieving bone ingrowth is extremely high, probably greater than 98%. Patient satisfaction with porous-coated implants has also been extremely high. Future problems revolve not about the stem or its porous surface, but about the bearing surface. Continued improvements in the articulating material should decrease long-term, wear-related complications. On this foundation, the evidence supports the use of extensively coated stems in both primary and revision arthroplasty.

REFERENCES

1. Bobyn JD, Pilliar RM, Cameron HU, et al. The optimum pore size for the fixation of porous-surfaced metal implants by the ingrowth of bone. *Clin Orthop* 1980;150:263–269.
2. Engh CA, Bobyn JD. The influence of stem size and extent of porous coating on femoral bone resorption after primary cementless hip arthroplasty. *Clin Orthop* 1988;231:7–28.
3. Engh CA, Bobyn JD, eds. *Biological fixation in total hip arthroplasty.* New Jersey: Slack, 1985.
4. Engh CA, Bobyn JD, Glassman AH. Porous coated hip replacement. The factors governing bone ingrowth, stress shielding, and clinical results. *J Bone Joint Surg* 1987;69B(1):45–55.
5. Engh CA, Glassman AH, Bobyn JD. Surgical principles in cementless total hip arthroplasty. *Tech Orthop* 1986;1:35–53.
6. Engh CA, Hooten JP Jr, Zettl-Schaffer KF, Ghaffarpour M, McGovern TF, Bobyn JD. Evaluation of bone ingrowth with proximally and extensively porous-coated AML prostheses retrieved at autopsy. *J Bone Joint Surg* 1995;77A:903–910.
7. Engh CA, Massin P, Suthers KE. Roentgenographic assessment of the biologic fixation of porous surfaced femoral components. *Clin Orthop* 1990;257:107–128.
8. Engh CA, McGovern TF, Bobyn JD, Harris WH. A quantitative evaluation of periprosthetic bone-remodeling after cementless total hip arthroplasty. *J Bone Joint Surg* 1992;74A:1009–1020.
9. Engh CA, McGovern TF, Schmidt LM. Roentgenographic densitometry of bone adjacent to a femoral prosthesis. *Clin Orthop* 1993;292:177–190.
10. Engh CA, O Connor D, Jasty M, McGovern TF, Bobyn JD, Harris WH. Quantification of implant micromotion, stress shielding, and bone resorption with porous-coated anatomic medullary locking femoral prostheses. *Clin Orthop* 1992;285:13–29.
11. Glassman AH, Engh CA, Culpepper WJ. Results of porous-coated total hip replacement in patients 50 years of age and younger. *Annual meeting of the American Academy of Orthopaedic Surgeons,* Atlanta, GA, February, 1996.
12. Judet R, Siguier M, Brumpt B, Judet T. A noncemented total hip prosthesis. *Clin Orthop* 1978;137:76.
13. Keaveny TM, Bartel DL. Effects of porous coating, with and without collar support, on early relative motion for a cementlesship prosthesis. *J Biomech* 1993;26:1355–1368.
14. Lord GA, Hardy JR, Kummer FJ. An uncemented total hip replacement: experimental study and review of 300 Madreporique arthroplasties. *Clin Orthop* 1979;141:2.
15. Maloney WJ, Bragdon C, Sychterz C, et al. Adaptive bone remodeling with the well-fixed cemented and cementless femoral components. *21st annual meeting of the Society Biomaterials Trans,* San Francisco, CA, 1995.
16. McGovern TF, Engh CA, Zettl-Schaffer KF, Hooten JP Jr. Cortical bone density of the proximal femur following cementless total hip arthroplasty. *Clin Orthop* 1994;306:145–154.
17. Moore AT. A metal hip joint: a new self-locking prosthesis. *South Med J* 1952;45:1015.
18. Sotereanos N, Engh CA, Glassman AH, Macalino GE, Engh CA Jr. Cementless femoral components should be made from cobalt chrome. *Clin Orthop* 1995;313:146–153.
19. Sychterz CJ, Engh CA. The influence of clinical factors on periprosthetic bone remodeling. *Clin Orthop* 1996;322:285–292.
20. Moreland JR, Bernstein ML. Femoral revision hip arthroplasty with uncemented, porous-coated stems. *Clin Orthop* 1995;318:141–150.
21. Lawrence JM, Engh CA, Macalino GE. Revision total hip arthroplasty. Long-term results without cement. *Orthop Clin North Am* 1993;24(4):635–644.

The Adult Hip, edited by J. J. Callaghan,
A. G. Rosenberg, and H. E. Rubash.
Lippincott–Raven Publishers, Philadelphia © 1998.

CHAPTER **65**

Hydroxyapatite Coating

William J. Donnelly, Michael A. R. Freeman, and Gareth Scott

Total hip arthroplasty is superior to all other surgical procedures for arthrosis or arthritis of the hip, to restore function and maintain quality of life (101). Despite the technologic advances that have occurred in total hip arthroplasty over the last three decades, the problems of late aseptic loosening and particulate wear debris continue to be stumbling blocks to achieving a permanent biologically integrated implant. Over the last decade, there have been extensive clinical studies and basic science research on the use of various methods of fixation of the prosthesis to the skeleton in an attempt to overcome the biomechanical and biologic problems of aseptic loosening, without increasing debris formation. Especially in younger, higher-demand patients, the accepted standard method of fixation using polymethylmethacrylate has demonstrated less than fully satisfactory survival results (20,29,30,62,70), and thus, in this group particularly, alternative methods of fixation have been sought.

W. J. Donnelly: Department of Orthopaedics, Princess Alexandria Hospital, Wilston, Brisbane, Queensland, Australia.

M. A. R. Freeman and G. Scott: Department of Orthopaedic Surgery, Royal London Hospital–University of London, London WIN 2DE, England.

To obtain reliable and reproducible permanent fixation in the absence of cement, it is thought that osteointegration of the implant with the surrounding bone (i.e., in the absence of an intervening layer of fibrous tissue) should occur. To obtain osteointegration, it appears that early stability of the implant must be achieved to avoid the immediate formation of a fibrous tissue interface at the bone–prosthesis junction. A number of methods of achieving this using noncemented femoral prosthesis fixation have been subjected to clinical trials with varied success.

Press-fit, porous-coated, and customized prostheses have all been examined in an attempt to achieve early stabilization followed by osteointegration in the absence of bone cement. The early press-fit components suffered from a lack of early mechanical stability, as even with the most precise surgical techniques, only a 10% to 20% initial bony contact could be achieved (74). The lack of bony contact promoted the formation of a fibrous membrane in areas of void, and thus it increased micromotion, bone resorption, and finally implant loosening.

Porous-coated surfaces were then developed in an attempt to encourage bony ingrowth, thus forming a microinterlock and providing a larger available surface area for ongrowth. The majority of the human implant retrieval studies have demonstrated that skeletal attachment by bony ingrowth is not always reliably achieved with porous-coated surfaces. Failure of bony ingrowth with an intervening layer of fibrous tissue between the bone and the implant has often been observed (7,24). Even where microinterlock was said to have been achieved with bone growth into the pores, a thin layer of fibrous membrane frequently separated the prosthesis from the bone. It may be supposed that this fibrous tissue layer might allow movement, the passage of particulate debris, loss of implant material as in bead shedding, and, ultimately, relatively high rates of failure. A porous coating is biologically passive, so that bone may (or may not) grow into the pores, depending on the local environment and stability.

In an attempt to achieve reproducible bone growth onto the implant, trials of bioactive and osteoconductive implant coatings have been carried out with calcium phosphate ceramics. The initial work with hydroxyapatite (HA) showed excellent early stability with early bony union of hydroxyapatite and hydroxyapatite-coated materials to the surrounding bony trabeculae. These encouraging results led to the introduction of hydroxyapatite-coated prostheses in hip surgery.

This chapter gives a brief overview of the history of hydroxyapatite-coated femoral and acetabular prostheses, and a discussion of the laboratory and clinical work behind the use and design of hydroxyapatite-coated implants. The clinical literature on the current usage and survivorship studies with hydroxyapatite femoral and acetabular components will be reviewed, and the theoretical problems encountered using hydroxyapatite-coated prostheses will be discussed.

EXPERIMENTAL STUDIES

Hydroxyapatite and Biocompatibility

Hydroxyapatite as an implant material was initially used for dental reconstructive surgery, providing a material filler or coating in the hope of achieving direct bony bonding and integration. Its excellent early results in this area led to its trial in the field of total joint arthroplasty as poor early results of noncemented hip prostheses highlighted the need for a more reliable method of implant fixation. Centers in the United Kingdom and continental Europe began work on the idea of using bioactive coatings, especially hydroxyapatite-coated implants, in an effort to achieve early stability and the long-term skeletal fixation necessary for bony integration (43,76). We believe, on the basis of unpublished reports, that similar work was also being undertaken at this time in Japan.

Although the great majority of work at this time showed hydroxyapatite to be nontoxic, noninflammatory, and nonallergenic (23,54,56,57), some concerns were raised by laboratory studies in which an inflammatory response to hydroxyapatite suspensions was recorded in rats (28,73). Additional work in canine models has demonstrated increased levels of gelatinase and interleukin-1 (factors both associated with osteolysis) in the membrane around well-fixed canine hydroxyapatite-coated prostheses (1,60). This problem has not been seen in the clinical setting with hydroxyapatite coatings in any form. A single histologic retrieval study (9) identifies hydroxyapatite debris, along with polyethylene and titanium debris, as a possible contributor to osteolysis. However, in this case it was impossible to quantify what part, if any, the hydroxyapatite particles played in inducing an osteolytic reaction when in the presence of other known osteolytic agents. A number of reports have identified the presence of hydroxyapatite particles within the cancellous bony structure without the incitement of any inflammatory reaction (3,37).

The lack of reactivity of host tissues to hydroxyapatite is further supported by the work of Klein et al. (59), who reported excellent biocompatibility with porous calcium phosphate cylinders in rabbit tibiae, as did Bucholz et al. (12) who filled metaphyseal defects in human tibial plateau fractures. Thus, from both the laboratory and clinical evidence available, it appears that calcium phosphate ceramics are biocompatible materials in both animals and humans.

Osteointegration with Hydroxyapatite

After showing no detrimental effects, much of the early research was directed at assessing the bonding and osteoconductive capacity of hydroxyapatite to bone.

With regard to the "adhesive" bond between hydroxyapatite and bone, Geesink et al. (43) inserted hydroxyapatite-coated titanium plugs into dog femora and tested the bone–hydroxyapatite interface strength; they demonstrated a pushout strength of 48.5 megapascals at 6 weeks and 54 MPa at 3 months, with no change in strength over the subsequent 2 years. Histology showed good filling of defects around the implant with bone, preservation of the hydroxyapatite coating, and no fragmentation of the hydroxyapatite coating at 2 years. The coating thickness had, however, decreased from 50 μm, to 10 to 30 μm in most places. As stated by Geesink et al., the shortcoming of this particular study was that the plugs were not mechanically loaded during their time of osteointegration.

At one time, it was thought that hydroxyapatite applied by plasma spray to titanium–aluminum–vanadium (titanium alloy; TiAlV) might form a chemical bond with titanium (47). It is now thought, however, that the bond is purely physical in nature and thus is dependent on the roughness of the substrate (36). In view of this, it is not surprising that similar attachment strengths to hydroxyapatite coatings have been demonstrated with TiAlV and with cobalt–chromium (CoCr) substrates of similar roughness (96). In both cases, the attachment strengths in tension and shear are about the same as the strength of hydroxyapatite itself. These strengths (in tension and shear), like those of most ceramics, are low (ranging from 20 to 50 MPa, depending on a number of factors including coating thickness and the method of application), and it is perhaps for this reason that, in bone, hydroxyapatite requires reinforcement with collagen to provide a composite material with adequate strength in tension and shear.

These considerations make it unlikely that an hydroxyapatite coating on metal could be relied upon to resist tensile and shear stresses applied cyclically over a period of years without risk of fatigue failure. It follows that the long-term clinical stability of hydroxyapatite-coated implants probably does not depend on hydroxyapatite acting over years as an adhesive between metal and bone, but rather on the presence of bone induced by hydroxyapatite to lie in direct contact with a rough metallic surface (Fig. 1).

With regard to osteoconduction, leading to the filling of gaps around an implant, a canine study was performed by Stephenson et al. (92). Titanium alloy plates, grooved on both sides with grooves of various sizes up to 5 mm wide by 3 mm deep, were implanted. One surface of the implant was coated with hydroxyapatite and the other simply shot blasted. It was demonstrated that at 4 and 8 weeks after insertion into the femoral condyles, on the side with the hydroxyapatite coating, bone filled the grooves, whereas on the TiAlV side, bone had grown in to a depth of only about 1 mm. Thus, the presence of hydroxyapatite was demonstrated to induce bone to fill relatively large voids when compared to a TiAlV surface. A number of elegant studies performed by Soballe (84,86,87) confirmed the osteoconductive effects of hydroxyapatite,

enabling bone to bridge gaps of 1 and 2 mm in both mechanically stable and unstable situations. A 1-mm gap around a titanium implant resulted in a 65% reduction in fixation strength when compared to an exact titanium press-fit, whereas no difference was found in the case of a hydroxyapatite-coated implant inserted with and without a gap at 4 weeks (89). The osteogenic effect of hydroxyapatite in enabling bone to bridge small gaps and achieve stable primary fixation is particularly important when one considers that for reasons related to surgical technique, implant design, and anatomic variations between patients, the amount of bone initially in direct contact with the implant occupies only very limited areas (74, 81). In the case of porous-coated prostheses, this may explain the relatively limited areas of bony ingrowth that have been reported, which are combined with larger areas of intervening fibrous membrane where presumably there has been no direct bone–prosthesis contact, nor the appropriate environment to induce bone to bridge the gap.

In summary, hydroxyapatite not only has a capacity to bond to bone but also to induce bone formation. It thus has the effect of filling gaps between an hydroxyapatite-coated implant and its skeletal bed. Viewed in this context, hydroxyapatite can be thought of as analogous to polymethylmethacrylate cement—they both fill gaps, hydroxyapatite by inducing bone formation, and polymethylmethacrylate by being pressurized into the periprosthetic spaces.

Experimental Studies of Loaded Hydroxyapatite-Coated Implants

Geesink et al. (43,47) performed experiments reproducing the physiologic situation in which the interface is repeatedly loaded using hydroxyapatite-coated and non-

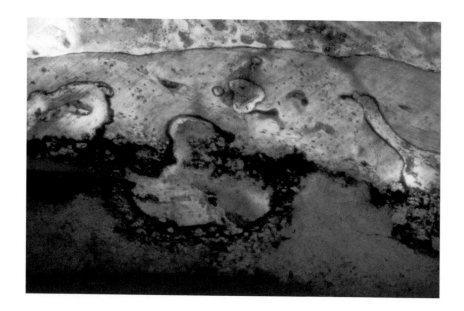

FIG. 1. The interface between an hydroxyapatite (HA)-coated prosthesis and bone, showing resorption of the HA, in a 57-year-old patient. Retrieved 4 years, 7 months after surgery. (Courtesy of Dr. A. J. Malcolm, Department of Pathology, Royal Victoria Infirmary, Newcastle upon Tyne, England.)

coated titanium canine total hip implants. Radiographic and histologic analyses of the implants were carried out at time intervals up to 2 years. Radiographically, a difference was evident from 6 weeks onwards between the hydroxyapatite-coated implants and the noncoated implants, with the former showing a complete lack of radiolucent lines and increased proximal bone density close to the implant. Histologically, the noncoated prostheses were coated with a fibrous tissue membrane from 3 weeks onwards. In contrast, the hydroxyapatite-coated stems consistently showed a "bone-plate" against the implant (usually by 3 weeks), which become stronger and more mineralized with time. Microscopy of the hydroxyapatite coating at 1 and 2 years showed some early resorption of the hydroxyapatite during the bone bonding period. There was no microscopic evidence of fragmentation or coating delamination.

Studies by Soballe et al. (84,88) using a canine model have confirmed more rapid and reliable early skeletal fixation using an hydroxyapatite-coated implant as compared with a porous implant. The ability of an hydroxyapatite-coated implant to encourage the filling of deliberately constructed gaps between cancellous bone and an hydroxyapatite-coated femoral stem subject to micromotion and cyclical loading has also been demonstrated by Soballe et al. (86).

Oonishi et al. (75) examined the bonding strength of hydroxyapatite-coated and non-hydroxyapatite-coated porous implants up to 12 weeks. The hydroxyapatite-coated implants showed a 4-times-greater interface strength than that of the uncoated specimens at 2 weeks, and they were twice as strong at 6 weeks. Twelve weeks after implantation, the strengths were similar. Oonishi et al. felt that the reason the bonding strengths became similar by 12 weeks was that the pull-out test was measuring the strength of the bone around the cylinders, and by this stage both were ingrown. The hydroxyapatite coating of the beads thus provided earlier and stronger fixation simply by accelerating the ingrowth, which, in this experiment, occurred over the first 12 weeks in uncoated specimens.

BIOLOGIC PROPERTIES OF HYDROXYAPATITE COATING

It is well established that although the composition and fabrication details of calcium–phosphate ceramics do not appear to affect their biocompatibility, they do affect the resorption and degradation of the material (2,67). Among these important variations are the Ca:P ratio, the crystallinity, the porosity, and, of course, the thickness of the hydroxyapatite coating. A number of pathways have been postulated for the resorption of the hydroxyapatite, including cell-mediated (osteoclastic resorption), mechanical (delamination or abrasion), and solution-mediated processes. These are affected by both the physical and the chemical composition of the coating material. Because of the variety of application techniques now in use, it is difficult to extrapolate the mechanical and biologic properties reported in one series directly to another series.

The calcium-to-phosphate ratio of calcium ceramics used by different investigators has varied considerably, with a ratio of around 1.67 currently being used for the coating of femoral stems (6,54,65). The crystalline-to-amorphous ratio is also of great importance: the higher the proportion of crystallinity, the slower the bony remodeling and resorption of the hydroxyapatite coating, so that a higher crystallinity is less bioactive but remains attached to the implant for a greater period. The porosity of the coating also affects the rate of dissolution: increased porosity results in a greater available surface area and thus in more rapid bioresorption (97).

The coating thickness affects the mechanical properties of the interface as hydroxyapatite ceramic is relatively weak in shear. Thus an increased coating thickness from 50 μm to 120 μm or 240 μm decreases the ability of an hydroxyapatite-coated implant to withstand shear fatigue (58), but it may prolong the life of the coat in the face of resorption if debonding does not occur.

As the number of human retrieval studies reported is now in excess of 60 (2), it is now possible to piece together a picture of the dynamics of hydroxyapatite-coated implants and how they are affected by the *in vivo* environment. However, because many of the retrievals are relatively short term and were obtained at the time of revision surgery performed because of femoral stem fracture, infection, or pain (i.e., not postmortem), caution is warranted in their interpretation. It should also be remembered, as mentioned, that the hydroxyapatite coating may vary from manufacturer to manufacturer (66).

A number of histologic retrieval studies have demonstrated the osteoinductive effect of hydroxyapatite coatings on early prosthesis fixation in humans, confirming the earlier experimental work in animals. Furlong and Osborn report on four postmortem specimens retrieved 10 days, 17 days, 7 weeks, and 19 weeks postoperatively, showing early fixation of the prosthesis by new bone (42). In the 10-day specimen, new bone formation on the prosthesis surface was demonstrated, with active osteoblasts laying down a layer of bone and osteoid that had reached a thickness of 40 to 100 μm, whereas in the 17-day specimen, "bilateral osteogenesis" was described, with new bone bridging a void from both the cancellous side and from the hydroxyapatite-coated surface itself.

In one case retrieved 3 weeks after implantation (10), new bone was observed along 10% of the hydroxyapatite surface of a femoral component, with osteoid present along an additional 20% of the surface. Hardy et al. (49) examined four hydroxyapatite-coated femoral stems retrieved within 9 months of implantation. In all cases, newly formed bone was observed overlying the hydrox-

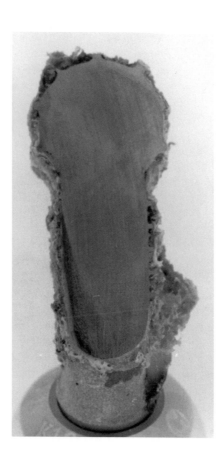

FIG. 2. A Freeman HA-coated femoral prosthesis revised to a Girdlestone's at 2 years for severe acetabular deficiency after shattering of the ceramic head. Extensive contact between the cancellous bone and the HA coating in the macroscopic specimen **(A)** and in the same specimen sectioned obliquely through the hydroxyapatite coating **(B)** is demonstrated.

A,B

yapatite with trabecular bridging, anchoring the prosthesis to the endosteal bone layer. In this series, good bony fixation was seen in a case of severe osteoporosis and in a case of infection, with no apparent deleterious effects on osteointegration. Soballe et al. (85) presented the histology of a retrieval specimen from an osteoporotic 98-year-old woman showing 48% of the hydroxyapatite surface covered by bone. Scanning electron microscopy showed direct contact between the hydroxyapatite and bone without any perceptible boundary between the newly formed bone and the hydroxyapatite ceramic. This suggests that the biologic response to hydroxyapatite-coated femoral stems is not affected by age or osteoporosis.

We have examined two retrieval specimens of Freeman hydroxyapatite-coated stems that were revised for infection and malposition. The histologic appearance in both was consistent with the findings described previously of excellent bony apposition and fixation at the time of revision (38) (Fig. 2).

A possible danger of an hydroxyapatite coating was identified by Bloebaum et al. (8), who reported on the histologic analysis of 14 patients and their retrieved hydroxyapatite-coated implants. Five of this group were revised for osteolysis. In these cases, hydroxyapatite, polyethylene, and metal particles were all present in the osteolytic regions of the periprosthetic tissue, along with an inflammatory infiltrate. The authors presented evidence for the migration of hydroxyapatite granules to the articular sur-

face, where they were found embedded in the polyethylene liner, suggesting a possible source of hydroxyapatite debris caused by third-body wear. Bloebaum et al. (8) stated that it was not possible to determine which of the three particles caused the osteolysis around the femoral stem and the subsequent component loosening.

There is no doubt from the evidence thus far provided by the histologic retrieval studies that, with time, the hydroxyapatite coating is removed from the prosthesis surface (Fig. 3). In a retrieval analysis, Bauer et al. (3) presented five hydroxyapatite-coated femoral stems retrieved from three patients at autopsy, with an *in situ* duration ranging from 5 to 25 months (mean, 12 months). They demonstrated the presence of remodeling canals in the hydroxyapatite coating with the resorption of bone and adjacent hydroxyapatite by osteoclasts in one specimen that was *in situ* for 9 months. In another case retrieved at 4.5 months after arthroplasty, granules of hydroxyapatite were demonstrated in the adjacent bone marrow, and on areas of the prosthesis the hydroxyapatite appeared to have entirely disappeared, leaving bone in direct contact with the metal stem (3). A variable amount of direct bony apposition to the femoral stem (32% to 78%) was reported, with the deposition of bone occurring most prominently in areas close to the endosteal surface.

Buma et al. (13) reported the histology of a bipolar hip prosthesis that was revised for severe mid-thigh pain at 4

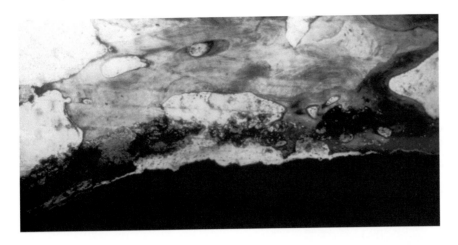

FIG. 3. The interface between an HA-coated prosthesis and bone in a 67-year-old patient, showing the separation of the HA from the metal. Retrieved 3 years, 2 months after surgery. (Courtesy of Dr. A. J. Malcolm, Department of Pathology, Royal Victoria Infirmary, Newcastle upon Tyne, England.)

years after implantation. In this study, histologic examination failed to reveal any trace of the hydroxyapatite coating persisting on the prosthesis, and there was trabecular bone closely adhering to the prosthetic contour. At the site of the bone–metal interface, titanium wear particles were found, both in the macrophages and in the surrounding bone. The cause of the pain in this patient was not determined.

Frayssinet et al. (37) reported the results of 10 *en bloc* retrievals from autopsy specimens of femoral prostheses from 5 days to 26 months after surgery. Two specimens were examined 2 years after insertion, and in one the hydroxyapatite coating was found to be almost totally removed, especially in the metaphyseal area. Some preservation of the coating was reported in areas partially protected by bony tissue covering the hydroxyapatite layer. Noted in these cases were good fixation and apposition of bone to the implant's titanium surface where it had once been covered by hydroxyapatite.

Although the picture is far from conclusive, at the present time it appears that hydroxyapatite coating promotes excellent (but not 100%) early osteointegration without the presence of an intervening fibrous membrane. Variable loss of the hydroxyapatite coating from the stem occurs over time, possibly leading to complete loss as early as 2 years after implantation. Thus, after use has been made of the "chemical induction" of bone onto the prosthesis, the long-term success of the implant must rely on the mechanical fixation produced by the interlock. This is achieved when bone replaces hydroxyapatite and then comes into direct contact with the underlying prosthesis. Long-term fixation cannot depend on adhesion between bone and hydroxyapatite. It seems likely that the amount of hydroxyapatite remaining on successful surviving implants, some of which are now approaching 10 years, is, at best, the same amount as that found in histologic retrievals after much shorter time periods. Indeed, it is probably significantly less.

In summary, it appears that hydroxyapatite acts not as an adhesive, but as a bioactive material promoting and accelerating direct contact between itself and bone over the course of the first postoperative weeks. Once this fixation has been achieved, the hydroxyapatite is gradually (i.e., over years) replaced by bone. The effectiveness of late fixation then depends on the material, the shape, and the surface finish of the implant itself, not on the hydroxyapatite.

PROSTHESIS DESIGN

Prosthetic Shape and Surface

The principles of hydroxyapatite-coated prosthesis design are the same as those of any other cementless prosthesis (39). The goal is to achieve early stability and long-term fixation to surrounding bone (Fig. 4).

A number of methods of creating surface asperities have been tried, with the aim of providing stability of the implant both at the time of implantation, before bone has had the opportunity to grow onto the hydroxyapatite coating, and in the long term, when the hydroxyapatite coating has been lost. Surface ridges can provide good macrointerlock and, when coated with hydroxyapatite, bone tends to grow into the grooves (92), providing excellent fixation (38,40,61). Hydroxyapatite coating of porous surfaces has also been demonstrated to provide good stability for osteointegration (75). Other possible ways of providing surface asperities include shot-blasting (35), electrical etching, and cast-in asperities. At the present time, it is unclear which of these configurations results in the best long-term clinical outcome.

Proximally or Fully Coated Prostheses

Both proximally and fully coated prostheses are currently being used, and differences in their survival rates or postoperative function have not yet been reported. Those who use stems with a proximal hydroxyapatite coating

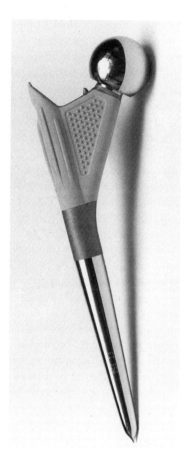

FIG. 4. The Freeman proximally HA-coated femoral prosthesis.

are attempting to avoid the proximal stress shielding that might occur with a distally fixed implant. On the other hand, the Furlong (H.-A.C.) prosthesis (41) uses a fully coated stem with the aim of providing the maximum possible area for bony attachment. To date, no remarkable proximal bone loss has been reported. This supports the finding, based on finite element analysis, that there is little advantage to be gained, with respect to the avoidance of proximal stress-shielding, by the use of a proximally coated instead of a fully coated prosthesis (100). Weinans et al. (100) reported a reduction from 54% to 50% in the amount of bone that might be resorbed proximally, comparing a proximally one-third-coated prosthesis to a fully coated one, respectively. Engh's experience with porous coating suggests that fully coated stems might produce radiographically visible stress shielding only when large-diameter (and therefore stiff) stems are used in osteoporotic femora. Only time will tell whether either the proximal or fully coated femoral prosthesis is superior in terms of survivorship or clinical results. Another factor to consider in the choice of proximal or full coating is the ease of extraction in the event of revision surgery. A proximally coated prosthesis has the advantage that it is easily removed with minimal bony destruction. In contrast,

access to the distal bone–prosthesis interface is virtually impossible without significant bony destruction.

THE CHOICE OF PROSTHETIC MATERIAL

Since the early days of total joint arthroplasty, the choice of material and method of manufacture of the femoral prosthesis has been of importance, with the method of failure of many early prostheses being catastrophic fatigue failure of the stem at its maximal stress concentration points. These problems have now been largely overcome thanks to better metallurgy and manufacturing techniques. However, the choice of metal or alloy is still important with regard to the bonding strength to the applied hydroxyapatite coating (and possibly the bone itself), stem elasticity, and the possibility of wear of exposed metal from abrasion by the surrounding bone.

Conflicting reports have been published as to whether or not the bond strength between titanium alloy (TiAlV) and hydroxyapatite is any stronger than that of other alloys such as chrome–cobalt (CrCo). Researchers at Plasma Biotal (Tideswell, Derbyshire UK, personal communication, 1995) have performed comparative bonding-strength tests on titanium and CrCo alloys, with varying thicknesses of hydroxyapatite. They reported a 20-MPa bond strength in these studies for both TiAlV and CoCr, and they showed that, with increasing thickness, the pull-off strength decreases. Others feel that a TiAlV substrate is preferable, because at the elevated temperatures used in plasma spraying, hydroxyapatite is thought to be more chemically reactive with titanium than with CrCo and thus may produce a chemical bond (45). However, there is significant variability in shear strength between different manufacturers' hydroxyapatite coatings (58).

The elasticity of the prosthesis is dependent both on the stem design and on the modulus of the material. The modulus of elasticity of CoCr (210 GPa) is approximately double that of titanium (110 GPa). As shown in both computer simulation (99) and animal experiments (11), there is a close relationship between stem stiffness and stress shielding. Stress-shielding and bone resorption are significantly less around a more flexible stem. Although this is important if trying to maximize fit and fill with a large bulky prosthesis, a similar decrease in elasticity can be achieved either by designing a stem in TiAlV (as opposed to CoCr) or by decreasing the diameter in CoCr by 2 mm. Finite element analysis studies have shown that as the stem stiffness and stress shielding decrease, the proximal interface stresses increase (53). Thus, although there are advantages in using a more flexible stem to avoid stress shielding, the potential increase in shear stresses proximally at the hydroxyapatite–prosthesis interface may pose a more serious problem. Thus, the clinical advantage of flexible stems in this situation, whether achieved by using a more flexible material or a stem of smaller diameter, is questionable (52).

Unfortunately, TiAlV has been shown to be susceptible to abrasive wear against bone, because it is a softer alloy than CoCr, and therefore there is a risk of increased metallic particulate debris and a possibility of osteolysis if any micromotion does occur between the stem and the surrounding bone (5). Furthermore, there is a potential link between Alzheimer's disease and long-term aluminum absorption (34,93), and aluminum may theoretically leach from a TiAlV prosthesis or from its particulate debris. Today, the most commonly used alloy for hydroxyapatite-coated prostheses still remains TiAlV, but the concerns expressed here have led the authors of this chapter to revert to the use of an hydroxyapatite-coated CoCr stem and acetabulum until these potential problems are settled.

THE NATURAL HISTORY OF THE HYDROXYAPATITE–METAL INTERFACE

The strength of the hydroxyapatite–metal interface is of importance in the short and long term. In the short term, a secure bond at this junction might be expected to prevent delamination of the hydroxyapatite coating and the possibility of third-body wear from particles that may migrate to the joint surface, as has been reported (8,15, 63). In the long term, the crucial issue is whether hydroxyapatite acts as a "glue," permanently anchoring the implant to the surrounding skeleton and thus being permanently subjected to cyclical shear and tensile stresses, with the consequential risk of fatigue (42,47,51), or whether it is resorbed and remodeled by invading haversian systems, thus eventually being replaced completely by bone interlocked directly with the metal implant (see Figs. 1,3). The method of application of the coating is of importance in achieving a strong final hydroxyapatite-metal interface bond. Plasma spraying currently attains the strongest fixation.

Manley et al. (66) evaluated the hydroxyapatite coating applied by four independent coaters. Although the chemical compositions were similar, crystallinity ranged from 35% to 50% and porosity ranged from 5% to 15%. Interface shear strength at 3, 6, and 12 weeks was performed on retrieved canine specimens and found to vary by more than 100% (2.6 to 6.3 MPa) at 3 weeks and 400% (2.6 to 10.5 MPa) at 12 weeks. Histologic differences at the tissue–implant interface were also noted at 12 weeks, with coating fragmentation occurring in 2 of the 4 coaters' specimens. It is postulated that variability in results from different studies may be related to differences in coating techniques.

If one takes the view that the hydroxyapatite is required to achieve permanent stability by acting as an adhesive, the surface geometry of the implant must be designed in such a way as to take advantage of the strength of the hydroxyapatite–metal interface in compression, while avoiding the interface being loaded in shear or tension, because under these conditions the fatigue strength of hydroxyapatite is significantly less. This can be achieved by providing either a macrointerlock with proximal ridges to counter rotational forces on the prosthesis, or a microinterlock with hydroxyapatite over a porous-beaded coating, as suggested by Oonishi et al. (75).

As it now appears (see preceding), the hydroxyapatite coating is progressively resorbed and replaced by bone in direct apposition to the metal stem (21). Thus, the eventual stability of the (originally) hydroxyapatite-coated prosthesis will once again depend on interlock between the bone and the prosthesis. Thus interlocking is needed to reduce tensile and shear forces at the bone–implant interface, whether one is relying on permanent hydroxyapatite adhesion or on direct contact of the metal stem to an adjacent layer of bone.

In summary, it appears probable that the incorporation of an hydroxyapatite-coated prosthesis spans three phases. In the first phase, starting at the moment of implantation and lasting about 3 to 6 weeks, the hydroxyapatite coat unites with the "injured" adjacent bone. Provided the prosthesis is sufficiently immobile in its osseous bed, this process ends with bony union. If, however, the initial press-fit is unstable, fibrous union might occur, leading ultimately to loosening. The first phase gives way to the second as union becomes complete. The implant is then fixed, partly by mechanical interlock at the "micro"-level and partly by adhesion between the prosthesis and hydroxyapatite and between the hydroxyapatite and bone. This phase may last for years, but, during it, the hydroxyapatite and the periprosthetic bone are remodeled, leading to a gradual replacement of the hydroxyapatite with living cancellous bone. The latter can form in direct contact with the surface of the implant, adding microinterlock with the surface roughness on the prosthesis to the already existing macrointerlock. In the third phase (i.e., when the preceding process is complete), fixation no longer depends on hydroxyapatite but instead is entirely attributable to mechanical micro- and macrointerlock.

CLINICAL RESULTS

Because hydroxyapatite-coated femoral components have now been used clinically for 10 years (41), a broad spectrum of medium-term clinical results of hydroxyapatite-coated femoral stems have been recently published (18,27,44,94) along with a number of short-term results. The results are encouraging, showing survival rates comparable to any cemented series and clinically overcoming the problems (e.g., thigh pain) experienced by the earlier

TABLE 1. *Summary of published hydroxyapatite (HA) femoral component clinical trial data*

Author (ref.)	HA hips (N)	Age (mean yr)	Male (%)	OA (%)	Follow-up (ave. yr)	Comp. study	Revision ASL (%)	Revision total (%)	Migration	Pain (%)	RLL (%)	Lysis (%)
Clinical/x-ray												
Geesink (46)	125	53	37	59	7	no	0	0	0 gross	4	0	0
Capello (18)	291	50	61	62	6	no	0.34	1.7	0 gross	8	0	0.34
Capello (17)	133	38	60.9	43	6	no	0	3	0 gross	2.3	4.5	
Thomas et al. (94)	50	58	62	100	5	no	0	0	NA	5.6	0	0
Dambreville et al. (27)	375	60	53	96	4	pc	0	0.3	NA	0.3	5.6	NA
McPherson et al. (69)	42	55	57.1	—	3	pc	2.4	2.4	NA	4.8	10	2.4
Petit (77)143	59.5	45.4	85	2+	no	0	0	0 gross	5.6	0.7	NA	
Tonino et al. (95)	222	62.7	36.5	75	2	no	0	1.8	NA	3.6	0	NA
Rossi et al.(80)	100	63	34	64	2+	no	0	1	NA	NA	21	NA
Mancini et al. (64)	135	62.7	48.1	72	2.2	no	0	0.7	0 gross	6	0.7	NA
Vidalain, ARTRO (98)	4770	59.2	58	71		no	0	0.33	NA	2	NA	0.5
Epinette (32)	1163	65.5	NA	80	303, 5 yr	no	0.1	1.6	NA	1.1	NA	0
RSA study												
Soballe et al. (90)	7	56.8	NA	—	1	ps	0	0	0.4 mm/yr	NA	NA	NA
Karrholm et al. (55)	23	56	91.7	69	2	c,pc	0	0	NA	NA	NA	NA
Kroon et al. (61)	26	51.9	61.5	92	1	pf,c	0	0	0.12 mm/yr	0	0	0

OA, osteoarthritis; comp., comparative; ASL, aseptic loosening; RLL, radiolucent lines; RSA, radiostereometry; pc, porous coat; ps, plasma spray; c, cemented; pf, press-fit.

generations of nonhydroxyapatite-coated, noncemented prostheses. This is also the experience of the authors of this chapter.

The results of these clinical and radiologic outcome analyses are summarized in Table 1 and will be discussed under the following headings: paired studies, survival studies, survival of the Freeman prosthesis, and survival in the younger patient.

The Effect of Hydroxyapatite Coating versus Press-Fit or Porous Coating in "Paired Series"

There have been a number of studies performed using prostheses of identical geometry, comparing a proximal hydroxyapatite coating with a porous-coated or press-fit prosthesis (22,27,48,55,61,69,90). These studies have demonstrated superior clinical and radiologic results for the hydroxyapatite-coated prostheses over either porous-coated or press-fit prostheses, with mean follow-up of 4 years or less. These studies report superior clinical results in terms of pain relief, functional ability, and radiologic evidence, and with regard to bone bonding to the prosthesis, the absence of radiolucent lines, and the absence of lytic lesions adjacent to the prosthesis in the

femoral canal. This suggests that the use of an hydroxyapatite coating enhances prosthetic fixation to the skeleton, limiting the effective joint space (82). The bone–prosthesis interface provides a relatively impermeable barrier, more efficiently preventing the ingress of particulate debris to any significant depth in the well-fixed stem than does either a press-fit or a porous-coated surface alone.

However, McPherson et al. (69) showed no difference in the clinical results at a minimum of 3 years, between a group of patients with hydroxyapatite-coated porous-coated femoral stems and a control group of non-hydroxyapatite-coated porous-coated femoral stems studied on a prospective randomized basis using matched groups. In the hydroxyapatite-coated group, follow-up roentgenograms showed relatively more bone remodeling and proximal cancellous hypertrophy. It should be noted that both groups had overall hip scores in excess of 95% good or excellent; the number of patients included was relatively small and the follow-up period was short. In addition, Karrholm et al. (55) reviewed a group of cemented, porous-coated, and hydroxyapatite-coated hips with clinical ratings and roentgen stereophotogrammetry (RSA). Only 35% of cemented stems demonstrated RSA, whereas 90% of hydroxyapatite and porous stems did.

Harris Hip Scores were significantly lower in the hydroxyapatite group: 81 points versus 94 in the cemented and 89 in the porous group.

Survival Studies of Hydroxyapatite-Coated Femoral Stems

There were no revisions for aseptic loosening in two published series with a mean follow-up of more than 5 years (46,94). A single case was revised in one further series (18).

The longest clinical survival series published to date is that by Geesink (46), who reported 125 hips in 100 patients with an average follow-up of 7 years (range, 6 to 8 years) using the Omnifit (Osteonics Corporation, Allendale, NJ) system. He reported excellent short- and medium-term clinical results with only 4% of cases having moderate pain at 12 months. In this study, no femoral stems were revised, and osteointegration occurred in all cases, with no radiologic evidence of aseptic loosening. A single case of excessive polyethylene wear resulting in acetabular osteolysis that required revision of the acetabular component at 5.5 years was reported in a young patient.

Capello (18) has presented the results of a multicenter study of the same prosthesis (Omnifit) in 291 hip replace-ments with a 5- to 7-year follow-up. In this series, one case has been revised for aseptic loosening and three for persisting pain, giving a combined clinical and mechanical failure rate of 1.7% at 5 to 7 years follow-up. They saw no case of intramedullary osteolysis (16,26).

Experience with Hydroxyapatite-Coated Prostheses

The authors of this chapter have been using a proximally hydroxyapatite-coated prosthesis since 1989 (see Fig. 4). (Prior to that, a prosthesis of similar geometry employing press-fit shot-blasted TiAlV fixation was used.) Cemented fixation of this prosthesis has been used continuously since 1983. Patients underwent clinical and radiologic examination, initially at 6 months, then annually till 3 years, and then every other year, and survival data was collected. Based on a standard radiographic series, using an Orthographics digitizing tablet (Orthographics, Salt Lake City, UT), vertical migration of the femoral stem was measured. Each x-ray was qualitatively examined for the presence of radiolucent lines, osteolysis, proximal osteoporosis, femoral neck resorption, and cortical hypertrophy (28b).

In this series of 115 hydroxyapatite-coated femoral stems (range, 2 to 7 years postoperatively; mean, 4 years), there have been no revisions for aseptic loosening. Two

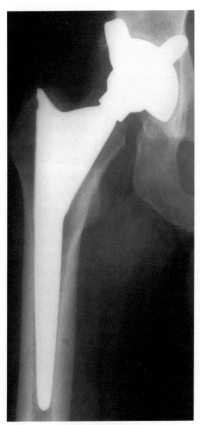 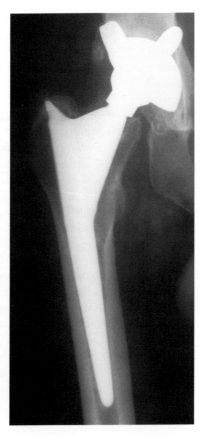

A,B

FIG. 5. Radiograph of an HA-coated femoral prosthesis at 3 months **(A)** and 7 years **(B)** after insertion.

stems have required removal: one for infection (see Fig. 2) and one as part of a Girdlestone conversion for a shattered ceramic femoral head (in a case of massive acetabular deficiency) versus a cemented survival of 222 out of 223 for this time period. Clinically, patients having hydroxyapatite-coated femoral prostheses had less postoperative pain than those with the similar press-fit shotblast TiAlV prosthesis and were indistinguishable from those with cemented prostheses. It is noteworthy that the population age of the hydroxyapatite-coated group of patients (mean, 52.0 yr; SD ± 11.9 yr) was significantly less than that of the cemented group (mean, 68.8 yr; SD ± 6.7 yr), which might have led to the expectation of a worse result in the former group. Radiographically, the hydroxyapatite-coated group showed fewer radiolucent lines ($p < .05$) than either the smooth press-fit or ridged press-fit stems (0%, 62%, and 38%, respectively, at 5 years). The incidence of radiolucent lines in the cemented group at 5 years was 9%. There was no evidence of osteolysis in the hydroxyapatite-coated group at any location other than at the level of neck resection. Thus, to date the hydroxyapatite-coated femoral stems have performed as well as or better than cemented stems, and significantly better than smooth or ridged shot-blasted TiAlV stems of similar geometry. Figure 5 shows radiographs of a typical hydroxyapatite-coated femoral prosthesis at 6 months and at 7 years, with good proximal fixation and no evidence of radiolucent lines or osteolytic lesions.

Survival of Hydroxyapatite-Coated Femoral Prostheses in the Younger Patient

Perhaps the main surgical indication for the use of a noncemented prosthesis is younger age. Both Capello (17) and Geesink (46) reported excellent results for total hip arthroplasty in the younger patient. The findings of the authors of this chapter have already been described.

Capello (17) presented, as a subgroup of his hydroxyapatite study group, the results of 133 hip replacements performed on a population aged from 18 years to 49 years (mean, 39 years), with a 5- to 7-year follow-up. In this group, there was a combined clinical and mechanical failure rate of 2.3%, with two cases revised for persisting pain and no cases for proven aseptic loosening. Of interest in this group was the high incidence of scalloping, perhaps a result of osteolysis, at the cut edge of the femoral neck (40%), with one case of definite intramedullary lysis. This may possibly reflect increased polyethylene wear debris caused by the high demands of the younger age group. The group had an average Harris Hip Score of 94, with 89% reporting no or only slight hip pain. Thus, for the specified time period, these results compare favorably to any other series of cemented or noncemented hip arthroplasties in the younger age groups.

Geesink (44) reported the 6-year results of 118 hydroxyapatite-coated total hip replacements in a group of patients aged 21 to 65 (mean, 53 yr). The survival rate at a mean of 6 years was 100% with an average Harris Hip Score of 98 after the first 3 years.

As already described, the authors of this chapter have obtained 100% survival (for aseptic loosening) at a maximum follow-up of 7 years (mean, 4 years) in 150 hydroxyapatite-coated prostheses in a population with a mean age of 52 years.

RADIOGRAPHIC ASSESSMENT

Migration Studies

Work has been performed comparing the migration of hydroxyapatite-coated femoral stems with press-fit TiAlV stems of similar geometry (40,61,83) and with porous-coated stems (55,90,91). The migration of hydroxyapatite-coated components was shown to be significantly less than that of either press-fit or porous-coated prostheses. This finding suggests that the hydroxyapatite-coated prosthesis should be less likely to require revision for aseptic loosening (40).

In our own experience (28b), there is no statistically significant difference in the migration of the hydroxyapatite-coated prostheses and cemented prostheses of similar geometry up to 6 years postoperatively. Both the cemented and the hydroxyapatite-coated stems have a significantly lower migration rate than do a series of smooth and ridged shot-blasted press-fit TiAlV stems of the same geometry ($p < .05$). The reduced migration of both the cemented and hydroxyapatite group correlated with a decreased rate of revision for aseptic loosening.

Radiolucent and Reactive Lines

Both radiodense and radiolucent lines are very rare around the hydroxyapatite-coated portion of femoral prostheses (see Table 1) (28b). This presumably reflects the almost invariable presence of a close bond between the hydroxyapatite and the surrounding bone.

Around the non-hydroxyapatite-coated portion of the prosthesis, thin radiodense lines can sometimes be distinguished from the prosthesis itself (33). Any implant (e.g., a nail) in the medullary canal becomes encapsulated in a thin plate of bone that is radiodense. If this radiodense "reactive" line is in contact with the implant, it cannot be detected radiographically. In the case of a proximally hydroxyapatite-coated and bonded femoral prosthesis, very small movements could be expected between the distal stem and the bone as a consequence of bending and/or axial compression in the diaphysis. Such movements will produce slight but visible separation between the reactive line and the prosthesis, but the intervening radiolucent line is too thin to be measured and the prosthesis *in toto* is not loose.

Radiolucent lines of measurable width (e.g., 1 to 2 mm) are common around press-fit implants, but they have not been seen, save rarely in one zone, around hydroxyapatite-coated prostheses (see Table 1).

Similarly, endosteal lysis is rare around hydroxyapatite-coated prostheses, but this may be a consequence of the relatively short follow-up time. "Spot-welds" have been reported (25), but they are rare in our experience. Intramedullary new bone beyond the tip of the stem (often referred to as pedestal formation) occurs occasionally, probably as a consequence of surgical interference with the canal beyond the prosthesis.

In our experience (unpublished), the incidence of both proximal osteoporosis and calcar resorption in hydroxyapatite-coated prostheses is minimal, being significantly less than that occurring in cemented femoral components measured at 5 years ($p < .05$). This may perhaps be explained by reference to Wolf's law, with proximal fixation, induced by the hydroxyapatite coating, resulting in increased stress transfer through the proximal femur, thus preserving bone stock or even increasing it.

Thus, although the interpretation of radiolucent and radiodense lines is imprecise (68), in general the use of an hydroxyapatite-coated prosthesis results in a stable prosthesis with good proximal bony ingrowth that may be able to form a seal, protecting the more distal endosteal bone from osteolysis and the consequences of wear debris.

THE HYDROXYAPATITE-COATED ACETABULAR COMPONENT

Reviews of the fate of cemented acetabular cups show aseptic loosening to be the greatest concern (14). As with noncemented femoral prostheses, the critical factor required for the survival of a noncemented acetabular component is initial stable skeletal fixation. This allows direct bone apposition to the prosthesis, rather than the development of an intervening fibrous tissue membrane. Numerous techniques have been suggested to obtain stable acetabular fixation, with varied success, including screw-in cups, pegged cups, inserting oversized implants, expanding cups, the use of stabilization screws, and porous coatings. However in contrast to the femoral bone–prosthesis interface, where significant shear forces occur, the acetabular cup is loaded mainly in compression, thus raising questions about the actual importance of a direct bone–prosthesis interface at the acetabulum.

Most authors have used metal-backed high-density polyethylene (HDP) and then sprayed the metal liner with hydroxyapatite. However, concerns have been raised regarding acetabular polyethylene thickness in metal-backed prostheses. Examination of cemented metal-backed acetabular sockets has revealed higher stresses and subsequently more wear than in cemented all-polyethylene components that have a thicker polyethylene layer (78). This has led to some concern that any metal-backed noncemented acetabular prosthesis with thinner polyethylene liners may generate more polyethylene wear debris than cemented all-polyethylene cups (79).

Comparative studies between acetabular components of identical geometry, with one group having a coating of hydroxyapatite, have been reported in the literature. Cartillier (19) reported the results of a retrospective multicenter trial of 2432 hydroxyapatite-coated and 1130 uncoated screw-in acetabular cups. The hydroxyapatite group was reported to have a failure rate of 0.53% (revised for malposition or infection) as compared to 8.14% in the uncoated group (revised for aseptic loosening). There was said to be no evidence of cup migration in any hydroxyapatite-coated prosthesis (although this observation might have been difficult to make on such a large number of prostheses). In those cases of hydroxyapatite-coated prostheses that were revised, histologic analysis revealed bony ongrowth in the absence of intervening fibrous tissue (19). However, neither the number of patients lost to follow-up, nor the method of follow-up, was reported, thus making conclusions difficult to draw in this particular study.

Measurement of proximal migration in two groups of identical textured, pegged CoCr acetabular components, one with an hydroxyapatite coating (69 hips) and the other uncoated (40 hips), was performed by Moilanen et al. (71). Radiographically, at 2 to 3 years there were fewer radiolucent lines in the hydroxyapatite-coated group, and there was a trend towards a smaller vertical migration rate (0.06 mm/yr) than in the noncoated group (0.08 mm/yr). The change in the inclination angle between the two groups differed significantly: the inclination in the hydroxyapatite group increased by 0.08°/year, and that in the noncoated group by 0.44°/year ($p = .023$). There was no difference clinically in this time period between the two groups. These findings suggest that an hydroxyapatite coating enhances the stability of the acetabular component.

Geesink (46) reported the results, at follow-up of 6 to 8 years, of 125 hydroxyapatite-coated hips in which a screw-in acetabular cup was used. There was a complete absence of radiolucent lines around hydroxyapatite-coated prostheses and no evidence of migration. One cup developed a radiolucent line in zone 1. In one case, a 23-year-old woman showed rapid progressive polyethylene wear with severe osteolysis at the bone implant junction. At the time of revision, the cause of the severe wear was ascertained to be femoral neck impingement upon the polyethylene lip. Hydroxyapatite particles could not be identified in the polyethylene liner.

Epinette and Edinin (personal communication, 1996) studied 107 Arc2f acetabular cups (a screw-in prosthesis with supplementary dome screws) in 104 patients (mean age, 63 years) with a minimum follow-up of 5 years. They found no instances of continuous three-zone radiolucency and no measurable migration at 5 years. They found an

TABLE 2. *Summary of hydroxyapatite-coated acetabular results*

Author (ref.)	Hips (N)	Age (mean yr)	Male (%)	Follow-up (ave. yr)	Comp. study	Revision ASL (%)	Revision total (%)	Migration	Pain (%)	RLL (%)	Lysis (%)
Capello et al. (16)	152	50	57	5.5	no	10.5	19.1	NA	2/152	NA	6
Geesink and Hoefnagels (44)	111	52	425	6.2	no	0	0.9	NA	0	NA	0.9
Epinette (32)	107	63	40	5.0	no	0	0	NA	0	NA	3
Cartillier (19)	2432	NA	NA	5	yes	0	0.5	0	0	NA	0
Duthoit et al. (31)	50	NA	NA	>6	yes	0	NA	0	NA	0	0
Moilanen et al. (71)	69			2	yes	—	—	0.06 mm/yr	NA	—	—

Comp., comparative; ASL, aseptic loosening; RLL, radiolucent lines.

incidence of acetabular osteolysis of 3%. No revisions were reported for aseptic loosening in this 5-year period.

In contrast to Epinette and Edinin, Capello (personal communication, 1995) studied 152 hydroxyapatite-coated metal-backed acetabular prostheses in a population with a mean age of 50. After follow-up of 5.5 years, 16 of 152 hips (10.5%) required revision for aseptic loosening (an overall revision rate of 19.1%). One explanation for the increased failure rate might be that the geometry differs from that in the previous series. Capello used a press-fit prosthesis that was spherical proximally and cylindrical distally, compared to the screw-in prostheses used by the previous authors. Capello's series, with the higher failure rate, possibly had a less stable macrointerlock than the ancillary screw-in immediate stabilization or the supplementary superior dome screws employed by the other reported designs (Table 2).

Thus, the short- to medium-term results of hydroxyapatite-coated acetabular cups appears promising, provided the basic design of the implant as a press-fit is good. The comparative studies show them to be an advance over the identical noncoated implants. The larger series show results comparable to those of cemented acetabular cups for the same period. However, as with the femoral prosthesis, the hydroxyapatite coating must eventually be resorbed and the integrity of the permanent fixation of the prosthesis will then depend on the design of the underlying prosthesis.

Hydroxyapatite Debris, Polyethylene Wear, and Osteolysis

Although the advantages of the osteoconductive properties of hydroxyapatite and its ability to stabilize the implant at an early stage have been well documented, concerns persist with regard to the long-term survival of the coating and its bond to the metallic substrate. These raise the risks of accelerated high-density polyethylene wear and of osteolysis caused by the hydroxyapatite debris.

Morscher (72) drew attention to the possibility of delamination of the hydroxyapatite coating, with the free particles lodging in the polyethylene acetabular liner and contributing to accelerated early wear caused by third-body abrasion of both the metal head and the polyethylene insert. In support of this view, Bloebaum et al. (8) demonstrated the presence of hydroxyapatite particles in the polyethylene insert in five cases revised for osteolysis out of 12 retrievals. The presence of hydroxyapatite particles in the polyethylene insert was found to correlate with scratching and burnishing on the superior regions of the articulating metal head and with excessive polyethylene wear. Similar work presented by Campbell et al. (15) demonstrated the presence of increased acetabular polyethylene scratching and increased burnishing of the corresponding titanium femoral heads in a group of retrieved hydroxyapatite-coated prostheses compared to a similar group of press-fit and cemented prostheses.

This report is contradicted by a number of studies. Hong et al. (50) suggested that free hydroxyapatite particles would be entirely confined by bony ongrowth, so that if separation occurred they would not be free to migrate to the articulating surface. In support of this view, a comparison of the surface roughness of 15 modular heads from retrieved hydroxyapatite-coated femoral stems compared with porous-coated and cemented femoral components was reported (4). Although all groups showed increased surface roughness over the initial manufacturer's specifications, the heads from the hydroxyapatite-coated group showed significantly less surface roughness, with fewer deep scratches than either the porous or cemented groups. Furthermore, analysis of the polyethylene liners from the patients with hydroxyapatite-coated stems showed no evidence of embedded ceramic particles. In the largest long-term series of hydroxyapatite-coated stems reported to date, Geesink (44) reported no radiographic evidence of increased polyethylene wear over normal values.

Dambreville and Lautridou (27) compared the mean annual polyethylene acetabular wear in a large series of porous-coated versus hydroxyapatite-coated femoral prostheses; they found no statistically significant difference between the two groups. The hydroxyapatite group actually had a smaller (though not statistically significant) mean annual polyethylene wear than did the porous-coated group. Moilanen et al. (71) compared the wear rate over 2 to 3 years in 69 hydroxyapatite-coated acetabular cups with that in 40 uncoated acetabular cups. They found no increase in the radiographically measured proximal linear wear in the hydroxyapatite-coated group over this period.

Thus, on balance, third-body wear caused by hydroxyapatite particles does not appear to be a clinical problem and indeed may be less of a problem than similar wear caused by detached metal beads or fragments of cement.

The other potential danger from free particles of hydroxyapatite is osteolysis associated with their possible resorption by macrophages. Although in one histologic study hydroxyapatite particles were noted in lytic bone cavities, they were accompanied by metal and polyethylene particles, so it was not possible to determine which of these was responsible for the osteolysis (9). In other reports of both animal and human studies, hydroxyapatite particles have been identified within histiocytes without osteolysis.

Intramedullary osteolysis is found (but not often) adjacent to hydroxyapatite-coated femoral stems. This probably reflects a tight seal around the implant formed by the ongrowth of bone onto the hydroxyapatite, which prevents polyethylene particles and other wear debris from accessing the bone–prosthesis interface and inducing lysis more distally around the stem. It also indicates that hydroxyapatite particles, if they are present, do not cause osteolysis. Thus, on present evidence, it seems unlikely that an hydroxyapatite coating causes osteolysis.

CONCLUSIONS

Hydroxyapatite coatings applied by plasma spray to orthopedic implants were first used clinically in 1985. Today, it is clear that the coating is biocompatible and that it induces bone to form on its surface. By doing this, the hydroxyapatite coat causes bone to fill residual gaps between the implant and the skeleton, interlocking with asperities on the implant surface as it does so. This process occurs rapidly—perhaps in as little as 3 weeks after implantation. Although newly formed bone adheres to the hydroxyapatite coat, it is likely that adhesion contributes little or nothing to the long-term fixation.

In the medium term (5 years), hydroxyapatite appears to produce very reliable femoral fixation: few if any implants appear to loosen aseptically, and survival and migration are equivalent to a cemented prosthesis. Certainly, an hydroxyapatite coat greatly improves the stability of an identical press-fit. Symptomatic results are similar to those achieved with cement, whereas radiolucent lines, neck resorption, and osteolysis appear less frequently.

Less information is available with regard to the acetabulum at any time period and to the femur at 5 to 10 years. Such as there is, it is similar to the early femoral findings.

Hydroxyapatite is lost from the prosthetic surface over the years to be replaced by bone in direct contact with metal. Thus, long-term fixation is dependent on interlock rather than adhesion. On the surface of the implant, asperities rather than porosities seem sufficient, although both have produced good clinical results.

It has been suggested that fragments of hydroxyapatite may become detached to cause wear and osteolysis. Although a number of retrieval studies have demonstrated hydroxyapatite particles in the articulating surface, the clinical significance of this is uncertain, as accelerated polyethylene wear has not been reported in up to 7 years of clinical follow-up, and osteolysis around an hydroxyapatite coating at current follow-up is rare.

In summary, an hydroxyapatite coating on a suitably designed prosthesis appears to be a very encouraging form of fixation, representing a technique as good as or better than polymethylmethacrylate up to 5, and perhaps 10, years after implantation.

REFERENCES

1. Anderson G, Greis PE. A histologic and biomechanical analysis of the membrane around a hydroxyapatite coated canine 01712626767 femoral prosthesis. *Trans Orthop Res Soc* 1992;397.
2. Bauer TW. Hydroxyapatite coatings: the histology of bone apposition and the mechanisms and consequences of coating metabolism. In: Epinette JA, Geesink RGT, eds. *Hydroxyapatite coated hip and knee arthroplasty*. Paris: Expansion Scientifique Française, 1995;136–141.
3. Bauer TW, et al. Hydroxyapatite-coated femoral stems. Histological analysis of components retrieved at autopsy. *J Bone Joint Surg Am* 1991;73(10):1439–1452.
4. Bauer TW, et al. An indirect comparison of third-body wear in retrieved hydroxyapatite-coated, porous, and cemented femoral components. *Clin Orthop* 1994;298:11–18.
5. Bischoff UW, et al. Wear induced by motion between bone and titanium or cobalt-chrome alloys. *J Bone Joint Surg Br* 1994;76(5):713–716.
6. Black J. Ceramics and composites. In: Black, ed. *Orthopaedic biomaterials in research and practice*, 1st ed. New York: Churchill Livingstone, 1988:191–211.
7. Bloebaum RD, et al. Postmortem comparative analysis of titanium and hydroxyapatite porous-coated femoral implants retrieved from the same patient. A case study. *J Arthroplasty* 1993;8(2):203–211.
8. Bloebaum RD, et al. Complications with hydroxyapatite particulate separation in total hip arthroplasty. *Clin Orthop* 1994;298:19–26.
9. Bloebaum RD, Dupont JA. Osteolysis from a press-fit hydroxyapatite-coated implant. A case study. *J Arthroplasty* 1993;8(2):195–202.
10. Bloebaum RD, et al. Retrieval analysis of a hydroxyapatite-coated hip prosthesis. *Clin Orthop* 1991;267:97–102.
11. Bobyn JD, et al. Producing and avoiding stress shielding: laboratory and observations of non-cemented total hip arthroplasty. *Clin Orthop* 1992;274:79–96.
12. Bucholz RW, Carlton A, Holmes R. Interporous hydroxyapatite as a bone graft substitute in tibial plateau fractures. *Clin Orthop* 1989;240:53–62.
13. Buma P, Gardeniers JWM. Tissue reactions around a hydroxyapatite-coated hip prosthesis. *J Arthroplasty* 1995;10(3):389–395.
14. Callaghan JJ, et al. Concerns and improvements with cementless metal-backed acetabular components. *Clin Orthop* 1995;311:76–84.
15. Campbell P, et al. Evidence of abrasive wear by particles from a hydroxyapatite coated hip prosthesis. *Trans Orthop Res Soc* 1993;224.
16. Capello WN. Hydroxyapatite in total hip arthroplasty: five-year clinical experience. *Orthopedics* 1994;17(9):781–792.
17. Capello WN. Primary THR in the younger age group: hydroxyapatite-coated femoral components at five to seven year follow-up. *Harris Hip Course* 1995.
18. Capello WN. Seven year clinical results of an HA-coated femoral

stem—A multicenter study. In: *Total hip and knee arthroplasty—Clinical issues in providing quality care*. Pinehurst, NC; 1995.

19. Cartillier JC. The contribution of hydroxyapatite: studies of implants of identical geometry with and without hydroxyapatite coating. In: Geesink RGT, Epinette JA, eds. *Hydroxyyapatite in hip and knee arthroplasty*. Paris: Expansion Scientifique Française, 1995;165–168.

20. Chandler HP, et al. Total hip replacement in patients younger than 30 years old. A five year followup study. *J Bone Joint Surg* 1981;63A: 1462.

21. Collier JP, et al. Loss of hydroxyapatite coating on retrieved, total hip components. *J Arthroplasty* 1993;8(4):389–393.

22. Cook SD, et al. Early clinical results with the hydroxyapatite-coated porous LSF total hip system. *Dent Clin North Am* 1992;36(1): 247–255.

23. Cook SD, et al. Hydroxyapatite-coated porous titanium for use as an orthopaedic biological attachment system. *Clin Orthop* 1988;230: 303–312.

24. Cook SD, Thomas KA, Haddad RJJ. Histologic analysis of retrieved human porous coated total joint components. *Clin Orthop* 1988; 234:90.

25. D'Antonio JA, et al. Early clinical experience with hydroxyapatite-coated femoral implants (see comments). *J Bone Joint Surg Am* 1992; 74(7):995–1008.

26. D'Antonio JA, Capello WN, Jaffe WL. Hydroxylapatite-coated hip implants. Multicenter three-year clinical and roentgenographic results. *Clin Orthop* 1992;285:102–15.

27. Dambreville A, Lautridou P. Comparison of two series of THR: hydroxyapatite versus porous coated. In: Epinette JA, Geesink RGT, eds. *Hydroxyapatite coated hip and knee arthroplasty*. Paris: Expansion Scientifique Française, 1995;169–175.

28. Dieppe PA, et al. Apatite deposition disease. A new arthropathy. *Lancet* 1976;7954:266–269.

28b. Donnelly WJ, et al. Radiological and survival comparisons of four methods of fixation of a proximal femoral stem. *J Bone Joint Surg Br* 1997;79(B):351–360.

29. Dorr LD, et al. Structural and cellular assessment of bone quality of proximal femur. *Bone* 1993;14:231–242.

30. Dorr LD, Luckett M, Conaty JP. Total hip arthroplasty in patients younger than 45 years. *Clin Orthop* 1990;260:215.

31. Duthoit E, Epinette JA, Carlier Y. The Arc 2f cup: biomechanics and interface: systematic study of HA-coated vs. porous textured components. In: Geesink RGT, Epinette JA, eds. *Hydroxyapatite coated hip and knee arthroplasty*. Paris: Expansion Scientifique Française, 1995; 176–182.

32. Epinette JA. HA-coated omnifit stems in primary hip replacement surgery: seven years' experience. In: Epinette JA, Geesink RGT, eds. *Hydroxyapatite coated hip and knee arthroplasty*. Paris: Expansion Scientifique Française, 1995;215–226.

33. Epinette JA, Geesink RGT. Radiographic assessment of cementless hip prostheses: ARA, a proposed new scoring system. In: Epinette JA, Geesink RGT, eds. *Hydroxyapatite coated hip and knee arthroplasty*. Paris: Expansion Scientifique Française, 1995;114–126.

34. Exley C, et al. Aluminium, beta-amyloid and non-enzymatic glycosylation. *FEBS Lett* 1995;364(2):182–184.

35. Feighan JE, et al. The influence of surface-blasting on the incorporation of titanium-alloy implants in a rabbit intramedullary model. *J Bone Joint Surg* 1995;77A(9):1380–1395.

36. Filiaggi MJ, Coombs NA, Pilliar RM. Characterization of the interface in the plasma-sprayed H.A. coating/Ti-6Al-4V implant system. *J Biomed Mater Res* 1991;25:1211–1229.

37. Frayssinet P, et al. Histological analysis of the bone–prosthesis interface after implantation in humans of prostheses coated with hydroxyapatite. *J Orthop Surg* 1993;7(3):246–253.

38. Freeman MA. Hydroxyapatite coating of prostheses (letter). *J Bone Joint Surg Br* 1992;74(6):933–934.

39. Freeman MAR. The fixation of prostheses without cement. In: Catterall A, ed. *Recent advances in orthopaedics*. Edinburgh: Churchill Livingstone, 1987;1–17.

40. Freeman MAR, Plante-Bordeneuve P. Can early migration predict late femoral prosthetic failure? *J Bone Joint Surg Br* 1994;76B:432–438.

41. Furlong R. Six years use of the unmodified Furlong hydroxyapatite ceramic coated total hip replacement. *Acta Orthop Belg* 1993;1: 323–325.

42. Furlong RJ, Osborn JF. Fixation of hip prostheses by hydroxyapatite ceramic coatings. *J Bone Joint Surg Br* 1991;73(5):741–745.

43. Geesink RG, de Groot K, Klein CP. Chemical implant fixation using hydroxyl-apatite coatings. The development of a human total hip prosthesis for chemical fixation to bone using hydroxylapatite coatings on titanium substrates. *Clin Orthop* 1987;225:147–170.

44. Geesink RG, Hoefnagels NH. Six-year results of hydroxyapatite-coated total hip replacement. *J Bone Joint Surg Br* 1995;77(4): 534–547.

45. Geesink RGT. *Hydroxyl-apatite coated implants*, 1st ed. Allondale, New Jersey: Osteonics, 1988;170.

46. Geesink RGT. Hydroxyapatite-coated total hip replacement: seven-year Omnifit results. In: Epinette JA, Geesink RGT, eds. *Hydroxyapatite coated hip and knee arthroplasty*. Paris: Expansion Scientifique Française, 1995;204–213.

47. Geesink RGT, De Groot K, Klein CPA. Bonding of bone to apatite-coated implants. *J Bone Joint Surg Br* 1988;70B(1):17–22.

48. Gouin F, et al. A comparative short term study of the same femoral implant with and without the addition of HA. In: Epinette JA, Geesink RGT, eds. *Hydroxyapatite coated hip and knee arthroplasty*. Paris: Expansion Scientifique Française, 1995;187–190.

49. Hardy DC, et al. Bonding of hydroxyapatite-coated femoral prostheses. Histopathology of specimens from four cases. *J Bone Joint Surg Br* 1991;73(5):732–740.

50. Hong L, Xu HC, de Groot K. Tensile strength of the interface between hydroxyapatite and bone. *J Biomed Mater Res* 1992;26(1):7–18.

51. Hoogendoorn HA, et al. Long-term study of large ceramic implants in dog femora. *Clin Orthop* 1984;187:281–288.

52. Huiskes R, Weinans H. Biomechanical aspects of hydroxyapatite coating on femoral hip prostheses. In: Epinette JA, Geesink RGT, eds. *Hydroxyapatite coated hip and knee arthroplasty* Paris: Expansion Scientifique Française, 1995;41–50.

53. Huiskes R, Weinans H, Van Reitbergen B. The relationship between stress shielding and bone resorption around total hip stems and the effect of flexible materials. *Clin Orthop* 1992;274:124–134.

54. Jarcho M. Calcium phosphate ceramics as hard tissue prosthetics. *Clin Orthop* 1981;157:259–278.

55. Karrholm J, et al. Micromotion of femoral stems in total hip arthroplasty. A randomized study of cemented, hydroxyapatite-coated, and porous-coated stems with roentgen stereophotogrammetric analysis. *J Bone Joint Surg Am* 1994;76(11):1692–705.

56. Kay JF, et al. Hydroxy-apatite-coated subperiosteal dental implants: design rationale and clinical experience. *J Prosth Dent* 1987;58(3): 339–343.

57. Kent JN, et al. HA coated and non-coated dental implants in dogs. In: *12th annual meeting of the Society of Biomaterials*. Minneapolis, 1986.

58. Kester MA, et al. Influence of thickness on the mechanical properties and bond strength of HA coatings applied to orthopaedic implants. *Trans Orthop Res Soc* 1991;16:95.

59. Klein CPAT, et al. Plasma sprayed coatings of tetracalciumphosphate, hydroxlyapatite and alpha-TCP on titanium alloy. An interface study. *Biomed Mater Res* 1991;25:53–65.

60. Klien AH, et al. A histologic, biomechanical, and mechanical analysis of the interface between bone and implant in a canine endoprosthesis model. *Trans Orthop Res Soc* 1992:552.

61. Kroon PO, Freeman MA. Hydroxyapatite coating of hip prostheses. Effect on migration into the femur. *J Bone Joint Surg Br* 1992;74(4): 518–522.

62. Malchau H, Herberts P, Ahnfelt L. Prognosis of total hip replacement in Sweden: followup of 92 675 operations performed 1978–1990. *Acta Orthop Scand* 1993;64:497–506.

63. Malcolm AJ. Cemented and hydroxyapatite coated hip implants—An autopsy retrieval study. In: Morrey BF, ed. *Biological, material, and mechanical considerations of joint replacement*. New York: Raven Press, 1993;39–50.

64. Mancini A, et al. HA-coated hip replacement systems: Italian experience of the Omniflex implant. In: Geesink RGT, Epinette JA, eds. *Hydroxyapatite coated hip and knee arthroplasty*. Paris: Expansion Scientifique Française, 1995;245–248.

65. Manley MT, ed. Calcium phosphate biomaterials: a review of the literature. In: Geesink RGT, Manley MT, eds. *Hydroxylapatite coatings in orthopaedic surgery*. New York: Raven Press, 1993.

66. Manley MT, Cook SD, Dalton JE. Compositional, mechanical, and histological comparison of hydroxyapatite coatings. In: *Trans Orthop Res Soc* 1993.

67. Manley MT, Edidin AA. Literature review of calcium phosphate bio-

materials. In: Geesink RGT, Epinette JA, eds. *Hydroxyapatite coated hip and knee arthroplasty.* Paris: Expansion Scientifique Française, 1995.

68. McCaskie A, et al. Radiological evaluation of the interfaces after cemented total hip replacement: interobserver and intraobserver error. *J Bone Joint Surg* 1996;78B(2):191–194.

69. McPherson E, et al. Hydroxyapatite-coated proximal ingrowth femoral stems. A matched pair control study. *Clin Orthop* 1995;315:223–230.

70. Mittelmeier H, Heisel J. Sixteen years' experience with ceramic hip prostheses. *Clin Orthop* 1992;282:64–72.

71. Moilanen T, et al. Hydroxyapatite coating of an acetabular prosthesis: effect on stability. *J Bone Joint Surg* 1996;78B:200–205.

72. Morscher EW. Editorials. *J Bone Joint Surg Br* 1991;73B(5):705–706.

73. Nagase M, Baker DG, Schumaker HR. Prolonged inflammatory reactions induced by artificial ceramics in the rat air pouch model. *J Rheumatol* 1988;15(9):1334–1338.

74. Noble PC, et al. The anatomical basis of femoral component design. *Clin Orthop* 1988;235:148–165.

75. Oonishi H, et al. The effect of hydroxyapatite coating on bone growth into porous titanium alloy implants. *J Bone Joint Surg* 1989;71B(2): 213–216.

76. Osborn JF. Biological behavior of the hydroxyapatite ceramic coating on the femur shaft of a titanium endoprosthesis--initial histologic evaluation of a human explant. (in German) *Biomedizinische Technik* 1987;32(7-8):177–183.

77. Petit R. The PRA prosthesis: biomechanical principles and clinical experience. In: Geesink RGT, Epinette JA, eds. *Hydroxyapatite coated hip and knee arthroplasty.* Paris: Expansion Scientifique Française, 1995;239–248.

78. Ritter MA. The cemented acetabular component of a total hip replacement. *Clin Orthop* 1995;311:69–75.

79. Robinson EJ, et al. Comparison of acetabular polyethylene wear in cemented versus cementless arthroplasty using the 3-D technique. *J Bone Joint Surg Br* 1995;77B(suppl 3):306.

80. Rossi P, et al. Short-term results of hydroxyapatite-coated primary total hip arthroplasty. *Clin Orthop* 1995;311:98–102.

81. Schimmel JW, Huiskes R. Primary fit of the lord cementless total hip. A geometric study in cadavers. *Acta Orthop Scand* 1988;59:638–642.

82. Schmalzried TP, Jasty M, Harris WH. Periprosthetic bone loss in total hip arthroplasty. Polyethylene wear debris and the concept of the effective joint space. *J Bone Joint Surg Am* 1992;74(6):849–863.

83. Scott G, Freeman MAR. Migration studies on cemented, press-fit and hydroxyapatite coated femoral stems. In: Geesink RGT, Epinette JA, eds. *Hydroxyapatite coated hip and knee arthroplasty.* Paris: Expansion Scientifique Française, 1995.

84. Soballe K, et al. Hydroxyapatite coating modifies implant membrane formation. Controlled micromotion studied in dogs. *Acta Orthop Scand* 1992;63(2):128–140.

85. Soballe K, et al. Histologic analysis of a retrieved hydroxyapatite-coated femoral prosthesis. *Clin Orthop* 1991;272:255–258.

86. Soballe K, et al. Gap healing enhanced by hydroxyapatite coating in dogs. *Clin Orthop* 1992;274:282–293.

87. Soballe K, et al. Hydroxyapatite coating converts fibrous tissue to bone around loaded implants. *J Bone Joint Surg Br* 1993;75(2): 270–278.

88. Soballe K, et al. Tissue ingrowth into titanium and hydroxyapatite-coated implants during stable and unstable mechanical conditions. *J Orthop Res* 1992;10(2):285–299.

89. Soballe K, et al. Fixation of porous coated versus HA coated implants. In: Geesink RGT, Epinette JA, eds. *Hydroxyapatite coated hip and knee arthroplasty.* Paris: Expansion Scientifique Française, 1995; 71–84.

90. Soballe K, et al. Migration of hydroxyapatite coated femoral prostheses. A roentgen stereophotogrammetric study. *J Bone Joint Surg Br* 1993;75(5):681–687.

91. Soballe K, et al. RSA studies on HA coated and porous coated implants. In: Geesink RGT, Epinette JA, eds. *Hydroxyapatite coated hip and knee arthroplasty.* Paris: Expansion Scientifique Française, 1995;105–109.

92. Stephenson PK, et al. The effect of hydroxyapatite coating on ingrowth of bone into cavities in an implant. *J Arthroplasty* 1991;6(1): 51–58.

93. Storey E, Masters CL. Amyloid, aluminum and the aetiology of Alzheimer's disease. *Med J Aust* 1995;163(5):256–259.

94. Thomas NP, et al. Medium term results of the Omnifit stem as proximally coated HA femoral prosthesis. In: Geesink RGT, Epinette JA, eds. *Hydroxyapatite coated hip and knee arthroplasty.* Paris: Expansion Scientifique Française, 1995;266–272.

95. Tonino AJ, et al. Hydroxyapatite-coated hip prostheses: early results from an international study. *Clin Orthop* 1995;311:211–225.

96. Tuke M. Personal communication, 1995.

97. Van Blitterswijk CA, et al. Variations in hydroxyapatite crystallinity: effects on interface reactions. In: Geesink RGT, Manley MT, eds. *Hydroxyapatite coatings in orthopaedic surgery.* New York: Raven Press, 1993.

98. Vidalain JP. The Corail THR system in primary hip arthroplasty: seven-year experience of the ARTRO group. In: Geesink RGT, Epinette JA, eds. *Hydroxyapatite coated hip and knee arthroplasty.* Paris: Expansion Scientifique Française, 1995;193–203.

99. Weinans H, Huiskes R, Grootenboer HJ. Effects of material properties of femoral hip components on bone remodelling and interface stresses. *J Orthop Res* 1992;10:845–853.

100. Weinans H, Huskies R, Grootenboer HJ. Effects of fit and bonding characteristics of femoral stems on adaptive bone remodelling. *J Biomech Eng* 1994;116:393–400.

101. Whiteside LA. Editorial comment. *Clin Orthop* 1994;298:2–3.

The Adult Hip, edited by J. J. Callaghan,
A. G. Rosenberg, and H. E. Rubash.
Lippincott–Raven Publishers, Philadelphia © 1998.

CHAPTER 66

Proximal Fixation of the Noncemented Stem

Lawrence D. Dorr and Mazen Said

THE PAST

The history of femoral stem designs incorporating proximal fixation provides a moving picture of cementless fixation development (Fig. 1). The concept of fixing the implant only into the proximal femur was popular because of a desire by orthopedic surgeons to load the femur in a manner that would be as physiological as possible. This required that the femur be loaded from the top to the bottom of the bone, rather than having fixation primarily concentrated in the diaphysis. In 1983 and 1984, when the first proximal fixation implants were introduced, the orthopedic community already was aware that the AML (Anatomic Medullary Locking, DePuy, Warsaw, IN) provided fixation primarily in the diaphysis, and that stress-shielded bone loss occurred proximally. Therefore, the original designs focused on achieving fixation in the metaphysis with no fixation surface available on a smooth diaphyseal stem.

The original bone ingrowth stems had no clinical history from which to gain information about correct design and surface level of fixation. The original designs were influenced as much by the metals used as by the philosophy of the designing surgeons. Titanium was favored by most people involved with the design of these implants, because it is a biologically inert metal and animal experiments had shown that it was attractive to bone (22,41,50). The problem that titanium presented in manufacturing was that the metal is notch-sensitive and the threat and fear of breakage predominated the distribution of porous coating placed on titanium. Therefore, the first titanium stems had only patched porous coating on the proximal surface, which left areas of smooth metal available as tracks for debris between the joint space and the femur diaphysis. Implants manufactured from cobalt–chrome alloys were able to use circumferential coating. Examples of the early titanium prostheses were the HGP (Harris-Galante Prosthesis, Zimmer, Warsaw, IN) and the APR (Anatomic Porous Replacement, Intermedics Orthopedics, Austin, TX). An example of a cobalt–chrome prosthesis with circumferential coating was the PCA (Porous Coated Anatomic, Howmedica, Rutherford, NJ).

Some companies elected not to use porous coating on titanium but to use another type of fixation surface. These fixation surfaces allowed a circumferential coating and were often extended onto the diaphyseal surface of the stem. An example of this type of surface would be the plasma spray on the Mallory-Head prosthesis (Biomet, Warsaw, IN). In Europe, the implants did not have a porous coating on titanium, but surface fixation was created by grit-blasting the metal, which produced a roughened surface. Examples of this type of prosthesis were the Zweymuller and CLS stems (Sulzer Medica, Winterthur, Switzerland).

The surgical technique for proximally fixed implants differed also from that used for diaphyseal fixed implants. The AML achieved fixation by reaming through the isthmus of the femur for a distance of 4 to 5 cm and achieving a tight fit of an implant that was at least 0.5 mm larger than the reamed hole. Conversely, proximally coated implants such as the APR and PCA would overream the diaphysis compared to the size of the stem in an attempt to force the primary fit, and, therefore, fix-

L. D. Dorr: Department of Orthopaedics, University of Southern California Hospital, Los Angeles, California 90033-4634.

M. Said: Department of Orthopaedics, Center for Implant Surgery, BNAI-ZION Medical Center, Haifa 31048 Israel.

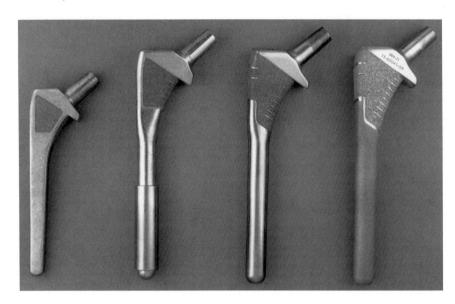

FIG. 1. The progression of the APR stem through the last 13 years of noncemented fixation. These stems illustrate the change in surface levels of fixation, as well as the geometry and the use of modularity.

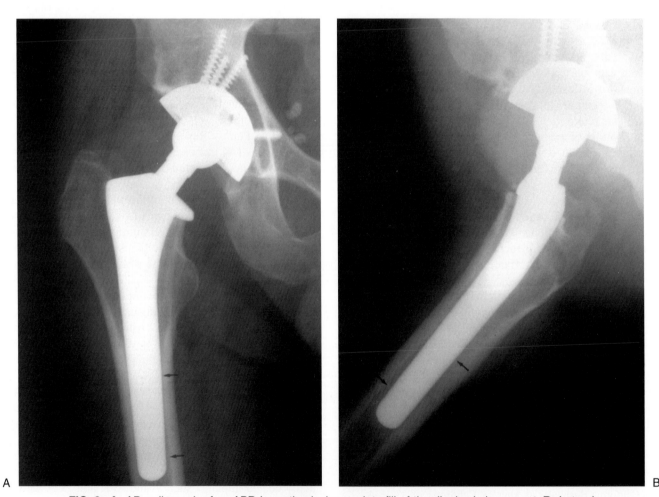

A   B

FIG. 2. A: AP radiograph of an APR-I prosthesis: incomplete fill of the diaphysis is present. **B:** Lateral radiograph of APR-I hip prosthesis demonstrating the anatomic shape of the stem and incomplete diaphyseal fill.

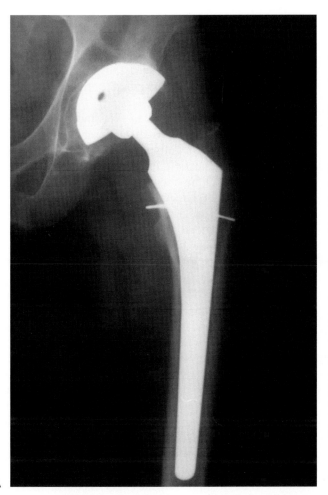
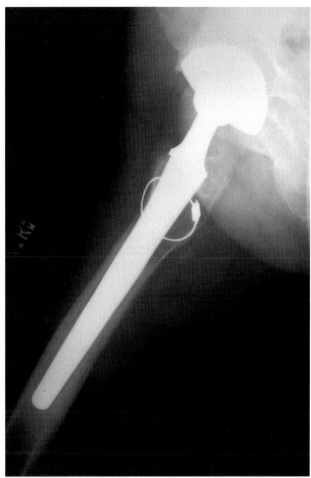

A

B

FIG. 3. A: AP radiograph of Omnifit HA (hydroxyapatite) hip prosthesis. **B:** Lateral radiograph of Omnifit HA prosthesis, which demonstrates the tapered prosthesis design.

ation of the implant into the proximal femur. This early surgical technique for proximally fixed implants resulted in a relatively high incidence of undersized implants, which caused a significant incidence of early loosening and failure of these hip replacements (10,13,21,29, 31–33,48). This error in surgical technique (and the resultant failures caused by it) was one of the factors contributing to the relatively high incidence of thigh pain and loosening noted with first-generation cementless implants that resulted in discouragement with these implants.

There were two different philosophies about the best design for achievement of proximal fit and fixation. One was the anatomic design employed by the APR and PCA (Fig. 2). The second was the tapered design employed by the Mallory-Head, the Omnifit (Osteonics, Allentown, NJ), and the European prostheses (Fig. 3). Subsequently, the tapered design has been used with the Taperloc (Biomet, Warsaw, IN) and the Natural Hip (Intermedics Orthopedics, Austin, TX). The anatomic design was favored by those who desired to achieve maximum fixation in the metaphysis and to concentrate as much off-

loading of the stem as possible in the metaphysis. The tapered design was favored by those who wanted the stability that could be provided by this design as it wedged itself into the femur (3,9,24,25,28,50). At the present time, with the current surface levels of fixation used, there has been little difference in regard to the percentage of fixation rates, the incidence of thigh pain, or revision rates for both of these geometrical designs (3,9,14,21,24, 28,29,32,37).

The experience with the early designs and techniques for the proximally fixed cementless stems resulted in improved understanding of the factors required for optimal fixation of a cementless stem. First, two levels of fixation were defined by the different geometries and different levels of surface coating. The true metaphyseal fixation was primarily confined to those stems with proximal patch porous coating and anatomic stems. The metaphyseal fixation in the original designs was felt to be satisfactory if it occurred with cancellous bone. Implant retrievals demonstrated that this cancellous fixation did provide bone ingrowth fixation to the porous coating (1,11,19,46). The second level of fixation was that which occurred with tapered stems and occurred in the high dia-physeal cortical bone, just below the lesser trochanter. This high diaphyseal fixation resulted in a spot weld fix-ation at this level and gave a firm cortical fixation. With the Mallory-Head stem and the Osteonics hydroxyap-atite-coated implant, the diaphyseal portion of the stem had a roughened or grit-blasted surface that promoted bone attachment to this portion of the stem also (Fig. 4). This further enhanced the endosteal bone attachment to the prosthesis.

A consequence of these early proximal fixation designs was thigh pain, which occurred for two reasons: inadequate fixation and the stiffness ratio between the stem and bone. The most common reason for thigh pain was the failure of adequate fixation. In active patients, the limited area of fixation provided by patch porous coating did not give sufficient stability of the implant against

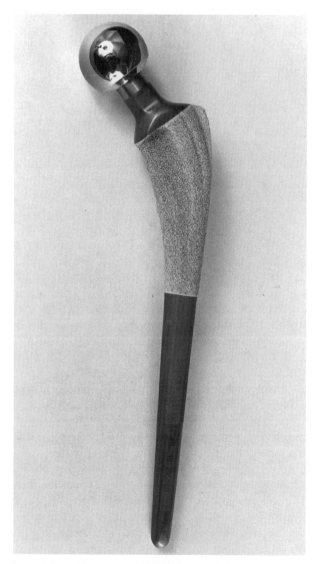

FIG. 4. The Mallory head stem, illustrating the proximal plasma spray coating with diaphyseal grit-blasted stem.

micromotion to prevent thigh pain. The evidence for this micromotion is seen radiographically by the appearance of radiolucent lines (Fig. 5). Radiolucent lines were fre-quently reported around the diaphyseal portion of the stem in implants with proximal porous coating and smooth distal stems (3,5,13,36,37).

After the initial experience in 1984 and 1985 with poor fit of these stems and the resultant loosening and pain, the surgical technique for fitting the prosthesis was changed. The surgical technique then demanded that a tight cir-cumferential fit of the smooth stem be obtained in the dia-physis. This tight circumferential fit required that the femur be reamed so that a fit in both the anterior–poste-rior and medial–lateral plane was obtained (Fig. 6). Better fixation was obtained with this new surgical technique, but the incidence of thigh pain was not necessarily decreased. The cause of thigh pain in these implants with satisfactory radiographic fixation was the stiffness ratio between the bone and the stem. Because the intramedullary canal is always wider on the lateral radi-ograph than the anteroposterior (AP) radiograph (Fig. 7), bone was necessarily reamed from the medial and lateral cortices to accommodate a tight circumferential fit. This reaming created an adverse stiffness ratio between the stem and the bone, and this adverse stiffness ratio resulted in increased pain and subsequently in an increased inci-dence of radiolucent lines (2,14,16,26,27,41).

The importance of the adverse stiffness ratio in these proximally coated designs with smooth diaphyseal stems can be illustrated by the experience with the APR-I. The ratio of the stiffness of the stem to the stiffness of the femur was compared in 117 hips. In simple terms, this ratio compares the size of the stem to the size of the femur. With a stem that has no fixation in the diaphysis, the differential deflection between either a too-flexible or a too-stiff stem and the bone may result in motion between the two, which has an impact on fixation. If the stiffness ratio is disparate between the stem and bone, the differential deflection of the more flexible structure may increase the interface shear stresses so that they exceed the frictional fit and cause interface instability, which leads to loosening. In fact, in this study, hips that had a stiffness ratio of 0.66 or greater did not demon-strate any bone ingrowth on radiographs. If the stiffness ratio of the stem to the femur was greater than 0.5, the fixation of the stem was statistically worse, as was the pain score for the patient ($p = .005$). Eighty-one hips had a stiffness ratio below 0.5, and 36 had a stiffness ratio greater than 0.5. The most important determining factor for a stiffness ratio greater than 0.5 was the amount of reaming that was done of the medial and lat-eral cortices as measured on the AP radiograph. The amount of reaming that was measured for those hips with a stiffness ratio less than 0.5 was 1.4 ± 0.9 mm. The amount of reaming for those hips with a stiffness ratio greater than 0.5 was 2.3 ± 1.5 mm ($p = .005$). On the lat-

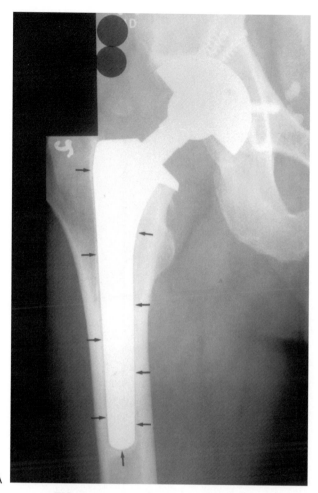 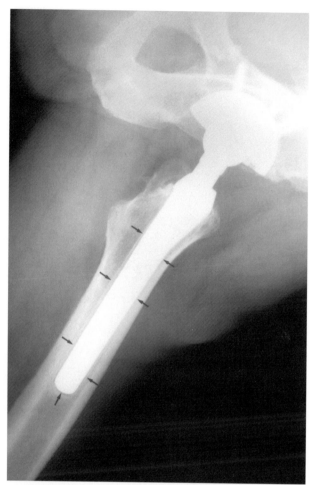

FIG. 5. A: AP radiograph of APR-I stem with radiolucent line around the entire stem, except the most medial surface and under the collar, where the stem is attached to the bone by the porous coating on its proximal medial surface and on the undersurface of the collar. **B:** Lateral radiograph with radiolucent line around the entire smooth portion of the stem with attachment of the bone at the proximal anterior and posterior surfaces where porous coating is on the surface of the stem.

eral radiograph, the reaming was less than 1.0 mm for both groups and there was no statistical difference. The reaming of the medial and lateral cortices is necessary to give the concentric fit in the diaphysis that provides the mechanical stability for the stem.

Because of this experience with the pain that occurred in patients who did not have a satisfactory implant fit, and because of the adverse results with excessive reaming of diaphyseal cortical bone, most orthopedic surgeons abandoned the use of cementless stems in hips in which the bone was not favorable. In the femoral bone types of Dorr et al. (12), this meant that some type B bones and all type C bones were cemented (Fig. 8). Proximal-coated cementless implants therefore began to have limited indications in hip arthroplasty.

A second consequence of these proximal-coated implants was the appearance of femoral diaphyseal osteolysis within the first 5 years after surgery (15,33,34, 39,44) (Fig. 9). This femoral focal osteolysis (11) was

most commonly observed in those implants with patch porous coating. Rarely was femoral focal osteolysis apparent in implants that had proximal circumferential coating (5,6,18). The appearance of this osteolysis was alarming and led to further abandonment of proximal-coated implants by some orthopedic surgeons. Notably, Dr. William Harris of Boston, who was one of the co-designers of the Harris-Galante prosthesis, became convinced that cementless fixation was not as effective as cemented fixation and recommended that all hip replacement surgeries be performed with bone cement for the femur.

The history of the APR again provides insight into the cause of focal osteolysis. Focal osteolysis is correlated to the occurrence of excessive polyethylene wear (13,15). Linear polyethylene wear of more than 0.2 mm per year or volumetric wear of more than 150 mm³ will result in a higher incidence of osteolysis. When linear wear is less than 0.1 mm per year, the incidence of osteolysis is only

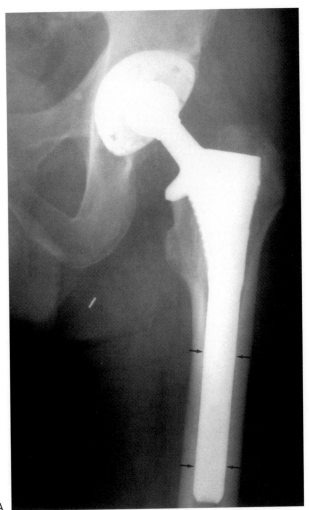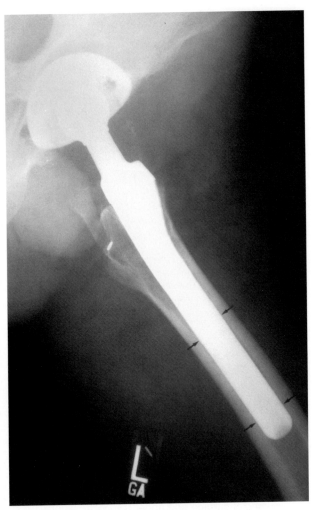

FIG. 6. A: AP radiograph of APR-IIT stem shows the improved fit of this geometry. There is a concentric fill of the diaphysis on both the AP and the lateral radiograph, giving a tight mechanical fit of the stem. **B:** Lateral radiograph of APR-IIT stem showing again the concentric mechanical fit of the stem in the diaphysis and the improved fit of this anatomic geometry in the femur.

4%. This correlation of increased osteolysis with linear wear of more than 0.2 mm per year has also been observed in cemented hips by Willert (47). In hips with the APR prosthesis, the occurrence of higher wear rates was directly related to the fixation of the stem. In a matched pair of patients with and without osteolysis, fixation was statistically significantly correlated with the amount of wear and the occurrence of osteolysis (15). Thirty-eight patients could be matched for age, sex, weight, bone type, and surgical technique with the APR-I. At 2 years after surgery there was no statistical difference in the amount of wear between these two groups of patients, one with osteolysis and one without. At 2 years, the linear wear in those hips with osteolysis was 0.21 mm and in those hips without osteolysis was 0.18 mm ($p = .68$). At this same 2-year time point, there was statistically better fixation as measured by the incidence and number of radiolucent lines for hips that *did not* develop

osteolysis. This statistical difference continued at the 5-year follow-up. In fact, the fixation in the hips that developed osteolysis became worse over time, whereas in the group without osteolysis the fixation remained stable. At the 5-year follow-up, the hips with osteolysis showed a volumetric wear of 185 mm^3 versus 96 mm^3 in those hips that did not develop osteolysis ($p = .0005$). The linear wear at 5 years was 0.3 mm in hips that developed osteolysis and 0.15 mm per year in hips that did not ($p = .0005$). The linear wear rate at 2 years in hips that did not develop osteolysis is higher on average than at 5 years because of the occurrence of initial run-in wear that occurs with all bearing surfaces. In this study, wear accelerated in those hips with poor stem fixation, indicating that poor stem fixation promotes increasingly greater wear. Increasingly greater wear results in an increased incidence of focal osteolysis. Therefore, one of the important factors required for a reduction in osteolysis is excellent and durable fixation of both the stem and the acetabular component.

With a stem that has no fixation in the diaphysis, the differential deflection between either a too-flexible or a too-stiff stem and the bone may result in motion between the two that impacts fixation. If the stiffness ratio is disparate between the stem and bone, the differential deflection of the more flexible structure may increase the interface shear stresses, so that they exceed the frictional fit and cause interface instability, which leads to loosening.

Clearly, these historical lessons with proximal-coated bone ingrowth femoral stems have taught us many of the criteria necessary for successful and durable fixation with bone ingrowth. The stem must be firmly fixed throughout its length and the choices for this fixation are either mechanical or biologic in the diaphysis. Wear must be controlled so that it does not exceed 0.1 mm of linear wear per year. The conflict between stiffness of the femur and stiffness of the stem must be resolved so that the bone remodeling is favorable for the fixation and durability of

the implant. In the remainder of this chapter we will examine the information available to us for determining the optimal stem design that will allow us to achieve proximal fixation and proximal load transfer.

THE PRESENT

The clinical experience with noncemented fixation in total hip arthroplasty to date has not been more successful than cemented total hip arthroplasty, and in some reports the results are even inferior (13,30–33,38,48). The clinical results of different types of femoral implants reported variable values, indicating variable concepts about implant material, geometry, and type of coating, and a specific philosophy and belief about type of fixation (5,6,14,18,21,30,48).

However, a great deal of information has been accumulated from both laboratory studies and clinical series in regard to the factors necessary for both optimal fixa-

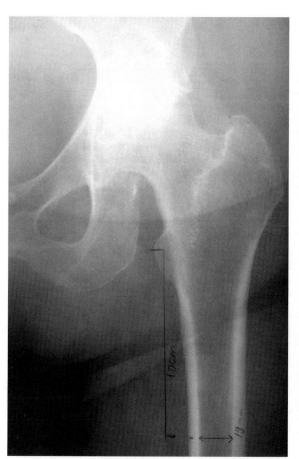 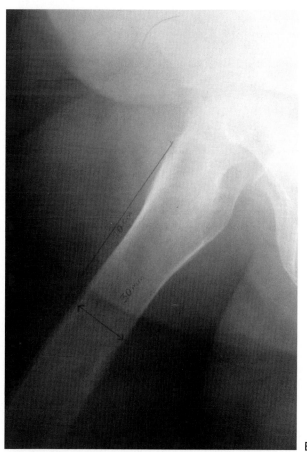

A   B

FIG. 7. A: The diameter of the intramedullary canal of this type C femur, measured at a point 10 cm from the lesser trochanter, is 16 mm using a ruler with 18% magnification. **B:** The intramedullary canal diameter of this type C bone as viewed on the lateral radiograph is 22 mm. This differential in the intramedullary canal diameter between the AP and lateral radiographs demonstrates the difficulty in achieving a concentric fit in the intramedullary canal as illustrated in (A) and (B) in a femur with this anatomy.

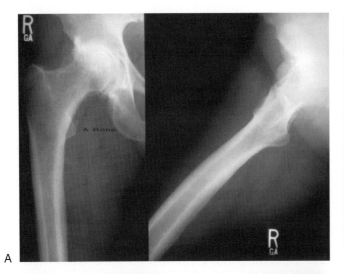

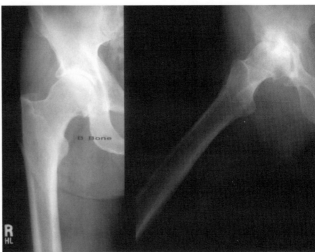

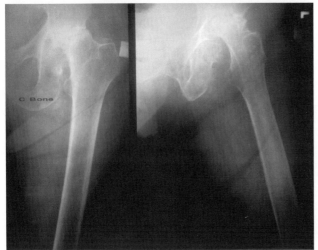

FIG. 8. A: Type A bone. The bone stock has thick cortices on both AP and lateral radiographs. On the AP radiograph, a funnel shape of bone is always present. On the lateral radiograph, the posterior cortex forms a posterior fin of bone that creates the isthmus on the lateral radiograph. The thick posterior cortex is the most metabolically active bone in the femur, and it is the first bone to resorb with metabolic or disuse osteoporosis. **B:** Type B bone. The funnel shape of the femur seen on the AP radiograph is lost, but the cortices remain thick. On the lateral radiograph, the posterior fin of bone is seen to be undergoing resorption, with scalloping and loss of thickness. The loss of this posterior cortex begins proximally and proceeds distally. The isthmus on the AP radiograph is widened as it is on the lateral radiograph in type B bone. **C:** Type C bone: an extreme example. The cortices are very thin, and on the lateral radiograph it is often very hard to define the cortex. In type C bone, there is no longer any posterior fin able to be observed and most often this bone will have a stovepipe type of appearance. Although type B bone is quite metabolically active, in type C bone the metabolism is burned out and the resorption is not as metabolically active as in type B bone.

tion and load transfer of the bone ingrowth femoral stem. The laboratory data have been generated from finite element analysis, studies of implant response in cadaveric bone, and implant retrievals from patients. From clinical series we have learned the response of both the patient and the hip to various stem design features that are designed to be primarily fixed in the proximal metaphyseal bone.

Laboratory research work is limited because of an inability to examine the condition of the artificial joint *in vivo*. The result of total hip arthroplasty in a patient occurs because the conditions are living bone and a dynamic process, whereas in the laboratory the conditions are those of dead bone and a static process. Laboratory data have been generated both by finite element analysis and cadaver studies. Huiskes has been the leader in the use of finite element analysis in studying the relationship of the stem and bone (24–26). His conclusion that stems that are too flexible can loosen because of high

proximal interface shear stress was supported clinically by the results of the Omniflex stem (7) (Osteonics, Allentown, NJ). He has studied the relationship of the level of fixation and load transfer (25–27). His results suggest a preference for a transitional level of fixation with proximal fixation the strongest, as opposed to the strongest fixation being in the diaphysis. With transitional levels of fixation, load transfer is more uniform and bone loss by stress-shielding is reduced. These data are supported clinically by the better bone remodeling of the Mallory-Head (3,37), Taperloc (24), and APR II (8,14) (Fig. 10) than is obtained with the AML.

Cadaver studies have also provided progress toward understanding the optimal design characteristics for a stem. Callaghan et al. (4) demonstrated superior torsional stability of an anatomic stem design versus a straight stem design. A tapered straight stem was not tested. Whiteside et al. (45) studied the importance of initial stem fit on stability. In a comparison of loose proximal

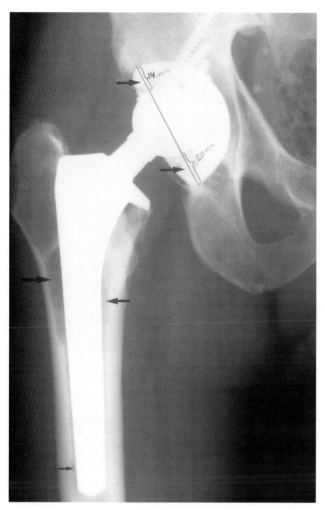

FIG. 9. AP radiograph of APR-I stem shows the wear present in the polyethylene of the socket, as well as focal osteolytic defects present in the femur.

and tight distal, versus loose distal and tight proximal, versus tight proximal and tight distal fits, the latter was clearly the best fit. A major weakness of these studies is that they were performed in cadaver bone, which does not have the compliance or viability of living bone. An important question is whether initial mechanical stability of the diaphyseal stem will be as durable as biologic fixation in the diaphysis. If mechanical stability is not as durable, then smooth diaphyseal stems should be abandoned.

The literature on clinical results of noncemented stems in the past 10 years provides information on the durability of mechanical versus biologic fixation. The APR-I stem has shown progressive loss of fixation after 5 years (13). This stem was implanted with the tight proximal, loose distal technique, and these clinical results support the laboratory findings of Whiteside (45). The HGP stem and the PCA stem had similar design philosophies to the APR-I and used similar overreaming techniques. The

HGP stem has also had progressive fixation loss (21,29, 31,50). PCA stem fixation failures have been reported as 8% to 15% in 4 to 6 years (10,21,29,32,33).

Rubash has recently reported excellent clinical success with the Multilock (Zimmer, Warsaw, IN) in patients less than age 65 with type A bone (Fig. 11) (43). The fixation in these 127 total hips was superb, with only four having radiolucent lines in the porous-coated zones, no pedestals, and no osteolysis (Table 1). The best clinical results for both thigh pain and radiographic fixation have been reported for the Mallory-Head stem and the Omnifit HA stem, which have biologic fixation in the diaphysis (3,6,20,37). Both the Mallory-Head stem and the Omnifit HA stem are tapered and have cortical contact in the metaphysis with a roughened surface on the diaphyseal stem which promotes diaphyseal bone attachment and stabilization of the stem. Mallory recently presented 9-year data that confirm the report by Mulliken et al. (37). D'Antonio recently presented 7-year data with no difference from his earlier report (9).

Stiffness of the stem also influenced clinical results. Bobyn et al. (2). found that a hollowed titanium stem produced bone remodeling in dogs that was superior that obtained from a solid cobalt–chrome stem. The incidence of thigh pain is reduced in the hollowed APR-II stem compared to the solid APR-II stem (8,14). Engh and Bobyn reported less stress-shielding in smaller-diameter AML stems (17). With the APR stems, we had better fixation, but there was more thigh pain with the solid APR-II stem than with the APR-I stem. The APR-II stem is longer than that of the APR-I to allow a fit in the femoral diaphyseal isthmus (see Fig. 1). Huiskes predicted this clinical result with a finite element study that showed that longer stems had higher flexural rigidity and concentrated more stress in the diaphysis (26). With both the APR-I (13) and APR-II stems (8,14), increasing stiffness not only increased thigh pain, but caused worse fixation. The use of a modular sleeve on the APR-II diaphyseal stem (see Fig. 1) increased the stiffness of the stem and the incidence of radiolucent lines. Eliminating use of the sleeve and hollowing the stem statistically reduced the occurrence of thigh pain and radiolucent lines (14).

The technical dilemma of a concentric mechanical fit of the stem has not been present for tapered stems that had biologic fixation in the diaphysis. The principle of the tapered stem has been to mechanically fit it into the femoral bone, ignoring the anatomy of the femur and wedging the stem into a tight fit so that there is mechanical stability. This wedge shape did not require a cylindrical diaphyseal stem and minimal reaming is necessary to prepare the diaphyseal canal. In fact, for the European tapered stems, the CLS and the Zweymuller, no reaming is usually performed and the femur is only broached and the implant malleted into position. In these stems the initial mechanical stability against torsion is provided by the wedged press-fit of the implant. The long-term stability

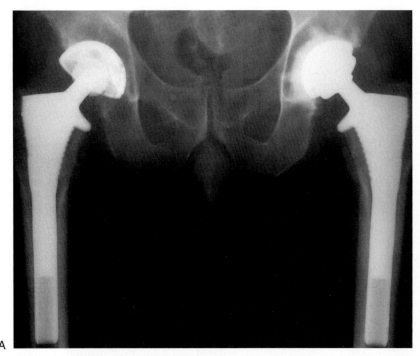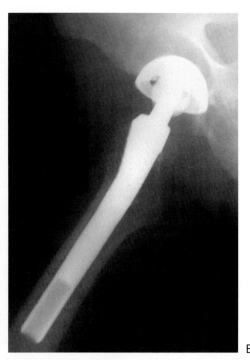

A

B

FIG. 10. A: AP pelvis of bilateral hip replacements 3 years postoperatively with the socket of the right hip being ceramic-on-polyethylene and the socket of the left hip being a Weber Metasul (Sulzer, Winterthur, Switzerland), a metal-on-metal articulation. The femoral stems illustrate the transitional fixation achieved with proximal porous coating and a tight distal mechanical fit. There is maintenance of the proximal metaphyseal bone without evidence of significant stress-shielding. The collar has maintained the medial neck cortical bone. This stem is smooth and reaming was done to match the fill on the AP and lateral radiographs so the medial and lateral cortices are thinned. **B:** A lateral radiograph of the right hip demonstrating the maintenance of the diaphyseal and metaphyseal bone and the fill of the bone by the stem.

of the implant is provided by the biologic fixation of the stem to the bone both in the metaphysis and in the upper diaphysis by the grit-blasted roughened metal surface.

Therefore, besides the difference in shape of the implants, the critical difference in these tapered implants has been the occurrence of diaphyseal biologic fixation. In a randomized study using the Mallory-Head prosthesis this concept of a tapered design with diaphyseal biologic fixation provided clinical results equivalent to cemented stems (3,37).

These laboratory and clinical studies have clarified the requirements for diaphyseal fixation of a cementless stem. Huiskes has shown the benefit of a transitional load transfer (27) and Whiteside the necessity of an initial tight proximal, tight distal fit (46). These studies support the concept of the proximal fixation class of implants for load transfer and bone remodeling. Laboratory studies suggest that mechanical stability of the stem in the diaphysis is satisfactory, but the clinical studies support biologic attachment, both for reduction of pain and durability.

In the metaphysis, the fit and fixation of the proximal stem should be to cortical bone. Implant retrieval by Engh has revealed the improved attachment of cortical

bone to the stem versus cancellous bone (19). Implant retrieval of the APR-I showed unpredictable attachment to cancellous bone in the metaphysis (1,19). Second, the cortical seal of the bone to metal provides the same protection against particulate infiltration into the diaphyseal femoral bones as does cement fixation. The importance of circumferential porous fixation was first suggested by Martell et al. when they reported results with the patched porous-coated HGP (34). With the APR-I with patched porous coating, the incidence of osteolysis in the diaphysis was 14% (13).

THE FUTURE

The knowledge gained from the past 10 years of laboratory studies and clinical use of bone ingrowth femoral stems has led us to conclude that the class of implants called proximal fixation should be reclassified as graduated load transfer implants. The characteristics of this group include a femoral stem that can provide graduated load transfer to the femoral bone without the clinical occurrence of thigh pain and with the expectation of long-term durability.

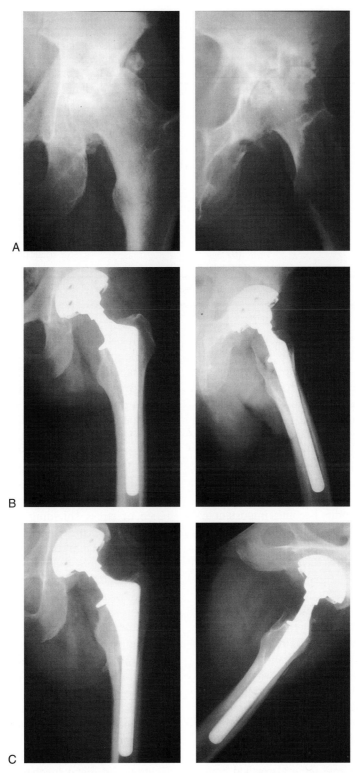

FIG. 11. A patient with an excellent Multilock uncemented prosthesis. **A:** Preoperative AP and lateral views of patient with type A bone. **B:** Immediate postoperative AP and lateral views. **C:** Four-year follow-up AP and lateral views.

TABLE 1. *Comparison of noncemented prosthesis for the femur and the acetabulum*

Author (ref.)	Prosthesis type	Follow-up (yr)	Femur			Acetabulum		
			Revised (%)	Loose (%)	Osteolysis (%)	Revised (%)	Loose (%)	Osteolysis (%)
Martell et al. (34)	HGP	5.6 (4.6–6.6)	4	9	8	1.7	1.7	0
Kim 1992 (31)	HGP	5.2 (5–5.5)	4.9	10	12	1.2	1.2	0
Kim 1993 (32)	PCA	6.3 (6.1–7.4)	3.4	6	24	1.7	2.6	8.6
Maric 1992 (33)	PCA	2.4 (1–4)	8	11	n.r.	0	0	0
Heekin (23)	PCA	6 (5–7)	1	5	18	2	6	
Dorr 1997 (13)	APR-I	6.7 (5–9)	11	21	41	3	0	1
Dorr 1996 (14)	APR-II	3.7 (2–5)	0.6	0	1.2	0	0	0
Mulliken et al. (37)	Mallory -Head	4.8 (4–6)	0	0	0	0	1.4	14 (around the screws)
D'Antonio 1996 (9)	Omnifit	6 (5–8)	1	0	0.5	17.0	11.9	7
Rubash 1996 (48)	Multilock	3.2 (2–6)	0 (97% ingrown)	0	0	1.0 (dislocation)	0	0

n.r., not regarded

The geometry of the stem must provide for initial mechanical stability that will permit biologic bony fixation to occur and will have stiffness relief that creates a favorable stiffness ratio between the stem and bone in the diaphysis. For a stem that is entirely smooth and relies on a frictional fit within the femoral bone, the stem shape is absolutely critical for both initial and long-term stability. However, for stems that will achieve bone ingrowth fixation to the femur, the rigidity of the stem shape as a mechanical entity is very important. The bone ingrowth stem of the future will achieve long-term fixation by biologic fixation and therefore rigidity becomes important to provide stiffness relief of the stem for more favorable long-term bone remodeling. Therefore, both tapered stems and anatomic-shaped stems have been and can be successful for the graduated load transfer concept.

We favor the anatomic-shaped stem because it allows a large proximal double-wedge geometry that ensures metaphyseal cortical fixation to the stem. By combining the cortical fixation of the stem with a medial porous-coated collar, the entire proximal femur can be sealed to cortical bone in a manner analogous to that which occurs with cement fixation. Perhaps more important, load transfer occurs into the cortical bone anteriorly and posteriorly by the cortical fixation to the stem and medially through the collar. With both the APR-I and APR-II stems, we have clearly demonstrated the superiority of the collar in maintaining proximal femoral cortical bone (8,13,14). The opinion of some surgeons is that stem implantation would be technically more difficult with an anatomic geometry and would require complex instrumentation and more stem size variability. With the APR anatomic hip system, these theoretical concerns have proved to not occur. The surgical technique is not more difficult or different with the anatomic-shaped stem than it is with the straight-tapered stem.

Stiffness relief must be present in a stem that will provide the graduated load transfer concept. Stiffness relief in the tapered stem is provided by the tapered shape of the stem. Stiffness relief in anatomic stems such as the APR can be provided by a slot in the stem, removing metal from the stem by the use of grooves, or by using a hollow stem. The flexural rigidity of the noncemented stem is approximately 3.6 times as high as a cemented stem in the mid-stem region (25). As a result, with these noncemented stems, distal interface stress transfer increases at the expense of proximal stress transfer, and the occurrence of stress shielding in the cortex increases. This explains the critical necessity for stiffness relief of the stem to a level that reduces the stiffness of the stem below that of the diaphyseal cortical bone. Stem length must be long enough to provide initial mechanical stability and this necessary length does increase the flexural rigidity, which again emphasizes the necessity for stiffness relief of this metal stem.

Fixation of the stem is the most important factor for good clinical results. Cemented stems have historically taught us this fact (38,49). The AML prosthesis with predictable distal diaphyseal fixation has confirmed the importance of fixation. It has become clear from the experience of the last 10 years that both proximal and distal fixation are needed (6,13,25,40,46). The controversy over the past 10 years has been whether proximal biologic fixation and distal mechanical fixation would be sufficient to achieve both predictable and durable fixation and maintain desirable stress transfer. Engh et al. have contended that this would not be possible and that they would opt for predictable fixation and ignore the bone remodeling consequences (18). At this time, we believe that this controversy is resolved and that optimal fixation occurs when both proximal metaphyseal and distal diaphyseal biologic fixation occur, but the fixation allows a more uniform stress transfer. Thus, we have named this concept graduated load transfer.

The laboratory data indicate that tight mechanical fixation provides excellent initial torsional stability and that this could be achieved either with a concentric fit of a smooth stem or, even better, with a concentric fit of a fluted stem (30). However, the clinical series have demonstrated a higher incidence of thigh pain and progressive loss of fixation in stems that have employed diaphyseal mechanical fixation (13,31,32). On the other hand, stems that employed proximal cortical fixation in combination with a roughened diaphyseal stem that promoted bone attachment to the stem have had no thigh pain and have demonstrated excellent durability to 10 years (3,6,20,37,50). Clearly, the concept of biologic fixation has proved superior to the concept of simply mechanical stability.

The question about fixation therefore becomes clarified in regard to the use of smooth distal shape with or without flutes. Although both ourselves with the APR-II and Rubash with the Multilock have obtained excellent results with a mechanical fit in type A bone, smooth distal stems with or without flutes are not predictable for pain relief and long-term durability for all bone types and shapes (43). Biologic fixation is required in the diaphysis. The question is how to obtain the proper amount of fixation in both the metaphysis and the diaphysis to ensure transitional stress transfer. The femoral bone biomechanically acts as a single unit and accordingly the load transfer and bone remodeling of the femoral bone without a stem responds to Wolfe's law. However, when a femoral stem is inserted into the femur there are now two separate units that differ from each other by structure, material, geometry, stiffness, and surface properties. The goal must be to achieve such conditions as to allow these two units to function and react as closely to one unit as possible. Huiskes and Bobyn term this phenomenon mechanical biocompatibility (21,31).

The conflict of interest between implant and bone stiffness, and load transfer, as correlated to the level of fixation, must be considered. Interface stresses in the proximal region must be reduced so that load transfer can be optimized in the metaphysis. In the metaphysis stem, stiffness cannot be reduced below that of the bone. As has been demonstrated by Engh in implant retrievals, the mineral content of the bone in the metaphysis will always be reduced by implantation of a stem (19). This fact underscores the absolute necessity for cortical fixation in the metaphysis by the stem, to permit load transfer into the metaphysis. Second, the diaphyseal stem must be flexible enough that the stiffness of this portion of the stem is not greater than that of the cortical diaphyseal bone. This diaphyseal stem flexibility will help to reduce bone resorption proximally.

The correct bone ingrowth cementless stem includes the following points: The implant geometry has to fit to cortical bone in the proximal femur, ensuring cortical contact mediolaterally and anteroposteriorly, it must fill the femoral canal sufficiently to allow initial mechanical stability and ultimate biologic fixation, it must have stiffness relief that prevents adverse stem bone stiffness ratios, and it must have a fixation surface that provides a transitional stress transfer from the proximal femur to the diaphysis. Technically, the implantation of the stem should be accomplished without reaming more than 1.5 mm of bone from the femoral diaphyseal mediolateral cortices. This means that the reamer should not engage bone over more than 1 to 2 cm of the femoral isthmus. Whiteside has indicated that this amount of contact in a stem that is undersized by 0.5 mm will provide satisfactory initial mechanical stability (42). With this technique, combined with a stem with stiffness relief, a favorable stem-to-bone stiffness ratio will occur and thigh pain should be eliminated. Transitional stress transfer can be achieved by ensuring cortical contact in the metaphysis, which will promote stress transfer in this area. In our experience, the addition of a porous-coated collar substantially improves this ability to load transfer. The proximal fixation may be enhanced by the adjunctive use of hydroxyapatite (6,20,35). Biologic fixation in the diaphysis can be obtained by a conundrum-grit-blasted surface, which permits bone attachment to the metal stem (Fig. 12). This biologic stability ensures long-term stability of the diaphyseal stem, which promotes long-term durability for the arthroplasty. These are the principles of graduated load transfer.

We have clinically tested these principles in a prospective randomized study that compared three groups of hips. One group received a proximally porous-coated APR stem that was grit-blasted on the diaphyseal portion of the stem; a second group had the proximal porous-coated stem with the addition of hydroxyapatite to the proximal porous coating and had a grit-blasted distal stem; and a third group of patients had cemented stems. For each of these arthroplasties, a noncemented bone ingrowth hemispherical socket was used. Thirty patients were entered into each group by a randomization scheme. At 2 years postoperatively, the data are definitive in support of this design concept for bone ingrowth fixation. There is no patient in the entire group of 90 who has thigh pain, whether the stem was cemented (30 patients). or noncemented (60 patients). The Harris Hip Score pain rating for each group is 42 points. The limp score for all 90 patients averages 10.5 of a possible 11 points. On SMA 36 patient assessment questionnaires, all patients believe they achieved their expectations with this surgery. These results are clearly superior to the previous results reported with the concept of proximal fixation with a smooth distal stem. The future is therefore clear that noncemented fixation will optimally be achieved using a graduated load transfer concept rather than the traditional proximally fixed concept.

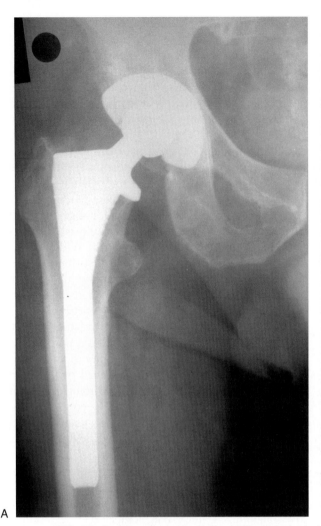
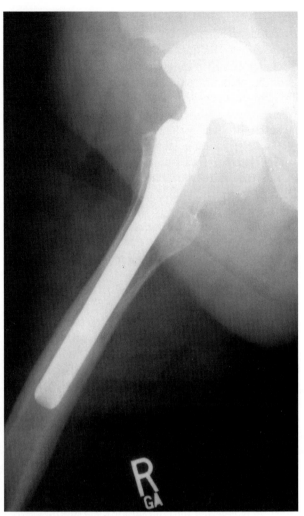

A

B

FIG. 12. A: AP radiograph of the APR grit-based stem seen in Figure 1. The stem does not require a concentric mechanical fit in the diaphysis, so reaming of diaphyseal bone is not necessary (compare to Figure 9). This 2-year postoperative radiograph demonstrates excellent maintenance of both proximal and distal bone illustrating that the grit-based stem does not prevent proximal loading of bone. The stem does not need to fill the intramedullary canal, because the metal has bone attachment that provides biologic rather than mechanical stability. This figure illustrates the concept of the graduated load transfer. **B:** Lateral radiograph of a 2-year postoperative APR grit-based stem shows excellent maintenance of metaphyseal and diaphyseal bone.

The results of our randomized study furthermore tend to support those who believe that noncemented fixation will ultimately replace cemented fixation for the stem. With the elimination of differences in clinical results with these stems, noncemented fixation becomes preferable because the fixation is indeed biologic. Furthermore, the surgery is technically easier, more forgiving, and can be performed more quickly. For all of these reasons, we believe that this evolution of proximal fixation into a graduated load transfer has elevated noncemented fixation into a predictable and reproducible technique that has clinical characteristics equivalent to cement fixation, and fixation characteristics superior to cement fixation.

REFERENCES

1. Bloebaum RD, Bachus KN, Rubman MH, Dorr LD. Postmortem comparative analysis of titanium and hydroxyapatite porous-coated femoral implants retrieved from the same patient. *J Arthroplasty* 1993;8: 203–211.
2. Bobyn JD, Glassman AH, Goto H, Krygier JJ, Miller JE, Brooks CE. The effect of stem stiffness on femoral bone resorption after canine porous-coated total hip arthroplasty. *Clin Orthop* 1990;261:196–213.
3. Burkart BC, Bourne RB, Rorabeck CH, Kirk PG. Thigh pain in cementless total hip arthroplasty. *Orthop Clin North Am* 1993;24(4): 645–653.
4. Callaghan JJ. The clinical results and basic science of total hip arthroplasty with porous-coated prostheses. *J Bone Joint Surg* 1993;75A: 299–310.
5. Callaghan JJ, Dysart SH, Savery CG. The uncemented porous coated anatomic total hip prosthesis. *J Bone Joint Surg* 1988;70A:337–346.
6. Capello WN. Femoral component fixation in the 1990's. Hydroxy-

apatite in total hip arthroplasty: five-year clinical experience. *Orthopedics* 1994;17:781–792.

7. Capello WN, Sallay PI, Feinberg JR. Omniflex modular femoral component. *Clin Orthop* 1994;298:54–59.

8. Cohen JL, Bindelglass DF, Dorr LD. Total hip replacement using the APR-II system. *Tech Orthop* 1991;6:40–58.

9. D'Antonio JA, Capello WN, Manley MT. Remodeling of bone around hydroxyapatite-coated femoral stems. *J Bone Joint Surg* 1996;78:1226–1234.

10. Dodge BM, Fitzrandolph R, Collins DN. Non-cemented porous-coated anatomic total hip arthroplasty. *Clin Orthop* 1991;259:16–24.

11. Dorr LD, Bloebaum R, Emmanual J, Meldrum R. Histologic, biochemical and ion analysis of tissue and fluids retrieved during total hip arthroplasty. *Clin Orthop* 1990;261:82–95.

12. Dorr LD, Faugere MC, Mackel AM, Gruen TA, Bognar B, Malluche NH. Structural and cellular assessment of bone quality of proximal femur. *Bone* 1993;14:231–242.

13. Dorr LD, Lewonowski K, Lucero M, Harris M, Wan Z. Failure mechanisms of APR-I cementless femoral stem. *Clin Orthop* 1997;334:157–167.

14. Dorr LD, Wan Z. Comparative results of a distal modular sleeve, circumferential coating, and stiffness relief using the APR-II. *J Arthroplasty* Vol. 11:4, June 1996.

15. Dorr LD, Wan Z. Natural history of femoral osteolysis with proximal ingrowth smooth stem implant. *J Arthroplasty* 1996;11:6.

16. Dujovne AR, Bobyn JD, Krygier JJ, Miller JE, Brooks CE. Mechanical compatibility of non-cemented hip prosthesis with the human femurs. *J Arthroplasty* 1993;8(1):5–21.

17. Engh CA, Bobyn JD, Glassman AH. Porous coated hip replacement. The factors governing bone ingrowth, stress shielding, and clinical results. *J Bone Joint Surg* 1987;69B:45–55.

18. Engh CA, Macalino GE. Porous coated total hip replacement. *Clin Orthop* 1994;298:89–96.

19. Engh CA, McGovern TF, Bobyn JD, Harris WH. A quantitative evaluation of periprosthetic bone-remodeling after cementless total hip arthroplasty. *J Bone Joint Surg* 1992;74A:1009–1020.

20. Geesink RGT, Hoefnagels NHM. Six-year results of hydroxyapatite-coated total hip replacement. *J Bone Joint Surg* 1995;77B:534–547.

21. Haddad R, Cook SD, Brinker MR. A comparison of three varieties of non-cemented porous-coated hip replacement. *J Bone Joint Surg* 1990;72B:2–8.

22. Head WC, Bauk DJ, Emerson RH. Titanium as the material of choice for cementless femoral components in total hip arthroplasty. *Clin Orthop* 1995;311:85–90.

23. Heekin RD, Callaghan JJ, Hopkinson WJ, Savory CG, Xenos JS. The porous-coated anatomic total hip prosthesis, inserted without cement. Results after 5–7 years in a prospective study. *J Bone Joint Surg* 1993;75A:77–91.

24. Hozack W, Rothman R. Taperloc femoral component, a 2–6 year study of the first 100 consecutive cases. *J Arthroplasty* 1994;9:489–493.

25. Huiskes R. The various stress patterns of press-fit, ingrowth and cemented femoral stems. *Clin Orthrop* 1990;261:27–38.

26. Huiskes R, Weinans H, Dalstra M. Adaptive bone remodeling and biomechanical design consideration. *Orthopedics* 1989;12:1255–1267.

27. Huiskes R, Weinans H, Van Rietbergen MS. The relationship between stress shielding and bone resorption around total hip stems and the effects of flexible materials. *Clin Orthop* 1992;274:124–134.

28. Huo MH, Martin RP, Zatorski LE, Keggiv KJ. Total hip arthroplasty using the Zweymuller stem implanted without cement. *J Arthroplasty* 1995;10:793–799.

29. Hwang SK, Park JS. Cementless total hip arthroplasty with AML, PCA and HGP prostheses. *Int Orthop* (SICOT) 1995;19:77–83.

30. Kendrick JB II, Noble PC, Tullos HS. Distal stem design and the torsional stability of cementless femoral stems. *J Arthroplasty* 1995;10(4):463–469.

31. Kim YH, Kim VE. Results of the Harris-Galante cementless hip prosthesis. *J Bone Joint Surg* 1992;74B:83–87.

32. Kim YH, Kim VEM. Uncemented porous coated anatomic total hip replacement. *J Bone Joint Surg* 1993;75B:6–13.

33. Maric Z, Karpman RR. Early failure of non-cemented porous coated anatomic total hip arthroplasty. *Clin Orthop* 1992;278:116–120.

34. Martell JM, Pierson RH, Jacob JJ, et al. Primary total hip reconstruction with a titanium fiber-coated prosthesis inserted without cement. *J Bone Joint Surg* 1993;75A:554–571.

35. McPherson EJ, Dorr LD, Gruen TA, Saberi MT. Hydroxyapatite coated proximal ingrowth femoral stems. A matched pair control study. *Clin Orthop* 1995;315:223–230.

36. Mont MA, Maar DC, Hungerford DS. Total hip replacement without cement for a non-inflammatory osteoarthritis in patients who are less than forty-five years old. *J Bone Joint Surg* 1993;75A:740–751.

37. Mulliken BD, Nayak N, Bourne RB, Rorabeck CH, Bullas R. Early radiographic results comparing cemented and cementless total hip arthroplasty. *J Arthroplasty* 1996;1:24–33.

38. Mulroy WF, Estok DM, Harris WH. Total hip arthroplasty with use of so-called second-generation cementing techniques. *J Bone Joint Surg* 1995;77A:1845–1852.

39. Otani T, Whiteside LA. Failure of cementless fixation of the femoral component in total hip arthroplasty. *Orthop Clin North Am* 1992;23(2):335–346.

40. Otani T, Whiteside LA, White SE. The effect of axial and torsional loading on strain distribution in the proximal femur as related to cementless total hip arthroplasty. *Clin Orthop* 1993;292:376–383.

41. Otani T, Whiteside LA, White SE, McCarthy DS. Effects of femoral component material properties on cementless fixation in total hip arthroplasty. *J Arthroplasty* 1993;8(1):67–74.

42. Otani T, Whiteside LA, White SE, McCarthy DS. Reaming technique of the femoral diaphysis in cementless total hip arthroplasty. *Clin Orthop* 1995;311:210–221.

43. Rubash H. Results of the multilock cementless prosthesis. *Personal communication.*

44. Smith E, Harris WH. Increasing prevalence of femoral lysis in cementless total hip arthroplasty. *J Arthroplasty* 1995;10:407–411.

45. Sugiyama H, Whiteside LA, Engh CA. Torsional fixation of the femoral component in total hip arthroplasty. *Clin Orthop* 1992;275:187–193.

46. Whiteside LA, White SE, Engh CA, Head W. Mechanical evaluation of cadaver retrieval specimens of cementless bone-ingrowth total hip arthroplasty femoral components. *J Arthroplasty* 1993;8(2):147–155.

47. Willert HG, Bertman H, Buchorn GH. Osteolysis in alloarthroplasty of the hip. The role of ultra-high molecular weight polyethylene wear particles. *Clin Orthop* 1990;258:95–107.

48. Woolson ST, Maloney WJ. Cementless total hip arthroplasty using a porous-coated prosthesis for bone ingrowth fixation. *J Arthroplasty* 1992;7:381–388.

49. Wroblewski BM. Cementless versus cemented total hip arthroplasty. *Orthop Clin North Am* 1993;24(4):591–597.

50. Zweymuller KA, Lintner FK, Semlitsch MF. Biologic fixation of a press-fit titanium hip joint endoprosthesis. *Clin Orthop* 1988;235:195–206.

The Adult Hip, edited by J. J. Callaghan,
A. G. Rosenberg, and H. E. Rubash.
Lippincott–Raven Publishers, Philadelphia © 1998.

CHAPTER 67

The Tapered Femoral Component

Richard H. Rothman and Peter F. Sharkey

Both the immediate and the long-term results of hip arthroplasty using a cemented femoral component, as measured by the critical criteria of safety, efficacy, and durability, are unquestionably outstanding. Proper stem design and good cement technique are prerequisites for ensuring extended longevity of the femoral component. The Charnley style of femoral stem implanted with optimal cement technique clearly has become the gold standard by which all other femoral components should be measured. Before implanting any modification of a cemented Charnley stem, the surgeon must be convinced that the outcomes of the operation will be improved by the change. This is indeed a daunting task when the long-term results of the Charnley femoral stem are critically reviewed.

Schulte et al. (33) reported the 20-year results of Charnley total hip arthroplasty performed by one surgeon. Astoundingly, the incidence of femoral revision in the 98 hips followed for 20 years was only 3%. Another 4% of the hips met radiographic criteria for loosening, but when the patients in the unrevised group were queried, 86% reported no pain and 14% had occasional, mild pain. McCoy et al. (26) reported that, at an average follow-up of 15.3 years, 87.5% of 35 Charnley hip arthroplasties were rated as clinically good or excellent. Two hips had been revised and two other femoral stems were radiographically loose. Another study (30) used survivorship analysis to determine the 17-year results of Charnley total hip replacement. Using revision as an endpoint, the success was 72% at 17 years. Kavanagh et al. (24) reported the Mayo Clinic experience with Charnley total

hip arthroplasty. The femoral component was radiographically loose in 26% of patients at 15 years. However, the revision rate was only 12.7%. Even the long-term results of properly performed cemented Charnley total hip arthroplasty in young patients are reasonably good. Joshi et al. (23) evaluated a group of patients younger than 40 at the time of arthroplasty. At 20 years, the probability of survival of the femoral component was 86%. (It may be noted that the results were considerably better for patients with a preoperative diagnosis of rheumatoid arthritis than for those with osteoarthritis.) Our own data (18) at Pennsylvania Hospital are similar to those reported by others (13,27,39,40). Survivorship of our 1041 Charnley total hip arthroplasties indicated that the probability of femoral component survival (defined by lack of need for revision) was 96% at 10 years.

In this chapter, the design rationale, implantation technique, and results of hip arthroplasty when an uncemented flat, tapered stem is utilized are discussed. The proof that an uncemented stem of any design is superior to the cemented Charnley stem is a difficult burden. Yet, the gratifying results we have achieved with a flat, tapered femoral stem has prompted us to continue recommendation of this uncemented implant in a wide variety of patients.

HISTORY OF THE FLAT, TAPERED STEM

The authors first became interested in an uncemented stem in the mid 1980s, when the results of cemented total hip arthroplasty, using early-generation cementing techniques, were being reported. At that time, there was a pervasive attitude of dissatisfaction with the long-term results of cemented hip arthroplasty, particularly in

R. H. Rothman and P. F. Sharkey: Department of Orthopaedic Surgery, The Rothman Institute, Thomas Jefferson University, Philadelphia, Pennsylvania 19107.

younger and more active patients (7–9,31,37,38), and cement disease was a major concern. Reviewing the literature of the time, we were prompted to choose a flat, wedge-shaped, tapered, uncemented implant for clinical trials. In 1986, Karl Zweymuller et al. (41), of the Orthopaedic University Clinic in Vienna, published the results of hip arthroplasty using a cementless titanium, flat, tapered stem. For implantation of this prosthesis, the femur was prepared by sequential rasping without reaming. These authors stated that their cardinal objective was to achieve maximal stable immediate fixation (both axial and rotational) in the metadiaphyseal region. Accordingly, stability was achieved by press-fitting the prosthesis into the osseous bed prepared by rasping only. This was a radical concept for achieving initial stability, compared to the prevailing methods of the time.

In the United States at that time, anatomically shaped stems were popular. Implantation of anatomic stems required complex shaping of the femoral canal to accommodate the implant. The goal was to configure the canal in such a way that it precisely matched the shape of the implant. This precise fit was considered essential for initial stability. However, this method of achieving initial stability was difficult, with a steep learning curve, and it might lead to frequent technical errors. In addition, the extensive canal preparation by modeling of the bone seemed unphysiologic.

Others were recommending the use of a collared prosthesis to achieve initial stability. Intuitively, it appears that the use of a collar may well provide initial axial stability, but it could also prevent press-fit of the component into the femur, resulting in rotational instability. Achieving rotational instability of the femoral component has since been proven to be a critical goal for successful uncemented hip arthroplasty (4,28,34).

At that time, Engh et al. (10,11) reported good results with a diaphyseal-fitting straight-stem implant. However, the stress shielding and bone loss of the proximal femur that they subsequently reported caused concern.

In this light, the results of Zweymuller et al. (42) were quite dramatic. Between 1979 and 1985, he had implanted 1225 cementless implants. In 1986, their results showed that only 10 reoperations had been necessary and these had included all causes, including infection. This was a revision rate of 0.8%, far better than any other large hip-arthroplasty series at that time. When the patients followed for more than 3 years were separately studied, 99.3% reported being very satisfied or largely satisfied with their new hips. Zweymuller et al. concluded that although these results were preliminary, they compared favorably with the early results realized with cementable prostheses.

In view of the commonly recognized problems associated with polymethylmethacrylate and reservations about the then-prevalent theories related to uncemented fixation, we embraced the design principles of Zweymuller et al. and sought an equivalent to the Zweymuller stem. In the mid 1980s, we began implantation of a simply designed femoral component called the Triloc (Depuy; Warsaw, IN). Canal preparation was simple and was felt to be a prerequisite to obtaining reproducible results. Initially, the component was used only in physiologically young, active patients who were considered at high risk for aseptic loosening using the cementing techniques of that time. In 1990, the early results of our experience with this implant were reported (16). The patients studied were young (average age, 51), predominantly male (by 3:1), and heavy (average weight, 187 pounds). The mean Charnley score for pain improved from 3.0 preoperatively to 5.7 postoperatively. With a minimum follow-up of 2 years, there were no revisions and no impending revisions, and no implant was definitely loose radiographically.

Despite excellent clinical success with the Triloc prosthesis, there was one significant design problem with the implant: the chrome–cobalt composition. In the mid 1980s, two major concerns related to uncemented implants were stress shielding of bone and the carcinogenic potential and systemic effects of chrome–cobalt exposure (3). Both these issues could be resolved by using an implant of titanium composition. The Taperloc femoral component (Biomet; Warsaw, IN) with its design similarities to the Triloc stem but composition of titanium seemed to be the ideal implant.

DESIGN RATIONALE

Based on the principles of Zweymuller et al. (42) and the clinical results reported utilizing the Zweymuller and Triloc stems, we began to use the Taperloc stem in 1987. The Taperloc prosthesis is designed with a flat, tapered wedge stem and no collar. It has titanium composition, modularity options, and a proximally plasma-sprayed porous surface. Reasons for choosing these design parameters are described in this section.

Achieving initial implant stability has been shown to be a critical factor for clinical and experimental osseointegration of the femoral stem (28). The flat, tapered wedge design was biomechanically tested in fresh-frozen human femora in our laboratories to determine initial stability (34). The implants were inserted using the same criteria as utilized clinically. The initial stability of the tapered implant when subjected to physiologic loads was dramatic and consistently good when compared to other uncemented designs (Table 1).

The initial stability of the uncemented implants was similar to that of a cemented control group, and this stability was compatible with the experimental requirements for bone ingrowth previously determined in a dog model (28). The excellent stability obtained with this prosthesis most likely relates to placement of a flat wedge in an

TABLE 1. *Initial stability of various uncemented implant designs*

Axial stability (3000 newton force)		
	Micromotion (microns)	
Design	Average	Range
Cemented control	29	11–67
Anatomic	111	106–116
Collared	34	10–90
Tapered wedge	28	10–46

Rotational stability (12 newton-meter force)		
	Micromotion (degrees $\times 10^3$)	
Design	Average	Range
Cemented control	0.113	0.039–0.324
Anatomic	1.177	0.307–2.396
Collared	0.113	0.037–0.158
Tapered wedge	0.095	0.037–0.158

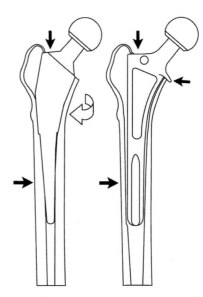

FIG. 2. The use of a collarless design allows complete seating of the prosthesis and achievement of rotational stability. A collar provides axial stability, but it has no inherent ability to provide rotational stability. Furthermore, the collar may prevent firm seating of the implant.

ovoid femoral canal. A rod-shaped stem placed in an ovoid and circularly reamed femoral canal can be seen intuitively to yield poor rotational stability, unless the implant–bone contact is intimate and extensive, such as is the case with the AML (Depuy; Warsaw, IN) prosthesis (Fig. 1). Additionally, insertion of the Taperloc stem does not require extensive reaming and, in fact, as will be described later in this chapter, a conical reamer is utilized only to open the femoral canal. No cortical reaming is undertaken. All other canal preparation is based on the use of sequentially sized broaches. Most of the cancellous bone in the canal is compacted until the bed assumes dimensions identical to the rasp and the corresponding implant. The implications are that the prosthesis is inserted into a canal that has been less physiologically stressed and that has a more intact endosteal blood supply than one prepared by reamers or other speed cutting tools.

Several of the early designs in uncemented hip arthroplasty advocated the use of collared femoral prostheses. The use of a collar clearly provides absolute axial stability if the collar comes into intimate contact with the strong calcar bone. Unfortunately, as collar–calcar contact occurs, rotational stability may be absent if the implant is not tightly fit into the prepared femoral bed. In biomechanical studies (4,34), the collared uncemented

implant has been shown to provide excellent initial stability with axial loading. However, the collar itself has no stabilizing effect against rotational forces. The collarless Taperloc implant allows for insertion until a stable endpoint is achieved (Fig. 2).

Fashioning an uncemented implant from titanium rather than chrome–cobalt has several definite advantages. Specifically, titanium is a very biocompatible material. In fact, bone will grow so intimately against a titanium surface that Albrektsson et al. (1) have coined the term *osseointegration*. This term suggests that bone has the ability to integrate into the surface of a titanium prosthesis. In fact, a chemical bond between the titanium and bone has even been proposed (1,6,42). Additionally, titanium implants, when compared to chrome–cobalt implants of similar design, have approximately half the modulus of elasticity. The tapered distal stem allows for a gradual transition in stiffness from the upper femur (Fig. 3). These features may help to account for the low incidence of thigh pain in patients fitted with a Taperloc implant. Finally, although uncemented chrome–cobalt implants have not been shown to cause an inordinately increased risk of malignancy, a theoretical concern remains.

Advocates of cemented fixation have espoused the view that all femoral components should be fixed with polymethylmethacrylate and that this decision should be made independent of age, weight, or sex of the patient and without regard to the diagnosis, inclusive of primary and revision operations (12,21). These proponents of cement fixation base their claim only partially on the low revision rates achieved with cemented femoral stems.

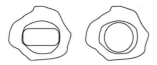

FIG. 1. A flat, wedge-shaped prosthesis in an ovoid femoral canal would be expected to provide better rotational stability than an implant with a design based on a round intramedullary rod.

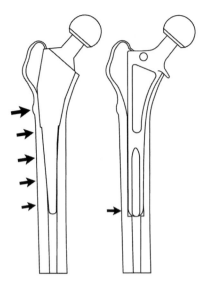

FIG. 3. The titanium composition and tapered-stem design of the Taperloc implant lower the modulus of elasticity of this prosthesis. The use of an implant with a rigid intramedullary rod design, particularly when made of chrome–cobalt, results in a more sudden transference of stress at the tip of the prosthesis.

Most now recognize that properly designed uncemented implants are also likely to yield outstanding short- (less than 2 years) and intermediate-term (2 to 5 years) results and that fixation is not the issue. A strong argument for cement has been based on the perceived high and increasing incidence of lysis associated with uncemented femoral components. Harris et al. (14) claimed that lysis of the femur about cementless components is progressive, and earlier in onset, higher in incidence, and more aggressive in extent than in cemented implants. The evidence for this belief lies in reports of significant osteolysis at 5- to 7-year follow-up utilizing several different uncemented implant designs. These studies have all been retrospective reviews without reasonably matched cemented controls. The uncemented hip replacements studied were implanted at a time when the relationship between polyethylene and wear was poorly understood. Many of the series of uncemented hips that have been reported evaluated implants with the potential for significant polyethylene wear from multiple causes: thin polyethylene, polyethylene sterilized with radiation in oxygen, liners that were incongruent with the metal backing, and titanium femoral heads.

It is apparent that osteolysis is a problem related to polyethylene wear and independent of the type of femoral fixation, cement, or bone ingrowth. However, in either case, cemented or uncemented, distal femoral osteolysis will occur if there is significant polyethylene wear and component loosening. This view is based on review of our own 5- to 8-year data for the Taperloc stem (19). We reviewed 103 primary uncemented hip arthroplasties that reflected our early experience with the Taperloc prosthe-

sis. The average follow-up was 6.08 years and the minimum follow-up was 5 years. The polyethylene in this series suffered from several design flaws, including inadequate thickness and incongruent liners. Furthermore, titanium heads were used. The incidence of osteolysis (greater than 25%) reflected these problems with polyethylene. However, remarkably, 100% of the significant, identifiable osteolysis occurred on the socket side of the hip, generally around screws that had been placed to augment initial stability of the metal shell. The incidence of distal femoral osteolysis was 0%. This may be related to the circumferential, closed-cell, porous coating of the Taperloc stem. Similar results have been reported with other circumferentially porous coated femoral stems (35). Distal femoral osteolysis is a function of excessive polyethylene wear and is associated with poor fixation of cemented and cementless components. There is no credible evidence at this time that cement unequivocally protects the femoral bone from osteolysis (20,22,32).

TECHNIQUE OF INSERTION OF THE TAPERLOC

A modification of the lateral-muscle-splitting approach to the hip described by Kevin Hardinge is frequently used to perform primary total hip arthroplasty. Although the trochanteric osteotomy as described by Sir John Charnley has been a dependable approach, providing excellent exposure with a very low complication rate, the Hardinge approach has been found to be an effective and useful alternative. The osteotomy has been reserved for certain patients who require greater exposure of the hip joint for satisfactory total hip replacement. Generally, the young muscular male patient, the obese patient, and the difficult reconstruction are selected for a trochanteric osteotomy. For most other patients in our practice, a total hip replacement is performed with a direct anterolateral (Hardinge) approach.

Once the acetabular component is inserted, the proximal femur is exposed. Hip arthroplasty is performed with the patient in the supine position, and, in order to expose the femur, the operative leg is placed in a position of modest external rotation and crossed over the opposite thigh. A laparotomy sponge is used to isolate the proximal femur, and the femur itself is elevated using a Mueller inferior acetabular retractor placed about the lesser trochanter. A second retractor, usually a Bennet, is placed beneath the greater trochanter to retract the posterior flap of soft tissue. This provides a generous exposure to the proximal femur. Forced rotation in abduction can lead to avulsion of the greater trochanter, so great care should be taken in osteoporotic elderly patients.

Next, the femoral canal is opened. First, excess soft tissue and cortical bone are excised from the tip of the greater trochanter, allowing access to the lateral aspect of

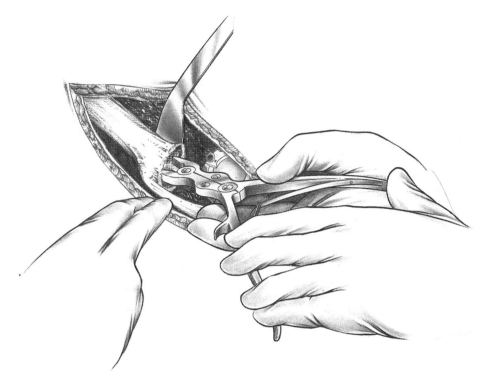

FIG. 4. Removal of cortical bridge and excessive soft tissue about the lateral aspect of the trochanter.

the trochanter (Fig. 4). This allows for reaming and broaching of the medial margin of the greater trochanter, and it avoids accidental varus positioning of the component. A straight stem curette is then introduced in the femoral canal in a neutral orientation (Fig. 5). Before inserting the curette, the surgeon should envision the direction and dimensions of the femur in both the anteroposterior and lateromedial planes. A fluted reamer is then introduced into the femoral canal along the path taken by the curette (Fig. 6). The reamer is inserted to a level based on templating of preoperative radiographs to estimate component size. The reamer is pushed slightly into varus and valgus to open up the canal. Minimal cancellous bone from the proximal femur is removed. Less cancellous bone is removed than the actual proportions of the implant. A femoral broach is then used to shape the fem-

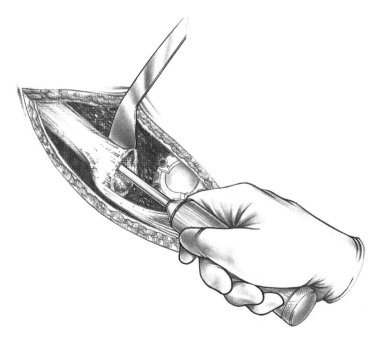

FIG. 5. Identification of the femoral canal with a small curette.

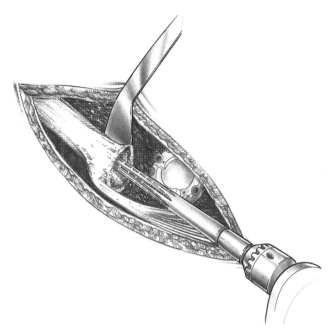

FIG. 6. Gentle insertion of a fluted power reamer.

oral canal to the exact dimensions of the actual prosthesis (Fig. 7). The broach is introduced in a neutral position (varus–valgus) and neutral version. Rotation is judged in relation to the position of the flexed leg.

Broaching is begun with a 7.5-mm broach and is progressively increased in 2.5-mm increments. Preoperative templating of radiographs is heavily relied on as a guide to the final size of the femoral component. The broach is introduced to its full depth, and, if resistance is met, broaching is continued with a series of small inward and outward taps. Broaching continues until full cortical seating has been accomplished. Full cortical seating can be determined by three parameters. First, there is a change in pitch as the broach becomes seated. Second, the surgeon notes that the implant fails to advance further in the canal. Finally, there is a change in the tactile sensation of the mallet as it strikes against the broach. As the surgeon gains experience with these criteria, full seating is readily determined and reproducible results are obtained.

Almost invariably, final sizing usually correlates to within one size of the preoperatively templated radiographs. If the size does not closely correlate with the preoperative assessment, this should serve as a warning sign and the femur should be carefully inspected for fracture. If a split of the femur is created, little resistance will be met as the implant passes into the canal, and no pitch change will occur. After the broach is seated, it serves as a trial prosthesis (Fig. 8).

The hip is reduced and stability and leg lengths are evaluated. Soft-tissue tension is evaluated by placing longitudinal traction on the leg while the hip is in a neutral position. In a typical man, less than 1 mm of distraction between the femoral head and socket is possible. In more supple women, 1 to 2 mm of distraction can be expected. Too much distraction indicates that the soft tissues are excessively loose or that leg length has not been restored. Several mechanisms may cause this soft-tissue laxity. For example, the cup may be placed too high in the pelvis, or the femoral component could be seated too low. This can

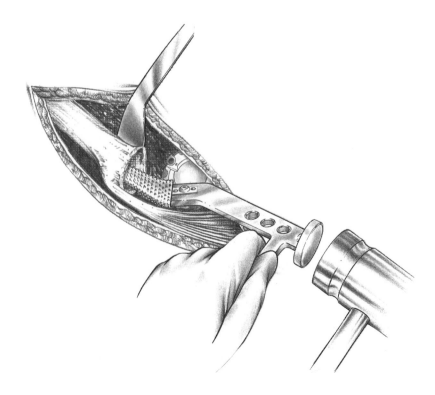

FIG. 7. Broaching the femur.

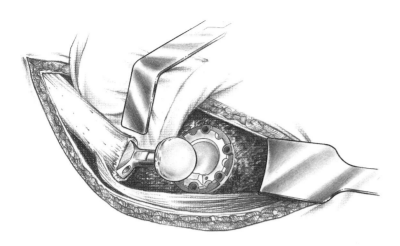

FIG. 8. Trial reduction using the broaches and trial head–neck sizes.

occur if the femoral neck is resected too low or if the chosen broach is too small and is seated too deeply into the canal. If the soft tissues are excessively tight, the cause is often related to a low position of the cup, retention of excessive femoral neck, or placing too large of a compo-

nent into the femur and having it get hung up before it is deeply seated. If the soft-tissue tension is appropriate, then the hip is checked for stability in both flexion and extension. The stability is checked with the hip flexed at 90° with adduction and internal rotation. If dislocation

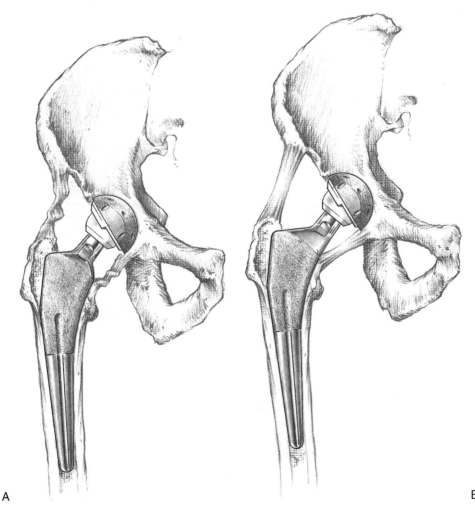

A   B

FIG. 9. Use of a lateral offset prosthesis increases soft-tissue tension without significantly increasing leg length.

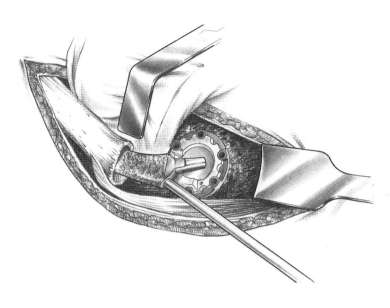

FIG. 10. Inserting the femoral prosthesis.

does occur, impingement may be present or the components could be malpositioned. With the hip in extension, stability is evaluated by external rotation and adduction.

Finally, leg lengths are evaluated. With a patient in the supine position, this is readily done. The limbs are placed in a neutral position and the medial malleoli are palpated and the leg lengths are estimated. We have found that this system is a precise and an easy way to determine leg lengths. If the hip is found to be unstable because of inadequate soft-tissue tension, then stability can be achieved by increasing the leg length. This is a satisfactory method if the limb is short. However, if the leg lengths are equal, then a lateral offset component is a better option. Use of the lateral offset often allows achievement of stability without inappropriate lengthening of the leg (Fig. 9). Stability, however, is more important than equal leg lengths and, therefore, unequal leg lengths should be accepted if this is the only way to gain stability. Using this technique, postoperative dislocation is a rare complication. After the appropriate components are chosen, the femoral prosthesis is inserted. The broach is removed with the extractor

and the femoral canal is copiously irrigated. Surgeons' gloves are always changed before inserting femoral and acetabular components. The appropriate-sized femoral component is placed in the femoral canal using an impactor (Fig. 10). Appropriate version is maintained during insertion of the prosthesis. The prosthesis is fully inserted by the same criteria as used for the broach. Again, three criteria are utilized: First, there is a pitch change as the mallet strikes the impactor; second, the implant fails to advance any further into the canal; and finally, there is a tactile sensation that the surgeon should feel as the implant becomes fully seated.

Once the component is inserted, a 22- or 28-mm trial femoral head is placed on the femoral component and a reduction is performed. Stability is again checked. Trials are done at this point because we often find that the depth of insertion of the broach and the actual implant may vary by a few millimeters. Because there is no collar on the prosthesis, it is inserted until it is fully seated. Achieving equal leg lengths is possible because of the wide range of neck lengths available. The hip is dislocated again, and,

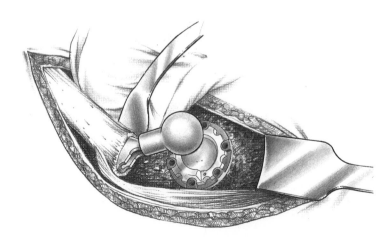

FIG. 11. Final reduction using a modular head–neck combination.

after the trial femoral head is removed, the Morse taper is thoroughly cleaned and dried. The appropriate-sized femoral head is then placed on the Morse taper and seated in position with light taps of an impactor. Retractors are removed, the socket is irrigated, and the acetabulum is carefully inspected to be sure no debris is present. Direct visualization of the acetabulum is mandatory during reduction of the prosthesis (Fig. 11). It is important to make sure that all debris is removed and that the capsule and other soft tissue are not trapped between the femoral head and socket. Stability and leg lengths are rechecked. The wound and components are then thoroughly cleaned and closure follows.

CLINICAL INDICATIONS AND RESULTS

Porous-coated implants designed for biologic fixation by bone ingrowth were introduced because of dissatisfaction with the long-term results associated with cemented hip arthroplasty, particularly in younger and more active patients. In the mid 1980s, Ranawat et al. (31) reported an almost 30% incidence of radiographic femoral loosening at the 5- to 10-year follow-up in patients between the ages of 40 and 60 at the time of arthroplasty. Collis (8), at about the same time, published the results of hip arthroplasty in patients under age 50. He studied 45 hips with arthritis, mainly caused by avascular necrosis, congenital dysplasia, or trauma, with an average follow-up of 7.5 years. The revision rate was 9%, but the incidence of radiographic femoral loosening was much higher. The average Postoperative Iowa Hip Rating was 92 points; however, because of the radiographic findings, deterioration of these results with time could be inferred. Dorr et al. (9) published results of hip arthroplasty in patients who were younger than 45 at the time of surgery, with follow-up averaging 4.5 years. The revision rate and impending failure rates were 19% and 45%, respectively. The question remains, how much has modern cement technique improved these results? Ballard et al. (2) recently reviewed a series of 42 arthroplasties performed with second-generation cement technique and a minimum 10-year follow-up. All patients were under age 50 at the time of the index operation. The femoral revision rate was 5%, and another 12% of stems were radiographically loose. These results are good, but not good enough to preclude examining alternative technology.

Cementless arthroplasty for the younger, more active patient has been performed long enough for several 5-year minimal follow-up series to be published. Clearly, implant design is critical because the results are so variable. High failure rates with uncemented stems of anatomic design and collared prostheses have been reported (5,15,36). On the other hand, Engh et al. (10,11) have reported good results with reliable, long-term fixation with a straight stem, fully porous-coated prosthesis.

In 1994, the 2- to 6-year results of arthroplasty for the first 100 Taperloc femoral components we implanted was published (17). Mean follow-up was 3.8 years and information was obtainable from 98 of the 100 patients in the study. Charnley pain and function scores rose from 3.0 and 2.8, respectively, to 5.5 and 5.4 after surgery. Evidence of bone ingrowth was 98% and there were no revisions. Results were considered excellent and equivalent to those obtainable with cement. This is particularly gratifying because this study population was young (average age, 56 years), active (only three patients with rheumatoid arthritis), and heavy (average weight 78 kg).

These excellent results with the Taperloc prosthesis led to an exploration of the limitations of this implant. With initial caution, the indications for implantation were extended to patients with relative osteopenia, such as those with rheumatoid arthritis, and also to elderly patients with osteoarthritis. The prosthesis was chosen for these patients not because of dissatisfaction with cement, but because of the advantages of the Taperloc implant: ease of insertion, shorter operative time, few technical errors, and reproducible results. In practices based at large residency hospitals, good cement technique is sometimes difficult to teach. The simplicity of inserting the Taperloc makes it almost universally possible to instruct residents and fellows on how to perform successful arthroplasty.

To assess the results of uncemented arthroplasty in patients who traditionally would have had a cemented procedure, 52 total hip arthroplasties in 41 patients with rheumatoid arthritis (25) were reviewed. Follow-up averaged 3.6 years with a range of 2 to 7 years. The average age of the patients was 56 years. The mean follow-up Charnley score for pain was 5.7. There were no intraoperative femoral fractures in this relatively osteopenic group and no femoral revisions. There was no definite radiographic loosening, and spot welds were noted in 98% of patients.

Octogenarians are another group for whom cementless arthroplasty would seem unconventional. An analysis of 64 cemented and 41 cementless femoral results in patients over age 80 was performed (28). Follow-up ranged from 2 to 5 years. Degenerative arthritis was the diagnosis for all patients studied and the demographics of the two groups were quite similar, including radiographic assessment of bone quality. The results of cemented total hip arthroplasty in the octogenarian population were excellent, but the results for uncemented total hip arthroplasty were quite similar. In this older age group, postoperative Charnley Scores for pain, function, and motion were 5.4, 4.3, and 5.4, respectively. This was not statistically different from a cemented control group. In our practice, uncemented total hip arthroplasty is now routinely performed for the elderly patient. Our extensive experience with the Taperloc prosthesis has provided us with data to make rational decisions about cemented ver-

TABLE 2. *Taperloc results based on preoperative diagnosis*

Category	Charnley Hip Score			Femoral revisions (%)	Radiographically loose stem (%)	Thigh pain (%)*	Distal femoral osteolysis (%)
	Pain	Function	Motion				
Young, active; osteoarthritis; N = 95; 2–6 yr follow-up							
Preoperative	3.0	2.7	3.1				
Postoperative	5.6	5.5	5.5	0	0	2	0
Rheumatoid arthritis; N = 52; 2–7 yr follow-up							
Preoperative	2.2	3.1	3.8				
Postoperative	5.7	5.0	5.4	0	0	6	0
Octogenarian; N = 41; 2–5 yr follow-up							
Postoperative	5.7	4.3	5.4	0	0	10	0

*Thigh pain was described as mild by all patients with this complaint.

sus cementless fixation of the femoral component. We now strongly believe that almost all patients with severe arthritis, regardless of age, weight, sex, or diagnosis, can have an excellent clinical result with a cementless implant of proper design. This statement stands in diametric opposition to those who advocate cement, but our consistently good results (in a very high-volume practice) validate this premise. Currently, we reserve the use of cement for the extremely osteopenic individual for whom a good press-fit cannot be achieved.

The results of uncemented total hip arthroplasty using the Taperloc prosthesis, stratified by preoperative diagnosis, are shown in Table 2.

CONCLUSIONS

This chapter is an argument for the use of the cementless tapered femoral prosthesis during total hip arthroplasty. Ultimately, though, decisions about implant choice can be made only when follow-up data become available. Longer-term data for the wedge-shaped Taperloc has recently been reviewed (19).

A 5- to 8-year follow-up is now available on 105 primary uncemented Taperloc femoral components and is shown in Table 3. The mean follow-up was over 6 years for the patients studied. The average age at follow-up was 61.2 years, the average weight 172.0 pounds, and there

were only five patients with rheumatoid arthritis. The femoral results were excellent. One femoral revision was performed to facilitate an acetabular revision, but the femoral revision rate for aseptic loosening was 0%. In addition, no femoral components had subsided or were felt to be loose radiographically.

Unfortunately, the acetabular revision rate was 11.4%, and acetabular cavitary lesions were identified in 25.5% of cases. Polyethylene wear and osteolysis were responsible for this failure rate. Despite the presence of particulate debris, there was only a 5% incidence of femoral osteolysis. However, the presence of osteolysis distal to the circumferential porous coating could not be radiographically identified. This coating may, therefore, act as a particulate seal.

If it were not for polyethylene wear and failure of the acetabular component, the revision rate for the Taperloc prosthesis, at 5- to 8-year follow-up, would be very low. This has prompted the continued and routine use of this femoral component. However, to lower the revision rate of the socket, the femoral head, the acetabular component, and polyethylene have been modified. Instead of titanium femoral heads, chrome—cobalt components are now used exclusively. The metal shell of the acetabular component has been modified so that the polyethylene seats firmly and is more congruent with the metal backing. The metal shell has also been modified to increase polyethylene thickness and to allow for use of a liner of

TABLE 3. *Follow-up (5 to 8 years) on the Taperloc femoral component*

Category	Charnley Hip Score			Femoral revisions (%)	Radiographically loose stem (%)	Thigh pain (%)	Distal femoral osteolysis (%)
	Pain	Function	Motion				
N = 105; 5–8 yr follow-up							
Preoperative	2.6	2.8	3.8				
Postoperative	5.5	5.2	5.6	1	0	3	0

uniform thickness (the older design had thicker polyethylene at the center that thinned as the rim was approached). In cases when the metal shell is small and polyethylene thickness would be less than 9 mm with a 28-mm head, a 22-mm head is substituted. Finally, the polyethylene is now sterilized in argon instead of the oxygen used previously. These modifications can be expected to diminish polyethylene wear and lower the incidence of arthroplasty failure and osteolysis.

If the rate of acetabular failure can be lowered, the 5- to 8-year results of arthroplasty with a Taperloc prosthesis would surpass the previously reported excellent results of the cemented Charnley total hip arthroplasty. This reasoning has prompted us to continue to routinely perform uncemented total hip arthroplasty using a tapered femoral component.

REFERENCES

1. Albrektsson T, Branemark PJ, Hansson HA, Lindstrom J. Osseointegrated titanium implants. *Acta Orthop Scand* 1981;52:155.
2. Ballard WT, Callaghan JJ, Sullivan PM, Johnston RC. The results of improved cementing techniques for total hip arthroplasty in patients less than fifty years old: a ten year follow-up study. *J Bone Joint Surg* 1994;76A:959.
3. Black J. Metallic ion release and its relationship to oncogenesis. In: Fitzgerald R, ed. *The hip: proceedings of the 13th open scientific meeting of The Hip Society.* St. Louis: CV Mosby, 1985;199.
4. Butler CA, Jones LC, Hungerford DS. Initial implant stability of porous coated total hip femoral components: a mechanical study. *Proceedings of the Orthopaedic Research Society 34th annual meeting.* Atlanta, Feb. 4-9, 1988.
5. Callaghan JJ, Dysart SH, Savory CG. The uncemented-porous coated anatomic total hip prosthesis: two year results of a prospective consecutive series. *J Bone Joint Surg* 1988;70A:337.
6. Carlsson L, Rostlund T, Albrektsson T, Branemark P. Osseointegration of titanium implants. *Acta Orthop Scand* 1986;57:285.
7. Chandler HP, Reinick FT, Wixson RL, McCarthy JC. Total hip replacement in patients younger than 30 years old: a 5 year follow-up study. *J Bone Joint Surg* 1981;63A:1426.
8. Collis DK. Cemented total hip replacement in patients who are less than fifty years old. *J Bone Joint Surg* 1984;66A:353.
9. Dorr LD, Takei GK, Conaty JP. Total hip arthroplasties in patients less than 45 years old. *J Bone Joint Surg* 1983;65A:474.
10. Engh CA, Bobyn JD. The influence of stem size and extent of porous coating on femoral bone resorption after primary cementless hip arthroplasty. *Clin Orthop* 1988;231:7.
11. Engh CA, Bobyn JD, Glassman AH. Porous coated hip replacement: the factors governing bone ingrowth, stress shielding and clinical results. *J Bone Joint Surg* 1987;69B:45.
12. Harris WJ. The case for cemented fixation of the femur in every patient. *Instr Course Lect* 1994;43:367.
13. Harris WH, McGann WA. Loosening of the femoral component after use of the medullary plug cementing technique: follow-up note with a minimum 5 year follow-up. *J Bone Joint Surg* 1986;68A:1064.
14. Harris WH, Smith EJ, Goetz DD. Bone cement as a seal protecting the femur from the ingress of particulate debris and femoral osteolysis. *Instr Course Lect* 1996;45:183.
15. Heekin RD, Callaghan JJ, Hopkinson WJ, Savory CG, Xenos JS. The porous coated anatomic total hip prosthesis, inserted without cement: results after five to seven years in a prospective study. *J Bone Joint Surg* 1993;75A:77.
16. Hozack WJ, Booth RE. Clinical and radiographic results with the Trilock femoral component—A wedge-fit porous ingrowth stem design. *Semin Arthroplasty* 1990;1:64.
17. Hozack W, Gardiner R, Hearn S, Eng K, Rothman R. Taperloc femoral component: a 2–6 year study of the first 100 consecutive cases. *J Arthroplasty* 1994;9(5):489.
18. Hozack WJ, Rothman RH, Booth RE, Balderston RA, Cohn JE, Pickens JT. Survivorship analysis of 1,041 Charnley total hip arthroplasties. *J Arthroplasty* 1990;5:41.
19. Hozack WJ, Rothman RH, Eng K, Mesa J. Primary total hip arthroplasty with a titanium plasma-sprayed prosthesis inserted without cement: a report of 105 cases with five to eight year follow-up. Submitted for publication.
20. Huddleston, H.D. Femoral lysis after cemented hip arthroplasty. J. Arthroplasty 3:285, 1988.
21. Jasty, M.J. Cemented fixation of the femur. Instructional Course Lectures. 43:373, 1994.
22. Jasty, M.J, Floyd, W.E, Schiller, A.L, Goldring, S.R, and Harris, W.H. Localized osteolysis in stable, non-septic total hip arthroplasty. *J Bone Joint Surg* 68A:912, 1986.
23. Joshi, A.B, Porter, M.L, Trail, I.A, Hunt, L.P, Murphy, J.C.M, and Hardinge, K. Long-Term Results of Charnley Low-Friction Arthroplasty in Young Patients. *J Bone Joint Surg* 75B:616, 1993.
24. Kavanagh, B.F, Dewitz, M.A, Ilstrup, D.M, Stauffer, R.N. and Coventry, M.B. Charnley total hip arthroplasty with cement: Fifteen - year results. *J Bone Joint Surg* 71(A): 1496, 1989.
25. McCallum, J.D, Hozack, W.J, Rothman, R.H, Mesa, J.J. and Eng, K. Uncemented total hip arthroplasty in rheumatoid arthritis: Two to seven year results. 1997 (submitted).
26. McCoy TH, Salvati EA, Ranawat CS, Wilson PD Jr. A fifteen-year follow-up study of one hundred Charnley low-friction arthroplasties. *Orthop Clin North Am* 1988;19:467.
27. Pavlov PW. A 15 year follow-up study of 512 consecutive Charnley-Muller total hip replacements. *J Arthroplasty* 1987;2:151.
28. Peyton RS, Bicalho PS, McGuigan FX, Hozack WJ, Rothman RH, Eng K. Uncemented total hip arthroplasty in octogenarians: comparison to an equivalent cemented group. 1997 (submitted).
29. Pilliar RM, Lee JM, Maniato Poulos C. Observations on the effect of movement on bone ingrowth into porous-surfaced implants. *Clin Orthop* 1986;208:108–113.
30. Ranawat CS, Atkinson RE, Salvati EA, Wilson PD. Conventional total hip arthroplasty for degenerative joint disease in patients between the ages of 40 and 60 years. *J Bone Joint Surg* 1984;66A:745.
31. Ranawat CS, Hangrai KK, Neves MC. A seventeen year survivorship study of Charnley total hip replacement. *Clin Exp Rheumatol* 1989;7 (suppl 3):153.
32. Rothman RH, Cohn JC. Cemented versus cementless total hip arthroplasty: a critical review. *Clin Orthop* 1990;254:153.
33. Schulte KR, Callaghan JJ, Kelley SS, Johnston RC. The outcome of Charnley total hip arthroplasty with cement after a minimum twenty-year follow-up: the results of one surgeon. *J Bone Joint Surg* 1993; 75A:961.
34. Sharkey PF, Albert TJ, Hume EL, Rothman RH. Initial stability of a collarless wedge-shaped prosthesis in the femoral canal. *Semin Arthroplasty* 1990;1:87.
35. Sharkey PF, Tvetden D, Barrack RL. Results of uncemented total hip arthroplasty with the LSF prosthesis: a five to eight year follow-up. Proceedings of the annual meeting of the American Academy of Orthopaedic Surgeons. New Orleans: 1994.
36. Smith EJ, Harris WH. Increasing rate of femoral lysis in cementless total hip arthroplasty. *J Arthroplasty* 1995;10:407.
37. Stauffer RN. Ten year follow-up study of total roentgenographic loosening of the components. *J Bone Joint Surg* 1982;64A:983.
38. Sutherland CJ, Wilde AH, Borden LS, Marks KE. A ten year follow-up of 100 consecutive Muller curved stem total hip replacement arthroplasties. *J Bone Joint Surg* 1982;64A:970.
39. Wejkner B, Stenport J. Charnley total hip arthroplasty: a ten- to 14-year follow-up study. *Clin Orthop* 1988;231:113.
40. Wroblewski BM. 15-21 year results of the Charnley low-friction arthroplasty. *Clin Orthop* 1986;211:30.
41. Zweymuller K. A cementless titanium hip endoprothesis system based on press-fit fixation: basis, research and clinical results. *Instr Course Lect* 1986;35:203.
42. Zweymuller KA, Lintner FK, Semlitsch MF. Biologic fixation of a press-fit titanium hip joint endoprosthesis. *Clin Orthop* 1988;235:195.

The Adult Hip, edited by J. J. Callaghan,
A. G. Rosenberg, and H. E. Rubash.
Lippincott–Raven Publishers, Philadelphia © 1998.

CHAPTER 68

Press-Fit Femoral Components

J. David Blaha

THE TRUE MEANING OF PRESS-FIT

Although the word is used frequently, there is considerable confusion about the meaning of press-fit. Thus, a chapter about this type of femoral component must begin with a definition.

The term *press-fit* originates in engineering, where it is used to denote a mechanical joining of two parts based on contact pressure (10). To achieve a press-fit, one of two members is made slightly oversized for a corresponding hole in the other member. Frequently, the part to be driven into the other is cooled, causing it to shrink (hence the term *shrink-fit,* which is a type of press-fit). When the two parts are forcibly driven together, there is controlled elastic deformation of both parts, with subsequent elastic recoil leading to high stresses over the area joining the two parts. Friction between the two pieces increases with the contact stress, leading to a mechanical joining. The high stress per area is a pressure-fit or press-fit joining of the two parts.

A nail driven into a block of wood is a familiar example of press-fit (Fig. 1). Usually, there is no hole drilled in the wood before the nail is inserted, but for particularly large nails a carpenter will often drill into the wood a hole slightly smaller than the diameter of the nail. When the nail is driven into place, the elastic recoil of the nail out-

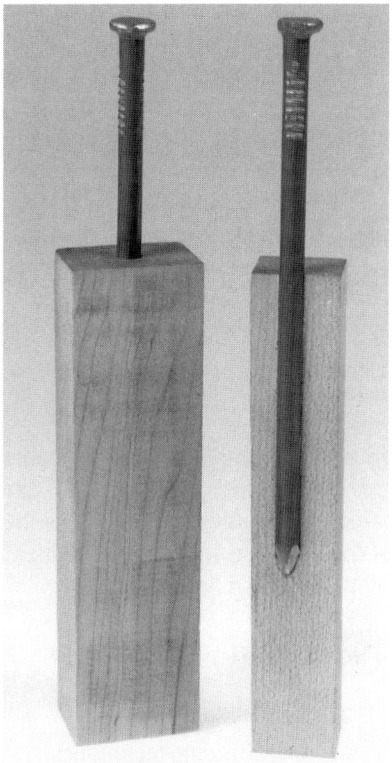

FIG. 1. A nail driven into a block of wood is an example of press-fit. For large nails, a carpenter drills a hole smaller than the diameter of the nail before inserting it. The elastic recoil of the wood toward the nail and that of the nail toward the wood lead to high contact pressure and stable joining of the nail with the wood.

J. D. Blaha: Department of Orthopaedics, West Virginia University, Morgantown, West Virginia 26506-9196.

ward into the wood, and the wood's recoil inward toward the nail, lead to high contact pressure and a stable joining of the nail with the wood.

Press-fit requires that the two materials to be joined be elastic and remain so over the period that the joining is expected to continue. If one of the pieces loses its elastic recoil, the high contact stresses will be lost and the joining of the parts will weaken or completely dissipate.

True Press-Fit in Bone

Bone is a viscoelastic material. This property of bone implies that its elastic recoil will become less with time. The amount that bone will "creep" or undergo stress–relaxation depends on its density: cortical bone has less viscoelastic behavior than cancellous bone (3,4). The fact that bone will relax and lose elasticity over time limits the amount of time over which a true press-fit can be maintained in bone. Once the initial press-fit dissipates, a prosthesis may move under load in the bone and either reestablish a press-fit or become loose.

COMMON USAGE OF *PRESS-FIT*

The advent of porous-ingrowth surfaces led to considerable confusion about the concept of press-fit. Porous-ingrowth prostheses were developed to be an alternative to the use of cement for fixation. A porous surface is a material or structure applied to the surface of an implant to promote interlock with the surrounding bone. The porous surface has interconnecting pores in its depth, and the intent is to have bone grow into and through the pores of the surface to interlock the porous structure of the surface with that of the bone. As porous-coated implants were being introduced, other implants were developed (or were already available) that did not have a porous surface specifically intended for interconnecting ingrowth, but which were intended for implantation without cement. Without regard for the true meaning of press-fit, these were termed press-fit implants. In this common usage, the term *press-fit* came to mean implant fixation without a porous surface and without cement. It is the confusion in the use of the term that leads to difficulties in comparing results with "press-fit" prostheses.

POROUS-INGROWTH VERSUS PRESS-FIT

The terms *porous-ingrowth* and *press-fit* are frequently used to indicate two different techniques. However, the two concepts are not mutually exclusive.

Surface Structure

Porous-ingrowth is one way to treat the surface of an implant so that bone will adapt to the surface and provide

long-term load transfer and fixation of the implant. Roughening the surface of the implant by corundum blasting or acid etching, grooving the surface for macro-interlock with bone, and application of hydroxylapatite are other means of surface treatment. The surface structure of an implant has nothing to do with the implant's press-fit nature.

Mechanical Joining

Press-fit is a means of mechanical joining of two objects. The joining is caused by driving an oversized object into an undersized hole. A smooth-surfaced implant may be press-fit if it is made to be oversized. A porous-surfaced or rough-surfaced implant may be press-fit if it is manufactured larger than the dimensions of the tools used to create the cavity into which it fits in the femur. Either smooth or nonsmooth implants can be made to be exact-fit if they are not deliberately made oversized.

The type of initial fixation (press-fit or exact-fit), the means to provide for continuing stability during viscoelastic relaxation and bone adaptation, and the surface treatment for bone attachment are independent of each other and make up the design rationale for a given implant system.

Osseointegration

Osseointegration is a term used to imply the direct apposition of bone to the surface of an implant without intervening tissue such a fibrous tissue. *Osseointegration* has been used by some to denote the bone apposition that occurs to implants that do not have a porous surface. For this chapter, the term may apply equally to any type of implant that supports direct apposition of bone to its surface regardless of subsurface interconnecting porosity.

DESIGNS FOR A PRESS-FIT FEMORAL-STEM IMPLANT

Because femoral stems are placed inside the femur, it is relatively easy to visualize the technique of placing a press-fit prosthesis. After resection of the top of the femur (i.e., the head and neck region), the canal is prepared with machining tools to make a cavity into which the prosthesis will be placed. The cavity is made just slightly smaller than the actual size of the prosthesis, so that when the prosthesis is placed, there will be deformation of the femur and of the prosthesis. As a result, there is elastic recoil of the two parts that leads to high contact forces (pressure) and creates the press-fit fixation. A short prosthesis designed not to fill the canal in its distal portion would have its press-fit fixation in the proximal bone. A longer prosthesis would have the possibility of press-fit in the upper diaphysis of the femur.

The joining of the prosthesis to bone would be complete after initial implantation were it not for the fact that bone is a viscoelastic material. With the constant stress of the oversized implant in the canal, the bone will undergo stress–relaxation and the contact forces with the implant will become less. If the prosthesis is long and press-fitted into the upper diaphysis, it might be possible to keep the implant stable by a proximal collar. However, for the short prosthesis to maintain a press-fit, the implant must take on a wedge shape so that, as stress–relaxation proceeds, axial load on the implant will cause slight migration of the implant further into the canal. This migration brings a larger cross section of the implant into the canal and causes the press-fit to be reestablished.

The proximal femur has relatively more cancellous bone and less cortical bone than the diaphysis, and it is more prone to viscoelastic relaxation than the diaphysis. An implant that establishes press-fit more proximally will have to be designed to accept more migration than one designed to have its press-fit more distally. In the extreme case, where the implant is very firmly press-fit into distal bone, little migration would be expected and the prosthesis could have a collar to contact the proximal femur. In the opposite extreme case, where press-fit is minimal distally and significant proximally, migration would be expected to be of sufficient magnitude that the implant should have no collar for proximal load transfer, lest the migration to reestablish press-fit be hindered by the collar.

The process of stress–relaxation and stability, through a collar or migration, to reestablish press-fit obviously cannot continue indefinitely. At some point, the implant must become stabilized by bone that in some way mechanically supports the implant and prevents further migration by transferring load from the implant to the bone. An implant must have some sort of macro- or microstructuring to allow the surrounding bone to mechanically accept the stresses from the interface and transfer them into the rest of the bone structure. Press-fit is not a method of permanent fixation of an implant to the bone, but it is rather a means of holding an implant stable enough to allow the bone to adapt to its presence and provide for long-term load transfer.

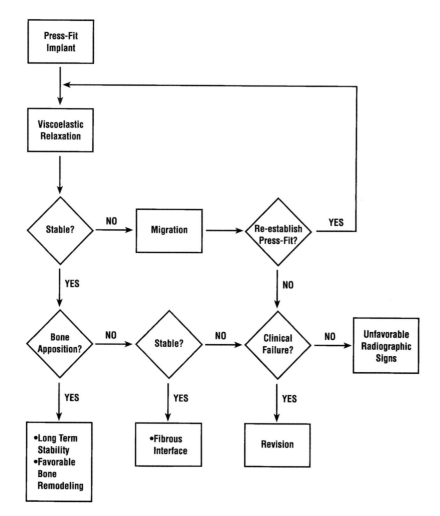

FIG. 2. Flow diagram of the concept of fixation of a cementless implant that was initially press-fit. In this scheme, the surface of the implant must accommodate bone apposition to achieve long-term fixation, but there is no requirement that the surface be porous.

The principles are then these: (a) establish press-fit, proximally, distally, or in combination, in the medullary canal of the femur; (b) allow for some migration of the implant consistent with the area in which the press-fit is obtained; and (c) provide for some means of bone attachment to the implant so that further migration can be eliminated by transfer of stress to the bone (Fig. 2).

CLINICAL EXPERIENCE WITH PRESS-FIT IMPLANTS

There have been many reports, mostly in the form of oral presentation, of press-fit femoral components. In some instances, the reports have been about devices that are truly press-fit, but in many cases the presentation is about an implant called press-fit using the more colloquial definition. This section about clinical experience will concern three prostheses, all called press-fit. All have been clinically successful.

Zweymuller Prosthesis

Karl Zweymuller introduced a tapered implant for press-fit fixation in 1979 (Fig. 3). The implant was not the first designed specifically for press-fit fixation and, in fact, Zweymuller had tried other cementless implants previously. The stem is wedge-shaped and is long enough to engage the upper diaphysis so as to have initial fixation with a press-fit at that level. The surface is roughened by corundum blasting (Fig. 4). There have been several design modifications over the years, but the principle of press-fit fixation (including a significant amount of load transfer in the upper diaphysis region) has been maintained since the introduction of the implant.

In recent years, there have been a few reports of use of the Zweymuller prosthesis presented in the orthopedic literature. Zweymuller et al. (12) reported that more than 40,000 patients had had the prosthesis implanted, and they showed histologic results from autopsy studies. The intimate approximation of bone to the implant suggests that with this implant, there was sufficient stability from press-fit to allow secondary bone apposition and osseointegration (Fig. 5).

Martin et al. (5) reported on 46 total hip arthroplasties in 46 patients using the Zweymuller stem, with minimum 3-year follow-up. They found 42 excellent, 3 good, and 1 fair result, with no revisions required. Radiographically, they found evidence of stable fixation in all hips and no osteolysis.

CLS Prosthesis

The CLS prosthesis is a three-dimensional taper (i.e., in the sagittal, coronal, and transverse planes) (Fig. 6). It is deliberately made small in its distal part so that it

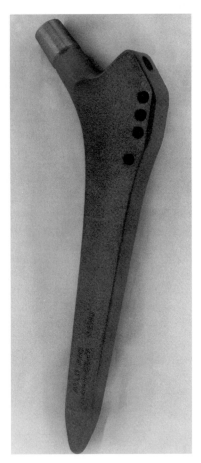

FIG. 3. The Zweymuller prosthesis is a straight, tapered wedge that is long enough to gain press-fit fixation in the upper diaphysis.

will not obtain a press-fit in the upper diaphysis. On the upper part of the prosthesis, there are grooves that contribute to the wedge-shaped geometry of the implant and also provide a larger surface area of the metal in contact with bone. The implant is made of titanium alloy and is treated by corundum blasting to have a roughness similar to that of the Zweymuller prosthesis. The implant has been in use for 13 years, so a significant number of patients have passed a potential 10-year follow-up.

Laboratory results show initial micromotion of the CLS implant after loading (6,9) This type of motion has often been presented as a negative because it might lessen ingrowth. Alternatively, for a truly press-fit prosthesis (particularly one that wedges in the canal proximally and not distally), such initial motion is important, as it represents further engagement of the stem taper with the bone. Such continuing engagement is an appropriate way to keep the implant stable, that is, through controlled subsidence particularly in viscoelastic bone.

Spotorno et al. (11) presented the results of the first 300 CLS stems used, implanted by the stem's designer (Fig. 7). At the 5- to 8-year follow-up, the mean Harris hip Score

FIG. 4. The surface of the Zweymuller prosthesis (and many others manufactured by Sulzer in Switzerland and other manufacturers elsewhere) is roughened by sandblasting with corundum (a fine sand made of aluminum oxide).

was found to be 94. There were seven revisions, two of which were for loosened femoral components. Two additional cases of loosening were suspected from radiographic review, giving a mechanical failure rate of 1.6%.

Robinson et al. (7) reported on 51 CLS stems with early follow-up of 2 to 4 years. No stem required revision and 6% had slight, occasional thigh pain. These authors found that 55% of cases had proximal-bone-density reduction, suggesting that the load transfer from this implant to the bone of the femur was more distal after osseointegration had taken place. A further report from Robinson et al. (8) at a mean 6-year follow-up showed continued satisfactory clinical results, with a survivorship prediction of 96% at 92 months. Six of the 57 hips in this study showed measurable subsidence, with the maximum being 4 mm. No femoral stem in this series was judged to be mechanically loose, either by clinical or by radiographic criteria.

Blasius et al. (1) documented the results from a multi-center study with an average 2-year follow-up of 1830 patients. Ninety-one percent of the cases had a good or excellent clinical result, and the incidence of femoral component loosening was less than 1%.

Omnifit Prosthesis

The Omnifit demonstrates the concept of press-fit and shows that press-fit is not distinct from porous coating.

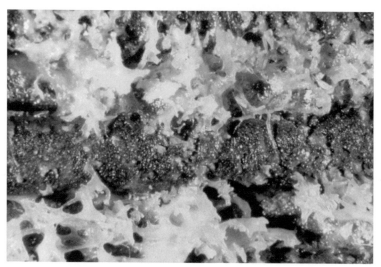
A

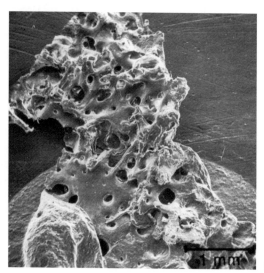
B

FIG. 5. A: Explanted prosthesis (in close-up view) shows cancellous bone adherent to the implant. **B:** Higher-power examination shows bone apposition to the implant.

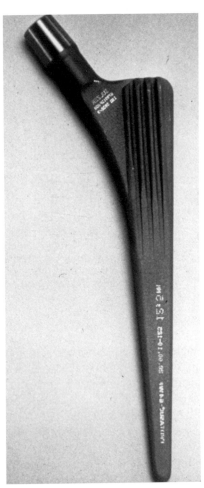

FIG. 6. The CLS prosthesis is a tapered wedge in all planes (i.e., coronal, sagittal, and transverse). It is designed to produce a press-fit in the upper portion of the femur.

This prosthesis has a double-wedge configuration proximally (coronal and sagittal) designed for press-fit in the metaphyseal portion of the femur (Fig. 8). Over the proximal one third of the stem, which is made from cobalt–chrome, there is a circumferential porous coating that provides both for surface roughness and interconnecting porosity in the depth of the coating.

Hellman and Capello (2) reported on 79 hips from a group of 111 hips, with an average follow-up of 101 months (range, 64 to 125). Ninety-six percent of the patients reported no or mild pain in the thigh, and no patients had activity-limiting thigh pain. Ninety-seven percent of patients had no or mild limp, and 93% required no support to walk. The aseptic revision rate in this group of patients was 2.5% (2 of 79) and the mechanical failure rate (i.e., those revised plus those radiographically loose) was 3.8% (3 of 79).

Review of the radiographs from this series demonstrated condensation of bone around the porous coating (especially at the junction of the coating and the distal part of the stem), and reactive lines about the uncoated part of the

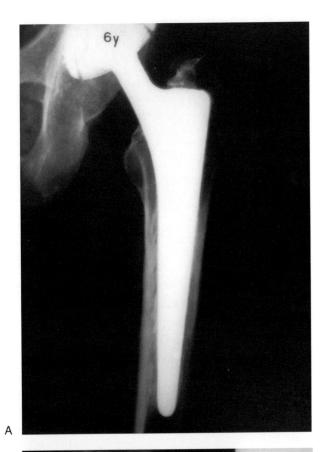

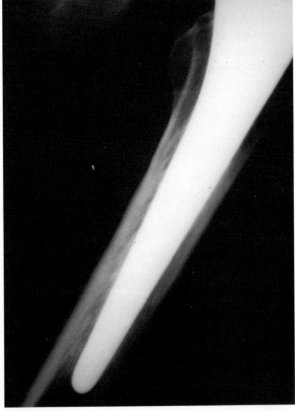

FIG. 7. Anteroposterior **(A)** and lateral **(B)** radiographs showing endosteal bone formation from the inner cortex to the roughened surface of the CLS stem.

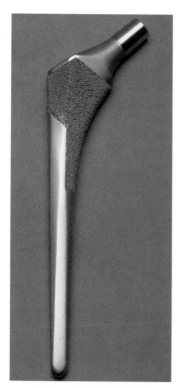

FIG. 8. The Omnifit prosthesis is a two-dimensionally tapered wedge that has proximal porous coating. Primary stability is achieved through press-fit, and secondary stability through bone apposition and ingrowth.

stem were common (21%). Three components moved in the canal (two shifted slightly into varus and one subsided minimally), but all stabilized and had excellent clinical results. There were two cases of intramedullary osteolysis, both associated with symptomatically loose stems, but, despite significant osteolysis associated with acetabular polyethylene wear, lesions were confined to the proximal femur (Gruen zones 1 and 7).

These results are equivalent to those with the Zwey-muller and CLS prostheses at similar time periods, which suggests that a similar mechanism of fixation is occurring. This prosthesis, like the others, is initially stabilized by press-fit (i.e., primary stability by press-fit), and in the long term it is fixed by bone apposition to (with growth into) the porous surface. The radiographic results suggest a subsidence-tolerant design that allows the implant to maintain stability should the initial press-fit dissipate.

Press-fit should not simply mean implantation without cement and without a porous coating. Rather, press-fit should refer to the engineering term *pressure-fit*, which is a means of joining two objects through high contact pressures. The surface configuration of an implant (porous, roughened, or smooth) does not relate to the press-fit nature of fixation for that implant.

If a prosthesis has a means of primary stability (press-fit), can tolerate loading while the bone undergoes viscoelastic relaxation, and has a surface to which bone can attach (whether a surface with interconnecting porosity or only surface roughness), that implant has a high probability of having a satisfactory result.

REFERENCES

1. Blasius K, Cotta, H, Schneider U, Thomsen M. CLS multicenter study—8 year results. *Z Orthop Ihre Grenzgeb* 1993;131:547–552.
2. Hellman EJ, Capello WN. Proximally coated stems. In: Sedel L, Cabanela M, eds. *Hip surgery: new materials and developments.* London: Martin Dunitz, 1996 *(in press).*
3. Lakes RS, Katz JL. Viscoelastic properties of wet cortical bone. I. Torsonal and biaxial studies. *J Biomech* 1979;12:657–678.
4. Lakes RS, Katz JL. Viscoelastic properties of wet cortical bone. II. Relaxation mechanisms. *J Biomech* 1979;12:679–687.
5. Martin RP, Huo MH, Zatorski L, Keggi KJ. Primary THR using a non-porous-coated, wedge-shaped stem implanted without cement: consecutive series, minimum 3-year follow-up. *Ortho Trans* 1994–1995;18:1168–1169.
6. McKellop H, Ebramzadeh E, Niederer PG, Sarmiento A. Comparison of the stability of press-fit hip prosthesis femoral stems using a synthetic model femur. *J Orthop Res* 9:297–305.
7. Robinson RP, Lovell TP, Green TM. Hip arthroplasty using the cementless CLS stem. A 2–4 year experience. *J Arthroplasty* 1994;9(2):177–192.
8. Robinson RP, Gaston RD, Green TM. Total hip arthroplasty using the CLS stem: a titanium alloy implant with corundum blast finish: results at a mean 6 years in a prospective study. *J Arthroplasty* 1996;11(3):286–292.
9. Schneider E, Kinast K, Eulenberger J, Wyder D, Eskilsson BS, Perren SM. A comparative study of the initial stability of cementless hip prostheses. *Clin Orthop* 1989;248:200–209.
10. Shigley JE. *Mechanical engineering design*, 3rd ed. New York: McGraw-Hill, 1977.
11. Spotorno L, Romagnoli S, Ivaldo N, Grappiolo G, Bibbiani E, Blaha JD, Gruen TA. The CLS system. Theoretical concept and results. *Acta Orthop Belgica* 1993;59(suppl 1):144–148.
12. Zweymuller CA, Lintner FK, Semlitsch MF. Biologic fixation of a press fit titanium hip joint endoprosthesis. *Clin Orthop* 1988;235:195–206.

The Adult Hip, edited by J. J. Callaghan, A. G. Rosenberg, and H. E. Rubash. Lippincott–Raven Publishers, Philadelphia © 1998.

CHAPTER 69

Custom Design and Robotic Insertion of Uncemented Femoral Prostheses

William L. Bargar

The clinical reports of cemented total hips from Charnley in the early 1960s were excellent, especially compared to earlier attempts at fixation. As this technique spread worldwide (and was modified), problems with aseptic loosening developed, and by the late 1970s, femoral component loosening, especially in young, active patients, was a major concern: cement was felt to be the weak link. Although cementless approaches to femoral component fixation pre-date the Charnley era, with the Judet brothers in the 1940s and Austin-Moore in the 1950s, their results were disappointing. Subsequently, porous-coated orthopedic implants were developed in the 1970s by Pilliar et al. (17) and Galante et al. (4), and the clinical application of this technology to porous-coated femoral components was introduced in the 1980s by Engh (3), Cameron (2), Hedley et al. (8), Tullos et al. (20), and Harris (7). Although these implants promised to eliminate the cement and provide perhaps permanent fixation of the implant to bone, the early reports of the first-generation porous-coated cementless femoral components in the mid 1980s did not equal the early results of cemented total hips (6). Thus began the debate (which continues today) of cementless versus cemented techniques. Problems that have been identified with uncemented femoral components include failure of ingrowth, intraoperative femoral fractures, thigh pain, stress shielding, and osteolysis.

VARIABILITY OF FEMORAL ANATOMY

Some of the problems associated with the use of cementless components can be attributed to the wide variation in size, shape, and orientation of the femoral canal. Noble et al. (16) measured a large number of cadaver femoral canals and found a great variation in the mediolateral and anteroposterior dimensions.

There is also significant variation in the ratio of proximal-to-distal canal size. Consider, for example, the various arcs, taper angles, curves, and offsets. The number of possible geometric combinations in the normal patient population is staggering. Attempting to fit the variable canal with an off-the-shelf implant is always a compromise between prosthesis availability and optimal fit.

Revision surgery creates more complexity. Added to these normal anatomic variations, the difficulties faced by the surgeon who performs a revision operation are compounded by distortion of the femoral canal caused by bone loss around the originally placed prostheses, as well as iatrogenic defects produced by removal of components and cement. All these factors have led a number of hip surgeons to look for better methods to improve the design of uncemented femoral prostheses.

W. L. Bargar: Department of Orthopaedics, University of California Davis School of Medicine, Sacramento, California 95816.

CUSTOMIZATION USING 3-D DATA FROM CT SCANS

In total hip replacement (THR), the ideal is to establish an optimal fit between the femoral prosthesis and the patient's bone. One way to reach this goal is to manufacture femoral prostheses individually for each patient. In other words, to make a prosthesis that would fit a specific patient rather than try to reshape the patient's bone to fit a ready-made prosthesis.

The method of customizing prostheses utilized by the author relies on the use of computerized tomography (CT) scan data for design. The advantages of CT scans over conventional roentgenography, include reduced distortion, digital accuracy with no magnification errors, and three-dimensional (3-D) information. Linking of such data to CAD/CAM technology shortens the time for design and manufacture and improves dimensional accuracy of the implant.

In practice, the CT scan image tape, as well as conventional roentgenograms, are sent to the manufacturer, who generates contour data using edge-detection software. This results in a computerized model of the endosteal and periosteal bone surfaces. If metal is present, as in revision cases, information about the endosteal surface immediately around the implant is lost as a result of scatter artifact, but the periosteal information is reliable (Fig. 1). Scaled true anteroposterior and Lauenstein (14) (modified frog-leg) roentgenograms with magnification markers are also sent. The design engineer creates a computer-assisted design (CAD) using parametric analysis of the CT and roentgenographic data (Fig. 2). In revision cases, the endosteal surface is estimated from roentgenograms. Magnification can be determined by comparing the CT scans with the roentgenograms, and appropriate corrections can be made. The design, with roentgenographic templates at the proper magnification, are sent to the surgeon for approval. After the surgeon and design engineer agree on any modification, the prosthesis with modular heads and a custom broach are fabricated and sent directly to the hospital.

Often, when a customized prosthesis results in an optimal fit to the bone, there is more-uniform stress transfer, increased initial stability of the prosthesis, greater chance of bone ingrowth, less thigh pain, decreased incidence of intraoperative femoral shaft fracture, and decreased stress shielding.

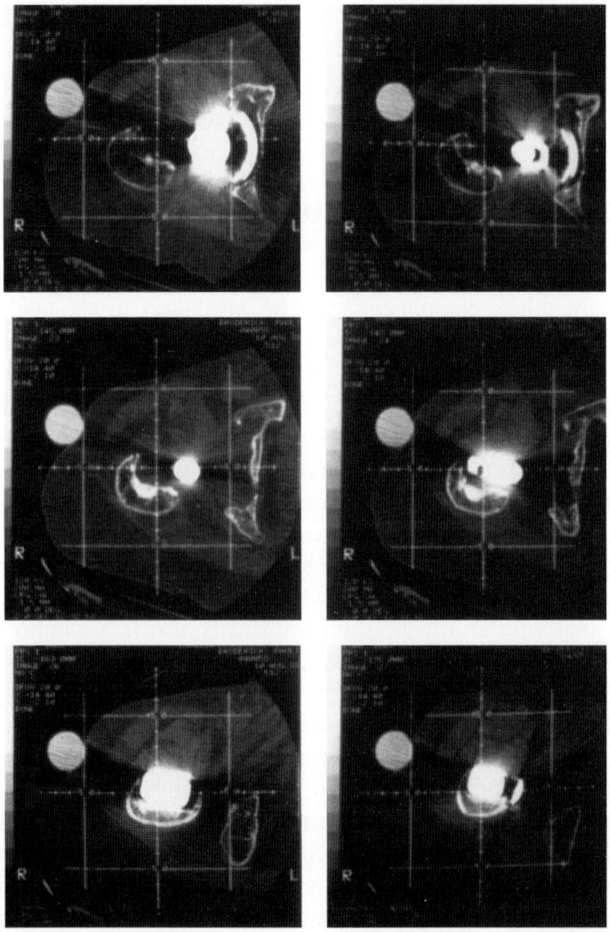

DESIGN RATIONALE FOR CUSTOM CEMENTLESS FEMORAL COMPONENTS

A set of prosthetic design rules for custom primary hip replacements has evolved, based on experience gained in preliminary cadaver and canine experiments and subsequently in operations in a clinical setting using the techniques discussed. The rules take into account the engineering limitations of design.

1. The prosthesis should be collarless (except in revisions) to allow uniform distribution of load to the femur.

2. It should have a modified rhomboidal cross section to maximize fit/fill, but it should maintain rotational stability.

3. The stem should be bowed when necessary to conform to the patient's bone.

4. The prosthesis should be insertable along a curved path, with no gaps between the prosthesis and the bone.

5. The prosthetic stem should have a cruciform cross section to reduce stiffness.

6. The stem length should be such that the stem has parallel contact with the walls of the femur over two to three internal canal diameters.

7. The proximal one third of the stem is porous coated or hydroxylapatite (HA) coated.

8. The stem is cylindrical (i.e., nontapered) to control bending loads but to allow transmission of all rotational and axial loads proximally.

9. The femoral head position should reproduce the patient's own head center, unless it is abnormal.

FIG. 1. CT showing metal scatter.

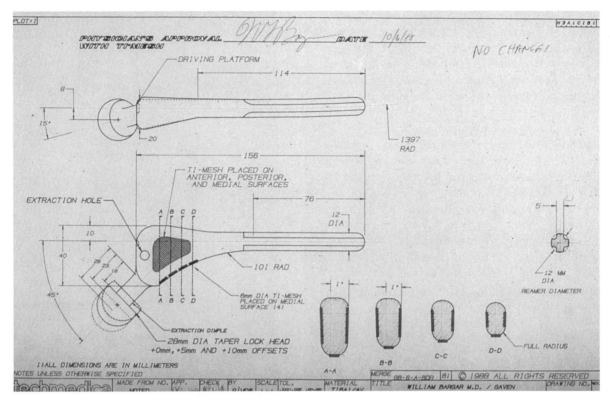

FIG. 2. Engineering drawing of custom implant.

These design rules evolved over a 3-year period from 1986 to 1989 (Fig. 3). The early designs had a longer stem reaching into the isthmus, and the proximal cross section was rectangular rather than rhomboidal as a result of initial manufacturing limitations. Later, the stem length was shortened and the diameter therefore increased by reaming to still achieve two to three internal canal diameters over which the walls were parallel. In revisions, however, the stem length was always chosen to be two to three canal diameters beyond any potential stress riser defects. The proximal body later became rhomboidal with an asymmetric anterior flare and a small lateral shoulder. In December 1989, the porous pads were abandoned in favor of an HA coating over a grooved surface.

RESULTS WITH CUSTOM PROSTHESES

Although no one would argue that customized prostheses will solve all the problems associated with THR, there is a place for them in selected cases, particularly in revision surgery. In 1989, the results of 48 THRs (25 primary

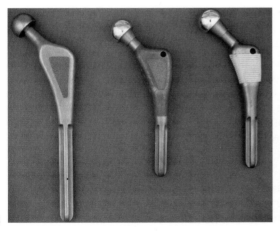

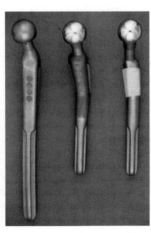

A,B

FIG. 3. Three custom implants, anteroposterior **(A)** and lateral **(B)** views.

and 23 revisions) performed using custom prostheses (and followed for a minimum of 2 years) were reported (1). Patients in whom custom prostheses had been used for the primary procedure had statistically higher Harris pain scores (i.e., less pain) than patients who received off-the-shelf prostheses. Patients who had undergone revision surgery with custom prostheses had lower Harris pain scores than those in the primary operation group, but 80% were still in the none or slight pain category. In the revision cases, custom implants decreased the need for bone grafting, and stability in host bone was achieved in situations where it would not have been possible to use off-the-shelf components without structural allografts. Recently, at the 1995 International Society for Technologies in Arthroplasty (ISTA) symposium in Puerto Rico, our minimum 5-year follow-up results using custom uncemented femoral components in both primary and revision cases were reported. These results are summarized in the next two sections.

Primary Cases

Seventy-two consecutive patients now have a minimum of 5 years of follow-up (range, 5 to 7 years). Selection criteria were patients with severe arthritis (degenerative joint disease, congenital dysplasia of the hip, rheumatoid arthritis, traumatic arthritis, juvenile rheumatoid arthritis), or avascular necrosis and either age under 65, weight over 200 lb (men) or 150 lb (women), or excessive activity. Four patients have been revised (three because of pad separation) and one was lost to follow-up, leaving 67 patients available for clinical evaluation.

The average Harris pain score at last follow-up is 40 ± 7 SD (maximum, 44). Ten patients (14%) have at least some activity-related thigh discomfort, but of these, 80% have only slight occasional pain with no compromise in activity. The average total modified Harris Hip Score is 89 ± 11 SD (maximum, 100). Radiographic analysis shows apparent ingrowth into at least one pad in 45 patients (63%) and no ingrowth in 5 (7%), and results are indeterminate in 22 (30%) (Fig. 4).

Of the four revisions, three were for late (more than 4 years) implant loosening caused by ingrowth pad separation (Fig. 5). At surgery, the pad was reported to be embedded in the bone. Histology confirmed excellent ingrowth into all separated pads. In addition, there are five patients (7%) with radiographic evidence of pad separation but with minimal symptoms. This makes a total ingrowth-pad-separation rate of 11% at 5 to 7 years. Other radiographic complications include two patients (3%) with distal osteolysis (one of whom has undergone a revision of the head and liner) and two patients with slowly progressive subsidence. There have been no dislocations or infections.

Clinical results are good to excellent despite ingrowth pad separation in 11% leading to a 5.5% revision rate.

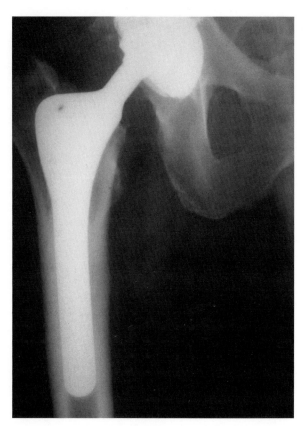

FIG. 4. Radiograph of successful primary porous-coated implant at the 5-year follow-up.

Excluding the pad pull-off cases (considered material failures), the results of this series compare favorably to the results of other cementless femoral components.

Since December 1989, ingrowth pads have been abandoned in favor of circumferential HA coating on a grooved surface. The results of a matched-group comparison of HA coating versus porous pads were recently reported. Twenty-nine HA-coated femoral stems used for primary total hip arthroplasty and followed for an average period of 62 months (range, 60 to 72) were compared with 30 porous-coated (PC) femoral stems that were followed for an average period of 64 months (range, 60 to 75). Patients in both groups were matched for age, sex, weight, primary diagnosis, and length of follow-up. All stems were titanium alloy (Ti) and were CT-based custom designs. Parametric design rules were identical for both groups. HA stems were coated over the proximal 3 cm, and PC stems had porous Ti mesh pads on the proximal anterior, medial, and posterior surfaces.

At follow-up, clinical evaluation was performed with the use of the Clinical Pain and Harris Hip scores. Radiographic evaluation utilizing anteroposterior and frog lateral views were performed, and patients were graded based on a modified Engh scale.

There have been two revisions for osteolysis and two for aseptic loosening in the porous group. No revisions

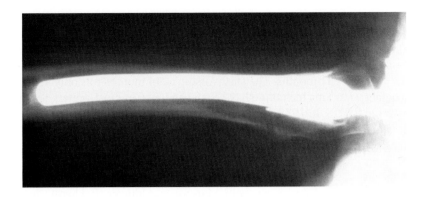

FIG. 5. Radiograph showing pad separation.

have been required in the HA group. Excluding the revisions in the porous group, comparison of the Clinical Pain and Harris Hip scores showed no statistical difference at mean follow-up of 62 and 64 months for the PC and HA groups, respectively (Wilcoxon Rank-sum test; p > .5). However, comparing the radiologic results, the groups are statistically different (chi square, p = .000). Osseointegration was present in 100% of the HA group, compared to 72% of the PC group. Only one case of osteolysis has been noted with the HA group.

Revision Cases

One hundred five consecutive patients needing revision hips received a custom implant 5 or more years ago (range, 5 to 9 years). Included were 56 men and 49 women. Average weight at surgery was 166 lb (range, 78 to 286). Average age was 60 years (range, 29 to 85). At surgery, all femoral reconstructions were completed without resorting to structural grafts. Leg-length discrepancy averaged 2 cm preoperatively (range, 0 to 7) and 0.7 cm postoperatively (range, 0 to 5). Ten patients have died and 14 were lost to follow-up, leaving 81 for complete analysis at 5 years.

Thirteen patients have required re-revision (four in the first 5 years): one had deep infection, one had osteolysis, seven had loosening, and four had pad pull-off with subsequent pain. Complications among all nonrevised patients included ten intraoperative femoral fissures, one late deep infection, two dislocations, and three cases of late ingrowth pad separation (classified as material, not design, failure).

At last follow-up of surviving hips, the average Harris Hip Score was 84.3 (range, 42 to 100) and the average pain score was 39 (range, 10 to 44). All cases with pad pull-off were clinically successful until this material failure occurred. Remaining implants are mechanically stable without progressive subsidence. Radiographic analyses of fixation demonstrate ingrowth in 62% of patients, are indeterminate in 16%, and demonstrate no ingrowth in 21% (Fig. 6). There was 95% prosthesis survival at 5 years. The incidence of pad failure was unacceptable, and

this method of fixation has since been abandoned in favor of circumferential HA coating.

Cost of Custom Implants

Initially, the cost of these implants was high (over $5000), but as with most new technologies, the cost has dropped, although it is still not in parity with off-the-shelf implants. Most custom implants today cost about $1000

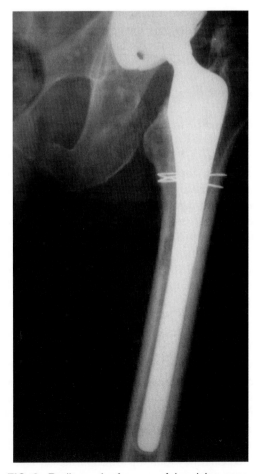

FIG. 6. Radiograph of successful revision case.

more than primary-type off-the-shelf implants, but their cost is equal to that of most revision-type off-the-shelf implants. In addition to the cost of the implant, there is the cost of the CT scan. The latter is an outpatient procedure, however, and is not part of the hospital costs.

The question, at least for primary implants, is whether this additional cost is worthwhile. This can be answered only by long-term survivorship and outcome data. Consider, however, an example of a failure in which the cost is estimated to be $50,000. If the additional $1000 spent initially could have prevented that failure, then an improvement of only 2% in the failure rate would justify the added expense.

Currently, because of cost issues and improvements in off-the-shelf designs for primary cases, it is advisable to use only custom implants when the degree of anatomic deformity is such that an off-the-shelf implant cannot meet our goals for implant fit or restoration of hip mechanics (see the algorithm in Fig. 11). In revision cases, the use of a custom-made implant is preferable in younger patients to avoid the potential problems of fretting and corrosion with modular implants and to avoid severe stress shielding with fully coated implants.

Experience with Custom Prostheses

Custom implants have been with us since the dawn of joint replacement surgery. Indeed, almost all implant designs have originated as custom prostheses. The usual indication for a custom implant is a clinical problem that cannot be solved by an off-the-shelf implant. Commonly, this is either in the arena of limb salvage or when severe deformity exists. In the mid 1980s, several surgeons in the United States and Europe began to apply the same idea of linking CT scan data for design, to CAD/CAM manufacturing for custom cementless femoral components to be utilized in all patients. This can be considered an extension of the usual indication.

The concept was first presented at a meeting in 1987 (5). It was first published in 1989 (1). At the same time, in the proceedings of the 1989 Hip Society meeting, Stulberg et al. (19) reviewed 73 primary custom-made uncemented implants inserted since July 1987. The early results were clinically equivalent to conventionally made implants, but there was less residual and recurrent thigh pain. The custom implants achieved 20% greater canal fit.

Also in that publication, Mulier et al. (15) reported their experiences in Belgium with custom implants made not from CT scan data but from molds of the intramedullary canal made at surgery. They reported over 800 consecutive procedures with good results. In a limited trial, no subjective difference was found with cemented Charnley total hip arthroplasties at 1 year. This technique was eventually introduced into the United States at several centers, but surgeons were unable to reproduce Mulier's results. In fact, in 1995, Lombardi et al. (13) reported failure of 21 of 74 patients using the intraoperative molding technique at a mean follow-up of 31 months. The survivorship at 44 months was only 45%. This technique has been abandoned at most centers.

In 1988, the International Society for the Study of Custom-made Prostheses (ISSCP) was formed. Multiple presentations have been made by European authors at these meetings, but their papers have not been published in English. Notable among the pioneers in Europe are Aubaniac and Argenson from Marseilles; Aldinger, Eckhardt, and Thumler from Germany; and Randelli from Italy. Most of these surgeons continue to use and refine their technique and report continued success (personal communication, Oct. 1996). The proceedings from the ISSCP meetings of 1991, 1992, and 1994 have been published by the British Journal of Bone and Joint Surgery in their Orthopaedic Proceedings (9–11) and in 1993 were published in the American Journal of Bone and Joint Surgery Transactions (12). In 1995, the name of the society was changed to the International Society for Technologies in Arthroplasty.

Some of the earliest contributions of applying CT scan data to design were made by Peter Walker. Although he first used the technique to design an off-the-shelf cementless prosthesis (Profile, DePuy Inc., Warsaw, Indiana) in the early 1980s, he and Robertson (18) published their concept of the design of custom hip stems prostheses using 3-D CT modeling in 1987. Since then, Walker has evolved the technique to the point that input from conventional radiographs can be linked to a library of CT data to design the implants. Although an engineer and not a surgeon, he continues to utilize his design and manufacturing technique for many surgeons in the United Kingdom and Europe and reports good results (personal communication, Oct. 1996).

Accuracy of Femoral Canal Preparation

Early on, it was recognized that the fit of custom femoral components was really a two-part problem. Not only must the implant be designed to best fit the femur, but to ensure optimal fit, the bone must be prepared with the same accuracy as the implant. Because the implants were designed and manufactured using CAD/CAM techniques, theoretically the 3-D information of the implant's shape could be utilized to machine a matching cavity in the bone. What was needed was a CAD/CAM machine in the operating room. However, these machines are very large and dirty, and the part to be machined must be placed in the device. The solution was a robotic arm that could be programmed to act like a CAD/CAM machine. Robotic arms are relatively small and are used in industry in ultra-clean environments similar to that of an operating room. If the patient's femur could be placed in a fixator anchored to the robot's base and a high-speed pneumatic cutting tool could be used as an end-effector, the robot could mill out the required shape.

DEVELOPMENT OF A SURGICAL ROBOT

Although the idea for the robot arose from experience with custom prostheses, it became evident that all cementless femoral components could benefit from a more precise femoral bone preparation. For preliminary studies of the efficacy of the robotic approach, however, custom prostheses that were unique for each patient could not be used, because they would introduce an additional variable. Therefore, to date all robot studies have been with noncustom, off-the-shelf components. Once the robot's efficacy has been established, it will be possible to link the two technologies of custom-fitting and robotics.

To accomplish robotic milling in surgery, the robot needed to be told *what* type and size of implant were to be used and also *where* in the bone the surgeon wanted the implant to fit. This required preoperative CT imaging of the bone and a way that the surgeon could preoperatively view the CT data and select the type, size, and position of the implant. Finally, the CT data and the surgeon's preoperative plan had to be registered to the robot and bone coordinate system in surgery.

We called our system ROBODOC. The ROBODOC project has evolved in five phases over a 10-year period.

Phase I (1986–1987): A laboratory feasibility study was conducted at the IBM Thomas J. Watson Research Center in Yorktown Heights, New York. A new computer language developed by IBM made it possible to program a robot that would perform a complex milling task unique for each patient.

Phase II (1987–1989): A 2-year study at the University of California (U.C.) Davis, funded by a grant from IBM, resulted in the development of the robotic system in the laboratory. Major hurdles in image processing and registration were overcome, making it possible to robotically machine femurs that were two orders of magnitude more accurate than those made with hand-held tools.

Phase III (1989–1991): Another 2-year study carried out at U.C. Davis and the Sacramento Animal Medical group facility brought the system into the surgical environment. Twenty-six total hip replacements were performed on dogs with hip dysplasia. All the animals recovered and appeared to have less pain and better function than dogs operated with conventional means.

Phase IV (1992–1993): To satisfy a Food and Drug Administration (FDA) requirement, robot-assisted THRs were performed on ten human patients. None of the patients suffered intraoperative complications. Postoperative evaluations were conducted by independent orthopedists, and postoperative review of roentgenograms by independent radiologists indicated satisfactory outcomes in all cases.

Phase V (1994 to present): A multicenter study with up to four sites in the United States and one in Europe. The U.S. sites make up a 300-patient randomized study (150 robot cases and 150 control cases) using three different implant systems.

Technique Employed in Robot-Assisted THR

Under local anesthesia, three titanium bone screws approximately 2 mm thick and 10 mm in diameter are implanted to serve as locator pins. One is placed in the greater trochanter, the other two in the distal femur (Fig. 7). The time of implantation can be from the afternoon or evening before THR surgery, or the same day as the operation. Implantation is avoided during the period from 7 days to 24 hours prior to operation because of concerns about the risk of infection.

After pin implantation, CT scans are made to capture the entire length of the femur and the locator pins. Tapes from the CT scans are loaded into the preoperative-planning work station, called ORTHODOC. The station consists of an IBM RS/6000 UNIX computer with color monitor, a nine-track drive for input, a cartridge tape drive for output, a keyboard, and a mouse (Fig. 8).

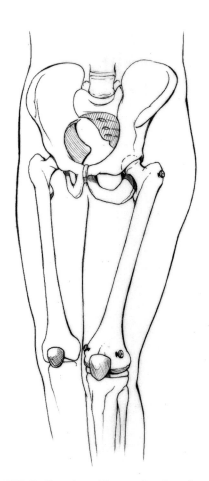

FIG. 7. Drawing of femur showing pins.

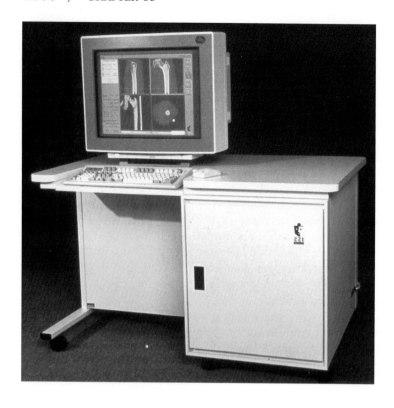

FIG. 8. Photo of ORTHODOC.

An ORTHODOC software program developed during phase II constructs three planar images of the femur, and a 3-D wire-frame image. The surgeon uses a mouse to manipulate and magnify the images and to display the femur in different planes (Fig. 9).

Two types of femoral prostheses are currently used: the Anatomic Medullary Locking prosthesis (AML, DePuy)

straight/distally fixed, and HA-Osteoloc (Howmedica) straight/proximally fixed. A third, Ranawat-Burstein (Biomet) anatomic/proximally fixed is scheduled to be added. Preoperatively, the surgeon chooses from a menu the type of implant that is most suitable and manipulates an image of the implant within an image of the bone, in all three dimensions. The final position and the type and

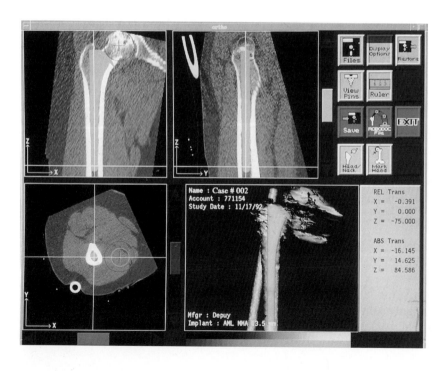

FIG. 9. Screen image on ORTHODOC.

size of the implant is based on the judgment of the surgeon.

In the operating room, patients are positioned in the lateral decubitus position. The extremity to be operated on is prepped and draped in the usual manner for a posterior approach, except that the femur, including the knee, is completely exposed. The lower leg is covered with a sterile stockinet. A sequential pneumatic compression thigh stocking has previously been placed on the opposite extremity.

The previous incision for placement of the greater trochanter locator screw is opened and extended to a formal posterolateral approach to the hip. The femoral neck is osteotomized approximately 5 mm proximal to the planned collar level. The robot will mill off the difference. The acetabular prosthesis is press-fit without cement, using conventional techniques.

The femur is then placed in a fixator that is attached through a sterile interface to the robot (Fig. 10). The locator pins are exposed and the robot guided to each pin. The robot probes the surface of the pin to determine the coordinates of the top center point. Interpin distances as found by the robot are compared to the interpin distances of the

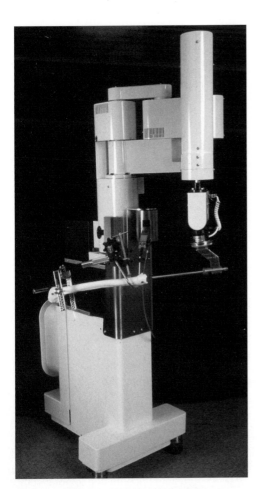

FIG. 10. Robot with fixator.

CT scan. These computations must agree to an acceptable level of precision before the operation continues. The robot's end-effector is changed to a specifically designed bit for the MIDAS Rex pneumatic high-speed burr. The robot then mills the inside of the femoral canal to the size and position of the implant that has been selected preoperatively on the work station. The robot is disconnected and the operation proceeds in the standard fashion with press-fit placement of the prosthesis, relocation of the joint, removal of the locator screws, and closure of the wound.

Interim Results of ROBODOC Multicenter Trial

The patients were evaluated using the modified Harris Hip Scale, the Hip Society Rating System, and the SF 36 Health Status Questionnaire. Surgical time, blood loss, length of stay, and complications were monitored. The 3-month-postoperative radiographs were reviewed by the principal investigator and independently by two reviewers in a blinded fashion. Each independent reviewer developed a rating scale using strict objective criteria to grade the fit, size selection, position, and reaming defects.

There have been 116 patients with 131 hips enrolled in the study to date. Of these, 127 hips (67 ROBODOC and 60 control) have completed a minimum 3-month follow-up, and 39 hips (21 ROBODOC and 18 control) have completed a 1-year follow-up. The modified Harris Hip Score at 3 months averaged 82.7 for the ROBODOC group and 82.6 for the control group (no significant difference). At the 1-year follow-up, the average score was 92.9 for the ROBODOC group and 89.6 for the control group. No statistically significant differences were noted at 3 months. At 1 year, more ROBODOC hips had excellent results and more fell into the no-pain category.

Average length of stay was not significantly different (7.2 days ROBODOC versus 6.5 days control). Surgical time was longer for the ROBODOC group (260 minutes for ROBODOC and 134 minutes for control, $p < .0001$). Average blood loss was also greater for the ROBODOC group (1275 cc ROBODOC versus 651 cc control, $p < .0001$). Analysis of these parameters by center showed significant variation.

SF-36 data were collected at 3 months and 1 year follow-up. The responses were similar at 3 months, but at 1 year higher ratings were seen in all categories for the ROBODOC group. The number of patients at 1 year was too small, however, for these differences to be statistically significant.

Postoperative complications were few. There were three intraoperative femoral fractures (cracks) in the control group and none in the ROBODOC group. There are no other significant differences in complications between groups.

For the AML cases, 25 hips (12 ROBODOC and 13 control) were reviewed radiographically. Although more ROBODOC hips showed improved radiographic results, the numbers were too small to show statistically significant differences. For the Osteoloc cases, 70 hips (38 ROBODOC and 32 control) were reviewed radiographically. Statistically significant differences were seen in fit, position, and size selection for the ROBODOC group.

Cost-Effectiveness of the ROBODOC System

Although no systems have been sold for non-FDA use in the United States, we project the cost for a complete system will be approximately $600,000. Placing a dollar figure on effectiveness is very difficult, if not impossible. The ROBODOC system does eliminate the need for surgical instrumentation for femoral preparation. In many implant systems, this represents several trays of instruments costing over $50,000. In addition, because the surgeon can pre-plan the exact size and type of implant needed, large inventories of implants are not required. These implants could be ordered direct, thereby eliminating the costs of distributors and local company representatives (20% to 30% of the cost of the implant). If the concept of the radiographic results serving as surrogate variables is accepted, then better long-term performance of cementless hip repairs performed with ROBODOC can be anticipated. This should result in decreased costs to society associated with longer productive employment, and fewer failures requiring costly revision surgery. Our data at this time do not support the conclusion of cost-effectiveness. Potential for this is seen, however, in this early interim report of the ROBODOC FDA multicenter trial.

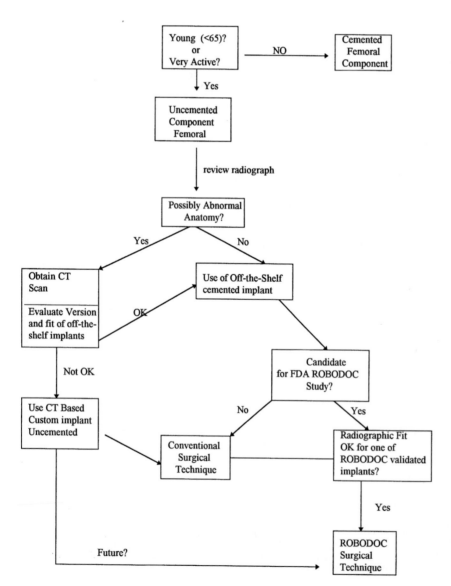

FIG. 11. Decision algorithm for use of custom uncemented femoral components and ROBODOC.

CONCLUSION

The development of CT-based custom femoral components and the development of a surgical robot for bone preparation share a common theme: use of CT scan image data and CAD/CAM techniques for design and insertion of cementless femoral components. By linking the fields of medical imaging with robotics, we can utilize the vast strides in information processing developed over the last 10 years to improve the accuracy and precision of prosthesis design and surgery.

These 10 years have also seen a significant improvement in the design and manufacturing of off-the-shelf implants. This raises the question, Who should receive a custom prosthesis and who can be adequately fit with an off-the-shelf prosthesis? This needs to be answered on a case-by-case basis, using the surgeon's discretion as to what is an adequate versus an optimal fit. Three-dimensional imaging and templating as is used in the ROBODOC system can help to answer this question.

Currently, it is appropriate to use an off-the-shelf cementless implant when the radiographs show what appears to be relatively normal anatomy (conventional radiographic templates of several designs are used to assess the adequacy of fit). If it does not appear that an acceptable fit can be achieved, a CT scan can be obtained and consideration given to the use of a custom implant. This algorithm is displayed in Figure 11. Using this algorithm, the author chooses a custom implant in approximately 20% of primary cementless cases and in over 50% of revision cases.

The potential application of surgical robotics is expanding rapidly. Its use is being investigated in revision of femoral components, total knee replacement, spinal instrumentation surgery, anterior cruciate ligament reconstruction, and osteotomies. Potential nonorthopedic applications include CT/MRI-guided soft-tissue biopsy, and ablative procedures and microsurgical procedures in the fields of ophthalmology, otolaryngology, and neurosurgery.

REFERENCES

1. Bargar WL. Shape the implant to the patient: a rationale for the use of custom-fit cementless total hip implants. *Clin Orthop* 1989;249:73–78.
2. Cameron HV. The results of early clinical treats with a microporous coated metal hip prosthesis. *Clin Orthop* 1982;165:188–190.
3. Engh CA. Hip arthroplasty with a Moore prosthesis with porous coating. *Clin Orthop* 1983;176:52–65.
4. Galante J, Rostoker W, Lueck R, Ray R. Sintered fiber metal composites as a basis for attachment of implants to bone. *J Bone Joint Surg* 1971;53A:101–114.
5. Greenwald S. *Current concepts in implant fixation.* Presented at a meeting of Mt. Sinai Medical Center, at Orlando, FL. December 11–13, 1987.
6. Haddad RJ, Cook SD, Thomas KA. Current concepts review: biologic fixation of porous coated implants. *J Bone Joint Surg* 1987;69A:1459–1466.
7. Harris WH. Current status of non-cemented implants in the hip. *Proceedings of the 14th open scientific meeting of the Hip Society.* St. Louis: CV Mosby, 1987;214–234.
8. Hedley AK, Gruen TA, Borden LS, Hungerford DS, Haberman E, Kenna RV. Two year follow-up of the PCA non-cemented total hip replacement in the hip. *Proceedings of the 14th open scientific meeting of the Hip Society.* St. Louis: CV Mosby, 1987;225–250.
9. ISSCP orthopaedic proceedings. *J Bone Joint Surg* 1992;74B(suppl 2).
10. ISSCP orthopaedic proceedings. *J Bone Joint Surg* 1993;75B(suppl 3).
11. ISSCP orthopaedic proceedings. *J Bone Joint Surg* 1995;77B(suppl 1).
12. ISSCP orthopaedic transactions. *J Bone Joint Surg* 1994;18(3).
13. Lombardi AV Jr, Mallory TH, Eberle RW, Mitchell MB, Lefkowitz, MS, Williams JR. Failure of intraoperatively customized non-porous femoral components inserted without cement in total hip arthroplasty. *J Bone Joint Surg Am* 1995;77(12):1836–1844.
14. Merrill V, ed. *Atlas of roentgenographic positions*, vol. 1, 3rd ed. St Louis: CV Mosby, 1967
15. Mulier JC, Mulier M, Brady LP, Steenhoudt H, Cauwe Y, Goossens M, Elloy M. A new system to produce intraoperatively custom femoral prosthesis from measurements taken during the surgical procedure. *Clin Orthop* 1989;249:97–112.
16. Noble PC, Alexander JW, Lindajl LJ, Yew DT, Granberry WM, Tullos HS. The anatomic basis of femoral component design. *Clin Orthop* 1988;235:148–165.
17. Pilliar RM, Cameron HU, Macmab I. Porous surface layered prosthetic devices. *Biomed Eng J* 1975;10:126.
18. Robertson DD, Walker PS, Granholm JW, Nelson PC, Weiss, PJ, Fishman EK, Magid D. Design of custom hip stem prostheses using three-dimensional CT modeling. *J Comput Assist Tomogr* 1987;11(5):804–809.
19. Stulberg SD, Stulberg BN, Wixon RL. The rationale, design characteristics, and preliminary results of a primary custom total hip prosthesis. *Clin Orthop* 1989;249:79–96.
20. Tullos HS, McCaskill BL, Dickey R, Davidson J. Total hip arthroplasty with a low-modulus porous coated femoral component. Progress report. *J Bone Joint Surg* 1984;66A:888–898.

The Adult Hip, edited by J. J. Callaghan,
A. G. Rosenberg, and H. E. Rubash.
Lippincott–Raven Publishers, Philadelphia © 1998.

CHAPTER **70**

The Asian Hip

Kunio Takaoka, Toyonori Sakamaki, Shigeru Yanagimoto, Tadami Matsumoto,
Nobuhiko Sugano, Susumu Saito, and Seneki Kobayashi

Japanese hips in the normal population and in patients with hip diseases are different from Western hips. In the first section of this chapter, anatomic features of the hip joint in Japanese normal adults and patients with hip disease are described. The physique of Japanese normal subjects and the dimensions of their hip joints are, on aver-

K. Takaoka and S. Kobayashi: Department of Orthopaedic Surgery, Shinshu University School of Medicine, Matsumoto, Japan.

T. Sakamaki and S. Yanagimoto: Department of Orthopaedic Surgery, Keio University School of Medicine, Tokyo, Japan.

T. Matsumoto: Department of Orthopaedic Surgery, University of Kanazawa School of Medicine, Kanazawa, Ishikawa, Japan.

N. Sugano: Department of Orthopaedic Surgery, Osaka University School of Medicine, Suita, Japan.

S. Saito: Department of Orthopaedic Surgery, Sumitomo Hospital, Osaka, Japan.

age, smaller than those of Western people. The Japanese acetabulum is steeper and shallower, and the investment of the femoral head is less. The predominant (60% to 70%) cause of hip disease in Japan is osteoarthrosis secondary to congenital dislocation or subluxation of the hip. The anatomic features of the Japanese hip joint may contribute to the frequent occurrence of the dysplastic hip. The majority of Japanese patients with hip disease have hypoplasia of the femoral neck and increased femoral anteversion.

In the second section, the etiology and characteristics of the dysplastic hip in Japan are described and compared with those of primary osteoarthrosis. A diagnosis of osteoarthrosis secondary to congenital subluxation or dislocation of the hip (i.e., the so-called dysplastic hip) was made according to the following criteria: history of congenital dislocation of the hip, joint subluxation indicated by a broken Shenton's line on radiographs made before development of advanced osteoarthrosis ("early" radiographs), and distinct hallmarks of this condition detected on radiographs or during hip surgery. Comparison of 291 dysplastic osteoarthrosis hips and 82 primary osteoarthrosis hips clarified the characteristics of dysplastic hips. Symptoms of osteoarthrosis in the dysplastic osteoarthrosis group began earlier in life and led to surgery at an earlier age than those in the primary osteoarthrosis group. Radiologically, the superolateral type (in the morphologic classification) and the hypertrophic type (in the classification based on the biologic response of the joint) were more common in the dysplastic osteoarthrosis group than in the other group.

In the third section, rotational acetabular osteotomy, a periacetabular osteotomy developed for osteoarthrosis secondary to a dysplastic hip and in widespread use in Japan, is introduced. Its advantages, indications, surgical technique, and results are detailed. Radiologic and clinical results of rotational acetabular osteotomies, performed in 292 hips followed for 70 months (range, 36 to 126 months) are reported. Sixty-five hips were radiographically classified in the preosteoarthrosis stage before surgery, 162 hips in the early stage with mild joint space narrowing, and 59 in the advanced stage with considerable joint space narrowing. Rotational acetabular osteotomy is a very useful operation for osteoarthrosis secondary to a dysplastic hip and provides excellent long-term results, especially, if done in preosteoarthrosis and early osteoarthrosis stages. In the advanced-stage group, the clinical results showed a tendency to deteriorate with time, a tendency especially evident in cases where the hips showed no widening of the joint space or improvement of the congruity between the acetabulum and the femoral head on the radiographs taken with abduction of the hip joint.

In the fourth section, dome pelvic (modified Chiari) osteotomy, another osteotomy developed in Japan for osteoarthrosis secondary to hip dysplasia, is also introduced. Its advantages, indications, surgical technique, results, and factors influencing the results are presented.

In the last section of the chapter, total hip arthroplasty with acetabular bone grafting is discussed. Such bone grafting is sometimes required in patients with osteoarthrosis secondary to a dysplastic hip. A literature review indicated that cemented total hip arthroplasty augmented by autogenous bone graft provides satisfactory results. A recent experience with cementless total hip arthroplasty augmented by autogenous bulk or cancellous chip grafts is documented in detail, including indications, surgical technique, and results. Autogenous bone grafting is a useful procedure to augment acetabular deficiency in cemented or cementless total hip arthroplasty for congenital hip dysplasia.

ANATOMIC FEATURES OF THE ASIAN HIP

Section Authors: Toyonori Sakamaki and Shigeru Yanagimoto

Values, such as those for the diameter of the femoral head, the overall length of the femur, and the offset of the femoral head, are slightly smaller for Japanese compared to Western populations. In addition to the external morphology of the femur, there are slight differences in the shape, width, and taper angle of the femoral cavity, and these factors must be taken into account when performing prosthetic replacement of the hip joint.

Morphologic Characteristics of the Japanese Hip Joint

Diseases of the hip joint in Japanese people are characterized by being largely associated with congenital dislocation of the hip and acetabular dysplasia. This tendency is also clear in the report of Hoaglund et al. (Table 1) (20). The incidence of the diseases affecting Japanese people and Caucasian Americans is quite different. Whether the morphologic characteristics of the hip joint of Japanese people contributes to the specific nature of their diseases has been discussed by many investigators. Various measurements related to the morphology of the femur and hip joint have already been obtained from dry femur specimens and plain x-ray findings, and the morphologic characteristics of Japanese people have been investigated by comparing the values obtained for Japanese and non-Japanese. We have divided our discussion of the morphology of the hip joint into a description of the morphology of the femur, and of the investment of the femoral head in the acetabulum.

TABLE 1. *Hip disease etiology in Japanese and American white patients*

	Japanese patients		American white patients	
	(N)	%	(N)	%
Dysplasia	92	46	9	4.5
CDH	28	14	0	0
Avascular necrosis	22	11	6	3
RA, AS	14	7	34	17
TB, infection	6	3	1	0.5
Trauma	3	1.5	0	0
Others	35	17.5	150	75
Total	200		200	

Distribution of hip diseases is quite different between Japanese and American white patients. Hip disease etiology in Japanese patients is largely associated with congenital dislocation of the hip and acetabular dysplasia.

CDH, congenital of the hip; RA, rheumatoid arthritis; AS, ankylosing spondylitis; TB, tuberculosis.

TABLE 2. *Measurements of the length of the femur and the diameter of the femoral head obtained from normal subjects*

Author (ref.)	Nationality	Cases (N)	Material/method	Femoral length (cm)	Head diameter (mm)
Onoue (48)	Japan	120	X-P	40.6	
Komatsu (30)	Japan	170	Cadaver		47.3*
Fuku (14)	Japan	28	CT scan	40.5	44.9
Fujii (13)	Japan	714	X-P		43.4
Trotter (68)		265	X-P	42.3	
Hoaglund (20)	Hong-Kong	500	X-P		46.6
Lavelle (32)	England	200	Cadaver	41.0	
Noble (47)	U.S.A.	200	Cadaver	43.7	46.1

The femurs of Japanese are on average about 5% smaller than those of non-Japanese.
* Includes cartilage portion.
X-P: radiography

Morphology of the femur. Measurements of the overall length of the femur and of the diameter of the femoral head obtained from normal subjects are shown in Table 2. Although there are differences according to the disease, the mean overall length of the femur of Japanese is approximately 40 cm, as opposed to about 42 cm in non-Japanese, and the mean diameter of the femoral head (bony portion) in Japanese is about 40 mm, versus around 46 mm in non-Japanese. Thus, the femurs of Japanese are on average about 5% smaller than the femurs of non-Japanese.

Morphology of the hip joint. The measurements of normal subjects reported by various investigators for the center edge (CE) angle and the Sharp angle of the covering of the femoral head are shown in Table 3. The mean CE angle and the mean Sharp angle in non-Japanese are both approximately 35°, whereas in Japanese the mean CE angle is about 32° and the sharp angle around 38°. The Japanese acetabulum is clearly steeper, and the investment of the femoral head smaller (13,14,53). In regard to sex differences, Fujii et al. (13) report acetabular dysplasia and poor femoral investment tend to be more common in women. Yoshida et al. (79) made three-dimensional measurements of the hip joint morphology of 62 normal Japanese subjects (21 men, 41 women)

using computed tomography (CT); they reported that Japanese women have a smaller anterior acetabular investment than Japanese men, suggesting that poor anterior acetabular investment is a cause of acetabular dysplasia.

Associations between anatomic features and clinical findings. The above findings clearly show that the femur of Japanese tends to be smaller than that of non-Japanese, reflecting their physique, so smaller sizing is needed in the production of artificial hips for Japanese. The acetabulum tends to be steeper and the investment of the head of the femur shallower in the hip joints of Japanese, with these tendencies even more pronounced in women. The anterior investment by the acetabulum is poor even when assessed on a horizontal plane. These anatomic features of the Japanese hip joint may be a factor in the frequent occurrence of congenital dislocation of the hip and acetabular dysplasia.

Three-Dimensional Morphology of the Japanese Femur

A correct grasp of the three-dimensional morphology of the femur is important when preparing artificial hip prostheses. Conventional measurement methods such as

TABLE 3. *Radiographic measurements (CE angle and Sharp angle) of normal subjects*

Author (ref.)	Country	Cases (N)	CE angle	Sharp angle
Sharp (57)	England	Male (50)		33°–38°
		Female (50)		33°–38°
Hoaglund (20)	Hong-Kong	Male (248)	35.9° ± 6.5°	
		Female (252)	35.8° ± 6.7°	
Fredensborg (12)	Sweden	Male (70)	35°	
		Female (70)	35°	
Nakamura (44)	Japan	Male (62)	32.3° ± 6.9°	37.3° ± 3.7°
		Female (65)	32.1° ± 6.5°	38.3° ± 3.4°
Fujii (13)	Japan	Male (340)	30.0° ± 6.2°	38.7° ± 3.3°
		Female (414)	27.8° ± 6.8°	41.5° ± 3.5°

The Japanese acetabulum is on average steeper, and the investment of the femoral head smaller than the non-Japanese acetabulum.
CE, center-edge.

plain radiographs lack the accuracy needed for measuring and understanding important parameters such as the three-dimensional morphology of the femoral cavity, femoral anteversion, and the offset of the head of the femur. We used CT scans to make three-dimensional measurements; our findings are reported here (14,77,78).

Three-dimensional measurement methods. We made CT scans of the proximal femur (slice thickness, 2 mm) at 1-cm intervals, input the cross-sectional images of the femur into a computer, and used the data to make three-dimensional measurements.

We determined the central axis of the femoral cavity in the proximal portion of the femur. It is important to establish the central axis of the bone cavity as the reference axis for the measurements. We determined the morphology of the tapering reamer that was most compatible with the proximal diaphyseal portion of the femoral cavity based on the cross-sectional images of the femur. The central axis of the tapered reamer was taken as representing the central axis of the proximal femoral cavity, and it was adopted as the reference axis for making the measurements.

A variety of parameters were measured:

1. Taper angle of the proximal femoral cavity: The taper angle of the tapered reamer was considered the taper angle of the proximal femoral cavity. The computer graphics technique employed in this study made it possible to measure the taper angle properly for the first time.
2. Femoral head offset: The femoral head offset was measured as the distance between the central axis and the center of the femoral head.
3. Femoral and transverse diameter: We determined the transverse diameter of the femur and the transverse diameter of the femoral cavity 2 cm below the lesser trochanter, using the mean inscribed circle and circumscribed circle of the inside diameter and outside diameter of the cortex.
4. Femoral anteversion: We used the tangent line connecting the posterior aspect of the medial and lateral femoral condyles as the base line, and we calculated the angle formed by the line that joined the central axis and the center of the femoral head.

Results and Discussion of the Three-Dimensional Measurements

Results of the measurements are shown in Table 4 (14,77,78). They are the first three-dimensional measurements ever obtained. The means and standard deviations of the various measurements in normal subjects and patients with osteoarthritis of the hip provide extremely important information for producing artificial femoral prostheses that are truly compatible with the morphology of the femoral cavity of Japanese. The data showed that

TABLE 4. *Computed tomography measurement data of Japanese hip*

	Patients with osteoarthritis	Normal hips
Cases (*N*)	52	28
Mean age	50.8 (18–86) yr	45.4 (14–79) yr
Femoral length	39.5 ± 2.4 cm	40.5 ± 2.4 cm
Femoral head diameter	46.0 ± 2.8 mm	44.9 ± 2.8 mm
Taper angle	3.8° ± 1.2°	4.9° ± 1.6°
Femoral head offset	37.0 ± 3.9 mm	41.1 ± 4.8 mm
Periosteal width	29.1 ± 2.0 mm	30.3 ± 2.6 mm
Endosteal width	15.7 ± 2.2 mm	16.3 ± 2.3 mm
Femoral anteversion	44.9° ± 14.9°	33.3° ± 11.2°

Japanese patients with osteoarthritis of the hip have hypoplasia of the femoral neck and increased femoral anteversion, reflecting the fact that osteoarthritis secondary to congenital dislocation of the hip and acetabular dysplasia accounts for the majority of cases.

Japanese patients with osteoarthritis of the hip have hypoplasia of the femoral neck and increased femoral anteversion, reflecting the fact that osteoarthritis secondary to congenital dislocation of the hip and acetabular dysplasia accounts for the majority of cases. Assessment of the relationships between measurements in normal subjects showed that sizing of the femur was almost perfectly proportional to other measurements. However, in patients with osteoarthritis of the hip, perhaps because of the variety of hypoplasia of the femoral neck, femoral head offset did not correlate with other measurements.

Conditions Required for Artificial Hip Joints Compatible with Japanese Patients

Based on these findings, the shape of artificial hip joints must meet the following conditions for compatibility in Japanese patients:

1. Smaller sizing is required than for non-Japanese.
2. Taking into consideration two facts, (a) that acetabular dysplasia accounts for the majority of hip disease, and (b) that the basic hip joint morphology of Japanese includes a steeper acetabulum and a smaller femoral head investment than that of non-Japanese, socket systems that provide firm fixation, even in patients with small acetabular investment of the femoral head, must be considered.
3. In regard to the stem of artificial hip joints, because the mean taper angle of the proximal femoral cavity is 4°, it would be preferable to consider 4° as the central value for the taper angle of the portion of the stem that corresponds to the diaphyseal portion. Stem sizing can be essentially proportional, but caution is required because the offset is short in some patients with osteoarthrosis of the hip.

DYSPLASTIC HIP: ETIOLOGY AND CHARACTERISTICS

Section Authors: Seneki Kobayashi and Kunio Takaoka

In a collaborative study on the long-term (10- to 20-year) performance of total hip replacements (THRs) (performed with N. S. Eftekhar at Columbia-Presbyterian Medical Center in New York City), we found that hips that underwent a primary THR differed between the Japanese hospital and the U.S. hospital both in demographic features of patients and in parameters assessed on radiographs (27,28). The Japanese patients weighed less on average than the American patients. The predominant underlying cause of hip disease was congenital subluxation or dislocation of the hip (i.e., the so-called dysplastic hip) in the Japanese group (69.7%), whereas it was primary osteoarthrosis (OA) (50.3%) in the U.S. group. In this section, we would like to describe characteristics of the dysplastic hip in Japan.

Definition of the Dysplastic Hip

When a patient had a history of congenital dislocation of the hip (treated or untreated), or when radiographs made before reaching the advanced stage of OA ("early" radiographs) show a 5-mm or more discrepancy in the constructed Shenton's line, it is easy to make the diagnosis of OA secondary to congenital subluxation or dislocation of the hip (i.e., dysplastic hip). Mild acetabular dysplasia without subluxation of the joint is not included in this category, because such a condition is not well established as a cause of OA (9). In addition to these criteria, we made the diagnosis of congenital subluxation or dislocation of the hip when we detected distinct hallmarks or stigmata of this condition on examination of radiographs or during surgery. The diagnosis was made even without history of congenital dislocation of the hip or without early radiographs. The diagnostic hallmarks included coxa valga, increased anteversion of the femoral neck, narrower femoral shaft compared with the contralateral unaffected side in a case of unilateral hip disease, and acetabular dysplasia that was obvious even after discounting changes due to OA. Primary OA was diagnosed when there was no history of preceding hip disorders and

when the joint was free from these gross developmental anatomic deformities.

Characteristics of the Dysplastic Hip

To clarify the characteristics of dysplastic hips, we performed a comparative study between OA secondary to congenital subluxation or dislocation, and primary OA of the hip. Between November 1992 and January 1994, 700 patients with OA of the hip attended our orthopedic outpatient clinic. Every case was searched for possible injuries, diseases, or deformities that might have been the cause of coxarthrosis. Although they had various stages of OA, 264 patients had 392 hips that were radiologically at the end stage of OA (Table 5), and they underwent THR. According to the aforementioned criteria, hip disease causes of the 392 hips with end-stage OA were as follows: congenital subluxation or dislocation (dysplastic hip), 291 hips (74%); primary OA, 82 hips (21%); and others, 19 hips (5%). Among the 291 hips that were diagnosed as OA secondary to congenital subluxation or dislocation, history of the primary disorder was clear only in 69 hips (24%), and in the other 222 hips (76%) the diagnosis was made by radiologic and/or operative findings. Among the 82 hips that developed primary OA, early radiographs (those made after cessation of growth and before developing advanced OA) were available in 16 hips (20%). The other 66 hips (80%) fit in none of the above-mentioned criteria for dysplastic hip, although early radiographs were not available.

Figure 1 shows the etiologic classification according to decades of patients' first visits to our department. The percentage of primary OA was 0% in the 1960s, 14% in the 1970s, 23% in the 1980s, and 35% in the 1990s. This increase in the percentage of primary OA with time may reflect the increase in the percentage of elderly people in the Japanese population and/or may follow the westernizing trend seen in the distribution of certain adult diseases in Japan (e.g., epidemiologic increases of coronary heart disease, colon cancer, and breast cancer).

Between the dysplastic OA group and the primary OA group, the following parameters were compared: gender, occupation, body weight, height, obesity (defined by body weight exceeding 120% of standard weight), age at

TABLE 5. *Radiologic assessments of osteoarthrosis of the hip (Japanese Orthopaedic Association)*

Stage	Joint space	Changes in bony structure	Changes in joint shape
Almost normal	Almost normal	Little	Little
Prearthrosis	Mild incongruity, no narrowing	Possible	Present
Early	Incongruity, partial narrowing	Osteopenia	Small osteophytes
Advanced	Incongruity, partial closure	Osteopenia, cysts	Osteophytes, double floor
End	Incongruity, extensive closure	Extensive osteopenia, large cysts	Remarkable osteophytes, thick double floor, acetabular destruction

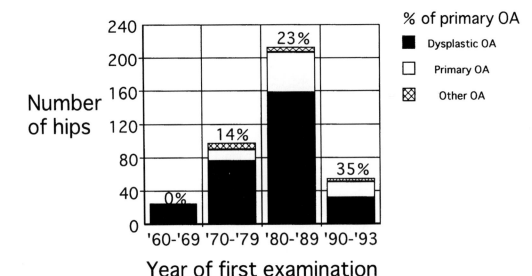

FIG. 1. Etiologic distribution according to decades of the first visits of patients to our department. The most predominant hip disease etiology was congenital subluxation or dislocation of the hip (i.e., the so-called dysplastic hip) in the Japanese patients. The percentage of primary OA (osteoarthrosis) has been increasing in the last four decades.

onset of hip pain, period between onset of hip pain and THR, age at the first examination at our department, period between the first examination and THR, age at surgery, unilateral or bilateral involvement of OA, and findings on radiographs made just before THR (Table 6). The four principal types of coxarthrosis were classified by morphology based on the site of the joint destruction and on the type of displacement of the femoral head: superolateral, concentric, medial, and destructive (34). We also classified three types of OA according to the biologic reaction of the joint to the disease: normotrophic, hypertrophic, and atrophic (4). We noted double floor formation and cystic changes on radiographs.

Although women were overrepresented in both groups, the percentage of men was lower in the dysplastic OA group than in the primary OA group. A lower percentage of laborers (most of them were women working on farms) was found in patients with dysplastic hips than in those with primary coxarthrosis. There was no difference in patient physique between the two groups. The average patient age at onset of pain in the dysplastic OA group was lower than that in the primary OA group. The average period between onset of pain and surgery was shorter in the dysplastic OA group than in the primary OA group, and so was the average period between the initial presentation of patients to our department and THR. The average patient age at surgery was lower in the dysplastic OA group than in the primary OA group. Symptoms of coxarthrosis in the dysplastic OA group began earlier in life and led to surgery at an earlier age than in those in the primary OA group. The incidence of bilateral disease was higher in the dysplastic OA group than in the primary OA group.

TABLE 6. *Comparison between coxarthrosis secondary to congenital subluxation or dislocation of the hip and primary coxarthrosis*

Parameter	Dysplastic OA (291 hips)	Primary OA (82 hips)
Male patients (%)	5	16*
Laborers (%)	43	56*
Body weight (kg)	52	53
Height (cm)	148	149
Obese patients (%)	21	20
Age at pain onset (yr)	48	59*
Years between pain onset and THR	11.8	7.9*
Age at first visit (yr)	56	64*
Years between first visit and THR	4.5	2.3*
Age at THR (years)	61	67*
Bilateral involvement (%)	73	56*
Radiologic findings:		
Morphology (S:C:M:D) (%)	91:1:0:9	60:6:7:27*
Biologic response (N:H:A) (%)	83:8:9	60:12:28*
Double floor formation (%)	84	55*
Cyst formation (%)	84	88

Symptoms of OA in the dysplastic OA group began earlier in life and led to surgery at an earlier age as compared with those in the primary OA group. Radiographically, the supero-lateral type in the morphologic classification and the hypertrophic type in the classification based on the biologic response of the joint were more common in the dysplastic OA group than in the other group.

* Statistically significant difference (*p* < .05), using T-test for averages and chi-square test for percentages.

OA, osteoarthrosis; THR, total hip replacement; S, supero-lateral; C, concentric; M, medial; D, destructive; N, normotrophic; H, hypertrophic; A, atrophic.

On radiographs, the superolateral type in the morphologic classification and the hypertrophic type in the classification based on the biologic response of the joint were more common in the dysplastic OA group than in the primary OA hips. The higher percentages of double floor formation in the dysplastic hips may reflect the higher incidence of hypertrophic OA in this group than in the other group.

Measurement of Early Radiographs in Primary OA

In the primary OA group, 16 hips (20%) had early radiographs that were used to make an assessment of the anatomic normalness of the hip joint. Five parameters of hip development, listed in Table 7 and illustrated in Figure 2, were measured concerning acetabular dysplasia. The presence of one or more pathologic values defined acetabular dysplasia. Slight deviation from an entirely normal anatomy (i.e., mild acetabular dysplasia without subluxation of the joint) was detected in ten hips (63%). None of the 16 hips showed a broken Shenton's line, protrusio acetabuli, or the pistol grip deformity of Stulberg et al. (61) (the femoral head tilt deformity) on early radiographs. Illustrative cases from both dysplastic and primary OA groups are shown in Figures 3 and 4.

Controversy on Definition of Primary OA

Traditionally, coxarthrosis has been separated into primary and secondary types, the former being OA developing in adult life after grossly normal growth of the hip and the latter term being applied where some major abnormality of the joint can be identified. Although we used this traditional etiologic classification of coxarthrosis, there has been a great controversy on this issue. Con-

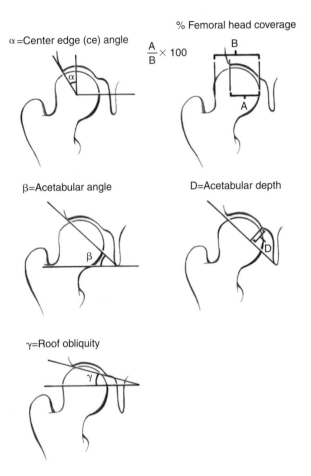

FIG. 2. Parameters of hip development concerning acetabular dysplasia. The presence of one or more pathologic values defined acetabular dysplasia.

genital subluxation and dislocation of the hip are well known to predictably lead to secondary OA (9,72–75). The hypothesis is advanced by some authors that most cases of primary OA are secondary to minor anatomic abnormalities of the hip (17,19,43,60). Acetabular dysplasia has been identified as a possible cause of OA in primary OA cases (33,34,75). However, the natural history of acetabular dysplasia in the absence of subluxation, which is defined by an intact Shenton's line on early radiographs, is difficult to predict and still controversial (9). Such hips were found in 63% in primary OA cases who had early radiographs in the present study. Further study is required on the fate of hips with acetabular dysplasia in the absence of subluxation.

Summary

Hips that underwent a primary THR differed between American and Japanese patients in demographic features of patients and in radiographic parameters. The most pre-

TABLE 7. *Exploration of anatomic features of hip joint on early radiographs*

Parameter	Author (ref.)	Pathologic range (condition)
Center-edge angle	Wiberg (75)	<20° (laterally displaced)
Acetabular angle	Sharp et al. (57)	≥43° (too steep)
Roof obliquity	Massie, Howorth (36)	>20° (too steep)
Femoral head coverage	Cooperman et al. (9)	<75% (insufficient coverage)
Acetabular depth	Stulberg et al. (61)	<15 mm (male) <14 mm (female) (too shallow)

These five parameters were measured to study acetabular dysplasia. Presence of one or more pathologic values defined acetabular dysplasia.

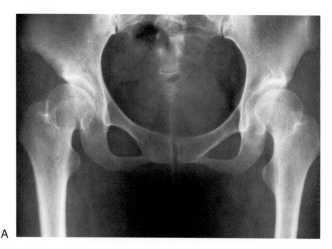
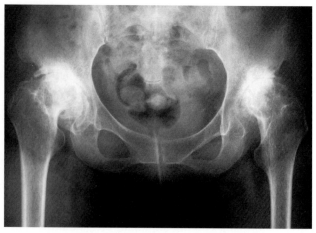

FIG. 3. Woman with bilateral dysplastic hips. **A:** Anteroposterior radiograph made at her first visit to our department at the age of 29 when bilateral hip pain started. Broken Shenton's lines on this early radiograph indicate subluxation of both hips. **B:** Anteroposterior radiograph made before bilateral total hip replacements performed when she was 52 years old. Both hips have developed end-stage osteoarthrosis.

dominant cause of hip disease was congenital subluxation or dislocation of the hip (i.e., the dysplastic hip) in the Japanese patients, whereas it was primary OA in the American cases. A diagnosis of OA secondary to congenital subluxation or dislocation of the hip was made according to the following criteria: history of congenital dislocation of the hip, joint subluxation indicated by a broken Shenton's line on radiographs made before development of advanced OA (early radiographs), and distinct hallmarks of this condition detected on radiographs or during hip surgery. In a study of hips undergoing a primary THR, the percentage of primary OA has been increasing in the last four decades, probably reflecting the increase in the elderly population and/or the westerniza-

tion trend seen in the distribution of certain adult diseases in Japan. Comparison between 291 dysplastic OA hips and 82 primary OA hips clarified characteristics of dysplastic hips. Symptoms of OA in the dysplastic OA group began earlier in life and led to surgery at an earlier age than those in the primary OA group. Radiographically, the superolateral type in the morphologic classification, and the hypertrophic type in the classification based on the biologic response of the joint were more common in the dysplastic OA group than in the other group. Mild acetabular dysplasia without subluxation of the joint was detected by measurements on early radiographs in 63% of 16 primary OA hips in which such radiographs were available. The natural history of acetabular dysplasia in

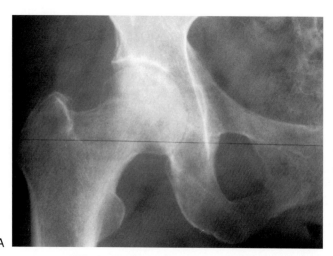
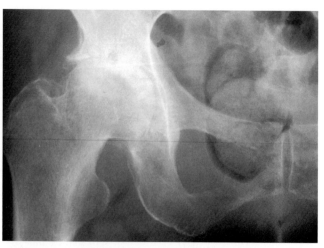

FIG. 4. Woman with primary osteoarthrosis of the right hip joint. **A:** Anteroposterior radiograph made at the first examination when she was 59 years old. Parameters of hip development measured on this early radiograph were within normal range. **B:** Anteroposterior radiograph made before surgery, which was performed only 9 months after the first examination. The hip has developed end-stage osteoarthrosis.

the absence of subluxation is still controversial and requires further research.

ROTATIONAL ACETABULAR OSTEOTOMY
Section Author: Tadami Matsumoto

Pelvic osteotomies for osteoarthrosis secondary to a dysplastic hip were established by Chiari (7), Sutherland and Greenfield (63), Tonnis (66), and Steel (58). On the other hand, periacetabular osteotomies preserving the pelvic ring were introduced by Eppright (11) and Wagner (70) in the West. In Japan, similar osteotomies were originated by Nishio (46) and Tagawa (45,64). The rotational acetabular osteotomy by Tagawa has come into wide use for early osteoarthrosis secondary to a dysplastic hip. Periacetabular osteotomies provide more extended shift of the acetabulum because they are performed closer to the joint than the pelvic osteotomies such as a triple osteotomy. Rotational acetabular osteotomy is one of the procedures that provide repositioning of the acetabulum with hyaline cartilage; furthermore, the osteotomy provides medialization by bone resection of the posteroinferior portion of the acetabulum. Rotational acetabular osteotomy makes it possible to normalize the coverage of the femoral head and inclination of the weight-bearing surface of the acetabulum, and to medialize the center of the femoral head. Rotational acetabular osteotomy has advantages in terms of the stability of the pelvis and labor, because it does not interrupt the pelvic ring.

Indications

Patients whose triradiate cartilage has not closed are not candidates for rotational acetabular osteotomy. Pre-osteoarthrosis, and osteoarthrosis in the early stage that shows good congruity on the anteroposterior (AP) radiographic view with abduction of the hip joint, are good indications for rotational acetabular osteotomy. In the advanced osteoarthrosis stage, the hip in which abduction of the hip joint makes the joint space wide and provides improvement of congruity between the acetabulum and the femoral head is a good candidate for rotational acetabular osteotomy. In some advanced cases, a radiograph with an anteriorly tilted pelvis is useful because it sometimes reveals improvement of the width and congruity of the joint space compared with the radiograph obtained with only abduction of the hip joint.

Surgical Technique

The patient is positioned in the true lateral position on the operating table, and the pelvis holder should be kept so as not to interfere with the taking of the intraoperative radiograph. The skin incision runs from craniad to caudad beginning at the top of the iliac crest, it travels down the thigh through the center between the anterior superior iliac spine and the anterior border of the greater trochanter, and it curves posteriorly, ending at the level of the lesser trochanter. This incision provides sufficient exposure to approach the hip joint anteriorly and posteriorly. The iliac origins of the tensor fasciae latae and gluteal muscles are detached anteriorly, and the greater sciatic notch is confirmed with an elevator. Then, the origin of the rectus femoris is exposed, cut, and reflected distally. The iliopsoas muscle is detached from the medial wall of the pelvis and the iliopectineal eminence is exposed. These procedures provide enough exposure for the osteotomy from the anterior and superior aspects of the hip joint. Next, the fasciae latae on the lateral aspect of the femur are excised, and the incision is extended superiorly in line with the fibers of the gluteus maximus, as in Moore's method. Stay sutures are inserted into the short rotator muscles, and then these are detached to expose the posterior aspect of the hip joint. The greater sciatic notch should be confirmed posteriorly, and the base of the ischium exposed. Then exposure for the hemispherical osteotomy is completed. The line of the osteotomy is placed 1.5 cm from the acetabular ridge in the superior aspect, just lateral to the iliopectineal eminence in the anterior aspect, and through the center between the greater sciatic notch and posterior acetabular ridge in the posterior aspect (Fig. 5).

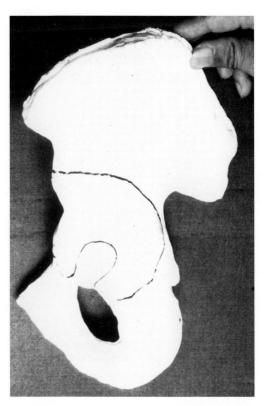

FIG. 5. Osteotomy line for the rotational acetabular osteotomy drawn on the lateral aspect of the pelvis. The osteotomy is performed with a specially curved osteotome.

The osteotomy is started from the superior aspect using a specially curved osteotome. The osteotome is directed superiorly and 30° from the perpendicular in the superior aspect (Fig. 6), posterolaterally and 20° from the perpendicular in the anterior aspect, and posteromedially and 25° from the perpendicular in the posterior aspect. Any penetration of the acetabular cartilage by the osteotome absolutely must be avoided. This is a key point for a successful result. After completion of the osteotomy, bone is removed from the inferoposterior portion to achieve medialization of the femoral head. Then, the acetabulum is rotated anterolaterally and the bone (2 × 3 cm) harvested from the external wall of the iliac wing is placed between the ilium and rotated acetabulum. Two Kirschner wires (diameter, 2 mm) are used for fixation of the rotated acetabulum and the pelvis. A radiograph is taken to confirm the position and congruity of the reestablished hip joint before wound closure. Holes are made in the iliac crest to reattach the fasciae latae to their original position. When the deformity of the femoral head is severe, the osteotomy produces incongruity of the hip

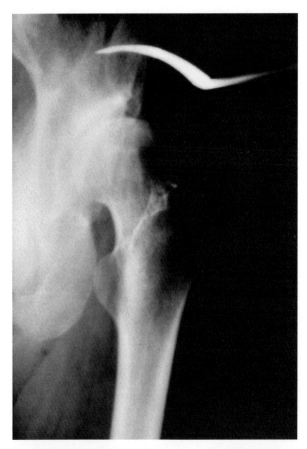

FIG. 6. Anteroposterior radiograph made during the rotational acetabular osteotomy to confirm the position and direction of the osteotome. It is taken when the osteotome is driven into the pelvis for the first time in the superior aspect of the acetabulum.

joint. In such cases, intertrochanteric osteotomy, usually valgus osteotomy, should be done to achieve good congruity. When the elevation of the greater trochanter is severe, distal transfer of the greater trochanter is occasionally performed. In most cases, elevation of the great trochanter does not affect the clinical results. Hypotensive anesthesia, maintained at approximately 80 mm Hg systolic artery pressure, is useful to reduce blood loss. Fewer homologous blood transfusions are needed when 400 mL autologous blood has been preserved prior to surgery. The average duration of surgery is approximately 2.5 hours, and the average blood loss is approximately 200 mL intraoperatively and 250 mL postoperatively (37).

Postoperative Management

A postoperative cast is not applied. The hip joint is maintained in abduction for several days after surgery. The patient is permitted out of bed in a wheel chair at 3 weeks after surgery. Partial weight bearing on two crutches is started at 5 or 6 weeks after surgery, and the Kirschner wires are removed at around 7 weeks. Usually, full weight bearing is allowed at 4 months after surgery, and muscle power of the abductors is restored to the preoperative level by 6 months after surgery.

Complications

In our experience, complications after this surgery are not common. Chondrolysis caused by penetration of the acetabular cartilage by the osteotome, nonunion, and necrosis of the rotated acetabulum have been reported in Japan (45), but these complications have not been seen in our series. Intraoperative massive bleeding occurred because of damage to a branch of the obturator artery in one case in which the patient's pelvis was severely deformed after a previous osteotomy. Only a few patients showed a transient lateral femoral cutaneous nerve palsy.

Results

Rotational acetabular osteotomies in 292 hips were performed from 1986 to 1992. The average age of the patients at the time of the operation was 33.1 years old (range, 14 to 48 years old). The average period of follow-up was 70 months (range, 36 to 126 months). Sixty-five hips were classified in the preosteoarthrosis stage on radiograph at the time of surgery, 162 hips in the early stage (i.e., mild joint space narrowing), and 59 in the advanced stage (i.e., considerable joint space narrowing). Radiographically, the center-edge angle was improved from -0.15° ± 10.7° preoperatively to 33.6° ± 8.4° postoperatively, and the angle of roof obliquity (36) was

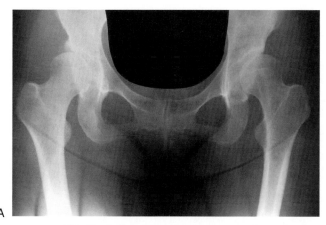
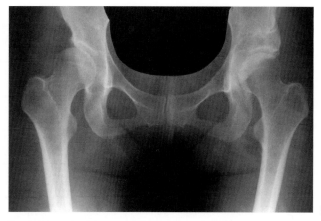

A   B

FIG. 7. A: Preoperative anteroposterior radiograph of both hips of a 22-year-old woman who underwent the rotational acetabular osteotomy in her left hip joint at the preosteoarthrosis stage. **B:** Anteroposterior radiograph made 7 years and 6 months after the osteotomy. Note the improvement in the center-edge angle and in the angle of roof obliquity. The femoral head has been medialized and shifted distally. There are no discernible signs of osteoarthrosis.

improved from 28.0° ± 8.9° preoperatively to 3.6° ± 6.8° postoperatively. The average medialization of the femoral heads was 3.5 mm, and the average caudal shift of the femoral head was 2.9 mm (Figs. 7,8).

For clinical evaluations, the Japanese Orthopaedic Association score (JOA score), which is similar to the Harris Hip Score, is used. The system consists of pain (40 points for no pain); walking ability (20 points for full function); range of motion (20 points for full range); and daily activities (20 points for full ability). The JOA score improved for the preosteoarthritis cases from 78.6 ± 10.3 points preoperatively to 98.6 ± 3.7 points at 3 years after surgery, with the score being maintained and the patient having no pain at the most recent examination. In the cases of early-stage osteoarthritis, the JOA score improved from 73.3 ± 11.4 points preoperatively to 97.3

± 5.5 points at 3 years after surgery, with this score also subsequently being maintained. In some cases in this group, however, flexion was slightly restricted. In the cases of advanced stage, the JOA score improved from 67.7 ± 10.2 points preoperatively to 90.0 ± 16.5 points at 3 years after surgery; the score fell to 83.3 ± 22.9 at the time of the most recent examination. The score tended to decrease gradually, and the standard deviation increased (Fig. 9).

Discussion and Conclusions

Rotational acetabular osteotomy is a very useful operation for osteoarthrosis secondary to a dysplastic hip and provides excellent long-term results, especially in pre-

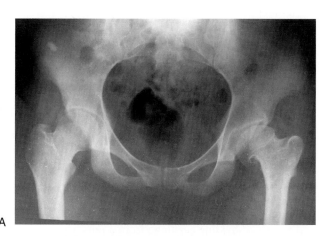
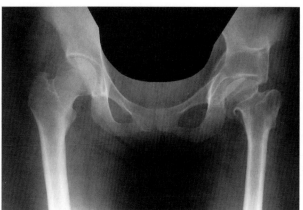

A   B

FIG. 8. A: Preoperative anteroposterior radiograph of both hips of a 31-year-old woman who underwent the rotational acetabular osteotomy in her left hip joint at the early stage of osteoarthrosis. **B:** Anteroposterior radiograph made 8 years after the osteotomy. Note the improvement in the anatomic features of the left hip joint (center-edge angle, acetabular angle, roof obliquity, and femoral head coverage). There is no progression of osteoarthrosis.

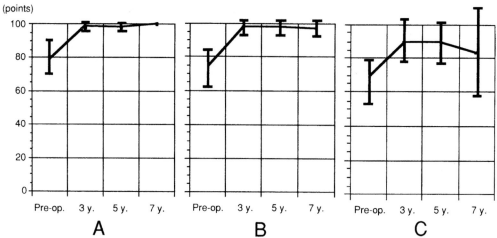

FIG. 9. The average Japanese Orthopaedic Association hip scores before surgery and 3, 5, and 7 years after the rotational acetabular osteotomy, according to the preoperatively determined radiologic stages of osteoarthrosis. Preosteoarthrosis **(A)**, early stage osteoarthrosis **(B)**, and advanced stage osteoarthrosis **(C)**. The postoperative improvement in the score has been maintained in patients who had preosteoarthrosis or early-stage osteoarthrosis before surgery (A and B). The score tended to deteriorate in cases with advanced osteoarthrosis.

osteoarthrosis and osteoarthrosis in the early stage. In the advanced stage, the clinical results showed a tendency to deteriorate with time, a tendency especially evident in patients whose hip showed no widening of the joint space or improvement of the congruity between the acetabulum and femoral head on the radiographs taken with abduction of the hip joint. However, in the advanced cases in which radiographs with anteriorly tilted pelvis revealed improvement of the width and congruity of the joint space, satisfactory results were obtained.

DOME PELVIC (MODIFIED CHIARI) OSTEOTOMY

Section Author: Nobuhiko Sugano

After first being described in 1953 (6), the Chiari medial displacement pelvic osteotomy became the widespread treatment of choice for congenital dislocation or subluxation of the hip and acetabular dysplasia for children and adults. The dome pelvic osteotomy was developed by Kawamura (1958) in Japan as a modification of Chiari's procedure (25). It was designed to improve the hip procedure by providing a dome-shaped bone shelf to support the femoral head. This is done by creating an arched rather than a flat acetabular surface when performing the osteotomy. In Chiari's original procedure, remodeling is ultimately necessary to recreate an acetabulum resembling the original articular surface (26). A decrease in remodeling time coupled with an increase in stability is the reason that some surgeons, including Chiari himself later on, prefer to fashion an arched rather than a flat acetabular roof (8,50). Furthermore, a faster remodeling time can help decrease the chances of post-

operative degenerative change (2). Unlike the original Chiari procedure, which uses an anterior approach, Kawamura believed the entire procedure can be conveniently performed through a lateral approach. If desired, a greater trochanter shift can be added easily to improve the abductor mechanism. In cases where the Chiari osteotomy is indicated, the dome pelvic osteotomy can be expected to provide better results.

After the subsequent introduction of the Salter and Pemberton pelvic osteotomies for childhood hip disorders (48,54,65,68), and of various periacetabular reorientation osteotomies for adult disorders (11,21,45,58,69), the number of indications for the dome and Chiari pelvic osteotomies has been significantly reduced. However, the dome osteotomy still holds an important place in the treatment of the patients described below.

Indications

Adolescents and adults with congenital subluxation of the hip and acetabular dysplasia, who are complaining of hip pain or persistent gross instability, are candidates for this treatment. In highly subluxated hips (with more than a half of the femoral head migrated proximally), the ilium may be too thin to produce a new roof and the osteotomy line may reach the sacroiliac joint. In such cases, other shelf procedures may work better (53). The acetabular reorientation osteotomies, which rely on shifting of naturally formed hyaline cartilage from a non-weight-bearing to a weight-bearing surface, are preferred in cases with minimal deformity of the femoral head and maintenance of the joint space. Although the presence of only minimal arthritic change on preoperative radiograph is preferable, the pelvic dome osteotomy can be performed even in the presence of severe degenerative changes in order to postpone joint replacement surgery in younger patients. It may provide increased bone stock in the acetabular side, which can facilitate later total hip arthroplasty. In some hips with a moderate loss of joint space, restoration is maintained, but others develop advanced arthrosis after surgery. Preoperative radiographic signs may not be sufficient to discriminate between these two groups, and in such cases, bone scintigraphy may provide useful information. If isotope uptake is localized only to the weight-bearing area, then the dome pelvic osteotomy may provide good results. However, if isotope uptake is present in both the weight-bearing and more medial non-weight-bearing areas of the joint, then the degenerative change is too advanced for this operation alone to be successful, and it may need to be combined with another procedure such as a femoral valgus osteotomy.

Dome pelvic osteotomy is also indicated for lateralization of the femoral head secondary to Perthes disease, and for insufficient coverage of the head resulting from postreduction avascular necrosis after treatment for developmental dysplasia of the hip. Also, it may be performed for unstable progressive subluxation in patients with neuromuscular disorders such as cerebral palsy or poliomyelitis.

Surgical Techniques

The patient is positioned on the operating table with the affected side upward. The skin incision is made longitudinally over the proximal femur, extending approximately 10 cm above and below the greater trochanter. The fascia is cut in line with the wound, between the gluteus maximus and the tensor fascia lata. With internal rotation of the extremity, the piriformis tendon is defined. The short rotators from the piriformis to the obturator externus are released from their insertion, leaving the quadratus femoris intact. The short rotator muscles are retracted until the sciatic notch is seen. After inserting an elevator between the capsule and the gluteus minimus, the greater trochanter is osteotomized in the direction of the elevator and is reflected superiorly with the attached muscles. Then, the upper aspect of the capsule of the hip joint and adjacent part of the iliac bone are exposed. The periosteum along the acetabular rim is incised and elevated until about 3 cm of the outer table of the iliac bone has been exposed. Three to five Steinmann pins of 4.5-mm diameter are then driven into the upper side of the exposed outer table of the ilium (Fig. 10) to hold the retracted gluteal muscles in place. The reflected head of the rectus femoris is sectioned from the capsule. With a periosteal elevator, the periosteum is incised along the anterior edge of the pelvis to the iliopectineal eminence. Likewise, the periosteum on the longitudinal arch of the

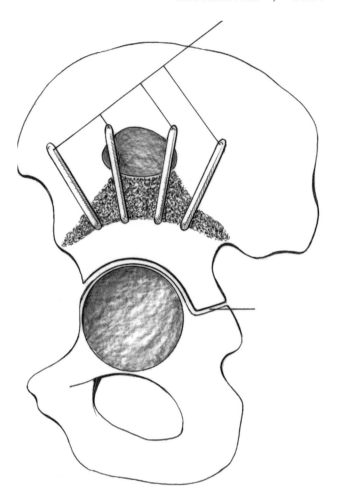

FIG. 10. Schematic representation of the dome pelvic (modified Chiari) osteotomy. The osteomatized greater trochanter has been reflected superiorly with the attached muscles. They are kept away from the upper aspect of the joint capsule with 4.5-mm Steinmann pins driven into the ilium. An arch-shaped osteotomy line is marked along the superior rim of the acetabulum. The pelvis is osteomatized from the osteotomy line at an angle of about 15° from the horizontal using an oscillating saw (Türk saw). After the osteotomy, the distal pelvic fragment is displaced medially until more than 80% of the femoral head is covered by the new dome-shaped roof.

sciatic notch is incised and the periosteum on the inner table is elevated using a malleable bowel retractor. While retracting the limb, the joint space is identified with a needle.

The hypertrophic joint capsule can sometimes make performing an osteotomy at the proper level difficult. In these cases, the superior portion of the capsule can be partially excised. A Kirschner wire of 2.5-mm diameter is then driven into the pelvis from the uppermost border of the capsule superomedially at an angle of approximately 15° from the horizontal. An x-ray is taken to verify the level and angle of the osteotomy. An arch-shaped osteotomy line is marked with an osteotome or a drill along the acetabular rim (see Fig. 10), and the pelvis is osteotomized to the inner table parallel to the guide wire using an oscillating saw (Türk saw). After the osteotomy is completed, the leg is forced into abduction and external rotation, which displaces the distal pelvic fragment medially. Medialization is performed until more than 80% of the femoral head is covered by the new roof. In the past, no internal fixation was used and a hip spica cast was applied for 3 weeks. Recently, however, internal fixation has become popular. Two Kirschner wires of 2.5-mm diameter are percutaneously driven into the ilium with the tips at the medial one-third border of the cut surface of the proximal fragment prior to displacement. The wires are then advanced 1.5 cm into the distal fragment after medialization. Varus or valgus osteotomy of the femur is added when the preoperative anteroposterior radiographs show better congruity in abduction or adduction, respectively. Using two AO cancellous screws, the greater trochanter is then reattached to the femur at a site 1 cm to 2 cm distal to its original position, to correct for the abductor shortening resulting from the osteotomy. Postoperatively, the Kirschner wires are removed after 3 or 4 weeks. Partial weight bearing is allowed at 6 weeks and full weight bearing at 12 weeks postoperatively.

Results

Results of Chiari's pelvic osteotomy reported in the last 10 years are shown in Table 8. Clinically, 51% to 93% excellent or good results were seen (2,3,5,16,22,30,38,41,49,50,75). The most consistent effect of this operation is the rapid and continued relief of pain. Although clinical deterioration occurs with a longer follow-up period and patients may eventually go on to replacement surgery, the

TABLE 8. *Results of Chiari pelvic osteotomy*

Authors (ref.)	No. of patients	Age at operation (mean yr) (range)	Follow-up period (mean yr) (range)	Clinical results	Radiologic results
Reynolds (50)	44	35 (18–55)	5.2 (2–13)	Excellent or good, 73%	n.a.
Graham et al. (16)	58	16 (7–45)	3.3 (1–12)	Excellent or good, 93%	Joint space narrowing, 7%
Calvert et al. (5)	49	19.8 (3–41)	14 (over 10)	Excellent or good, 65%	Osteoarthritis (OA) score, 0.7 preop. 2.7 at final 53% new OA change
Høgh, Macnicol (22)	68	19 (3–41)	10 (2–18)	Pain relief, 87%	OA progressed with time
Betz et al. (3)	24	n.a. (10–22)	n.a. (3–20)	Excellent or good, 88%	n.a.
Rejholec et al. (49)	104	n.a. (3–45)	18 (n.a.)	Pain free, 40% Pain of lumbosacral spine, 15% Pain of hip joints, 48%	No upward migration, 62%
Windhager et al.[a] (75)	236 Group A, 215 Group B, 21	14.1 (2.6–51.3)	A, 24.8 (20.0–34.2) B, 15.4 (6–28)	Excellent or good, 51%	Progression of OA None, 5%
Lack et al.[b] (30)	100	38 (30–59)	15.5 (10–21)	Good, 75%	Progression of OA THA, 20% 2–19 years postoperatively
Matsuno et al.[c] (38)	100	21 (10–51)	9.3 (6–14.8)	Excellent or good, 78%	Progression of OA None, 80%
Anwar et al.[c] (1)	101	30 (15–55)	8.3 (5–14)	Excellent or good, 92%	Progression of OA None, 91%
Migaud et al. (41)	90	34 (16–59)	6 (2–15)	Excellent or good, 79%	Progression of OA None, 82% THA, 12%

[a] Chiari performed 91% of the operations between 1953 and 1967.
[b] All the operations were performed by Chiari between 1968 and 1977.
[c] Dome pelvic (modified Chiari's) osteotomy through a transtrochanteric lateral approach.

operation can benefit patients for 15 to 20 years in many cases (76).

Upon review of the literature, several technical factors are important in achieving good results. Placement of the osteotomy cut is critical. An osteotomy that is begun too inferior may lead to increased stress at the site of the new roof, and poor results can be expected. Likewise, a cut placed too high or too horizontal may lead to poor results, but this can be corrected with bone grafting of the large voids created when it occurs. Also, the curved osteotomy line of Kawamura has demonstrated superior results to the original straight cut (26). Displacement of the fragment by more than two thirds is usually needed to sufficiently cover the femoral head. These requirements can be fulfilled more consistently through the lateral approach. Overall, using the dome pelvic osteotomy, the surgeon can reliably create an osteotomy with a congruent roof and adequate coverage in a more standardized way than the original Chiari procedure.

The Trendelenburg sign is often seen in cases in which a Chiari osteotomy was indicated. It is seldom eliminated after the Chiari osteotomy unless accompanied by a trochanteric shift (3,50,76). The dome pelvic osteotomy is advantageous because the trochanteric shift is performed concomitantly. More than 1 cm of shift has been reported to be effective in preventing a postoperative Trendelenburg sign and progression of degenerative change.

Sciatic nerve injury and delayed union or nonunion of the osteotomy site are possible complications of the Chiari osteotomy. However, these can be avoided by using meticulous surgical technique and careful observation allowed by the wider field of vision provided by the lateral transtrochanteric approach.

Radiologically, many parameters of hip dysplasia such as the center-edge angle and acetabular head index are improved to within the normal range and can be maintained if the operation was performed correctly. Improvement of degenerative change was seldom observed by this procedure. Preoperative degree of degenerative change and age at operation are related to outcome. Severe joint space narrowing and age over 45 are associated with a poor outcome. In advanced stages of osteoarthritis, a combined femoral osteotomy should be considered.

Given that the articular surface created through remodeling is fibrocartilage at best, durability against the weight-bearing forces is unreliable. Even in hips with no sign of osteoarthritis preoperatively, a long-term follow-up of Chiari's original series showed appearance of degenerative change in 90% of cases followed for over 20 to 34 years (76). The rate of osteoarthritic change may seem quite high, but when compared to conservative treatment for similar grades of hip dysplasia, it is clear that the Chiari osteotomy can prevent or delay the osteoarthritic change. Although a long-term follow-up study of over 20 years is not yet available for the dome pelvic osteotomy, mid-term results have been excellent (2,38) and long-term results showing significant improvement over the Chiari series are expected.

TOTAL HIP ARTHROPLASTY WITH ACETABULAR BONE GRAFTING FOR CONGENITAL HIP DYSPLASIA
Section Author: Susumu Saito

Japanese patients who require surgical treatment of the hips generally have specific problems, which differ from those of American or European patients. First, osteoarthrosis, the predominant hip disease, is mostly secondary to antecedent congenital dysplasia or dislocation of the hip. Second, the patients are relatively young. Finally, they have relatively short stature and light body weight. Hoaglund et al. (21) reported a comparative study of hip diseases in the Japanese and the white American patients. They pointed out that osteoarthritis in 80% of the Japanese patients was secondary to congenital dysplasia or dislocation of the hip, whereas that was found in only 5.7% of white American patients. The mean age of Japanese patients was approximately two decades younger than that of white Americans. From this perspective, the Japanese experience in hip surgery has differed.

Degree of Dysplasia

There is a broad spectrum of disease severity, from mild dysplasia to complete dislocation of the hip. The acetabulum is characterized by abnormal sloping and in some cases by a severely dysplastic structure. The femoral intramedullary canal is also dysplastic, smaller, and straighter. There is increased femoral neck anteversion. We adopted Crowe's classification system (10). According to the amount of subluxation, dysplastic hips can be classified into four groups: group 1, less than 50% subluxation; group 2, 50% to 75% subluxation; group 3, 75% to 100% subluxation; and group 4, more than 100% subluxation.

Long-term Results of Cemented Total Hip Arthroplasty for Congenital Hip Dysplasia

Total hip arthroplasty is a challenging surgical procedure (1,10,21,58). Distorted hip anatomy requires complex reconstruction techniques to obtain sufficient containment and stable fixation of components. Various methods to compensate for the deficient acetabular bone stock have been described, including reconstruction using small sockets with cemented augmentation (39), cemented sockets with structural bone graft (18), and

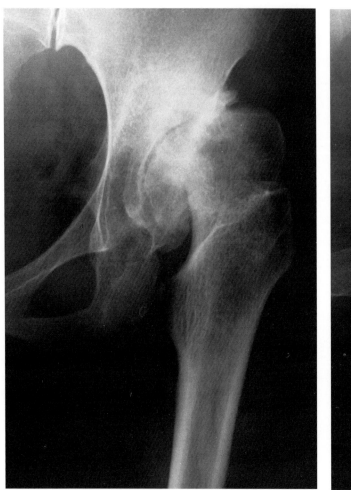
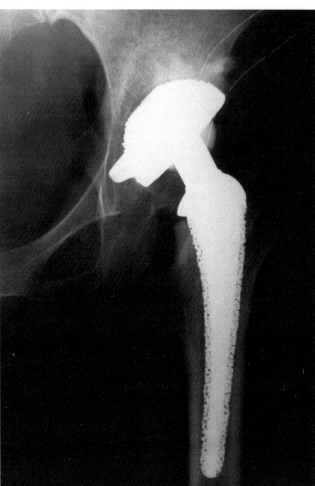

A

B

FIG. 11. Radiographs of a 43-year-old woman. **A:** She suffered from osteoarthrosis secondary to congenital hip dysplasia (Crowe group 3). **B:** A cementless Lübeck prosthesis was implanted with cancellous chip grafting for the deficient acetabulum. **C:** Four years after surgery, both components were stable and cancellous chip grafts showed incorporation and excellent remodeling. The hip score improved from 9 (pain, 2; mobility, 4; function, 3) to 18 (pain, 6; mobility, 6; function, 6).

cementless socket placement using small components at a "high hip center" (56). Among these three methods, bone grafting of the dysplastic acetabulum was first reported by Harris et al. (18) and is now widely recognized to be a useful procedure. They used large bone graft from the excised femoral head, and reported satisfactory short-term results. Long-term follow-up data, however, showed high failure rates of sockets. At a mean follow-up period of 7 years, 20% of sockets were loose (15), and at a mean follow-up period of 12 years, 46% were loose and 20% required revision (43). They concluded that the use of bulk corticocancellous autogenous grafts could not be recommended. Because of the criticism of large bone grafts by Harris et al. (18), several authors have used smaller grafts, which showed better long-tern results. Marti et al. (35) reported an 11% socket loosening rate and 8% revision rate in 63 primary total hip arthroplasties at a mean follow-up of 10 years. Inao et al. (24) reported

a 15% socket loosening rate and no revisions required in 20 total hip arthroplasties at a mean follow-up period of 8.4 years. Anwar et al. (1) reported 34 hips with neglected congenital dislocation (Crowe group 4) at a mean follow-up period of 9.4 years. The radiologic loosening rate of the socket was noted to be 23.5%, and there was a revision rate of 11%. In the Japanese literature, Iida et al. (23) clearly demonstrated that the smaller graft provided a lower loosening rate of the socket, and that the long-term survival rate of total hip arthroplasty augmented by bone grafts was significantly higher than that of the first 100 low-friction arthroplasty series, where acetabular bone grafting was not performed. These data indicate that acetabular augmentation by small bone grafts improves long-term survival of the socket. Recently, cementless total hip arthroplasty with structural acetabular grafting and porous socket has been performed and has showed satisfactory short-term results (58).

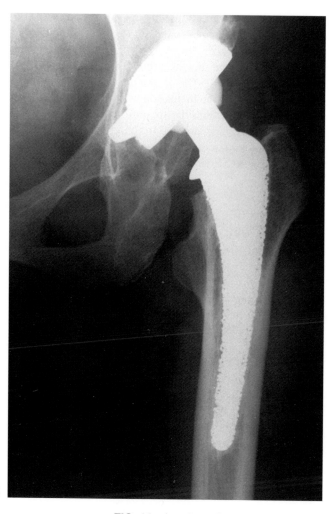

C

FIG. 11. *(continued)*

For group 4 hips, a conventional cemented total hip arthroplasty system is used. In the Lübeck system, the stem and metal socket of the implants are made of cobalt–chrome–molybdenum alloy, and the whole surface of the implant contacting bone has a spongy metal structure similar to cancellous bone. A polyethylene liner component and a modular alumina ceramic head, 28 mm in diameter, are used (63).

Surgical Procedure for Total Hip Arthroplasty with Bone Grafting

In Crowe group 1, 2, or 3 dysplasia, a posterolateral approach is used. The greater trochanter is usually not osteotomized. The cementless socket is placed at or near the true acetabulum, where the maximum bone stock is available. This provides the most satisfactory biomechanical results. A slightly high placement of the socket is usually used, because an increase less than 2 cm in the position does not increase the loosening rate of the cemented socket (52). In most cases, acetabular reaming should be performed deeply, until the medial wall of the pelvis appears, so as to provide good containment of the socket by viable bone (Fig. 11). Preoperative planning is extremely important to achieve optimal positioning and maximal bony coverage of the socket. The socket is placed at 40° to 50° of abduction and 15° of anteversion. When there is a lack of sufficient bony coverage of the socket, autogenous bulk or cancellous chip grafting from the resected femoral head is indicated regardless of the extent of bony defect. Bulk graft is fixed with two AO cortical screws, and cancellous chip grafts are impacted and fixed with fibrin glue.

On the femoral side in Crowe group 1, 2, or 3 hips, the femur has a sufficient intramedullary canal to insert the standard stem of the Lübeck system. In a small number of patients whose proximal femur shows a marked anteversion more than 60°, we use a cemented stem with an anteversion of 10°. Because the osteoarthritis secondary to congenital hip dysplasia frequently shows a huge osteophyte in the anterior portion of the acetabulum, it should be resected by chisel to avoid the postoperative restriction of motion and reduce the risk of dislocation. Postoperatively, the patient requires crutches for 6 weeks, and then full weight bearing is permitted.

In Crowe group 4 hips, cemented total hip arthroplasty is indicated. We prefer the Bioceram total hip prosthesis (Kyocera Corporation, Kyoto, Japan), because of its wide variation of components and alumina ceramic head (62). Osteotomy of the greater trochanter is required to provide wide exposure. The true acetabulum is severely dysplastic. The socket is again placed near the true acetabulum, where the maximal thickness and anteroposterior width of bone stock are obtained. It is preferable to ream the acetabulum cavity up to the medial wall so that coverage

On the femoral side, the loosening rate was almost the same as that usual for total hip arthroplasties, ranging from 0% to 16% (24,29,35,42). Even in Crowe group 4 hips where a straight and narrow femoral stem was predominantly used, femoral loosening was rated at 8.8% (1).

Indications of Total Hip Arthroplasty with Bone Grafting

Treatment of congenital hip dysplasia in an adult depends on the severity of the disease, the stage of the secondary arthritic changes, the age of the patient, available bone stock, and the functional goals of the patient. Total hip arthroplasty is generally indicated for severe osteoarthritis of the hip, which causes a painful and disabling condition or limits the walking ability of the patients.

The authors prefer the cementless total hip using a spongy metal Lübeck hip prosthesis (S+G Implants, Lübeck, Germany) for Crowe group 1, 2, or 3 dysplasia.

of the socket with the host bone is maximized. Autogenous bulk bone grafts are fixed to the superolateral bony defect with two AO cortical screws. In hips with complete dislocation, a large bone graft is required to cover not only the superolateral but also the anterior and posterior bony defect despite the use of a small socket. A small socket, 42 or 44 mm in diameter, is usually used, because of the small skeletal features of Japanese patients. The femur must be shortened at or below the level of the lesser trochanter, to provide easy reduction. Such shortening of the femur is performed to leave lateral cortex, which provides maximal contact to the greater trochanter. A straight stem is usually inserted. Lengthening of the limb should be less than 3 cm because of the risk of sciatic nerve palsy. The iliopsoas must be released. Reattachment of the osteotomized greater trochanter can be fixed by a three-wire technique, but currently we use fixation with a cable system to avoid trochanteric nonunion.

Postoperatively, the patient requires crutches for 3 months and then full weight bearing is permitted. In patients with bilateral congenital dislocation of the hip, total hip arthroplasty is indicated for both hips, because total hip arthroplasty in only one hip will create a marked leg-length discrepancy.

Results of Cementless Total Hip Arthroplasty Augmented by Bone Grafting

Forty-six hips in 39 patients who underwent cementless total hip arthroplasty with autogenous bone grafting in our clinic were followed from 2 to 5.8 years, with an average of 2.9 years. The spongy metal Lübeck hip prosthesis was implanted in all hips. Bulk graft was used in ten hips and cancellous chip grafts obtained from the resected femoral head was used in 36 hips. All hips were diagnosed with osteoarthritis secondary to congenital dysplasia or dislocation of the hip. According to the classification system proposed by Crowe et al. (3), there were 25 hips in group 1, 11 hips in group 2, 7 hips in group 3, and 3 hips in group 4. Patient age at surgery ranged from 40 to 70 years, with an average of 56 years.

The mean of the Merle d'Aubigne and Postel hip score (18 points for normal hip) (40) improved from 9.4 (pain, 1.6; mobility, 4.5; function, 3.3) before surgery to 17.0 (pain, 5.9; mobility, 5.5; function, 5.6) at final evaluation. All hips were rated as excellent (65%) or good (35%). Thigh pain was recognized in only three hips and spontaneously disappeared within 2 years after surgery.

Radiologically, there were no socket migrations or circumferential radiolucent lines. All bone grafts achieved radiologic union, which, on average, occurred at 12 months in bulk grafts and at 5 months in cancellous chip grafts (see Fig. 11c). Cancellous chip grafts showed excellent remodeling by 13 months after surgery, as assessed by the presence of trabeculation. Cancellous

chip grafts also showed bony densification in 64% of the cases, and there was an absence of radiolucent lines at the graft–socket interface. However, bulk grafts revealed partial remodeling near the host bone only, and apparent radiolucent lines in 50% of the cases. Resorption of grafts and ectopic bone formation were mild and found in about 30% of cases. On the femoral side, there were no hips that showed migration or circumferential radiolucent lines. All stems were assessed as having optimum fixation according to Silber and Engh (58).

Conclusions

Osteoarthritis in Japanese patients who require surgical treatment is mostly secondary to antecedent congenital hip disease such as congenital dysplasia or dislocation. These patients require surgical treatment at a relatively young age. Cemented total hip arthroplasty augmented by autogenous bone graft provided satisfactory results. Recently, cementless total hip arthroplasty with bone graft has been performed and has shown satisfactory short-term results. These results, using a spongy metal Lübeck prosthesis, augmented by autogenous bulk or cancellous chip grafts, are encouraging. Autogenous bone grafting is a useful procedure to augment acetabular deficiency in cemented or cementless total hip arthroplasty for a dysplastic hip.

REFERENCES

1. Anwar MM, Sugano N, Masuhara K, Kadowaki T, Takaoka K, Ono K. Total hip arthroplasty in the neglected congenital dislocation of the hip. A 5- to 14-year follow-up study. *Clin Orthop* 1993;295:127–134.
2. Anwar MM, Sugano N, Matsui M, Takaoka K, Ono K. Dome osteotomy of pelvis for osteoarthritis secondary to hip dysplasia. *J Bone Joint Surg* 1993;75B:222–227.
3. Betz RR, Kumar SJ, Palmer CT, MacEwen GD. Chiari pelvic osteotomy in children and young adults. *J Bone Joint Surg* 1988;70A:182–191.
4. Bombelli R. *Osteoarthritis of the hip: classification and pathogenesis, the role of osteotomy as a consequent therapy*, 2nd ed. New York: Springer-Verlag, 1983.
5. Calvert PT, August AC, Albert JS, Kemp HB, Catterall A. The Chiari pelvic osteotomy. A review of the long-term results. *J Bone Joint Surg* 1987;69B:551–555.
6. Chiari K. Beckenosteotomie als Pfannendachplastik. *Wien Med Wochenschr* 1953;103:707–714.
7. Chiari K. Ergebnisse mit der Beckenosteotomie als Pfannendachplastik. *Z Orthop* 1955;87:14–26.
8. Chiari K. Medial displacement osteotomy of the pelvis. *Clin Orthop* 1974;98:55–71.
9. Cooperman DR, Wallensten R, Stulberg SD. Acetabular dysplasia in adult. *Clin Orthop* 1983;175:79–85.
10. Crowe JF, Mani VJ, Ranawat CS. Total hip replacement in congenital dislocation and dysplasia of the hip. *J Bone Joint Surg* 1979;61A:15–23.
11. Eppright RH. Dial osteotomy of the acetabulum in the treatment of dysplasia of the hip. *J Bone Joint Surg* 1975;57A:1172.
12. Fredensborg N. The CE angle of normal hips. *Acta Orthop Scand* 1976;47:403–405.
13. Fujii G, Sakkurai M, Funayama K, et al. Radiological studies on the hip joint in adults Japanese. *Seikeigeka* 1994;45:773–780.

14. Fuku H. Cementless hip prosthesis design: a basic study and analysis of the proximal femur in normal Japanese people. *J Jpn Orthop Assoc* 1994;68:763–773.

15. Geber SD, Harris WH. Femoral head autografting to augment acetabular deficiency in patients requiring total hip replacement. A minimum 5-year and an average 7-year follow-up study. *J Bone Joint Surg* 1986;68A:1241–1248.

16. Graham S, Westin GW, Dawson E, Oppenheim WL. The Chiari osteotomy. A review of 58 cases. *Clin Orthop* 1986;208:249–258.

17. Harris WH. Etiology of osteoarthritis of the hip. *Clin Orthop* 1986;213:20–33.

18. Harris WH, Crothers O, Oh I. Total hip replacement and femoral head bone-grafting for severe acetabular deficiency in adults. *J Bone Joint Surg* 1977;59A:752–759.

19. Hermodsson I. The development of coxarthrosis: a radiological follow-up of patients operated upon. *Radiologe* 1983;23:378–384.

20. Hoaglund FT, Yau CM, Wong WL. Osteoarthritis of the hip and other joints in southern Chinese in Hong-Kong. *J Bone Joint Surg* 1973;55A:545–557.

21. Hoaglund FT, Shiba R, Newberg AH, Leung K. Disease of the hip. A comparative study of Japanese Oriental and American white patients. *J Bone Joint Surg* 1985;67A:1376–1383.

22. Høgh J, Macnicol MF. The Chiari pelvic osteotomy. A long-term review of clinical and radiographic results. *J Bone Joint Surg* 1987;69B:365–373.

23. Iida H, Nakayama Y, Matsusue Y, Nakamura T. Long-term results of total hip arthroplasty with acetabular bone graft. *Seikei Saigai Geka* 1995;38:1293–1299.

24. Inao S, Gotoh E, Ando M. Total hip replacement using femoral neck bone to graft the dysplastic acetabulum. Follow-up study of 18 patients with old congenital dislocation of the hip. *J Bone Joint Surg* 1994;76B:735–739.

25. Kawamura B. Transverse pelvic osteotomy for congenital dislocation of the hip. *Nippon Iji Shinpou* 1958;1977:109.

26. Kawamura B, Hosono S, Yokogushi K. Dome osteotomy of the pelvis. In: Tachdjian MO, ed. *Congenital dislocation of the hip.* New York: Churchill Livingstone, 1982;609–623.

27. Kobayashi S, Eftekhar NS, Terayama K. Predisposing factors in fixation failure of femoral prostheses following primary Charnley low friction arthroplasty: a 10- to 20-year followup study. *Clin Orthop* 1994;306:73–83.

28. Kobayashi S, Eftekhar NS, Terayama K, Iorio R. Risk factors affecting radiological failure of the socket in primary Charnley low friction arthroplasty: a 10- to 20-year followup study. *Clin Orthop* 1994;306:84–96.

29. Kobayashi S, Terayama K. Radiology of low-friction arthroplasty of the hip. A comparison of socket fixation techniques. *J Bone Joint Surg* 1990;72B:439–443.

30. Komatsu I. Morphological studies of the upper end of the femur: measurements of the diameter of the femoral head and neck. *J Jpn Orthop Associ* 1986;60:755–762.

31. Lack W, Windhager R, Kutschera HP, Engel A. Chiari pelvic osteotomy for osteoarthritis secondary to hip dysplasia: indications and long-term results. *J Bone Joint Surg* 1991;73B:229–234.

32. Lavelle JL. An analysis of the human femur. *Am J Anat* 1974;141:415–426.

33. Lloyd-Roberts GC. Osteoarthritis of the hip: a study of the clinical pathology. *J Bone Joint Surg* 1955;37B:8–47.

34. Marks JS, Stewart IM, Hardinge K. Primary osteoarthrosis of the hip and Herberden's nodes. *Ann Rheum Dis* 1979;38:107–111.

35. Marti RK, Schüller HM, Steijn MJA. Superolateral bone grafting for acetabular deficiency in primary total hip replacement and revision. *J Bone Joint Surg* 1994;76B:728–734.

36. Massie WK, Howorth MB. Congenital dislocation of the hip: part I. Method of grading results. *J Bone Joint Surg* 1950;32A:519–531.

37. Matsumoto T. Measures against bleeding in the operation of the hip joint. *Hip Joint* 1992;18:308–310.

38. Matsuno T, Ichioka Y, Kaneda K. Modified Chiari pelvic osteotomy: a long-term follow-up study. *J Bone Joint Surg* 1992;74B:470–478.

39. McQueary FG, Missouri S, Johnston RC. Coxarthrosis after congenital dysplasia. Treatment by total hip arthroplasty without acetabular bone-grafting. *J Bone Joint Surg* 1988;70A:1140–1144.

40. Merle d'Aubigne R, Postel M. Functional results of hip arthroplasty with acrylic prosthesis. *J Bone Joint Surg* 1954;36A:451–475.

41. Migaud H, Duquennoy A, Gougeon F, Fontaine C, Pasquier G. Outcome of Chiari pelvic osteotomy in adults. 90 hips with 2–15 years' follow-up. *Acta Orthop Scand* 1955;66:127–131.

42. Mulroy RD, Harris WH. Failure of acetabular autogenous grafts in total hip arthroplasty. Increasing incidence: a follow-up note. *J Bone Joint Surg* 1990;72A:1536–1540.

43. Murray RO. The aetiology of primary osteoarthritis of the hip. *Br J Radiol* 1965;38:810–824.

44. Nakamura S, Ninomiya S, Nakamura T. Primary osteoarthritis of the hip joint in Japan. *Clin Orthop* 1989;241:190–196.

45. Ninomiya S, Tagawa H. Rotational acetabular osteotomy for the dysplastic hip. *J Bone Joint Surg* 1984;66A:430–436.

46. Nishio A. Open reduction by acetabular shift for congenital dislocation of the hip. *J Jpn Orthop Assoc* 1956;30:482–484.

47. Noble PC, Alexander JW, Lindahl LJ, Yew DT, Granberry WM, Tullos HS. The anatomical basis of femoral component design. *Clin Orthop* 1988;235:148–165.

48. Onoue Y. A study on the prevent intramedullary nails for the femoral fractures. *J Jpn Orthop Associ* 1977;51:315–329.

49. Pemberton PA. Pericapsular osteotomy of the ilium for the treatment of congenital subluxation and dislocation of the hip. *J Bone Joint Surg* 1965;47A:65–86.

50. Rejholec M, Stryhal F, Rybka V, Popelka S. Chiari osteotomy of the pelvis: a long-term study. *J Pediatr Orthop* 1990;10:21–27.

51. Reynolds DA. Chiari innominate osteotomy in adults. Technique, indications and contra-indications. *J Bone Joint Surg* 1986;68B:45–54.

52. Saito M, Saito S, Ohzono K, Ono K. The osteoblastic response to osteoarthritis of the hip. Its influence on the long-term results of arthroplasty. *J Bone Joint Surg* 1987;69B:746–751.

53. Saito S, Noma K, Fujii A. Acetabular dysplasia in female adults. *J Central Japan Orthop* 1974;17:115–117.

54. Saito S, Takaoka K, Ono K. Tectoplasty for painful dislocation or subluxation of the hip. Long-term evaluation of a new acetabuloplasty. *J Bone Joint Surg* 1986;68B:55–60.

55. Salter RB. Innominate osteotomy in the treatment of congenital dislocation and subluxation of the hip. *J Bone Joint Surg* 1961;43B:518–539.

56. Schutzer SF, Harris WH. High placement of porous-coated acetabular components in complex total hip arthroplasty. *J Arthroplasty* 1994;9:359–367.

57. Sharp IK. Acetabular dysplasia: the acetabular angle. *J Bone Joint Surg* 1961;43B:268–272.

58. Silber DA, Engh CA. Cementless total hip arthroplasty with femoral head bone grafting for hip dysplasia. *J Arthroplasty* 1990;5:231–240.

59. Steel HH. Triple osteotomy of the innominate bone. *J Bone Joint Surg* 1973;55A:343–350.

60. Solomon L. Patterns of osteoarthritis of the hip. *J Bone Joint Surg* 1976;58B:176–183.

61. Stulberg SD, Cordell LD, Harris WH, Ramsey PL, MacEwen GD. Unrecognized childhood hip disease: a major cause of idiopathic osteoarthritis of the hip. In: Amstutz HC, ed. *The hip: proceedings of the third open scientific meeting of the Hip Society.* St Louis: CV Mosby, 1975;212–228.

62. Sugano N, Nishii T, Nakata K, Masuhara K, Takaoka K. Polyethylene sockets and alumina ceramic heads in cemented total hip arthroplasty. A 10-year study. *J Bone Joint Surg* 1995;77B:548–556.

63. Sugano N, Saito S, Takaoka K, Ohzono K, Masuhara K, Saito M, Ono K. Spongy metal Lübeck hip prostheses for osteoarthritis secondary to hip dysplasia. A 2-6-year follow-up study. *J Arthroplasty* 1994;9:253–262.

64. Sutherland DH, Greenfield R. Double innominate osteotomy. *J Bone Joint Surg* 1977;59A:1082–1091.

65. Tagawa H. The treatment of coxarthrosis in adolescents and young adults. *Hip Joint* 1975;1:108–114.

66. Teuffer AP, Noguera JG. Experience with innominate osteotomy (Salter) and medial displacement osteotomy (Chiari) in the treatment of acetabular dysplasia: preliminary report of 82 operations. *Clin Orthop* 1974;98:133–136.

67. Tonnis D. Eine neue Technik der Dreifachosteotomie Zur Schwenkung dysplastischer Huftpfanen bei Jungendlichenund Erwachsenen. *Z Orthop* 1981;119:253–265.

68. Trotter M, Peterson RR. Transverse diameter of the femur: on roentgenograms and on bones. *Clin Orthop* 1967;62:233.

69. Utterback TD, MacEwen GD. Comparison of pelvic osteotomies for the surgical correction of the congenital hip. *Clin Orthop* 1974;98:104–110.

70. Wagner H. Osteotomies for congenital hip dislocation. In: Evarts CM, ed. *The hip: proceedings of the 4th open scientific meeting of the hip society.* St Louis: CV Mosby, 1976;45–66.

71. Wagner H. Experiences with spherical acetabular osteotomy for the correction of the dysplastic acetabulum. In: Hastings DE, ed. *Acetabular dysplasia; skeletal dysplasia in children. Progress in orthopaedic surgery 2.* New York: Springer, 1978;131–145.

72. Wedge JH, Wasylenko MJ. The natural history of congenital dislocation of the hip: a critical review. *Clin Orthop* 1978;137:154–162.

73. Wedge JH, Wasylenko MJ. The natural history of congenital disease of the hip. *J Bone Joint Surg* 1979;61B:334–338.

74. Weinstein SL. Natural history of congenital hip dislocation (CDH) and hip dysplasia. *Clin Orthop* 1987;225:62–76.

75. Wiberg G. Studies on dysplastic acetabula and congenital subluxation of the hip joint: with special reference to the complication of osteoarthritis. *Acta Chir Scand* 1939;83(suppl 58):53–68.

76. Windhager R, Pongracz N, Schönecker W, Kotz R. Chiari osteotomy for congenital dislocation and subluxation of the hip: results after 20 to 34 years follow-up. *J Bone Joint Surg* 1991;73B:890–895.

77. Yanagimoto S. Basic study of cementless hip prosthesis design: analysis of the proximal femur in Japanese patients with osteoarthritis of the hip. *J Jpn Orthop Assoc* 1991;65:731–744.

78. Yanagimoto S, Sakamaki T. Basic study of hip prosthesis design: analysis of shape of the femoral medullary canal in Japanese subjects by computed tomographic scanning. In: Imura S, Akamatu I, Azuma H, Sawai K, Tanaka S, eds. *Hip biomechanics.* Tokyo: Springer-Verlag, 1993;289–302.

79. Yoshida H, Sakamaki T, Izumida R, et al. Analysis of the normal hip by computed tomography. *Hip Joint* 1993;19:406–411.

The Adult Hip, edited by J. J. Callaghan,
A. G. Rosenberg, and H. E. Rubash.
Lippincott–Raven Publishers, Philadelphia © 1998.

CHAPTER 71

Early Complications and Their Management

Craig G. Mohler and Dennis K. Collis

Total hip replacement (THR) is an increasingly popular operation for management of the painful arthritic hip, with an estimated 200,000 patients undergoing this operation per year in the United States alone (120). After any major surgical procedure, complications can occur. Complications after THR are important not only to patients and their surgeons, but also to third-party payers and managed care organizations.

SYSTEMIC COMPLICATIONS

Mortality

Total hip replacement is most frequently performed in elderly patients, many of whom have preexisting medical conditions. An analysis of patients undergoing THR in an Australian study (99) demonstrated that 71% had one or more serious medical problems identified prior to surgery.

As with any procedure of this magnitude in an elderly population, there is a risk of death after surgery. A National Institutes of Health Consensus conference in

1982 estimated the risk of death after THR to be less than 1% (108). Analysis of Medicare claims data between 1983 and 1985 reveals an overall mortality of 0.95% in the first 30 days after THR. As would be expected, increasing age is associated with an increased risk of mortality. Patients between 66 and 69 years of age had a perioperative mortality rate of 0.34% after THR, compared to a mortality rate of 3.75% in patients aged 85 years and older (173). Female sex was associated with a statistically significant decrease in mortality, as was the indication for surgery. Patients in whom THR was performed for arthritis or failed THR had a lower mortality rate than patients undergoing THR for hip fracture (0.95% versus 6.2%) (173). Although the mortality after THR is higher than with other orthopedic operations such as arthroscopy, the overall mortality rate of 0.95% after THR in the Medicare population is lower than that of elderly patients undergoing carotid endarterectomy (9.8%) and prostatectomy (3.3%) (171,178).

Perioperative mortality after THR in the United Kingdom shows similar trends for increasing mortality with age and decreased mortality in women. The risk of death after THR in hospitals in the Oxford Regional Health Authority was 2.5 times higher in the first 90 days after surgery compared to the remainder of the first postoper-

C. G. Mohler and D. K. Collis: Orthopaedic and Fracture Clinic, Sacred Heart Medical Center, Eugene, Oregon 97401.

ative year. The most common causes of perioperative death were ischemic heart disease and venous thromboembolic events (137). No difference in mortality rates between community hospitals and teaching hospitals could be detected.

The influence of newer anesthetic techniques on the mortality after total joint replacement was examined at the Hospital for Special Surgery by Sharrock et al. (142). They demonstrated a drop in the mortality rate after THR from 0.36% to 0.1% over a 10-year period from 1981 to 1991. The threefold reduction in mortality was attributed in part to modern medications and nursing, and improved surveillance of deep venous thrombosis, as well as improvements in anesthetic techniques, including better perioperative monitoring and a shift towards regional anesthetic techniques.

Pulmonary Complications

Pulmonary complications are among the most common problems encountered in the perioperative period. Although the incidence of respiratory complications is higher after abdominal or thoracic surgery, respiratory problems do occur after THR. Some common perioperative pulmonary complications after THR include atelectasis, pulmonary edema, and pneumonia. Marrow embolization resulting in cardiopulmonary problems is a less common complication relatively unique to THR.

Preoperative Assessment

Prior to any major surgery such as THR, it is important to identify patients at risk for perioperative pulmonary complications. Patients with chronic obstructive pulmonary disease (COPD) and abnormal pulmonary function studies have a 70% postoperative pulmonary complication rate (151). Obese patients and patients who smoke more than one pack of cigarettes per day are also at higher risk for pulmonary problems after surgery (113,169). Finally, advanced age is associated with an increased risk of postoperative pulmonary complications, probably as a result of age-related effects on lung elastic tissues (161). Spirometry is useful to assess lung volumes, and preoperative arterial blood gas measurements can be used to serve as a baseline for comparison after surgery, particularly if spirometry results are abnormal. Preoperatively, cessation of smoking and reduction of excessive weight help decrease the risk of pulmonary complications. Administration of bronchodilators and breathing exercises prior to surgery can be valuable in patients with COPD, as can treatment of intercurrent lung infections with antibiotics. Patients who are malnourished prior to surgery (as is common in COPD) exhibit respiratory muscle weakness and abnormal ventilatory responses; therefore, assessment of nutritional status and correction of any nutritional deficiencies can have substantial benefit (5,6).

The Role of Anesthetic Techniques

General anesthesia has numerous diffuse effects on the respiratory system. Alterations in bronchopulmonary mucociliary function and increased pulmonary secretions combined with decreased lung compliance and depressed cough reflexes promote alveolar collapse and atelectasis (24,123). The duration of general anesthesia also influences the development of respiratory problems after surgery. Procedures lasting longer than 3 hours (such as revision THR) have a threefold higher rate of pulmonary complications after surgery (82). Although these changes occur to some extent in all patients after general anesthesia, the presence of preexisting pulmonary disease greatly magnifies their clinical significance (118).

Regional anesthesia (spinal or epidural) has been shown to reduce several morbidity parameters after surgery, including pulmonary problems. Compared to general anesthesia, regional anesthesia tends to minimize alterations in lung volumes and presumably other parameters of lung function as well (134). A randomized prospective trial of epidural versus general anesthesia in elderly patients undergoing THR showed a significant drop in the postoperative arterial PaO_2 in patients in the general anesthesia group (66). Regional anesthesia may also be of benefit in patients with difficult airway problems (such as the unstable rheumatoid cervical spine) (142). Numerous studies demonstrate a reduction in deep venous thrombosis and pulmonary embolism in patients undergoing total joint replacement surgery with regional anesthesia, probably related to improved lower extremity blood flow and reduced venous stasis (35,87,141).

Although regional anesthetic techniques are not without complications [including hypotension, neurologic injury, and rare toxic effects of anesthetic agents (17)], spinal and epidural anesthesia are less stressful metabolically than general anesthesia (134,182). It seems logical to suggest regional anesthesia with light sedation over general anesthesia in those patients most at risk for pulmonary problems after surgery.

Common Postoperative Pulmonary Problems

Common pulmonary problems after surgery include atelectasis, pulmonary edema, and pneumonia. These disorders typically present with some degree of pulmonary insufficiency, including tachypnea, fever, cough, and tachycardia. The differential diagnosis is aided by auscultation, chest radiography, and analysis of arterial blood gas measurements.

Atelectasis, or alveolar collapse, is exceedingly common after general anesthesia and results from a decrease in the functional residual capacity caused by altered ventilatory patterns (monotonous, shallow breathing) and retained secretions. The incidence of clinically significant atelectasis after THR has been estimated to be between 2% to 7% (34,44). Atelectasis is less common after THR than after other major surgeries such as abdominal and thoracic procedures. More rapid mobilization after THR has probably resulted in a decreased rate of this complication compared to earlier studies.

Clinically, atelectasis can present a variable picture ranging from no overt symptoms to severe respiratory insufficiency. Atelectasis is the most common cause of fever after surgery, at least in the initial 24 to 48 hours (118). Auscultation reveals decreased lung sounds over the lung bases, and chest radiography usually shows consolidation of lung segments. The treatment of atelectasis is aimed at restoration of alveolar ventilation through incentive spirometry and cough–deep breathing exercises and administration of supplementary oxygen.

Pulmonary edema is caused by an increase in lung water resulting in decreased lung functional residual capacity and alveolar collapse. The resultant intrapulmonary shunting leads to ventilation–perfusion mismatch and coupled with decreased lung compliance results in pulmonary insufficiency. The causes of pulmonary edema can be subdivided into two main categories: (a) cardiogenic (e.g., heart failure resulting from excessive fluid administration during and after surgery) and (b) noncardiogenic (resulting from disorders causing pulmonary capillary endothelial damage). In cardiogenic pulmonary edema, pump failure caused by depressed or injured myocardium leads to increased pulmonary capillary pressures and pulmonary edema. In noncardiogenic pulmonary edema, injury to pulmonary capillary endothelium causes transudation of fluid into interstitial and peribronchial spaces and eventually into alveolar spaces. The clinical syndrome of noncardiogenic pulmonary edema, termed adult respiratory distress syndrome (ARDS), has been described in various disorders including shock, sepsis, pneumonia, inhaled chemical irritants, and the fat embolism syndrome. The fat embolism syndrome, which has been reported after total hip and knee replacement (19,63,75,149), is characterized by central nervous system depression, petechiae, and varying manifestations of pulmonary insufficiency, including hypoxemia and pulmonary edema. Pulmonary insufficiency in the fat embolism syndrome has been ascribed to both mechanical (blockage of pulmonary capillaries by fat globules) and biochemical causes (release of chemically toxic free fatty acids) (85). Although numerous studies (21,46,111,125,172) document embolization of fat and marrow contents during cemented THR, the incidence of pulmonary edema and ARDS after cemented THR is quite low. Cardiovascular complications associated with polymethylmethacrylate (PMMA) are covered in more

detail in the section on postoperative cardiac complications in this chapter.

Pulmonary edema clinically presents much like atelectasis with fever, dyspnea, and cough. The degree of tachypnea is often greater with pulmonary edema because of the decreased lung compliance. The development of ARDS with severe pulmonary capillary congestion and intrapulmonary shunting is heralded by progressive refractory hypoxemia despite supplementary oxygen. Radiographically, pulmonary edema causes diffuse increases in lung density with a so-called white-out from confluent infiltrates in ARDS (170).

Cardiogenic pulmonary edema is treated by improving myocardial contractility with digitalis and reducing excessive lung water with diuretics, in addition to administration of supplementary oxygen (54). The use of pulmonary artery catheterization can help assess pulmonary vascular pressures and cardiac output, and it can be useful to distinguish cardiogenic from noncardiogenic pulmonary edema. Noncardiogenic pulmonary edema is treated by reducing excessive lung water using diuretics while maintaining intravascular volume by the administration of colloid solutions or blood products. Efforts must be made to identify and treat the cause of abnormal pulmonary capillary permeability in ARDS, such as treatment of sepsis and removal of chemical irritants. In ARDS, mechanical ventilation, including use of positive end-expiratory pressure (or PEEP), may be necessary to improve gas exchange (170). The mortality from ARDS can be as high as 50%, usually because of superimposed sepsis or cardiac problems (9,170).

Pneumonia can be difficult to diagnose in the postoperative period. The incidence has been estimated to be as high as 10% in elderly patients after THR (143). Pneumonia can arise *de novo* or can be superimposed on all other postoperative pulmonary complication, such as atelectasis or pulmonary edema. Postoperative pneumonia results from impairment of lung mechanisms that clear secretions (e.g., depressed cough reflex resulting from narcotics) and aspiration of infected secretions. Colonization of the upper respiratory tract with enteric bacteria occurs in nearly 100% of patients with major pulmonary problems after surgery (36). Typically, patients present with fever and a productive cough. Chest radiography shows patchy consolidation of lung fields, and sputum examination and culture can reveal organisms in 50% of cases. Treatment consists of vigorous tracheobronchial toilet and intravenous antibiotics. Usually broad-spectrum empirical antibiotic coverage is initiated in nosocomial pneumonia, with adjustments based on culture results (36).

Cardiac Complications

Cardiac complications occur after THR with a reported incidence from 2% to 10% (44,89,143). This section discusses preoperative cardiac assessment of patients undergoing THR and common postoperative cardiac problems, including angina and myocardial infarction, congestive heart failure, and arrhythmias. The cement implantation syndrome and cardiac complications related to the use of PMMA are also examined.

Preoperative Assessment

Total hip replacement is usually a procedure performed to relieve pain from arthritis, and as such it is an elective procedure. The risks of noncardiac surgery in patients with heart disease can be substantial and risk/benefit analysis can be very important prior to planned THR.

Analysis of cardiac risk factors in a large series of patients undergoing noncardiac surgery has allowed identification of factors that predict an adverse patient outcome (61,168) (Table 1). Analysis of preoperative data from 1001 patients over age 40 identified nine risk factors for adverse cardiac events, which were then assigned points after multivariate analysis. Patients were then stratified into four risk classes with differing rates of cardiac complications. The risk of significant cardiovascular complications was 1% for class I (0 to 5 points) and the risk increased to 7% for class II (6 to 12 points). For patients in the class III risk group (13 to 25 points), the risk of cardiac complications was 13%, and in the high risk class IV group (26+ points), the risk of cardiac complications was 78%, with a 56% cardiac mortality rate. This multifactorial index of cardiac risk for noncardiac surgery has been validated in subsequent studies (184) and enables the calculation of risk for a significant cardiac event such as myocardial infarction, congestive heart failure, or a lethal arrhythmia after surgery.

In patients with cardiovascular risk factors, consultation with an internist or cardiologist prior to surgery can help assess and manage cardiac problems. Electrocardio-

TABLE 1. *Calculation of multifactorial cardiac risk index*

Variable	Points
S3 gallop or jugular venous distension	11
Myocardial infarction in past 6 months	10
Premature ventricular contractions (more than 5/minute)	7
Rhythm other than sinus on preoperative EKG	7
Age over 70 years	5
Emergency operation	4
Intraperitoneal, intrathoracic, or aortic operation	3
Suspected critical aortic stenosis	3
Poor general medical condition[a]	3

[a]Includes electrolyte abnormalities, abnormal arterial blood gases, renal insufficiency, abnormal liver status, or bedridden patient.

(Reproduced with permission from Weitz H, Goldman L. Non-cardiac surgery in the patient with heart disease. *Med Clin North Am* 1987;71:413–432.)

graphy (EKG) should be performed preoperatively in patients over age 40 and in patients with a history of ischemic heart disease, as patients with an abnormal resting EKG (demonstrating ischemia or previous myocardial infarction) are at higher risk of myocardial reinfarction after surgery (150). In patients with EKG changes suggestive of ischemia, exercise EKG (treadmill testing) is indicated. Because most patients undergoing THR are unable to exercise maximally because of their hip disease, radioisotope imaging with a thallium-dipyridamole scan can be useful to document areas of ischemia. A positive treadmill or radioisotope scan is an indication for cardiac catheterization (54).

The Role of Anesthetic Techniques

General anesthesia has significant, diffuse effects on the mechanical and electrical properties of the heart. Inhalational anesthetics depress cardiac contractility in a dose-dependent fashion, as do some barbiturates. Negative inotropic effects of anesthetic agents are offset by the sympathetic response caused by surgical stimulation, which also tends to blunt the peripheral vasodilation caused by general anesthetic agents (24,168). Regional anesthetic techniques have minimal effects on the myocardium, although peripheral resistance tends to be lowered. Conflicting data exist regarding the cardiac benefits of choosing regional over general anesthesia. Some studies comparing regional to general anesthesia have shown lower rates of myocardial infarction and cardiovascular failure when regional anesthetic techniques are used (134,182). However, a recent randomized prospective study comparing regional to general anesthesia in lower extremity vascular procedures failed to show a difference in cardiac complications between the two types of anesthesia, leading the authors to conclude that despite the anticipated advantages of regional anesthesia, there was no significant difference in cardiac endpoints between it and general anesthesia (15,60). Few studies have compared anesthetic techniques and cardiac complications after THR. In a retrospective study, Sculco and Ranawat found fewer cardiac complications after spinal compared to general anesthesia for THR (135). In a prospective series of patients randomized to receive either regional or general anesthesia for THR, a higher rate of postoperative hypoxemia was seen in patients after general anesthesia, with one death from myocardial infarction. There were no cardiac complications in the regional anesthesia group (66). Changes in mortality after total joint replacement at the Hospital for Special Surgery over a 10-year period were studied by Sharrock, who found a decrease in mortality from cardiac problems in the second 5 years of the study. This drop in cardiac mortality was attributed to changes in anesthetic technique, including improved intraoperative monitoring and extensive utilization of epidural anesthesia (142).

The peripheral vasodilation accompanying epidural anesthesia has been used successfully to produce controlled intraoperative hypotension for total joint procedures, resulting in reduced blood loss (139). A mean arterial blood pressure of 60 mm Hg has been shown to be the optimum level of hypotension to reduce blood loss using this technique (140). Such hypotension requires aggressive monitoring with arterial and central venous pressure lines, and it may be contraindicated in patients with ischemic or valvular heart disease, particularly aortic stenosis (1,168).

Problems Related to Polymethylmethacrylate

Complications occurring intraoperatively during cemented total hip arthroplasty related to cement have been reported since the early 1970s (63,74,149). The incidence of hypotension noted after insertion of PMMA during early studies of total hip replacements has been reported to range from 33% to 100% (69). More recent studies have shown a lower incidence of such hypotension. Acute hypotension (defined as significant when a drop in systolic blood pressure of 20 mm Hg of mercury occurs after insertion of cement) was noted in 4.8% of cemented THRs performed in a study at the Hospital for Special Surgery, compared to an incidence of 0% after insertion of uncemented stems (138). Cardiovascular changes occurring during insertion of PMMA range from hypotension to cardiac arrest. Cardiac arrest, although uncommon, has been reported to occur after both primary and revision total hip arthroplasties performed with both standard and long-stem cemented components (41,114).

The etiology of cement-related hypotension has been a source of debate for many years. Possible causes cited in the literature are listed in Table 2.

Initially, methylmethacrylate monomer was implicated as a causative factor in cement-related hypotension. Intravenous administration of monomeric methylmethacrylate in experimental animals produces profound peripheral vasodilation (116). However, measurements of peak methylmethacrylate venous levels obtained from intraoperative blood samples after femoral component insertion with cement are far lower than that required to produce hypotension experimentally (42,69). Other experimental

TABLE 2. *Possible causes of cement-related hypotension*

1. Cement-related myocardial depression (96)[a]
2. Monomer toxicity (42,94,116)
3. Anaphylatoxin release (10)
4. Prostaglandin release (172)
5. Embolization of fat and marrow debris (20,21,46,63,111, 172)

[a]Numbers in parentheses are references.

studies (94) have shown that injection of supraphysiologic amounts of monomer (approximately 5 times that encountered during THR) failed to have any cardiopulmonary effects, and that doses of approximately 100 times that encountered during THR were required to produce cardiac arrest (67). Although toxic when injected intravenously in large doses, methylmethacrylate monomer probably is not the chief mediator of cement-related cardiovascular problems.

Anaphylatoxin release has been suggested as another cause of hypotension that occurs with insertion of cemented hip prostheses. Bengston et al. (10) studied a group of patients selected to have either cemented or uncemented insertion of femoral components. In the cemented group, reduced activity of whole complement and decreased levels of complement proteins were found in association with an increase in anaphylatoxins C3a and C5a. Because anaphylatoxins are potent mediators of vascular permeability, it is postulated that the release of such anaphylatoxins might explain cardiovascular changes that occur with insertion of PMMA.

Abundant clinical and experimental evidence now exists implicating embolization of marrow contents as a significant cause of acute hypotension during insertion of cemented femoral components. Both laboratory (20,111) and postmortem clinical data (63) have demonstrated fat and marrow contents in pulmonary capillaries after insertion of cemented femoral components. Orsini et al. (111) in a dog model examined the influence of intramedullary pressure by recording peak intramedullary pressures during insertion of bone cement into the canine femur. The dogs were randomized into three groups: a group receiving noncemented implants, a group in which bone wax was used to generate high intramedullary pressures, and a group in which bone cement was inserted to generate high intramedullary pressures. In the bone cement group, peak intramedullary pressures of over 800 mm Hg were generated, resulting in significantly more pulmonary embolization of marrow contents than that seen in the noncemented group. Intramedullary pressures as high as 575 mm Hg have been reported intraoperatively during THR in humans (157).

Pulmonary embolization of marrow contents (including air, fat, and bone marrow) causes diffuse physiologic responses (85). The embolization of such contents contributes to hypotension through both a mechanical effect and the initiation of a chemical cascade, including release of prostaglandins (20). During experimental cemented bilateral arthroplasty in dog models, a significant drop in mean blood pressure occurred within 3 minutes of component insertion, accompanied by a marked increase in pulmonary vascular resistance and by a decrease in systemic vascular resistance immediately after prosthesis insertion. A significant decrease in cardiac output also occurred, which returned to baseline about 5 minutes after component insertion (172). These experimental hemodynamic measurements have been confirmed by clinical reports of monitored cardiac arrests occurring during cemented long-stem femoral component and total knee component insertion (19,114).

Intraoperative transesophageal echocardiography performed during cemented THR demonstrates a snow flurry of echogenic material in the right atrium immediately after component insertion (80,159). Placement of a venting hole in the shaft of the femur, thus preventing the rise of pressure in the medullary space during cement insertion, results in a decreased frequency of this phenomenon, implicating embolization of marrow contents as the cause of these emboli. Erath et al. performed a study in which intraoperative transesophageal echocardiography, hemodynamic measurements, and pulmonary ventilation perfusion scanning was performed during THR (46). Thirty-five study patients underwent either cemented or noncemented hip arthroplasty. A statistically significant increased number of right atrial echogenic particles, duration of echogenesis, and total venous embolism was noted in the cemented group. The mean cardiac output was lower in the cemented group, who also demonstrated higher pulmonary arterial pressures and pulmonary vascular resistance after insertion of cemented femoral prostheses compared to the noncemented group (46).

Clinically, intraoperative cardiovascular changes occurring during cemented THR are seen within 30 minutes after insertion of cement (115). The most common clinical finding is a transient decrease in arterial oxygen tension (109). Pulmonary shunt (the proportion of cardiac output passing through the lungs without participating in gas exchange) has been calculated to be 28% higher after femoral component insertion with cement, a finding that persists for 48 hours after surgery (125). Kallos demonstrated a significant drop in arterial oxygen tension shortly after cement insertion which recovered within 10 minutes. Venting of the femoral shaft (presumably preventing embolization of marrow contents) resulted in lower drops in arterial oxygen tension (75). Clinically significant hypotension (defined as a drop in systolic blood pressure of at least 20 mm Hg) (138) occurs less commonly, with an incidence of approximately 5% during cemented THR. Several prospective studies (46,75,109) have not shown significant hypotension in association with insertion of PMMA. Patients who seem to be at particular risk for cardiovascular complications after insertion of PMMA include elderly patients, patients with underlying malignant disease, and preexisting cardiac or pulmonary disease (115). Insertion of a long-stem femoral component into a previously unoperated canal (as is done for treatment of a periprosthetic femur fracture) may also predispose the patient to cement-related cardiovascular complications.

Modern technique for insertion of cemented femoral components includes the use of high-pressure pulsatile lavage, thorough curettage of the femoral canal, and insertion of two or more packs of cement into a plugged canal, which is then pressurized to ensure cement penetration into the cancellous bone interstices (97). High-volume, high-pressure pulsatile lavage cleanses the femoral canal of marrow debris, allowing penetration of liquid PMMA. Additionally, and perhaps more important, such lavage removes marrow contents that might otherwise be embolized to the lung, resulting in cardiovascular complications. Experimentally, meticulous pulsatile lavage has been shown to eliminate significant decreases in arterial oxygen tension and pulmonary shunt fraction, while eliminating the increases in pulmonary vascular resistance and pulmonary artery pressures (144) that occur when cement is inserted without lavage, and reducing the number of fat microemboli in the lungs to one-quarter that seen without lavage (21). Thus, high-pressure, high-volume pulsatile lavage is essential when performing modern cemented THR. Patients who might be at risk for cardiovascular-related complications during cement insertion should be identified preoperatively. Maintenance of arterial oxygenation through supplementary oxygen and adequate volume replacement is essential during surgery. Patients at risk for cardiovascular complications benefit from invasive hemodynamic monitoring and vasopressors, which should be readily available at the time of cement insertion (115). Cement pressurization must be carried out with great care and it may be necessary to decrease the amount of pressurization carried out in patients with underlying cardiovascular or pulmonary disease. When inserting a long-stem femoral component, consideration may be given to placement of a venting hole distal to the femoral isthmus (114).

Common Postoperative Cardiac Problems

Common postoperative cardiac problems after surgery include angina pectoris, myocardial infarction, congestive heart failure, and arrhythmias. This section will briefly discuss these problems, outlining diagnostic and therapeutic stratagems; however, as with other medical complications, such problems are more fully dealt with in medical and subspecialty texts, and their ultimate management should be directed by an internist or medical specialist.

The incidence of ischemic heart disease, including angina pectoris and myocardial infarction, is between 0.59% and 1.37% after THR (44,89). Angina and myocardial infarction result from an imbalance between myocardial oxygen supply and demand. The resulting ischemia produces a decrease in cardiac contractility, resulting in reduced stroke volume and ejection fraction. With myocardial infarction, there may be additional areas of hypokinesis or akinesis of the ventricles. Classically, angina pectoris and myocardial infarction present with crushing substernal chest pain, radiating to the neck or one or both arms. Typically, the duration of angina is brief, whereas myocardial infarction may present with chest pain lasting for over 30 minutes with accompanying systemic symptoms such as nausea and diaphoresis. Postoperatively, chest pain may not be a prominent symptom of myocardial ischemia because administration of narcotics and sedatives may blunt or obscure chest pain. Other findings such as sudden hypotension, dyspnea, and signs of congestive heart failure in patients with a preoperative history of ischemic heart disease should alert the physician to the possibility of myocardial ischemia. It is recommended that postoperative EKGs be obtained routinely on patients with a previous history of ischemic heart disease or on those who exhibit unexplained cardiovascular complications. Myocardial infarction is diagnosed electrocardiographically by findings of Q waves or ST-T segment changes; however, the presence of preexisting bundle branch block can prevent the typical electrocardiographic changes seen after myocardial infarction (4). Serial cardiac enzymes are also used to diagnose myocardial infarction. Typically, elevations of the MB isoenzyme of creatine kinase and the LD-1 and LD-2 isoenzymes of lactate dehydrogenase occur after myocardial infarction. However, surgical trauma to skeletal muscle, as occurs during THR, can also result in significant elevation of serum levels of LD, CK, and CK-MB. Wukich et al. (181) prospectively examined the effects of THR on the levels of total CK, LD, and their isoenzymes. They found no significant increase in the LD-1 and LD-2 isoenzymes as a result of surgery, but significant increases in both total CK and its isoenzyme CK-MB were reported. The CK-MB isoenzyme fraction, even if elevated after THR, did not exceed 5% of the total CK activity in patients without myocardial infarction. Thus, although there is an increase in the CK-MB isoenzyme attributable to hip surgery, if the fraction exceeds more than 5% of the total CK activity it should not be attributed to the trauma of hip surgery alone. If cardiac complications occur after hip surgery, the cardiac consultant must be apprised of these enzymatic changes, as a false-positive diagnosis of myocardial infarction may be made if the enzyme changes are interpreted according to standards set for nonsurgical patients (181).

Angina should be treated by administration of sublingual nitroglycerine and maintenance of blood pressure through volume replacement. Preoperative cardiac medications must be promptly instituted after surgery, particularly beta-blockers (112). Patients with sustained angina during the postoperative period should be immediately transferred to a monitored unit. Appropriate measures should be taken to confirm the diagnosis of infarction, including serial EKGs and cardiac enzyme analyses. Detailed treatment of myocardial infarction is beyond the scope of this chapter; however, recognition of infarction and appropriate consultation is often the responsibility of the operating surgeon. It is well to remember that there is a 25% to 43% incidence of cardiac death after postsurgical myocardial infarction (181).

Congestive heart failure (CHF) has been reported to occur in up to 10% of elderly patients after THR (143). Congestive heart failure is caused by a depressed contractile state of the myocardium, resulting in a diminished ability of the heart to carry out its normal pumping function. CHF presents with symptoms of dyspnea and orthopnea, with physical examination findings of distended neck veins, pulmonary rales, and a third heart sound heard on auscultation. CHF can be difficult to diagnose in the immediate postoperative period because many of its symptoms and signs are common to other postoperative disorders (atelectasis, for example). Chest radiography typically shows an enlarged cardiac silhouette and increased pulmonary interstitial fluid. Invasive cardiac monitoring (right heart catheterization) typically demonstrates elevated pulmonary capillary wedge pressures. However, if this is not available, prompt improvement after intravenous administration of furosemide may help to confirm the diagnosis (49,53).

Congestive heart failure is not uncommon in patients with preexisting cardiac problems and diminished cardiac reserves who receive large volumes of fluids and blood after surgery. CHF is treated with the use of intravenous morphine and loop diuretics, such as furosemide. The administration of intravenous digoxin to enhance myocardial contractility is helpful, particularly in patients with atrial fibrillation (49). If heart failure worsens despite treatment, then transfer to an intensive care unit for invasive monitoring may be desirable.

Cardiac arrhythmias may be asymptomatic or may produce symptoms varying from palpitations to syncope. Superventricular tachycardia, including atrial fibrillation, has been estimated to occur in 4.8% of patients after THR (73). Patients at increased risk for arrhythmias after surgery include those with a previous history of arrhythmias such as atrial fibrillation, conduction disturbances recognized on preoperative electrocardiograms (including left anterior hemiblock and atrial premature contractions), and elderly patients. Cardiac arrhythmias are more common in patients with ischemic heart disease and those taking certain medications, including digoxin. The arrhythmias may produce hemodynamic instability and even sudden death. Analysis of pre- and postoperative EKGs is essential to diagnose arrhythmic disturbances of the heart. Arrhythmias may produce cardiovascular instability, particularly uncontrolled atrial fibrillation in patients with hypertrophic cardiomyopathy and aortic stenosis (49). Atrial arrhythmias, including atrial fibrillation, are common postoperatively and are more common in patients with congestive heart failure, preexisting lung disease, and in those patients 70 years old or older. Atrial fibrillation, the most dangerous postoperative atrial arrhythmia, should be treated to control cardiac rhythm and prevent heart failure. Premature ventricular contractions (PVCs) arise from ectopic ventricular foci and when isolated should not be treated; however, certain types of PVCs (so-called malignant PVCs), including those occurring more frequently than ten per minute and occurring in pairs or triplets, are more dangerous and require antiarrhythmic therapy. Ventricular tachycardia and ventricular fibrillation are, of course, potentially lethal, and demand prompt therapy with intravenous lidocaine and, in the case of ventricular fibrillation, cardiopulmonary resuscitation. Atrioventricular block, resulting from blocking of the sinoatrial impulses into the ventricle, represents a continuum of varying severity. Complete heart block requires identification of the underlying cause (including digoxin intoxication) and placement of a pacemaker (54).

Gastrointestinal Complications

Complications involving the gastrointestinal tract occur with an incidence ranging from 1.2% to 4.6% after THR (44,89). The most common of these complications is postoperative paralytic ileus, but other more serious complications such as gastrointestinal bleeding may complicate the postoperative course.

Patients at risk for gastrointestinal bleeding after THR include those with a history of peptic ulcer disease (which is estimated to occur in up to 10% of the population) (148) and patients who have previously used nonsteroidal anti-inflammatory drugs (NSAIDs). As a mainstay of treatment of arthritic disorders, NSAIDs are the most frequently prescribed medication in the United States (7). Although relatively safe, use of these agents may produce severe complications, including gastric and duodenal ulcerations and gastrointestinal bleeding. Upper gastrointestinal endoscopy reveals ulcerations in the stomach and/or duodenum in 30% of patients on chronic NSAID therapy (58). NSAIDs cause mucosal gastrointestinal ulcerations through both local and systemic components. Many NSAIDs, particularly aspirin, are weak organic acids and have an ulcerative effect when they penetrate gastric mucosa (130,148). NSAIDs block the production of prostaglandins through inhibition of cyclooxygenase, which promotes acid production and ulcer formation. The risk of NSAID-induced gastrointestinal ulceration is increased in the elderly and is more frequent during the first month of therapy (64).

Patients with chronic liver disease, such as cirrhosis, are at increased risk of complications after THR, including bleeding and infection. The presence of encephalopathy, coagulopathy (prothrombin time greater than 16 seconds), ascites, serum albumin less than 3 mg/dL, and bilirubin levels greater than 2 mg/dL place the patient with chronic liver disease at risk for surgical mortality of over 35% (55).

The preoperative assessment of patients with chronic liver disease, especially those with a history of severe disorders such as cirrhosis, include biochemical tests of the liver and measuring serum electrolytes, serum alkaline phosphatase, bilirubin, albumin, and liver enzymes. Patients with a previous history of hepatitis should undergo screening for type A, type B, and non-A/non-B hepatitis. Because screening of patients prior to autologous blood deposition usually includes serologic studies for viral hepatitis, such studies may be the first indicator that a patient has had viral hepatitis.

Although in the majority of cases elective surgery is not recommended in patients with liver failure, occasionally in emergencies such as deep infection or periprosthetic fracture, surgery will be required. Preoperative consultation with an internist and/or gastroenterologist is essential in managing patients pre- and postoperatively with chronic liver disease, especially in the setting of liver failure. Coagulopathy secondary to depletion of vitamin K–dependent clotting factors responds to administration of vitamin K in malnutrition, but this is often not effective in patients with chronic liver failure. Administration of fresh frozen plasma immediately prior to surgery should be performed to bring the prothrombin time to within 3 seconds of normal (53).

Treatment of ascites and fluid overload, including careful administration of diuretics and salt restriction, should be undertaken. Malnutrition in association with chronic liver disease should be treated prior to elective surgery by administration of nutritional supplements, being careful to avoid protein supplementation, which may precipitate hepatic encephalopathy (53).

Perioperative management of patients with peptic ulcer disease, including those with NSAID-induced ulcerations, includes administration of H_2-receptor antagonists such as cimetidine and ranitidine, or acid pump inhibitors such as omeprazole, which should be administered prophylactically to prevent bleeding (101). Administration of antacids to keep the gastric pH greater than 3.5 has also been shown to be effective in preventing gastrointestinal bleeding in patients at risk for this complication after surgery (121).

Cessation of NSAIDs prior to surgery is desirable, although these agents may be used successfully to treat postoperative pain in combination with opioid analgesics. Ketorolac (Toradol) is a relatively new NSAID, which is available in injectable form. It is commonly used to supplement narcotic analgesia after orthopedic surgery. It is indicated for short-term (up to 5 days) management of pain, as longer courses of treatment have been associated with gastrointestinal ulcerations as have doses exceeding 30 mg per day (37,81). Ketorolac is contraindicated in patients with a previous history of peptic ulcer disease or gastrointestinal bleeding.

Common Postoperative Problems

Gastrointestinal bleeding is a major potential gastrointestinal complication after surgery. Upper gastrointestinal bleeding is usually manifested by hematemesis or melena, whereas the passage of bright red blood per rectum usually indicates a lower gastrointestinal site. Postoperative gastric hemorrhage is usually secondary to preexisting peptic ulcer disease, stress ulceration, and Mallory-Weiss esophageal tears resulting from postoperative vomiting (62). The most common cause of lower gastrointestinal bleeding is diverticular disease followed by polyps and carcinoma (156).

Generally in patients who present with either upper or lower GI bleeding, initial steps should be undertaken to stabilize the patient, including insertion of large-bore intravenous lines and occasionally central venous pressure monitoring lines for administration of fluids. Intravascular volume should be restored with crystalloid, with blood transfusion reserved for patients with severe hypotension and concomitant medical problems, such as coronary artery disease. A nasogastric tube should be inserted in all patients and the aspirate tested for blood.

In general, management of gastrointestinal bleeding should be undertaken by an internist and/or general surgeon. Further treatment of upper GI bleeding includes medical therapy with antacids and H_2-receptor antagonists, and occasionally administration of vasoconstrictors such as vasopressin in patients with hemorrhage from esophageal varices (62). Upper GI endoscopy is commonly carried out for gastrointestinal bleeding, with an accuracy of 90%. Lower gastrointestinal bleeding may require lower gastrointestinal tract endoscopy. After THR, it is prudent to administer prophylactic antibiotics prior to any type of upper or lower gastrointestinal invasive procedure (160).

Paralytic or adynamic ileus commonly occurs after abdominal surgery, but it can also occur after THR. Ileus typically presents much like intestinal obstruction with nausea, vomiting, and abdominal distention. It is commonly associated with medications such as opioids and anticholinergics, which may be administered in the postoperative period. In patients with postoperative ileus, it is important to rule out a true bowel obstruction by performance of a diagnostic study such as abdominal flat plate films, lower gastrointestinal bowel contrast studies, or colonoscopy. If intestinal obstruction is ruled out, the ileus is treated by nasogastric suction, with careful attention to electrolyte abnormalities and fluid balance, and removal of offending medications, which may precipitate ileus. Serial abdominal radiographs should be obtained in cases of massive colonic distention to determine the risk of cecal perforation (62).

Diarrhea is probably less common in the postoperative period than constipation, usually because of the constipating effects of narcotic medications administered after surgery. The most common cause of postoperative diarrhea is related to antibiotic administration (62). Pseudomembranous colitis, caused by *Clostridium difficile,* is one of the most severe complications of antibiotic administration after surgery. Antibiotic-associated diarrhea usually begins about 3 days after the institution of antibiotic therapy and can present with symptoms of abdominal pain and fever as well as diarrhea. Stools may be grossly bloody. The diagnosis of pseudomembranous colitis is made by identifying *C. difficile* toxin in stool samples. Antibiotic-associated diarrhea should be treated by cessation of broad-spectrum antibiotics and administration of oral vancomycin (62).

Renal and Urinary Complications

Renal and urinary complications after THR cover a spectrum of problems, from metabolic complications and deep hip infection in the perioperative period in patients with chronic renal failure, to probably the most common complication occurring after THR, urinary retention.

Patients with preexisting renal insufficiency are at high risk for multiple complications after THR. The degree and severity of these complications are directly related to the residual glomerular filtration rate (GFR). Patients with moderate to severe renal failure (GFR less than 25 mm per minute) are at especially high risk for complications such as bleeding, infection, nutritional deficiency, and electrolyte abnormalities after surgery (18,93). Nonfatal complications can occur after surgery in as many as 60% of patients who are dialysis dependent (93). Patients on hemodialysis undergoing THR are at higher risk for both aseptic and septic loosening. Naito and co-workers (106) found a 35% mechanical failure rate after cemented THR in dialysis patients, a complication ascribed to the well-known bone mineral density changes (renal osteodystrophy) occurring in hemodialyzed renal patients. Lieberman and co-workers, reviewing renal dialysis patients undergoing THR, found a 19% deep infection rate in this patient group (88).

Aseptic necrosis of the femoral head occurs commonly after renal transplantation as a result of steroid use for immunosuppression. Cemented THR performed on renal transplantation patients, in contrast to hemodialysis patients, has a failure rate comparable to THR performed in patients who are not renal transplant recipients. In a series from Minnesota, Cheng and co-workers reported 5- and 10-year survivorships at 91% and 78%, respectively, in a group of renal transplant recipients whose average age at the time of surgery was 33 years (25). Although most transplant recipients are relatively young, a reduced life expectancy makes this patient population more comparable to older patients. Uncemented THR has also been shown to perform well in this patient population, with a lower incidence of loosening compared to cemented THR in one study (104). Although renal function may be normal after transplantation, care must be taken to manage fluids and electrolytes appropriately, as transplant-related complications have been reported after THR (38).

Urinary retention is extremely common after THR. The incidence of retention requiring urinary catheterization after THR ranges from 0.8% to 35% (45,122). Risk factors indicating a likelihood of postoperative urinary retention in men after total hip arthroplasty were examined by Redfern et al. (122) who found that patients with a peak urinary flow rate less than 17 mL/sec had a statistically significant likelihood to develop postoperative urinary retention. Waterhouse et al., in a prospective study of urinary retention after THR found that in their male population, a history of previous urinary problems (including previous prostatectomy), evidence of urinary flow obstruction (measured on urine flowmetry) and an inability to pass urine into a urinal while supine were predictive of postoperative urinary retention (166). Walts and co-workers in contrast found that the most important factor in their series leading to postoperative urinary retention was the use of epidural morphine for postoperative pain management (163). Male sex appears to be another risk factor for urinary retention, although there is a higher incidence of preoperative bacteriuria in female patients (22).

Common Postoperative Renal/Urinary Problems

Electrolyte imbalances, most commonly hyponatremia, can occur in the postoperative period after THR. The incidence of postoperative hyponatremia (defined as serum sodium less than 130 Eq/L) is high (26). Postoperative hyponatremia occurs either in the setting of diminished total body sodium and water (such as in patients taking diuretics preoperatively), which has been reported after THR (68) or in cases of excessive fluid administration after surgery. In the latter setting, administration of hypotonic solutions in combination with increased vasopressin secretion after surgery (which promotes renal tubular water resorption), results in hyponatremia.

Patients with hyponatremia may be asymptomatic or exhibit a variety of signs and symptoms ranging from lethargy and confusion to coma. Hyponatremia should be considered in the differential diagnosis of confusion in the postoperative period. The diagnosis is made by serum electrolyte measurements and the cause of the hyponatremia may be elucidated by measurement of urine electrolytes (12).

Hyponatremia is treated by restriction of free water, and in certain cases, administration of hypertonic saline solution, which must be managed carefully to prevent cerebral edema (12).

Chronic Renal Failure

As previously noted, patients with chronic renal failure are at increased risk for multiple complications during and after surgery, including bleeding, cardiovascular complications, and infection (18). The risk of complications rises in inverse proportion to the fall of GFR. Patients with renal insufficiency undergoing THR should be apprised of these risks, and consultation with a nephrologist is appropriate before proceeding with surgery. Management of chronic renal failure is beyond the scope of this text and should be undertaken by an internist or nephrologist. Dialysis-dependent patients should be dialyzed within 24 hours prior to surgery to manage hypervolemia and hyperkalemia (18). Recombinant human erythropoietin has been shown to be effective in treating the anemia that commonly occurs in chronic renal failure, and it may also be useful in reversing the platelet dysfunction seen in uremic patients (23,48). Patients should be transfused before surgery if the hematocrit does not rise above 25%, and transfusion should be done while the patient is undergoing dialysis to remove excessive potassium present in stored blood. Strict attention should be paid in the postoperative period to fluid balance and hydration in these tenuous patients. Also, in dialysis-dependent patients, resumption of a normal dialysis schedule should proceed within 48 hours after surgery to treat the hyperkalemia that commonly occurs after surgery. Finally, universal precautions should be used in the operating room as well as when removing drains and dressings after surgery because of the very high prevalence of hepatitis B antigen in the dialysis population (155).

Urinary Retention

As previously noted, urinary retention is a common postoperative complication after THR, with an incidence ranging from 0.8% to 35%. Risk factors predicting postoperative urinary retention include a previous history of urologic disease (such as benign prostatic hyperplasia or previous prostate surgery), diminished urinary peak flow rates indicative of obstruction (122), an inability to urinate into a urinal when supine (166), and the use of epidural morphine anesthesia (163). Bladder atonia resulting from urinary retention promotes incomplete emptying of the bladder and predisposes the patient to urinary tract infection. Urinary retention after THR can have serious consequences. In patients requiring bladder catheterization after THR, Wroblewski and del Sel found a 6.2% incidence of deep hip infection, compared to an expected incidence of 0.5% at their institution. In addition, almost 35% of their male patients required prostatectomy after THR for acute urinary retention, with a mortality rate of 8.6% (180). A careful history and physical examination (including a rectal prostatic examination) may help identify male patients at risk for urinary retention, allowing appropriate urologic consultation before hip surgery. Prostatic or bladder surgery, if contemplated, should be performed well before any elective hip surgery.

Concerns about urinary tract infections and their association with indwelling catheters has led many surgeons to adopt a *pro re nata* in-and-out catheterization protocol rather than utilizing indwelling bladder catheters. Although bacteriuria commonly occurs within 72 hours after insertion of an anchored indwelling catheter, use of short-term (less than 48 hours) catheterization has been shown to reduce the incidence of postoperative urinary retention without increasing the incidence of urinary tract infection. Michelson and co-workers studied a randomized group of 100 total joint arthroplasty patients who had either a short-term indwelling catheter or a *pro re nata* intermittent catheterization and found a 27% incidence of urinary retention in the indwelling catheter group (after removal of the catheter) compared to a 52% incidence in the intermittent catheterization group, a statistically significant difference (95). There was no significant difference in the rate of postoperative urinary tract infection. Oishi and co-workers, in a similar nonrandomized study comparing indwelling to intermittent catheterization, reported postoperative urinary retention rates of 7% and 84%, respectively (110). Carpiniello et al., in a study of women undergoing total joint replacement, found use of an indwelling catheter for 24 hours resulted in a urinary retention rate of 4%, compared to a 57% rate in those treated with intermittent catheterization (22). Ritter et al., reporting on a comparison of bladder management protocols after total joint replacement, found, as did other authors, that no significant difference in urinary tract infection rates existed when short-term indwelling catheters were compared to intermittent catheterization (127). They suggested that insertion of an indwelling catheter in the operating room offered several advantages, including optimal aseptic technique and decreased emotional and physical trauma to the patient. Intraoperative indwelling catheterization also enables precise measurement of urinary output intraoperatively and in the postoperative period (127).

It is clear from the data in the literature that insertion of a short-term, anchored indwelling catheter markedly decreases the incidence of urinary retention without an increase in the urinary tract infection rate. Commonly, there is a large diuresis in the first 2 or 3 days after surgery, and an indwelling catheter helps prevent the frequently intermittent catheterizations necessary after surgery in noncatheterized patients. It has been the authors' practice to remove indwelling catheters within 48 hours after surgery when patients are more mobile and are able to use a urinal or bedside commode. Short-term use of antibiotic prophylaxis targeted against common urinary tract pathogens while the patient is catheterized appears to reduce the incidence of infection (132). It is the authors' practice to continue oral antibiotic prophylaxis for at least 1 day after removal of the urinary catheter. Long-term use of such prophylaxis may, however, result in selection of more resistant organisms and is not recommended (132).

Pharmacologic manipulation of the bladder to avoid urinary retention without catheterization has been utilized after total joint replacement. Alpha-adrenergic blockers, such as prazosin, relax the smooth musculature of the bladder and promote bladder emptying. Peterson and co-workers found a statistically significant decrease in urinary retention after administration of prazosin after total joint arthroplasty in male patients (119). Unfortunately, alpha-adrenergic blockers may cause hypotension, which may make administration of such drugs difficult or dangerous in the immediate postoperative period.

Urinary Tract Infections

Urinary tract infections have been reported to occur at rates as high as 26% after THR (143). Prior to surgery, any history of previous urinary tract infection should be elicited. The utility of preoperative routine urinalysis as a screening study has been questioned, with a cost-effectiveness analysis revealing an extremely low incidence of urinary tract abnormalities in patients undergoing non-prosthetic knee surgery (83). This study showed that only an estimated 4.6 wound infections would be prevented by routine urine screening in their population studied, at a screening cost of $1.5 million per infection (83). However, although data at present are not entirely conclusive, all patients undergoing prosthetic joint surgery should have a routine urinalysis, and if screening detects signs of urinary tract infection (more than 25 white blood cells per high-power field), a urine culture and antibiotic-sensitivity tests should be performed. If a urinary tract infection is detected preoperatively, culture-specific antibiotics should be administered, preferably at least 2 weeks prior to surgery. It has been the authors' practice to administer a dose of intravenous aminoglycocide (with adjustment for renal function) in addition to routine prophylactic antibiotics immediately prior to surgery in patients with a positive urinalysis or urine culture.

Postoperative Mental Status Changes

Every physician caring for a patient after THR is familiar with mental status changes that can occur after surgery. THR is commonly performed in patients older than 65 years of age, and it is this group that is most at risk for postoperative confusion. The rate of acute confusional states in elderly hospitalized patients approaches 50% (176). The rate of postoperative confusion can range from 23% to 44% in patients after hip fracture, but it appears to be somewhat lower in THR patients. Sheppeard and co-workers noted prolonged confusion in 26% of their elderly patients series after THR (143). Patients with mental confusion are more susceptible to complications after surgery, such as pressure ulcerations, wound hematomas, falls, and prosthetic dislocations, and they are more likely to require prolonged hospitalization compared to nonconfused patients (11,65,92). Risk factors for postoperative confusion after THR include age over 70 years, history of substance abuse, poor cognitive status, abnormal preoperative serum electrolytes, severe underlying medical disease, visual or auditory impairment, preoperative depression, and a history of anticholinergic medication use (antidepressants and narcoleptics) (11,92,98). By categorizing risk factors, clinicians can stratify patients into risk groups for the development of delirium, and a clinical prediction rule for delerium using points assigned to various risk factors has been developed and validated in a large study of patients undergoing noncardiac surgery (92).

Prior to any elective hip surgery, risk factors for postoperative confusion must be identified and measures undertaken to rectify correctable problems. Appropriate general medical or psychiatric consultation should be obtained with attention paid to simplification of drug regimens, adjustment of neuroleptic medications, and treatment of substance abuse problems. Attention should be paid to postoperative pain medications, and doses of narcotics should be decreased in elderly, frail patients. Although some studies (66) have suggested that regional anesthesia is associated with less cognitive dysfunction than general anesthesia, more recent studies have not confirmed this supposition. Recent randomized controlled studies comparing regional to general anesthesia for total hip and knee replacement (71,177) and hip fracture fixation (11,13) have failed to show a difference in the rates of postoperative cognitive dysfunction between the two types of anesthesia. Preoperative medications should not include anticholinergic drugs (scopolamine or atropine), which may precipitate confusion in high-risk patients. Prevention of hypotension intraoperatively may help prevent postoperative mental status problems as well, as severe perioperative blood pressure drops can contribute to this problem (65).

Common Postoperative Mental Status Problems

Delirium may be the most common postoperative mental status problem to occur in the postoperative elderly patient. It is defined as a transient organic mental syndrome characterized by a global disorder of cognition and attention, a reduced level of consciousness, abnormally increased or reduced psychomotor activity, and a disturbed sleep–wake cycle (90). Its presentation is familiar to all physicians caring for elderly patients. It includes restlessness, insomnia, hallucinations, difficulty in thinking, and slurring of speech. Fluctuations in attention, perception, orientation, and intellectual functioning may

occur, and lucid periods may alternate with periods of confusion. Disturbance of the sleep–wake cycle is characteristic of delirium, with drowsiness during the day and fragmented, shortened sleep at night. A hyperactive form of delirium may occur with agitation, restlessness, and belligerence, or the delirious patient may be hypoalert and withdrawn. Delirious, agitated patients may remove drains or indwelling catheters and are more susceptible to prosthetic dislocations and trochanteric separation after THR (143).

Delirium may be caused by any number of organic factors, including primary intracranial disease, systemic diseases affecting the brain, exogenous toxic substances (such as narcotics), and withdrawal from sedative/hypnotic drugs. Dementia, another organic mental syndrome causing global cognitive impairment, may be distinguished in that delirium is usually acute in onset with a fluctuating course, whereas the onset of dementia is usually insidious and features such as hallucinations and agitation are absent. However, it is important to note that delerium may arise in a patient with preexisting underlying dementia. The most common cause of delirium in elderly patients is intoxication from medications, particularly from anticholinergic drugs. Electrolyte imbalances, especially hyponatremia and systemic infections, commonly result in delirium. Virtually any major organ system dysfunction can result in delirium, and it is worth remembering that delirium may be a presenting symptom in such serious medical problems as pneumonia or myocardial ischemia. Postoperative pain medications, even when administered in therapeutic doses, may cause delirium in elderly patients.

The diagnosis of delirium in the postoperative period includes review of pre- and postoperative medications and identification of substance abuse, if possible. After performance of a careful history and physical examination (including a mental status exam), laboratory studies should be obtained, including serum electrolytes and blood gases. A chest radiographs and EKG should also be obtained, and if laboratory and other studies do not offer an obvious diagnosis, then computed tomography (CT) or magnetic resonance imaging (MRI) of the head may be obtained to rule out intracranial pathology. In the elderly, the cause for delirium can usually be identified in 80% to 90% of patients (91).

Treatment of delirium centers around identification and treatment of the underlying cause. While the underlying disorder is treated, adequate fluid and nutrition should be ensured. Treatment of agitation may be lifesaving and includes the use of sedatives, such as haloperidol, and soft restraints. In patients withdrawing from sedative/hypnotic drugs, the use of benzodiazadine drugs in a withdrawal protocol is recommended. Abductor pillows or braces may be necessary for prevention of prosthetic dislocation in agitated patients.

WOUND PROBLEMS

Wound Drainage

Total hip replacement involves creation of a substantial wound with implantation of a large amount of foreign material. Primary wound healing is of paramount importance to the total joint surgeon, as complications related to wound healing range from prolonged wound drainage to perhaps the most dreaded complication after THR—deep wound infection.

Preoperatively, factors that may predispose the patient to poor wound healing should be identified. Malnutrition is a prevalent and often unrecognized problem in elderly patients. Gherini et al. (59) assessed delayed wound healing after THR and its relationship to malnutrition and found a statistically significant association between low preoperative serum transferrin levels and delayed wound healing. They did not find a significant association between serum albumin and total lymphocyte count in delayed wound healing, and they suggested using preoperative transferrin levels to identify those patients at risk for poor wound healing secondary to malnutrition.

The operative field should be shaved immediately prior to surgery in the holding area before entering the operating theater. We prefer a 10-minute prep, using iodophor paint followed by cleansing of the skin with isopropyl alcohol to defat the skin, allowing for better adherence of subsequently applied iodophor-impregnated drapes. The surgeon should be present during prepping and draping to ensure absolutely sterile technique. In primary cases, 1 gram of cefazolin, or vancomycin for cephalosporin-allergic patients, is administered intravenously 30 minutes prior to surgery. The restriction of personnel traffic during surgery is critical in the prevention of infection. In 1971, the senior author established a protocol to control infection in a conventional operating room, including both the institution of strict operating room discipline and restriction of personnel traffic. In a consecutive series of 298 THRs performed using this protocol and prophylactic antibiotics, no deep infections were reported (29). In addition to preoperative prophylactic antibiotics and control of intraoperative environmental factors, the authors also prefer the use of body exhaust systems to control bacterial shedding from personnel.

Surgical technique should emphasize careful handling of tissues and expeditious, but not rapid or hurried, surgical technique. Meticulous hemostasis both during surgery and at the conclusion to prevent wound hematoma and seroma formation cannot be overemphasized. Wound closure should also be meticulous. The authors prefer a Charnley-type bolster dressing with wires inserted into the subcutaneous tissues, which are then tied down over sponge bolsters. This method is especially useful in obese patients in whom subcutaneous wound closure is difficult.

Closed wound drainage, once standard, has become a rather controversial topic, particularly in the era of cost containment. The routine use of suction drainage theoretically reduces the incidence of wound hematomas, therefore decreasing the incidence of postoperative wound drainage and possibly infection. However, multiple, well-controlled randomized studies (8,27,128) have shown that postoperative wound drainage offers no distinct advantages. Ritter and co-workers performed a randomized prospective study of 415 total joint replacements in which wound drainage was used in 215. No wound drainage was utilized in the remaining 200 joint replacements. No statistically significant difference was noted between the drained and nondrained groups in the incidence of wound swelling and drainage. They recorded a cost savings of $21,500 when drains were not used and felt that the use of postoperative drains offered no advantage in the outcome of primary total joint replacement surgery (128). Beer and co-workers (8), evaluating 100 total joint replacements in which half of the surgical wounds were drained, found no significant difference between drained and nondrained wounds in the incidence of wound swelling or persistent drainage. Cobb (27), in a randomized study of wound drainage in hip fracture surgery, found an increased incidence of wound complications in the drained wounds, with no wound healing problems documented in the nondrained group. Currently, the authors utilize drains in selected cases after THR, including anticoagulated patients and obese patients.

Drains, if utilized, are removed at 24 hours after surgery, as studies have shown that continued presence of drains beyond 24 hours after THR does not reduce the likelihood of hematoma formation and can lead to bacterial contamination (40,174).

The initial wound dressing change is performed at 48 hours after surgery by the operating surgeon. At this point, wound healing is assessed and a sterile dressing applied and maintained until the patient's discharge. The presence of wound drainage is cause for concern. Persistent wound drainage after THR is a known risk factor for deep infection (154). Bloody drainage emanating from the wound at the initial dressing change is usually a result of hematoma formation and is cause for concern. If drainage is copious and free-flowing, anticoagulants are discontinued and the patient is returned to the operating room promptly for evacuation of the hematoma. Aspiration at the bedside for treatment of wound hematomata after THR is ineffectual and not recommended. A postoperative wound hematoma represents an ideal culture medium for bacterial organisms, and it is the authors' belief that these should be aggressively treated to prevent infection. Yellow serous drainage emanating from the wound is not uncommon after THR, especially in obese patients. There are no firm guidelines available for treatment of serous wound drainage after THR. It has been the authors' experience that this drainage usually ceases within 3 to 4 days after surgery. If serous weeping develops, prophylactic anticoagulation is discontinued and the wound drainage cultured. It has been our practice to maintain the patient on intravenous antibiotics until wound drainage has ceased. The wound is examined daily and the patient is not discharged until the drainage has stopped.

Early or stage I postoperative infections (defined as those occurring within the first month after surgery) are easily recognized and present with typical findings of acute infection, including purulent drainage, erythema, warmth, and swelling accompanied by pain and fever (30,51). Wound cellulitis accompanied by drainage can occur without deep infection. Such superficial infections, defined as those superficial to the fascia lata, are treated by early debridement. The patient is returned to the operating room and the hip joint is aspirated and the fluid cultured after sterile prepping and draping, but before exposure of the surgical wound. The wound should then be explored and the relationship of the infection to the fascia lata determined. Cultures should be obtained from the surgical wound and then a thorough debridement carried out. If the infection is superficial to the fascia lata, the wound is packed open and sterile dressing changes at the bedside carried out for the next 3 to 4 days, while culture-specific intravenous antibiotics are maintained. The patient is then returned to the operating room for repeat debridement and wound closure. Patients with superficial infections are usually maintained on oral antibiotics for another 4 to 6 weeks.

Early deep sepsis after THR (stage 1) can be defined as a deep infection of the operative wound that occurs within the first month after surgery. Such infections include the infected deep hematoma, superficial infection that progresses to a deep infection, and the typical fulminant postoperative infection (50). These infections by definition penetrate beneath the fascia lata to involve the prosthetic joint. Patients at risk for deep infection include those with rheumatoid arthritis (who have an infection rate roughly double that of nonrheumatoid patients) (131). Patients who require corticosteroid administration (e.g., those with systemic lupus erythematosis) and those with diabetes mellitus are also at increased risk for infection after THR (107). It has also been suggested that immune competence decreases with age, which may make elderly patients more susceptible to deep infection (102). The diagnosis of a postoperative wound infection is easily established by the observation of purulent material draining from a painful red wound. Laboratory tests that can be helpful include determination of a complete blood count with differential, sedimentation rate, and C-reactive protein (57). The microbiology of periprosthetic hip infections is dominated by gram-positive organisms

(*Staphylococcus aureus, Staphylococcus epidermidis,* and streptococcal species), which account for over two thirds of the organisms isolated from periprosthetic deep wound infections (50,56,57).

The treatment of early stage 1 infection after THR is surgical. Aggressive deep debridement of the wound should be carried out promptly with dislocation of the hip and removal of the polyethylene liner of the acetabular component (if a modular component was utilized) for a more complete debridement. The acetabular liner should be exchanged, and the components retained. In stage 1 infections, in contrast to stage 2 or chronic infections, the components may be retained with a reasonable chance for cure. Criteria that must be met for retention of the components include short (less than 3 to 4 weeks) duration of infection, cultures that show gram-positive organisms sensitive to antibiotics, and well-fixed components (57). Appropriate antibiotics should be administered intravenously, based on culture and sensitivity results. The recommended duration of parenteral antibiotic therapy after debridement with retention of components after early periprosthetic wound infection varies from 4 to 6 weeks (57).

The results of postoperative deep wound infections with debridement and retention of the components combined with parenteral antibiotics are much better than those noted with similar treatment for established chronic infections or hematogenous infections (3). Tsukyama et al. (158) recently reported the results of a detailed study of deep infections after THR. In this series, there was a 71% success rate in treating early postoperative wound infections with retention of the components, debridement, and treatment with antibiotics. The authors unexpectedly found that almost all failures in the early infection group treated with debridement and retention of the components occurred in hips in which the femoral prosthesis was inserted without cement. They suggested that porous coating provided a sanctuary for bacteria and recommended that porous-coated implants be removed at the time of debridement in patients with an early postoperative deep infection.

Failure of treatment of early deep wound sepsis with debridement, and retention of components necessitates more extensive procedures, including two-stage exchange arthroplasty (56).

NEUROVASCULAR INJURIES

Fortunately, neurovascular injuries are uncommon complications of THR. However, they are certainly very devastating both to the patient and the surgeon. The most important aspect of avoiding injury to any of the neurovascular structures is a sound knowledge of the normal anatomy and a recognition of the changes from normal that can occur with either the primary or the revision situation.

Vascular Injury

The incidence of vascular injury associated with THR is quite rare, in the 0.1% to 0.2% range (105). The small incidence is counterbalanced by the great enormity of this complication, particularly if one of the major vessels is injured.

Anatomy. The external iliac artery and vein run obliquely from the L5-S1 region down the medial border of the psoas muscle anterior with the vein running anterior and lateral to the vein. The amount of psoas muscle interposed between the vessels and the bony anterior column decreases along the arcuate line. The muscle actually becomes tense at the anterior superior quadrant. The vein remains medial and posterior to the artery until it is more distal, when it runs more medial and inferior to the artery along the medial border of the psoas. It is interposed between the anterior bony column and the parietal peritoneum and is relatively immobile along the pelvic rim. After passing under the inguinal ligament, the external iliac artery becomes the common femoral artery where it courses directly anterior and medial to the hip capsule, separated here only by the iliopsoas tendon. At this point, the artery is lateral to the vein; therefore, it is more susceptible to injury. Approximately 3.5 cm below the inguinal ligament, the profundus femoral artery arises from the lateral side of the femoral artery and passes posteriorly to lie between the pectineus and the adductor longus. The lateral femoral circumflex artery arises from the lateral side of the proximal profunda femoral artery and passes laterally beneath the sartorius and rectus femoris. The medial circumflex artery usually arises from the posterior medial profundus artery, but it may also arise from the femoral artery itself. The medial circumflex winds around the femur between the pectineus and the psoas muscle external to intertrochanteric line.

The obturator artery and vein transverse the lateral or quadrilateral surface of the pelvis. Lateral to the vessels, the obturator muscle and fascia separate them from the quadrilateral surface and the anterior quadrant of the acetabulum. They lie in contiguity to the superior and lateral aspect of the obturator foramen where they exit the true pelvis by the obturator canal. This is again a point where they are fixed and relatively nonmobile. The gluteal and internal pudendal vessels are the terminal branches of the anterior division of the internal iliac artery. They exit the pelvis between the piriformis and coccygeus muscles and are closest to the posterior bony column at the level of the ischial spine. They curve around the ischial spine to reenter the pelvis through the lesser sciatic notch.

Another major branch of the arterial tree is made up of the superior gluteal vessels, which are branches of the posterior division of the anterior iliac artery. The superior gluteal vein and artery run closest to the posterior column as they exit through the superior aspect of the sciatic notch. Again, at this point they are quite fixed to the pelvis above the pyriformis muscle.

Clearly, this descriptive anatomy indicates that the areas of most likely injury are where the vessels are fixed or closest to the bony anatomy, because during hip replacement the surgeon is working directly on the bony anatomy. The most serious injuries, those that might result in a significant catastrophic hypotension, are to the iliac vessels and the femoral artery. Injury to these vessels requires almost immediate surgical attention to prevent the patient's demise. Wasielewski et al. described quadrants that are formed by a line from the anterosuperior iliac spine dividing the acetabulum in equal halves (164). This line is bisected by a perpendicular forming four quadrants, and the anterosuperior quadrant is defined as the most dangerous. Any penetration of the bony floor of the acetabulum in the anterosuperior quadrant can endanger the external iliac artery and vein as well as the obturator artery and vein (76,164). The bony pelvis is much thinner anteriorly than posteriorly and therefore represents the greatest danger area. The other major area of vascular concern is anterior to the anterior column where the femoral artery can clearly be injured by any penetrating instrument when working within the confines of the pelvis, or it could be injured by retractor placement if the retractors are not kept close to the bony surface.

In the revision situation, if the acetabular component migrates either superiorly or centrally, vascular structures are more at risk, and the surgeon must take special caution in these situations. Preoperative arteriograms may be necessary to specifically outline the arterial relationship to the bony pelvis or displaced prosthetic components, particularly if the socket has migrated medially. Delayed injury to the iliac vessels has been reported as a result of implant migration (16,124,136).

Nerve Injury

The incidence of nerve palsy after primary THR range from 0% to 3% (43,70,147,183) and from 2.9% to 7.6% (43,70,84,133) after revision hip surgery. The majority of these injuries are to the sciatic nerve, most frequently the peroneal division (43), but the tibial division can also be injured. The incidence of palsy of the femoral nerve is reported to be approximately 0.1% to 0.2% (145,153).

Anatomy. The sciatic nerve, which comprises the sacral plexus roots of L4-L5, S1, S2, and S3, lies anterior to the pyriformis muscle, just proximal to its exit from the pelvis through the greater sciatic notch. It passes over the posterolateral surface of the posterior acetabular column, then descends behind the greater trochanter, between it and the ischial tuberosity, crossing over the obturator internus and quadratus femoris. It is at the point of its most fixed bony attachment, passing out of the sciatic notch, that it is most subject to injury. The next relatively fixed point is around the fibular head and it is also subject to injury at this area. It has been noted that the peroneal branch of the sciatic nerve is more susceptible to injury than the tibial branch. The common peroneal branch of the sciatic nerve is located more laterally, which makes it more vulnerable, and the tibial branch of the sciatic nerve contains more connective tissue than the peroneal branch, which may allow it to undergo more traction or elongation before causing neural compromise (43).

Sciatic Nerve Injury

Sciatic nerve injuries are the most common peripheral nerve injury to occur after THR. Risk factors for sciatic nerve injuries include revision hip surgery, congenital dislocation of the hip, lengthening with or without lateral displacement of the proximal femur, and female sex (43,70,133).

The causes of sciatic nerve palsies after THR include direct trauma, excessive tension as a result of intraoperative lengthening of the extremity, ischemia, injury from heat of polymerization of PMMA, and compression by wound hematoma and from dislocation of the femoral component (43,70,147,167). Forty percent of sciatic nerve palsies result from unexplained causes. Of known causes, almost 50% are related to lengthening and lateral displacement of the extremity, with 22% occurring from direct injury (retractor injury, cautery burn or reamer injury) and 20% occurring from bleeding complications (including compression from large wound hematomas) (52,165).

The prognosis for recovery from sciatic nerve palsies associated with THR is variable. Most authors report at least some recovery unless the nerve is severely damaged or transected. Schmalzreid et al. (133) reviewed a group of patients in whom nerve palsies occurred after THR and found that the extent of recovery was correlated directly with degree of neural damage. All patients in whom some neural recovery was documented immediately after surgery or prior to discharge from the hospital gained normal or near normal function. Patients who had severe dysesthesias had a poor recovery. Edwards et al. (43) in a review of patients with both stretch-induced and direct injury nerve palsies, found that patients in whom the nerve was directly injured had a better prognosis than patients in whom the nerve was injured by lengthening of the extremity. They recommended limiting leg lengthening to less than 4 cm in THR, as their study showed that sciatic nerve palsy developed only when lengthening exceeded this amount.

Femoral Nerve Injury

The femoral nerve forms from the branch of the second, third, and fourth lumbar nerves within the pelvis,

overlies the iliopsoas muscle, and passes into the thigh through the femoral triangle. This triangle lies directly anterior and medial to the hip joint, and within this space the femoral nerve is most likely to be injured. The borders of the triangle are the inguinal ligament, the sartorius muscle, and the adductor longus muscle. The floor of the triangle consists of the iliopsoas and pectineus muscle, as well as the roof of the overlying anterior fascia. This space is relatively unyielding, and therefore this is the area of potential injury either by retraction, manipulation, or hematoma. Again, any screw placement or penetration of the bony anterior, inferior, and anteroinferior quadrants of the acetabulum risks injury to this nerve. In contrast to the sciatic nerve, retractor placement seems to be the most significant risk factor in damaging the femoral nerve. Femoral nerve palsies have also been reported after correction of hip flexion contractures (84) and from extravasation of cement (117). The femoral nerve can be injured basically by the same mechanisms that cause injury to the sciatic nerve. The nerve is reported to be at increased risk of injury during anterior and anterolateral approaches to the hip joint (145).

A review of femoral nerve injuries by Simmons et al. (145) demonstrated that most femoral nerve injuries are caused by retractor placement. A cadaveric dissection performed as part of this study illustrated this point, showing that the tendinous portion of the iliopsoas muscle affords little protection from compression or retraction of the nerve by an interior retractor (145). The prognosis for recovery of femoral neuropathies, much like sciatic neuropathies, is correlated with the mechanism of injury. Stretch-induced femoral neuropathies (167) do not recover as well as those induced by direct compression from anterior retractor placement. Simmons et al. reported complete recovery in all ten patients in their study in whom femoral nerve injury occurred from retractor placement (145).

Nerve Injury Treatment

The treatment of sciatic or femoral nerve injuries that occur after surgery is, of course, dependent on the cause of the injury. If a nerve palsy is encountered immediately after surgery, flexion of the hip and knee can help relieve the stretch on the femoral and sciatic nerves and should be done immediately in the recovery room. The wound should be inspected, as development of a large wound hematoma may have caused pressure on the sciatic nerve. The postoperative radiographs should be reviewed and limb lengthening, if present, noted and measured.

Almost 50% of nerve palsies after THR are due to unknown causes. If no easily identifiable cause (wound hematoma, leg lengthening) is identified, then observation of postoperative nerve palsies is appropriate treatment. Serial nerve conduction studies obtained during the postoperative period can help document recovery. As noted previously, nerve palsies resulting from direct injury, such as from retractor placement tend to have a good prognosis for recovery.

In patients in whom leg lengthening has occurred and is felt to be the cause of the nerve palsy, acute shortening of the limb can be carried out by exchanging the modular head/neck (if present) for a shorter construct.

Patients with nerve palsies from large wound hematomas benefit from immediate decompression of the hematoma. Fleming et al. (52), in a study of nerve palsies resulting from wound hematomas, demonstrated recovery in four patients who underwent prompt surgical decompression of the hematoma. The one patient in their study who was treated expectantly with observation had a poor result.

Somatosensory-Evoked Potentials

Somatosensory-evoked potential (SSEP) is a technique that can be used to monitor peripheral nerve function intraoperatively. Initially used intraoperatively during spinal surgery (72), it has been used as a tool to detect injury to the sciatic nerve. Such monitoring can be useful during revision THR, because of the increased incidence of sciatic nerve injury during this procedure. Subclinical nerve injury is quite common during THR as described by Weber and co-workers (167) who found in a prospective study that 21 out of 30 patients undergoing THR had electromyographic evidence of nerve compromise during surgery, with only two patients exhibiting clinical findings.

Theoretically, the use of SSEP monitoring intraoperatively would be useful to detect nerve injuries during THR, particularly during revision surgery. Stone et al. reported on the use of SSEP during THA in 50 patients, 39 of whom underwent primary THR and 11 of whom underwent revision surgery (152). Twelve instances of temporary sciatic nerve compromise were detected during surgery, three from retractor placement during acetabulum preparation, one from acetabular reamer contact, six during femoral reaming, and two secondary to excessive lengthening of the limb after trial reduction. The authors recommended the use of SSEP during revision surgery, as the incidence of intraoperative nerve compromise detected by intraoperative monitoring was 36% in the revision setting compared to 15% in primary procedures (152).

Black et al. (14) used SSEP monitoring to detect intraoperative sciatic nerve compromise during 100 consecutive THR procedures, of which 23 were revision surgeries. The peroneal nerve at the fibular neck was monitored to measure sciatic nerve function. Eighteen patients exhibited changes consistent with sciatic nerve injury. Femoral reaming and prosthesis reduction was the most common surgical event associated with intraoperative changes. Two patients exhibited postoperative sciatic nerve palsies. The incidence of postoperative sciatic nerve palsies detected during intraoperative monitoring was not less than that noted after surgery without monitoring (2.0% versus 2.6%). Because of the this comparison and the cost of monitoring patients, SSEP monitoring was not felt to be indicated for routine procedures, although the authors did feel that monitoring during high risk procedures such as revision THR was of value.

Although theoretically the use of SSEP monitoring would be useful to detect nerve injuries during THR, no study in the literature has shown that monitoring prevents nerve injury. At this time, SSEP monitoring remains an experimental technique and a research tool, but it does not represent the standard of care needed to prevent nerve palsies in hip surgery.

Obturator Nerve Palsies

Obturator nerve palsies are extremely rare, fortunately, because the diagnosis is also difficult. Consistent groin pain after THR, some evidence of intrapelvic cement extrusion intrapelvically, or a clinical examination showing obturator muscle weakness and positive electromyographic findings are needed to confirm the diagnosis (165).

CONTRALATERAL LIMB PROBLEMS

Complications in the contralateral limb after total hip arthroplasty are rare but have been reported. Smith et al. (146) in 1989, reported on six patients who suffered contralateral limb problems after total hip arthroplasty. In five patients, a revision procedure was performed. Each patient was operated on in the lateral decubitus position and the operative time ranged from 3 to over 8 hours. Complications noted on the contralateral side included complete nerve palsy involving the femoral and peroneal nerves in five patients. One patient suffered a contralateral popliteal artery occlusion that necessitated below-the-knee amputation. Rhabdomyolysis from crush injury to contralateral limb musculature developed in four patients, causing acute renal failure in one patient.

The authors identified several factors that they felt may have contributed to the problem, including the use of hypotensive anesthesia, the extent and duration of the operation, the possibility that the operated limb might place excessive pressure on the contralateral limb during anterior dislocation, and the placement of the pelvic clamps used for lateral positioning of the patient. The authors prospectively monitored pressures in the femoral triangle in a group of patients in the lateral position using a manometer, and they correlated these pressures with pulse oximetry measurements of blood flow to the contralateral limb. They found that excessive pressure in the pelvic triangle from the pelvic clamp resulted in loss of the normal oximetric wave form, which was restored upon release of the clamp. Also noted was an increase in pressure in the femoral triangle with anterior dislocation of the hip and crossing the operative limb over the contralateral (down) limb (146).

The authors recommended identifying patients at risk for this complication prior to THR, including those with preexisting contralateral limb problems (such as peripheral vascular disease), overweight patients, and those undergoing lengthy procedures, and recommended that visual checks of the contralateral limb should be performed at intervals during THR.

Lachiewicz et al. (79) also reported six cases of contralateral limb involvement during THR. He observed a similar phenomenon of rhabdomyolysis with mild oliguria and nerve palsies in a group of patients undergoing lengthy revision THR procedures. In contrast to the series reported by Smith et al. (146), the authors felt that the dependent leg problems observed in their study were secondary to a crush-type injury to the contralateral gluteal muscle compartment. The authors observed swollen gluteal compartments on the contralateral side after surgery; compartment pressure measurements performed in one patient confirmed the diagnosis of compartment syndrome. Fasciotomy was performed in one patient with rapid resolution of symptoms, but in the remaining five patients compartment release was not performed. All patients in this group had recovery of urine output and sciatic nerve function. The authors recommended careful positioning of the patient on the operating table and aggressive intravenous hydration for prophylaxis against acute renal failure if myoglobinuria develops.

EARLY INSTABILITY

Early instability can be defined as those hips that dislocate within 3 months after THR. The overall incidence of early instability ranges between 1% and 3% (77,78,179). Early dislocations, compared to late dislocations, are more commonly a result of soft-tissue laxity prior to healing of the pseudocapsule around the hip. One series of dislocations after THR showed that the greatest risk for dislocation occurred in the first 5 weeks after surgery (77), and another series demonstrated that 70% of dislocations after THR occurred within the first month after surgery (175). Risk factors fall into several categories. There is a definite predilection in the female population to postoperative dislocation, some studies reporting dislocation rates roughly double that in the male population (77,78,179). There do not appear to be any height or weight risk factors for postoperative dislocation. Preoperative diagnosis of congenital dislocation of the hip similarly has a very low correlation with the inci-

dence of postoperative dislocation. The most significant preexisting factor resulting in postoperative dislocations is prior hip surgery. Some studies report an incidence of under 1% in primary THRs, and a dislocation rate up to 20% after revision THR (175). After performance of 10,500 THRs at the Mayo Clinic, an incidence of dislocations of 2.2% in primary procedures was noted with an incidence of 4.8% after revision surgery (179).

Factors under the Surgeon's Control

There appears to be a distinct difference between dislocations after different types of surgical approaches. Most series report that the dislocation rate after a posterior surgical approach to the hip is 2 to 3 times greater than that seen after an anterior approach (100,129,179). In a large Mayo Clinic series, a postoperative dislocation rate of 2.3% with the anterior approach was reported, compared to a dislocation rate of 5.8% with a posterior approach (179).

Many surgeons feel that a larger femoral head diameter reduces the incidence of dislocation. In fact, the 32-mm head was introduced by Müller in an attempt to decrease the incidence of postoperative dislocation seen with the Charnley prosthesis, which featured a 22-mm head diameter (33). In theory, a smaller head size would be more likely to dislocate because the head must travel a shorter distance before dislocation occurs, and because the neck impinges on the socket edge more easily than with a larger-diameter head (2). However, clinical studies have failed to confirm this theoretical supposition (179). No clear clinical data exist demonstrating a correlation between head size and hip instability.

Increased femoral offset is another prosthetic variable that may influence hip dislocation. Increased femoral offset increases the abductor moment arm, increases soft-tissue tension, and may decrease the incidence of postoperative dislocations. Fackler and Poss (47) demonstrated a statistically significant increase in dislocation rate when femoral offset was decreased by insertion of a femoral component with a valgus neck–shaft angle. They also found a significant decrease in the distance from the center of the femoral head to the tip of the greater trochanter in hips with postoperative dislocations.

The most important factor under the surgeon's control is the position of the components. Cup orientation is critically important, and paradoxically can be extremely difficult to assess intraoperatively. A safe zone of acetabular component orientation was described by Lewinnek et al. (86), who recommended a lateral opening of the cup of 40° plus or minus 10° and an anteversion of 15° plus or minus 10° to decrease the incidence of postoperative dislocation. A statistically significant increased incidence of instability was noted if cup orientation was placed outside of this so-called safe zone. Acetabular component orientation has been considered by some to be the most important variable leading to postoperative dislocation. Cups placed in retroversion or excessive abduction are associated with an increased incidence of postoperative dislocations (31,77,109). The surgical approach may influence positioning of the acetabular component, as it has been demonstrated that the surgeon tends to place the acetabular component in 5° to 7° less anteversion with the posterior approach. Therefore, great care must be taken when using the posterior approach to properly antevert the acetabular component because of the increased incidence of dislocations after the posterior approach (179). It has also been demonstrated that acetabular component orientation is influenced by variations in patient positioning. If the device used to hold the patient in the lateral decubitus position allows the pelvis to rotate forward, unrecognized acetabular component retroversion can occur (100). There is little doubt that cups that are in neutral anteversion, and certainly those that are retroverted, have an increased tendency to dislocate, although a malpositioned cup does not necessarily dictate that a dislocation will occur. Cups exhibiting lateral openings on the anteroposterior (AP) plane greater than 50° also have a predilection for dislocation.

Numerous acetabular component designs available today incorporate an elevated rim on the liner, which, in theory, may decrease the incidence of postoperative dislocations. First utilized by Charnley (45), an extended posterior lip on the acetabular component was introduced to decrease the incidence of posterior dislocations with the Charnley prosthesis. Cobb and co-workers (28) reviewed a large series of THRs performed at the Mayo Clinic to determine the efficacy of an augmented acetabular component. Between 1985 and 1991, 5167 THRs were performed at their institution; with 2469 augmented acetabular components and 2698 standard acetabular components. The 2-year probability for dislocation in hips with an augmented acetabular liner was 2.19%, compared to a 3.85% dislocation rate in hips with a standard acetabular component, a difference that was statistically significant. They also found that the acetabular component with the elevated rim provided increased stability when the results were analyzed according to the operative approach, sex of the patient, mode of fixation of the acetabular component, and type of procedure (primary versus revision). Caution must be used when interpreting these results, because the long-term effects of such enhanced stability are unknown. Concern must be raised about the potential for increased wear resulting from impingement of the femoral neck against the elevated rim. Such wear has been demonstrated at the time of revision of THR featuring elevated rim acetabular components (103). An additional concern with the elevated-rim acetabular component is the potential for an increased rate of cup loosening because of increased rotatory torque applied to the acetabular component. Theoretical

concerns regarding wear and loosening with elevated-rim acetabular components have led some authors (28) to recommend against the routine use of this practice.

With regard to the femoral component, unequivocally excessive anteversion or retroversion may lead to component dislocation. The most common error is excessive femoral anteversion (47). Many contemporary uncemented femoral components feature built-in femoral anteversion, which should caution the surgeon to guard against additional anteversion during component insertion.

Hips that remain stiff in the postoperative period and do not regain a significant range of motion have little likelihood of dislocation. However, hips that flex beyond 120° have a possibility of dislocation, both because of capsular laxity and because of femoral neck impingement on the cup (100).

One final factor that is critical to the incidence of dislocation is the mental status of the patient during the postoperative period. Proper instruction in total hip precautions, both preoperatively and during the postoperative period, is an essential part of the perioperative regimen. A patient unable to avoid flexion beyond 90° because of mental confusion is more likely to dislocate posteriorly after THR performed from a posterior approach. Similarly, after an anterior approach to the hip, patients must limit external rotation and adduction. Patients who have significant mental confusion may need to have a brace or cast placed about the hip to protect against dislocation for the first 6 weeks after surgery.

Diagnosis

The diagnosis of dislocation in THR is relatively simple. In general, there is a history of a sudden change in position of the hip, the patient experiences pain, and shortening of the affected limb is noted. Commonly with posterior dislocations, there is shortening, adduction, and internal rotation of the limb. With anterior dislocations, usually external rotation of the limb is noted, often without significant shortening. Although radiographs are not essential to establish the diagnosis, an AP pelvis and true cross-table lateral of the hip confirm the dislocation and its direction.

Treatment

The treatment of a dislocated THR consists of expedient reduction. Unlike traumatic dislocation of a normal hip, a dislocated THR is not a true emergency, but expedient reduction is necessary for the patient's comfort. Occasionally, dislocations can be reduced in the emergency room under intravenous sedation, but it is probably safest to undertake reduction in the operating room under anesthesia. Mobilization of the hip after dislocation depends on the cause of the dislocation and the position of the components. An unusual situation precipitating dislocation, such as a fall in a compliant patient, may be treated by reduction followed by protected ambulation. Most surgeons prefer some type of immobilization after dislocation, either with a pantaloon spica cast or a commercially available hip spica brace. Success rates ranging from 63% to 83% have been reported after cast or brace immobilization for dislocated THR (39,126). The incidence of redislocation after reduction of a dislocation occurring in the early period after THR is low, ranging from 20% to 30% (77). However, this is dependent on component orientation. If the acetabular component or femoral component is malpositioned, then early surgical treatment may be necessary to prevent further dislocations. Daly and Morrey (32) reported on surgical treatment of recurrent dislocations and found that reoperation was successful in approximately 70% of procedures aimed at correction of malpositioned components. A lower rate of success was documented in procedures when the cause of the instability was not clearly defined (32).

Postoperative THR dislocations are an unpleasant experience for the patient and the surgeon, and the best treatment is prevention by careful proper surgical technique and pre- and postoperative teaching of THR precautions.

REFERENCES

1. Aken HV, Miller ED. Deliberate hypotension. In: Miller RD, ed. *Anesthesia*, 4th ed. New York: Churchill-Livingstone, 1994;1481–1505.
2. Amstutz HC, Markolf K. Design features in total hip replacements. In: *The Hip*. St Louis: CV Mosby, 1974;111–122.
3. Amstutz HC, Cass Z. Management of the septic total hip replacement. *The Hip*. St Louis: CV Mosby, 1977;152.
4. Arensberg D. Coronary atherosclerotic heart disease. In: Lubin MF, Walker HK, Smith RB, eds. *Medical management of the surgical patient*, 2nd ed. Boston: Butterworth, 1988;101–107.
5. Arora NS, Rochester DF. Respiratory muscle strength and maximal voluntary ventilation in undernourished patients. *Am Rev Respir Dis* 1982;126:5–8.
6. Bartlett RH. Pulmonary insufficiency. In: Wilmore DW, Cheung LY, Harken AH, Holcroft JW, Meakins JL, eds. *Care of the surgical patient*, 2nd ed. New York: Scientific American, 1988;VII:6–12.
7. Baum LB, Kennedy DL, Forbes MB. Utilization of non-steroidal anti-inflammatory drugs. *Arthritis Rheum* 1985;28:686–692.
8. Beer KJ, Lombardi AV, Mallory TH, Vaughan BK. The efficacy of suction drains after routine total joint arthroplasty. *J Bone Joint Surg* 1991;73A:584–587.
9. Bell RC, Coalson JJ, Smith JD, Johanson WG. Multiple organ system failure and infection in the adult respiratory distress syndrome. *Ann Intern Med* 1983;99:293–298.
10. Bengtson A, Larsson M, Gammer W, Heideman M. Anaphylatoxin release in association with methylmethacrylate fixation of hip prostheses. *J Bone Joint Surg* 1987;69A:46–49.
11. Berggren D, Gustafson Y, Eriksson, et al. Postoperative confusion after anesthesia in elderly patients with femoral neck fracture. *Anesth Analg* 1987;66:497–504.
12. Berl T, Schrier RW. Disorders of water metabolism. In: Schrier RW, ed. *Renal and electrolyte disorders*, 4th ed. Boston: Little Brown, 1992;1–88.
13. Bigler D, Adelhoj B, Petring OU, Pederson NO, Busch P, Calhke P.

Mental function and morbidity after acute hip surgery during spinal and general anesthesia. *Anaesthesia* 1985;40:672–676.
14. Black DL, Reckling FW, Porter SS. Somatosensory-evoked potential monitored during total hip arthroplasty. *Clin Orthop* 1991;262:170–177.
15. Bode RH, Lewis KP, Zarich SW, et al. Cardiac outcomes after peripheral vascular surgery. *Anesthesiology* 1996;84:3–13.
16. Brentlinger A, Hunter JA. Perforation of the external iliac artery and ureter presenting as acute hemorrhagic cystitis after total hip replacement. *J Bone Joint Surg* 1987;69A:620–622.
17. Brown DL, Wedel DJ. Spinal, epidural and caudal anesthesia. In: Miller RD, ed. *Anesthesia*, 3rd ed. New York: Churchill Livingstone, 1990;1377–1402.
18. Burke JF, Francos GC. Surgery in the patient with acute or chronic renal failure. *Med Clin North Am* 1987;71:489–497.
19. Byrick RJ, Forbes D, Waddell JP. A monitored cardiovascular collapse during cemented total knee replacement. *Anesthesiology* 1986;65:213–216.
20. Byrick RJ, Kay JC, Mullen JBM. Pulmonary marrow embolism: a dog model simulating dual component cemented arthroplasty. *Can J Anesth* 1987;34:336–342.
21. Byrick RJ, Bell RS, Kay JC, Waddell JP, Mullen JBM. High volume, high pressure pulsatile lavage during cemented arthroplasty. *J Bone Joint Surg* 1989;71A:1331–1336.
22. Carpiniello VL, Cendron M, Altman HG, Malloy TR, Booth R. Treatment of urinary complications after total joint replacement in elderly females. *Urology* 1988;32:186–188.
23. Cases A, Escolar G, Reverter JC, et al. Recombinant human erythropoietin treatment improves platelet function in uremic patients. *Kidney Internat* 1992;42:668–672.
24. Chambers D. Effects of anesthetic agents and techniques on body systems. In: Lubin MF, Walker HK, Smith RB, eds. *Medical management of the surgical patient*. Boston: Butterworth, 1988;64–77.
25. Cheng EY, Klibanoff JE, Robinson HJ, Bradford DS. Total hip arthroplasty with cement after renal transplantation. *J Bone Joint Surg* 1995;77A:1535–1542.
26. Chung HM, Kluge R, Schrier RW, Anderson RJ. Postoperative hyponatremia. A prospective study. *Arch Intern Med* 1986;146:333–336.
27. Cobb JP. Why use drains? *J Bone Joint Surg* 1990;72B:993–995.
28. Cobb TK, Morrey BF, Ilstrup DM. The elevated rim acetabular liner in total hip arthroplasty. Relationship to postoperative dislocation. *J Bone Joint Surg* 1996;78A:80–87.
29. Collis DK, Steinhaus K. Total hip replacement without infection in a standard operating room. *J Bone Joint Surg* 1976;58A:446–450.
30. Coventry MB. Treatment of infections occurring in total hip surgery. *Orthop Clin North Am* 1975;6:991–1003.
31. Coventry MB, Beckenbaugh RD, Nolan DR, Ilstrup DM. Total hip arthroplasty. A study of postoperative course and early complications. *J Bone Joint Surg* 1974;56A:273–284.
32. Daly PJ, Morrey BF. Operative correction of an unstable total hip arthroplasty. *J Bone Joint Surg* 1992;74A:1334–1343.
33. Dall DM, Grobbelaar C, Learmouth ID, Dall G. Charnley low friction arthroplasty of the hip. *Clin Orthop* 1986;211:85–90.
34. Daniel NN, Coventry MB, Miller WE. Pulmonary complications following total hip arthroplasty with Charnley prosthesis as revealed by chest radiographs. *J Bone Joint Surg* 1972;54A:282.
35. Davis FM, Laurenson VG, Gillispie WJ, Wells JE, Foate J, Newman E. Deep vein thrombosis after total hip replacement. A comparison between spinal and general anesthesia. *J Bone Joint Surg* 1989;71B:181–185.
36. Demling RH, Wolfort S. Early postoperative pneumonia. In: Wilmore DW, Cheung LY, Harken AH, Holcroft JW, Meakins JL, eds. *Care of the surgical patient*, 2nd ed. New York: Scientific American, 1993;IX(7):1–13.
37. De Andrade JR, Maslanka M, Maneatis T, Bynum L, Burchmere M. The use of ketorolac in the management of postoperative pain. *Orthopedics* 1994;17:157–166.
38. Dodeo S, Gibbens CLMH, Emerton M, Simpson AHRW. Total hip replacement in renal transplant recipients. *J Bone Joint Surg* 1995;77B:299–302.
39. Dorr LD, Wolf AW, Chandler RW, Conaty JP. Classification and treatment of dislocations of total hip arthroplasty. *Clin Orthop* 1983;173:151.

40. Drinkwater CJ, Neil MJ. Optimum timing of wound drain removal following total joint arthroplasty. *J Arthroplasty* 1995;10:185–189.

41. Duncan JAT. Intraoperative collapse or death related to use of acrylic bone cement in hip surgery. *Anesthesia* 1989;44:149–153.

42. D'Hollander A, Monteney E, Houghe L, et al. Cardiovascular effects of methylmethacrylate monomer. *Surg Gynecol Obstet* 1979;149:61–64.

43. Edwards BN, Tullos HS, Noble PC. Contributory factors and etiology of sciatic nerve palsy in total hip arthroplasty. *Clin Orthop* 1987;218:136–141.

44. Eftekhar NS, Kiernan HA, Stinchfield FE. Systemic and local complications following low friction arthroplasty of the hip joint. *Arch Surg* 1976;111:150–155.

45. Eftekhar NS. Dislocation and instability complicating low friction arthroplasty of the hip joint. *Clin Orthop* 1976;121:120–125.

46. Erath MH, Weber JG, Abel MD, et al. Cemented versus noncemented total hip arthroplasty. Embolism, hemodynamics and intrapulmonary shunting. *Mayo Clin Proc* 1992;67:1066–1074.

47. Fackler CD, Poss R. Dislocation in total hip arthroplasty. *Clin Orthop* 1980;151:169–178.

48. Faris PM, Ritter MA, Abels RI. The effects of recombinant human erythropoietin on perioperative transfusion in patients having a major orthopedic operation. *J Bone Joint Surg* 1996;78A:62–72.

49. Felner JM. Congestive heart failure. In: Lubin MF, Walker HK, Smith RB, eds. *Medical management of the surgical patient*. Boston: Butterworth, 1988;121–124.

50. Fitzgerald RH, Randall KR, Brown WJ, Nasser S. Treatment of the infected total hip arthroplasty. *Curr Opin Orthop* 1994;5:26–30.

51. Fitzgerald RH. Infected total hip arthroplasty: diagnosis and treatment. *J Am Assoc Orthop Surg* 1995;3:249–262.

52. Fleming RE, Michelsen CB, Stinchfield FE. Sciatic paralysis: A complication of bleeding following hip surgery. *J Bone Joint Surg* 1979;61A:37–39.

53. Friedman LS, Maddrey WC. Surgery in the patient with liver disease. *Med Clin North Am* 1987;71:453–476.

54. Fullerton DA, Harken AH. Cardiac insufficiency. In: Wilmore DW, Cheung LY, Harken AH, Holcroft JW, Meakins JL, eds. *Care of the surgical patient*. New York: Scientific American, 1988;VII:1–10.

55. Garrison RN, Cryer HM, Howard DA, et al. Clarification of risk factors for abdominal operations in patients with hepatic cirrhosis. *Ann Surg* 1984;199:648–655.

56. Garvin KL, Fitzgerald RH, Salvati EA, Brause BD, Nercessian OA, Wallrich SL, Ilstrup DM. Reconstruction of the infected total hip and knee arthroplasty with gentomyicin-impregnated Palacos bone cement. *Instr Course Lect* 1993;42:293–302.

57. Garvin KL, Hanssen AD. Current concepts review: infection after total hip arthroplasty—past, present, and future. *J Bone Joint Surg* 1995;77A:1576–1588.

58. Geis GS, Stead H, Wallemark LB, Nicholson PA. Prevalence of mucosal lesions in the stomach and duodenum due to chronic use of NSAIDs in patients with RA or OA. *J Rheumatol* 1991;18(S):11–14.

59. Gherini S, Vaughn BX, Lombardi AV, Mallory TH. Delayed wound healing and nutritional deficiencies after total hp arthroplasty. *Clin Orthop* 1993;293:188–195.

60. Go AS, Brower WS. Cardiac outcomes after regional or general anesthesia [editorial]. Do we have the answer? *Anesthesiology* 1996;84:1–2.

61. Goldman L. Cardiac risks and complications of noncardiac surgery. *Ann Intern Med* 1983;98:504–513.

62. Gordon S, Chatzinoff M, Pekin SR. Medical care of the surgical patient with gastrointestinal disease. *Med Clin North Am* 71:433–452.

63. Gresham GA, Kuczynski A, Rosborough D. Fatal fat embolism following replacement arthroplasty for transcervical fractures of the femur. *Br Med J* 1971;2:617–619.

64. Griffin MR, Piper JM, Daugherty JR, Snowden M, Ray WA. Nonsteroidal anti-inflammatory drug use. Increased risk for peptic ulcer disease in elderly persons. *Ann Intern Med* 1991;114:257–263.

65. Gustafson Y, Berggren D, Brannstrom B, et al. Acute confusional states in elderly patients following femoral neck fracture. *J Am Geriatr Soc* 1988;36:525–530.

66. Hole A, Terjesen T, Breivik H. Epidural versus general anesthesia for total hip arthroplasty in elderly patients. *Acta Anaesth Scand* 1980;24:278–287.

67. Homsy CA, Tullos HS, Anderson MS, Differante NM, King JW. Some physiologic aspects of prosthesis stabilization with acrylic polymer. *Clin Orthop* 1972;83:317–328.

68. Hornick P, Allan P. Acute hyponatremia following total hip replacement. *Br J Clin Pract* 1990;44:776–777.

69. James ML. Anaesthetic and metabolic complications. In: Ling RSM, ed. *Complications of total hip replacement*. Edinburgh: Churchill Livingstone, 1984;1–18.

70. Johanson NA, Pellici PM, Tsairis P, Salvati EA. Nerve injury in total hip arthroplasty. *Clin Orthop* 1983;175:214–222.

71. Jones MJT, Piggot SE, Vaughan RS, et al. Cognitive and functional competence after anesthesia in patients over 60: controlled trial of general and regional anesthesia for elective hip or knee replacement. *Br Med J* 1990;300:1683–1687.

72. Jones SJ, Edgar MA, Ransford AD, Thomas NP. A system for the electrophysiological monitoring of the spinal cord during operations for scoliosis. *J Bone Joint Surg* 1983;65B:134–139.

73. Kahn RL, Hargelt MJ, Urquhart B, Sharrock NE, Petersen MG. Supraventricular arrhythmias during total joint arthroplasty. Incidence and risk. *Clin Orthop* 1993;296:265–269.

74. Kallos T, Enis JE, Gollam F, Davis JH. Intramedullary pressure and pulmonary embolism of femoral intramedullary contents in dogs during insertion of bone cement and a prosthesis. *J Bone Joint Surg* 1974;56A:1363–1367.

75. Kallos T. Impaired arterial oxygenation associated with use of bone cement in the femoral shaft. *Anesthesiology* 1975;42:216.

76. Keating EM, Ritter MA, Faris PM. Structures at risk for medially placed acetabular screws. *J Bone Joint Surg* 1990;72A:510–511.

77. Khan MA, Brakenbury PH, Reynolds ISR. Dislocation following total hip arthroplasty. *J Bone Joint Surg* 1981;63B:214–218.

78. Kristiansen B, Jorgensen L, Holmich P. Dislocation following total hip replacement. *Arch Orthop Trauma Surg* 1985;103:375–377.

79. Lachiewicz PF, Latimer HA. Rhabdomyolysis following total hip arthroplasty. *J Bone Joint Surg* 1991;73B:576–579.

80. Lafont ND, Kustucki WM, Marchand MN, Buogaerts JG. Embolism detected by transesophageal echocardiography during hip arthroplasty. *Can J Anesth* 1994;41:850–853.

81. Lanza FL, Kavlin DA, Yee JP. A double blind placebo-controlled endoscopic study comparing the mucosal injuries seen with an orally and parenterally administered new nonsteroidal analgesic ketorolac tromethamine at therapeutic and super-therapeutic doses. *Am J Gastroenterol* 1987;92:939.

82. Latimer RG, Dickman M, Day WC, Gunn ML, Schmidt CD. Ventilatory patterns and pulmonary complications after upper abdominal surgery determined by preoperative and postoperative computerized spirometry and blood gas analysis. *Am J Surg* 1971;122:622–632.

83. Lawrence VA, Gafni A, Gross M. The unproven utility of the preoperative urinalysis: economic evaluation. *J Clin Epidemiol* 1989;42:1185–1192.

84. Lazansky MG. The debit side of total hip replacement. *Clin Orthop* 1973;95:96–103.

85. Levy D. The fat embolism syndrome. *Clin Orthop* 1990;261:281–287.

86. Lewinnek GE, Lewis JC, Taur R, Compere CZ, Zimmerman JR. Dislocations after total hip replacement. *J Bone Joint Surg* 1978;60A:217–220.

87. Lieberman JR, Juo M, Hanway J, Salvati EA, Sculco TP, Sharrock NE. The prevalence of deep venous thrombosis with hypotensive epidural anesthesia. *J Bone Joint Surg* 1994;76A:341–348.

88. Lieberman JR, Fuch MD, Haas SB, Garvin KL, Golgupta R, Pellicci PM, Salvati EA. Hip arthroplasty in patients with chronic renal failure. *J Arthroplasty* 1995;10:191–195.

89. Ling RSM. Systemic and miscellaneous complications. In: Ling RSM, ed. *Complications of total hip replacement*. Edinburgh: Churchill Livingstone, 1984;201–212.

90. Lipowski ZJ. Delirium in the elderly patient. *New Engl J Med* 1989;320:578–582.

91. Lipowski ZJ. Transient cognitive disorders (delirium, acute confusional states) in the elderly. *Am J Psychiatry* 1983;140:1426–1436.

92. Marcantonio ER, Goldman L, Mangione CM, et al. A clinical prediction rule for delerium after elective non-cardiac surgery. *JAMA* 1994;271:134–139.

93. Mars RL. Chronic renal failure. In: Lubin MF, Walker HK, Smith RB, eds. *Medical management of the surgical patient*, 2nd ed. Boston: Butterworth 1988;343–347.

94. McLaughlin RE, Difazio C, Hakala M, et al. Blood clearance and

acute pulmonary toxicity of methylmethacrylate in dogs after simulated arthroplasty and intravenous injection. *J Bone Joint Surg* 1973; 55A:1621–1628.

95. Michelson JD, Lotke PA, Steinberg ME. Urinary bladder management after total joint replacement surgery. *New Engl J Med* 1988;319: 321–326.

96. Mir GN, Lawrence WJ, Autian J. Toxicological and pharmacological actions of methylmethacrylate monomers. 1. Effects on isolated perfused rabbit heart. *J Pharm Sci* 1975;62:778–782.

97. Mohler CG, Kull LR, Martell JM, Rosenberg AG, Galante JO. Total hip replacement with insertion of an acetabular component without cement and a femoral component with cement. *J Bone Joint Surg* 1995;77A:86–96.

98. Monks R. Cognitive and sensory defects. In: Wilmore DW, Cheung LW, Harken AH, Holcroft JW, Meakins JO, eds. *Care of the surgical patient*, 2nd ed. New York: Scientific American, 1988;VII(10):3–13.

99. Morand EF, Littlejohn GO. Medical problems in joint replacement patients. A retrospective study of 243 total hip arthroplasties. *Med J Aust* 1989;152:408–411.

100. Morrey BF. Instability after total hip arthroplasty. *Orthop Clin North Am* 1992;23:237–248.

101. Morris SJ. Peptic ulcer disease. In: Lubin MF, Walker HK, Smith RB, eds. *Medical management of the surgical patient*, 2nd ed. Boston: Butterworth, 1988;189–196.

102. Murasko DM, Goonewardene IM. T-cell function in aging: mechanisms of decline. *Ann Rev Gerentol Geriatr* 1990;10:71–96.

103. Murray DW. Impingement and loosening of the long posterior wall acetabular component. *J Bone Joint Surg* 1992;74B:377–379.

104. Murzic WJ, McCollum, DE. Hip arthroplasty for osteonecrosis after renal transplantation. *Clin Orthop*, 1994;299:212–219.

105. Nachbur B, Meyer RP, Verkkala K, Zurcher R. The mechanisms of severe arterial injury in surgery of the hip joint. *Clin Orthop* 1979; 141:122–133.

106. Naito M, Ogata K, Shiota E, Nakamoto M, Goya T. Hip arthroplasty and hemodialysis patients. *J Bone Joint Surg* 1994;76B:428–431.

107. Nassar S. Prevention and treatment of sepsis in total hip replacement surgery. *Orthop Clin North Am* 1992;23:265–277.

108. NIH Consensus Conference. Total hip-joint replacement in the United States. *JAMA* 1982;248:1817.

109. Nolan DR, Fitzgerald RH, Beckenbaugh RD, Coventry NB. Complications of total hip arthroplasty treated by reoperation. *J Bone Joint Surg* 1975;57A:977–981.

110. Oishi CS, Williams VJ, Hanson PB, Schneider JE, Colwell CW, Walker RH. Perioperative bladder management after primary total hip arthroplasty. *J Arthroplasty* 1995;10:732–736.

111. Orsini EC, Byrick RJ, Mullen JBM, Kay JC, Waddell JP. Cardiopulmonary function and pulmonary microemboli during arthroplasty using cemented or non-cemented components. *J Bone Joint Surg* 1987;69A:822–832.

112. Pantano JA, Lee YC. Acute propranolol withdrawal and myocardial contractility. A study of effects in normal man. *Arch Intern Med* 1976; 867–871.

113. Pasulka PS, Bistrian PR, Benotti PN, Blackburn GL. The risks of surgery in obese patients. *Ann Intern Med* 1986;104:540–546.

114. Patterson BM, Healey JH, Cornell CN, Sharrock NE. Cardiac arrest during hip arthroplasty with a cemented long-stem component. *J Bone Joint Surg* 1991;73(1):271–277.

115. Patterson BM, Lieberman JR, Salvati EA. Intraoperative complications during total hip arthroplasty. *Orthopedics* 1995;18:1089–1095.

116. Peebles DJ, Ellis RH, Stride SDK, Simpson BRJ. Cardiovascular effects of methylmethacrylate cement. *Br Med J* 1972;1:349–351.

117. Pess GM, Lusskin R, Waugh TR, Baltista AE. Femoral neuropathy secondary to pressurized cement in total hip replacement treatment by decompression and neurolysis. *J Bone Joint Surg* 1987;69A:623–625.

118. Peters RM. Respiratory function. In: Davis JM, Drucker WR, Foster RS, et al., eds. *Clinical surgery*. St Louis: CV Mosby, 1987;145–175.

119. Peterson MS, Collins DN, Selakovich WG, Finkbeiner AE. Postoperative urinary retention associated with total hip and total knee arthroplasties. *Clin Orthop* 1991;269:102–108.

120. Praemer A, Furner S, Rice DP. Medical implants and major joint procedures. In: *Musculoskeletal conditions in the United States*. Park Ridge, IL: American Academy of Orthopaedic Surgeons, 1992; 125–142.

121. Priebe HJ, Skillman JJ, Bushnell BS, et al. Antacid versus cimetidine in preventing acute gastrointestinal bleeding. *N Engl J Med* 1983;308:1571–1575.

122. Redfern TR, Machin DG, Parsons KF, Owen R. Urinary retention in men after total hip arthroplasty. *J Bone Joint Surg* 1986;68A: 1435–1438.

123. Rehder K, Sessler AD, Marsh HM. General anesthesia and the lung. *Am Rev Respir Dis* 1975;112:541–563.

124. Reiley MA, Bond D, Branick RJ, Wilson EH. Vascular complications following total hip arthroplasty. *Clin Orthop* 1984;186:23–28.

125. Ries MD, Lynch F, Rauscher LA, Richman J, Mick C, Gomez M. Pulmonary function during and after total hip replacement. Findings in patients who have insertion of a femoral component with and without cement. *J Bone Joint Surg* 1993;75A:581–587.

126. Ritter MA. Dislocation and subluxation of the total hip replacement. *Clin Orthop* 1976;121:92–94.

127. Ritter MA, Faris PM, Keating EM. Urinary tract catheterization protocols following total joint arthorplasty. *Orhopedics* 1989;12: 1085–1087.

128. Ritter MA, Keating EM, Faris PM. Closed wound drainage in total hip or total knee replacements. *J Bone Joint Surg* 1994;76A:35–38.

129. Roberts JM, Fu FH, McClain EJ, Ferguson AB. A comparison of the posterolateral and anterolateral approaches to total hip arthroplasty. *Clin Orthop* 1983;187:205–210.

130. Saag KG, Cowdery JS. Nonsteroidal anti-inflammatory drugs. Balancing benefits and risks. *Spine* 1994;19:1530–1534.

131. Salvati EA, Robinson RP, Zeno SM, et al. Infections rates after 3175 total hip and total knee arthroplasties performed with and without a horizontal unidirectional filtered air flow system. *J Bone Joint Surg* 1982;64A:525–535.

132. Schaeffer HA. Catheter-associated bacteriuria. *Urol Clin North Am* 1986;13:735–747.

133. Schmalzreid TP, Amstutz HC, Dorey FJ. Nerve palsy associated with total hip replacement. *J Bone Joint Surg* 1991;73A:1074–1080.

134. Scott NB, Kehlet H. Regional anesthesia and surgical morbidity. *Br J Surg* 1988;75:299–304.

135. Sculco TP, Ranawat C. The use of spinal anesthesia for total hip replacement arthroplasty. *J Bone Joint Surg* 1975;57A:173–177.

136. Scullin JP, Nelson CL, Beven EG. False aneurysm of the left external iliac artery following total hip arthroplasty. Report of a case. *Clin Orthop* 1975;113:145–149.

137. Seagroatt V, Tan JS, Goldacre M, Bulstrode C, Nugent I, Gill L. Elective total hip replacement. Incidence, emergency readmission rate and postoperative mortality. *Br Med J* 1991;303:1431–1435.

138. Sharrock NE, Sanborn KV, Urquhart B, Mineo R, Kahn R. Acute hypotension following insertion of femoral prostheses during total hip replacement. *Anesth Analg* 1990;70:368.

139. Sharrock NE, Mineo R, Urquhart B. Haemodynamic effects and outcome analysis of hypotensive extradural anesthesia in controlled hypertensive patients undergoing total hip arthroplasty. *Br J Anaesth* 1991;67:17–25.

140. Sharrock NE, Mineo R, Urquhart B, Salvati EA. The effect of two levels of hypotension on intraoperative blood loss during total hip arthroplasty performed under lumbar epidural anesthesia. *Anesth Analg* 1992;76:580–584.

141. Sharrock NE, Ranawat CS, Urquhart B, Peterson M. Factors influencing deep vein thrombosis following total hip arthroplasty under epidural anesthesia. *Anesth Analg* 1993;76:765–771.

142. Sharrock NE, Cazan MG, Hargett MJ, Williams-Russo P, Wilson PD. Changes in mortality after total hip and knee arthroplasty over a ten-year period. *Anesth Analg* 1995;80:242–248.

143. Sheppeard H, Cleak DK, Ward DJ, O'Connor BT. A review of early mortality and morbidity in elderly patients following Charnley total hip replacement. *Arch Orthop Trauma Surg* 1980;97:243–248.

144. Sherman RMP, Byrick RJ, Kay JC, Sullivan TR, Waddell JP. The role of lavage in preventing hemodynamic and blood gas changes during cemented arthroplasty. *J Bone Joint Surg* 1983;65A:500–506.

145. Simmons C, Izant TH, Rothman RH, Booth RE, Balderston RA. Femoral neuropathy following total hip arthroplasty. *J Arthroplasty* 1991;6:559–566.

146. Smith JW, Pellicci PM, Sharrock N, Mineo R, Wilson PD. Complications after total hip arthroplasty. The contralateral limb. *J Bone Joint Surg* 1989;71A:528–535.

147. Solheim LF, Hgen R. Femoral and sciatic neuropathies after total hip arthroplasty. *Acta Orthop Scand* 1980;51:531–534.

148. Soll A. Gastric, duodenal, and stress ulcer. In: Sleisenger MH, Fordtran JS, eds. *Gastrointestinal disease*, 5th ed. Philadelphia: WB Sanders, 1993;580–652.

149. Spengler DM, Costenbader M, Bailey R. Fat embolism syndrome following total hip arthroplasty. *Clin Orthop* 1976;121:105–107.

150. Steen PA, Tinker JH, Tarhan S. Myocardial reinfarction after anesthesia and surgery. *JAMA* 1978;239:2566–2570.

151. Stein M, Koota GM, Simon M, Frank HA. Pulmonary evaluation in surgical patients. *JAMA* 1962;181:765–770.

152. Stone RG, Weeks LE, Hajdu M, Stinchfield FE. Evaluation of sciatic nerve function during total hip arthroplasty. *Clin Orthop* 1985;201: 26–31.

153. Sunderland S. *Nerves and nerve injury*, 2nd ed, Edinburgh: Churchill Livingston, 1978.

154. Surin VV, Sundholm K, Backman L. Infection after total hip replacement. With special reference to a discharge from the wound. *J Bone Joint Surg* 1983;65B:412–418.

155. Szmuness W, Prince AM, Grady GF, et al. Hepatitis B infection. A point prevalence study in 15 US hemodialysis centers. *JAMA* 1974; 227:901–906.

156. Tedesco FJ, Waye JD, Raskin JB, et al. Colonoscopic evaluation of rectal bleeding. A study of 304 patients. *Ann Intern Med* 1978;89:907–909.

157. Tronzo RG, Kallos T, Wyche MQ. Elevation of intramedullary pressure when methyl-methacrylate is inserted in total hip arthroplasty. *J Bone Joint Surg* 1974;56A:714–718.

158. Tsukyama DT, Estrada R, Gustilo RB. Infection after total hip arthroplasty. A study of the treatment of one hundred and six infections. *J Bone Joint Surg* 1996;78A:512–523.

159. Ulrich C, Burri C, Worsdorfer O, Heinrich H. Intraoperative transesophageal two-dimensional echocardiography in total hip replacement. *Arch Orthop Trauma Surg* 1986;105:274–278.

160. Vanderhofft JE, Robinson RP. Late infection of a bipolar endoprosthesis following endoscopy. *J Bone Joint Surg* 1994;76A:744–745.

161. Wahba WM. Influence of aging on lung function. Clinical significance of changes from age twenty. *Anesth Analg* 1983;62:764–776.

162. Walan A, Bader J-P, Claussen M, et al. Effect of omeprazole and rantidine on ulcer healing and relapse rates in patients with benign gastric ulcer. *N Engl J Med* 1989;320:69–75.

163. Walts LF, Kaufman RD, Moreland JR, Weiskopf M. Total hip arthroplasty. An investigation of factors related to postoperative urinary retention. *Clin Orthop* 1985;194:280–282.

164. Wasielewski RC, Cooperstein LA, Kruger MP, et al. Acetabular anatomy and the transacetabular fixation of screws in total hip arthroplasty. *J Bone Joint Surg* 1990;72A:501–508.

165. Wasielewski RC, Crossett LS, Rubash HE. Neural and vascular injury in total hip arthroplasty. *Orthop Clin North Am* 1992;23:219–235.

166. Waterhouse N, Beaumont AR, Murray K, Staniforth T, Stone MH. Urinary retention after total hip replacement. A perspective study. *J Bone Joint Surg* 1987;69B:64–66.

167. Weber ER, Darbe JR, Coventry MB. Peripheral neuropathies associated with total hip arthroplasty. *J Bone Joint Surg* 1976;58A:66–69.

168. Weitz H, Goldman L. Noncardiac surgery in the patient with heart disease. *Med Clin North Am* 1987;71:413–432.

169. Wellman JJ, Smith BA. Respiratory complications of surgery. In: Lubin MF, Walker HK, Smith RB, eds. *Medical management of the surgical patient*. Boston: Butterworth, 1988;155–161.

170. Wellman JJ, Smith BA. Adult respiratory distress syndrome in the surgical patient. In: Lubin MF, Walker HK, Smith RB, eds. *Medical management of the surgical patient*. Boston: Butterworth, 1988; 175–186.

171. Wennberg JE, Roos N, Sola L, Jaffe R. Use of claims data systems to evaluate health care outcomes. Mortality and reoperation following prostatectomy. *JAMA* 1987;257:933.

172. Wheelwright EF, Byrick RJ, Wigglesworth DF, et al. Hypotension during cemented arthroplasty. Relationship to cardiac output and fat embolism. *J Bone Joint Surg* 1993;75B:715–723.

173. Whittle J, Steinberg EP, Anderson GF, Herbert R, Hochberg MC. Mortality after elective total hip arthroplasty in elderly Americans. *Clin Orthop* 1993;295:119–126.

174. Willett KM, Simmons CD, Bentley G. The effect of suction drains after total hip replacement. *J Bone Joint Surg* 1988;70B:607–610.

175. Williams JF, Gottesman MJ, Mallory TH. Dislocation after total hip arthroplasty. Treatment with an above-knee hip spica cast. *Clin Orthop* 1982;171:53–58.

176. Williams-Russo P, Urquhart BL, Sharrock NE, Charlson ME. Postoperative delerium. Predictors and prognosis in the elderly orthopedic patient. *J Am Geriatr Soc* 1992;48:759–767.

177. Williams-Russo P, Sharrock NE, Mattis S, Szatrowski TP, Charlson ME. Cognitive effects after epidural vs general anesthesia in older adults. A randomized trial. *JAMA* 1995;274:44–50.

178. Winslow CM, Solomon DH, Chassin MR, Coswcoff J, Merrick NJ, Brook RH. The appropriateness of carotid enderarterectomy. *N Engl J Med* 1988;318:721.

179. Woo RYG, Morrey BF. Dislocations after total hip arthroplasty. *J Bone Joint Surg* 1982;64A:1295–1306.

180. Wroblewski BM, del Sel HJ. Urethral instrumentation and deep sepsis in total hip replacement. *Clin Orthop* 1980;146:209–213.

181. Wukich DK, Callaghan JJ, Graeber GM, Martyak T, Savory CG, Lyon JL. Cardiac isoenzyme values after total joint arthroplasty. *Clin Orthop* 1989;242:232–240.

182. Yeager MP, Glass DD, Neff RK, Brinck-Johnsen T. Epidural anesthesia and analgesia in high risk surgical patients. *Anesthesiology* 1987; 66:729–736.

183. Zechmann JP, Reckling FW. Association of preoperative hip motion and sciatic nerve palsy following total hip arthroplasty. *Clin Orthop* 1989;241:197–199.

184. Zeldin R. Assessing cardiac risk in patients who undergo noncadiac surgical procedures. *Can J Surg* 1984;27:402.

The Adult Hip, edited by J. J. Callaghan,
A. G. Rosenberg, and H. E. Rubash.
Lippincott–Raven Publishers, Philadelphia © 1998.

CHAPTER 72

Late Complications and Their Management

Brian G. Evans

Total hip arthroplasty (THA) has revolutionized the treatment of end-stage arthritic conditions of the hip. However, success is not seen in all patients and complications can occur both in the early perioperative period and later. This chapter will review complications occurring after the early perioperative period.

HETEROTOPIC OSSIFICATION

Heterotopic ossification (HO) is the formation of bone tissue within what are normally soft tissues. The specific sequence of events leading to HO remains to be defined. However, there appears to be a metaplasia of local fibroblasts into osteoblastic cells that produce bone. The stimulus for this transformation may be growth factors such as bone morphogenetic protein. These factors may be released into the local tissues by trauma from the surgical approach or the reaming of the femur or acetabulum. Although HO commonly occurs after surgery or trauma, it can also occur without local trauma, such as after spinal or head injury (29). All forms of HO are histologically identical, representing true bone formation, not simply calcification of the soft tissue. HO can occur in 10% to 90% of cases after total hip arthroplasty. The formation of this tissue commonly has little effect on the clinical result. However, in 2% to 10% of patients, the bone formation can be extensive, resulting in restriction of motion and pain (Fig. 1).

B. G. Evans: Department of Orthopaedic Surgery, Georgetown University Medical Center, Washington, D.C. 20007-2197.

The first radiographic manifestations of HO can usually be detected between 3 and 6 weeks postoperatively. By 12 weeks postoperatively, most of the bone that is going to form will be evident, whereas the radiodensity will increase in time as the tissue matures. The immature bone is associated with an elevation in the serum alkaline phosphatase level and increased uptake on the technetium-99-methylene diphosphonate (^{99}Tc-MDP) bone scan. However, a slow increase in the volume of bone present can continue for up to 1 year. Final maturation of the bone can take between 2 and 5 years (59). Maturation of the bone is determined by a stable appearance on serial radiographs, normal serum alkaline phosphatase, and uptake on the bone scan similar to other areas of bone.

Etiology and Risk Factors

Although the specific sequence of events leading to HO remains unclear, many risk factors have been identified for the formation of HO. These can be divided into either patient- or technique-related factors (Table 1). Although all of the listed factors place the patient at risk to develop HO, previous HO at the site of a THA is associated with as high as a 90% probability of occurrence of HO with contralateral surgery without prophylaxis (21). Patients with hypertrophic osteoarthritis or diffuse idiopathic skeletal hyperostosis (DISH) are also likely to have an increased risk of HO forming after THA (32). Ankylosing spondylitis has also been associated with an increased risk of HO. For example, Bisala and associates found extensive HO formation in 39% of patients not receiving prophylaxis (8). However, HO

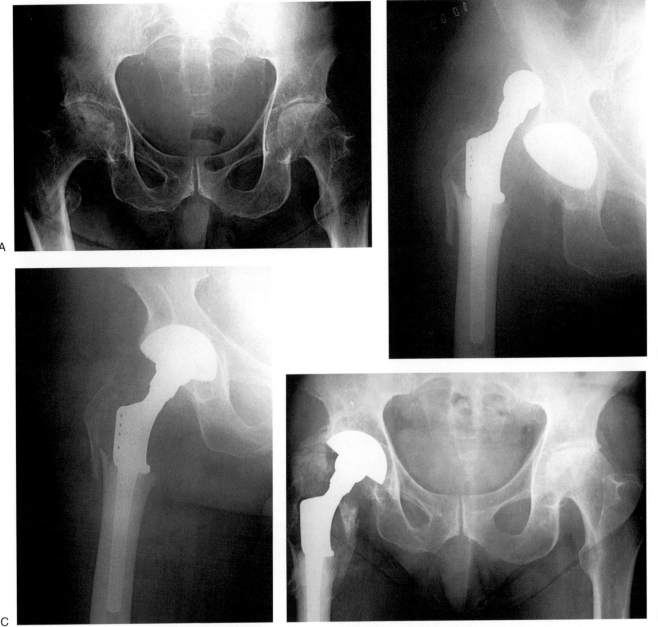

FIG. 1. A: This 53-year-old man, with a history of alcohol abuse and stage III avascular necrosis of both hips, sustained an intertrochanteric fracture of the right hip. **B:** He had a calcar replacement total hip arthroplasty to treat the fracture and the avascular necrosis. A dislocation occurred postoperatively. **C:** After reduction, the trochanteric fragment is noted to be proximally migrated. **D:** At 8 months postoperatively, the patient is pain free, ambulates with a cane because of increasing pain in the left hip, and has 70 degrees of flexion with grade 4 HO.

was noted postoperatively in only 11% of patients after THA by Kilgus and associates (51). Thus, HO has not been found to be consistently common after THA in ankylosing spondylitis.

Men have demonstrated a higher rate of postoperative HO than women (54). Men have also been associated with a greater volume of HO formed than women (95). The risk of developing HO is increased in patients who have had prior surgery or trauma to the hip (54). Pritchett

and associates recommend perioperative prophylaxis for all patients having THA after acetabular fracture (82).

In addition to patient factors, surgical factors play a role in the development of HO. Surgical trauma to the soft tissues, and bone debris from the reaming of the femoral and acetabular beds, can promote the formation of HO. Arthroplasties that are more complex with longer operative times have been associated with an increased rate of HO postoperatively (84). Although it has been

TABLE 1. *Risk factors for formation of heterotopic ossification*

Patient factors
Hypertrophic osteoarthritis
Diffuse idiopathic skeletal hyperostosis
Ankylosing spondylitis
Advanced age
Male sex
Previous heterotopic ossification
Previous trauma to the hip

Technique factors
Surgical approach
Trochanteric osteotomy
Femoral fracture
Prolonged operative time
Anesthesia
Postoperative hematoma
Dislocation
Infection
Method of component fixation

claimed that the anterior and transtrochanteric approaches are associated with an increased rate of HO compared to posterior approaches (7), several studies have not supported this assertion, demonstrating no significant difference in the rate of HO on the basis of surgical approach (24,72,85).

The type of prosthesis used has also been a source of concern for the development of HO. Maloney and associates demonstrated an increased rate of HO after the use of noncemented stems compared to a similar group of patients receiving cemented stems with identical noncemented acetabular reconstruction (65). Noting the opposite, Lieberman and associates found an increased rate of HO after cemented THA in patients with OA (62). Others, However, have not been able to determine a difference in the rate of HO based on the type of component fixation (23,93). Postoperative complications such as hematoma and dislocation may also lead to an increased rate of HO (5). This may be related to greater injury to the soft tissues around the hip when these events occur.

The large number of factors possibly resulting in HO, and the large variation in the rate of HO between studies make comparison difficult. In addition, factors such as deep venous thrombosis (DVT) prophylaxis also play a role. Pagnani and associates demonstrated a significant decrease in the rate of HO in a group of patients receiving aspirin for DVT prophylaxis compared to a group receiving coumadin (77).

Classification

Several classifications of HO have been described (37,75). The most commonly used, the Brooker classification (12), describes four grades. Grade 1 consists of isolated islands of bone in the soft tissues. In grade 2, exostoses extend from either the pelvis, the femur, or both, with a separation of more than 1 cm (Fig. 2). In grade 3, the exostoses are separated by less than 1 cm (Fig. 3). Grade 4 represents radiographic ankylosis of the hip (Fig. 4). Grades 1 and 2 and many cases of grade 3 HO are associated with few clinical symptoms. However, clinical symptoms are commonly present in patients with grade 4. Extensive HO can result in restricted range of motion and, rarely, clinical ankylosis of the hip. In this subgroup of patients, resection of the bone can be beneficial, but the rate of recurrence without prophylaxis can be high.

Prophylaxis

Prevention of HO in the high risk patient is the most effective method to obtain an excellent clinical result after arthroplasty. All patients should receive meticulous surgical technique to minimize surgical trauma to the soft tissues and to minimize contamination of the soft tissues with particulate bone debris, which may promote HO. Beyond this, there are two therapeutic limbs for prophylaxis: pharmacologic and radiation therapy.

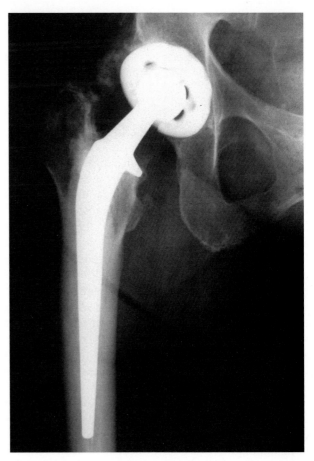

FIG. 2. Grade 2 heterotopic ossification 1 year after total hip arthroplasty in a 65-year-old woman.

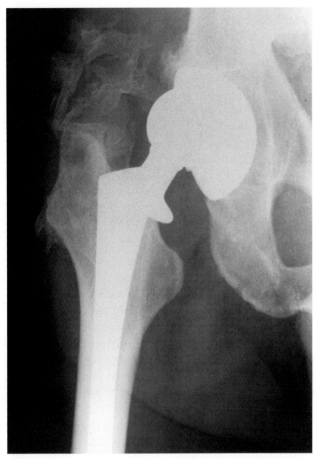

FIG. 3. Grade 3 heterotopic ossification 5 years after total hip arthroplasty in a 72-year-old man.

Pharmacologic Prophylaxis of HO

Two principal classes of medications have been utilized as prophylaxis historically: nonsteroidal anti-inflammatory drugs (NSAIDs) and diphosphonates. Diphosphonates were initially recommended because they were found to inhibit the mineralization of bone and appeared to be effective in preventing the formation of HO (26). However, it has been demonstrated that while diphosphonates delay the radiographic appearance of HO, they do not prevent the local formation of unmineralized bone matrix. Ossification of the osteoid is inhibited as long as the medication is administered. However, when the diphosphonate is stopped, the osteoid ossifies and the HO appears both clinically and radiographically (100). Thus, diphosphonates are no longer recommended as a prophylactic agent for HO.

Nonsteroidal anti-inflammatory drugs function through the inhibition of prostaglandin production and other cellular mediators. The specific mechanism leading to inhibition of HO is poorly understood. However, multiple studies have documented the beneficial effect of these drugs in the prevention of HO (Table 2). The most

widely studied NSAID for the prophylaxis of HO is indomethacin. However, many NSAIDs have been studied for their effectiveness as prophylactic agents against HO. The optimal dosage and length of therapy have yet to be determined. Many early series used a 6-week course of therapy on an empiric basis. However, several studies now demonstrate a 2-week course of therapy to be effective prophylaxis (see Table 2). The shortest course found effective was described by Pritchett, who found six doses of Ketorolac postoperatively to be effective prophylaxis after THA (83). NSAID therapy is commonly initiated on the first postoperative day. Delay beyond 5 to 7 days can limit the effectiveness of the prophylaxis (96).

Concern has been raised regarding the inhibition of bone ingrowth by NSAIDs. Keller and associates found the administration of indomethacin to attenuate the increase in bone ingrowth into a porous titanium implant in rabbits (48). In a similar study utilizing a cobalt–chromium implant, Trancik and associates demonstrated a reduction in bone ingrowth with aspirin, ibuprophen, and indomethacin (103). The response was noted to be

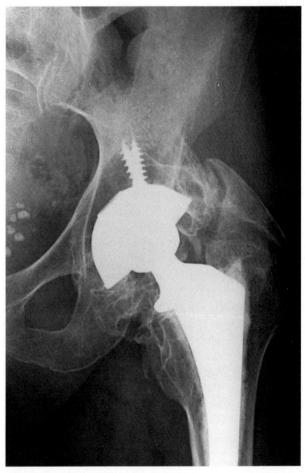

FIG. 4. Grade 4 heterotopic ossification 4 years after total hip arthroplasty in an 81-year-old woman. Her postoperative course was complicated by a stroke.

TABLE 2. *The effect of nonsteroidal anti-inflammatory drugs (NSAIDs) for prophylaxis of HO*

Author (ref.)	NSAID	Duration of treatment	Effectiveness
Ahrengart (2)	Ibuprophen	10 da	No effect
Burssens et al. (14)	Tenoxicam 10 mg/da	6 wk	2/27 grade 3
	Tenoxicam 20 mg/d	6 wk	1/26 grade 3
	Placebo	6 wk	5/27 grade 3
Gebhur et al. (30)	Naproxen	8 da	3/27 any HO
	Untreated	8 wk	12/23 any HO
Hoikka et al. (42)	Flurbiprofen	3 wk	3/32 any HO
	Placebo	3 wk	14/31 any HO
Huk et al. (43)	Aspirin	2 wk	0% grade 3 or 4
	Indomethacin	2 wk	0% grade 3 or 4
Kjaersgaard-Anderson et al. (55)	Indomethacin	2 wk	1/19 any HO
	Placebo	2 wk	11/22 any HO
Kjaersgaard-Anderson and Ritter) (56	Indomethacin	2 wk	0/13 any HO
	Aspirin	6 wk	1/33 grade 1 HO
Pritchett (83)	Ketorolac	2 da	0/152 severe HO
	Untreated		11/151 severe HO
Tozun et al. (102)	Indomethacin	4 wk	0/29 significant HO
	Untreated		8/27 significant HO
Wahlstrom et al. (106)	Diclofenac	6 wk	1/46 any HO
	Placebo	6 wk	35/47 any HO

monly used after THA for DVT prophylaxis, such as coumadin, heparin, or low-molecular-weight heparin, may lead to excessive postoperative bleeding or hematoma formation if used with NSAIDs. Kristensen and associates did not note any increase in bleeding complications postoperatively when combining indomethacin with low dose heparin in the early postoperative period (58). However, when used in conjunction with hypotensive epidural anesthesia, aspirin alone has been found to be excellent prophylaxis for both DVT and HO after THA (43).

Radiation Therapy as HO Prophylaxis

Radiation therapy has been repeatedly demonstrated to be effective as prophylaxis for HO (Table 3). The specific mechanism of the inhibition is not fully understood. However, it is known that radiation therapy affects cells that are actively dividing and therefore it most likely prevents the metaplasia of the local soft-tissue cells that produce osteoid matrix. On a theoretical basis, therefore, therapy should be instituted in the early postoperative period prior to the formation of osteoid matrix. This has been borne out in clinical studies that demonstrate reduced effectiveness of the therapy if instituted more than 3 to 7 days postoperatively (20).

Radiation initially was administered postoperatively in 1000 to 2000 cGy total dose in five to ten fractions (18). Recent data demonstrate effective therapy can be delivered with a does of 700 to 800 cGy in single-dose therapy (27,39,88). Healy et al. established a lower threshold

dose related and did not significantly reduce ingrowth at 2 weeks compared to a control group. A clinical study with porous-ingrowth total hip arthroplasty was unable to demonstrate any compromise in early fixation resulting from the use of NSAIDs for HO prophylaxis (53).

Two other areas of concern more significantly impacted the use of NSAIDs in the early postoperative period. The first was the side-effects of these medications. The most commonly observed is gastrointestinal intolerance. Other effects such as central nervous system depression, headache, and renal insufficiency combined with gastrointestinal intolerance have contributed to as many as 20% of patients discontinuing therapy prior to completion of the regimen (89). This form of prophylaxis is contraindicated for patients with a history of peptic ulcer disease, renal insufficiency, liver compromise, or allergic reaction or intolerance to NSAIDs.

The NSAIDs also have an inhibitory effect on platelet adhesion. This effect can potentially lead to increased postoperative bleeding if initiated after surgery. In addition, platelet inhibition may not be desirable with some forms of prophylaxis for DVT. Medications that are com-

TABLE 3. *Effectiveness of radiation therapy as prophylaxis for HO*

Author	Dose	Fractions	Results
Kennedy et al. (49)	1000 cGy	5	7/32 any HO
Healy et al. (39)	700 cGy	1	2/34 grades 2 and 3
Healy et al. (40)	550 cGy	1	12/19 any HO
	700 cGy	1	9/88 any HO
Fingeroth and Ahmed (27)	600 cGy	1	3/45 grade 2 or 3
Schai et al. (88)	600 cGy	1	0/17 HO
Maloney et al. (64)	7.5 Gy	3	0/15 grade 3 or 4
Pelligrini et al. (80)	800 cGy	1	21% any HO
	1000 cGy	5	21% any HO
Seegenschmeidt et al. (91)	7 Gy preop	1	2/23 x-ray failure
	17.5 Gy postop	5	1/21 x-ray failure
Gregoritch et al. (34)	8 Gy, <4 hr preop	1	2% grade 3 or 4
	8 Gy, <48 hr postop	1	5% grade 3 or 4

dose, noting reduced effectiveness with a single dose of 550 cGy (40). Therapy is commonly administered through anteroposterior portals to avoid the incision. If cemented components were inserted, no specific shielding is necessary for the implant. However, if a trochanteric osteotomy was utilized, the osteotomy site should be shielded. When porous ingrowth components are utilized, shielding is necessary to protect the prosthesis–bone interface from radiation, which may prevent the inhibition of ingrowth (101). Alternatively, a rectangular portal can be oriented to expose the tissue between the pelvis and the proximal femur. Use of the rectangular portal has been associated with a 31% rate of extraportal ossification (80).

Seegenschmeidt and associates studied a randomized group of patients comparing 7 Gy single-dose preoperative therapy versus five fractions of 3.5 Gy postoperatively (91). No clinically significant HO developed in either group. Pelligrini and associates also performed a randomized trial comparing pre- versus postoperative radiotherapy (34,79). The groups received 8 Gy either less than 6 hours prior to the procedure or less than 51 hours after the procedure. No significant difference was noted between the two groups in appearance of HO, functional outcome, or fixation as judged from radiographs. Three trochanteric nonunions were noted in the preoperative group. The preoperative dosing eliminated the potential pain and difficulty in transporting patients in the early postoperative period while maintaining efficacy.

Radiation therapy has not been associated with delayed wound healing if the incision is excluded from the portal. As radiation therapy does not have any effect on bleeding, there is no concern of interaction or alteration in the selection of DVT prophylaxis postoperatively. In addition, the therapy can be completely administered while the patient is hospitalized. This eliminates the concern of patient tolerance or compliance with the therapy. These are distinct advantages of radiation therapy for HO prophylaxis. The disadvantages are the need for careful shielding or exclusion of porous-coated surfaces and trochanteric osteotomy sites. The induction of a local sarcoma from radiation therapy is another concern. However, two reviews of radiation therapy–induced sarcomas found no secondary sarcomas in patients receiving less than 3000 cGy over less than 3 weeks (9,52). The current low-dose protocols are well below this level with a lower threshold for efficacy at approximately 700 to 800 cGy.

Treatment of HO

The majority of patients who develop HO have no functional deficit. However, patients who develop grade 3 or 4 HO will manifest a reduction in the range of motion of the hip. Patients may also have a significant amount of pain associated with extensive HO. If the pain is unresponsive to conservative measures, resection of the HO should be considered. Restriction of the range of motion alone is infrequently an indication for resection. An additional indication for resection of HO may occur at the time of revision surgery in patients who have preexisting extensive HO.

Resection of HO should be delayed until the bone is mature (usually 6 to 12 months after the last surgery) to reduce the risk of recurrence (25). Maturity is assessed by review of plain radiographs to determine if the lesion is stable between serial radiographs. The HO should have the radiographic appearance of mature bone. Additional studies that can be beneficial are bone CT scan and the serum alkaline phosphatase. The bone scan will demonstrate uptake similar to that of the uninvolved bone of the pelvis when the HO is mature. The serum alkaline phos-

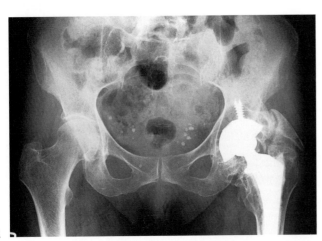 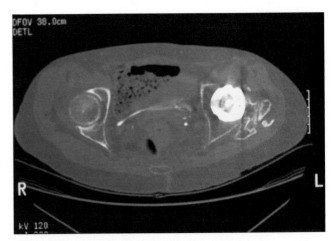

FIG. 5. A: The AP pelvic radiograph of the patient in Figure 4. **B:** CT illustrates the posterior location of the HO extending from the posterior rim of the acetabulum. A small island of heterotopic bone is also located just posterior to the greater trochanter. This study can assist in preoperative planning for resection of the heterotopic bone.

phatase should be normal. Preoperative planning may be aided by the use of computed axial tomography (CAT) scan images to improve assessment of the location and volume of HO to be resected (Fig. 5).

Resection of the HO should be as atraumatic as possible to maintain the integrity of the remaining soft tissues and to reduce the risk of recurrence. Consideration should be given to obtaining an intraoperative radiograph to verify that all HO has been resected. All patients undergoing resection of HO around a THA should have prophylaxis to prevent or minimize recurrence. Prophylaxis can be in the form of NSAIDs, such as indomethacin, or radiation therapy, as outlined above.

LOCAL MALIGNANCY

Joint replacement requires the insertion of artificial implants constructed of metals and plastic. Although these materials have been demonstrated to be biocompatible in bulk form, they may be harmful in particulate or ionic form. Periarticular osteolysis and bone resorption is becoming an increasing problem, resulting in revision surgery (38), with a growing volume of data demonstrating the central role of particulate polymeric and metallic debris in the production of osteolysis (13,108). This debris has been documented to travel to regional lymph nodes, and it can result in increased metal levels detected in the patients serum and urine (45–47).

The metals and polymers utilized in the production and fixation of orthopedic implants can induce malignancy (15,70,94,98). Chromium salts, cobalt, iron, nickel, beryllium, cadmium, zinc, and titanium have been shown to induce tumors in laboratory animals (70,71,92). Industrial exposure to metals such as nickel and chromium has been associated with an increased incidence of pulmonary malignancies (22). These agents may induce malignant degeneration by alteration of the cellular DNA or because of the physical characteristics of the material (10,28). The potential, therefore, exists for debris from an arthroplasty to result in either local or distant malignancy.

Local malignancy has been documented in several papers (Table 4). Martin and associates summarized 15 cases of tumor at the site of an implant, including eight total joint replacements (67). In the case presented by Martin and associates, increased levels of metal were detected in the tumor tissue. Brien and associates also measured the metal levels in an osteosarcoma at the site of a THA (11). Increased levels of chromium, nickel, and barium were detected in the local tissues. Seventeen cases of local malignancy have been reported around total joint replacements. Eight cases were malignant fibrous histiocytoma or fibrosarcoma. In addition, the majority of the cases involved the use of cobalt–chromium implants. No definitive conclusions regarding the risk of local malignancy can be drawn from these cases. However, it does give rise to concern. Three of the cases were in patients with the Mckee-Farrar implants, with a metal-on-metal articulation. New devices with metal–metal articulations may eliminate polyethylene debris but may create other unanticipated complications. A central tumor registry would be beneficial to assist in identifying these cases and perhaps determine the risk or relationship of local malignancy after total joint replacement.

Several studies have documented the distant spread of debris from a total hip arthroplasty (17,41). Jacobs and associates have identified increased levels of metal in the urine of patients with well-functioning titanium alloy total hip replacements (45). This increased exposure to metal particles and metal ions may increase the risk of distant malignancy as well as a local tumor. Gillespie and associates studied the incidence of distant tumors in patients after total hip replacement (31). The authors reviewed the records of 1358 individuals who had had a total hip replacement from 1966 to 1973. They then correlated these patients with the New Zealand Cancer Registry and the Register of Deaths over the period from 1966 to 1983. The rate of cancer in the THA population was then compared to the general population extracted from data published by the New Zealand Health Statistics Centre, yielding a total follow-up of 14,286 person-years for the study population with 164 cancers recorded. The results for all cancers revealed a decreased rate of cancer in the THA population at less than 10 years follow-up [107 cancers observed versus 143.8 cancers expected ($p < .01$)]. However, after 10 years follow-up there was a significant increase in cancer rate in the THA population [57 observed versus 36 expected ($p < .01$)]. Considering specific tumors, the authors noted a reduced risk of cancer of the breast and colon. An increase was noted in the incidence of tumors of the lymphatic and hemopoietic systems [21 observed versus 12 expected, ($p < .05$)]. The most significant increase was in the first year postoperatively [5 observed versus 1 expected ($p < .01$)]. However, even if these tumors in the first year were excluded, the increased rate of lymphatic and hemopoietic tumors remained elevated ($p < .05$). The authors concluded that the risk of lymphatic and hemopoietic tumors may be increased due to either the underlying diseaseor the medical treatment for arthritis prior to joint replacement, or as a response to the surgery and THA implants. However, the authors stressed that the risk of malignancy remains low. The risk of developing a tumor of the lymphatic or hemopoietic system was 2 out of 1000 in the general population over 10 years, compared to 6 out of 1000 in the THA population.

Nyren and associates performed a similar study correlating the Swedish Inpatient Register with the Swedish Cancer Register (76). A cohort of 39,154 patients were identified and 327,922 person-years were covered in the

TABLE 4. *Local malignancy as a complication of THA*

Author (ref.)	Location	Implant	Interval from insertion to identification of tumor (yr)	Tumor	Materials
Arden and Bywaters (4)	Femur	Mckee-Farrar THA	2.5	Fibrosarcoma	Cobalt–chromium
Bago-Granell et al. (6)	Femur	Cemented Charnley-Müller THA	2	Malignant fibrous histiocytoma	n.a.
Pennen and Ring (81)	Femur	Uncemented ring prosthesis	5	Osteosarcoma	Cobalt–chromium
Ryu et al. (87)	Acetabulum	Uncemented THA	15 mo	Sarcoma	Alumina, cobalt-chromium
Weber (107)	Tibia	Cemented TKA	4.5	Epitheiloid sarcoma	Cobalt–chromium
Swann (97)	Femur	Cemented McKee-Farrar	4	Malignant fibrous histiocytoma	Cobalt–chromium
Case Records of MGH (16)	Femur	Austin Moore THR	3.5	Giant cell tumor malignancy	n.a.
Martin et al. (67)	Femur	Cemented Charnley-Müller THA	10	Osteosarcoma	Cobalt–chromium
Lamovec et al. (60)	Femur	Cemented Charnley-Müller THA	12	Synovial sarcoma	Stainless steel
Brien et al. (11)	Femur	Cemented Charnley THA	8	Osteosarcoma	Stainless steel
Nelson et al. (73)	Femur	Cemented Müller THA	10	Malignant fibrous histiocytoma	Cobalt–chromium
Troop et al. (104)	Femur	Multiple THAs	15	Malignant fibrous histiocytoma	Multiple
Haag et al. (35)	Femur	Weber-Huggler THR	10	Malignant fibrous histiodytoma	n.a.
Kolstad et al. (57)	Femur	Freeman-Swanson TKR	3 mo	Adenocarcinoma	Cobalt–chromium
Tait et al. (99)	Gluteal region	Charnley-Müller THR	11	Malignant fibrous histiocytoma	Cobalt–chromium
van der List et al. (105)	Distal femur	Charnley-Müller THR, Aufranc-Turner THR	15	Malignant epithelioid haemangio-endothelioma	Cobalt–chromium
Rushforth et al. (86)	Acetabulum	McKee-Farrar THR	6 mo	Osteosarcoma	Cobalt–chromium
Jacobs et al. (44)	Femur	Noncemented THA	5 mo	Malignant fibrous histiocytoma	Titanium alloy
Aboulafia et al. (1)	Femur	Endoprosthesis with chronic infection	2	Malignant fibrous histiocytoma	Cobalt–chromium

MGH, Massachusetts General Hospital; n.a., information not given.

study period. The authors noted an overall increase in cancer risk of 3%. No significant difference was noted in the rate of bone or connective tissue tumors (bone tumors, 6 observed versus 4 expected; connective tissue tumors, 28 observed versus 26 expected). Increased risks were noted for kidney cancer, prostate cancer, and mel-anoma. No significant increase was noted for hemato-poietic or lymphatic tumors. The authors concluded that the risk of cancer after THA is negligible from a public health perspective. Mathiesen and associates studied a smaller population in Sweden of 10,785 individuals and 58,437 person-years over the study period 1974 to 1989

(68). They found no relationship between THA and lymphatic or hematopoietic tumors in their population.

The incidence of local malignancies reported is minute compared to the number of THAs currently implanted (3,36). The risk of systemic or distant malignancy also appears to be low. However, continued close observation is necessary as the technology evolves. New techniques, new implants, and new articulations must be carefully followed to accurately assess the safety of these new developments.

STRESS FRACTURES

Stress fractures can occur when relatively high repetitive stress is applied to normal bone, and insufficiency fractures occur when relatively normal repetitive stress is applied to weakened bone. They commonly occur in patients who have an increase in either load or activity. For example, military recruits typically develop stress fractures in the metatarsals 2 to 3 weeks after the initiation of training. The bone, in response to the new level of stress, remodels by first removing bone through osteoclastic action to prepare for new bone deposition. However, after bone has been removed and prior to deposition, the bone is weakened and subject to fracture even with normal activities. These fractures can be nondisplaced and difficult to identify on radiographs, and occasionally they are detected only after callus begins to form. Bone scans or magnetic resonance imaging (MRI) may be able to demonstrate these lesions in the absence of changes on plain radiographs.

Significant alterations in the stress pattern delivered to the femur and acetabulum occur after THA. In addition, osteoporosis is common in the elderly patient population. These two factors alone or in combination can predispose a patient to a stress or other fracture after THA (33,69). The incidence of this late complication is unknown. However, the differential diagnosis of the patient with pain after THA should include stress fractures.

Few reports exist in the literature describing stress fractures. Marmour published a case with a stress fracture of the pubic ramus (66). This occurred in an 80-year-old patient 1 year after THA. The patient had pain with motion of the hip and with weight bearing. Radiographs demonstrated a radiolucent line about the acetabular component, suggesting loosening. The patient had a medical evaluation to rule out metastatic disease to the pelvis, but the author did not indicate if a bone scan had been obtained. Repeat radiographs 1 month later revealed a healing stress fracture of the pubic ramus. The patient's symptoms subsequently improved and she returned to her previous ambulatory status without pain.

Launder and Hungerford published an additional case of a pubic stress fracture after THA (61). This case involved a 46-year-old woman with rheumatoid arthritis who had received medical therapy with prednisone, cytoxin, aspirin, gold salts, and penicillamine. The patient had a THA for 6 years without symptoms. She noted gradually increasing pain after getting out of a car. Her pain progressed until she could no longer bear weight. She had pain with motion of the hip and in the groin. Radiographs and medical work up were initiated to rule out loosening or infection. Radiographs obtained at the time of an arthrogram demonstrated an incomplete fracture of the superior pubic ramus. The fracture subsequently went on to heal and the patient returned to a pain-free status.

In addition to fractures in the pubic rami, fractures can occur in the sacrum in osteoporotic patients. These can occur in patients without prior surgery as well as in patients after THA (Fig. 6). Three cases were reported by Lourie referred to as spontaneous osteoporotic fracture of the sacrum (SOFS). The fractures were in elderly osteoporotic patients. The patients complained of severe incapacitating pain in the low back, leg, and groin without antecedent trauma or injury. The patients were neurologically intact and without tension signs. However, severe pain to palpation over the sacrum was a common feature. Plain radiographs were commonly negative. Bone scan revealed diffuse uptake in the sacrum and tomography demonstrated the fracture in all three of the patients. The patients were treated with activity restricted to tolerance and pain control, followed by gradual mobilization. Two of the fractures healed without sequelae; the third patient died of an aspiration pneumonia.

Newhouse and associates reviewed a series of 17 patients (74). The majority presented with severe pain in the back, buttock, or groin without trauma or with a minor injury. Ten patients had a fracture of the pubic ramus as well. The fractures were rarely evident on plain radiographs. Bone scan and CT were diagnostic in all patients. The patients without severe medical disease resolved with the use of non-narcotic analgesic medications, rest, and gradual return to ambulation. The time to pain-free independent ambulation was 11 months (range, 4 to 24 months).

Stress fractures can also occur in the femur. Lotke and associates published a report of two cases of femoral stress fracture in association with a cortical window after revision THA (63). These cases demonstrated gradual onset of thigh pain after revision THA. No history of acute trauma was present in either case. The pain began 12 and 6 months after the revision surgery. Plain radiographs were positive in one patient. Bone scans were positive in both patients. The patients were evaluated for infection and loosening and neither was identified. One patient was treated in a spica cast for 12 weeks with resolution of symptoms and pain-free ambulation 18 months after the fracture. The second patient was treated initially with restricted weight bearing. This failed to alleviate the symptoms after 8 weeks. The patient then underwent

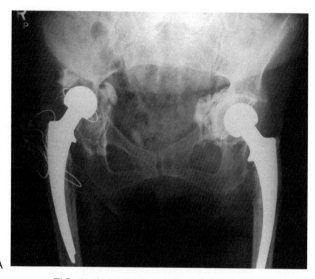

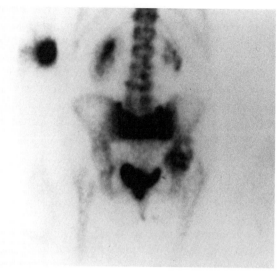

FIG. 6. A: The AP pelvic radiograph of an 82-year-old woman with a history of osteoporosis and previous lumbar compression fractures. She had had a bilateral total hip replacement 10 years previously. Although she had noted the gradual increase in right hip pain, while riding in a car 2 weeks prior to presentation, she developed the rapid onset of severe incapacitating pain in the buttock and right hip. She was unable to bear weight. No acute fractures are noted. Comparison with previous radiographs obtained 1 year ago demonstrated no change in component position of either THA. **B:** A ^{99}CT MDP bone scan posterior view revealed a typical diffuse uptake in the sacrum consistent with a sacral insufficiency fracture. The patient was treated conservatively with restriction of activities and pain control. Her symptoms improved and at 3 months after the fracture she had returned to her previous ambulatory sta-

open bone grafting, followed by 12 weeks of spica immobilization. Follow-up at 24 months after fracture revealed the patient to have pain-free ambulation and radiographs demonstrated healing.

These cases emphasize the need to bypass stress risers in the femur to reduce the stress concentration at these sites (78,90). Patients suspected of a femoral or pelvic stress fracture should also be evaluated for the more common entities of loosening or infection. Bone scans, tomography, and CT can be helpful in the diagnosis of stress fractures. When evaluating patients with THA and severe pain prior radiographs are very helpful in the differentiation of loosening from other causes of pain in the hip, buttock, and groin. Pelvic and sacral fractures can be conservatively treated with pain control and gradual mobilization as tolerated. The data regarding femoral stress fractures are scanty. These patients may benefit from surgical intervention to assist healing and prevent progression to an unstable fracture.

LATE INSTABILITY

Many factors can impact the rate of dislocation, such as prior hip surgery, component malposition, trochanteric nonunion, weak myofascial sleeve, operative approach, component design, and postoperative range of motion. The majority of dislocations occur early after surgery (50). Woo and Morrey noted 59% of dislocations

occurred by 3 months postoperatively and 77% had occurred by 1 year (109). However, they found that 6% of dislocations occurred 5 years after surgery. Coventry and Scanlon documented a dislocation rate of 0.4% from 5 to 10 years after hip replacement (18).

Khan et al. noted that a dislocation that occurred beyond 5 weeks postoperatively had a higher rate of recurrent dislocation than patients with the initial dislocation in the first 5 weeks (50). This phenomenon was also noted by Woo and Morrey (109). Coventry and Scanlon specifically addressed the problem of late dislocation (18), reviewing 32 THAs in 32 patients whose initial dislocation occurred between 5 and 10 years postoperatively. No significant relationship between the number of surgeries to the hip prior to THA, the approach, trochanteric union, or loosening with late dislocation were seen. The data suggested that this group of patients had a greater range of motion, 97° of flexion compared to 91°, than the general population of hip arthroplasty patients. In addition, it was noted that this group had an increased incidence of radiographic acetabular loosening. Coventry and Scanlon noted that 44% of patients required additional surgery: six needed acetabular revision and four needed revision of both components, two required exploration with excision of ectopic bone or scar, and two required an open reduction of the hip. One hip with a trochanteric nonunion had the trochanter repaired at the time of component revision. Dislocation had recurred in two THAs after surgery.

Daly and Morrey reviewed the results of operative correction of an unstable THA (19). Comparing dislocations that occurred after 5 years with those that occurred earlier, they found no difference in the success of operative correction. Dislocation had recurred in 39% of patients after operative correction. The authors noted that the operative stabilization was the most successful if a precise determination of the cause of the instability is made and appropriate correction performed.

SUMMARY

Total hip arthroplasty is extremely successful for the relief of pain and restoration of function, resulting from arthritic conditions of the hip. Complications can and do occur after THA, many arising in the early postoperative period. However, it is important to remember that complications can occur late after THA. Long-term follow-up is necessary to identify and treat these complications. In addition, long-term follow-up is also essential to detect complications related to wear and wear debris, as discussed in other chapters. Induction of primary sarcoma at the site of THA is a concerning complication. Although the incidence appears to be low, continued surveillance may be beneficial to detect and treat this complication early. In summary, many of the late complications can be prevented and the morbidity minimized by careful assessment of the patient preoperatively, by meticulous surgical technique, and by appropriate postoperative management.

REFERENCES

1. Aboulafia AJ, Littelton K, Shmookler B, Malawar MM. Malignant fibrous histiocytoma at the site of hip replacement in association with chronic infection. *Orthop Rev* 1994;23(5):427–432.
2. Ahrengart L. Periarticular heterotopic ossification after total hip arthroplasty. *Clin Orthop* 1991;263:49–58.
3. Apley AG. Malignancy and joint replacement: the tip of the iceberg *(editorial)*. *J Bone Joint Surg* 1989;71B(1):1.
4. Arden GP, Bywaters EGL. Tissue reaction. In: Arden GP, Ansell BM, eds. *Surgical management of juvenile chronic polyarthritis.* London: Academic Press, 1978;269–270.
5. Azcarate JR, dePablos J, Cornejo F, Canadell J. Postoperative dislocation: a risk factor for periprosthetic ectopic ossifications after total hip replacement. *Acta Orthop Belg* 1986;52:145.
6. Bago-Granell J, Morris E, Aguirre-Canyadell M, Nardi J, Tallada N. Malignant fibrous histiocytoma of bone at the site of total hip arthroplasty. A case report. *J Bone Joint Surg* 1984;66B(1):38–40.
7. Bischoff R, Dunlap J, Carpenter L, Demouy E, Barrack R. Heterotopic ossification following uncemented total hip arthroplasty. Effect of the operative approach. *J Arthroplasty* 1994;9(6):641–644.
8. Bisla RS, Ranawat CS, Inglis AE. Total hip replacement in patients with ankylosing spondylitis with involvement of the hip. *J Bone Joint Surg* 1976;58A:233–238.
9. Brady LW. Radiation-induced sarcomas of bone. *Skeletal Radiol* 1979;4:72.
10. Brand KG. Foreign body induced sarcomas. In: Becker FF, ed. *Cancer, a comprehensive treatise*, vol 1. New York: Plenum Press, 1975; 485–511.
11. Brien WW, Salvati EA, Healey JH, Bansal M, Ghelman B, Betts F. Osteogenic sarcoma arising in the area of a total hip replacement. a case report. *J Bone Joint Surg* 1990;72A(7):1097–1099.
12. Brooker AF, Bowerman JW, Robinson RA, Riley LH. Ectopic ossification following total hip replacement: incidence and a method of classification. *J Bone Joint Surg* 1973;55(A):1629–1632.
13. Buly RL, Huo MH, Salvati EA, Brien WH, Bansal M. Titanium wear debris in failed cemented total hip arthroplasty: an analysis of 71 cases. *J Arthroplasty* 1992;7(3):315–323.
14. Burssens A, Thiery J, Kohl P, Molderez A, Haazen L. Prevention of heterotopic ossification with tenoxicam following total hip arthroplasty: a double blind, placebo-controlled dose-finding study. *Acta Orthop Belg* 1995;61(3):205–211.
15. Carter RL, Roe FJC. Induction of sarcomas in rats by solid and fragmented polyethylene: experimental observations and clinical implications. *Br J Cancer* 1969;23:401–407.
16. Case Records of the Massachusetts General Hospital: Case 38-1965. *N Engl J Med* 1965;273:494–504.
17. Case CP, Langkamer VG, James C, Palmer MR, et al. Widespread dissemination of metal debris from implants. *J Bone Joint Surg* 1994; 76B(5):701–712.
18. Coventry MB, Scanlon DW. The use of radiation therapy to discourage ectopic bone. *J Bone Joint Surg* 1981;63(A):201.
19. Daly PJ, Morrey BF. Operative correction of an unstable total hip arthroplasty. *J Bone Joint Surg* 1992;74A(9):1334–1343.
20. DeFlitch CJ, Strker JA. Postoperative hip irradiation in prevention of heterotopic ossification: causes of treatment failure. *Radiology* 1993; 188(1):265–270.
21. Delee J, Ferrari A, Charnley J. Ectopic bone formation following low friction arthroplasty of the hip. *Clin Orthop* 1976;121:53.
22. Doll R. Cancer of the lung and nose in nickel workers. *Br J Indust Med* 1958;15:217–223.
23. Duck HJ, Mylod AG. Heterotopic bone in hip arthroplasties. Cemented versus noncemented. *Clin Orthop* 1992;282:145–153.
24. Errico TJ. Fetto JF, Waugh TR. Heterotopic ossification. Incidence and relation to trochanteric osteotomy in 100 total hip arthroplasties. *Clin Orthop* 1984;190:138–141.
25. Fahmy NRM, Wrobelewski BM. Recurrance of ectopic ossification after excision in Charnley low friction arthroplasty. *Acta Orthop Scand* 1982;53:799.
26. Finerman GAM, Stover SL. Heterotopic ossification following hip replacement or spinal cord injury: two clinical studies with EHDP. *Bone* 1981;3:337.
27. Fingeroth RJ, Ahmed AQ. Single-dose 6 Gy prophylaxis for heterotopic ossification after total hip arthroplasty. *Clin Orthop* 1995;317: 1313–140.
28. Friend SH, Horowitz JM, Gerber MR, et al. Deletions of a DNA sequence in both retinoblastoma and mesenchymal tumors: organization of the sequence and its encoded protein. *Proc Natl Acad Sci USA* 1987;84:9059–9063.
29. Garland DE, Blum CE, Waters RL. Periarticular heterotopic ossification in head-injured adults. *J Bone Joint Surg* 1980;62A(7): 1143–1146.
30. Gebhur P, Soelberg M, Orsnes T, Wilbek H. Naproxen prevention of heterotopic ossification after hip arthroplasty: a prospective control study of 55 patients. *Acta Orthop Scand* 1991;62(3):226–229.
31. Gillespie WJ, Frampton CMA, Henderson RJ, Ryan PM. The incidence of cancer following total hip replacement. *J Bone Joint Surg* 1988;70B(4):539–542.
32. Goel A, Sharp DJ. Heterotopic bone formation after hip replacement: the influence of the type of osteoarthritis. *J Bone Joint Surg* 1991; 73B:255–257.
33. Green DL. Complications of total hip replacement. *South Med J* 1976; 69(12):1559–1564.
34. Gregoritch SJ, Chadha M, Pelligrini VD, Rubin P, Kantorowitz DA. Randomized trial comparing preoperative versus postoperative irradiation for the prevention of hererotopic ossification following prosthetic total hip replacement: preliminary. 1997.
35. Haag M, Adler CP. Malignant fibrous histiocytoma in association with hip replacement. *J Bone Joint Surgery Br* 1989;71B:701.
36. Hamblen DL, Carter RL. Sarcoma and joint replacement *(editorial)*. *J Bone Joint Surg* 1984;66B(1):625–627.
37. Hamblen DL, Harris WH, Rottiger J. Myositis ossificans as a complication of hip arthroplasty. In: Procedings of the British Orthopaedic Association. *J Bone Joint Surg* 1961;53(B):764.
38. Harris WH. The problem is osteolysis. *Clin Orthop* 1995;311:46–53.
39. Healy WL, Lo TC, Covall DJ, Pfeifer BA, Wasilewski SA. Single-dose

radiation therapy for the prevention of heterotopic ossification after total hip arthroplasty. *J Arthroplasty* 1990;5(4):369–375.

40. Healy WL, Lo TC, Desimone AA, Rask B, Pfeifer BA. Single-dose irradiation for the prevention of heterotopic ossification after total hip arthroplasty: a comparison of doses of five hundred and fifty and seven hundred centigray. *J Bone Joint Surg.*

41. Hicks DG, Judkins AR, Sickel JZ, Rosier RN, et al. Granular histiocytosis of pelvic lymph nodes following total hip arthroplasty: the presence of wear debris, cytokine production and immunologically activated macrophages. *J Bone Joint Surg.*

42. Hoikka V, Lindholm TS, Eskola A. Flurbiprophen inhibits heterotopic bone formation in total hip arthroplasty. *Arch Orthop Trauma Surg* 1990;109(4):224–226.

43. Huk OL, Evans BG, Lieberman JR, Pellicci PM, Sculco TP, Salvati EA. Aspirin versus indomethacin versus coumadin for the prevention of deep venous thrombosis and their effect on heterotopic ossification. Presented at the 64th meeting of the American Academy of Orthopaedic Surgeons.

44. Jacobs JJ, Rosenbaum DH, Hay RM, Gitelis S, Black J. Early sarcomatous degeneration near a cementless hip replacement: a case report and review. *J Bone Joint Surg* 1992;74B(5):740–744.

45. Jacobs JJ, Skipor AK, Black J, Urban RM, Galante JO. Release and excretion of metal in patients who have a total hip replacement component made of titanium base alloy. *J Bone Joint Surg* 1991;73A(10):1475–1486.

46. Jacobs JJ, Urban RM, Gilbert JL, Skipor AK, et al. Local and distant products from modularity. *Clin Orthop* 1995;319:94–105.

47. Jones DA, Lucas HK, O'Driscoll M, Price CHG, Wibberley B. Cobalt toxicity after McKee hip arthroplasty. *J Bone Joint Surg* 1975;57B: 289–296.

48. Keller JC, Trancik TM, Young FA, St. Mary E. Effects of indomethacin on bone ingrowth. *J Orthop Res* 1989;7:28–34.

49. Kennedy WF, Gruen TA, Chessin H, Gasparini G, Thompson W. Radiation therapy to prevent heterotopic ossification after cementless total hip arthroplasty. *Clin Orthop* 1991;262:185–191.

50. Khan MAA, Brakenbury PH, Reynolds ISR. Dislocation following total hip replacement. *J Bone Joint Surg* 1981;63B(2):214–218.

51. Kilgus DJ, Namba RS, Gorek JE, et al. Total hip replacement for patients who have ankylosing spondylitis: the importance of heterotopic bone and the durability of fixation of cemented components. *J Bone Joint Surg* 1990;72A:834–839.

52. Kim JH, Chu FC, Woodard HQ, Melamed MR, Huvos A, Cantin J. Radiation-induced soft-tissue and bone sarcoma. *Radiology* 1978; 129:501.

53. Kjaergaard-Anderson P, Sletgard J, Gjerloff C, Lund F. Heterotopic bone formation after noncemented total hip arthroplasty: location of ectopic bone and the influence of postoperative antiinflammatory treatment. *Clin Orthop* 1990;252:156.

54. Kjaersgaard-Anderson P, Hougaard K, Linde F, Christiansen SE, Jensen J. Heterotopic bone formation after total hip arthroplasty in patients with primary or secondary coxarthrosis. *Orthopaedics* 1990; 13(11):1211–1217.

55. Kjaersgaard-Anderson P, Nafei A, Teichert G, Kristensen O, et al. Indomethacin for the prevention of heterotopic ossification: a randomized controlled study in 41 hip arthroplasties. *Acta Orthop Scand* 1993;64(6):639–642.

56. Kjaersgaard-Anderson P, Ritter MA. Short-term treatment with nonsteroidal antiinflammatory medications to prevent heterotopic bone formation after total hip arthroplasty: a preliminary report. *Clin Orthop* 1992;279:157–162.

57. Kolstad K, Hogstorp H. Gastric carcinoma metastasis to a knee with a newly inserted prosthesis: a case report. *Acta Orthop Scand* 1990; 61:369–370.

58. Kristensen SS, Pedersen P, Pedersen NW, Schmidt SA, Kjaersgaard-Andersen P. Combined treatment with indomethacin and low-dose heparin after total hip replacement. A double blind placebo controlled clinical trial. *J Bone Joint Surg* 1990;72B:44.

59. Kromann-Andersen C, Scherff Sorensen T, Hogaard K, Zdravkovic D, Frigaard E. Ectopic bone formation following Charnley hip arthroplasty. *Acta Orthop Scand* 1980;51:633.

60. Lamovec J, Zidar A, Cucek-Plenicar M. Synovial sarcoma associated with total hip replacement: a case report. *J Bone Joint Surg* 1988; 70A(10):1558–1560.

61. Launder WJ, Hungerford DS. Stress fracture of the pubis after total hip arthroplasty. *Clin Orthop* 1981;159:183–185.

62. Lieberman IH, Moran E, Hastings DE, Bogoch ER. Heterotopic ossification after primary cemented and noncemented total hip arthroplasty in patients with osteoarthritis and rheumatoid arthritis. *Can J Surg* 1994;37(2):135–139.

63. Lotke PA, Wong RY, Ecker ML. Stress fracture as a cause of chronic pain following revision total hip arthroplasty: report of two cases. *Clin Orthop* 1986;206:147–150.

64. Maloney WJ, Jasty M, Willett C, Mulroy RD, Harris WH. Prophylaxis for heterotopic bone formation after total hip arthroplasty using low-dose radiation in high risk patients. *Clin Orthop* 1992;280:230–234.

65. Maloney WJ, Krushell RJ, Jasty M, Harris WH. Incidence of heterotopic ossification after total hip replacement. Effect of the type of fixation of the femoral component. *J Bone Joint Surg* 1991;73(A): 191–193.

66. Marmor L. Stress fracture of the pubic ramus simulating a loose total hip replacement. *Clin Orthop* 1976;121:103–104.

67. Martin A, Bauer TW, Manley MT, Marks KE. Osteosarcoma at the site of a total hip replacement: a case report. *J Bone Joint Surg* 1988; 70A(10):1561–1567.

68. Mathiesen EB, Ahlbom A, Berman G, Lindgren JU. Total hip replacement and cancer: a cohort study. *J Bone Joint Surg* 1995;77B(3): 345–350.

69. McElfresh EC, Coventry MB. Femoral and pelvic fractures after total hip arthroplasty. *J Bone Joint Surg* 1974;56A(3):483–492.

70. Memoli VA, Urban R, Alroy J, Galante GO. Malignant neoplasms associated with orthopaedic implant materials in rats. *J Orthop Res* 1986;4:346–355.

71. Merritt K, Brown SA, Sharkey NA. Blood distribution of nickel, cobalt, and chromium following intramuscular injection into hamsters. *J Biomed Mater Res* 1984;18:991–1004.

72. Morrey BF, Adams RA, Cabanela ME. Comparison of heterotopic ossification after anterolateral, transtrochanteric and posterior approaches for total hip arthroplasty. *Clin Orthop* 1984;188:160–167.

73. Nelson JP, Phillips PH. Malignant fibrous histiocytoma associated with total hip replacement: a case report. *Orthop Rev* 1990;19(12): 1078–1080.

74. Newhouse KE, El-Khoury GY, Buckwalter JA. Occult sacral fractures in osteoporotic patients. *J Bone Joint Surg* 1992;74A(10):1472–1477.

75. Nollen AJC, Sloof TJJH. Para-articular ossifications after total hip replacement. *Acta Orthop Scand* 1973;44:230.

76. Nyren O, McLaughin JK, Gridley G, Ekbom A, Johnell O, Fraumeni JF, Adami H. Cancer risk after hip replacement with metal implants: a population-based cohort study in Sweden. *J Natl Cancer Inst* 1995; 87(1):28–33.

77. Pagnani M, Pellicci P, Salvati EA. Effect of aspirin on heterotopic ossification after total hip arthroplasty in men who have osteoarthrosis. *J Bone Joint Surg* 1991;73(A):924.

78. Pellicci PM, Wilson PD, Sledge CB, Salvati EA, Ranawat CS, Poss R. Revision total hip arthroplasty. *Clin Orthop* 1982;170:34.

79. Pelligrini VD, Gregoritch SJ. Preoperative irradiation for prevention of heterotopic ossification following total hip arthroplasty. *J Bone Joint Surg* 1996;78A(6):870–881.

80. Pelligrini VD, Konski AA, Gastel JA, Rubin P, Evarts CM. Prevention of heterotopic ossification with irradiation after total hip arthroplasty: radiation therapy with a single dose of eight hundred centigray administered to a limited field. *J Bone Joint Surg* 1984;66B(5):632–634.

81. Penman HG, Ring PA. Osteosarcoma in association with total hip replacement. *J Bone Joint Surg* 1984;66B(5):632–634.

82. Pritchett JW, Bortel DT. Total hip replacement after central fracture dislocation of the acetabulum. *Orthop Rev* 1991;20(7):607–610.

83. Pritichett JW. Ketorolac prophylaxis against heterotopic ossification after hip replacement. *Clin Orthop* 1995;314:162–165.

84. Riegler HF, Harris CM. Heterotopic bone formation after total hip arthroplasty. *Clin Orthop* 1976;117:209.

85. Roberts JM, Fu FH, McClain EJ, Ferguson AB. A comparison of the poaterolateral and the anterolateral approaches to total hip arthroplasty. *Clin Orthop* 1984;187:205.

86. Rushforth GF. Osteosarcoma of the pelvis following radiotherapy for carcinoma of the cervix. *Br J Radiology* 1974;47:149–152.

87. Ryu RKN, Bovill EG Jr, Skinner HB, Murray WR. Soft-tissue sarcoma associated with aluminum oxide ceramic total hip arthroplasty: a case report. *Clin Orthop* 1987;216:207–212.

88. Schai P, Brunner R, Morscher E, Schubert KH. Prevention of heterotopic ossification in hip arthroplasties by means of an early single-dose radiotherapy (6 Gy). *Arch Orthop Trauma Surg* 1995;114(3):153–158.

89. Schmidt SA, Kjaersgaard-Anderson P, Nielsen JB. The use of indomethacin to prevent the formation of heterotopic bone formation after total hip replacement: a randomized double blind clinical trial. *J Bone Joint Surg* 1988;70(A):834.
90. Scott RD, Turner RH. Avoiding complications with long stem total hip replacement arthroplasty. *J Bone Joint Surg* 1975;57A:722.
91. Seegenschmeidt MH, Martus P, Goldman AR, Wolfel R, et al. Preoperative versus postoperative radiotherapy for prevention of heterotopic ossification (HO): first results of a randomized trial in high risk patients. *Int J Radiat Oncol Biol Phys.*
92. Sinbaldi K, Rosen H, Liu SK, DeAngelis M. Tumors associated with metallic implants in animals. *Clin Orthop* 1976;118:257–266.
93. Slatgard J, Kjaersgaard-Anderson P, Gjerloff C, Lund F. Heterotopic ossification following noncemented porous coated total hip replacement. *Acta Orthop Scand* 1988;59(suppl 227):39.
94. Snow ET. Metal carcinogenisis: mechanistic implications. *Pharmacol Ther* 1992;53(1):31–65.
95. Søballe K, Christensen F, Kristensen SS. Ectopic bone formation after total hip arthroplasty. *Clin Orthop* 1988;228:57.
96. Sodemann B, Persson PE, Nilsson OS. Prevention of periarticular heterotopic ossification following total hip arthroplasty: clinical experience with indomethacin and ibuprophen. *Arch Orthop Trauma Surg* 1988;107:329.
97. Swann M. Malignant soft-tissue tumour at the site of a total hip replacement. *J Bone Joint Surg* 1984;66B(5):629–631.
98. Swanson SAV, Freeman MAR, Heath JC. Laboratory testing on total joint replacement implants. *J Bone Joint Surg* 1973;55B:759–773.
99. Tait NP, Hacking PM, Malcolm AJ. Case reports: malignant fibrous histiocytoma occuring at the site of a previous total hip replacement. *Br J Radiol* 1988;61:73–76.
100. Thomas BJ, Amstutz HC. Results of the administration of diphosphonate for the prevention of heterotopic ossification after total hip arthroplasty. *J Bone Joint Surg* 1985;67(A):400.
101. Thomas BJ. Heterotopic bone formation after total hip arthroplasty. *Orthop Clin North Am* 1992;23(2):347–358.
102. Tozun R, Pinar H, Yesiller E, Hamzaoglu A. Indomethacin for the prevention of heterotopic ossification after total hip arthroplasty. *J Arthroplasty* 1992;7(1):57–61.
103. Trancik TM, Mills W, Visson N. The effect of indocin, aspirin and ibuprophen on bone ingrowth into a porous coated implant. *Clin Orthop* 1989;249:113–121.
104. Troop JK, Mallory TH, Fisher DA, Vaughn BK. Malignant fibrous histiocytoma after total hip arthroplasty: a case report. *Clin Orthop* 1990;253:297–300.
105. van der List JJJ, van Horn JR, Sloof TJJH, ten Cate LN. Malignant epithelioid hemangioendothelioma at the site of a hip prosthesis. *Acta Orthop Scand* 1988;59:328–330.
106. Wahlstrom O, Risto O, Djerf K, Hammerby S. Heterotopic bone formation prevented by diclofenac: prospective study in 100 arthroplasties. *Acta Orthop Scand* 1991;62(5):419–421.
107. Weber PC. Epitheliod sarcoma in association with total knee replacement: a case report. *J Bone Joint Surg* 1986;68B(5):824–826.
108. Willert HG, Bertram H, Buchhorn GH. Osteolysis in alloarthroplasty of the hip: the role of ultra-high molecular weight polyethylene wear particles. *Clin Orthop* 1990;258:95–107.
109. Woo RYG, Morrey BF. Dislocation after total hip arthroplasty. *J Bone Joint Surg* 1982;64A(9):1295–1306.

Complex Total Hip Arthroplasty

The Adult Hip, edited by J. J. Callaghan,
A. G. Rosenberg, and H. E. Rubash.
Lippincott–Raven Publishers, Philadelphia © 1998.

CHAPTER 73

Total Hip Arthroplasty in the Management of Congenital Hip Dislocation

William H. Harris

Osteoarthritis of the hip secondary to developmental hip dysplasia or developmental hip dislocation covers a wide spectrum of challenges to the reconstructive hip surgeon. Cases with mild deformation represent virtually no difference from the surgery typical for the standard primary total hip replacement. At the other extreme, the problems presented by severe forms of acetabular hypoplasia (femoral underdevelopment, gross anatomic abnormalities, total dislocation, major leg-length discrepancies, and a high-riding greater trochanter) lie at the extremes of the challenges presented for total hip replacement surgery (Fig. 1).

Understanding these differences, being able to recognize the magnitude of the problems, and marshaling the skills and techniques required to solve them are crucial for the appropriate management of this widely varied form of osteoarthritis.

A variety of classifications have been offered to identify and subdivide the complexity of the problems presented by osteoarthritis secondary to developmental dysplasia and dislocation (4,16). To define the inherent difficulties in the reconstructions, and to alert the sur-

geon to the potential pitfalls associated with such reconstructions, we have used, as have Hartofilakidis et al. (14), the following simple and effective classification: (a) dysplasia, (b) subtotal dislocation, (c) total dislocation (Fig. 2).

The definitions of groups (a) and (c) are relatively straightforward. In mild or moderate dysplasia, the acetabular development approximates a normal hip but clearly shows hypoplasia and/or malformation of the acetabulum and/or the femoral head. However, there is a distinct and recognizable relationship between the femoral head and the acetabulum, despite the fact that they are not necessarily normal or congruent. Some amount of contact exists between the articular surface of the femoral head and the articular surface of the hypoplastic, deformed acetabulum. In these cases, usually the bone stock is only marginally compromised. In general, there are less severe leg-length discrepancies, the greater trochanter is less severely displaced from its normal relationship, and the length of the abductors, although perhaps reduced, is not severely so.

At the other extreme, the situation associated with a total dislocation on a developmental basis of the hip is far more severe. There is no articulation between the femoral head and the acetabular recess. The limb is frequently severely shortened. The abductor muscles are distinctly abnormal, both in length and in direction. Serious problems exist in

W. H. Harris: Department of Orthopaedic Surgery, Massachusetts General Hospital, Harvard Medical School, Boston, Massachusetts 02114.

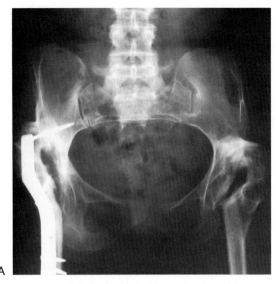
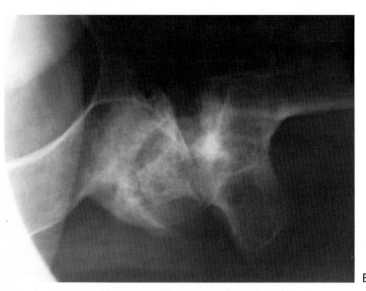

A   B

FIG. 1. A: AP radiograph of the hips and pelvis of a 33-year-old woman with severe bilateral developmental dislocations of the hip and marked femoral deformity secondary to bilateral subtrochanteric osteotomy. **B:** True lateral radiograph of the left hip showing the severe deformity in the lateral view of the subtrochanteric deformity.

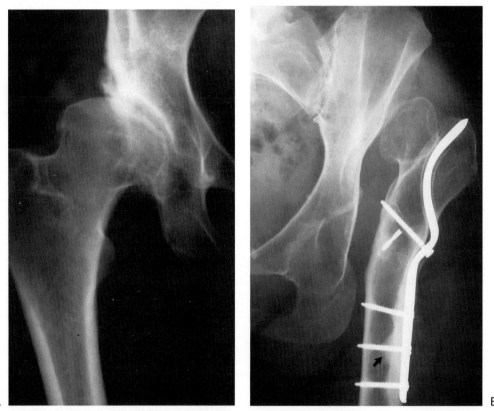

A   B

FIG. 2. A: AP radiograph of the hips and pelvis of a 37-year-old woman with mild dysplasia of the acetabulum. **B:** AP radiograph of the left hip of a 43-year-old woman with total dislocation of the left hip on a congenital basis and residual deformity from subtrochanteric osteotomy with internal fixation.

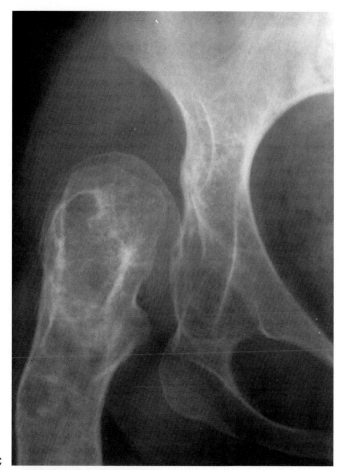

C

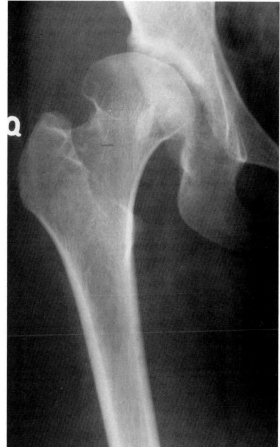

D

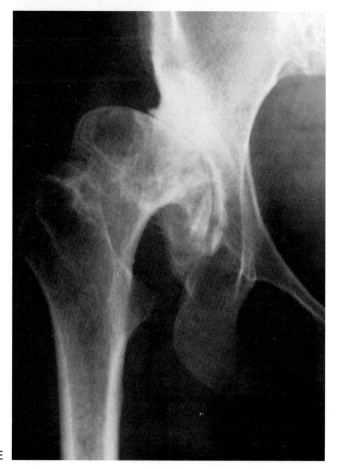

E

FIG. 2. *Continued.* **C:** AP radiograph of the right hip of a 26-year-old woman with Ollier's disease who also had a subtotal dislocation of a hip (developmental). Note that the location of the femoral head is opposite the region where the anlage of the lateral portion of the acetabulum resides. The presence of the head in this position has compromised further the acetabular volume by inhibiting the development of the lateral portion of the acetabulum. **D:** AP radiograph of the left hip of an 18-year-old woman with hypoplasia of the right hip (developmental). Note that this stage would be classified as dysplasia, rather than subtotal or total dislocation. **E:** AP radiograph of the right hip of the same person shown in Figure 2D, 23 years later. Note that the subsequent migration of the femoral head (noting the severity of the process and the evolutionary change) would now place the patient in the category of subtotal dislocation.

obtaining sufficient pelvic bone stock to support the acetabular reconstruction. Because the socket reconstruction almost always must be done at the level where the normal acetabulum should have developed, however hypoplastic that area is, the problems associated with lengthening the limb to achieve such acetabular replacement are complex. They involve dealing with the length of the femur, the reattachment of the greater trochanter, the redirection and lengthening of the abductor muscles, and the avoidance of traction injury to the sciatic nerve. Also, in these cases, but not exclusively in these cases, the medullary canal of the femur is commonly extremely small.

Between these two groups lie those patients who have a subtotal dislocation. In these patients there is still some residual relationship between the femoral head and the acetabulum, although the direct contact between femoral head articular surface and acetabular articular surface may be markedly reduced or markedly distorted. Frequently, the femoral head is substantially subluxed laterally, the acetabular contour is quite sloping, and the mechanics of the joint are severely compromised. In some cases of subtotal dislocation, the femoral head has been sufficiently displaced laterally and away from the articular surface of the acetabulum that, in fact, the presence of the femoral head has interfered with the development of the cartilaginous anlage of the lateral aspect of the acetabulum, leading to a marked truncation of lateral acetabular development. Alternatively, certain cases of subtotal dislocation may be the result of progressive erosion of the lateral aspect of the acetabulum in a patient who started out in the dysplastic category but whose hip became a subtotal dislocation in association with progressively developing osteoarthritis, increasing degrees of lateral subluxation, and erosion of the lateral portion of the acetabular bone stock.

It is quite important to appreciate that certain instances in the subtotal dislocation category may be associated with anatomic distortions that can, at times, make these reconstructions even more difficult than in patients with a total dislocation. The reason for this is that in a total dislocation, the femoral head does not block the cartilaginous anlage of the lateral portion of the acetabulum. As a result, there are some instances of total dislocation in which there is a greater mass of pelvic bone stock available for the acetabular reconstruction than in some of the severe instances of subtotal dislocation. Equally so, the late, severe erosive destruction of the lateral portion of the acetabulum secondary to the osteoarthritic process can seriously compromise pelvic bone stock even though in some of these cases at a younger age, sufficient bone had been present to have allowed a quasi-normal acetabular reconstruction.

The anatomic considerations associated with these developmental abnormalities constitute the central issues in the complexity of these reconstructions. To reemphasize, the difficulties may range from minimal to severe.

SPECIAL CONSIDERATIONS FOR THE INDICATIONS FOR SURGERY

As a general rule, the indications for reconstructive surgery in this group of patients do not differ substantially from the indications in cases with more normal anatomy. The vast majority of patients want the surgery primarily for pain relief, with a second criterion being substantial interference with ordinary functioning in the activities of daily living. For many patients, severe limp, major leg-length discrepancy, compromise in knee function, and compromise in the function of the lumbar spine add to the impetus toward surgery.

However, several special features apply here. The first is that a number of these patients begin to encounter significant loss of joint space or significant symptoms at a relatively early age, secondary to the developmental abnormality. In an effort to avoid total hip replacement surgery in patients who are young, it is important to assess carefully all of the methods of extending the longevity of the existing hip prior to doing a total hip replacement. This includes all of the usual modes of conservative management of osteoarthritis of the hip, including weight reduction, anti-inflammatory medications, the use of support, heat, and rest. Even more important for a number of these patients is the value of early intervention if osteotomy of the hip is a suitable alternative. This may be a femoral osteotomy, an acetabular osteotomy, or both. If successful osteotomy can be carried out, many years of very satisfactory function can be obtained, substantially delaying the need to do a total hip replacement in the younger patient.

Of special importance is the recognition that patients with bilateral total dislocation of the hip generally do not require reconstructive surgery. The vast majority of such adult patients walk poorly with severe limps but have relatively little or even no pain, require no support, and can function quite satisfactorily for many years or decades. Thus, caution should be exercised in assessing these patients for total hip replacement surgery. The mere presence of a severe limp in such cases is often not sufficient indication to warrant the complexities of such surgery.

On the other hand, it also needs to be clearly stated that a small percentage of such patients, even those in their fifties and sixties, will develop disabling pain, even though for 50 or 60 years they functioned quite well with bilateral total hip dislocations. If this occurs, they then become candidates for the complex surgery.

Another special factor in the indications for total hip replacement surgery in the severe forms of this type of arthritis is a clear recognition of the increased risk of serious complications and the increased complexity of the surgery. These two factors often tilt the balance against recommending surgery in patients who have moderate symptoms, which in the presence of normal anatomy and a relatively straightforward total hip reconstruction would constitute sufficient indication for the operation. Because such issues as the requirement for major bone grafting to provide additional pelvic bone stock, nonunion of the greater trochanter, sciatic nerve palsy, increased risk of loosening of the acetabular or femoral component, femoral nerve palsy, and division of the profunda femoris artery are more common in the surgery of the severe cases of developmental dysplasia and dislocations, the specific indications for surgery should be clear in the minds of both the patient and the surgeon.

General Comments on the Complexities Arising from the Unique Anatomic Abnormalities in These Cases

Among the distinctive anatomic abnormalities that complicate the surgery are both those distortions of the normal anatomy from the developmental abnormality, and those additional distortions that are the result of previous operations perfrmed in the management of the primary abnormality. Specifically, the severe proximal displacement of the femoral head relative to the normal location of the acetabulum means that the direction of the abductor muscles, instead of being lateral and distal, may be severely altered, even becoming nearly horizontal in direction (Fig. 3). Failure to recognize this can lead to substantial confusion in identifying the appropriate tissue planes and anatomic structures during the surgery. The hip capsule, in the presence of total dislocations, has an hourglass configuration, extending from the rim of the hypoplastic acetabulum, narrowing to a small aperture, and then enlarging to surround the totally dislocated femoral head.

Even more hazardous are abnormal locations of both the femoral nerve and the profunda femoris artery. The femoral nerve, instead of taking its customary distal lateral course, may, in fact, in its upper branches, reverse directions and, after leaving the pelvis, proceed in a craniad direction as well as laterally. This renders it vulnerable to traction injury during retraction of the medial structures, which customarily would not cause any damage to the femoral nerve whatsoever. Similarly, the proximal displacement of the femur leads to an aberrant position of the profunda artery, subjecting it to laceration at the inferior margin of the acetabulum in a region that is usually free of major arterial structures.

Because the optimal position for the location of the reconstructed acetabulum in the vast majority of cases (90% or more) is at the level where the normal acetabulum should develop, the management of a high total dislocation may require excision of a substantial amount of the proximal portion of the femur. If one attempts to reduce a total dislocation into the socket at the level of the normal acetabulum without shortening the femur, the risk of sciatic palsy is quite high. Two methods exist for achieving that shortening of the femur. One is to

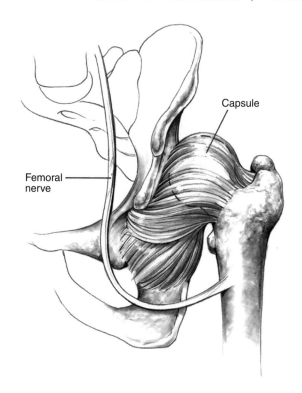

FIG. 3. Drawing of the left hip of a totally dislocated hip (developmental) shows three important characteristics: (a) because the femoral head is so high, the femoral nerve takes an abnormal course (thus, the nerve is subject to a high risk of traction injury); (b) the hip capsule has an hourglass configuration secondary to the deformity associated with the complete dislocation; and (c) the length and direction of the abductor muscles from the wing of the ilium to the greater trochanter are substantially distorted.

osteotomize the greater trochanter and excise a portion of the proximal femur, even down as low as below the lesser trochanter (Fig. 4A). The second is to carry out a subtrochanteric segmental resection of the femur, translocating distally the proximal metaphyseal portion of the femur including the greater trochanter and then obtaining union between proximal metaphyseal area and the remaining diaphyseal region (Figs. 4B,5).

It is of interest, and sometimes surprise, that although one shortens the actual length of the *femur* in this process, the *limb* itself may be lengthened because the femoral head now articulates with the acetabular component at the level of where the normal hip should have developed.

In considering those cases with more severe abnormalities, however, particularly the cases with subtotal and total dislocations, four key issues dominate the surgical planning, the surgery itself, and the incidence of postoperative complications. They are (a) hypoplasia of the acetabulum, (b) hypoplasia and distortion of the femur, (c) restoration of abductor function, and (d) dealing with leg-length abnormalities.

A   B

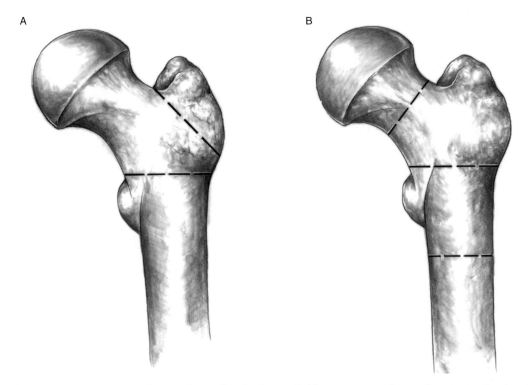

FIG. 4. Two general approaches to shortening the femur. **A:** The greater trochanter is osteotomized and the metaphyseal region is excised along the head and neck. **B:** The metaphyseal region and the greater trochanter are preserved, but an intertrochanteric/subtrochanteric transverse segment of the diaphysis is removed.

Hypoplasia of the Acetabulum

The key problem is obtaining bony support for the acetabular reconstruction. Nine out of ten times, the best place for the acetabular reconstruction is where the normal hip joint should have developed, *even though* that area may be severely hypoplastic. The anatomy of the pelvis is such that the greatest mass of bone occurs at that location in almost all cases. Rarely, there will be another, better location, such as on the wing of the ilium, but these occasions usually occur only after a shelf procedure or other prior reconstructive surgery has been done. Although the vast majority of cases provide the greatest bone mass at the level of the normal acetabulum, of course, even this may be deficient.

The ideal is to expose that portion of the pelvis and optimize the bone stock available there to support the acetabular component. Obviously, if there is reduced acetabular bone stock, then the first solution to the problem in most instances is to use a small acetabular component. We commonly do reconstructions with an acetabular component of 40 mm outside diameter (OD). Larger is better, because it allows a greater thickness of polyethylene, but the 40-mm OD sockets have provided excellent long-term success for many patients. A mandatory concomitant of the use of a small acetabular component is the use of a small femoral head. Our rule is that for sockets smaller than 50 mm OD, a 22-mm head is preferable.

This is generally compatible with satisfactory reconstruction and simultaneous maintenance of polyethylene thickness of adequate amount. One of the incorrect decisions commonly made by inexperienced surgeons in reconstructing hips with major deficiencies of acetabular bone stock is the use of a femoral component with a large femoral head.

On the issue of cement versus cementless sockets under circumstances of limited acetabular bone stock, our preference has been to use the cementless acetabular component fixed with screws. Generally, there is not sufficient bone stock to risk trying to use a press-fit in the very hypoplastic sockets. The risk of fracture under these circumstances may be prohibitive. On the contrary, one could argue in favor of cementing so that the reduction of the polyethylene thickness caused by the thickness of the metal shell is obviated. In reality, however, the thickness of the metal shell and the thickness of the required layer of cement are roughly equal. Therefore, fixation can be achieved with a cementless modular component fixed with screws, and the same thickness of polyethylene will be obtained as with a cemented acetabular component. Experience over the first decade with the use of such sockets showed that the clinical behavior of well-designed cementless sockets is at least the equivalent of cemented ones in the older age group (19) and distinctly preferable in those aged 50 years and under (17), and the incidence of major radiolucent lines developing behind the cement in the pelvis is greater with cement than with cementless implants (20). Because many of these patients require this total hip replacement at a young age, and because hemispherical cementless sockets fixed with screws have a better record than cemented sockets in the young, we generally use cementless sockets (17).

In those primary operations with only a moderate reduction in acetabular bone stock, conventional techniques can be used in most instances and the deficiency in bone stock can be accommodated simply by using smaller acetabular components. However, paramount among the critical requirements for successful reconstruction of the acetabulum is the need to establish that the apex of the acetabular recess is more craniad (or higher) than the lateral lip of the acetabulum. If this is not done, the risk of the acetabular component breaking loose in a lateral direction (socket breakout) is increased. Thus, in reconstructing a sloping or shallow acetabulum, it is important to preserve the lateral-most portion of acetabular bone stock and to carve or ream medial to that to create an apex to the acetabular recess that is higher (more craniad) than the lateral lip.

If at all possible, it is wise to leave the medial portion of the acetabulum intact. Others have recommended, at times, a deliberate fracture of the medial wall with surgically created protrusio, to center the acetabular reconstruction in the available iliac bone (5). General experience has shown that this is adverse and that other techniques of increasing the coverage are preferable.

It is now uncommon to need to augment the bone stock by bulk structural grafting. When needed, this can be done with a femoral head autograft or femoral head allograft, either bolted to the lateral portion of the wing of the ileum at the region of the acetabular margin or grafted within the acetabular recess (1,7,8,10–12). However, long-term results have shown that a high proportion of these structural bulk acetabular grafts fail, whether they are femoral head autografts, femoral head allografts, distal femoral structural allografts, or proximal tibial grafts (21).

The temporal history of such bulk structural grafts is important. They rarely fail during the first 5 years. Thus, the initial results are quite gratifying. However, the failure rate rises rapidly thereafter. Our recent study of bulk structural femoral autografts and allografts used in acetabular reconstructions showed that after 15 years, 60% of the sockets were loose (21). In this application, femoral head autografts did better than femoral head allografts. Nearly two thirds of all the acetabular components that had been cemented into such bulk grafts were loose, but in the case of femoral head allografts, 60% had already required revision, whereas the corresponding figure for femoral head autografts was 30%. Our current recommendations are to use such grafts only as a last resort (21). If they are necessary, they can be a great asset. However, if one can

obtain sufficient support from intact, viable host bone, the outlook is substantially better.

Step one in obtaining sufficient support is to use smaller acetabular components. The definition of adequate support is generally believed to be that about 70% of the cementless acetabular hemisphere be covered with intact viable host bone. It has been clearly demonstrated that 30% of the lateral portion of the acetabular component need not be covered with bone. This remaining 30% can be covered with particulate bone graft, preferably autologous but acceptably allograft, and, if the rest of the acetabular component is rigidly fixed to the pelvis, it would generally obtain bony ingrowth. The particulate graft will unite to the host and provide additional support, although probably not bony ingrowth for the acetabular component.

On the other hand, bulk structural allografts, which occupy 30% or less of the lateral surface of the acetabular component, have a high success rate. They have this high success rate probably because they are not necessary (22).

If bulk grafting (either bulk autografting or allografting) is required, the techniques that have been well worked out and fully described (1,7–12) should be used. Some have recommended using screws to fix the bulk graft to the wing of the ilium. That is successful at times, but the incidence of nonunion is distinctly higher with screws than with the use of bolts. Nonunion of the graft to the host is uncommon but in severe cases, where the ilium is quite hypoplastic, screws have little purchase into the thin supra-acetabular portion of the ilium. It is in these circumstances that bolts have the greatest holding power and, consequently, a reduced incidence of nonunion. The greater the proportion of support for the acetabular component that can be achieved by intact viable host bone, the greater the stability and the higher the probability of long-term success. At the other extreme, bulk grafts have provided as much as 90% of the support of the acetabular component.

It has been argued that graft failure is related to the direction of the trabeculae of the graft material, suggesting that if the trabeculae are oriented in their normal anatomic relationship, collapse is less likely (1). Because all of these grafts, autogenous or allografts, are avascular, that argument appears unlikely. In spontaneous avascular necrosis of the femoral head, in association with steroids, in association with alcohol intake, or with dislocation of the hip that remains unreduced for several days, the trabeculae of the femoral head are oriented in an absolutely normal direction. Nevertheless, they collapse.

Suggestions that the distal femoral bulk structural allografts or autografts, or the proximal tibial autografts or grafts, in the configuration of a upside-down 7 have higher duration of survival may be premature. Because few of the bulk grafts used to augment acetabular bone stock for total hip replacements fail prior to 5 years, 8- or 10-year data would be necessary to establish that any of these other graft types are preferable. No such data exist.

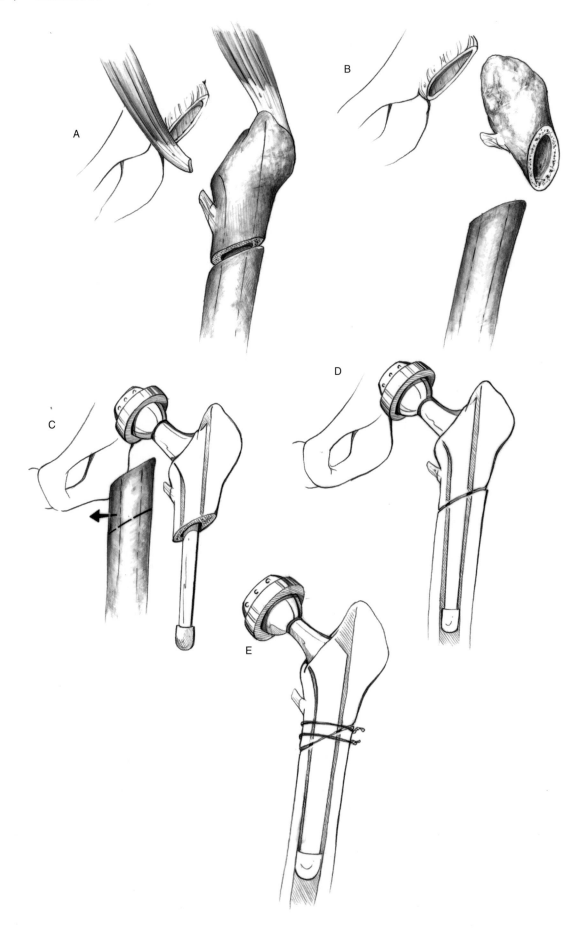

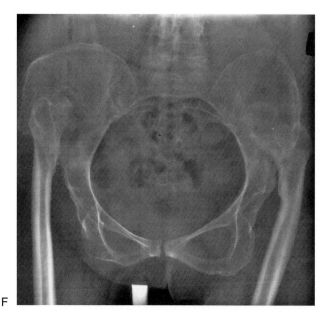

F

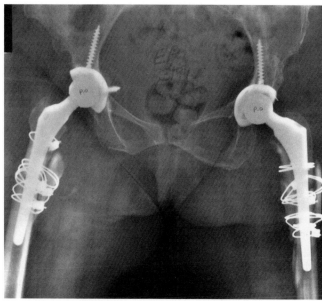

G

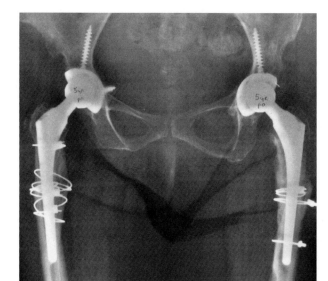

H

FIG. 5. Technique of subtrochanteric osteotomy for total hip arthroplasty in patients with total congenital hip dislocation as proposed by Capello. The patient must have 90° of hip flexion preoperatively to allow the subtrochanteric femoral osteotomy site to be opposed. After the hip is exposed, the femoral neck is osteotomized and the psoas tendon is released. An oblique subtrochanteric osteotomy is then performed. **A:** The femoral shaft is exposed, the proximal femur is broached for the implant to be utilized, and the distal femur is reamed to accept the prosthesis. **B:** The implant is inserted into the proximal fragment and the appropriate amount of the distal femoral segment is resected to obtain arthroplasty stability, restore leg length, and prevent sciatic nerve stretching. **C:** The femoral component with the proximal femur is opposed to the distal fragment and, as demonstrated by the *arrow*, may be rotated to reduce the excessive anteversion that is present in many cases of congenital dysplasia of the hip. **D:** The subtrochanteric osteotomy site is secured with wire or cables and can be augmented with cortical strut allografts. **E:** This approach eliminates the need for a transtrochanteric osteotomy. The case of a 70-year-old woman with total congenital hip dislocation where this approach was utilized is illustrated. Preoperative **(F)**, postoperative **(G)**, and 5-year follow-up **(H)** radiographs are presented. (Case provided by Dr. William Capello, Indiana University.)

Because these other forms of bulk corticocancellous grafts have a shorter-term history, they are enthusiastically supported by some authors. This information will be tested during years 5 through 10. The fundamental fault appears to be the fatigue failure of a dead corticocancellous material underload over a long period of time. The structural deficiency of such grafts in the absence of blood supply is made worse by the weakening in the graft associated with creeping substitution.

One additional point about bulk grafting is clear. The experience of using a *cementless* acetabular component in cases in which less than 60% of the surface of the acetabular component is in contact with intact, viable host bone has been less satisfactory. If a graft that covers more than 40% of the acetabular component is needed, it

is prudent to cement the acetabular component into the host and the graft, rather than put a cementless component into a dead bulk graft.

Management of the Hypoplastic or Distorted Femur

As is true on the acetabular side, the mild cases of developmental dysplasia that lead to osteoarthritis requiring a total hip replacement do not provide much of a challenge for the femoral reconstruction. At the other extreme, severe difficulties arise from issues such as marked hypoplasia of the femur, a very small medullary canal, and severe distortion of the femur on a developmental basis or on the basis of previous intertrochanteric or subtrochanteric osteotomies (see Fig. 1). In addition, recall that in many severe cases, the femoral component must be placed solely in the diaphysis of the femur, rather than across the metaphysis into the diaphysis. This frequently means that the femoral component must be straight, short, and quite small. The ordinary contours of most cemented and cementless femoral components, which take advantage of the transition from metaphyseal to diaphyseal areas in the proximal femur, are not appropriate. The attempt to use such prostheses can lead to fracture of the femur. For these cases a *straight, short* femoral component is required, whether the fixation is with cement or cementless.

A separate issue arises in the use of cementless components in the extremely small femurs. The diameter of the femoral component required may be very narrow, perhaps 8 or 9 mm at most. The inherent weakness of some cementless femoral components secondary to the porous surface and low fatigue strength may be a concern about the long-term fatigue resistance of such small implants. Although cemented implants may have an even smaller diameter in order to provide for an adequate layer of cement mantle, they are made of superalloys and do not suffer the weakening effect of the porous outer layer. Among the other special problems associated with dysplastic femurs is distortion of the geometry of the medullary canal, including reversal of the normal asymmetry of the mediolateral width of the femoral canal compared to the anterior-posterior width of the femoral canal (Fig. 6).

Similarly, severe difficulties can arise from a marked varus or valgus deformity, particularly secondary to a previous subtrochanteric osteotomy. In some of these cases, it is necessary to recreate the osteotomy and reestablish a more normal alignment, simultaneously with the total hip replacement procedure. Equally, some of the femurs in these cases have such excessive anteversion that proper orientation of the femoral component can be a problem. For cemented stems, this problem can usually be readily handled by simply reducing the excessive anteversion by placing the stem within the cement mass. For cementless stems, the problem may be more difficult. In extreme cases, some have recommended a subtrochanteric osteotomy to permit reduction of the anteversion by external rotation of the metaphyseal fragment on the diaphyseal one, and then the insertion of the cementless stem (Fig. 7) (15). Other cementless femur advocates have recommended the use of modular stems in these circumstances.

Restoration of Abductor Function

The next major hurdle is the restoration of abductor function. If the femoral head is distorted or reduced in height, as is common in growth disturbances associated with avascular necrosis secondary to the treatment of developmental dislocation or dysplasia, the greater trochanter may reside more craniad than the center of rotation of the femoral head. In many instances, this can be corrected simply by choosing an appropriate location and length of the femoral component so that the femoral head of the prosthesis is restored to a more craniad position relative to the greater trochanter. However, in total dislocations and in severe subluxations, it is often necessary to advance the greater trochanter distally. This is particularly true in cases in which the upper portion of the femur has to be shortened to allow the reduction of the hip to take place at the level of the locus of the normal hip center. In these instances, reattachment of the greater trochanter can become a difficult task.

This difficulty often translates into the specific issue of obtaining sufficient length of the abductors to allow the trochanter to reside at its new position, substantially further distal than its lifetime location. This problem is substantially facilitated by placing the femur in wide abduction, either at the time of reattachment of the greater trochanter to the diaphyseal portion of the femur if it has been osteotomized, or at the time of attempted reattachment of the metaphyseal segment containing the trochanter to the diaphyseal segment, after excision of a subtrochanteric segment of the femur. It is also facilitated by a complete capsulectomy and by excision of all of the scar tissue, either spontaneously formed or resulting from previous surgery, which tends to inhibit the mobilization and stretching of the abductor muscles.

Equally so, the severe anatomic rearrangement necessary for such reconstructions commonly calls for release of the iliopsoas muscle and at times release or distal transposition of that portion of the gluteus maximus muscle that inserts into the proximal portion of the femur.

Other alternatives available for the management of short abductor musculature are more severe. One is the creation of a Z-plasty within the substance of the abductors as they approach their insertion into the greater trochanter. This clearly lengthens the abductors, but it weakens them. Similarly, an abductor slide can be performed by removing all of the abductors subperiosteally from the ileum and advancing them after the trochanter has been reattached and the limb is placed in wide abduction. In so doing, the entire abductor mass is advanced on the superior gluteal neurovascular leash. The most proximal portion of the abductors is thus moved distally and laid back against the bare portion of the wing of the ileum. Because this provides no initial stability, it is necessary for these patients to be placed in spica casts for 6 weeks while the abductors reattach to the ileum. This drastic procedure reestablishes continuity of the abductors between the ileum and the advanced position of the greater trochanter, but it also compromises abductor power. Either of these two alternatives should be considered only as a last resort.

A very interesting feature of the problem of obtaining sufficient length of the abductor musculature to allow advancement of the greater trochanter to a more normal

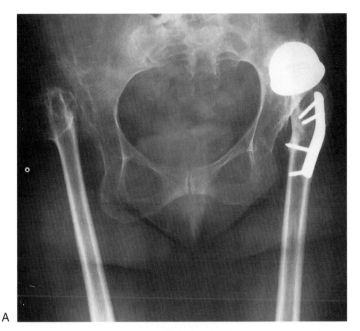

A

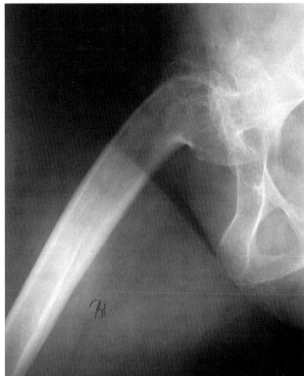

B

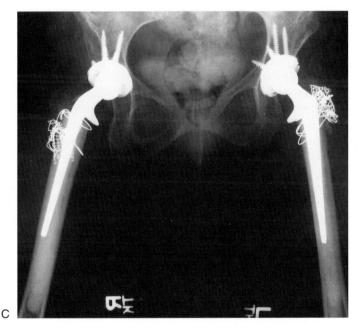

C

FIG. 6. A: AP radiograph of the hips and pelvis of a 43-year-old woman with bilateral total dislocations of the hips (developmental). She has had a cup arthroplasty on the left as well as a subtrochanteric osteotomy. This view of the proximal portion of the right femur shows a very narrow medullary canal. **B:** The frog lateral view shows that, in this dimension, this width of the femoral canal is much wider, twice as wide as the medial-lateral width. **C:** The AP radiograph of the hips and pelvis after her reconstruction show hybrid total hip replacements on both sides. Cementless acetabular components have been fixed to the pelvis with screws. There is excellent bony coverage of the acetabular component. Very small straight congenital dysplasia of the hip precoat components were required for insertion into the diaphysis of each femur. Trochanteric osteotomies were done. Subtrochanteric resection of a portion of the femoral metaphysis was necessary to allow reduction of the reconstructed femur into the newly established acetabular component. In both instances, the greater trochanter was advanced to the lateral aspect of the shaft of the femur and reattached using trochanteric mesh and circumferential wires.

position is an understanding of how the abductors actually function in cases with total dislocation. Judging the apparent length of the abductor from the anatomic location of the origin of the abductors to the location of the greater trochanter as represented on an anteroposterior (AP) radiograph, one would expect the abductors to be very short indeed, and quite tight. Generally speaking, this is not so. They may be tight, but they are usually far more flexible and longer than that simple anatomic consideration would suggest. The reason for this lies in the fact that in a hip that is completely dislocated, when the

patient sits down, the abductors are stretched by the relative displacement of the greater trochanter in the act of flexing the hip. Thus, sitting constantly stretches the abductors well beyond their resting length in the standing position. This flexibility eases the problem of advancing the greater trochanter.

Conversely, when one is faced with the unusual circumstance in which a totally dislocated hip is very stiff, difficulty in getting the abductors stretched enough to complete the reconstruction are substantially worsened. This stiffness or marked limitation of motion may be secondary to

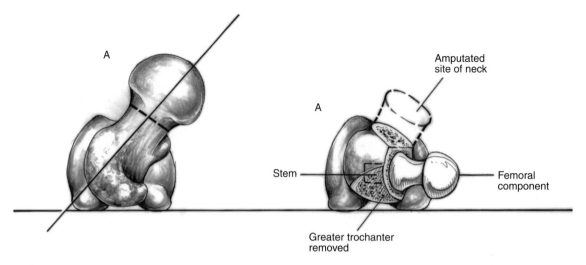

FIG. 7. At times, femoral neck anteversion is severe in congenital hip dislocation. The greater trochanter is located posteriorly in addition to a narrowing of the femoral shaft. **A:** The amputated site of the neck. **B:** The site of removal of the greater trochanter. An attempt is made to keep the femoral component in the neutroversion plane; nevertheless, a slightly anteverted position of the stem may be selected to allow insertion. This compromise is the exception to the rule, which may be carefully considered in severe narrowing and anteverted femurs. (From Eftekhar NS. *Total hip arthroplasty*. St. Louis, MO: Mosby Yearbook, 1993;955.)

the underlying pathology of the developmental abnormality of the hip, or it may be secondary to previous surgery in the region of the hip. It is wise to pay special attention to a high-riding dislocated hip that is stiff. Reestablishment of the abductor power will be far more complex.

To advance the trochanter in complex cases, all the capsule should be removed and any fibrous bands should be eliminated; this reduces the elasticity of the abductor mass. The greater trochanter should be moved distally as far as it can reach and then the femur must be brought into wide abduction to approximate the lateral surface of the femoral shaft to the greater trochanter. To reattach the trochanter in cemented total hip replacements, we prefer to use three vertical wires passing through the medullary canal and two horizontal wires placed circumferentially, to attach the greater trochanter. The three vertical wires, after passing through the medullary canal, go through drill holes in the greater trochanter. The two horizontal wires pass through drill holes in the lesser trochanter if it is still present and surround the upper portion of the femur, passing through the greater trochanter to be tied laterally (Fig. 8). Patients with this type of reconstruction must use protected weight bearing for 3 months. Longer protection is occasionally necessary if union is delayed. Special care must also be given to be sure that wires passing through the medullary canal are well out of the way at the time of the insertion of the cemented femoral stem.

When a cementless stem is used, it is generally considered unwise to have wires pass through the medullary canal, because of the issue of fretting. Rather, circumferential wires are used, generally two passing through the lesser trochanter and a third passing distal to the lesser

trochanter. These wires then pass through drill holes in the greater trochanter.

The bed to receive the trochanter upon the femur should be free of all muscle and fibrous tissue. Firm and direct apposition should be achieved with the wiring. Often after the greater trochanter has been osteotomized, it is wise to use trochanteric mesh (13) to support the small or osteoporotic piece of the greater trochanter during the wiring process. The mesh allows the wires to be tightened aggressively but prevents them from cutting through the trochanteric fragment.

At times, it is necessary to abduct the newly reconstructed hip as much as 60° to approximate the greater trochanter to the lateral portion to the lateral portion of the shaft of the femur. This will produce an apparent leg lengthening, which may require the use of a lift temporarily on the opposite side. Generally, this apparent leg-length discrepancy spontaneously reduces over time as the abductors stretch out.

Rarely, instances occur in which there is no remaining greater trochanter, or it is so small or fragmented that it cannot serve as a vehicle to unite the distal portion of the abductors to the femur. Under these circumstances, it is wise to place the femur in wide abduction and sew the abductors directly to the fascia lata as far distal as possible. These patients must then be non-weight bearing and in wide abduction for 6 weeks to allow the insertion of the abductors to heal. Generally, this requires a spica cast. Functionally, in general, these patients who have the abductors sewn into the fascia lata will require the use of a cane, but the tethering of the abductors into the fascia lata is a distinct asset in reducing the risk of dislocation.

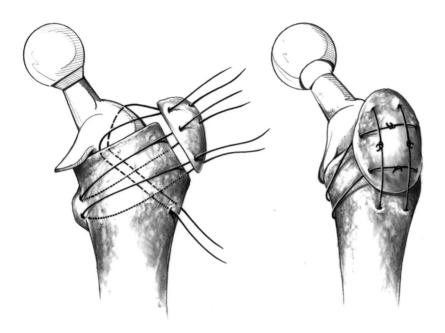

FIG. 8. Trochanteric wiring technique.

Postoperatively, once the greater trochanter has united, physical therapy is often helpful to optimize abductor function. In general, sidelying abduction against gravity is the preferred exercise. Once that has been achieved satisfactorily, additional strength can be generated by doing sidelying abduction exercises against gravity while wearing a 1-pound or 2-pound ankle weight.

Leg-Length Adjustment

Leg-length adjustment can be a complex issue in severe cases of developmental subtotal or total dislocation requiring total hip replacement. If the bone stock at the level of the normal acetabulum is adequate and if the subluxation is mild, restoration of leg length can be achieved in the usual ways by adjusting both the size and location of the acetabular component and the length of the femoral neck and size of the femoral head. However, with complete dislocation, and particularly if the acetabular hypoplasia is severe, the only recourse is to carry out the reconstruction at the level where the normal hip should have developed. Then, to reduce the femoral head without producing a sciatic palsy, it becomes necessary to shorten the femur.

In most such instances, despite the fact that the femur is being shortened, the limb itself is being lengthened because the femoral head no longer rides high on the ilium. The dominant issue here is to obtain the optimal leg length without incurring a sciatic palsy. In such instances, accurate techniques of being able to measure leg lengths intraoperatively at the beginning and subsequent stages are imperative. One such mode of doing this has been described by Woolson and Harris (24). Although instances have been reported of achieving substantially

more leg lengthening (3), the general experience has been quite convincing that efforts to gain more than 2 or 2.5 cm of leg length carries a high risk of encountering sciatic difficulties.

Several other factors are also important in the leg length question. A critical assessment is the presence of pelvic tilt. Many patients with severe arthritis secondary to developmental hip disease have an extensive pelvic tilt. This tilt may be the result of an adduction deformity on the ipsilateral side, an abduction deformity on the contralateral side, or lumbosacral changes. This pelvic tilt can lead to a substantial apparent leg-length discrepancy even if the true leg lengths were equal. These considerations can lead to a series of complexities in correcting both the true and the apparent leg lengths. If, for example, the patient has a severe fixed lumbosacral problem that causes the pelvic tilt, making the leg lengths equal may not be ideal. The lumbar osteoarthritis may prevent resolution of the pelvic tilt, and even if the true leg lengths are created equal by the operation, the patient would still walk with an apparently short leg. In all cases of a leg-length discrepancy, the lateral flexibility of the lumbar spine, and the presence or absence of adduction and adduction deformities, must be correlated with both true and apparent measurements of any leg-length discrepancy.

SURGICAL TECHNIQUES

Incisions

Although any one of a variety of hip incisions is used by different authors, the majority of such surgery is carried out by using a Kocher-Langenbach incision or a direct lateral incision. Rarely do other incisions represent such a specific advantage that they would be preferable.

In cases of total dislocation, the distorted anatomy may make the surgical approach unfamiliar and even dangerous. Commonly, identification and osteotomy of the greater trochanter are vital in establishing proper orientation for the surgeon and correlation of the distorted anatomy. Once the hip capsule is opened, the examining finger can pass within the capsule from the dislocated femoral head down toward the true acetabulum, through the hourglass constriction. This is frequently the safest and at times the only way to identify where the true acetabulum is located. Commonly, release of the iliopsoas tendon from the lesser trochanter is a distinct advantage, and then progressively a complete capsulectomy can be carried out.

Preparation of the Acetabulum

To obtain optimal exposure of the hypoplastic acetabulum in a patient with total dislocation of the hip (developmental), it is often necessary to pass one cobra retractor over the anterior column under the iliopsoas muscle, into the iliac fossa. Then a second cobra retractor is passed across the inferior aspect of the acetabulum and the tip of that cobra retractor may have to penetrate through the obturator fascia. With this instrument in place, all the medial structures can be reflected medially, providing the key exposure of the hypoplastic true acetabulum. At first, the true acetabulum is often hard to locate because it lies so deep and so far medial in the wound and because it is obscured by the hip capsule and pulvinar which lie in abnormal relationships to the mouth of the socket (Figs. 9,10).

Throughout all of this medial dissection and retraction of the soft tissues medially to expose the anterior rim of the acetabulum, great care must be taken not to retract any further medially than is required, because of the danger of a traction lesion to the femoral nerve. This risk is accentuated by the aberrant position of the femoral nerve in cases of total dislocation.

Once the trochanter has been reflected craniad, the entire capsule has been excised, and the true acetabulum exposed, it is possible to make an estimate of the amount of femur that must be removed in order to obtain reduction of the head of the femoral prosthesis into the reestablished acetabulum. Although this cannot be determined exactly, a first estimate can be obtained. Excision of a large portion of the proximal part of the femur or, in the alternate technique, excision of a segment of subtrochanteric diaphysis can be carried out. These excisions should be conservative so that at a later time in the procedure more precise cuts can be made to effect the correct amount of shortening of the femur. My preference is to excise the metaphyseal area rather than do the subtrochanteric area. In the technique involving sub-

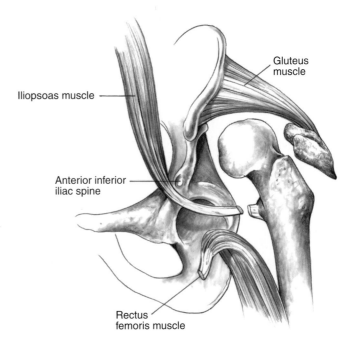

FIG. 9. An exploded view of the acetabulum showing the release of the iliopsoas, the release of the greater trochanter, and the release of the rectus in a patient with total dislocation of the hip.

trochanteric resection, osteotomy of the trochanter is not carried out, because the metaphyseal area including the greater trochanter will be advanced distally. Using either technique, removal of the unwanted bone increases the exposure and creates an increased freedom for the rest of the surgery.

Acetabular Reconstruction

After clearing the pulvinar and fat from the true acetabulum, assessment is made of the available bone stock. This includes palpation of the thickness of the anterior column between the index finger placed in the iliac fossa underneath the iliopsoas muscle and the thumb in the acetabular recess, and by similar palpation of the thickness of the posterior column. This information is used to determine how much bone can be removed while still maintaining sufficient bone stock to provide integrity for the reconstruction. If, for example, the posterior column is substantially thicker than the anterior column, as is commonly the case, the reamers should be directed to remove more bone from the thicker posterior column during the process of enlarging the acetabular recess.

In severe cases, it is often necessary to start with very small reamers such as 36 or 38 mm OD. Carefully and gradually, the acetabular recess is enlarged, hoping, in these severe cases, to create a hemispherical recess of 40 or 42 mm in diameter fully containing the cementless acetabular component. If this can be achieved, standard

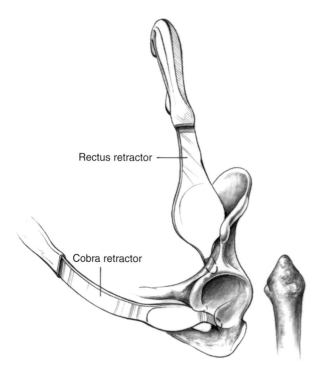

Rectus retractor

Cobra retractor

FIG. 10. The rectus retractor is placed over the anterior margin of the acetabulum, providing medial exposure in that region, and a Cobra retractor is placed into the obturator fossa, showing how that portion of the deeply buried acetabulum in a congenitally dislocated hip can be exposed.

techniques can be used to introduce the hemispherical porous-coated cementless acetabular component in the optimal attitude of 45° of abduction and 20° or 30° of anteversion, and fix that acetabular component with screws. A minimum of two screws is required.

With severe hypoplasia of the acetabulum, the placement of these screws is important. One area of thick bone is the strong mass leading from the acetabulum to the inferior portion of the sacroiliac joint. A second prominent area of bone is that thickened area of the wing of the ilium leading toward the iliac tubercle.

Because the options for the placement of screws into strong bone in the ilium are limited, it is wise to use a socket with multiple screw holes. That way, the options are increased for choosing the best location for the screws. An index finger should be passed through the sciatic notch to identify that region carefully as a guide to screw placement, and to protect the sciatic nerve during screw placement. All of the advice about conservative placement of the screws in the anteromedial region of the acetabulum (23) must be assiduously observed. As noted above, the OD of the acetabular component will determine what head size is required. Our rule is that any acetabular component less than 50 mm OD makes the use of a 22-mm-diameter head advisable.

In many of the difficult reconstructions in this patient population, the complexity of the acetabular reconstruction

hinges on major deficiency of the *lateral* portion of the acetabulum. This is true in many instances of subtotal dislocation and some instances of severe dysplasia. In these cases, there may well be sufficient bone stock anteriorly and posteriorly, with the major deficiency being lateral.

In most of these cases, it is possible to convert a sloping acetabulum to one in which the apex of the hemispherical recess is higher than the most lateral portion of bone (the lateral lip) by crafting the surgery on the acetabulum to achieve this configuration. Generally, the optimal approach is to identify the most lateral portion of acetabular bone stock and preserve it while deepening the acetabulum medial to the lateral lip. In severe cases, this may require hand crafting with acetabular gouges, but it can be done using acetabular reamers. If the reamer chosen is smaller than the general dimensions of the acetabular recess, then reaming can be directed medially and superiorly while leaving the lateral lip intact and unreamed. Once the appropriate contour of the dome of the acetabulum has been created, the acetabular recess can be progressively enlarged, maintaining the apex higher than the lateral lip and not compromising the structural integrity of the lateral lip.

If this can be achieved and the acetabulum is enlarged to an acceptable size (40 mm OD or greater), the acetabular reconstruction can be carried out without additional grafting.

Two circumstances may exist that do not fit this description. In the first, one can obtain an acetabular recess of sufficient volume to encompass an acetabular component of sufficient size but not completely. Here, the guidelines are clearly established. As noted above, it is acceptable to have 30% of the lateral portion of the porous surface of the acetabular component uncovered by bone. If 70% of the porous surface is in contact with viable host bone and the acetabular component is rigidly fixed, excellent bony ingrowth and stability can reliably be achieved despite the uncovered portion. It is prudent to add particulate bone graft over the exposed portion to enlarge the bone mass in that region and provide some additional structural support after the graft unites.

In those circumstances of even greater severity of deficiency of bone stock laterally, additional dilemmas arise. If less than 70% of the acetabular component is covered, usually bulk structural grafting will be necessary. In the case of a primary total hip replacement, it is wise to use the existing femoral head if it is structurally sound. If it is not, or if one is doing a revision operation, an allograft must be used. A femoral head allograft is probably as appropriate as any other source of graft, despite some short-term data that would suggest that other graft sources might be better.

The graft should be shaped to contour closely to the lateral portion of the wing of the ilium after exposure of that cortex by stripping off the abductor muscles. The closer the contour of the graft to the contour of the iliac wing, the better the fit, the greater the stability, and the higher the probability of obtaining union.

The best results in terms of bone union have been achieved fixing the graft to the pelvis with bolts (11,12). A key issue here is that, in many instances, the supra-acetabular portion of the ilium is so hypoplastic that screws may not achieve good purchase. Bolts, on the other hand, can provide excellent fixation even if this region of the bone is thin.

The attachment of the bolt to the nut can be achieved either through a separate incision along the iliac crest, which allows access to the iliac fossa and the quadrilateral space, or by using a nut carrier on the index finger, which is passed into the iliac fossa underneath the iliopsoas muscle from the lateral wound (8–11).

Once the graft is fixed to the wing of the ilium, additional reaming of the acetabular recess can establish continuity of the contour of the recess from the intact viable host bone to the adjacent graft.

At this stage, important decisions need to be made about the most appropriate technique to be used. Evidence appears clear that if a major portion of the structural support must be achieved by the dead graft, cementless fixation is inappropriate. Cement should be used to fix the acetabular component. There is general agreement that if the aggregate supporting structure is 50% dead graft, cement should be used. As discussed, if 70% support can be achieved from the host bone, a cementless socket works well. The decision in terms of those cases with host bone covering more than 50% but less than 70% remains less certain.

An additional technical point of importance in these cases is the fact that the bulk of the graft may in fact redirect the angle of the abductor muscles as they leave the pelvis and approach the femur, and that they may, in fact, complicate reattachment of the greater trochanter.

Preparation of the Femur

If the technique of using an osteotomy of the greater trochanter and resection of the proximal portion of the femur to provide the shortening of the femur is used, at this stage the medullary canal of the femur is opened using the Charnley awl, and it is prepared to receive the femoral component. Because the metaphyseal portion of the femur has been removed, the femoral component will generally need to be small and straight. Our preference is for the CDH Precoat femoral component. Alternatives are a CDH design of a cementless femoral component, generally extensively porous-coated and straight and small, or proximally porous-coated, with or without additional hydroxyapatite. Some surgeons advocate modular components, and in small canals where porous-coated stems would be a mechanical compromise, hydroxyapatite macrolock stems can be utilized.

In the use of a cemented femoral component, the critical features are preparation of the medullary canal, pressurization of the cement, porosity reduction of the cement, assurance of appropriate anteversion, and both proximal and distal centralization to ensure the establishment of a uniform minimum cement mantle thickness. Although some have advocated a polished surface on the cemented femoral stem (7) instead of a smooth surface or a bonded surface, recent evidence shows that even the polished surface bonds to bone cement (J. Davies and W. H. Harris, unpublished data). In addition, the previous concept that the polished femoral stem can subside within the cement mantle over distances greater than 0.5 mm through the process of creep in cement has recently been shown to be incorrect (22).

In those femoral canals that are very small or abnormally shaped, it is often possible to enlarge the femoral canal sufficiently by drilling. This can be very helpful in permitting the use of a larger femoral component (cemented or cementless), and an excellent cement mantle can still be obtained in cemented cases. The optimal cement mantle thickness has been shown to be about 2.5 mm. In very severe cases, this thickness is not possible and one should aim to obtain 1.5 mm of uniform mantle thickness of the cement. The deleterious effects of thinner cement mantles, or of defects in the cement mantle, are clearly established (18). Defects in the cement mantle should be studiously avoided, using the techniques mentioned.

In cases of severe hypoplasia of the femur, the medullary canal may be so small that custom-made implants as small as 7, 8, or 9 mm in diameter may be needed, whether they are for cementless or cemented use. In cementing the femoral component in such difficult cases, the use of a distal centralizer and proximal centralization using two fins underneath the collar of the prosthesis in the shape of a V greatly facilitate optimizing the cement mantle. With such small femoral components, the distal centralizer must be of the napkin-ring style rather than the style that inserts into a hole in the distal tip of the stem.

In the techniques using a subtrochanteric intercalary wire resection of the femur without osteotomy of the greater trochanter, preparation of the femur involves adjusting the pieces to optimize the disparity in cross-sectional diameter, between the distal surface of the proximal portion and the proximal surface of the distal portion of the femur. It is possible to rotate the metaphyseal segment versus the diaphyseal segment to reduce excessive anteversion. If one is using a cementless femoral component, particular care must be taken to ensure rotatory stability of the component and the two fragments in the reapproximation of the femur across the removed segment. This is more easily done with an extensively porous-coated implant than with a proximally porous-coated implant, but success has been reported with proximally porous-coated implants as well (15).

When the medullary canal has been prepared, a trial reduction is attempted. If it is not possible to achieve the reduction, or if, in the process of achieving it, it appears that the sciatic nerve is being placed under excessive stretch (and this can be judged either by visualization or palpation of the sciatic nerve during the attempted reduction), the femur must be shortened further. If the initial transection of the metaphyseal area of the femur was carried out above the lesser trochanter, further resection is needed either through or below the lesser trochanter. If the proximal portion of the femur must be resected substantially below the lesser trochanter, then disruption of a portion of the insertion of the gluteus maximus into the femur is commonly encountered. When only part of this insertion is disrupted, the proximal portion of the insertion of the maximus into the femur can be doubled over and sewn to the distal portion. If all of the insertion is disrupted, sometimes it is necessary to reflect that portion of the gluteus maximus that inserts into the proximal femur separately and reattach it to the femoral cortex.

Restoration of Abductor Function

Once trial reduction can be achieved, range of motion and stability can be checked, and an assessment can be made of the capacity to bring the greater trochanter into contact with the lateral femoral cortex. This is facilitated by freeing the greater trochanter and abductors from all surrounding capsule, scar, and short external rotators so that the greater trochanter can be mobilized as far distally as possible. Then, the femur is brought into maximal abduction so that contact can be made. It is commonly necessary to abduct the femur 50° or 60°.

If additional mobilization is required to reapproximate the greater trochanter to the shaft of the femur, it will be necessary to use a prosthesis with a shorter neck.

Only in instances in which all of these methods have failed should adoption of one the previously mentioned alternatives, such as Z-plasty of the abductors, abductor slide, or sewing the abductors into the fascia lata with the leg in wide abduction, be considered.

POSTOPERATIVE CARE

With straightforward reconstructions and even complex reconstructions with massive grafting or fragile trochanteric reattachments, mobilization can generally begin 1 or 2 days postoperatively. If the leg has been placed in wide abduction to reattach the greater trochanter, it is commonly necessary to overcome the apparent leg-length discrepancy by adding a lift to the shoe on the opposite side. Progression from the use of a walker to crutches can proceed rapidly and most of these patients are able to leave the hospital in 4 or 5 days.

Crutches are usually needed for 3 months in cases in which the greater trochanter has been osteotomized, for 3 to 6 months in instances of intercalary bone resection in the subtrochanteric area, and for 6 months to protect bulk grafts and allow them to have a high probability of uniting. Otherwise, the postoperative program is not very different from a conventional total hip replacement.

ACKNOWLEDGMENT

Supported by the William H. Harris Foundation, WACC 533, Massachusetts General Hospital, Boston, Massachusetts 02114.

REFERENCES

1. Chandler HP, Pennenberg B. *Bone stock deficiency in total hip replacement*. Thorofare, NJ: Slack, 1988;47–102.
2. Cooper RA, McAllister CM, Borden LS, Bauer TW. Polyethylene debris-induced osteolysis and loosening in uncemented total hip arthroplasty. A cause of late failure. *J Arthroplasty* 1992;7:285–290.
3. Coventry MB. Total hip arthroplasty in the adult with complete congenital dislocation. In: Evarts CM, ed. *The hip*. St. Louis: CV Mosby, 1976;77–87.
4. Crowe JF, Mani VJ, Ranawat CW. Total hip replacement in congenital dislocation and dysplasia of the hip. *J Bone Joint Surg* 1979;61A:15–23.
5. Dunn HK, Hess WE. Total hip reconstruction in chronically dislocated hips. *J Bone Joint Surg* 1976;58A:838–845.
6. Fowler JL, Gie GA, Lee AJ, Ling RS. Experience with the Exeter total hip replacement since 1970 [published erratum appears in *Orthop Clin North Am* 20: preceding 519]. *Orthop Clin North Am* 1988;19:477–489.
7. Gross AE, Allan DG, Catre M, Garbuz DS, Stockley I. Bone grafts in hip replacement surgery. The pelvic side. *Orthop Clin North Am* 1993;24:679–695.
8. Harris WH. Allografting in total hip arthroplasty: in adults with severe acetabular deficiency including a surgical technique for bolting the graft to the ilium. *Clin Orthop* 1982;162:150–164.
9. Harris WH. Autografting and allografting in aseptic failure of total hip replacement. In: Welch RB, ed. *The hip*. St. Louis: CV Mosby, 1984;286–295.
10. Harris WH. Total hip replacement for osteoarthritis secondary to congenital dysplasia or congenital dislocation of the hip. *Int Orthop* 1978;2:127–128.
11. Harris WH, Crothers OD. Autogenous bone grafting using the femoral head to correct severe acetabular deficiency for total hip replacement. In: Evarts CM, ed. *The hip*. St Louis: CV Mosby, 1976;161–185.
12. Harris WH, Crothers O, Oh I. Total hip replacement and femoral-head bone-grafting for severe acetabular deficiency in adults. *J Bone Joint Surg* 1977;59A:752–759.
13. Harris WH, Jones WN. The use of wire mesh in total hip replacement surgery. *Clin Orthop* 1975;106:117–121.
14. Hartofilakidis G, Stamos K, Ioannidis TT. Low friction arthroplasty for old untreated congenital dislocation of the hip. *J Bone Joint Surg* 1988;70B:182–186.
15. Holtgrove JL, Hungerford DS. Primary and revision total hip replacement without cement and with associated femoral osteotomy. *J Bone Joint Surg* 1989;71A:1487–1495.
16. Lazansky MG. Low-friction arthroplasty for the sequelae of congenital and developmental hip disease. *Instr Course Lect* 1974;23:194–200.
17. Martell JH, Galante JO, Pierson RH, Jacobs JJ, Rosenberg AG, Maley M. Esperienza clinica con artroprotesi totale d'anca primaria non cementata. *Chir Organi Mov* 1992;77:383–396.
18. Mulroy WF, Estok DM II, Harris WH. Total hip arthroplasty with so-called second generation cementing techniques. A 15 year average follow-up. *J Bone Joint Surg* 1995;77A:1845–1852.
19. Schmalzreid TP, Harris WH. The Harris-Galante porous-coated acetabular component with screw fixation. Radiographic analysis of eighty-three primary hip replacements at a minimum of five years. *J Bone Joint Surg* 1992;74A:1130–1139.

20. Schmalzried TP, Harris WH. The hybrid total hip replacement. A 6.5 year follow-up study. *J Bone Joint Surg* 1993;75B:608–615.

21. Shinar AA, Harris WH. Average sixteen year fate of bulk structural acetabular auto- and allografts in total hip arthroplasty. *J Bone Joint Surg Am* 1997 (accepted).

22. Verdonshot N. Biomechanical failure scenarios for cemented total hip replacement. ISBN 90-9008649-8 CIP-Gegevnes Koninklijke Biblio-theek, Den Haag. *PhD thesis at the Catholic University of Nijmegen.* Nijmegen, The Netherlands. 1995;59–102.

23. Wasielewski RC, Cooperstein LA, Kruger MP, Rubash HE. Acetabular anatomy and the transacetabular fixation of screws in total hip arthro-plasty. *J Bone Joint Surg* 1990;72A:501–508.

24. Woolson ST, Harris WH. A method of intraoperative limb length mea-surement in total hip arthroplasty. *Clin Orthop* 1985;194:207–210.

The Adult Hip, edited by J. J. Callaghan,
A. G. Rosenberg, and H. E. Rubash.
Lippincott–Raven Publishers, Philadelphia © 1998.

CHAPTER 74

Complex Primary Acetabular Replacement

Thomas P. Vail and Donald E. McCollum

The goal of acetabular reconstruction is to achieve a lasting functional outcome for a patient undergoing hip arthroplasty. Optimal function is dependent on restoring hip joint mechanics, achieving secure fixation and coverage of the implant, and managing both bone and soft-tissue abnormalities (Table 1). Recognition of factors that may complicate the surgical technique or outcome of acetabular reconstruction is essential. The purpose of this chapter is threefold. First, factors that make acetabular reconstruction difficult will be outlined, with emphasis on preoperative assessment. Second, options for treatment of difficult acetabular reconstructive problems will be reviewed in detail. Third, prognostic indices for specific clinical situations will be highlighted.

The technical challenges in acetabular reconstruction fall under the headings of difficult exposure such as in ankylosis or protrusio acetabuli, bone loss such as in congenital dysplasia or reconstruction after fracture, and qualitative bone deficits such as in radiation necrosis or metabolic bone disease. However, in most clinical situations, complex acetabular reconstruction will include a combination of technical challenges. For example, difficulty in exposure is expected when operating on a stiff hip. The hip may be stiff for a variety of reasons, including medial migration of the hip center, previous trauma,

or a history of irradiation. Likewise, acetabular bone deficiency makes stable implant fixation difficult to achieve, in addition to complicating exposure. Bone that is biologically impaired may not achieve ingrowth into a porous implant or maintain a stable interface with cement. In addition, bone that is biologically impaired may also be structurally inadequate. Examples of clinical situations where bone may be both biologically and structurally impaired include protrusio acetabuli from a variety of causes (Table 2), previously irradiated bone, and bone that has been devitalized secondary to prior trauma or internal fixation.

Successful acetabular reconstruction requires familiarity with potential problems and access to the tools required to deal with those problems. Thoughtful preoperative planning is required, along with knowledge of details regarding the published experience with particular disease entities. In particular, the surgeon must determine optimal socket placement, what type of fixation might work best, what size component is required, whether bone graft or a customized implant is required, and how the exposure of the acetabulum can be achieved. The best

T. P. Vail and D. E. McCollum: Department of Orthopaedic Surgery, Duke University Medical Center, Durham, North Carolina 27710.

TABLE 1. *Principles of acetabular reconstruction*

1. Restore hip mechanics, center of rotation
2. Restore acetabular integrity
3. Ensure acetabular component coverage
4. Secure rigid graft fixation
5. Secure rigid prosthesis fixation

TABLE 2. *Causes of acetabular protrusio*

Ankylosing spondylitis
Idiopathic
Infection
Metabolic bone disease
Osteomalacia
Osteoporosis
Paget's disease
Rheumatoid arthritis
Rickets
Trauma
Tumor

time to make those determinations is during the preoperative assessment.

PREOPERATIVE ASSESSMENT OF THE DIFFICULT PRIMARY ACETABULUM

Meticulous preoperative planning is an essential step in complex primary acetabular reconstruction. During the preoperative evaluation of the patient and the radiographs, the surgeon should begin to formulate a plan for carrying out the surgical procedure. In patients with abnormal bony anatomy or soft-tissue contracture, one can anticipate how the position of the pelvis may change on the operating table, and how the bony anatomy will affect placement of the acetabular arthroplasty. Often it is extremely difficult to judge the orientation of the face of the acetabulum at the time of surgery. Determination of the optimal center of rotation of the acetabulum, and assessment of bone defects preoperatively will also facilitate the operative procedure.

Acetabular Orientation

Physical examination is the key to identifying bony deformity and contracture of soft tissue that might affect acetabular component position. Plain radiographs with Judet views will usually suffice to further delineate anatomy. Unusual or distinctly abnormal bony anatomy may necessitate the use of computerized tomography.

Acetabular component position is critical for postoperative stability and may have a relationship with wear. Every effort should be made to ensure that the acetabular prosthesis is positioned properly while on the operating table by placing the leg through a methodical check of stability with care to note positions of either impingement or subluxation. Relying on an elevated wall on the socket for stability is risky because the elevated liner can actually lead to a decreased safe range of motion (48) and early loosening if impingement occurs (53).

The placement of the acetabular prosthesis in the correct position will depend directly on the orientation of the bony acetabulum. The orientation of the face of the acetabulum is a primary function of the topographical bony anatomy of the pelvis, and a secondary function of the peripelvic soft tissue (36,54). Congenital dysplasia of the hip (CDH) is an example of a condition with dramatic primary topographical changes in acetabular version and inclination. In CDH, the bony anatomy is abnormal. The acetabulum is often shallow and steeply inclined in CDH, and the anteversion varies significantly from patient to patient (5). Associated capsular contracture, adduction contracture, and leg-length discrepancy can also be present in CDH. These soft-tissue abnormalities can superimpose changes in acetabular orientation. Conditions in which soft-tissue contracture may lead to secondary changes in acetabular orientation include scoliosis, hyperlordosis of the lumbar spine, inflammatory arthritis, and other causes of leg-length inequality. The orientation of the acetabulum will change as the patient moves from the operating table to the upright position. McCollum and Gray (48) have pointed out that the normal pelvis on the operating table in the lateral decubitus position has a decreased lumbar lordosis and a downward obliquity to the operative side. The surgeon can underestimate anteversion, and overestimate the amount of cup abduction if this position is not noted. Likewise, soft-tissue contractures can result in changes in acetabular position from the apparent position on the operating table to the actual position during stance. A fixed adduction contracture will elevate the pelvis to the adducted side (35). A flexion contracture will functionally shorten an extremity. If the adduction contracture is not corrected, the acetabular inclination in stance may be greater than it appears on the operating table. The presence of fixed contracture of soft tissue with pelvic obliquity should be noted preoperatively, and specifically managed surgically to avoid component malposition.

Center of Rotation

Placement of the acetabular component in the correct anatomic location is critical for restoration of normal biomechanics in cases of bone loss with displacement of the center of rotation. The center of rotation can be displaced superiorly, medially, and laterally in certain bone loss situations. The aim in the management of an abnormal center of rotation is to restore the normal lever arm for the abductor muscles of the hip (Fig. 1), as well as the normal joint reactive forces. In developmental dysplasia of the hip, where the center of rotation may be elevated and laterally displaced, normal joint mechanics can be established by placing the hip in the paleoacetabulum (45). However, this must be weighed against the requirement for large bone grafts or cement augmentation (24,51,52). Russotti and Harris (67) have reported acceptable clinical results in patients treated with proximal positioning of the acetabular component without lateral displacement in cir-

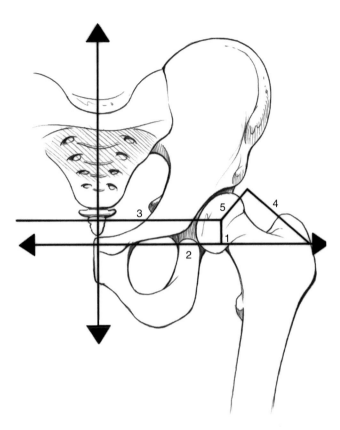

coordinate system that utilizes x and y axes centered on the acetabular teardrop can be placed over a radiograph. Linear distances from the teardrop to the center of rotation of the hip in the x and y planes can be recorded and followed (22).

Acetabular Bone Defects

Acetabular bone defects in primary hip surgery can arise from numerous causes covered in this chapter including trauma, congenital dysplasia, and those causes of acetabular protrusio listed in Table 2. Evaluation and understanding of acetabular bone defects will aid in determining the best approach to the hip, whether bone graft might be required, and the appropriate equipment to have available.

Evaluation of anterior and posterior bone defects will require Judet views of the pelvis in addition to standard radiographic views. In cases of large defects, or in the presence of medial migration of the femoral head where

FIG. 1. This diagram of the pelvis shows the lever arms for the rotational moments around the hip joint. The abductor moment arm is shown as distance 5. Because the abductor musculature (distance 4) must work to oppose the forces of gravity acting at the midline of the pelvis (distance 3), it is important to restore the normal lever arm of the abductor muscles. Without adequate force generation by the abductor muscles, the pelvis will drop to the opposite side during single-leg stance.

cumstances where major bone loss has occurred. With regard to acetabular protrusio, Crowninshield et al. (12) have stated that cortical bone stresses on the medial wall of the acetabulum are increased if the acetabular component is placed medially, and that they can be reduced if the component is placed in a more normal lateral position. Several authors have correlated clinical success in total hip arthroplasty for acetabular protrusio with placement of the acetabulum at the normal center of rotation (3,31,33,49,62,63,68,69).

Ranawat et al. (62) developed a method to locate the correct anatomic position of the acetabulum in deformed hips that facilitates preoperative templating. Figure 2 is a diagram of a normal pelvis showing the placement of Ranawat's triangle. Other commonly used measures of hip joint position are also shown. The acetabular teardrop may be the most useful landmark for following progression of acetabular protrusion. The acetabular teardrop varies little with slight degrees of pelvic obliquity (22). A

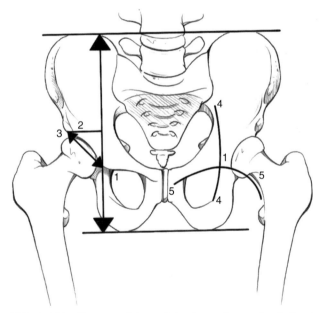

FIG. 2. This diagram of the pelvis shows the method of calculating the anatomic position of the acetabulum described by Ranawat et al. (62). Parallel horizontal lines are drawn at the levels of the ischial tuberosities and the iliac crests. These lines are connected by a perpendicular line that passes through a point (1) located 5 mm medial to the intersection between Shenton's line (5) and Kohler's lines (4). A second point (2) is located on the perpendicular line superior to point 1, at a distance equal to one fifth of the pelvic height measured between the two horizontal lines. From point 2, another perpendicular line is drawn laterally to point 3, which equals the distance between 1 and 2. The isosceles triangle between 1, 2, and 3 locates the acetabulum of a normal hip, with the line 2-3 passing through the subchondral bone of the acetabulum.

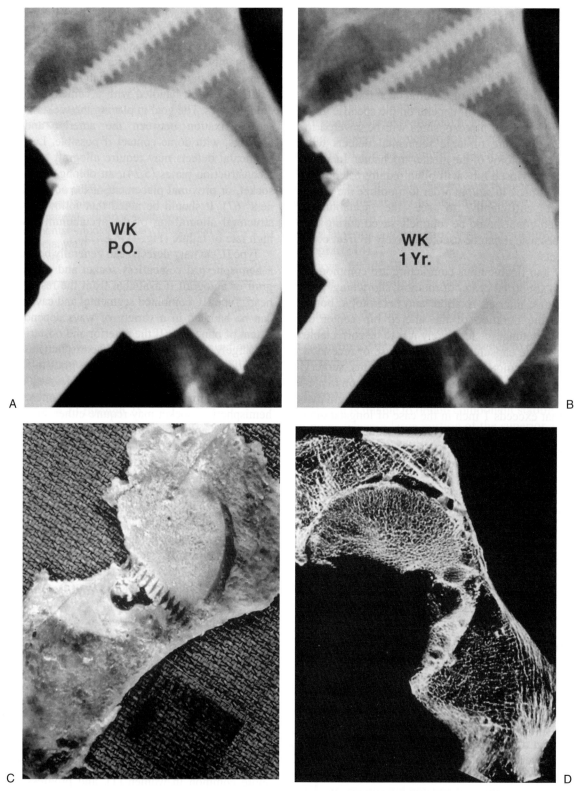

FIG. 4. A case of combined structural and morselized allograft retrieval. Postoperative **(A)** and 1-year follow-up **(B)** radiographs of acetabular reconstruction prior to patient's death. Cross section of specimen **(C)**, specimen radiograph **(D)**,

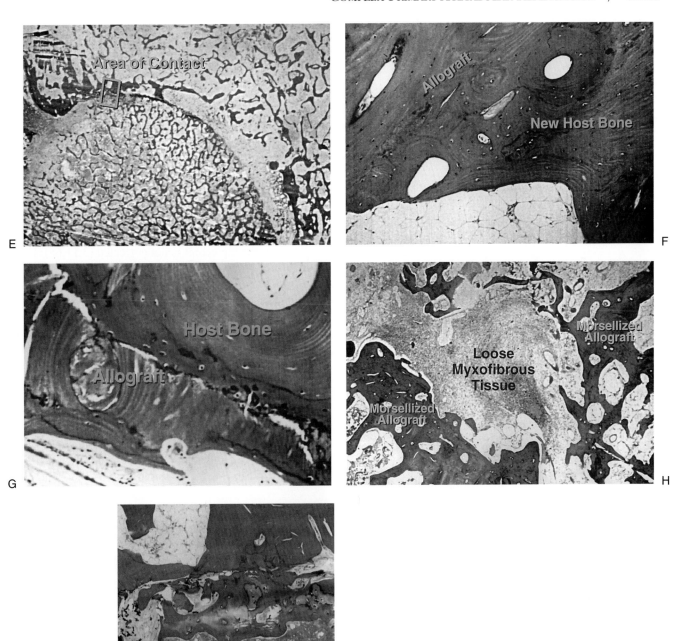

FIG. 4. *Continued.* and histologic specimen **(E)** demonstrate some areas of graft incorporation to host bone (superior-lateral) and areas of medial gaps. Various microscopic histologic sections demonstrate areas of allograft host bone incorporation **(F)**, partial incorporation with fracture **(G)**, and nonincorporation **(H,I)**. (Courtesy of Charles A. Engh, Sr.)

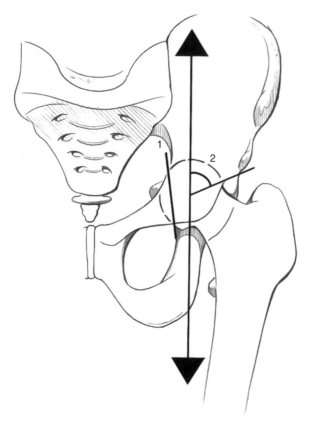

FIG. 5. The diagnosis of acetabular protrusio can be made if the femoral head migrates medial to Kohler's line (1). The normal center-edge angle (2) averages 36° (71). The angle is increased as acetabular protrusio progresses.

These techniques include the use of support rings, bulk autogenous graft with a cemented socket, morselized graft with a cemented socket either with or without a supporting metallic mesh, cement augmentation without bone graft, medial bone graft and a bipolar socket, and a fixed cementless socket with medial bone graft. Sotelo-Garza and Charnley (69) reported on the low friction technique for treatment of protrusio in 1978, comparing the use of a cemented socket with or without slices of autogenous femoral-head bone graft placed medially. The authors concluded that there was no difference in the results whether a bone graft or cement alone had been used. However, other authors have concluded that loosening may be accelerated when cement alone is used, especially when the hip center is not corrected (3,11,68). In a more recent report from Wrightington (34), medial bone graft was recommended to allow correct lateralization and to protect the thin medial wall from the thermal effects of polymerization of polymethylmethacrylate. In addition, Jasty and Harris (29,39) reported that patients with defects through the central acetabular wall had an unacceptably high rate of acetabular component loosening when mesh alone was used without bone graft. If a cemented socket is chosen, a flanged cup can make appropriate placement of the relatively small cup into the larger cement mantle easier to achieve (19) (Fig. 9).

The use of a supporting mesh in conjunction with medial bone graft and a cemented socket for treatment of painful protrusio (Fig. 10) was reported by McCollum et

a rate approximately twice that of femoral head collapse, and that 29 of 36 patients (71%) with protrusio were on steroids.

There is general agreement that the center of rotation should be restored from its abnormal medial position to a more normal lateral position, despite a large variety of surgical techniques for reconstruction (3,21,22,33,43,49, 62,68,69). Dorr and Ranawat (62) emphasized that normalization of the hip center had implications for the long-term fixation of the implant and for the development of radiolucent lines. Clinical observations correlate with the laboratory observation that in a protruded acetabulum, cortical bone stresses on the medial part of the pelvic wall increase with medial placement of the acetabular component (12) (Figs. 6,7). In addition, Borden and Greenky (5) pointed out that because the migration of the femoral head is generally both medial and superior, the depth of the socket is oblong in shape (Fig. 8). The oblong shape of the socket will require careful reaming to create convergence of the acetabular rim without preferentially reaming the superior rim and causing a secondary superior segmental defect.

A variety of surgical techniques have been described to treat the acetabular deficiency associated with protrusio.

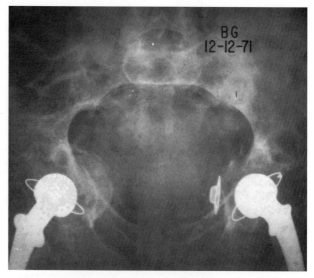

FIG. 6. This radiograph shows a case of bilateral protrusio acetabuli. On the right, the patient was treated with a cemented total hip and medial bone grafting. On the left hip, the patient had medial placement of the socket supported by cement, but no bone graft. (Reprinted with permission from McCollum DE, Nunley JA. Bone grafting in acetabular protrusio: a biologic buttress. In: *The hip: proceedings of the sixth open scientific meeting of the Hip Society,* St. Louis, MO: CV Mosby, 1978;133.)

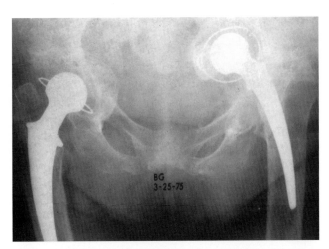

FIG. 7. The 3-year and 3-month follow-up radiographs on the patient in Figure 6. Note that the right hip, which received bone graft, has not shown progression of protrusio. However, the left hip, treated with medial placement of the socket and no bone graft, has shown marked progression of the protrusio acetabuli. (Reprinted with permission from: McCollum DE, Nunley JA. Bone grafting in acetabular protrusio: a biologic buttress. In: *The hip: proceedings of the sixth open scientific meeting of the Hip Society*, St. Louis, MO: CV Mosby, 1978;133.)

al. (49) in 32 patients with 2 to 8 years of follow-up, and later at 10.9 to 17.4 years of follow-up (21). A cortico-cancellous graft was used with Gelfoam at its periphery to prevent cement extrusion, followed by a fine Vitallium (Howmedica Inc., Rutherford, NJ) mesh and a cemented acetabular prosthesis. If the medial wall was found to be completely absent, a protrusio ring was used. No patient in the early report showed progression of the protrusion either in the early postoperative period while the graft was healing or after radiographic incorporation of the graft. At the later follow-up report, the Harris hip rating had dropped an average of 17 points to 72 points, but the technique had been effective in arresting the progression of protrusio acetabuli in 90% of the patients (Fig. 11). In Ranawat and Zahn's (63) report on 23 patients (27 hips) treated with a medial bone graft and a cemented socket and followed for a mean of 3.5 years, none of the hips showed further protrusion, but 11% of the patients showed cement–bone demarcation in three acetabular zones. The authors concluded that for protrusio acetabuli of greater than 5 mm, autogenous bone graft was successful in providing good hip function. No mesh or accessory means of containing cement was used or felt to be necessary.

Heywood (33) described a technique for acetabular arthroplasty using a solid bone graft fashioned from the autogenous femoral head and used to support the medial in conjunction with a cemented prosthesis. Nine cases, reported at 3 months to 2 years of follow-up, showed no complications and radiographic consolidation as demon-

strated by tomography. The Heywood technique has also been used in conjunction with a porous, cementless metal socket. Ebert et al. (17) reported that 24 hips followed for 3 to 9 years demonstrated graft consolidation without subsequent radiolucencies or graft resorption.

Particulate or morselized bone graft has also been used to treat protrusio in conjunction with a cemented socket (42), a bipolar socket (8,50,74), and a noncemented, porous metal socket (24) (Fig. 12). The particulate bone graft is simply placed against the deficient medial wall and reverse-reamed to provide a firm platform over which the socket is placed. The uncemented, porous socket is dependent on solid rim fixation and viable bone at the periphery of the acetabulum (Fig. 13). Although autogenous and homologous particulate graft seem to consolidate well behind a fixed cup that is either cemented or cementless, the results with a bipolar cup are mixed. Wilson and Scott (74) reviewed 22 hips with protrusio acetabular deformity in 14 patients who were treated with a bipolar socket hemiarthroplasty combined with medial wall bone grafting and followed for 36 to 76 months. No patient had groin pain and 17 hips displayed less that 3 mm of migration, although five hips had 3 to 7 mm of migration. Of note is the fact that the authors used a bipolar shell sized 1 to 2 mm larger than the last reamer used. In a series of 18 acetabular reconstructions

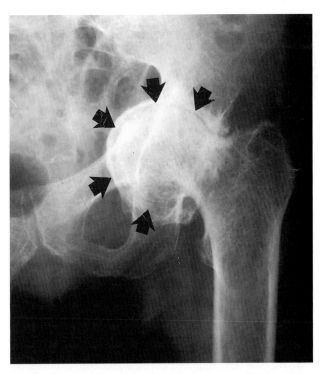

FIG. 8. The *arrows* outline the oblong shape of the acetabulum in protrusio acetabuli. The socket is oblong in shape because the migration is both medial and superior. This asymmetric shape should be noted when attempting to ream the acetabulum so that eccentric reaming does not lead to a superior segmental deficiency.

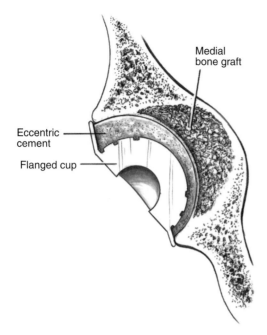

FIG. 9. The use of a flanged cup can help ensure appropriate inferior and medial placement of the cup within a large cement mantle when a cemented cup with medial bone graft is selected as treatment.

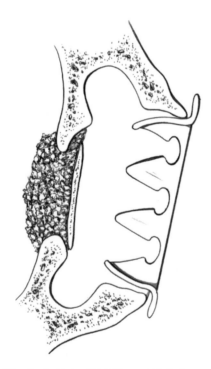

FIG. 10. The technique of treating acetabular protrusio utilized by McCollum (49). The original technique included a wafer of bone from the femoral head placed medially. The wafer technique was replaced with particulate bone graft. A protrusio ring was used with a cemented socket for medial wall deficiency. Subsequently, a noncemented socket has been used with particulate graft.

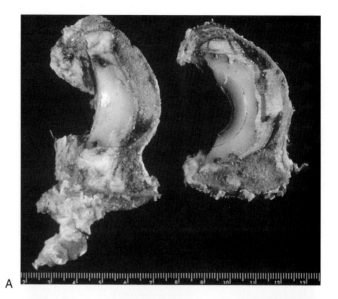

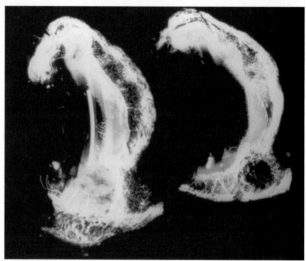

FIG. 11. Autopsy retrieval of patient with morselized graft, Gelfoam, and cemented component in a case of acetabular protrusio. Note the partial graft incorporation on gross specimen **(A)** and section **(B)** radiographs.

(13 cavitary, 5 combined deficiencies), Brien et al. (8) reported graft resorption and a high rate of failure using the bipolar prosthesis. In a larger report from the Mayo Clinic (50) using a bipolar with a mixed group of graft types and a preponderance of revision cases, there was a 27% complication rate (primarily related to the revision procedures), and the majority of the hips showed some graft resorption. However, 83% of the patients reported clinical improvement.

In summary, the use of medial bone graft that consists of either autogenous bone or a combination of autograft and allograft behind either a cemented or cementless, porous socket with restoration of the hip center of rotation is the best technique for acetabular reconstruction in acetabular protrusio. When an adequate rim of bone is

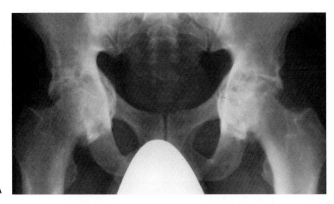
A

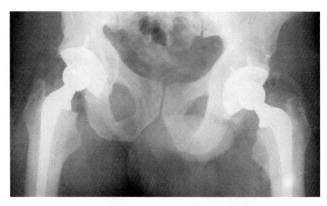
B

FIG. 12. The preoperative **(A)** and postoperative **(B)** radiographs of a patient with ankylosing spondylitis and acetabular protrusio. **(A)** shows restoration of the normal center of rotation of the hip by using a noncemented socket secured on the acetabular rim, and supported medially by autogenous bone graft.

available to allow the use of a cementless socket, there may be an additional benefit of fewer radiolucent lines at early follow-up when compared to a cemented socket. However, ingrowth probably does not occur in the areas where bone graft is opposite porous coating (Fig. 14) (23,32).

Ankylosis

Conversion of an ankylosed hip to a total hip arthroplasty is a technical challenge for the surgeon, mainly because of the difficult exposure (58). Patient education is also important because the recovery can be difficult, particularly if the abductor mechanism is atrophic or absent. Whereas relief of low back pain is an attainable goal, many patients will show only minimal functional improvements, with persistent limp and weakness of the hip girdle muscles. A successful outcome after conversion of ankylosed hip to an arthroplasty is dependent on the diagnosis or etiology of the ankylosis (whether spontaneous or surgically created), the indications for operation, the length of time between fusion and arthroplasty, and the age of the patient. In particular, the arthroplasty failure rate has been high in patients under 50 years of age with a history of previous surgery (41,70).

The indications for conversion from an ankylosed hip to an arthroplasty include pain in the low back and ipsilateral knee, a need for improved mobility, and limb-length discrepancy. Back pain in these patients is a

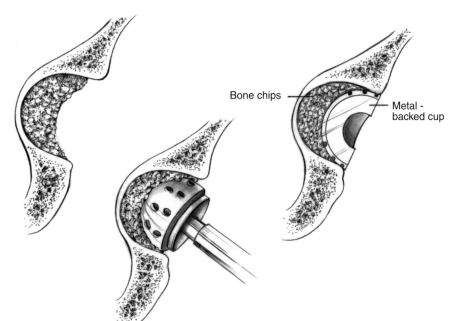

Bone chips

Metal-backed cup

FIG. 13. Corticocancellous bone chips can be molded to fit the defect and the metal socket by *(left)* placing the chips, *(middle)* reaming with the reamer 1 to 2 mm smaller than the socket chosen and rotated in reverse, and *(right)* placing the metal-backed cup into the defect with secure rim contact.

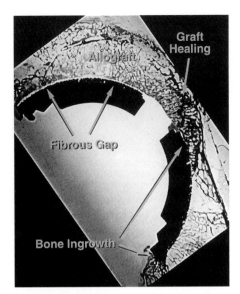

FIG. 14. Histologic section of autopsy retrieval from acetabulum where superiomedial allograft was used along with an uncemented acetabular component. Fibrous gap is noted at the junction of the allograft bone and porous-coated acetabular component. The junction between allograft and host bone has united and bone ingrowth has occurred inferiorly where host bone is opposed to the acetabular component porous surface. (Courtesy of Charles A. Engh, Sr.)

mechanical, nonradicular type of pain. The knee pain can be frequently associated with ligamentous instability. In particular, patients with longstanding adduction contracture at the hip will develop valgus instability at the knee, with associated medial collateral ligament laxity. Patients with spontaneous fusion generally fall into two categories: infections of childhood (Figs. 15,16), and degenerative arthritis. Kilgus et al. (41) reported that the most common diseases leading to arthrodesis or ankylosis include hematogenous bacterial infection, posttraumatic arthritis, ankylosing spondylitis, tuberculous infection, and postoperative infection.

The technique for exposure of the ankylosed hip generally requires osteotomy of the greater trochanter (if it is present) for exposure of the femoral neck and acetabulum. The femoral neck must then be cut *in situ*. Exposure can be difficult because of distorted bony anatomy and contracture of surrounding soft tissues. Ankylosis resulting from childhood pyarthrosis is frequently associated with extensive scar formation and limb shortening. The shortening of the limb is related both to the absence of the joint space and to early cessation of growth. These factors make restoration of length difficult, if not impossible, to achieve. Attempts at lengthening more than 1 inch in conversion of an ankylosed hip resulting from a childhood pyarthrosis may lead to sciatic nerve injury. Amstutz and Sakal (2) reported leg lengthening of up to 6 cm without complication, and Hardinge et al. (27) noted a maximum increase of 4 cm.

As with most degenerative conditions requiring acetabular reconstruction, the goal in this group of patients should be to place the center of rotation of the hip in the anatomic location. The anatomic location is the most favorable with regard to joint mechanics (11), and it places the residual abductor muscles at their greatest mechanical advantage. However, the strength of the abductor muscles postoperatively seems to be related to preoperative muscle mass as well as to the placement of the hip center (41,46).

Kilgus et al. (41) reviewed 41 fused hips in 38 patients that were converted to total hip arthroplasty. The most frequent indication for surgery was progressively debilitating low back or hip pain, functional deficit caused by hip malposition, or knee problems. The postoperative flexion arc averaged 87 degrees, and limbs were lengthened an average of 2.5 cm. Postoperative muscle strength was noted to improve up to 2 years after surgery. Pain was relieved, mobility improved, and dependence on walking aids decreased. Failures were caused by sepsis in four patients, femoral component loosening in four patients, and acetabular component malposition in one patient. The authors noted that the failures were predominantly in patients younger than 50 at the time of arthroplasty, those with a history of two or more previous surgeries, and those with a history of hip injury. However, older patients with a history of spontaneous ankylosis as a result of

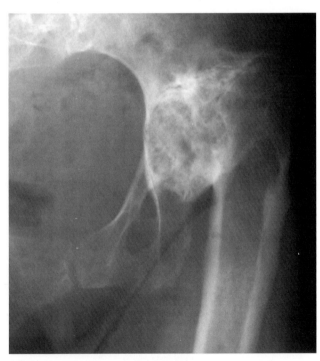

FIG. 15. An ankylosed hip in a 61-year-old woman with a history of a childhood pyarthrosis. The patient presented with a chief complaint of nonradiating low back pain and limited hip movement.

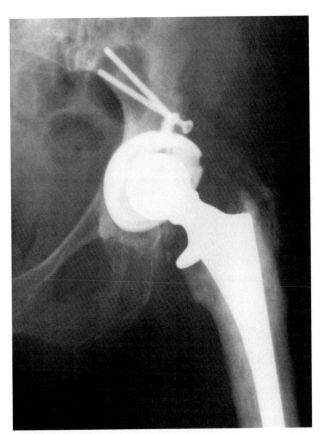

FIG. 16. The postoperative radiograph of the patient in Figure 15 illustrates reconstruction of a superior rim deficiency utilizing autogenous bone graft and a noncemented socket. The acetabular component has been placed in the anatomic location. Note that the greater trochanter is nearly absent in this case.

childhood sepsis without previous surgery did particularly well.

Other authors have reported that patients can be more dependent on walking aids, such as crutches, after conversion from a fused hip to an arthroplasty (64). Nevertheless, patients were found to be grateful for increased mobility and ease of sitting. Poor results with regard to the hip score are associated with advanced age at the time of fusion and duration of the arthrodesis. Hardinge et al. (27) reported the poorest range of motion postoperatively in old cases of infantile sepsis, thought to be caused by depression of growth of the proximal femur and related musculature. In a review of 80 total hip arthroplasties in 74 patients, Strathy and Fitzgerald (70) reported only one failure in the 20 hips of 15 patients who had a spontaneous ankylosis. However, 20 (33%) of the 60 hips of the 60 patients who had a surgical ankylosis had complications associated with the arthroplasty, including loosening, infection, and dislocation. Postoperative infection has been associated with previous surgery (7). Reconstruction in the case of arthrodesis is also discussed in the chapter on hip arthrodesis.

ACETABULAR RECONSTRUCTION AFTER FRACTURE

Acetabular reconstruction after fracture incorporates many of the concepts covered in other sections within this chapter. Ankylosis, scarring, tethering of the sciatic nerve, sciatic nerve palsy, retained hardware in the operative field, fracture nonunion, and large segments of necrotic bone can complicate treatment. One of the basic tenets of dealing with a difficult acetabular reconstruction in this setting is to give the fracture adequate time to heal. It is easier to resurface a healed acetabular malunion than an unstable nonunion. Primary arthroplasty at the time of fracture is uncommon but may be indicated in the older patient (11).

Proper preparation requires having the tools to remove retained hardware if it precludes placement of the acetabular arthroplasty. Tools include standard equipment used for placement of screws and plates, and an available high-speed, metal-cutting burr. In general, hardware that is not in the way of the acetabular reconstruction is not removed

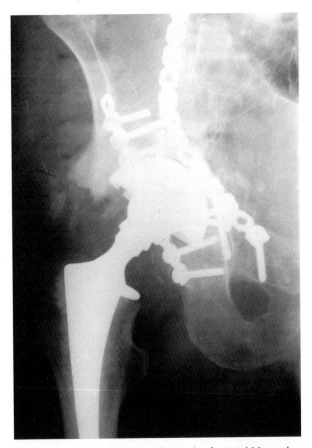

FIG. 17. This postoperative radiograph of a total hip replacement, done as a late reconstruction after an acetabular fracture, shows that the majority of the hardware remains in place. Screws and plates that come into contact with the acetabular component, however, must be removed. There has been some heterotopic bone formation at the acetabular rim.

(Fig. 17). As is the case with any stiff or ankylosed hip, trochanteric osteotomy or trochanteric slide may be required to achieve exposure, but this is not routinely done unless indicated.

In a classic article on this topic, Harris (28) described the use of mold arthroplasty for treatment of traumatic arthritis of the hip after dislocation and acetabular fracture. Pritchett and Bortell (60) reported on 19 patients, average age 49 years, with total hip replacement after central fracture dislocation of the acetabulum, followed for a minimum of 2 years. Patients were treated with low dose irradiation to discourage heterotopic ossification postoperatively. No component loosening, infection, dislocation, or heterotopic bone was noted. The average follow-up Harris Hip Score was 84. Other mid-term reports of cementless hemispherical cups placed after acetabular fracture indicate minimal radiolucencies and no migration of the cups, with radiographic healing of associated bone grafts (40). These results seem to be superior to the use of cemented arthroplasty after previous acetabular fracture where the loosening rate has been reported as high as 53% at similar length of follow-up (65). However, a recent report by Dan Mears (personal communication, 1996) did demonstrate higher loosening rates with uncemented acetabular components used in cases of previous central fracture dislocation treated by open reduction and internal fixation. The etiology could be ischemia from the trauma and dissection at the time of reduction and fixation.

ACETABULAR RECONSTRUCTION AFTER PELVIC IRRADIATION

Radiation therapy treatment has the potential for skeletal complications (7,9,10,61,71). Irradiation of the pelvis can complicate acetabular reconstruction by adversely affecting the vascularity and structural integrity of bone. Osteonecrosis of the pelvis (15), with resultant bony collapse and progressive acetabular protrusion (26,30), are recognized complications of pelvic irradiation. The radiation-induced changes in bone are both vascular and cellular (20,72). Vascular changes can vary from minimal change to fibrosis and hyalinization of the media of blood vessels. In addition, radiation can make bone hypocellular with marrow fibrosis, leading to osteopenia (20) and susceptibility to fracture (10,13) and infection (Fig. 18). Radiation changes in bone are thought to be dose related, with an initial threshold at 3000 rads and cell death occurring at 5000 rads (6,37). Higher doses in fewer fractionations may also cause more damage (71).

Radiation changes in the pelvis can be recognized radiographically by the presence of osteopenia. Subsequent changes can be mixed or sclerotic, with associated soft-tissue calcifications (Fig. 19) and radiation enteritis (13). Focal lytic areas in long bones after irradiation have also been described (57). The radiographic appearance must be correlated with clinical findings, as previously irradiated bone has the potential for malignant transformation (6).

A high rate of acetabular loosening has been reported after total hip replacement in previously irradiated hips using both cemented and cementless components. Massin and Duparc (47) reported 52% acetabular loosening at a mean follow-up of 69 months in 56 patients (71 hips). Patients in this series received an average of 5500 rads during radiation therapy. The high rate of failure was thought to be caused by mechanical insufficiency of irradiated periacetabular bone. In a subsequent group of 22 patients, acetabular reinforcement rings were used. At a mean length of follow-up of 40 months, the aseptic loosening rate was 19%, with two additional cases of septic loosening. Jacobs et al. (38) reported on early failure of acetabular components inserted without cement after previous pelvic irradiation. Nine acetabular components in eight patients were reviewed at an average of 37 months after surgery. Four of the nine acetabular components were found to have failed at an average of 25 months after insertion. The failed hips received an average dose of radiation of 5551 rads.

In summary, radiation treatment to the pelvis has potential impact on implant longevity and the rate of complications in acetabular reconstruction. The sequellae of radiation therapy, such as soft-tissue fibrosis, radiation enteritis, marrow fibrosis, and focal bone necrosis, can add technical complexity to surgical procedures. Severe bone destruction, soft-tissue injury, or vascular insufficiency secondary to irradiation may lead the surgeon to consider non-operative treatment, or treatment other than acetabular arthroplasty. The surgeon should be aware of the long-term, progressive effects of radiation so that the patient can be adequately counseled on reasonable expectations after surgery.

SUMMARY

Primary acetabular reconstruction can become complicated in the presence of a difficult exposure, a quantitative bone deficit, or a qualitative bone deficit. The preoperative assessment of deformity and the awareness of potential complications will significantly impact the probability of a successful surgical outcome. The choice of surgical technique will depend on the need to restore the normal mechanics of the hip joint and deficient bone stock.

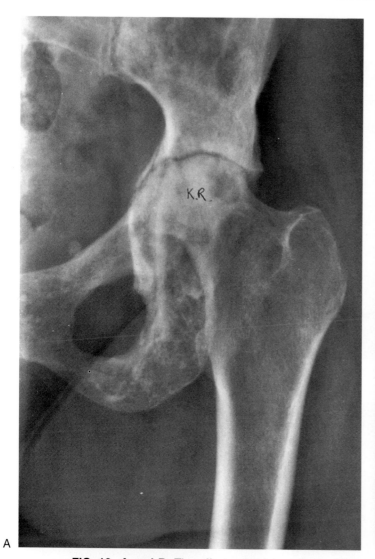

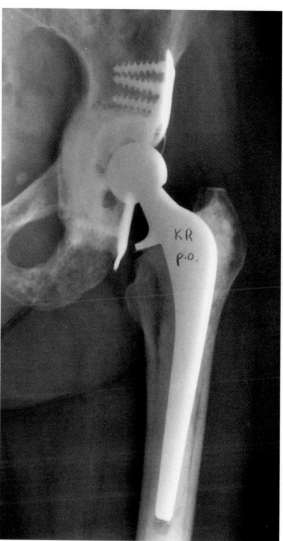

A

B

FIG. 18. A and B: The effects of pelvic radiation. The patient, a 47-year-old woman who had breast cancer, received radiation treatment of 6000 to 7000 rads to the hip joint area for metastatic disease. The radiograph shows a mixed sclerotic, lytic pattern of the bone with femoral head collapse, medial acetabular wall fracture, and soft-tissue calcification **(A).** Cemented acetabular reinforcement rings, such as the one shown in Figure 10, should be considered in such cases.

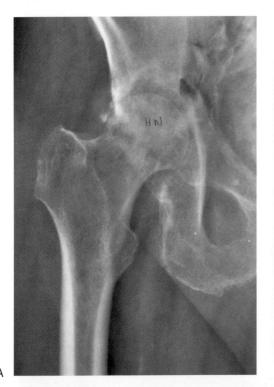

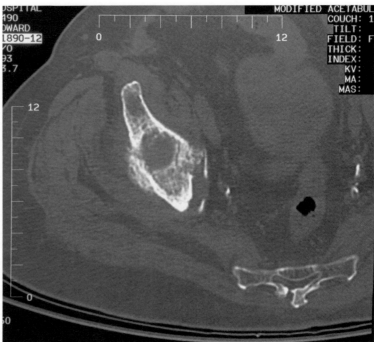

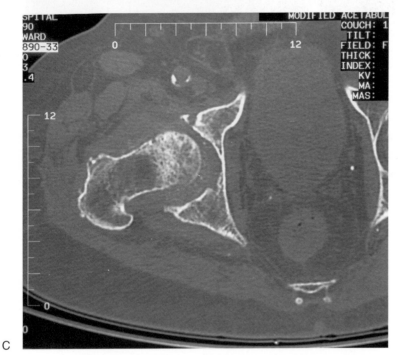

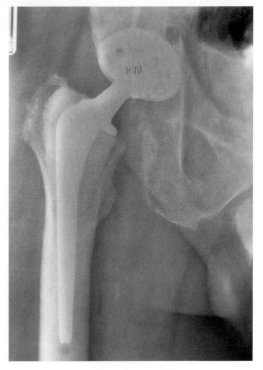

FIG. 19. This 76-year-old man with a history of prostatic carcinoma sustained a pathologic fracture of the acetabulum after treatment with 5000 rads of irradiation to the hip joint area for metastatic disease **(A)**. A computed tomographic (CAT) scan section **(B)** through the dome of the acetabulum shows the healing fracture at 6 months after its occurrence. A second CAT scan section **(C)** shows minimal postir-radiation changes within the posterior column inferiorly. At the time of surgery, the bone in the acetab-ular area was grossly healthy, with normal-appearing vascularity and a visibly healing fracture. There-fore, a cementless socket was chosen for treatment **(D)**.

REFERENCES

1. Alexander C. The aetiology of primary protrusio acetabuli. *Br J Radiol* 1965;38:567–580.

2. Amstutz HC, Sakal DN. Total joint replacement for ankylosed hips. *J Bone Joint Surg* 1975;57A:619.

3. Bayley JC, Christie MJ, Ewald FC, Kelley K. Long term results of total hip arthroplasty in protrusio acetabuli. *J Arthroplasty* 1987;2:275.

4. Berry DJ, Muller ME. Revision arthroplasty using an anti-protrusio cage for massive acetabular bone deficiency. *J Bone Joint Surg Br* 1992;74(5):711–715.

5. Borden LS, Greenky SS. The difficult primary total hip replacement. Acetabular problems. In: Steinberg ME, ed. *The hip and its disorders*. New York: WB Saunders, 1991;1007–1019.

6. Bragg DG, Shidnia H, Chu FC, Higinbotham NL. The clinical and radiographic aspects of radiation osteitis. *Radiology* 1970;97:103–111.

7. Brewster RC, Coventry MB, Johnson EW Jr. Conversion of the arthrodesed hip to a total hip arthroplasty. *J Bone Joint Surg* 1975;57A:27.

8. Brien WW, Bruce WJ, Salvati EA, Wilson PD, Pellicci PM. Acetabular reconstruction with a bipolar prosthesis and morselized bone grafts. *J Bone Joint Surg Am* 1985;72:1230–1235.

9. Chan Sl, Kagan R, Streeter OE Jr, Ryoo MC. Outcome of care. Complications from radiation therapy treatment. *Am J Clin Oncol* 1993;16:81–85.

10. Csuka M, Brewer BJ, Lynch KL, McCarty DJ. Osteonecrosis, fractures, and protrusio acetabuli secondary to x-irradiation therapy for prostatic carcinoma. *J Rheumatol* 1987;14:165–170.

11. Coventry MB. The treatment of fracture dislocation of the hip by total hip arthroplasty. *J Bone Joint Surg* 1974;56A:1128–1134.

12. Crowninshield RD, Brand RA, Pedersen DR. A stress analysis of acetabular reconstruction in protrusio acetabuli. *J Bone Joint Surg* 1983;65A:495.

13. Dalinka MK, Vazzeo JP Jr. Complications of radiation therapy. *CRC Crit Rev Diagn Imaging* 1985;23:235–267.

14. D Antonio JA, Capello WN, Borden LS, Bargar WL, Bierbaum BF, Boettcher WG, Steinberg ME, Stulberg SD, Wedge JH. Classification and management of acetabular abnormalities in total hip arthroplasty. *Clin Orthop* 1989;243:126.

15. Deleeuw HW, Pottenger LA. Osteonecrosis of the acetabulum following radiation therapy. A report of two cases. *J Bone Joint Surg* 1988;70A:293–299.

16. Duthie RB, Harris CM. A radiographic and clinical survey of the hip joint in seropositive rheumatoid arthritis. *Acta Orthop Scand* 1965;40:346.

17. Ebert FR, Hussain S, Krackow KA. Total hip arthroplasty for protrusio acetabuli: a 3- to 9-year follow up of the Heywood technique. *Orthopedics* 1992;15(1):17–20.

18. Edelstein G, Murphy WA. Protrusio acetabuli: radiographic appearance in arthritis and other conditions. *Arthritis Rheum* 1983;26:1511.

19. Eftekhar NS. Specific conditions and variations: Protrusio acetabuli. In: Eftekhar NS, ed. *Total hip arthroplasty*. St. Louis, MO: Mosby, 1993;1033–1067.

20. Ergun G, Howland WJ. Postradiation atrophy of mature bone. *CRC Crit Rev Diagn Imaging* 1980;12:225–243.

21. Gates HS III, McCollum DE, Poletti SC, Nunley JA. Bone grafting in total hip arthroplasty for protrusio acetabuli. *J Bone Joint Surg* 1990;72(A):248–251.

22. Gates HS III, Poletti SC, Callaghan JJ, McCollum DE. Radiographic measurements in protrusio acetabuli. *J Arthroplasty* 1989;4(4):347–351.

23. Greis PE, Kang JD, Silvaggio V, Rubash HE. A long term study on defect filling and bone ingrowth using a canine fiber metal total hip model. *Clin Orthop* 1992;274:47–59.

24. Gross AE, Allan DG, Catre M, Garbuz DS, Stockley I. Bone grafts in hip replacement surgery. The pelvic side. *Orthop Clin North Am* 1993;24(4):679–695.

25. Haentjens P, de Boeck H, Handelberg F, Casteleyn PP, Opdecam P. Cemented acetabular reconstruction with the Muller support ring. A minimum five-year clinical and roentgenographic follow-up study. *Clin Orthop* 1993;290:225–235.

26. Hall FM, Mauch PM, Levene MB, Goldwtein MA. Protrusio acetabuli following pelvic irradiation. *AJR* 1979;132:291–293.

27. Hardinge K, Williams D, Etienne A, et al. Conversion of fused hips to low friction arthroplasty. *J Bone Joint Surg* 1977;59B:385.

28. Harris WH. Traumatic arthritis of the hip after dislocation and acetabular fractures: treatment by mold arthroplasty. *J Bone Joint Surg* 1969;51A:737.

29. Harris WH. Management of the deficient acetabulum using cementless fixation without bone grafting. *Orthop Clin North Am* 1993;24(4):663–665.

30. Hasselbacher P, Schumacher HR. Bilateral protrusio acetabuli following pelvic irradiation. *J Rheumatol* 1977;4:189–196.

31. Hastings DE, Parker SM. Protrusio acetabuli in rheumatoid arthritis. *Clin Orthop* 1975;108:76.

32. Heekin RD, Engh CA, Vinh T. Morselized allograft in acetabular reconstruction: a post-mortem retrieval analysis. *Clin Orthop* 1995;319:184–190.

33. Heywood AWB. Arthroplasty with a solid bone graft for protrusio acetabuli. *J Bone Joint Surg* 1980;62B:332.

34. Hirst P, Esser M, Murphy JC, Hardinge K. Bone grafting for protrusio acetabuli during total hip replacement. *J Bone Joint Surg* 1987;69B:229.

35. Hoikka V, Ylikoski M, Eskola A, Santavirta S. Inclination of the acetabular cup in erect posture radiographs. *Orthopedics* 1993;16(12):1321–1323.

36. Horne G. Preoperative assessment of the acetabulum. *Orthop Clin North Am* 1993;24(4):655–661.

37. Howland WJ, Loeffler RK, Starchman DE, Jognson RG. Postirradiation atrophic changes of bone and related complications. *Radiology* 1975;117;677–685.

38. Jacobs JJ, Kull LR, Frey GA, Gitelis S, Sheinkop MB, Kramer TS, Rosenberg AG. Early failure of acetabular components without cement after previous pelvic irradiation. *J Bone Joint Surg* 1995;77A:1829–1835.

39. Jasty M, Harris WH. Results of total hip reconstruction using acetabular mesh in patients with central acetabular deficiency. *Clin Orthop* 1988;237:142–149.

40. Karpos PAG, Christie MJ. THA following acetabular fracture using cementless acetabular components: 4 to 8 year results. Presented to *The fifth fall meeting of the Association for Arthritic Hip and Knee Surgery*. November, 1995.

41. Kilgus JD, Amstutz HC, Wolgin MA, Dorey FJ. Joint replacement for ankylosed hips. *J Bone Joint Surg* 1990;72A:45.

42. Kinzinger PJ, Karthaus RP, Slooff TJ. Bone grafting for acetabular protrusion in hip arthroplasty. 27 cases of rheumatoid arthritis followed for 2–8 years. *Acta Orthop Scand* 1991;62(2):110–112.

43. Knight JL, Fujii K, Atwater R, Grothaus L. Bone-grafting for acetabular deficiency during primary and revision total hip arthroplasty. A radiographic and clinical analysis. *J Arthroplasty* 1993;8(4):371–382.

44. Kwong LM, Jasty M, Harris WH. High failure rate of bulk femoral head allografts in total hip acetabular reconstructions at 10 years. *J Arthroplasty* 1993;8(4):341–346.

45. Laforgia R, Specchiulli F, Miolla L, Solarino GB. Total hip replacement in the paleoacetabulum: biomechanical considerations. *Ital J Orthop Traumatol* 1991;17(3):345–350.

46. Lubahn JE, Evarts CMCC, Feltner JB. Conversion of ankylosed hips to total hip arthroplasty. *Clin Orthop* 1980;153:146.

47. Massin P, Duparc J. Total hip replacement in irradiated hips: a retrospective review of 71 cases. *J Bone Joint Surg* 1995;77B:847–852.

48. McCollum DE, Gray WJ. Dislocation after total hip arthroplasty. Causes and prevention. *Clin Orthop* 1990;261:159–170.

49. McCollum DE, Nunley JA, Harrelson JM. Bone grafting in total hip replacement for acetabular protrusion. *J Bone Joint Surg* 1980;62(A):1065.

50. McFarland EG, Lewallen DG, Cabanela ME. Use of bipolar endoprosthesis and bone grafting for acetabular reconstruction. *Clin Orthop* 1991;(268):128–139.

51. McQueary FG, Johnston RC. Coxarthrosis after congenital dysplasia. Treatment by total hip arthroplasty without acetabular bone-grafting. *J Bone Joint Surg* 1988;70(A):1140–1144.

52. Mulroy RG Jr, Harris WH. Failure of acetabular autogenous grafts in total hip arthroplasty. *J Bone Joint Surg* 1990;72(A):1536–1540.

53. Murray DW. Impingement and loosening of the long posterior wall acetabular implant. *J Bone Joint Surg Br* 1992;74(3):377–379. Comment in: *J Bone Joint Surg Br* 1993;75(1):162–163.

54. Murray DW. The definition and measurement of acetabular orientation. *J Bone Joint Surg Br* 1993;75(2):228–232.

55. Oh I, Harris WH. Design concepts, indications, and surgical technique for use of the protrusio shell. *Clin Orthop* 1982;162:175–184.

56. Otto AW. *Seltene Biobachtungen zur Anatomie. Physiologie und Pathologie gehorig*, 2nd ed. Berlin, 1824.
57. Paling MR, Herdt JR. Radiation osteitis: a problem of recognition. *Radiology* 1980;137;339–342.
58. Perugia L, Santori FS, Mancini A, Manili M, Falez F. Conversion of the arthrodesed hip to a total hip arthroplasty. Indications and limitations. *Ital J Orthop Traumatol* 1992;18(2):145–153.
59. Pomeranz MM. Intrapelvic protrusion of the acetabulum (Otto pelvis). *J Bone Joint Surg* 1932;14:663–686.
60. Pritchett JW, Bortel DT. Total hip replacement after central fracture dislocation of the acetabulum. *Orthop Rev* 1991;20(7):607–610.
61. Prosnitz LR. Radiation complications for Hodgkin's disease and seminoma: assessing the risk:benefit ratio. *Int J Radiat Oncol Biol Phys* 1988;15:239–241.
62. Ranawat CS, Dorr LD, Inglis AE. Total hip arthroplasty in protrusio of rheumatoid arthritis. *J Bone Joint Surg* 1980;62(A):1059–1065.
63. Ranawat CS, Zahn MG. The role of grafting in correction of protrusio acetabuli by total hip arthroplasty. *J Arthroplasty* 1986;1(2):131–137.
64. Reikeras O, Bjerkreim I, Ragnhild G. Total hip arthroplasty for arthrodesed hips: 5 to 13 year results. *J Arthroplasty* 1995;10(4):529–31.
65. Romness DW, Lewallen DG. Total hip arthroplasty after fracture of the acetabulum. Long term results. *J Bone Joint Surg* 1990;72B(5):761–764.
66. Rosson J, Schatzker J. The use of reinforcement rings to reconstruct deficient acetabula. *J Bone Joint Surg Br* 1992;74(5):716–720.
67. Russotti GM, Harris WH. Proximal placement of the acetabular component in total hip arthroplasty. A long-term follow-up study. *J Bone Joint Surg Am* 1991;73(4):587–592.
68. Salvati EA, Bullough P, Wilson PD Jr. Intrapelvic protrusion of the acetabular component following total hip replacement. *Clin Orthop* 1975;111:212–227.
69. Sotelo-Garza A, Charnley J. The results of Charnley arthroplasty of the hip performed for protrusio acetabuli. *Clin Orthop* 1978;132:12.
70. Strathy GM, Fitzgerald RH Jr. Total hip arthroplasty in ankylosed hip: a ten-year follow-up. *J Bone Joint Surg* 1988;70A:963.
71. Thames HD Jr, Withers HR, Peters LJ, Fletcher CH. Changes in early and late radiation responses with altered dose fractionation: implications for dose-survival relationships. *Int J Radiat Oncol Biol Phys* 1982;8:219–226.
72. Warren S. The histopathology of radiation lesions. *Physiol Rev* 1944;24:225–238.
73. Wiberg G. Studies on dysplastic acetabula and congenital subluxation of the hip joint: with special reference to the complications of osteoarthritis. *Acta Chir Scand* 1939;83:Suppl 58.
74. Wilson MG, Scott RD. Bipolar socket in protrusio acetabuli. *J Arthroplasty* 1993;8(4):405–411.

The Adult Hip, edited by J. J. Callaghan,
A. G. Rosenberg, and H. E. Rubash.
Lippincott–Raven Publishers, Philadelphia © 1998.

CHAPTER 75

Complex Primary Femoral Replacement

Andrew H. Glassman

Total hip replacement (THR) is considered complex when the likelihood of intraoperative technical difficulties, perioperative complications, or premature failure is greater than usual. The purpose of this chapter is to identify conditions that render primary femoral arthroplasty technically complex, to describe the specific challenges encountered during THR in each of these conditions, and to outline the surgical techniques that have been developed to deal with these problems.

Optimal reconstruction of the arthritic hip requires careful attention to intraosseous considerations, (e.g., the relationship between the components and recipient bones) and to extraosseous considerations (e.g., the spatial relationship between the acetabulum and the proximal femur). A variety of congenital, developmental, and acquired conditions manifest as alterations in femoral anatomy, bone quality, or both. These abnormalities impact primarily upon intraosseous considerations. It must be remembered that many of the conditions to be discussed also affect acetabular reconstruction, which is covered elsewhere in this book. The demands that these conditions impose upon acetabular arthroplasty must be kept in mind when planning femoral arthroplasty, to optimize extraosseous relations (e.g., leg length, offset, and stability against dislocation). Also, these conditions are frequently accompanied by soft-tissue abnormalities that must be addressed during reconstruction.

LEG-LENGTH DISCREPANCY

General

Leg length after routine or complex THR is a major concern for both surgeon and patient. Most often, the preoperative discrepancy is minimal and does not in itself present

A. H. Glassman: Joint Replacement Program, National Hospital Medical Center, Arlington, Virginia 22206.

technical demands sufficient to render a case complex. The point at which leg-length concerns become problematic is difficult to define precisely, but the following general principles and specific situations should be kept in mind.

Most challenging cases involve the need to lengthen an extremity while avoiding the well-known complications associated with this undertaking. The mechanical consequences of excessive lengthening include a vaulting limp, pelvic obliquity, and low back pain (20,21,40,44,70). The principal physiologic consequence is postoperative nerve palsy, for which excessive leg lengthening is the most common identifiable cause (15,53,65,66). The amount that a limb can be lengthened during THR without incurring nerve injury is uncertain (34,53). A range of 2 to 3 cm is commonly cited (1,63,72). Sunderland (62) states that acute lengthening of a peripheral nerve by as little as 6% of its length may result in severe nerve injury, suggesting that the absolute amount of lengthening possible may be less in shorter individuals. The etiology and age at onset of hip disease also influence the amount of lengthening possible. Individuals who have reached skeletal maturity prior to the onset of hip disease will have developed normal nerve length and should tolerate full restoration of limb length in the face of shortening beyond the 2 to 3 cm mentioned. An example would be posttraumatic arthritis after central fracture/dislocation in an adult. In contrast, a patient who suffered childhood sepsis with physeal arrest may tolerate far less lengthening. The risk of overlengthening the limb is particularly high in certain situations that must be recognized. The most obvious example is moderate to severe developmental dysplasia with subluxation or dislocation. Acetabular reconstruction with the prosthetic socket in the anatomic (low) position may require a femoral shortening procedure to avoid excessive lengthening of the sciatic nerve, if not the limb. More subtle but equally challenging is extreme coxa vara. The surgical management of both conditions is discussed later.

The need to shorten the extremity during THR is far less common. Trochanteric advancement may be required to avoid compromise of abductor function and dislocation, especially if the limb is shortened 2 cm or more (72).

The management of patients with pelvic obliquity requires careful consideration. Attempts to correct an apparent leg-length discrepancy in the presence of long-standing fixed pelvic obliquity generally results in excessive leg lengthening or shortening, aggravates mechanical low back pain, and is poorly tolerated. The most important factors in the successful management of complex leg-length problems are careful preoperative planning and surgical technique.

Preoperative Evaluation

True leg-length discrepancy (TD) arises from shortening of the component bones or cephalad displacement of the femoral head relative to the true acetabulum. It is most commonly measured as the distance between the anterior superior iliac spine (ASIS) and the distal aspect of the ipsilateral medial malleolus. Factors contributing to spurious measurements must be recognized. Locating the ASIS can be quite difficult, especially in obese patients (1,73), and may be impossible if the patient has had prior pelvic osteotomy. Full-length scanograms are helpful in such cases (73) but not economically feasible for routine use. Unilateral or asymmetric contractures of the hip or knee must be recognized. Hip flexion contractures are reconciled by sitting the patient up until both thighs lie flat on the exam table. A unilateral knee flexion contracture is accommodated by placing a padded bolster beneath the knees until both are equally flexed. The magnitude of a unilateral abduction contracture should be measured and the opposite limb placed in an equal amount of abduction. In the absence of asymmetrical contractures, a patient with a TD usually exhibits a compensatory, reversible scoliosis, with its apex directed toward the shortened limb. If the scoliosis is purely secondary and flexible, a lift equal to the measured TD placed under the short extremity should level the pelvis and correct the scoliosis. This is confirmed with a standing pelvic radiograph with the lift in place (1). As an additional test, pelvic obliquity and scoliosis secondary to leg-length discrepancy are eliminated when the patient is in the sitting position. Apparent leg lengths are measured from the umbilicus to the medial malleolus of each leg. In the presence of a TD, an apparent discrepancy (AD) of similar magnitude will exist.

If an AD is found in the absence of a TD, or if there is a significant difference in the magnitude of the two types of discrepancy, a fixed pelvic obliquity is present. This will not disappear when the patient is examined in the seated position, or when the TD is corrected with a lift. The presence of fixed pelvic obliquity can also be confirmed using standing radiographs. A fixed scoliotic deformity that does not resolve on bending films is generally found.

Preoperative templating is covered elsewhere in this text, but several points should be emphasized. Acetabular component position is largely dictated by the patient's anatomy, and socket position is therefore templated first. Because much more latitude is possible on the femoral side, leg-length discrepancies are reconciled by femoral component selection and positioning after the cup position is established. The level of neck resection and depth of femoral component seating are planned to optimize the extraosseous relations, but in so doing, the intraosseous "fit and fill" of the stem will be altered. The level of neck resection determines the depth of seating of the femoral component and therefore the component size required. With modular femoral heads, the surgeon can choose a preferred level of femoral neck resection and subsequently correct leg length with various lengths of heads.

Different combinations of neck resection and femoral head length can yield the same leg length, but each results in a different amount of femoral offset (Fig. 1). For example, a patient with coxa valga can be managed by combining a high neck resection, a larger femoral component, and a shorter prosthetic head (see Fig. 1B). In cases of coxa vara, a low neck cut, a smaller femoral component, and a long prosthetic head may be combined to restore both leg length and offset (see Fig. 1C). However, sacrifice of the femoral neck results in diminished torsional stability of the implant. The use of a longer head and neck segment also increases the stresses placed on the prosthetic neck. Adequate femoral head length may require a skirt about the base of the head, which can lead to reduced range of motion, impingement, and dislocation. Hence, it is recommended that in extreme cases of coxa vara, an implant with adequate inherent offset be selected (49).

Preoperative planning for cases of moderately severe developmental dysplasia with subluxation may be difficult and inconclusive. It has been demonstrated that placement of the prosthetic acetabular component in the so-called high position (i.e., in the false acetabulum) results in more predictable fixation at intermediate follow-up (52) than structural grafting of the false acetabulum followed by cup fixation in the anatomic position. It may, however, be impossible to predict whether the cup can be contained adequately in the false acetabulum using plain radiographs alone, and the surgeon should be prepared to perform bone grafting if necessary. The significance with regard to femoral arthroplasty is that femoral shortening is rarely required if the acetabular component is placed high.

Surgical Management

Optimization of leg length requires the ability to perform accurate intraoperative measurements before and after arthroplasty. A variety of techniques and devices have been developed to accomplish this. Direct comparison of leg lengths is possible only when the procedure is performed with the patient supine, as advocated by Charnley (10). When the lateral decubitus position is used, indirect measurement techniques must be employed. All rely on assessment of changes in the length of the operative limb before and after arthroplasty. These techniques are reliable if appropriate attention is given to the following details. First, the patient must be securely fastened to the operating table, as minor shifts in position during surgery will significantly affect limb measurement. Several stabilization systems, designed specifically for hip surgery, are now commercially available. Next, the operating table must be level during all measurements. Most tables feature leveling devices or can be fitted with them. Finally, the operative limb must be placed in the same position during initial and final measurements. Hip flexion is best controlled by positioning the extremity parallel to the dependent, non-operative limb, which is secured to the table with stockinette (Fig. 2). Hip rotation and abduction/adduction are more difficult to reproduce postarthroplasty after contractures are released and offset and anteversion are altered. Most devices for the intraoperative measurement of limb length rely on measurement of the distance between fixed points on the ilium and the femur (27–29,37,44,72,73). The change in this distance after component implantation is adjusted to equal the preoperative discrepancy. A device that also measures femoral offset is preferred.

The nature and severity of the discrepancy should be considered when selecting the optimal surgical approach. When lengthening or shortening of 2 cm or more is planned, trochanteric osteotomy and repositioning should be considered. The author's preferred technique in such cases is the sliding trochanteric osteotomy (23). The pertinent feature of this approach is the creation of a longer,

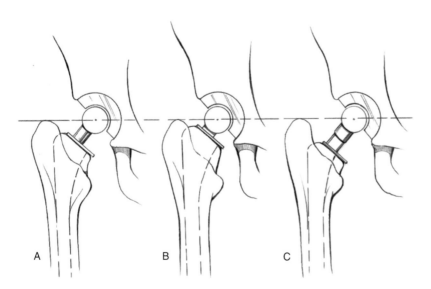

FIG. 1. The same leg length can be achieved using various combinations of neck resection level and modular head length, with each producing a different amount of offset. **A:** In the normal femur, leg length and offset are reestablished with a standard neck resection and medium length modular head. **B:** A higher neck resection level and larger prosthesis combined with a short modular head yields the same leg length but reduced offset. This combination would be appropriate in cases of coxa valga. **C:** Coxa vara can be managed using a low neck resection level, a smaller prosthesis, and a longer neck length, yielding the same leg length and increased offset.

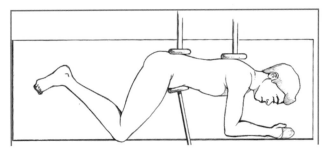

FIG. 2. Author's preferred method of positioning and securing the patient to the operating table in the lateral decubitus position.

thinner, more vertically oriented trochanteric fragment than is the case with a standard osteotomy. This facilitates proximal or distal translation and fixation during closure (Fig. 3). Formal exposure of the sciatic nerve from the greater sciatic notch to the tendinous insertion of the gluteus maximus is indicated when lengthening is to exceed 2 cm, or in cases of prior trauma or infection when adhesions may bind the nerve or alter its natural course.

The management of soft-tissue contractures varies. Hip flexion, external rotation, and abduction contractures generally do not require formal releases (1). A complete capsulectomy usually suffices. Fixed adduction contractures may require percutaneous adductor tenotomy. If an

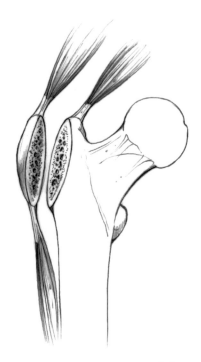

FIG. 3. Schematic depiction of the sliding trochanteric osteotomy. Note that the osteotomy is more vertically oriented than a standard osteotomy, creating a longer, thinner fragment. The origin of the vastus lateralis remains attached to the trochanteric segment.

iliotibial band contracture exists, as evidenced by a positive Ober's test, Z-lengthening may be required. Flexion contractures occasionally require iliopsoas lengthening or release.

Intraoperatively, changes in leg length are achieved by combining adjustments of neck resection level, femoral component seating, and the length of head and neck segment selected, as described in the previous planning section. Femoral offset, abductor tension, and stability against dislocation must also be respected. The so-called shuck test wherein the prosthetic neck is grasped and the limb is pistoned to assess abductor tension and hip stability should not be relied on. Once leg length and offset are acceptable as determined by the use of the measuring devices, the hip should be put through a physiologic range of motion. Posterior stability is tested with the hip in extreme flexion and again with the hip held in 90 degrees of flexion in combination with adduction and internal rotation. Anterior stability is tested with the hip in extension and external rotation. Inadequate stability despite optimum leg length and offset is addressed by removal of osteophytes, changes in femoral or acetabular version, trochanteric advancement, or a combination of these. Deliberate overlengthening of up to 1 cm can occasionally be justified and is in general well tolerated. Care is taken to avoid excessive abductor tension, which may predispose to trochanteric nonunion or abduction contracture.

The sciatic nerve should be carefully inspected and palpated for the development of tension during trial reduction and dislocation, and as the hip is placed through a range of motion. Studies have demonstrated the potential value of monitoring somatosensory evoked potentials (SSEPs) from the sciatic nerve or its divisions during THR (5,65). This method is far more sensitive in detecting physiologic responses and potential nerve damage than clinical judgment alone. However, a significant reduction in the incidence or severity of nerve palsies from the routine use of this costly technique has not been demonstrated (5). It is therefore recommended that such monitoring be reserved for certain high risk cases, such as severe developmental dysplasia, planned lengthening of 2 cm or more, or cases with significant prior surgery, infection, or trauma.

EXCESSIVE FEMORAL ANTEVERSION

Excessive femoral anteversion or antetorsion (13) may be idiopathic or associated with recognized conditions such as developmental dysplasia or juvenile rheumatoid arthritis. With regard to total hip replacement, excessive femoral anteversion impacts primarily upon the extraosseous aspects of the arthroplasty. If uncorrected, excessive anteversion predisposes to impingement of the prosthetic neck or greater trochanter posteriorly, limitation of external rotation, and anterior dislocation. The intraosseous aspects of the procedure are also affected in that standard cemented or cementless components may be impossible to insert in acceptable position.

Pathoanatomy

Controversy remains as to the normal amount of anteversion found in the adult femur, largely because of the use of differing anatomic landmarks and measuring techniques. Using the plane of the posterior femoral condyles as the distal reference axis, most authors report normal adult values of femoral anteversion in the range of 13° to 16° (13,17,74). Torsion may occur in the neck, metaphysis, or femoral shaft (13). In most instances, there is no obvious distortion of the metaphysis or subtrochanteric area of the femur. It is important to note that the greater trochanter may be situated in an extreme posterior position. Excessive anteversion associated with specific disease entities such as congenital dysplasia and juvenile rheumatoid arthritis may be accompanied by a constellation of other anatomic disturbances as discussed elsewhere in this and other chapters.

Preoperative Planning

Clinically, most cases of exaggerated femoral anteversion are subtle, noted incidentally at the time of surgery, and accommodated by minor adjustments in femoral insertion. Truly pathologic anteversion (antetorsion) is most commonly encountered in congenital dysplasia and is therefore anticipated at the time of diagnosis. In other cases, excessive anteversion is suspected from an intoeing gait, increased internal rotation, and limited external rotation. Clinical measurement of femoral rotation is measured with the patient in the prone position, with the hips in full extension if possible (36). In extreme cases, internal rotation may be as great as 90°, although the arthritic process may limit this significantly.

The degree of excessive anteversion can usually be quantified using standard roentgenograms (13,17). An approximate measure of anteversion is obtained on a true lateral radiograph by measuring the angle of the femoral neck relative to the shaft (Fig. 4). In practice, this technique usually suffices to confirm the presence of excessive anteversion and to alert the surgeon to the potential need for special implants or surgical techniques. Although rarely necessary, computerized tomography is currently the method of choice for precise measurement of rotational deformity (13,64).

Either cemented or cementless femoral component fixation may be used. However, caution must be exercised in committing to a single implant based on what appears to be a satisfactory intraosseous fit during preoperative tem-

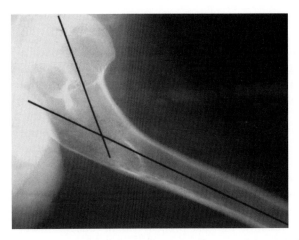

FIG. 4. The degree of femoral anteversion can be approximated on a true lateral radiograph of the proximal femur.

plating. An implant that provides optimal "fit and fill" in the metaphyseal area on templating of the anteroposterior roentgenogram usually cannot be retroverted sufficiently to correct excessive anteversion during surgery. If cemented fixation is preferred, straight stems with reduced metaphyseal segments should be available. Among cementless stems, anatomic proximally coated designs with dedicated right and left implants should be avoided, as they allow for very little intraoperative adjustment of anteversion (Fig. 5A). In contrast, an axisymmetric design with an anteverted neck may be used in reverse [e.g., an anteverted stem for a left hip may be used on the right (in effect, a retroverted neck)] (see Fig. 5B). Other options include extensively porous-coated stems with undersized metaphyseal segments or modular stems that allow for adjustment of anteversion independently of metaphyseal filling. Rarely, a custom stem may be indicated. Finally, the coexistence of other anatomic abnormalities may merit consideration of a subtrochanteric derotational osteotomy.

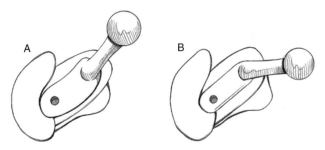

FIG. 5. Selection of cementless prosthetic design for use in cases of excessive femoral anteversion. **A:** Anatomic proximally coated stems should be avoided for this application, as an optimum fit does not allow for adjustment in anteversion. **B:** An axisymmetric stem with an anteverted neck may be used in reverse (e.g., a right stem can be used in a left femur to compensate for excessive femoral anteversion).

Surgical Technique

In most cases, any standard surgical approach to the hip will suffice. Trochanteric osteotomy and repositioning should be considered when the greater trochanter is abnormally posterior.

Although preparation of the femur is implant specific, most hip surgeons agree that the femoral component should be inserted in approximately 15° of anteversion (42). When preparing the femur for cemented stem insertion, serial broaching is undertaken beginning with the smallest size and correcting the excessive anteversion. Removal of competent cancellous bone is to be avoided. Commonly, the last broach will be one or more size smaller than that which the femur could accommodate in the excessively anteverted position. If adequate correction of anteversion cannot be achieved with the smallest broach, either a straight cemented stem intended for congenital dysplasia of the hip (CDH) or another alternative must be selected. In most cemented stem systems, broaches are sized to provide for a uniform cement mantle of approximately 2 mm when the corresponding stem is used. Thus, during stem insertion, the surgeon must maintain the same rotational orientation as that used for the broach and must resist the temptation to further retro-

vert the stem to gain more correction. As Charnley pointed out (10), attempts to avoid femoral component anteversion or deliberate retroversion of a cemented stem lead to a thin cement mantle posteriorly, with subsequent cement splitting and early loosening.

Preparation for the use of a cementless stem generally entails axial reaming followed by broaching. Reaming is done in the routine fashion. Broaching is subject to considerations similar to those described for cemented stems. The surgeon begins with the smallest broach, inserted in an acceptable degree of anteversion, and then proceeds with larger broaches. In contrast to cemented technique, cancellous bone need not be preserved and, in fact, it is preferable for the porous surface to be in direct contact with cortical bone. Thus, anteversion may be corrected by sculpting of the endosteal cortex with a high-speed burr, especially posteromedially. The largest broach that can be inserted in an acceptable degree of anteversion may be smaller than that templated and may fill the metaphyseal region poorly, especially anteromedially. Biologic fixation is critically dependent on immediate implant stability. Thus, if a proximally coated stem designed for metaphyseal filling and ingrowth is used, the rotational stability of a such a stem when metaphyseal filling is poor must be critically assessed. A straight-stemmed

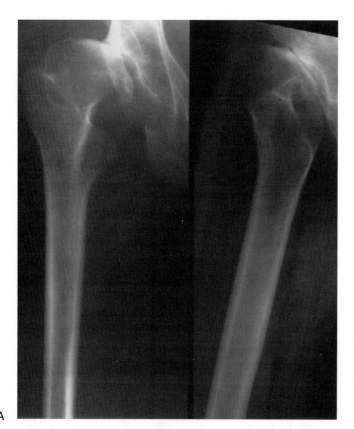 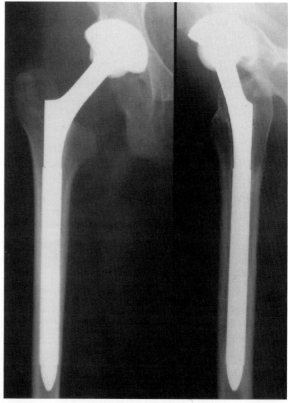

A

B

FIG. 6. A custom "bent rod" extensively porous-coated stem may be used to achieve any desired angle of version. **A:** Preoperative radiographs of patient with moderately severe developmental dysplasia and excessive anteversion. **B:** Postoperative radiographs after THR using a bent rod.

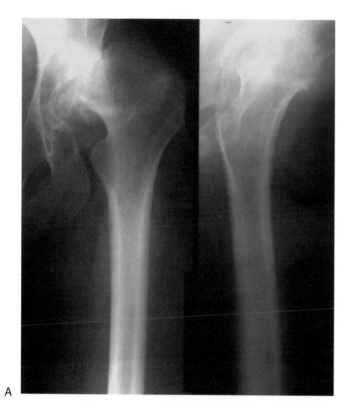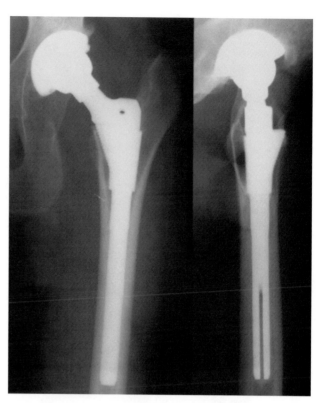

A   B

FIG. 7. A modular stem may also be used to achieve the desired degree of anteversion. **A:** Preoperative anteroposterior and lateral views demonstrating dysplasia and excessive femoral anteversion. **B:** Postoperative radiographs after THR with a modular stem. Note the anteversion of the modular sleeve and considerably less anteversion of the prosthetic neck.

design with distal flutes or splines to augment rotational stability may be useful for this application.

An alternative is the use of an extensively porous-coated straight-stemmed implant. Such stems are available with reduced metaphyseal segments that allow for greater correction of anteversion. Initial rotational stability and subsequent biologic fixation are achieved in the diaphysis. As such, in extreme cases, the posteromedial neck may actually be slotted to accommodate the metaphyseal portion of the implant. A variant of the standard extensively coated stem that is actually a "bent rod" with no metaphyseal segment is also available (Fig. 6).

Yet another option is the use of a modular stem. Several currently available designs feature metaphyseal segments or sleeves in various sizes to optimize proximal "fit and fill." The neck and stem segment can then be rotated relative to the metaphyseal segment to the desired degree of version (Fig. 7) and locked into place (9). Such stems may be regarded as off-the-shelf custom implants. Finally, a true custom implant based on three-dimensional computerized tomography (3,31) or intraoperative molds (46) may be employed.

Although most cases of excessive femoral anteversion can be managed using the techniques described, it may be preferable in certain cases to employ a subtrochanteric derotational osteotomy. The archetype is severe develop-mental dysplasia with high dislocation, marked anteversion, and a posteriorly situated greater trochanter, especially if the need for femoral shortening is anticipated. Derotational osteotomy for excessive anteversion alone is rarely indicated. The author's preferred method for osteotomy is that described by Capello (personal communication). In this technique (Fig. 8), the initial surgical approach is posterior, followed by resection of the femoral neck. The femur is then provisionally prepared with appropriate reaming and broaching. Although various femoral components may be used, cementless implants circumvent the difficulties of cement escape and interposition at the osteotomy site. Among cementless stems, cylindrical designs with features providing distal rotational stability (e.g., extensively coated or fluted designs) are particularly well suited for this application. After initial femoral preparation, the broach is positioned over the femur and the osteotomy is performed in the subtrochanteric area, at the level corresponding to the junction of the proximal triangular and distal cylindrical portions of the broach. An oblique. step-cut, or transverse osteotomy can be employed. Although the latter two provide improved rotational control of the fragments, creating a second oblique shortening derotational osteotomy is technically challenging. After the osteotomy is performed, the proximal segment of the femur is mobilized

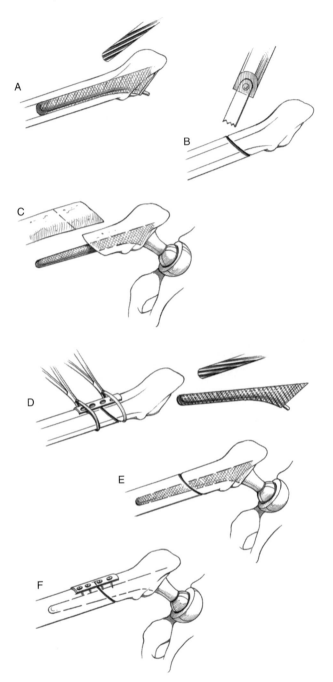

FIG. 8. Steps in the performance of a subtrochanteric shortening osteotomy.

anteriorly and superiorly, in essence flipping the cut end proximally. This may require release of the iliopsoas tendon. Excellent exposure of the acetabulum is provided for cup insertion. The broach or trial is reinserted into the proximal femur but not into the distal fragment and the prosthetic head is reduced. The cut ends of the femur are then allowed to bayonet beside one another. Traction is applied to the femur until proper length is achieved, and the level of the shortening osteotomy is marked. Generally, the shortening is done at the proximal end of the dis-

tal fragment. Further shortening of the proximal segment may compromise rotational stability of the implant within it. The proximal segment is derotated into the appropriate degree of anteversion and the end of the broach or trial is inserted into the distal femoral fragment. Leg length, offset, and stability against dislocation are then tested. If these are acceptable, the osteotomy is provisionally fixed with a bone plate and clamps. Final preparation of the femur is then undertaken, including repeat reaming and broaching. This step is critical for two reasons. First, after femoral shortening, the initial preparation will not extend far enough distally. Second, additional femoral reaming may be required to achieve the necessary endosteal bite over 4 to 5 cm of the distal fragment, dictating the use of a larger diameter implant. After final preparation, the femoral component is inserted. If an oblique or step-cut osteotomy is used, supplemental fixation is usually not required. Fixation with a small plate is recommended after transverse osteotomy. With either, bone grafting of the osteotomy site with morselized femoral head autograft is recommended. In addition to cases of severe acetabular dysplasia (Fig. 9), subtrochanteric osteotomy in this fashion is applicable with or without shortening and/or derotation to cases of subtrochanteric deformity from various causes. Examples include femoral bowing in association with various dysplasias, and angular deformity after previous osteotomy or fracture malunion.

JUVENILE RHEUMATOID ARTHRITIS (JUVENILE CHRONIC ARTHRITIS)

General

Juvenile rheumatoid arthritis (JRA) is defined as the onset of inflammatory polyarticular arthritis prior to the age of 16 years. The reported incidence of hip involvement varies between 10% and 63.5% of patients (32,33). The hip has been cited as the single most important cause of lost mobility in these patients (43,51). Although the interval between disease onset and the need for hip surgery can be 10 years or more (71), the majority of patients are still adolescents and therefore skeletally immature at the time of surgery. Total hip replacement is justified despite extreme youth on the basis of severe disability and the built-in restraints imposed by polyarticular lower extremity disease. In addition, many patients have a shortened life expectancy as a result of systemic organ involvement (39). Stiffness, contractures, and resultant limited mobility rather than pain are the most commonly reported indications for THR (7,38,54,67,71), and the majority of series report gratifying clinical if not radiographic results in this regard. Management of these patients demands a multidisciplinary approach involv-

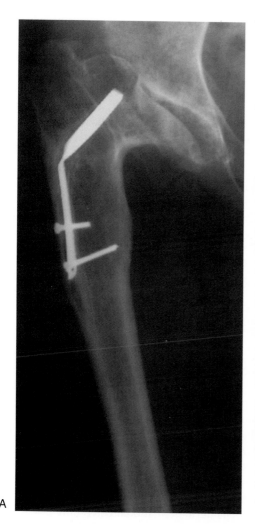
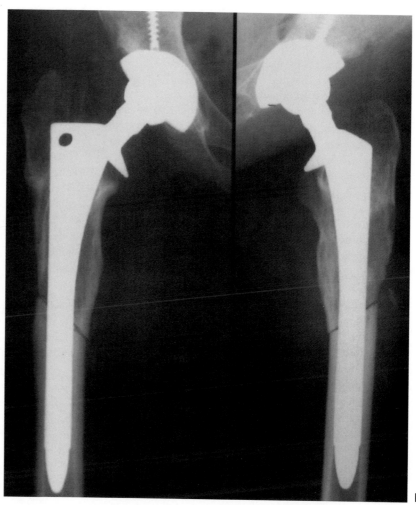

A   B

FIG. 9. Severe developmental dysplasia, managed with a shortening, derotational subtrochanteric osteotomy. **A:** Severe dysplasia and secondary osteoarthritis after intertrochanteric osteotomy during childhood. High subluxation of the femoral head and retained blade plate are present. **B:** Immediate postoperative films after oblique, shortening, and derotational osteotomy using an extensively porous-coated stem.

ing the pediatrician, rheumatologist, anesthesiologist, child psychologist, therapists, and family (51,54). Patient motivation and maturity should be critically assessed before arthroplasty is undertaken (54).

Pathoanatomy

Abnormalities in bony architecture and quality are common in JRA. Their origins are multifactorial. Growth disturbances result in deformities of the pelvis and the femur. Both the acetabular cavity and the femoral head may be extremely hypoplastic. Significant protrusio acetabuli, subluxation, or ankylosis may be present (32,38). The normal proportionality between the femoral metaphysis and diaphysis is often lost. In general, the metaphysis is disproportionately large relative

to the femoral canal, which can be quite small. In addition, the femoral canal is often disproportionately wide in the anteroposterior dimension and relatively narrow from medial to lateral (51,67). Abnormal bowing of the femur may be present. Excessive femoral anteversion can be dramatic, in the range of 60° to 80° (54). As a rule, bone quality is severely compromised. This is attributable to disuse as well as to the chronic steroid therapy frequently necessary to control symptoms of inflammation. The proximal femur, particularly the greater trochanter and the femoral neck, are usually the most severely affected (67). Hypervascularity of the marrow cavity has also been noted (71). Soft-tissue contractures, sometimes of a dramatic nature, are commonplace. Most major muscle groups about the hip are involved, typically the flexors, adductors, and external rotators.

Preoperative Planning

Careful preoperative planning is particularly important to the success of THR in the patient with JRA. A team approach ensures that the patient is optimally prepared medically and psychologically. Cervical spine involvement (autofusion of cervical segments, atlantoaxial instability), mandibular hypoplasia, and stiffness of the temporomandibular joint render endotracheal intubation extremely difficult (51,54). If general anesthesia is chosen, capabilities for fiberoptic intubation should be in place (51). Spinal anesthesia may be preferred (54).

Templating and provisional implant selection must be done prior to the scheduling of surgery to ensure availability of nonstandard components. In a series of 64 THRs in patients with JRA, Scott and co-workers (54) reported the need for such components in one half of cases. Custom components were required in 11% of cases reported in one series (71) and in 12.3% of cases in another (69).

Acetabular templating provides a reference for planning leg length and offset, and it is therefore essential for determining the level of femoral neck resection and prosthetic neck length. Also, marked acetabular hypoplasia may dictate the use of a miniature all-polyethylene cemented socket to achieve adequate polyethylene thickness. Thus, femoral components with 22-mm heads should be available.

The optimal choice of femoral component fixation for these patients is unclear. Adequate clinical data regarding the long-term performance of cementless femoral component fixation for JRA are at present unavailable. The use of cementless stems in the face of such poor bone quality has been questioned by some (71) and cautiously employed by others (55,67). Given the variety of femoral deformities seen in this disease, it may be difficult or impossible to achieve immediate implant stability while avoiding femoral fracture using standard cementless components. Modular or custom implants may be preferable if cementless fixation is chosen. Conversely, competent cancellous bone, critical to the long-term success of modern cementing techniques, is often deficient in patients with JRA (56), and endosteal hypervascularity may compromise cementing technique (71). Cemented femoral components have been used in the majority of reported series, and most authors stress the need for a broad implant inventory, including miniature and microminiature stems. As mentioned, the femoral diaphysis may have an ovoid cross-sectional configuration, and templating must therefore be performed on both anteroposterior and lateral roentgenograms. Medial-lateral narrowing of the canal may require the use of a narrow cylindrical stem. A true lateral of the proximal femur or axial computed tomography is used to assess the degree of femoral anteversion (67). Femoral bowing is measured and, if extreme, a corrective osteotomy is planned.

Exposure

Poor bone quality coupled with severe contractures make adequate soft-tissue release imperative to avert fracture from vigorous retraction. Trochanteric osteotomy is often required to prevent uncontrolled avulsion or to gain adequate exposure of the femoral canal (54). A complete capsulectomy should be performed. In general, the short external rotators are released. The iliopsoas, adductors, and the tendinous insertion of the gluteus maximus may also require release. In the presence of protrusio acetabuli or ankylosis, femoral neck resection prior to dislocation of the femoral head lessens the risk of fracturing the osteopenic proximal femur. Extensive releases potentiate the risk of nerve palsy from excessive leg lengthening (54). Thus, the sciatic nerve should be exposed and observed during trial reduction.

Technical Details of Femoral Arthroplasty

The degree of femoral anteversion is estimated in relationship to the transcondylar plane of the distal femur with the knee flexed to 90°. If possible, the metaphysis and neck are prepared in approximately 15° of anteversion. If this cannot be accomplished without violating the confines of the femoral neck, several options exist. A modular cementless component with adjustable anteversion can be used (9). Alternatively, the neck is deliberately violated and an extensively porous-coated stem that relies on diaphyseal fixation is used. Other options include a subtrochanteric derotational osteotomy (24,30) or the use of a custom prosthesis. In cases of extreme anteversion, the greater trochanter is generally situated posteriorly. Unless a subtrochanteric derotational osteotomy is used, the greater trochanter should be removed and repositioned laterally to optimize abductor function. When a cemented component is used, the details of contemporary cement preparation and delivery should be strictly followed.

Complications

In addition to the usual risks shared with the general population, patients with JRA undergoing THR are prone to specific complications. These patients often regain the ability to ambulate after prolonged periods of confinement to bed or wheelchair and are at risk for fractures adjacent to or distant from the hip. Cage et al. (7) reported three femoral fractures during recreational activities among 29 patients after THR.

Some series indicate an increased risk of infection and problems with wound healing. Severt et al. (56) noted a 5.3% incidence of deep sepsis, and problems with wound healing in another 19% of 75 primary cemented THRs. Others (38) do not note an increase in either of these problems. Nerve palsies after extensive soft-tissue releases have been mentioned. Scott et al. (54) reported three sciatic and one femoral nerve palsy in their series of 64 hips.

Results

The radiographic results of cemented stems in JRA vary widely among reported series (Table 1). Five such series comprising 293 THRs in 167 patients were reviewed (38,39,54,69,71). The mean age was 19.1 years, and the mean follow up 8.1 years (range, 1.7 to 18 years). The mean incidence of femoral component loosening or failure was 14.7% (range, 3.2% to 35.7%). Interestingly, there is no trend toward improved results when earlier series are compared with more recent ones. There is consensus among the authors in two regards. The first is that radiographic results tend to deteriorate more rapidly with time than those of the general population when similar cementing techniques are used. This has been attributed to the continued remodeling and increased turnover of immature bone in these young patients (39,51,67,69), as well as the poor initial bone quality. The other point of agreement is that good clinical results and functional improvement are maintained despite radiographic deterioration (7,38,39,71).

There is little information regarding the use of cementless femoral components in this population. Severt and Cracchiola (55) reported favorable results using cementless components in 40 hips affected by rheumatoid arthritis, seven of which were the juvenile form. There were no radiographic failures at 2- to 6-year follow-up.

TOTAL HIP REPLACEMENT AFTER ARTHRODESIS

General

Both spontaneous fusion after childhood sepsis and surgical fusion for various conditions are less common since the advent of modern antimicrobial therapy and total hip replacement, respectively. Furthermore, most arthrodesed hips are well tolerated (8,58,59) and only a small proportion require further surgery. In two large series conducted in the mid 1970s, conversion of an arthrodesed hip to a total hip arthroplasty comprised 4% of all THRs in one (2), and 0.6% of THRs in the other (26). Nonetheless, hip surgeons still encounter patients in whom conversion is appropriate. Spontaneous fusion in rheumatic disease, particularly ankylosing spondylitis (68), continues to be one indication. More important, decompensation of other joints as a result of surgical fusion may occur as late as 60 years postoperatively (2,4,41), and these patients will continue to present to the hip surgeon. Finally, as Sponseller et al. (58) aptly described, "Temporal and cultural changes, including knowledge of people with total hip replacement, have increased patient expectation and decreased patient acceptance of arthrodesis." In their 1984 series, 13% of patients with arthrodesis were sufficiently dissatisfied that conversion was undertaken.

Indications

The indications for conversion to THR can be divided into two categories: cases with fibrous ankylosis/nonunion and those with solid fusion. Pseudarthrosis rates after surgical attempts at arthrodesis range between 0% and 10% in the contemporary literature (8). Brewster et al. (6) reported a series of 33 cases in which a surgical fusion was attempted and conversion to THR was eventually required. Painful pseudarthrosis, present in 19 cases (57.6%), was the most common indication for THR. Hardinge et al. (26), in a series including both spontaneous and surgical fusions, cited painful pseudarthrosis as the indication for THR in only 29.6% of cases. Certainly, pain isolated to the affected hip should prompt an investigation for nonunion (plain or computerized tomography, fluoroscopic examination). The treatment of pseudarthrosis is dependent on several factors. For failed surgical fusion, the most important consideration is the time elapsed since the attempt. If the nonunion occurs during the immediate postoperative period and the indications for fusion were appropriate, then repeat fusion may be the treatment of choice. For longstanding nonunion with deformity and/or symptoms in other joints (see later), THR may be considered. Traumatic disruption of the fusion mass or femoral neck fracture after fusion is subject to the same considerations. Hardinge et al. (26) reported five proximal femoral fractures among 29

TABLE 1. *Radiographic results of cemented stems in JRA*

Author (ref.)	Hips (N)	Patients (N)	Age (yr, mean)	Follow-up (yr, mean/range)	Stem loosening or failure (%)
Scott et al. (54)	64	38	n.a.	n.a.	6.2
Lachiewicz (38)	62	34	26	6/2–11	3.2
Learmonth et al. (39)	14	7	16	8.5/4–11	35.7
Witt et al. (71)	96	54	16.75	11.5/5–18	27.1
Williams and McCullough(69)	57	34	16.4	4.6/1.7–9	10.5

patients who had undergone remote surgical fusion for osteoarthritis. All were converted to THR. Similarly, fracture through the fused hip was the indication for conversion to THR in 5 of 46 patients (10.9%) reported by Reikeras et al. (50).

In the presence of a solid arthrodesis, ipsilateral hip pain is unusual and, if present, should raise the possibility of infection. Far more commonly, patients with a solid fusion seek treatment for pain in other joints, deformity, and functional disability such as difficulty sitting or driving (35). Gore et al. (22) described the compensatory changes during gait in patients with unilateral hip fusion. These include increased pelvic rotation in both the sagittal and transverse planes, increased motion of the contralateral hip, increased flexion of the ipsilateral knee, and increased abduction/adduction moments of the ipsilateral or contralateral knee. With time, these joints become symptomatic and develop degenerative changes. The most common complaint prompting conversion of a fused hip to a THR is mechanical low back pain (2,25,35,41,50). Back pain was cited as the most prominent symptom in 75.6% of patients in one series (41), and it was the major indication for conversion in 56.5% of cases in another (50). Multilevel arthritic changes have been noted in the lumbosacral spine of patients at a mean follow-up of 32.9 years (2). Malposition of the fused hip in excessive abduction appears to be a major contributing factor (8).

Knee pain after hip fusion is also extremely common. Ipsilateral knee symptoms appear to be more common with hip adduction (25), whereas contralateral knee pain is more likely with excessive abduction. All patients in the series of Amstutz and Sakai (2) had some degree of ipsilateral knee instability. In the majority (94%), instability was medial-lateral. Anteroposterior instability was present in 25%, and pain was noted by 43.8%. Ipsilateral frontal plane knee deformity is often present and is related to the position of the fused hip. Excessive hip abduction generally results in varus deformity, and adduction, in valgus deformity.

Contralateral hip pain after hip arthrodesis occurred in 7.3% to 33.7% of three large series (8,25,35). Contributing factors include increased dependence for support, exaggerated motion (22), and higher joint reactive force secondary to relative adduction (to compensate for limb shortening on the fused side). Contralateral hip pain may add to the constellation of symptoms favoring conversion of the fused hip, but it is rare as an isolated finding, and it often requires THR on that side as well. In a long-term follow-up of 28 hips, Callaghan et al. (8) found loss of at least one half the joint space of the contralateral hip in ten cases (35.7%). Six required THR.

Most patients with longstanding hip fusion suffer from a combination of the above problems. Kilgus and co-workers (35) cited generalized loss of function from immobility or malposition of the fused hip as the second most common indication for conversion to THR (after low back pain). Only 10% were fused in a position considered acceptable.

Pathoanatomy

With rare exceptions, the anatomy about the hip after arthrodesis is significantly altered. The nature and extent of the abnormalities present depends on the original diagnosis, patient age at the time of fusion, and whether the fusion was spontaneous or surgically created. Distortions or deficiencies of both soft tissue and bone may be extreme.

Soft-tissue contractures are the rule (35,50). Their direction and severity are dictated by the position of the fused hip. The periarticular tissues may be infiltrated or replaced by dense scar tissue (60), especially in cases of prior infection. Abductor insufficiency results from inadequate childhood development, disuse atrophy (60), stripping from the ilium during surgical fusion, and degeneration and fibrosis (4). In addition, surgically created extra-articular arthrodesis may result in partial or total replacement of the abductors and short external rotators with bone (see Fig. 9).

A broad spectrum of bony abnormalities is possible. Cases of spontaneous fusion after tuberculous or pyogenic infection may exhibit significant loss of both femoral and acetabular bone stock. The problem is magnified by patient youth at disease onset, which is often before puberty (25). Physeal arrest results in limb shortening and underdevelopment or absence of the greater and lesser trochanters and proximal metaphysis (2,25). Lubahn et al. (41) reported total absence of the greater trochanter in 22.2% (4 of 18) hips undergoing conversion from arthrodesis to THR. Subtrochanteric or intertrochanteric osteotomies performed in conjunction with surgical arthrodeses result in angular deformities of the femoral shaft.

Preoperative Planning

Careful preoperative planning is of particular importance to ensure that a variety of implant options are available at the time of surgery. A primary operative plan and one or more alternative plans should be established. Bone graft, appropriate instrumentation, and adequate blood to execute each of the possible plans should be available. The presence, size, position, and condition of the greater trochanter is noted. Radiographs should be carefully assessed for the presence of any remaining joint space.

Surgical Management

Conversion from arthrodesis to THR presents a multitude of technical challenges (35,50). Exposure may be quite difficult as a consequence of the primary disease process and prior surgical intervention, as mentioned. No single approach is optimal for all cases. Trochanteric osteotomy has been strongly advocated by some (2,6,25,35), although others (50) report satisfactory exposure using either the posterior or direct lateral approach. If trochanteric osteotomy is performed, care should be taken to minimize stripping of the abductors from the ilium, preserving as much of their blood supply as possible (35). One should anticipate difficulty in identifying the normal anatomic landmarks (2). The sciatic nerve should be identified and protected, and if necessary, exposed.

Any existing internal fixation devices must be removed (Fig. 10). Cortical bone may cover side plates fixed to the proximal femur. If possible, this bone should be removed as a single piece, preserving its soft-tissue attachments and therefore its blood supply. It may subsequently be reattached to the femur as a vascularized strut graft. Screws through such plates are often firmly osseointegrated. Stripping or breakage of the screw heads is common during attempts at their removal. A high-speed drill and metal-cutting burrs are used to remove such heads, and the remaining shanks are removed with an appropriately sized trephine.

Exposure and adequate mobilization of the femur is especially challenging after extra-articular arthrodeses, whether iliofemoral (Hibbs, Charnley) or ischiofemoral (Kirkaldy-Willis, Brittain) (14). These generally involve bicortical or tricortical grafts slotted into the proximal femur and the pelvis, and take-down of such fusion masses may be extremely difficult. Selection of the proper level of femoral neck resection is critical. Amstutz (2) cites two cases in which the resection level was too high and violated the pelvis, resulting in fractures of the pubis and ischium. He recommends placement of guide pins into the pelvis and proximal femur, followed by intraoperative radiographs prior to osteotomy.

After removal of the bony fusion mass, scarring and soft-tissue contractures must be addressed to adequately expose the acetabulum and proximal femur, correct deformities, and reestablish leg length. Adductor tenotomy was required in at least half of the cases reported in two series (2,35). The iliopsoas also commonly requires release (26). After adequate mobilization of the proximal femur, the acetabulum should be meticulously exposed. Any bone within the acetabular cavity, whether a remnant of the femoral head or greater trochanter, should be carefully assessed. If, for example, a successful intra-articular fusion has been performed, the intra-articular bone mass can be used for acetabular component fixation. If a nonunion exists, or if the fusion was purely extra-articular, then all bone and soft tissue within the acetabulum must be removed before preparing it for the prosthetic

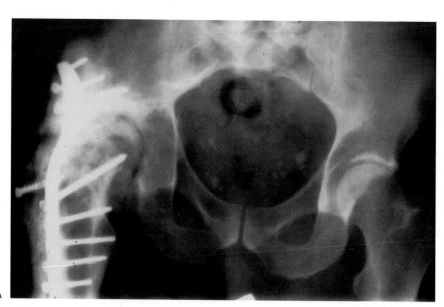

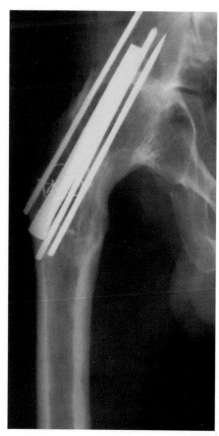

A

B

FIG. 10. The abductors and external rotators may be largely replaced by bone after extra-articular arthrodesis. **A:** Side plates *in situ* for several years may be largely intraosseous and difficult to remove. **B:** The removal of pins, screws, and nails may also be challenging.

socket. Defects of the acetabular rim may require structural grafting. Contained, cavitary defects are generally manageable with morselized grafting. The author's preference is for the use of porous-coated hemispheric acetabular components in such cases, unless a substantial portion of the prepared rim and cavity is occupied by bone graft. As discussed below, it may be preferable to employ a design compatible with the use of a constrained (i.e., captured) liner.

A major challenge during femoral reconstruction is establishing stable implant fixation despite abnormalities of proximal femoral architecture and bone quality. Absence of the normal proximal metaphyseal flare may dictate the use of custom or modular femoral stems. Amstutz et al. (2) reported the need for nonstandard, extra-small, or straight-stemmed components in one half of cases. Angular deformities after inter- or subtrochanteric osteotomy may require corrective osteotomy (24,30). Stress risers created by screw holes or cortical plates should be bypassed using long-stemmed prostheses, cortical strut allografts, or both. Either cemented or cementless fixation may be employed. If cementless fixation is chosen for a patient in whom the normal proximal metaphyseal flair is absent, an extensively porous-coated straight-stemmed implant should be considered. When cemented fixation is employed, bony defects left by removed hardware must be sealed to obtain adequate cement containment and pressurization.

Another major objective of femoral arthroplasty is the restoration of satisfactory hip mechanics, the components of the which include leg length, offset, stability against dislocation, and abductor function. Although equalization of leg lengths is a desirable goal for both patient and surgeon, several precautions must be taken. First, equalization may be impossible for those patients in whom disease onset occurred prior to skeletal maturity. Careful attention must be given to sciatic nerve tension during trial reduction in such cases. In addition, excessive lengthening may render it difficult or impossible to reattach the greater trochanter. It is far preferable to leave the leg shorter and achieve stable trochanteric fixation without excessive abductor tension. Similar consideration should be given to the degree of inherent femoral component offset. Although lateralized stems may improve stability against dislocation, they can in certain cases compromise trochanteric reattachment by increasing abductor tension.

Even without significant limb lengthening, restoration of abductor function may represent a formidable technical challenge, especially if the hip has been fused in significant abduction and the muscles have become shortened (2). Worse still, the abductors may have been detached during arthrodesis leaving a "bald" trochanter, or they may be replaced by bone or scar tissue. In nearly all cases, there is some compromise of abductor vascularity. Besser (4) has described tearing of the abductor

muscles during attempts at trochanteric fixation. When the normal abductor mechanism cannot be restored, an abductor myoplasty should be performed (4) by suturing the proximal femur to the tensor fascia lata anteriorly and the gluteus maximus and iliotibial band posteriorly. The sutures are tightened but not tied and hip stability is critically assessed. If the hip remains unstable, a constrained cup liner should be used (2). Such patients should be immobilized in either a spica cast or hip abduction brace for 6 weeks postoperatively, and they must undergo prolonged physical therapy thereafter.

Results

The clinical results after conversion of fused hips to conventional THR are in general described as very gratifying. The most commonly cited sources of patient satisfaction include relief of low back pain, correction of leg-length discrepancy and deformity, improved mobility, and increased sitting comfort. Relief of low back pain is the most predictable benefit, with 73% to 92.3% of patients reporting complete or near complete relief in the series reviewed (2,25,26,35,41). Improvement or elimination of leg-length discrepancy is also quite predictable and has been described as one of the most appreciated changes after conversion (26). Corrections of several centimeters of true shortening have been reported. Equally important is the correction of apparent discrepancies secondary to pelvic obliquity, malposition, and contractures. Predictably, improvements in range of motion are reported in all series. Motion, however, never equals that of the normal hip or of hips after routine primary THR. Final range of motion appears related to the degree of preoperative deformity and is generally most limited in the direction opposite the deformity (35). The ultimate range of motion achieved is inversely related to the duration of the fusion (2), and it is worst in cases where spontaneous fusion occurs after infection (26).

Abductor function after THR is less predictable. Most authors report improved strength over a protracted period of at least 2 and possibly as long as 5 years postoperatively (25,35,50). Nonetheless, patients must be informed that the hip will always suffer some residual weakness (8,25). In one series (50), none of 46 patients with hip fusions required external support preoperatively. After conversion to THR, 78.3% required one or two crutches and 87% demonstrated a positive Trendelenburg sign at follow-up of 5 to 13 years. Other series (2,25,41) report similar results and cite residual weakness as a major source of patient dissatisfaction. As Hardinge et al. (25) state, "The patient would have thus exchanged a stiff but strong limb for one that was mobile and longer, but weaker overall, without, in many cases, an improvement in overall function." Thus, conversion solely to increase hip mobility, in the absence of significant pain or deformity, should be approached with great caution, and only after frank discussion with the patient. Abductor function after THR appears to be better in patients surgically fused as adults after full development of the abductors and greater trochanter, than in patients with spontaneous fusion after childhood sepsis (6).

Although ipsilateral knee pain may improve after conversion to THR, approximately one third of patients in most series continue to experience pain (2,26,35). This is particularly so if instability is present preoperatively.

The reported radiographic results after conversion to THR vary widely in the literature, in part because of the diversity of case material, the reasons for fusion and subsequent conversion, the length of follow-up, and the prostheses employed. Strathy and Fitzgerald (60) compared the results of 19 cases with spontaneous fusions to those of 40 surgical fusions at a mean of 10.4 years (range, 9 to 15 years) after conversion to cemented THR. They reported significantly better results after spontaneous fusion—one failure resulting from late infection and no mechanical failures—compared to the surgically fused hips in which the mechanical failure rate was 22.5%. They did not distinguish femoral versus acetabular failure. In contrast, Hardinge et al. (25) reported excellent results in 112 patients converted to cemented THR, including 39 patients with spontaneous fusions and 73 with surgical fusions. Only one stem (0.9%) was loose at mean follow up of 8.15 years (range, 2 to 19 years). Kilgus et al. (35) reported a mechanical failure rate of 7.9% among 38 cemented hips at mean follow up of 7 years (range, 2 to 16.5 years). All failures were femoral, including two cases of aseptic loosening and one stem breakage. They commented on the excellent appearance of the acetabular bone–cement interface and attributed this to cancellization of the subchondral bone. Little information is available regarding the results of cementless THR after hip fusion. Reikeras et al. (50) compared the results of 39 cemented and seven cementless THRs at mean follow-up of 8 years (range 5 to 13 years). Eight cemented stems failed by aseptic loosening (20.5%), but this was attributed to suboptimal stem design in six cases. In contrast, only one cementless stem (7.1%) was loose. There were no reported failures of either cemented or cementless cups.

Complications

With few exceptions, the reported incidence of serious complications after conversion of arthrodesed hips to THR is higher than for routine primary procedures. The most significant complications include deep infection, dislocation, and nerve palsy.

Among series reviewed, the incidence of deep infection ranges from 1.9% to 15.3% (2,6,25,35,60). The infection rate after surgical fusion is significantly higher than for spontaneous fusion in all series in which the two types are compared.

The incidence of dislocation is slightly increased in most series, with a reported range of 1.7% to 6.25% (2,6,35,41,60). Hardinge et al., however, reported no dislocations in two series of patients (25,26). They regularly maintained patients at bed rest for up to 3 weeks after surgery.

Nerve palsy after conversion to THR has been reported to occur in 1.8% to 13.4% of cases (2,25,26). Most injuries involve the sciatic or peroneal nerve, although Amstutz (2) reported four femoral nerve palsies among 112 cases (3.6%).

TOTAL HIP REPLACEMENT AFTER PROXIMAL FEMORAL FRACTURE OR FAILED INTERTROCHANTERIC OSTEOTOMY

General

It is estimated that total hip replacement will be necessary in approximately 15% of cases after internal fixation for femoral neck fracture, usually because of nonunion or avascular necrosis (47,61). THR after intertrochanteric fracture is indicated for progression of preexistent osteoarthritis, the development of posttraumatic osteoarthritis, nonunion, perforation of the acetabulum by an internal fixation device, or, rarely, avascular necrosis of the femoral head (47). In a review of the literature, Mehlhoff et al. (45) cited rates of nonunion of 5% to 15%, and of avascular necrosis, 7% to 12%, after internal fixation of femoral neck fractures. For intertrochanteric fractures, the complication rates were 2% to 5% for nonunion, 2% to 12% for device penetration of the acetabulum, and 3% to 12% overall failure.

Total hip replacement after failed intertrochanteric osteotomy is included in this section because the indications (e.g., progression of osteoarthritis), pathoanatomy, and technical considerations are nearly identical to cases of prior intertrochanteric fracture. In one large series (57), conversion to THR was required in 22% of cases of prior medial displacement osteotomy.

Pathoanatomy

Disturbances of proximal femoral anatomy are usually minimal after femoral neck fracture, although in cases of basilar fracture, the neck may be deficient. After intertrochanteric fracture, significant abnormalities of the greater and lesser trochanters and metaphysis are often present (Fig. 11). Either trochanter may be displaced, or rotated, often in more than one plane. The femoral neck may be angulated in the frontal plane, frequently into excessive valgus, and retroverted or anteverted on lateral radiographs. Significant limb shortening is common. The

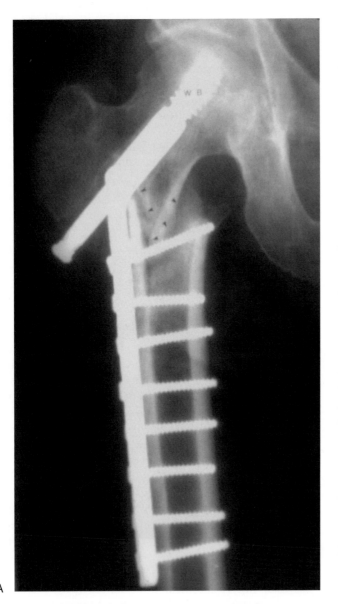

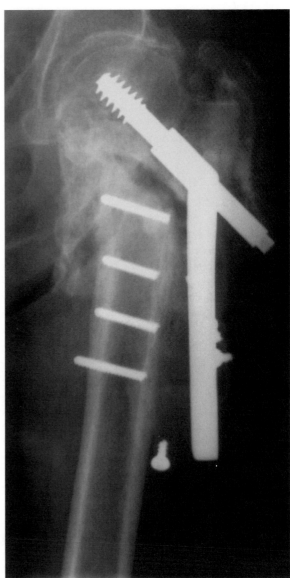

A   B

FIG. 11. A: Significant abnormalities of the proximal femur after internal fixation of an intertrochanteric fracture. **B:** Broken screws require the use of hollow trephines for removal.

intertrochanteric area may be translated relative to the distal metaphysis. Sizable medial displacement of the distal portion of the canal was noted in 75% of cases in one series (45). When a medial displacement osteotomy is employed at the time of fracture fixation (11), a spike of the proximal medial femoral cortex will occupy the metaphysis and may interfere with canal preparation. Internal fixation devices induce remodeling changes in surrounding bone. The trabecular bone of the metaphysis and neck surrounding pins, blade plates, and lag screws is converted into a sclerotic neocortex. Screw holes vacated after hardware removal represent stress risers and exit routes for cement (16,45,47). The lateral cortex beneath side plates is often thinned as a result of stress shielding. Nonunion of the trochanters results in retraction of the iliopsoas or abductors.

Preoperative Planning

Considerations during preoperative planning include the timing and method of hardware removal, implant selection in the face of distorted anatomy and bone defects, and the treatment of malunions or nonunions of the trochanters or intertrochanteric area.

If possible, the manufacturer of any internal fixation device should be identified from prior records so that appropriate instrumentation is available for removal. In certain cases, it may be advantageous to remove internal fixation devices as a separate procedure, with or without grafting of bony defects, and to undertake THR at a later date (18,48,49). This approach is most appropriate if hardware removal is difficult or is expected to create large bone defects. It is also advisable if infection is suspected despite a negative or equivocal preoperative evaluation (49).

Either a cementless or a cemented femoral component may be used, depending on the circumstances and surgeon preference, with each having potential merits and drawbacks. In general, no special prostheses are required in cases of prior femoral neck fracture (45). In contrast, femoral component selection for cases of prior intertrochanteric fracture or osteotomy can be challenging. If cementless fixation is chosen, it may be difficult to obtain an acceptable fit using a standard implant. Options include a corrective osteotomy or a custom or modular component. With cemented implants, fit may also be problematic. A special double-curved osteotomy stem is useful in certain cases (18). In addition, provisions must be made to limit the escape of cement through defects. With cemented or cementless fixation, a stem of adequate length to bypass stress risers left after hardware removal should be selected, or strut grafting of the cortex above and below the stem tip is planned. If an intertrochanteric nonunion is to be treated by skewering it with the prosthetic stem, a collared prosthesis should be used to help maintain compression across the fracture site. As an alternative, the un-united proximal metaphyseal segment may be replaced with a calcar replacement-type prosthesis (45). Particulate bone graft to fill defects and treat nonunions, and possibly cortical strut allografts should be available.

Surgical Management

The optimal surgical approach is selected on a case-by-case basis. If the greater trochanter is malunited, a trochanteric osteotomy to allow for subsequent repositioning is advised. A possible exception is the presence of an intertrochanteric nonunion, in which case trochanteric osteotomy may devascularize the proximal metaphyseal segment. When a side plate is present, the vastus lateralis must be elevated to allow removal. Hardware removal is often complicated by bony overgrowth or screw breakage (18). A complete capsulectomy and sufficient soft-tissue release is performed to allow dislocation with minimal force. The hip should be dislocated prior to the removal of internal fixation devices to minimize the risk of fracture through screw holes (47).

A provisional neck resection is performed in routine fashion. Reaming or broaching must be approached cautiously. The sclerotic tracks left by multiple pins, compression screws, or blade plates are not easily penetrated by blunt-tipped intramedullary reamers or broaches, both of which may be deflected eccentrically. Difficulties in femoral reaming were reported in 34.1% of cases in one series of failed intertrochanteric osteotomies converted to THR (18). It is advisable to open the femoral canal with a high-speed burr before using the standard instrumentation. Canal preparation after corrective osteotomy or in the presence of an intertrochanteric nonunion is facilitated by provisional reduction and fixation of the femur with a plate and clamps. Even so, it may be very difficult to control the proximal segment. In all cases with femoral distortion, reaming and/or broaching is undertaken cautiously and continued just until initial resistance is met. The instrument is left in place and biplanar check radiographs are obtained to assure proper alignment. Malalignment can usually be corrected by using a high-speed burr to remove endosteal bone deflecting the instrument. When preparing the femur for a long-stem prosthesis, check films also reduce the risk of distal perforation. Screw holes and other defects should be tightly packed with morselized graft. A novel alternative has been suggested by Patterson and co-workers (47), wherein the screws removed from the side plate are shortened with a bolt cutter and reinserted into the cortical holes during cementing. They are then removed and the holes packed with graft. This method assumes the plate and screws have not previously loosened and stripped the holes.

When managing intertrochanteric nonunions and cases requiring corrective osteotomy, the proximal segment must be rigidly fixed to either the remaining femur or the femoral component or, ideally, to both. The stability of the proximal segment is critically assessed with the broach or trial prosthesis in place. If questionable, internal fixation with a small plate is performed. If cement is used, the fragments must be apposed accurately enough to prevent interposition or escape of cement. When contemplating the use of a cementless femoral component, the principles of biologic fixation must be respected. Specifically, bone ingrowth requires immediate mechanical stability between the ingrowth surface and adjacent bone. A proximally porous-coated stem can therefore be used only if it is rigidly press-fitted in the metaphysis. Furthermore, a design that achieves rotational stability in the diaphysis with flutes or splines is preferred. If there is any question regarding cementless implant stability in the metaphysis, an extensively porous-coated stem should be used and the nonunion or osteotomy site internally fixed. As with any nonunion, all scar tissue and sclerotic bone should be removed. Morselized grafting of the site is recommended. If the lateral cortex is extremely thin secondary to a side plate, cortical strut allografting should be considered. The same is true if a short-stemmed prosthesis is chosen and stress risers (e.g., screw holes) are present at the level of the stem tip.

Results

Few studies limited to the results of THR in the above conditions are available. Mehlhoff et al. (45) compared the results of cemented THR in 14 previous intertrochanteric fractures to those of 13 cases of femoral neck fractures at a minimum of 2 years. They emphasized the high incidence of technical difficulties and perioperative complications in the former group as opposed to the latter. In the intertrochanteric fracture group, femoral fracture or perforation occurred in 15.4% and dislocation in 23.1%. Neither complication was observed in any of the femoral neck fractures, although one (7.1%) developed a deep infection. No radiographic results were provided. Franzen et al. (19) reported considerably less favorable results for secondary THR after femoral neck fracture. Among 84 cases, nine failed prior to the 5-year follow-up because of recurrent dislocation (four), infection (two), loosening (two), or cup failure (one). Complications included dislocation in 5.9% and deep infection in 2.4%. The femoral component loosening rate at 5 years was 18.2%. When compared to a group of primary THRs using similar cementing technique, the age- and sex-adjusted risk of prosthetic failure was 2.5 times greater in the fracture group, although the excess risk was confined to patients over 70 years of age.

Studies of THR after intertrochanteric osteotomy also demonstrate an increased risk of complications as compared to primary THR. Ferguson et al. (18) reported the results of cemented THR for failed intertrochanteric osteotomy in 305 cases, including 215 followed for 5 years. Intraoperative technical difficulties were encountered in 23% of cases, including femoral fracture in 2.3%. Late infection occurred in 3.2%. Without canal plugging or cement pressurization, 19.5% of stems were considered probably loose, 11.4% possibly loose, and 12.1% were definitely loose and revised. In contrast, Soballe et al. (57) reported only one femoral component mechanical failure (a stem fracture) among 112 cemented THRs performed for failed intertrochanteric osteotomies. Apart from an increased risk of intraoperative femoral fracture (5.2%), their results were comparable to a group of 262 primary cemented THRs.

SUMMARY

Primary femoral arthroplasty is considered difficult in several commonly encountered conditions. A select few have been discussed. Although the abnormalities to be dealt with vary widely among them, the principles involved in their successful surgical management are strikingly similar. An effort has been made to emphasize these principles. Specifically, a thorough knowledge of the pathoanatomy of each condition is essential. Abnormalities known to accompany each diagnosis are thus anticipated. The surgeon dealing with these problems must be familiar with currently available implants and the appropriate techniques for their insertion. Careful and

timely preoperative templating optimizes component selection and ensures the availability of the preferred implant and one or more back-ups, appropriate instrumentation, and bone graft if needed. The surgeon must be thoroughly familiar with a variety of surgical approaches, as well as with adjunctive surgical techniques such as bone grafting, corrective osteotomy, soft-tissue releases, and abductor myoplasty. Finally, one must be cognizant of the increased risk of specific perioperative complications associated with each condition so that proper preoperative precautions and postoperative monitoring are observed.

Numerous other conditions rendering primary hip replacement difficult (e.g., dwarfism, osteogenesis imperfecta, and Paget's disease) have not, for space considerations, been discussed. It is hoped that the principles delineated in this chapter and summarized above will be found useful in these conditions as well.

REFERENCES

1. Abraham WD, Dimon JH. Leg length discrepancy in total hip arthroplasty. *Orthop Clin North Am* 1992;201–209.
2. Amstutz HC, Sakai DN. Total joint replacement for ankylosed hips. *J Bone Joint Surg* 1975;57A:619–625.
3. Bargar W. Shape the implant to the patient: a rationale for the use of custom-fit cementless total hip implants. *Clin Orthop* 1989;249:73–78.
4. Besser MIB. A muscle transfer to replace absent abductors in the conversion of a fused hip to a total hip arthroplasty. *Clin Orthop* 1982;162:173–174.
5. Black LL, Reckling FW, Porter SS. Somatosensory-evoked potential monitoring during total hip arthroplasty. *Clin Orthop* 1991;262:170–177.
6. Brewster RC, Coventry MB, Johnson EW. Conversion of the arthrodesed hip to a total hip arthroplasty. *J Bone Joint Surg* 1975;57A:27–30.
7. Cage DJ, Granberry WM, Tullos HS. Long term results of total hip arthroplasty in adolescents with debilitating polyarthropathy. *Clin Orthop* 1992;283:156–162.
8. Callaghan JJ, Brand RA, Pederson DR. Hip arthrodesis. A long-term follow-up. *J Bone Joint Surg* 1985;67A:1328–1335.
9. Cameron HU. The 3-6 year results of a modular noncemented low-bending stiffness hip implant. A preliminary study. *J Arthroplasty* 1993;8:239–243.
10. Charnley J. *Low friction arthroplasty of the hip. Theory and practice.* New York: Springer-Verlag, 1991.
11. Dimon JH, Hughston JC. Unstable intertrochanteric fractures of the hip. *J Bone Joint Surg* 1967;49A:440–447.
12. Dunlap CK, Shands AR, Hollister LC, Gall S, Streit HA. A new method for determination of torsion of the femur. *J Bone Joint Surg* 1953;35A:289–311.
13. Eckhoff DG. Effect of limb malrotation on malalignment and osteoarthritis. *Orthop Clin North Am* 1994;25:405–414.
14. Edmonson AS, Crenshaw AH, eds. *Campbells operative orthopaedics*, 6th ed. St. Louis: CV Mosby, 1980.
15. Edwards BN, Tullos HS, Noble PC. Contributory factors and etiology of sciatic nerve palsy in total hip arthroplasty. *Clin Orthop* 1987;218:136–141.
16. Eschenroeder HC Jr, Krakow KA. Late onset femoral stress fracture associated with extruded cement following hip arthroplasty. *Clin Orthop* 1988;236:210–213.
17. Fabray G, MacEwen GD, Shands AR. Torsion of the femur: a follow-up study in normal and abnormal conditions. *J Bone Joint Surg* 1973;55A:1726–1738.
18. Ferguson GM, Cabanela ME, Ilstrup DM. Total hip arthroplasty after failed intertrochanteric osteotomy. *J Bone Joint Surg* 1991;76B:252–257.

19. Franzen H, Nilsson LT, Stromqvist B, Johnsson R, Herrlin K. Secondary total hip replacement after fractures of the femoral neck. *J Bone Joint Surg* 1990;72B:784–787.
20. Friberg O. Clinical symptoms and biomechanics of the lumbar spine and hip joint in leg length inequality. *Spine* 1983;8:643–651.
21. Giles LGF, Taylor JR. Low back pain associated with leg length inequality. *Spine* 1981;6:510–521.
22. Gore DR, Murray MP, Sepic SB, Gardner GM. Walking patterns of men with unilateral surgical hip fusion. *J Bone Joint Surg* 1975;57A:759–765.
23. Glassman AH, Engh CA, Bobyn JD. A technique of extensile exposure for total hip arthroplasty. *J Arthroplasty* 1987;2:11–21.
24. Glassman AH, Engh CA, Bobyn JD. Proximal femoral osteotomy as an adjunct in cementless revision total hip arthroplasty. *J Arthroplasty* 1987;2:47–63.
25. Hardinge K, Murphy JCM, Frenyo S. Conversion of hip fusion to Charnley low-friction arthroplasty. *Clin Orthop* 1986;211:173–179.
26. Hardinge K, Williams D, Etienne A, MacKenzie D, Charnley J. Conversion of fused hips to low friction arthroplasty. *J Bone Joint Surg* 1977;59B:385–392.
27. Harris WH. Total hip replacement for failed endoprostheses and sup arthroplasty: technical considerations. *Instr Course Lect* 1974;23:154.
28. Harris WH. A new approach to total hip replacement without osteotomy of the greater trochanter. *Clin Orthop* 1975;106:19.
29. Harris WH. Revision surgery for failed, nonseptic total hip replacement. The femoral side. *Clin Orthop* 1982;170:8–20.
30. Holtgrew JL, Hungerford DS. Primary and revision total hip replacement without cement and with associated femoral osteotomy. *J Bone Joint Surg* 1989;71A:1487–1495.
31. Huo MH, Salvati ER, Lieberman JR, Burstein RH, Wilson PD Jr. Custom designed femoral prostheses in total hip arthroplasty done with cement for severe dysplasia of the hip. *J Bone Joint Surg* 1993;75A:1497–1504.
32. Isdale IC. Hip disease in juvenile rheumatoid arthritis. *Ann Rheumat Dis* 1970;29:603–608.
33. Jacqueline F, Boujot A, Cant L. Involvement of the hips in juvenile rheumatoid arthritis. *Arthritis Rheum* 1961;4:500–513.
34. Johanson NA, Pellicci PM, Tsairis P, Salvati EA. Nerve injury in total hip arthroplasty. *Clin Orthop* 1983;179:214–222.
35. Kilgus, DJ, Amstutz HC, Wolgin MA, Dorey FJ. Joint replacement for ankylosed hips. *J Bone Joint Surg* 1990;72A:45–54.
36. Kling TF, Hensinger RN. Angular and torsional deformities of the lower limbs in children. *Clin Orthop* 1983;176:136–147.
37. Knight WE. Accurate determination of leg length during total hip replacement. *Clin Orthop* 1977;123:27.
38. Lachiewicz PF, McCaskill B, Inglis AE, Ranawat CS, Rosenstein BD. Total hip arthroplasty in juvenile rheumatoid arthritis: two to eleven year results. *J Bone Joint Surgery* 1986;68A:502–508.
39. Learmonth ID, Heywood AWB, Kaye J, Dall D. Radiologic loosening after cemented hip replacement for juvenile chronic arthritis. *J Bone Joint Surg* 1989;71B:209–212.
40. Love BRT, Wright K. Leg length discrepancy after total hip joint replacement. *J Bone Joint Surg* 1983;65B:103.
41. Lubahn JD, Evarts CM, Feltner JB. Conversion of ankylosed hips to total hip arthroplasty. *Clin Orthop* 1980;153:146–152.
42. McCollum DE, Gray WJ. Dislocation after total hip arthroplasty. *Clin Orthop* 1990;261:159–170.
43. McCullough CJ. Surgical management of the hip in juvenile chronic arthritis. *Br J Rheum* 1994;33:178–183.
44. McGee HMJ, Scott JHS. A simple method of obtaining equal leg length in total hip arthroplasty. *Clin Orthop* 1984;194:269–270.
45. Mehlhoff T, Landon GC, Tullos HS. Total hip arthroplasty following failed internal fixation of hip fractures. *Clin Orthop* 1991;269:32–37.
46. Mulier JC, Mulier M, Brady LP, Steenhoudt H, Cauwe Y, Goosens M, Elloy M. A new system to produce intraoperatively custom femoral prosthesis from measurements taken during the surgical procedure. *Clin Orthop* 1989;249:97–112.
47. Patterson BM, Salvati EA, Huo MH. Total hip arthroplasty for complications of intertrochanteric fracture. *J Bone Joint Surg* 1990;72A:776–777.
48. Petty W. Total hip arthroplasty: operative technique. In: Petty W, ed. *Total joint replacement*. Philadelphia: WB Saunders, 1991;272.
49. Poss R. Complex primary total hip arthroplasty: the difficult femur. *Instr Course Lect* 1995;44:281–286.
50. Reikeras O, Bjerkreim I, Gundersson R. Total hip arthroplasty for arthrodesed hips. 5 to 13-year results. *J Arthroplasty* 1995;10:529–531.
51. Ruddlesdin C, Ansell BM, Arden GP, Swann M. Total hip replacement in children with juvenile chronic arthritis. *J Bone Joint Surg* 1986;68B:218–221.
52. Russotti GM, Harris WH. Proximal placement of the acetabular component in total hip arthroplasty. *J Bone Joint Surg* 1991;75A:587–592.
53. Schmalzried TP, Amstutz HD, Dorey FJ. Nerve palsy associated with total hip replacement. *J Bone Joint Surg* 1991;73A:1074–1087.
54. Scott RD, Sarokhan AJ, Dalziel R. Total hip and total knee arthroplasty in juvenile rheumatoid arthritis. *Clin Orthop* 1984;182:90–98.
55. Severt R, Craccchiola A III. Uncemented total hip replacement in rheumatoid arthritic diseases: two to six year follow-up. *Orthop Trans* 1990;14:581.
56. Severt R, Wood R, Craccchiola A III. Long term follow-up of cemented total hip arthroplasty in rheumatoid arthritis. *Clin Orthop* 1991;265:137–145.
57. Soballe K, Boll KL, Kofod S, Holsebro BS, Kristensen SS. Total hip replacement after medial-displacement osteotomy of the proximal part of the femur. *J Bone Joint Surg* 1989;71A:692–697.
58. Sponseller PD, McBeath AA, Perpich M. Long-term follow-up of hip arthrodesis performed in young patients. In: Welch RB, ed. *The hip. Proceedings of the twelfth open scientific meeting of the Hip Society.* St. Louis: CV Mosby, 1984:43–53.
59. Sponseller PD, McBeath AA, Perpich M. Hip arthrodesis in young patients. A long-term follow-up study. *J Bone Joint Surg* 1984;66A:853–859.
60. Strathy GM, Fitzgerald RH. Total hip arthroplasty in the ankylosed hip. *J Bone Joint Surg* 1988;70A:963–966.
61. Stromqvist B, Hansson LI, Nilsson LT, Thorgren KC. Hook-pin fixation in femoral neck fractures: a two year follow up study of 300 cases. *Clin Orthop* 1987;218:58–62.
62. Sunderland S. *Nerves and nerve injury.* Edingurgh: Churchill Livingstone, 1978.
63. Turula KB, Friberg O, Lindholm TS, et al. Leg length inequality after total hip arthroplasty. *Clin Orthop* 1986;202:163–168.
64. Visser JD, Jonkers A, Hillen B. Hip joint measurements with computerized tomography. *J Pediatr Orthop* 1982;2:143–151.
65. Wasielewski RC, Crossett LS, Rubash HE. Neural and vascular injury in total hip arthroplasty. *Orthop Clin North Am* 1992;23:219–235.
66. Weber ER, Daube JR, Coventry MB. Peripheral neuropathies associated with total hip arthroplasty. *J Bone Joint Surg* 1976;58A:66–69.
67. Wedge JH, Commisky DJ. Primary arthroplasty of the hip in patients younger than 21 years. *Instr Course Lect* 1995;44:275–280.
68. Welsh RB, Charnley J. Low-friction arthroplasty of the hip in rheumatoid arthritis and ankylosing spondylitis. *Clin Orthop* 1970;72:22–32.
69. Williams WW, McCullough CJ. Results of cemented total hip replacement in juvenile chronic arthritis. A radiologic review. *J Bone Joint Surg* 1993;75B:872–874.
70. Williamson JA, Reckling FW. Limb length discrepancy and related problems following total hip joint replacement. *Clin Orthop* 1978;134:135–138.
71. Witt JD, Swan M, Ansell BM. Total hip replacement for juvenile chronic arthritis. *J Bone Joint Surg* 1991;73B:770–773.
72. Woolson ST. Leg length equalization during total hip replacement. *Orthopaedics* 1990;13:17–21.
73. Woolson ST, Harris WH. A method of intra-operative limb length measurement in total hip arthroplasty. *Clin Orthop* 1985;194:207–210.
74. Yoshioka Y, Cooke TDV. Femoral anteversion. Assessment based on functional axes. *J Orthop Res* 1987;5:86–91.

The Adult Hip, edited by J. J. Callaghan,
A. G. Rosenberg, and H. E. Rubash.
Lippincott–Raven Publishers, Philadelphia © 1998.

CHAPTER 76

Hip Fractures Treated by Arthroplasty

Patrick A. Meere, Paul E. DiCesare, and Joseph D. Zuckerman

The outcome of internal fixation of displaced hip fractures is associated with specific complications such as osteonecrosis, malunion, and fixation failure (9,167, 169). In a meta-analysis of 106 reports of outcomes after displaced fractures of the femoral neck, Lu-Yao et al. found that at the 2-year follow-up, the probability of nonunion and osteonecrosis were 33% and 16%, respectively (124). Within this time period, the probability of a second operation ranged from 20% to 36%. The most common secondary procedure was conversion of a failed internal fixation to arthroplasty. The relative risk of reoperation after internal fixation in this time period was found to be 2.6 times greater than that for primary endoprosthetic replacement (124). Considering these morbidity rates and the number of surgical re-interventions associated with internal fixation, several authors have proposed primary prosthetic replacement of the femoral head in the treatment of selected cases of displaced hip fractures (9,38,93,124,167,168,169).

Historical Development

Hip fractures have historically been associated with significant mortality and morbidity (169,172,185). Prior to the advent of endoprosthetic replacement, the majority of displaced hip fractures were treated by internal fixation (9). This remains the standard of care for younger

patients. In elderly patients, however, the rate of complications (nonunion, osteonecrosis) associated with the internal fixation of displaced femoral neck fractures led to the development of primary prosthetic replacement. As a result, the indications for prosthetic replacement have evolved over the last three decades; however, definitive indications for open reduction and internal fixation (ORIF) versus primary prosthetic replacement have not been agreed upon. The debate about the optimal treatment for the so-called unsolved fracture persists to this day, partly because of the relative lack of controlled prospective clinical studies.

Prior to the early 1970s, prosthetic replacement for displaced femoral neck fractures in the elderly was limited to uncemented unipolar arthroplasties. The clinical experience with the Moore and Thompson hemiarthroplasties has been widely reported by several authors (2,14,50, 65,71,92,112,122,143,146,156,195). The Austin-Moore prosthesis was designed for use without bone cement, using a fenestrated stem to allow "self-locking" of the prosthesis in the proximal femur. The Thompson prosthesis was designed for a more extensive neck resection and did not use a fenestrated stem (206).

Cemented bipolar hemiarthroplasties evolved as a response to specific complications of unipolar endoprostheses, namely acetabular erosion and high impact forces on the acetabulum. The original designs were those of Bateman (11) and Giliberty (67), both in 1974. This design class had the theoretical advantage of increased range of motion and relatively easier conversion to a total arthroplasty (3,7,11,67,68,155,192,193). Although the early clinical results were favorable, the longer-term

P. A. Meere, P. E. DiCesare, and J. D. Zuckerman: Department of Orthopaedic Surgery, Hospital for Joint Diseases, New York, New York 10003.

complications of femoral stem loosening, acetabular erosion, decreased joint motion, pain, and hip function prompted a reevaluation of the clinical performance of bipolar hemiarthroplasties (14,50,65,71,92,112,122,143, 146,156,195).

As a response to these significant complications, including a high revision rate to total joint arthroplasty, increasing consideration was given to the initial management of acute displaced femoral neck fractures by primary total hip arthroplasty. The clinical performance of this method of treatment has been the subject of numerous reviews (24,33,36,43,65,73,168,186). The functional outcome of total hip arthroplasties in this specific trauma-patient population was shown to be different from that found in primary elective cases in the treatment of osteoarthritis. As will be discussed, the rate of complications from dislocation and aseptic loosening is higher in the posttraumatic population (24,33,43,168,186).

Current Status

The standard of care for undisplaced femoral neck fractures in the elderly and for all femoral neck fractures in the younger age group remains primary internal fixation.

In elderly patients with a displaced femoral neck fracture, with adequate bone stock and a moderate to high level of demand, the choice of treatment is based on a careful analysis of the so-called patient-and-fracture factors. In otherwise active healthy patients with displaced fractures, internal fixation is the preferred option. In debilitated patients with medical comorbidities and lower activity level, primary prosthetic replacement is preferred. In the presence of preexisting arthritis, metabolic bone disease, or a pathologic process involving the acetabulum, total hip arthroplasty is preferred. The incidence of postoperative complications is less in these special cases partly as a result of a lower level of demand.

A controversy remains as to the implant of choice: unipolar versus bipolar prostheses. The mechanical efficiency of bipolar devices at preventing acetabular erosion and protrusio has not been consistently confirmed, and many studies have documented a gradual lessening of the inner joint motion over time (48,97,155,193).

ACUTE FEMORAL NECK FRACTURES

The accepted treatment of nondisplaced or minimally displaced femoral neck fractures is by closed or open reduction and internal fixation, regardless of age (Fig. 1). An exception is made in cases of preexisting symptomatic degenerative hip disease. In these cases and in the presence of neoplastic disease, the mode of treatment by primary total hip arthroplasty is probably preferred.

Displaced femoral neck fractures may be treated differently because of the increased incidence of healing

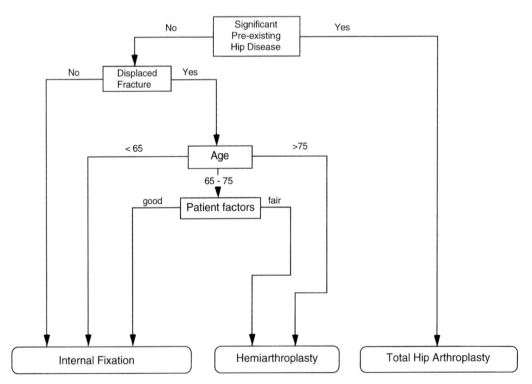

FIG. 1. Treatment algorithm for acute femoral neck fractures.

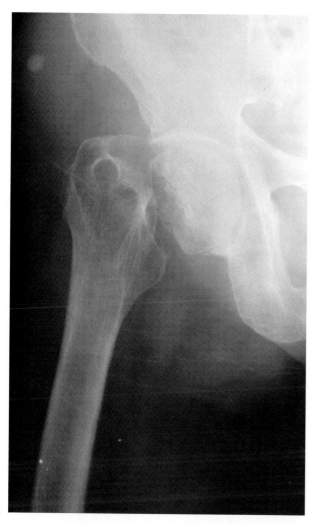
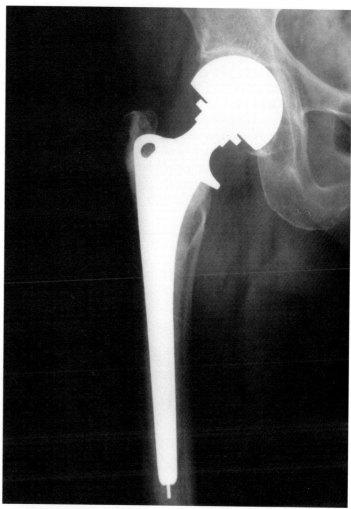

FIG. 2. A: Anteroposterior (AP) radiograph of an acute displaced femoral neck fracture in a 92-year-old woman. **B:** Postoperative radiograph showing a cemented unipolar hemiarthroplasty.

complications. Additional considerations include the quality of the bone stock, the age of the patient, and the expected activity level. Some authors have recommended the use of physiologic age rather than chronologic age as an assistive tool in determining optimal individual treatment (160). However, physiologic age lacks specific criteria. Although age categories overlap, a consensus appears to treat younger patients, particularly those with a high activity level and good quality bone stock, by internal fixation (38,151,160). Primary prosthetic replacement is preferred for older patients (Fig. 2) with limited activity and poor quality bone stock. The remaining intermediate age group should be assessed carefully for both patient factors and fracture factors as described by Zuckerman et al. (206). Patient factors include the age of the patient, ambulatory ability, functional status, mental status, ability to participate in a rehabilitation program, and associated medical problems. The fracture fac-

tors include the amount of displacement, extent of osteoporosis, degree of comminution, and age of the fracture.

Implants

Unipolar Implants

The original design of the unipolar hemiarthroplasty used for displaced femoral neck fractures had the following features: a solid polished unipolar head with a collared, straight, fenestrated stem designed for noncemented use. The best-known design of this type was the Austin-Moore prosthesis. A second design was the Thompson prosthesis, characterized by a solid unipolar head and a collared, shorter, curved, nonfenestrated stem. Although the original design was for use without cement, the development of cement fixation in the late 1960s led to its use with the Thompson prosthesis because of the curved, nonfenestrated stem.

D'Arcy and Devas reported their experience with the cemented Thompson prosthesis in a series of 361 femoral neck fractures (39). The average age in the series was 81 years; 156 patients (161 hips) were followed for 3 years, with a satisfactory outcome reported for 82% of patients. They noted that the majority of unsatisfactory results were in patients younger than 75 years of age. The 1-month mortality was significant (12.9%). The major complications noted were acetabular erosion and pain. Radiologic evidence of acetabular erosion was identified in 11%, infection in 4.7%, femoral shaft penetration in 2%, and dislocations in 2%.

Whittaker et al. reported a series of 160 hemiarthroplasties using both the Moore and Thompson prostheses (198). The rate of acetabular joint-space narrowing at 4 years was 25%, with 5% exhibiting significant protrusio. The incidences of problems at 5 years or more were 64% and 24%, respectively. Philips reported a series of 241 patients with displaced femoral neck fractures treated by primary cemented Thompson hemiarthroplasty (155). The average age was 79.6 years. At 3 to 14 years of follow-up, 72 cases were available for clinical and radiographic review. A strong correlation was found between the incidence of acetabular erosion and the level of physical activity. Complete acetabular erosion was found in 34 of 38 hips (89%) of active patients and in none in the remaining 34 inactive patients. The severity of erosion was also noted to increase with time in the active group, resulting in increased pain. A 44% revision rate was reported in the active subgroup. A comparable rate of revision in active patients was found in a study by Kofoed and Kofod (109). This study reported a rate of revision of 55% using the Austin-Moore hemiarthroplasty.

The morbidity and mortality reported with the use of unipolar prostheses is variable and reflects the many confounding variables encountered in this patient population.

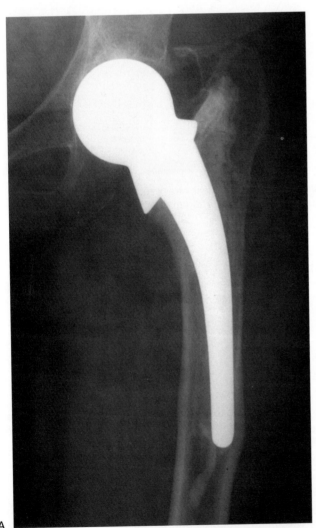 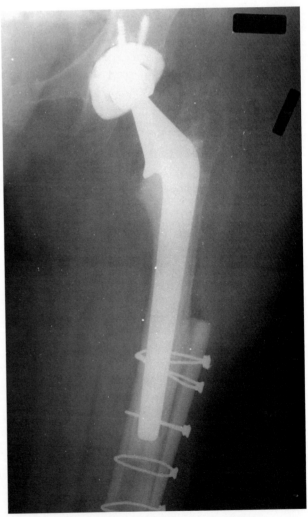

FIG. 3. A: AP radiograph of a 16-year-old cemented unipolar endoprosthesis demonstrating acetabular protrusio and aseptic loosening. **B:** After conversion to THR and fixation of the distal periprosthetic fracture.

Nather et al. reported on a series of 110 patients with a mean age of 78 years treated by primary prosthetic replacement using either a Moore or Thompson implant (143). The 1-year mortality was 15%. The overall complication rate was 13%, with dislocations in 2.7% and infections in 4.5% of patients. Jalovaara et al., in a study on the quality of life after hemiarthroplasty for displaced femoral neck fractures, concluded that the Moore prosthesis was associated with serious complications that interfered with functional and social rehabilitation (98).

Holt et al., in a study on functional outcomes after over 1000 femoral neck fractures, concluded that the best predictors were age and pre-injury mobility (91). The 1-year mortality was 11.3% and fractures treated by internal fixation were noted to have a lower mortality than the noncemented hemiarthroplasty group. Marcus et al. reported on 97 Austin-Moore prostheses with an average follow-up of 26 months (130). The dislocation rate was 3% and the 3-month mortality was 7%. There is evidence to show that functional outcomes deteriorate with time (69).

Studies have consistently shown that acetabular wear increases significantly over time (Fig. 3). In an histologic analysis of 12 elderly patients undergoing revision of hemiarthroplasty to total replacement, Dalldorf et al. found considerable degeneration of acetabular cartilage as compared to an age-matched control group (41). The progression in the severity of the degeneration correlated with the age of the implant. All six patients with a hemiarthroplasty in place for longer than 5 years and with a stable femoral component demonstrated near complete loss of cartilage (41).

In the elderly population undergoing primary prosthetic replacement, one of the most significant complications is dislocation. Not only is this a functional problem, but it has also been associated with an increased risk of mortality. Blewitt et al. reviewed 20 cases of dislocation in a series of 1000 consecutive hemiarthroplasties (13). The 6-month mortality in these 20 patients was 65%. Maxwell and Turner reviewed 13 patients who required reduction under anesthesia for dislocation of an Austin-Moore prosthesis (132). The 1-month mortality was 69%. In a comparative study between bipolar and unipolar prostheses, Drinker and Murray found a rate of dislocation of 8.9% and 7.5%, respectively (48). The authors noted that although the incidence was comparable, the outcomes of reduction were quite different. Whereas all Thompson dislocations were reducible by closed means, 5 of the 9 bipolar dislocations required open reduction (48).

Bipolar Implants

The development of the bipolar hemiarthroplasty was based in part on the clinical experience with the unipolar hemiarthroplasty. As discussed, the most significant complication of unipolar hemiarthroplasties was the progressive acetabular wear and concomitant pain. Over time,

this erosion could result in acetabular protrusio. Based on Charnley's pioneering arthroplasty principles, two bipolar designs emerged in the early 1970s: the Bateman and the Giliberty bipolar hemiarthroplasties. The femoral stem and head were essentially identical to the current total hip arthroplasty stem. The second component consisted of an outer metallic shell of the same diameter as a unipolar implant. Within this shell, a polyethylene inner bearing was encased with an inner-joint bearing-surface matching the femoral head diameter. In the case of the Bateman, this inner diameter was set at 22 mm as per Charnley's low friction arthroplasty theory, whereas the Giliberty design used a 32-mm head.

The theoretical advantage of the bipolar design was to dissipate the joint forces through the inner bearing surfaces, thereby decreasing the rate of superior acetabular erosion and the incidence of pain. In addition, it was speculated that the combined arc of motion of the dual joint should reduce the incidence of dislocation, because most of the motion should take place at the inner articulation. The third anticipated advantage was an easier conversion to a total hip arthroplasty, because the femoral component was already present (Fig. 4).

In 1979, Drinker and Murray compared the clinical performance of 101 Bateman bipolar hemiarthroplasties with 160 cemented Thompson unipolar hemiarthroplasties (48). At the 3-year follow-up, the Harris Hip Scores were similar (77.5 and 76.4, respectively). There was no statistical difference in the overall morbidity and mortality between the two groups. Although the incidences of complications were similar, the study found that dislocations of the bipolar hemiarthroplasties were much less likely to be successfully reduced by closed means. Five of nine Bateman dislocations went on to open reduction compared to none of 12 for the Thompson group. The issue of the relative range of motion of the bipolar components was studied in a subset of 13 cases. The relative sagittal axis motion between the inner and outer bearing surfaces was found to be less than predicted and worsened with time when comparing the 2- and 4-year measurements. This loss of the bipolar motion did not translate into a lesser functional score, however, because the subgroup's mean Harris Hip Score at 3.4 years was 93 (48).

Different authors have addressed the issue of range of motion. In a study of 20 bipolar prostheses 3 months after implantation, Verberne demonstrated that inner bearing motion was less than 20% of total hip excursion (193). Philips performed a fluoroscopic study of 100 bipolar prostheses 1 year after implantation (155). Twenty-four hips had normal acetabular cartilage, whereas 76 had degenerative changes. In the first group, bipolar motion was present in 80%. In the degenerative group, only 25% of the hips displayed bipolar motion. The effect of head size on range of motion was analyzed by Brueton et al. (21). Seventy-five cases were divided into two groups based on head size. The 22-mm group showed primarily

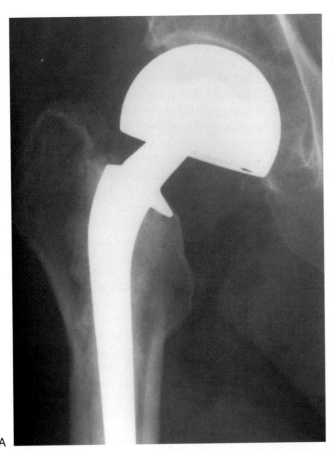
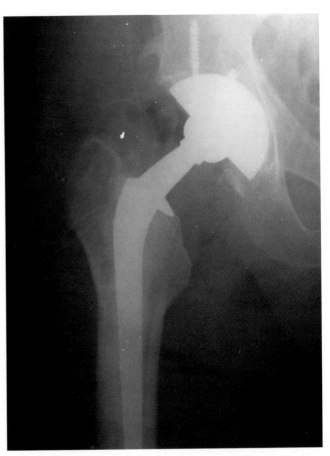

A   B

FIG. 4. A: AP radiograph of a clinically painful hip treated with a cemented bipolar hemiarthroplasty, demonstrating no significant femoral loosening. **B:** After conversion of the bipolar implant to a noncemented acetabular arthroplasty.

intraprosthetic motion (inner-bearing), whereas the 32-mm group demonstrated predominantly extraprosthetic motion (outer-bearing).

Numerous studies have focused on the clinical performance of the bipolar hemiarthroplasties. Langan (115) expressed cautious support for the Giliberty prosthesis on the basis of 65 cases with short-term follow-up of 19 months. Although he noted a loss of the inner joint motion, the functional score was good to excellent. Long and Knight reported on the clinical outcome of 156 cases with a mean age of 79 years and average follow-up of 29 months. The functional outcome and incidence of complications were comparable to those of unipolar hemiarthroplasties (123). Contrary to other studies, however, the range of motion under weight-bearing conditions was shown to be almost entirely at the inner bearing. The dislocations were difficult to manage by closed methods. The cause of the dislocations was ascribed to postoperative positioning, component separation and improper implant sizing. This study concluded that there were no demonstrable advantages over the unipolar implants.

Other studies have reported a decrease in acetabular erosion and component loosening, improved functional outcomes, and the persistence of inner bearing motion. Overgaard et al. reported a series of 171 displaced femoral neck fractures in 168 patients with a physiologic age greater than 75 years (150). The mortality rate at 1 year was 22%. There were four immediate dislocations and no late dislocations. The reoperation rate was 4%. At the 6-year follow-up, 62 patients were alive. Of this group, only four had weight-bearing pain, three had subsidence, and none showed radiologic evidence of protrusio. James and Gallannaugh reported no evidence of acetabular erosion in 323 patients followed for over 7 years (99). Bochner et al. reported their experience with bipolar arthroplasties (Bateman, modified Bateman, and Osteonics) in a consecutive series of 120 hemiarthroplasties, of which 90 patients were followed for at least 2 years (14). In the following group, 91% were pain free and 92% demonstrated satisfactory power and motion. A subgroup of 26 cases were analyzed radiologically 6 months after implantation, using standard (weight-bearing) radiographs. This analysis demonstrated persistence of motion at both joint bearing levels. In a later study, Goldhill et al. reported on a series of 246 patients with an average of 78 years and a range of follow-up between 1 and 6 years (71). Dislocations occurred in 0.9% (successfully treated by closed reduction) and the revision rate was 0.4% (not caused by wear). There was no evidence of significant acetabular wear or femoral component loosening.

On the basis of the reports noted, questions remain as to whether the bipolar design provides superior clinical outcomes. Numerous studies have attempted to address this point in comparative studies. Eiskjaer et al. in 1993 reported on a total of 679 cases, composed of 202 Austin-Moores, 209 trunion-bearing Christiaensens, and 268 cemented Hasting bipolar hemiarthroplasties (50). The cumulative prosthesis survival at 5 years was 90%, and at 10 years 85%. Survivorship analysis demonstrated that most of the cases requiring revision to a total hip arthroplasty occurred within 4 to 5 years after surgery. The authors noted that age and type of prosthesis did have a significant impact on component survival. Significantly fewer failures were found with the bipolar cemented component and with patients under 75 years of age.

Yamagata et al., in their classic study, reviewed 1001 cases of hip hemiarthroplasties (202). There were 682 unipolar and 319 bipolar design cases. The groups were matched with respect to age (mean, 74 years) and sex (68% female). However, only 62% of the series were femoral neck fractures; other diagnoses included osteonecrosis and osteoarthritis. The results of the multivariate analysis of the anticipated prosthesis survivorship demonstrated a 13.7% probability of reoperation at 8 years for bipolar components as opposed to 22.9% for unipolars. The increased acetabular wear identified with unipolar designs correlated with the length of time since the operation, the bone quality, and the quality of the press-fit (uncemented femoral components). The authors concluded that unipolar designs (fixed head endoprostheses) showed less femoral loosening but greater acetabular wear at a follow-up of more than 2 years. Although the bipolar group appeared to have a lesser reoperation rate, this superior prosthetic survival rate was primarily a reflection of cement fixation regardless of design. The recommended indications for the bipolar design were in younger, physically active patients, whereas the unipolar design was recommended for older, less active patients.

Primary Total Hip Arthroplasty

The primary treatment of acute displaced femoral neck fractures by total hip arthroplasty remains very controversial. Most authors would agree that there are limited indications for primary total hip arthroplasty after femoral neck fractures. These include preexisting osteoarthritis, rheumatoid arthritis, and degenerative arthritis secondary to Paget's disease. However, other investigators have used total hip arthroplasty for displaced femoral neck fractures in healthy, active patients in the absence of preexisting degenerative changes. The results have been, at best, inconsistent.

In an early report on the clinical performance of primary total hip replacement in 112 acute femoral neck fractures, Sim and Stauffer concluded that this treatment was best reserved for the previously active elderly patient (168). This series included 16 cases with associated hip disease; significant osteoporosis was present in 67%. Medical complications were numerous (21%) and included five pulmonary emboli. The surgical complication rate was 22% and included an infection rate of 0.9%. Twelve dislocations (10.7%) were reported, of which two were nonreducible by closed means. At a mean follow-up of only 22 months, radiographs did not demonstrate any evidence of definite or probable loosening. The functional outcome was considered good at the 1-year follow-up in 85 patients; 81% reported no pain, whereas 17.6% reported mild discomfort. Almost 70% of the patients regained their pre-fracture level of activity.

Taine and Armour's retrospective review of 163 cases of primary total hip arthroplasties for displaced femoral neck fractures demonstrated a significant incidence of medical and surgical complications (186). The incidence of medical complications was 30%; dislocations occurred in 12% of cases. Most dislocations occurred early and there was a significant correlation with the use of the posterior approach. In the 57 cases followed for 42 months, the functional score (Harris Hip Score) was good or excellent in 61%.

Patient selection in total hip arthroplasties for acute femoral neck fractures is of great importance as shown in the study of Delamarter and Moreland, where the functional results and pain relief were found to be better than with hemiarthroplasties and comparable to elective total hip arthroplasties (43). In this study of 27 patients (average age of 72 years and mean follow-up of 3.8 years), there were no dislocations, reoperations, or deep infections. Of importance in this study is that 82% of cases demonstrated moderate to severe acetabular degenerative changes, and 30%, severe osteoporosis. Fifteen cases had associated hip disorders. The authors attributed the exceptional clinical outcome to the prompt and aggressive management of medical complications and to the experience of the surgeons.

Considerably poorer results were reported by Greenough and Jones in their retrospective study of 37 patients undergoing primary total hip arthroplasty for displaced femoral neck fractures (73). None of the patients had preexisting hip disease. At a mean follow-up of 56 months, 49% of patients had had or were scheduled for revision surgery. Radiologic loosening was present in an additional 11%. The dislocation rate was 8%. The authors concluded that this mode of treatment was unacceptable in the younger, active patient without preexisting hip disease.

The main conclusions from the review of the current literature is that the use of total hip arthroplasty in displaced femoral neck fractures is indicated in selected patients with preexisting hip disease. Under these circumstances, the functional outcome, rate of complications, and morbidity are comparable if not superior to hemiarthroplasty.

Surgical Technique

Approach

The surgical approach utilized has been reported to impact on the dislocation rate, infection rate, duration of surgery, and surgical blood loss. The posterior approach has been associated with a greater dislocation rate (28,95,188,200). However, it remains the most common approach utilized. In the setting of spastic hemiplegia, the posterior approach should be avoided because of the potential for instability with flexion and adduction (206). The anterior or direct lateral approach combined with selective release of contractures is favored to maximize stability in severe cases of spastic hemiplegia. Staeheli et al., in their review of 48 patients with Parkinson's disease treated primarily by prosthetic replacement, found no significant correlation between outcome and surgical approach (175).

The approach used may also affect the rate of infection. In the presence of urinary or bowel incontinence, the posterior approach has been associated with an increased infection rate (26,75,200,206).

Cemented versus Noncemented Fixation

Although the initial hip fracture endoprostheses were designed for noncemented use, the current use of state-of-the-art femoral component designs has led to the use of cemented fixation as the preferred technique. Numerous reports have documented the improved outcomes of cemented implants (12,57,191).

Emery et al. reported on a prospective randomized (cement versus noncemented) series of 53 bipolar hemiarthroplasties with a mean follow-up of 17 months (52). No significant differences were found in the rate of postoperative complications, operative time, blood loss, or mortality. The noncemented group, however, reported greater pain and dependency on walking aids (52). In a study by Lennox et al., in 207 patients reviewed at an average of 19 months after surgery, the mortality was higher in the noncemented group. In addition, patient satisfaction was highest in the cemented hemiarthroplasty group (116). In 1995, Christie et al., in a randomized series of 24 patients, reported a decrease in the risk of embolic phenomena in cemented hemiarthroplasties with the use of thorough intramedullary lavage prior to cementing (30). Finally, Lo et al., in a review of 451 cases with at least a 2-year follow-up, confirmed a higher func-

tional score in the cemented group and found no significant difference in mortality or mortality (122).

The literature is misleading in that the specific implant type of a given study group is often poorly defined. The spectrum for the noncemented group ranges from the original fenestrated stem to the press-fitted or distally filling coated modern implants. The cemented group shows similar heterogeneity from first-generation to third-generation techniques. There appears to be no documented evidence regarding accelerated acetabular erosion or increased rate of infection with the use of cement. Overall, the advantage of immediate mechanical stabilization in the typical elderly patient and the absence of significant difference in morbidity and mortality tend to favor the use of cemented fixation of the femoral component.

Special Situations

Preexisting Hip Disease

The occurrence of a femoral neck fracture in the presence of moderate to advanced underlying arthritis is a relatively rare phenomenon. Once arthritic ankylosis has developed, the most common site for fracture is in the intertrochanteric and subtrochanteric level. However, early or mild degenerative changes may be encountered much more commonly. In a series of femoral neck fractures reported by Colhoun et al., 21% of fractures were found to have some degree of osteoarthritis (35). Other authors have noted a 3% to 8% incidence of rheumatoid arthritis patients in series of femoral neck fractures (102, 183).

Stromqvist et al. compared the clinical outcome of internal fixation of displaced and nondisplaced fractures in a rheumatoid population and a comparison group (183). For nondisplaced fractures, the incidence of complications (loss of fixation, nonunion, late segmental collapse) in the rheumatoid group was 1 of 5, compared with 6 of 27 in the comparison group. In the displaced fracture group, however, the rate of complications in the presence of rheumatoid arthritis was 19 of 20 (95%), with 14 cases requiring conversion to total hip arthroplasty. The complication rate in the comparison group was 53%.

Although some authors have reported variable success with hemiarthroplasty in the presence of preexisting osteoarthritis, the current trend favors primary total hip arthroplasty as the treatment of choice in the setting of preexisting symptomatic osteoarthritis or rheumatoid arthritis.

Parkinson's Disease

The management of hip fractures in patients with Parkinson's disease has been a subject of controversy. Historically, high rates of complications have been reported with internal fixation as well as with primary prosthetic replacement. Dislocation rates of up to 37% were reported by Coughlin and Templeton when a posterior approach was used (37). However, Eventor also using a posterior approach, reported a complication rate of only 3% (55). Mortality has also been reported to be higher than in a comparison group. The incidence of hip fractures associated with Parkinson's disease has actually increased as a result of newer pharmacologic agents (175). In the Mayo Clinic series of 49 patients with displaced femoral neck fractures reported by Staeheli et al., the outcome obtained with primary prosthetic replacement for displaced fractures was favorable. The most common complications were medical (urinary tract infection and pneumonia), and the rate of dislocation was very low (2%). This is in contrast to earlier reports of dislocation rates of up to 37% (37,95). The surgical approach did not appear to play a critical role. Staheli et al. recommended primary prosthetic replacement but did indicate that adductor tenotomy should be performed in the presence of contracture (to improve stability) and that meticulous medical and nursing care was necessary to minimize morbidity (175).

In patients with Parkinson's disease, primary prosthetic replacement is the treatment of choice for displaced femoral neck fractures in older patients and in patients with poorly controlled disease. In younger, more active, and well-controlled patients, reduction and internal fixation is preferable. Nondisplaced fractures should also be treated by internal fixation followed by early mobilization.

Renal Osteodystrophy

The pathophysiology of chronic renal failure leads to secondary hyperparathyroidism and renal osteodystrophy. This diffuse metabolic osteoporosis is compounded in the elderly with age-related involutional osteoporosis. The compromised bone quality thus predisposes to hip fractures, whereas the underlying renal failure predisposes to medical and surgical complications. The ratio of femoral neck fractures to intertrochanteric fractures was 3:1 in one study of 48 fractures. In this study by Thornhill and Creasman, the average age was 62 years (189). The intertrochanteric fractures were all treated by ORIF with a uniformly successful rate of union. However, the femoral head fractures treated by ORIF had a failure rate of 31% and those treated by primary prosthetic replacement had a revision rate of 33% (5 out of 15 patients).

In a smaller series, Chalmers and Irvine had a 100% failure rate using internal fixation in five femoral neck fractures with hyperparathyroidism; two cases were secondary to chronic renal failure (27).

The current recommendations for the management of femoral neck fractures in secondary hyperparathyroidism and chronic renal failure are to treat these injuries by primary prosthetic replacement. An anterior or anterolateral approach may be preferable to minimize the risk of dislocation, because these patients are in semi-recumbent chairs for prolonged periods during dialysis. In addition, careful hemostasis is necessary, because these patients require anticoagulation during dialysis. Therefore, if possible, dialysis should be performed just before surgery and then 48 hours after surgery to minimize the effect of the anticoagulation.

Previous Cerebrovascular Accident

Patients who have a cerebrovascular accident are at higher risk for hip fractures. These are most commonly femoral neck fractures, which can be sustained at the time of the stroke from an associated fall or they may occur later as the result of falls on the affected side because of weakness and balance problems. Additional predisposing factors for fractures include the development of ipsilateral poststroke osteoporosis, hemiplegic spasticity, and contractures (usually hip flexion–adduction).

In a 1960 report on this problem, Soto-Hall found a fracture incidence of 9% in his series (174). His biomechanical analysis of the deforming forces at the fracture site led him to recommend release of contractures about the hip prior to anatomic reduction and internal fixation. Without such releases, the internal fixation would be subjected to bending moments about the fracture site fulcrum from the imbalanced, spastic hip musculature, potentially resulting in fixation failure. However, he did not provide outcome data to support this approach. In contrast, the majority of published reports on this topic favor primary prosthetic replacement as the treatment of choice for femoral neck fractures in spastic hemiplegia (174).

As in the case of Parkinson's disease, the degree of spasticity and muscular imbalance is variable. Our preferred approach for mild cases with nondisplaced femoral neck fractures is anatomic reduction and internal fixation. In displaced fractures with mild spasticity, the protocol previously described is used with a careful evaluation of both patient and fracture factors. In the presence of severe spasticity, displaced and nondisplaced femoral neck fractures should be treated by primary prosthetic replacement. Technical considerations include the use of an anterior or direct lateral approach and the selective release of flexion–adduction contractures.

Paget's Disease

This metabolic bone disease of uncertain etiology has been the subject of considerable research, but questions remain about the potential for fracture healing. The healing potential is known to vary depending on the stage of the disease at the time of injury. Although once thought to heal at a normal rate, most authors now agree that there is significant delay in bone healing with respect to age-matched controls (136,139,177,194). The most common proximal femoral fracture associated with Paget's disease is at the intertrochanteric and subtrochanteric level. However, the frequency of femoral neck fractures has been reported to vary from 7% to 22% (10,47,76,114,144).

The unacceptably high rate of failure of internal fixation has been documented by several authors (10,76,144). Failure of non-operative management was also established in a series by Grundy, reporting a 100% nonunion rate in 11 patients with both operative and non-operative management (76). Dove reported a 75% failure rate with internal fixation in contrast to 78% painless ambulation when a cemented endoprosthesis was used (47). Similar results were reported by Stauffer and Sim in a smaller series (177).

The current recommendation for displaced femoral neck fractures in patients with Paget's disease is primary prosthetic replacement. The decision to convert to a total hip arthroplasty must be based on the level of preexisting symptomatic involvement of the acetabulum. With mild symptoms and mild radiologic changes, a cemented hemiarthroplasty is preferred. When definite preexisting symptoms or significant Paget's disease of the acetabulum is present, total hip arthroplasty is the treatment of choice. Technical considerations include the significant deformity of the proximal femur, management of hypersclerotic bone, and the potential for bleeding.

Arthroplasty for Failed Internal Fixation

Several studies have looked at the clinical outcome of arthroplasty after either failure of internal fixation of femoral neck fractures or for osteonecrosis with collapse (Fig. 5). The incidence of osteonecrosis after internal fixation ranges in the literature from 5% to 15% for nondisplaced femoral neck fractures and from 9% to 35% for displaced femoral neck fractures (119,129). The predisposing factors implicated in the development of this com-

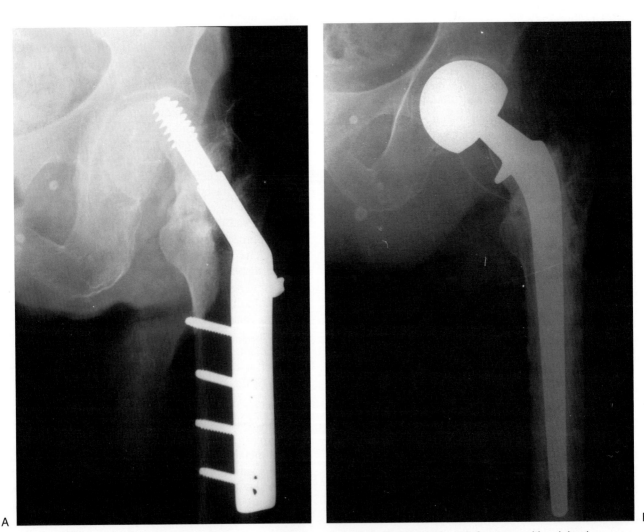

FIG. 5. A: AP radiograph showing loss of fixation of a displaced femoral neck fracture, with minimal acetabular degenerative changes. **B:** After conversion to cemented unipolar arthroplasty.

plication include the adequacy of the reduction, the delay of treatment, and the surgical placement of the instrumentation used (8,29,61,119,129). In a 1964 study, Garden analyzed the effect of malreduction on late segmental collapse (61). Using a specific alignment index, he determined that the incidence of osteonecrosis increased as the alignment became more unsatisfactory; mild deviations resulted in a 6.6% incidence of collapse, whereas moderate and severe deviations resulted in 65% and 100% incidences of late segmental collapse, respectively.

Of importance is the fact that only a subgroup of radiologically proven osteonecrosis cases will progress to worsening clinical symptoms requiring revision to a prosthetic replacement. Barnes et al. found that 30% of their patients with late segmental collapse became significantly disabled (8). The rate of conversion to a prosthetic replacement is 35% to 40% (29,34,176,182).

Numerous comparative analyses have been made comparing secondary arthroplasty with other treatment approaches. Franzen et al. reported on 84 secondary total hip arthroplasties for failed osteosynthesis of femoral

neck fractures and compared the clinical outcome to that for primary hip arthroplasty for osteoarthritis (59). The follow-up period ranged from 5 to 12 years. The main conclusion was that the results obtained were superior to those reported for primary arthroplasty for femoral neck fractures. This comparison, however, was based on the specific reports of Taine and Armour (12% revision rate at 3.5 years) (186) and Greenough and Jones (42% revision at 5 years in patients under 70 years old) (73). The authors also commented that the age- and sex-adjusted risk of prosthetic failure was 2.5 times greater after failure of internal fixation, but that this increased risk applies only to patients older than 70 years of age. Of the 33 survivors, six (18%) showed evidence of radiologic loosening at last follow-up. Mehlhoff et al. compared secondary arthroplasty with primary arthroplasty in a retrospective study of 27 patients (133). The salient conclusions were that, for femoral neck fractures, the clinical outcome was comparable, but that primary arthroplasty of intertrochanteric fractures yielded much poorer results with a higher rate of complications.

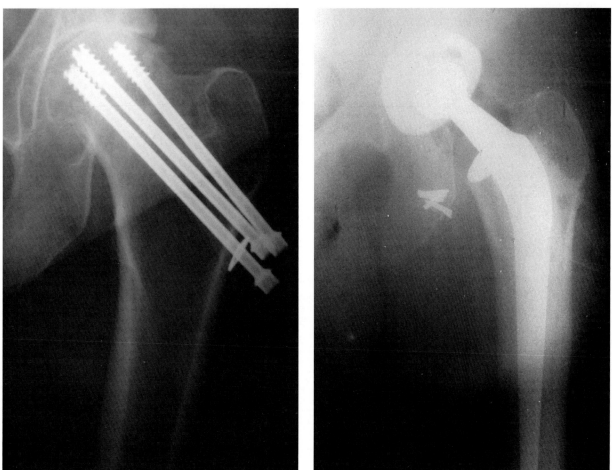

A
B

FIG. 6. A: AP radiograph showing degenerative arthritis after treatment of a subcapital femoral fracture by internal fixation (cannulated screws). **B:** After conversion to total hip arthroplasty (hybrid type).

In a 1991 study, Nilsson et al. compared the functional outcome of matched groups (28 patients, each with 5 years of follow-up) treated by secondary arthroplasty versus primary internal fixation (145). On the basis of a standardized health profile questionnaire, the authors showed superiority of the osteosynthesis group with respect to sleep, housework, hobbies, and general function.

Another report from Nilsson et al. in 1994 looked at the functional outcome of secondary arthroplasty versus primary hemiarthroplasty for femoral neck fractures (146). The matched hemiarthroplasty group consisted of 33 patients treated with a noncemented Austin-Moore prosthesis. The secondary arthroplasty group was as reported in their previous comparative study; the mean follow-up was 7 years (range, 4 to 12 years). On the basis of the results of the Nottingham Health Profile Questionnaire, the authors concluded that secondary arthroplasty treatment was superior in long-term functional capacity, specifically with respect to walking ability.

These studies support the current position that in the majority of femoral neck fractures, the treatment of choice remains either anatomic reduction and internal fixation or hemiarthroplasty. Total hip arthroplasty should be reserved for acute femoral neck fractures that occur in the presence of preexisting symptomatic degenerative disease. Total hip arthroplasty remains an excellent treatment for failed internal fixation, either for loss of fixation, nonunion, or osteonecrosis with collapse (Fig. 6).

ACUTE INTERTROCHANTERIC FRACTURES

Intertrochanteric hip fractures result from either direct forces (impact at the area of the greater trochanter) or indirect forces (transmitted along the axis of the femur to the intertrochanteric area), usually as a consequence of a patient falling from standing height (86,121). These fractures are located distal to the femoral neck and the anatomic limits of the hip joint capsule. Because the cancellous bone in this region is primarily well vascularized, the complications of nonunion and osteonecrosis associated with intracapsular hip fractures are rare after intertrochanteric fractures. As a result, the indication for primary unipolar, bipolar, or total joint arthroplasty is much more limited (Fig. 7).

The incidence of intertrochanteric fractures is dependent on age, sex, and geographic location. Numerous studies have reported an increased incidence of intertrochanteric fractures with advancing age for either sex (56,60,85). Early reports had suggested that patients sustaining intertrochanteric fractures had an average age of approximately 75 years, 10 years older than patients sustaining femoral neck fractures (32,54,140,149,159). More recent reports have not verified this finding (45). In a review of patients over 65 years old at the Hospital for Joint Diseases since 1985, the mean age for patients with intertrochanteric fractures was 79.4 years compared to a mean age of 78.6 years for patients with femoral neck fractures. The incidence of intertrochanteric fractures has

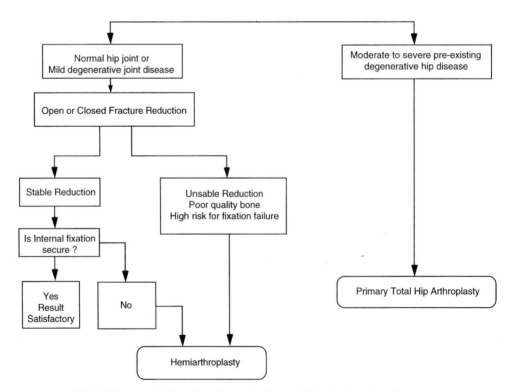

FIG. 7. Treatment algorithm for acute femoral intertrochanteric fractures.

been reported to increase eightfold for men and fivefold for women over 80 years of age (60). The female-to-male ratio for intertrochanteric fractures ranges from 2:1 to 8:1 (31,40,85,121,166,181). In the United States, the incidence of intertrochanteric fractures for patients over 65 years is sex dependent, with more women (age-adjusted incidence of 63.4/100,000) than men (age-adjusted incidence of 34/100,000) sustaining fractures (135). Intertrochanteric fracture rates also vary with geographic location, with the highest reported rates outside the United States occurring in Israel (41/100,000) (118), followed by Sweden (overall incidence, 35/100,000 for patients over 65 years of age) (85), England (27/100,000) (108), and Spain (17/100,000) (121). Mortality rates for patients sustaining intertrochanteric fractures are similar to the morality rate for patients sustaining femoral neck fractures (45,105,138,197). The advanced age of the population sustaining intertrochanteric fractures is associated with a higher incidence of degenerative hip disease, resulting in a subset of patients in whom primary prosthetic replacement should be considered.

The classification system of Evans (1949), based on the stability of the fracture pattern and the ability to convert an unstable fracture pattern to a stable reduction, has been the most widely accepted (53). This classification system is useful for both understanding the fracture patterns and determining treatment. A fracture is determined to be stable if the posteromedial cortical buttress is intact. An unstable fracture pattern is identified by posteromedial cortical comminution in the region of calcar femorale. These unstable fractures can be converted to stable fractures, however, if medial cortical opposition can be obtained. The reverse obliquity fracture pattern in this classification system is inherently unstable as a result of the propensity for medial displacement of the femoral shaft. Kyle (113) later refined the Evans classification system and described four main fracture types: type I (stable, two-part nondisplaced fracture); type II (stable fracture pattern, displaced into varus with a small lesser trochanteric fragment, but with an intact posteromedial cortex); type III or four-part fracture (unstable fracture, displaced into varus with posteromedial cortical comminution and a greater trochanteric fracture); and type IV (unstable fracture similar to type III fractures with subtrochanteric fracture extension). The reverse obliquity fracture pattern was not described in this classification system but should also be included as described previously (201).

For patients being considered for primary prosthetic replacement, the fracture patterns are important because they may determine the type of femoral component to be used and whether planned internal fixation of either the greater or lesser trochanteric fragments should be performed at arthroplasty. In general, one should use a femoral component of the calcar replacement design rather than lengthening the neck of the femoral compo-

nent. Longer femoral necks will function to lateralize the femur in relation to the patient's center of gravity, thereby increasing loosening forces on the hip as well as increasing the incidence of trochanteric bursitis.

Treatment

Early restoration of the patient's preinjury activity level is the primary goal in the treatment of intertrochanteric fractures in the elderly. If this is not achieved, such patients are at risk for many complications (54,104,113), including decubiti, urinary tract infection, joint contractures, pneumonia, and thromboembolic disease. In the absence of preexisting degenerative hip disease, all patients should be managed operatively by open or closed fracture reduction and internal fixation to avoid the complications associated with prolonged recumbency. Patients with preexisting symptomatic degenerative hip disease should be managed by primary total joint arthroplasty (Fig. 8); those patients with mild or no degenerative hip disease, and in whom a stable fracture reduction and secure internal fixation cannot be obtained, can be managed by hemiarthroplasty.

Prosthetic Replacement

More technical considerations exist when performing primary prosthetic replacement for acute intertrochanteric fractures than in replacement for displaced femoral neck fractures. The location of femoral neck fractures allows for routine placement of the femoral component because the distal portion of the femoral neck is intact, providing excellent support for the prosthesis. In addition, the greater trochanter–abductor mechanism is intact. However, in primary prosthetic replacement for comminuted intertrochanteric fractures, the choice of femoral component must take into account the loss of the calcar femorale and must allow for reattachment of the greater trochanter to restore the function of the hip abductors. As a result, prosthetic replacement for intertrochanteric fractures requires more extensive surgery than open or closed reduction with internal fixation, with increased blood loss, increased surgical and anesthetic time, and the potential for increased complication rate. Some studies suggest that the potential advantages of primary prosthetic replacement include earlier full weight bearing, an expedited functional recovery, and a reduced length of hospital stay (72,178).

Many studies have reported satisfactory results using either a unipolar or a bipolar endoprosthesis in the management of acute intertrochanteric fractures in the absence of preexisting degenerative hip disease (53,60, 75,161,178,179). Haentjens and co-workers reported on 100 patients over 75 year of age treated with either a cemented primary bipolar arthroplasty (91 patients) or

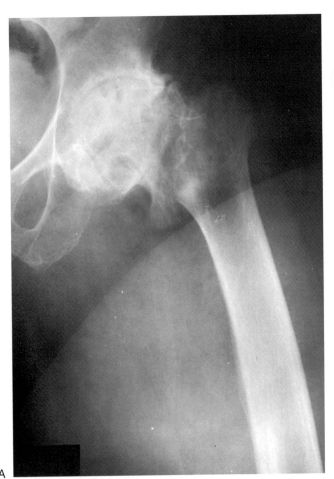
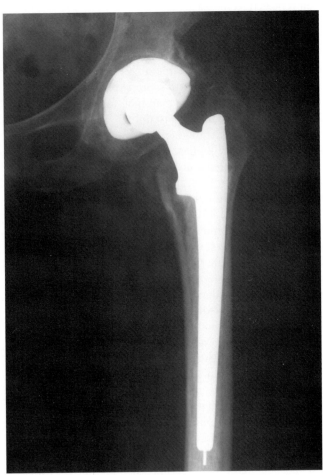

A   B

FIG. 8. A: AP radiograph showing an intertrochanteric femoral fracture with preexisting degenerative arthritis of the hip. **B:** After treatment with primary calcar replacement total hip arthroplasty (hybrid type).

total hip arthroplasty (9 patients) for unstable intertrochanteric and subtrochanteric fractures (60). Excellent to good results were noted in 78% of patients; however, 44% of those patients who had undergone total hip arthroplasty sustained a dislocation, compared to 3.3% in the bipolar group. Hip dislocation was also associated with an increased incidence of pressure sores and pulmonary complications. Other complications included loss of greater trochanter fixation in four cases, one fracture distal to the femoral component, and one pseudoarthrosis of the femur enveloping the femoral stem.

Haentjens and co-workers also reported on a prospective study comparing the results of 37 consecutive patients over 75 years of age who were managed by either bipolar arthroplasty or internal fixation (78). They concluded that the arthroplasty group had an easier and faster rehabilitation, with a lower incidence of decubiti, pulmonary infection, and atelectasis, which they attributed to earlier return to full weight bearing. A 5% dislocation rate was noted in the arthroplasty group. Stern and Angerman reported their results of a series of 105 com-

minuted intertrochanteric fractures treated by insertion of a Leinbach (calcar replacement) prosthesis followed for an average of 8.1 months (178). They concluded that unrestricted full weight bearing decreased hospital stay and reduced the incidence of secondary operations, thrombophlebitis, pulmonary embolus, decubiti, and pneumonia. Harwin and colleagues reported on the results of 58 elderly patients with acute unstable intertrochanteric fractures treated with a bipolar Bateman-Leinbach prosthesis (84). At an average follow-up of 28 months, they noted that morbidity and mortality were similar to those of a group treated with internal fixation. Ninety-one percent of patients could ambulate prior to hospital discharge. These authors stressed the importance of an anterolateral approach to decrease the risk of hip dislocation. Other authors have reported results of primary arthroplasty in smaller cohorts of patients. Good or fair results were reported in 32 of 34 cases by Rosenfeld and co-workers (161). Stern and Goldstein reported that 86% patients became ambulatory with a walker by 10 days postoperatively (179). Stern and

Angerman reported that 94% of 105 patients managed with primary endoprosthesis regained their prefracture ambulatory status (178). Green and co-workers, reporting on the use of a bipolar head–neck prosthesis in 20 elderly patients, emphasized restoration of leg length and hip capsule repair to decrease the risk of dislocation (72). At a mean follow-up of 13.2 months, 12 of 16 surviving patients were ambulatory, and there were no dislocations or infections; however, 25% of patients reported residual pain. It is important to note that in these reports of prosthetic replacement for acute intertrochanteric hip fractures, patient cohorts were primarily the most debilitated patients with the most unstable fracture patterns.

In the absence of preexisting degenerative hip disease, the indication for hemiarthroplasty may be the elderly, debilitated patient with a comminuted, unstable intertrochanteric fracture in severely osteoporotic bone. However, many patients who fit these criteria have been successfully treated by internal fixation. A more precise indication for primary hemiarthroplasty is an elderly patient with a comminuted unstable intertrochanteric fracture that cannot be converted to a stable reduction, or one in which secure internal fixation cannot be achieved. Precise analysis of the hip radiographs and classification of the fracture pattern is critical for preoperative planning of primary hemiarthroplasty. Although the decision may be made intraoperatively if stable internal fixation cannot be achieved, it is preferable to plan for primary hemiarthroplasty preoperatively, because a change in plan during surgery will result in prolonged operative and anesthetic time and increased blood loss. Changing plans intraoperatively is nevertheless preferable to accepting a malreduced fracture reduction and inadequate internal fixation that can result in early loss of fixation and the need for reoperation.

At the Hospital for Joint Diseases, primary hemiarthroplasty has been performed infrequently for treatment of acute intertrochanteric fractures. In a cohort of 200 consecutive intertrochanteric fractures (45% were classified as unstable), only three cases were treated by primary hemiarthroplasty (in only one case was the plan changed intraoperatively). In the absence of preexisting hip disease, it is very difficult to predict preoperatively which unstable fractures are best managed with primary hemiarthroplasty. In the authors' opinion, almost all intertrochanteric fractures can be adequately treated with sliding hip screw fixation if the procedure is performed with careful attention to the principles of fracture reduction and proper insertion of the device. In those few cases of elderly patients who have loss of fixation, conversion to a hemiarthroplasty or total hip arthroplasty can provide satisfactory results (17,79,107).

Postoperative management should be aimed at early mobilization of the patient and unrestricted weight bearing. Both medical and surgical complications should be anticipated after intertrochanteric fractures, because many of these elderly patients have preexisting medical problems. The mortality rate and postoperative complications such as urinary tract infections, decubiti, cardiopulmonary problems, and deep venous thrombosis occur at a rate similar to patients with femoral neck fractures (45,54,135,197). Wound infection has been reported to occur in less than 3% of cases (87,147,187). Patients at greater risk for postoperative infection are those who present with urinary tract infection or decubitus ulcers, have a prolonged operating time, have impaired cognition interfering with proper wound care, urinary and/or fecal incontinence, and close proximity of the surgical incision to the perineum (149).

Failed Internal Fixation

Paramount to achieving a successful result from internal fixation is stable fracture reduction achieved by proper insertion of the sliding hip screw device. Complications such as nonunion, malunion, or implant failure are more probable (a) if during internal fixation, the sliding hip screw is placed into the anterosuperior femoral head; (b) if reaming is improperly performed, thus creating a second channel; (c) if stable reduction cannot be attained; (d) if there is excessive collapse of the fracture, exceeding the sliding capacity of the device; (d) if imperfect screw-barrel engagement prevents sliding; or (e) if poor bone quality prevents secure fracture fixation. Nonunion after internal fixation is uncommon, occurring in less than 2% of cases (53,113,131,142,166,199).

If fixation failure occurs with loss of fracture reduction, resulting in a mal- or nonunion, the treatment options are (a) to accept the deformity; (b) to attempt a second open reduction and internal fixation, which may require augmentation with methylmethacrylate; and (c) to convert to either a hemiarthroplasty (bipolar or unipolar) or total hip arthroplasty (17,79,107) (Fig. 9). As a general rule, acceptance of deformity should be reserved only for nonambulatory patients who are poor surgical risks. If reoperation is indicated, conversion to a hemiarthroplasty or total hip arthroplasty is preferred to a second attempt at internal fixation because the osteoporosis, comminution, and previous surgery will significantly interfere with the surgeon's ability to obtain secure internal fixation and leading to fracture healing (131). Total joint arthroplasty in this setting is indicated for posttraumatic osteoarthrosis, perforation of the acetabulum by the internal fixation device, or (uncommonly) for femoral head osteonecrosis. Implant selection for these patients is usually a cemented calcar femoral stem with either a bipolar or unipolar head. If preexisting acetabular degeneration is noted or has occurred during the interval between internal fixation and arthroplasty (e.g., in cases where the sliding hip screw has cut out of the femoral head and damaged the acetabulum), the acetabulum

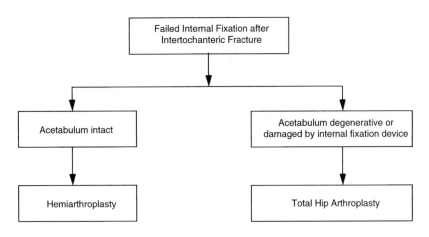

FIG. 9. Treatment algorithm for failed internal fixation of femoral intertrochanteric fractures.

should also be replaced with either a cemented or a non-cemented component. An important technical note reported by Patterson and co-workers (153) is that after removing a sliding hip screw device, the holes in the femoral cortex may act as stress risers, predisposing to spiral femur fractures during hip range of motion, hindering cement pressurization, or leading to intrusion of cement that interferes with subsequent cortical bone remodeling. These authors recommend replacing the removed screws in the cortical holes until they are flush with the endosteal surface and then cementing the femoral component, followed by screw removal after the cement has polymerized, and finally filling the holes with cancellous bone obtained during femoral canal preparation.

Few papers have addressed the results of hip arthroplasty after failed internal fixation of intertrochanteric fractures. Haentjens and co-workers reported the results of nine elderly patients who were treated by salvage hip arthroplasty after failed internal fixation of either intertrochanteric or subtrochanteric hip fractures (79). Mean time to reoperation was 7 months, and the clinical results were fair to excellent in all patients at a mean follow-up of 41 months. The authors stressed that restoration of function with early walking and full weight bearing are responsible for these good clinical results. Stoffelen and colleagues reported on 12 patients who experienced failed internal fixation and were treated by an endoprosthesis (180). The mean time to reoperation was 6 months, and all patients had a satisfactory result at a mean follow-up of 32 months. These authors stressed that endoprosthesis appears to be a valuable method to salvage failed internal fixation of intertrochanteric fractures in the elderly. Kim and co-workers reported on seven patients (mean age, 35 years) who had neglected unstable intertrochanteric fractures and were treated with a long-stem cementless porous-coated hemiarthroplasty (106). At a mean follow-up of 45 months, the average Harris Hip Score was 96, and all patients had fracture consolidation.

The majority of patients with an intertrochanteric femoral fracture should be managed operatively by open or closed fracture reduction and internal fixation. In the presence of preexisting symptomatic degenerative hip disease, the treatment of choice is primary total joint arthroplasty. Hemiarthroplasty may be indicated in patients with mild or no degenerative hip disease and in whom a stable fracture reduction and secure internal fixation cannot be obtained.

CONCLUSION

The treatment of choice in the majority of hip fractures remains either anatomic reduction and internal fixation or hemiarthroplasty. Total hip arthroplasty should be reserved for acute displaced femoral neck and intertrochanteric fractures that occur in the presence of preexisting symptomatic degenerative disease. Total hip arthroplasty remains an excellent secondary treatment for failed internal fixation either for loss of fixation, nonunion, or osteonecrosis with collapse.

REFERENCES

1. Altchek M. Avoiding dislocation in prosthetic hip replacement. *Orthop Rev* 1993;22(5):644–646.
2. Anderson LD, Hamsa WR Jr, Waring TL. Femoral-head prostheses. a report of three hundred and fifty-six operations and their results. *J Bone Joint Surg* 1964;46A:1049–1065.
3. Anderson PR, Milgram JW. Dislocation and component separation of the Bateman hip endoprosthesis. *JAMA* 1978;240:2079–2080.
4. Arnold WD, Lyden JP, Minkoff J. Treatment of intracapsular fractures of the femoral neck, with special reference to percutaneous Knowles pinning. *J Bone Joint Surg* 1974;56A:254–262.
5. Asai T, Nagaya I, Miyake N, Kondo K, Tsukamoto M. The treatment of intracapsular hip fractures with total hip arthroplasty in rheumatoid arthritis. *Bull Hosp Joint Dis* 1993;53(2):29–33.
6. Askin SR, Bryan RS. Femoral neck fractures in young adults. *Clin Orthop* 1976;114:259–264.
7. Barmada R, Siegel IM. Postoperative separation of the femoral and acetabular components of a single-assembly total hip (Bateman) replacement. Report of two cases. *J Bone Joint Surg* 1979;61A: 777–778.

8. Barnes R, Brown JT, Garden RS, Nicoll EA. Subcapital fractures of the femur. *J Bone Joint Surg* 1976;58B:2–241976.

9. Barnes R, Brown JT, Garden RS, Nicoll EA. Subcapital fracture of the femur: a prospective review. *J Bone Joint Surg Br* 1976; 58B:2–24.

10. Barry HC. Fractures of the femur in Paget's disease of bone in Australia. *J Bone Joint Surg* 1967;49A:1359–1370.

11. Bateman JE. Single-assembly total hip prosthesis. Preliminary Report. *Orthop Dig* 1974;2:15–22.

12. Beals RK. Survival following hip fracture. Long follow-up of 607 patients. *J Chronic Dis* 1972;25:235–244.

13. Blewitt N, Mortimore S. Outcome of dislocation after hemiarthroplasty for fractured neck of the femur. *Injury* 1992;23(5):320–322.

14. Bochner RM, Pellicci PM, Lyden JP. Bipolar hemiarthroplasty for fracture of the femoral neck. *J Bone Joint Surg* 1988;70A:1001–1010.

15. Bogoch E, Ouellette G, Hastings D. Failure of internal fixation of displaced femoral neck fractures in rheumatoid patients. *J Bone Joint Surg* 1991;73B(1):7–10.

16. Boyd HB, Griffin LL. Classification and treatment of trochanteric fractures. *Arch Surg* 1949;58:853–866.

17. Boyd HB, Lipinski SW. Nonunion of trochanteric and subtrochanteric fractures. *Surg Gynecol Obstet* 1957;104:463–470.

18. Bray TJ, Smith-Hoefer E, Hooper A, et al. The displaced femoral neck fracture: internal fixation versus bipolar endoprosthesis. Results of a prospective randomized comparison. *Clin Orthop* 1988;230:127–140.

19. Bray TJ, Templeman DC. Fractures of the femoral neck. In: Chapman MW, ed. *Operative orthopaedics*, vol 1. Philadelphia: JB Lippincott, 1988;341–352.

20. Broos PL. Hip fractures in elderly people: the surgical treatment in Leuven, Belgium. *Acta Chir Belg* 1994;94(3):130–135.

21. Brueton RN, Craig JS, Hinves BL, Heatley FW. Effect of femoral component size on movement of the two-component hemiarthroplasty. *Injury* 1993;24(4):231–235.

22. Brummer R. *Natural course in nailed fractures of the femoral neck. A 5-year prospective investigation.* 1983;(in preparation).

23. Byers PD, Hoaglund FT, Purewal GS, Yau AC. Articular cartilage changes in Caucasian and Asian hip joints. *Ann Rheumat Dis* 1974;33: 157–161.

24. Cartlidge IJ. Primary total hip replacement for displaced subcapital femoral fractures. *Injury* 1982;13:249–253.

25. Ceder L, Svensson K, Thorngren KG. Statistical prediction of rehabilitation in elderly patients with hip fractures. *Clin Orthop* 1980;152: 185–190.

26. Ceder L, Lindberg L, Odberg E. Differentiated care of hip fracture in the elderly. *Acta Orthop Scand* 1980;51:157–162.

27. Chalmers J, Irvine GB. Fractures of the femoral neck in elderly patients with hyperparathyroidism. *Clin Orthop* 1988;229:125–130.

28. Chan RN, Hoskinson J. Thompson prosthesis for fractured neck of the femur. *J Bone Joint Surg Am* 1975;57B:437–443.

29. Christie J, Howie C, Armoir P. Fixation of displaced femoral neck fractures: compression screw fixation versus double divergent pins. *J Bone Joint Surg* 1988;70B:199–201.

30. Christie J, Robinson CM, Singer B, Ray DC. Medullary lavage reduces embolic phenomena and cardiopulmonary changes durung cemented hemiarthroplasty. *J Bone Joint Surg Br* 1995;77(3):456–459.

31. Cleveland M, Bosworth DM, Thompson FR. Intertrochanteric fractures of the femur. *J Bone Joint Surg* 1947;29:1049–1067.

32. Cleveland M, Bosworth DM, Thompson FR. Management of the trochanteric fracture of the femur. *JAMA* 1948;137:1186–1190.

33. Coates RL, Armour P. Treatment of subcapital femoral fractures by primary total hip replacement. *Injury* 1980;11:132–135.

34. Cobb AG, Gibson PH. Screw fixation of subcapital fractures of the femur: a better method of treatment. *Injury* 1986;17:259–264.

35. Colhoun EN, Johnson SR, Fairclough JA. Bone scanning for hip fracture in patients with osteoarthritis; brief report. *J Bone Joint Surg* 1988;70B:848.

36. Collis DK. Cemented total hip replacement in patients who are less than fifty years old. *J Bone Joint Surg Am* 1984;66A:353–359.

37. Coughlin L, Templeton J. Hip fractures in patients with Parkinson's disease. *Clin Orthop* 1980;148:192–195.

38. Cuckler JM, Tamarapalli JR. An algorithm for the management of femoral neck fractures. *Orthopaedics* 1994;17(9):789–792.

39. D'Arcy J, Devas M. Treatment of fractures of the femoral neck by replacement with the Thompson prosthesis. *J Bone Joint Surg* 1976; 58B(3):279–286.

40. Dahl D. Mortality and life expectancy after hip fractures. *Acta Orthop Scand* 1980;51:163–170.

41. Dalldorf PG, Banas MP, Hicks DG, Pellegrini VD Jr. Rate of degeneration of human acetabular cartilage after hemiarthroplasty. *J Bone Joint Surg* 1995;77A(6):877–882.

42. Davy DT, Kotzar GM, Brown RH, Heiple KG, Goldberg VM, Heiple KG Jr, Berilla J, Burstein AH. Telemetric force measurements across the hip after total arthroplasty. *J Bone Joint Surg* 1988;70A:45–50.

43. Delamarter R, Moreland JR. Treatment of acute femoral neck fractures with total hip arthroplasty. *Clin Orthop* 1987;218:68–74.

44. Devas M, Hinves B. Prevention of acetabular erosion after hemiarthroplasty for fractured neck of femur. *J Bone Joint Surg* 1983; 65B(5):548–551.

45. Dias JJ, Robbins JA, Steingold RF, Donaldson LJ. Subcapital vs intertrochanteric fracture of the neck of the femur: are there two distinct subbpopulations? *J R Coll Surg Edinb* 1987;32:303–305.

46. Dorr LD, Glousman R, Hoy ALS, et al. Treatment of femoral neck fractures with total hip replacement versus cemented and non cemented hemiarthroplasty. *J Arthroplasty* 1986;1:21–28.

47. Dove J. Complete fractures of the femur in Paget's disease of bone. *J Bone Joint Surg* 1980;62B:12–17.

48. Drinker H, Murray WR. The Universal proximal femoral endoprosthesis. A short-term comparison with conventional hemiarthroplasty. *J Bone Joint Surg* 1979;61A:1167–1174.

49. Eiskjaer S, Ostgard SE. Risk factors influencing mortality after bipolar hemiarthroplasty in the treatment of fracture of the femoral neck. *Clin Orthop* 1991;270:295–300.

50. Eiskjaer S, Ostgard SE. Survivorship analysis of hemiarthroplasties. *Clin Orthop* 1993;286:206–211.

51. Ekelund A, Rydell N, Nilsson OS. Total hip arthroplasty in patients 80 years of age and older. *Clin Orthop* 1992;281:101–106.

52. Emery RJ, Broughton NS, Desai K, Bulstrode CJ, Thomas TL. Bipolar hemiarthroplasty for subcapital fracture of the femoral neck. A prospective randomised trial of cemented Thompson and uncemented Moore stems. *J Bone Joint Surg* 1991;73B:322–324.

53. Evans EM. The treatment of trochanteric fractures of the femur. *J Bone Joint Surg* 1949;31B:190–203.

54. Evans EM. Trochanteric fractures. *J Bone Joint Surg* 1951;33B: 192–204.

55. Eventor I, Moreno M, Geller E, Jardiman R, Salama R. Hip fractures in patients with Parkinson's syndrome. *J Trauma* 1983;23:98–101.

56. Finsen V, Benum P. Changing incidence of hip fractures in rural and urban areas of central Norway. *Clin Orthop* 1987;218:104–110.

57. Follaci FM, Charnley J. A comparison of the results of femoral head prosthesis with and without cement. *Clin Orthop* 1969;62:156–161.

58. Frankel VH, Burstein AH, Lygre L, Brown RH. The telltale nail. In: Proceedings of The American Academy of Orthopaedic Surgeons. *J Bone Joint Surg* 1971;53A:1232.

59. Franzen H, Nilsson LT, Stromqvist B, Johnsson R, Herrlin K. Secondary total hip replacement after fractures of the femoral neck. *J Bone Joint Surg* 1990;72B:784–787.

60. Gallagher JC, Melton LJ, Riggs BL, Bergtrath E. Epidemiology of fractures of the proximal femur in Rochester, Minnesota. *Clin Orthop*

61. Garden RS. Malreduction and avascular necrosis in subcapital fractures of the femur. *J Bone Joint Surg* 1971;53B:183–197.

62. Garden RS. Low-angle fixation in fractures of the femoral neck. *J Bone Joint Surg Br* 1961;43B:647–663.

63. Garden RS. Reduction and fixation of subcapital fractures of the femur. *Orthop Clin North Am* 1974;5:683–712.

64. Garroway RY, Ordway CB, Kleiman RS. Endoprosthetic replacement of the femoral head. A retrospective study comparing cement fixation with press fit fixation. *Contemp Orthop* 1984;9:41–45.

65. Gebhard JS, Amstutz HC, Zinar DM, Dorey FJ. A comparison of total hip arthroplasty and hemiarthroplasty for treatment of acute fracture of the femoral neck. *Clin Orthop* 1992;282:123–131.

66. Gerber C, Strehle J, Ganz R. The treatment of fractures of the femoral neck. *Clin Orthop* 1993;292:77–86.

67. Giliberty RP. A new concept of a bipolar endoprosthesis. *Orthop Rev* 1974;3:40–45.

68. Giliberty RP. Hemiarthroplasty of the hip using a low-friction bipolar endoprosthesis. *Clin Orthop* 1983;175:86–92.

69. Gill DR, Wilson PD, Cheung BY. Southland Hospital's experience with the Austin Moore hemiarthroplasty. *N Z Med J* 1995;108(9):173–174.

70. Gingras MB, Clarke John, Evarts CMcC. Prosthetic replacement in femoral neck fractures. *Clin Orthop* 1980;152:147–157.

71. Goldhill VB, Lyden JP, Cornell CN, Bochner RM. Bipolar hemiarthroplasty for fracture of the femoral neck. *J Orthop Trauma* 1991; 5(3):318–324.

72. Green S, Moore T, Proano F. Bipolar prosthetic replacement of unstable intertrochanteric hip fractures in the elderly. *Clin Orthop* 1986; 224:169–177.

73. Greenough CG, Jones JR. Primary total hip replacement for displaced subcapital fracture of the femur. *J Bone Joint Surg* 1988;70B:639–643.

74. Gregory RJ, Wood DJ, Stevens J. Treatment of displaced subcapital femoral fractures with total hip replacement. *Injury* 1992;23(3): 168–170.

75. Grossling HR, Hardy JH. Fracture of the femoral neck: a comparative study of methods of treatment in 400 consecutive cases. *J Trauma* 1969;9:423–429.

76. Grundy M. Fractures of the femur in Paget's disease of bone. *J Bone Joint Surg* 1970;452B:252–263.

77. Haentjens P, Casteleyn PP, De Boeck H, Handelberg F, Opdecam P. Treatment of unstable intertrochanteric and subtrochanteric fractures in elderly patients. Primary biopolar arthroplasty compared with internal fixation. *J Bone Joint Surg* 1989;71:1214–1225.

78. Haentjens P, Casteleyn PP, Opdecam P. Primary bipolar arthroplasty or total hip arthroplasty for the treatment of unstable intertrochanteric and subtrochanteric fractures in elderly patients. *Acta Orthop Belg* 1994;60(suppl 1):124–128.

79. Haentjens P, Casteleyn PP, Opdecam P. Hip arthroplasty for failed internal fixation of intertrochanteric and subtrochanteric fractures in the elderly patient. *Arch Orthop Trauma Surg* 1994;113:222–227.

80. Hammer AJ. Intertrochanteric and femoral neck fractures in patients with Parkinsonism. *South Afr Med J* 1991;79(4):200–202.

81. Harris WH. Traumatic arthritis of the hip after dislocation and acetabular fractures: treatment by mold arthroplasty. An end result study using a new method of result evaluation. *J Bone Joint Surg Am* 1969; 51A:737–755.

82. Harris WH, Rushfeldt PD, Carlson CE, Scholler J-M, Mann RW. Pressure distribution in the hip and selection of hemiarthroplasty. In: *The hip: proceedings of the third open scientific meeting of The Hip Society*. St. Louis, MO: CV Mosby, 1975;93–98.

83. Harrlngton KD. The use of methylmethacrylate as an adjunct in the internal fixation of unstable comminuted intertrochanteric fractures in osteoporotic patients. *J Bone Joint Surg* 1975;57A:744–750.

84. Harwin SF, Stern RE, Kulick RG. Primary Bateman-Leinbach bipolar prosthetic replacement of the hip in the treatment of unstable intertrochanteric fractures in the elderly. *Orthopedics* 1990;13: 1131–1136.

85. Hedlund R, Lindgren U, Ahlbom A. Age and sex specific incidence of femoral neck and trochanteric fractures. *Clin Orthop* 1987;222: 132–139.

86. Hedlund R, Lindgren U. Trauma type, age and gender as determinants of hip fractures. *J Orthop Res* 1987;5:242–246.

87. Hedstrom SA, Lidgren L, Sernbo I, Torholm C, Onnerfalt R. Cefuroxime prophylaxis in trochanteric hip fracture operations. *Acta Orthop Scand* 1987;58:361–364.

88. Higgins RW, Hughes JL. Preliminary results of eighty-one hip replacements with the Bateman endoprosthesis. *Orthop Trans* 1983;7:411–412.

89. Hodge WA, Carlson KL, Fijan RS, Burgess RG, Riley PO, Harris WH, Mann RW. Contact pressures from an instrumented hip endoprosthesis. *J Bone Joint Surg* 1989;71A(9):1378–1386.

90. Holmberg S. Life expectancy after total hip arthroplasty. *J Arthroplasty* 1992;7(2):183–186.

91. Holt EM, Evans RA, Hindley CJ, Metcalfe JW. 1000 femoral neck fractures: the effect of pre-injury mobility and surgical experience and outcome. *Injury* 1994;25(2):91–95.

92. Hui AC, Anderson GH, Choudhry R, Boyle J, Gregg PJ. Internal fixation or hemiarthroplasty for undisplaced fractures of the femoral neck in octagenarians. *J Bone Joint Surg Br* 1994;76(6):891–894.

93. Hunter GA. Displaced fractures of the femoral neck—Internal fixation or hemiarthroplasty? *Instr Course Lect* 1980;29:1–4.

94. Hunter GA. Should we abandon primary prosthetic replacement for fresh displaced fractures of the neck of the femur? *Clin Orthop* 1980;152:158–161.

95. Hunter GA. The rationale for internal fixation and against hemiarthroplasty. In: *The hip: proceedings of the eleventh open scientific meeting of The Hip Society*. St. Louis, MO: CV Mosby, 1983;34–41.

96. Hunter GA. The results of operative treatment of trochanteric fractures of the femur. *Injury* 1974–1975;6:202–205.

97. Izumi H, Torisu T, Itonaga I, Masumi S. Joint motion of bipolar femoral prostheses. *J Arthroplasty* 1995;10(2):237–243.

98. Jalovaara P, Virkkunen H. Quality of life after primary hemiarthroplasty for femoral neck fracture. Six year follow-up of 185 patients. *Acta Orthop Scand* 1991;62(3):208–217.

99. James SE, Gallannaugh SC. Bi-articular hemiarthroplasty of the hip: a 7-year follow-up. *Injury* 1991;22(5):391–393.

100. Johnson JTH, Crothers O. Nailing versus prosthesis for femoral-neck fractures. A critical review of long-term results in two hundred and thirty-nine consecutive private patients. *J Bone Joint Surg* 1975;57A: 686–692.

101. Jonsson B, Johnell O, Redlund-Johnell I, Sernbo I. Function 10 years after hip fracture. 74 patients after internal fixation. *Acta Orthop Scand* 1993;64(6):645–646.

102. Julkunen H. Medical aspects in the treatment of femoral neck fractures with rheumatoid arthritis. *Scand J Rheumatol* 1974;3:13.

103. Juttman JW, Quist J, Kroesen JH. Which approach for femoral head replacement? *Neth J Surg* 1991;43(3):258–260.

104. Kaufer H, Matthews LS, Sonstegard D. Stable fixation of intertrochanteric fractures. *J Bone Joint Surg* 1974;56A:899–907.

105. Kenzora JE, McCarthy RE, Lowell JD, Sledge CB. Hip fracture mortality. *Clin Orthop* 1984;186:45–56.

106. Kim YH, Oh JH, Koh YG. Salvage of neglected unstable intertrochanteric fractures with cementless porous-coated hemiarthroplasty. *Clin Orthop* 1992;277:182–187.

107. Knight WM, DeLee JC. Nonunion of intertrochanteric fractures of the hip: a case study and review. *Orthop Trans* 1982;16:438.

108. Knowelden J, Buhr AJ, Dunbar O. Incidence of fractures in persons over 35 years of age. *Br J Prev Soc Med* 1964;18:130.

109. Kofoed H, Kofod J. Moore prosthesis in the treatment of fresh femoral neck fractures. *Injury* 1982;14:531–540.

110. Koval KJ, Zuckerman JD. Hip fractures. I. Overview and evaluation and treatment of FNFs. *J Am Assoc Orthop Surg* 1994;2:141–149.

111. Krein SW, Chao EYS. Biomechanics of bipolar hip endoprostheses. *J Orthop Res* 1984;2:356–368.

112. Kwok DC, Cruess RL. A retrospective study of Moore and Thompson hemiarthroplasty: a review of 599 surgical cases and an analysis of the technical complications. *Clin Orthop* 1982;169:179–185.

113. Kyle RF, Gustilo RB, Premer RF. Analysis of 622 intertrochanteric hip fractures: a retrospective study. *J Bone Joint Surg* 1979;61A:216–221.

114. Lake M. Studies of Paget's disease (osteitis deformans), *J Bone Joint Surg* 1951;32B:323–335.

115. Langan Peter. The Giliberty bipolar prosthesis. A clinical and radiographical review. *Clin Orthop* 1979;141:169–175.

116. Lennox IA, McLaughlan J. Comparing the mortality and morbidity of cemented and uncemented hemiarthroplasties. *Injury* 1993;24(3): 185–186.

117. Lestrange NR. The Bateman UPF prosthesis. A 48-month experience. *Orthopedics* 1979;2:373–377.

118. Levine S, Makin M, Menszel J, Robin G, Naor E, Steinberg R. Incidence of fractures of the proximal end of the femur in Jerusalem. *J Bone Joint Surg* 1970;52A:1193–1202.

119. Linde F, Anderson E, Hvass I, Madsen F, Pallesen R. Avascular femoral head necrosis following fracture fixation. *Injury* 1986;17: 159–163.

120. Lindsey RW, Cahill D. Late disassembly of a bipolar prosthesis without cup dislocation. *Contemp Orthop* 1984;9:29–37.

121. Lizaur-Utrilla A, Orts AP, Del Campo FS, Barrio JA, Carbonell PG. Epidemiology of trochanteric fractures of the femur in Alicante, Spain 1974-1982. *Clin Orthop* 1987;218:24–31.

122. Lo WH, Chen WM, Huang CK, Chen TH, Chiu FY, Chen CM. Bateman bipolar hemiarthroplasty for displaced intracapsular femoral neck fractures: uncemented vs cemented. *Clin Orthop* 1994;302:75–82.

123. Long JW, Knight W. Bateman UPF prosthesis in fractures of the femoral neck. *Clin Orthop* 1980;152:198–201.

124. Lu-Yao GL, Keller RB, Littenberg B, Wennberg JE. Outcomes after displaced fractures of the femoral neck. A meta-analysis of 106 published reports. *J Bone Joint Surg* 1994;76A(1):15–25.

125. Luthje P. Incidence of hip fracture in Finland. *Acta Orthop Scand* 1985;56:223–225.

126. Lyritis GP, Johnell O. Orthopaedic management of hip fracture. *Bone* 1993;14(suppl 1):S11–7.

127. Makin M. Osteoporosis and proximal femoral fractures in the female elderly of Jerusalem. *Clin Orthop* 1987;218:19–23.

128. Malhotra R, Arya R, Bhan S. Bipolar hemiarthroplasty in femoral neck fractures. *Arch Orthop Trauma Surg* 1995;114(2):79–82.

129. Manniger J, Kazar G, Fekete G, Nagy E, Zolczer L, Frenyo S. Avoidance of avascular necrosis of the femoral head following fractures of the femoral neck by early reduction and internal fixation. *Injury* 1985;16:437–448.

130. Marcus RE, Heintz JJ, Pattee GA. Don't throw away the Austin Moore. *J Arthroplasty* 1992;7(1):31–36.

131. Mariani EM, Rand JA. Nonunion of intertrochanteric fractures of the femur following open reduction and internal fixation. *Clin Orthop* 1987;218:81–89.

132. Maxwell HA, Turner PG. Dislocation of the Austin Moore hemiarthroplasty: is closed manipulation justified? *J R Coll Surg Edin*b 1994;39(6):370–371.

133. Mehlhoff T, Landon GC, Tullos HS. Total hip arthroplasty following failed internal fixation of hip fractures. *Clin Orthop* 1991;269:32–37.

134. Melton LJ, llstrup DM, Riggs BL, Beckenbaugh RD. Fifty year trend in hip fracture incidence. *Clin Orthop* 1982;162:144–149.

135. Meyn MA, Hopson C, Jayasankar S. Fractures of hip in the institutionalized psychotic patient. *Clin Orthop* 1977;122:128–134.

136. Milgram JW. Orthopaedic management of Paget's disease of bone. *Clin Orthop* 1977;127:63–69.

137. Miller K, Atzenhofer K, Gerber G, Reichel M. Risk prediction in operatively treated fractures of the hip. *Clin Orthop* 1993;293:148–152.

138. Miller CW. Survival and ambulation following hip fracture. *J Bone Joint Surg* 1978;60A:930–934.

139. Moore AT. Metal hip joint. A new self-locking vitallium prosthesis. *South Med J* 1952;45:1015–1019.

140. Morris HD. Trochanteric fractures. *South Med J* 1941;34:571–578.

141. Muhr C, Tscherne H, Thomas R. Comminuted trochanteric femoral fractures in geriatric patients: the results of 231 cases treated with internal fixation and acrylic cement. *Clin Orthop* 1979;138:41–44.

142. Mulholland RC, Gunn DR. Sliding screw plate fixation of intertrochanteric femoral fractures. *J Trauma* 1972;12:581–591.

143. Nather A, Seow CS, Iau P, Chan A. Morbidity and mortality for elderly patients with fractured neck of femur treated by hemiarthroplasty. *Injury* 1995;26(3):187–190.

144. Nicholas JA, Killoran P. Fracture of the femur in patients with Paget's disease. *J Bone Joint Surg* 1965;47A:450–461.

145. Nilsson LT, Franzen H, Stromqvist B, Wiklund I. Function of the hip after femoral neck fractures treated by fixation or secondary total hip replacement. *Int Orthop* 1991;15(4):315–318.

146. Nilsson LT, Jalovaara P, Franzén H, Niinimäki T, Strömqvist B. Function after primary hemiarthroplasty and secondary total hip arthroplasty in femoral neck fracture. *J Arthroplasty* 1994;4:369–374.

147. Norden CW. A critical review of antibiotic prophylaxis in orthopedic surgery. *Rev Infect Dis* 1983;5:928–932.

148. Nordin BEC, Polley KJ. Metabolic consequences of the menopause: a cross-sectional longitudinal, and intervention study on 557 normal postmenopausal women. *Calcif Tissue Int* 1987;41(suppl 1).

149. Norton PL. Intertrochanteric fractures. *Clin Orthop* 1969;66:77–81.

150. Overgaard S, Jensen TT, Bonde G, Mossing NB. The uncemented bipolar hemiarthroplasty for displaced femoral neck fractures. Six-year follow-up of 171 cases. *Acta Orthop Scand* 1991;62(2):115–120.

151. Papandrea RF, Froimson MI. Total hip arthroplasty after acute displaced femoral neck fractures. *Am J Orthop* 1996;25(2):85–88.

152. Parker MJ. Internal fixation or arthroplasty for displaced subcapital fractures in the elderly? *Injury* 1992;23(8):521–524.

153. Patterson BM, Salvati EA, Huo MH. Total hip arthroplasty for complications of intertrochanteric fracture. A technical note. *J Bone Joint Surg* 1990;72A(5):776–777.

154. Phillips TW. Thompson hemiarthroplasty and acetabular erosion. *J Bone Joint Surg* 1989;71A(6):913–917.

155. Phillips TW. The Bateman bipolar femoral head replacement. A fluoroscopic study of movement over a four-year period. *J Bone Joint Surg* 1987;69B(5):761–764.

156. Pritchett JW, Bortel DT. Parkinson's disease and femoral neck fractures treated by hemiarthroplasty. *Clin Orthop* 1992;279:310–311.

157. Protzman RR, Burkhalter WE. Femoral-neck fractures in young adults. *J Bone Joint Surg* 1976;58A:689–695.

158. Pun WK, Ip FK, So YC, Chow SP. Treatment of displaced subcapital

159. Riska EB. Trochanteric fractures of the femur. *Acta Orthop Scand* 1971;42:268–280.

160. Robinson CM, Saran D, Annan IH. Intracapsular hip fractures. Results of management adopting a treatment protocol. *Clin Orthop* 1994;302:83–91.

161. Rosenfeld RT, Schwartz DR, Alter AH. Prosthetic replacement for trochanteric fractures of the femur. *J Bone Joint Surg* 1973;55A:420.

162. Rydell NW. Forces acting on the femoral head-prosthesis. *Acta Orthop Scand* 1966;889(suppl).

163. Saito N, Miyasaka T, Toriumi H. Radiographic factors predicting nonunion of displaced intracapsular femoral neck fractures. *Arch Orthop Trauma Surg* 1995;114(4):183–187.

164. Salvati EA, Wilson PD Jr. Long-term results of femoral head replacement. *J Bone Joint Surg* 1973;55A:516–524.

165. Salvati EA, Artz T, Aglietti P, Asnis SE. Endoprostheses in the treatment of femoral neck fractures. *Orthop Clin North Am* 1974;5:757–777.

166. Sarmiento A, Williams EM. The unstable intertrochanteric fracture: treatment with a valgus osteotomy and I-beam nail-plate. *J Bone Joint Surg* 1970;52A:1309–1318.

167. Sikorski JM, Barrington R. Internal fixation versus hemiarthroplasty for the displaced subcapital fracture of the femur. A prospective randomized study. *J Bone Joint Surg* 1981;63B(3):357–361.

168. Sim FH, Stauffer RN. Management of hip fractures by total hip arthroplasty. *Clin Orthop* 1980;152:292–297.

169. Skinner P, Riley D, Ellery J, et al. Displaced subcapital fractures of the femur: a prospective randomized comparison of internal fixation, hemiarthroplasty and total hip replacement. *Injury* 1989;20:291–293.

170. Skinner PW, Powles D. Compression screw fixation for displaced subcapital fracture of the femur: success or failure? *J Bone Joint Surg Br* 1986;68B:78–82.

171. Snorrason F, Karrholm J, Holmgren C. Fixation of cemented acetabular prostheses. The influence of preoperative diagnosis. *J Arthroplasty* 1993;8(1):83–90.

172. Soreide O, Skjaerven R, Alho A. The risk of acetabular protrusion after prosthetic replacement of the femoral head. *Acta Orthop Scand* 1982;53:791–794.

173. Soreide O, Lillestol J, Alho A, Hvidsten K. Acetabular protrusion following endoprosthetic hip surgery. A multifactorial study. *Acta Orthop Scand* 1980;51:943–948.

174. Soto-Hall R. Treatment of transcervical fractures complicated by certain common neurological conditions, *Instr Course Lect* 1960;17:117–120.

175. Staeheli JW, Frassica FJ, Sim FH. Prosthetic replacement of the femoral head for fracture of the femoral neck in patients who have Parkinson disease. *J Bone Joint Surg* 1988;70A:565–568.

176. Stappaerts KH, Broos PL. Internal fixation of femoral neck fractures: a follow-up study of 118 cases. *Acta Chir Belg* 1987;87:247–251.

177. Stauffer RN, Sim FH. Total hip arthroplasty in Paget's disease of the hip. *J Bone Joint Surg* 1976;58A:476–478.

178. Stern MB, Angerman A. Comminuted intertrochanteric fractures treated with a Leinbach prosthesis. *Clin Orthop* 1987;218:75–80.

179. Stern MB, Goldstein TB. The use of the Leinbach prosthesis in intertrochanteric fracture of the hip. *Clin Orthop* 1977;128:325–331.

180. Stoffelen C, Haetjens P, Reynders P, Casteleyn PP, Broos P, Opdecam P. Hip arthroplasty for failed internal fixation of intertrochanteric and subtrochanteric fractures in the elderly patient. *Acta Orthop Belg* 1994;60(suppl 1):135–139.

181. Stover CN, Fish JB, Heap WR. Open reduction of trochanteric fracture. *NYS J Med* 1971;71:2173–2181.

182. Stromqvist B, Hansson LI, Nilsson LT, Thorngren KG. Hook-pin fixation in femoral neck fractures: a two-year follow-up study of 300 cases. *Clin Orthop* 1987;218:58–62.

183. Stromqvist B, Kelly I, Lidgren L. Treatment of hip fractures in rheumatoid arthritis. *Clin Orthop* 1988;228:75–78.

184. Stromqvist B, Nilsson LT, Thorngren KG. Femoral neck fracture fixation with hook-pins. 2-year results and learning curve in 626 prospective cases. *Acta Orthop Scand* 1992;63(3):282–287.

185. Swiontkowski MF, Winquist RA, Hansen ST Jr. Fractures of the femoral neck in patients between the ages of twelve and forty nine years. *J Bone Joint Surg* 1984;66A:837–846.

186. Taine WH, Armour PC. Primary total hip replacement for displaced

subcapital fractures of the femur. *J Bone Joint Surg Br* 1985;67B: 214–217.

187. Tengve B, Kjellander J. Antibiotic prophylaxis in operations on trochanteric femoral fractures. *J Bone Joint Surg* 1978;60A:97–99.

188. Testa NN, Mazur K. Heterotopic ossification after direct lateral approach and transtrochanteric approach to the hip. *Orthop Rev* 1988;18:965–971.

189. Thornhill TS, Creasman C. Hip fractures in patients with renal failure. Presented at the *52nd meeting of the American Association of Orthopaedic Surgeons*, 1985, Jan 24.

190. Tooke SM, Favero KJ. Femoral neck fractures in skeletally mature patients, fifty years old or less. *J Bone Joint Surg* 1985;67A:1255–1260.

191. Tressler HA, Johnson EW. Cited in: Sledge CB, ed. *The hip. Proceedings of the fifth open scientific meeting of the Hip Society*. St. Louis, MO: CV Mosby, 1977; 124.

192. Van Demark RE Jr, Cabanela ME, Henderson ED. The Bateman endoprosthesis. 104 arthroplasties. *Orthop Trans* 1980;4:356–357.

193. Verberne GHM. A femoral head prosthesis with a built-in joint. A radiological study of the movements of the two components. *J Bone Joint Surg* 1983;65B(5):544–547.

194. Watson-Jones R. *Fractures and joint injuries*, 4th ed, Baltimore: Williams & Wilkins, 1955.

195. Welch RB. The rationale for primary hemiarthroplasty in the treatment of fractures of the femoral neck in elderly patients. *Hip* 1983;42–50.

196. West WF, Mann RA. Evaluation of the Bateman self-articulating femoral prosthesis. *Orthop Trans* 1979;3:17.

197. White BL, Fisher WD, Laurin CA. Rate of mortality for elderly patients after fracture of the hip in the 1980s. *J Bone Joint Surg* 1987;69A:1335 –1340.

198. Whittaker RP, Abeshaus MM, Scholl HW, Chung SMK. Fifteen years' experience with metallic endo-prosthetic replacement of the femoral head for femoral neck fractures. *J Trauma* 1972;12: 799–806.

199. Wilson H, Rubin BD, Helbig FEJ, Fielding JW, Unis GL. Treatment of intertrochanteric fractures with Jewett nail: experience with 1,015 cases. *Clin Orthop* 1980;148:186–191.

200. Wood MR. Femoral head replacement following fracture: an analysis of the surgical approach. *Injury* 1979-80;11:317–320.

201. Wright LT. Oblique subcervical (reverse intertrochanteric) fractures of the femur. *J Bone Joint Surg* 1947;29:707–710.

202. Yamagata M, Chao EY, Ilstrup DM, et al. Fixed-head and bipolar hip endoprostheses: a retrospective clinical and roentgenographic study. *J Arthroplasty* 1987;2:327–341.

203. Zindrick MR, Daley RJ, Hollyfield RL, et al. Femoral neck fractures in the geriatric population: the influence of perioperative health upon the selection of surgical treatment. *J Am Geriatr Soc* 1985;33: 104–108.

204. Zuckerman JD. The internal fixation of intracapsular hip fractures: a review of the first hundred years. *Orthop Rev* 1982;11:85–95.

205. Zuckerman JD. Trauma hip in orthopaedic knowledge update III. *Am Assoc Orthop Surg* Jan 1990.

206. Zuckerman JD, ed. *Orthopaedic injuries in the elderly. Hip fractures*. Urban & Schwarzenberg, 42–92.

The Adult Hip, edited by J. J. Callaghan,
A. G. Rosenberg, and H. E. Rubash.
Lippincott–Raven Publishers, Philadelphia © 1998.

CHAPTER 77

Management of Periprosthetic Fractures

Brad L. Penenberg

Femoral fracture in the presence of a total hip arthroplasty (THA) component can be one of the most challenging problems in orthopedic surgery. Inadequate treatment can be disastrous and often requires the use of high-risk salvage procedures in an attempt to restore even limited locomotion in the affected limb. Fortunately, appropriate treatment can permit the maintenance of satisfactory quality of life.

Various fracture classifications have been offered over the years. Perhaps the simplest and best recognized is that of Bethea et al. (1), who separated these fractures into types A, B, and C based on location and degree of comminution. Johanssen et al. (8), like Bethea et al., considered the significance of fracture location, particularly as it related to the likelihood of prosthesis loosening and fracture healing. Kelley (9) emphasized the importance of fracture pattern, the region involved, and prosthesis fixation. Each system addressed periprosthetic fracture within the context of the state of the art of THA at the time.

Kelley's (9) classification of periprosthetic femur fractures, based on timing (intraoperative versus postoperative), location, degree of severity, and implant stability, is very useful. Fracture management, however, will be dis-

cussed not only with regard to the use of standard techniques, but also in the context of expanding clinical experience with newer techniques. Over the last few years, for example, we have acquired increased confidence in the use of different types of uncemented long-stem femoral components for use in fractures associated with THA components (2). In addition, we have begun to understand the applications and the limitations of the use of structural femoral allograft bone for segmental reconstruction and as onlay fixation plates (5,7,10–12,14–16).

The designation of fractures as simple or complex is given based on the likelihood of implant stability. In the case of simple periprosthetic femur fractures, implant fixation is less likely to be compromised and management usually requires only fracture fixation. On the other hand, complex fractures, because of more extensive bone involvement or the presence of moderate comminution, often require component revision.

Successful management depends first on accurate determination of the extent of the fracture; second, on its influence on implant stability; and third, on understanding the nature and applicability of available treatment options.

In general, the preferred method of treatment is surgical unless the patient is a poor surgical risk. The general approach to conservative management typically involves

B. L. Penenberg: Los Angeles, California 90048.

4 to 6 weeks of skeletal traction, followed by the use of a cast brace. Non-operative management, although associated with a high rate of union (13), exposes the patient to the usual risks of recumbency as well as the greater likelihood of mal-union (1)

INTRAOPERATIVE METAPHYSEAL FRACTURES

Simple Metaphyseal Fractures

Simple metaphyseal fractures (Fig. 1),which occur most commonly upon insertion of uncemented femoral components, are occasionally missed intraoperatively and are identified only on postoperative films by prosthesis subsidence associated with a mildly displaced metaphyseal fragment. You will recognize these fractures 100% of the time if you (a) keep the entire circumference of the calcar in view during prosthesis insertion (this can be accomplished by removing any obstructing soft tissue, using a femoral neck retractor/elevator, and continually cleaning and drying the surface of the calcar during prosthesis insertion) and (b) note whether the actual implant

seats deeper than the trial, or if there is suddenly a less firm end point than was noted with the trial. It has been the author's experience that this is indicative of fracture. Although all periprosthetic fractures cannot be avoided, being aware of a fracture as soon as it occurs can minimize displacement, permit the use of minimal fixation, and result in minimal disruption of the usual intraoperative and postoperative course. For proximally filling femoral components with a higher propensity for fracture, a prophylactic cerclage wire applied before broaching and implantation of the component may prevent such fractures.

The least problematic type of intraoperative metaphyseal fracture occurs with the opening of a seam (1 mm or less) in the metaphysis at, or just prior to, final seating of the implant. To identify the extent of the fracture, the soft tissue is cleared from the calcar down along the metaphysis until the lowermost edge of the fracture is seen. If there is no separation of the fracture, and approximately 1 cm of calcar height remains, a cerclage wire is placed around the calcar and usual postoperative management is carried out (Fig. 2). Wire(s) may need to be placed on or below the lesser trochanter if only minimal calcar is present. A large-diameter Luque wire (double stranded)

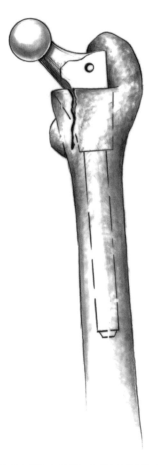

FIG. 1. Intraoperative metaphyseal fracture—simple.

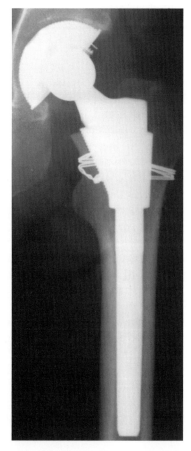

FIG. 2. Minimally displaced calcar fracture was treated with two large-diameter, double-stranded Luque wires.

works well when placed above and below the lesser trochanter.

If the seam has opened (i.e., the fracture has separated more than 1 mm), consideration should be given to backing out the prosthesis and anatomically reducing the fracture. Cerclage wire(s) may then be applied and the prosthesis replaced. If there is any question regarding implant or fracture stability, additional wire fixation may be required. In the case of a modular prosthesis, the implant size may be increased (if bone stock allows) in either length or diameter, for greater distal press-fit. Conversion to a cemented prosthesis should be considered if the above techniques are not suitable. If the fracture line extends to the lesser trochanter or below, wire placement must be adjusted accordingly. In general, the most distal wire should come to within 1 cm of the distal extent of a relatively stable metaphyseal fracture.

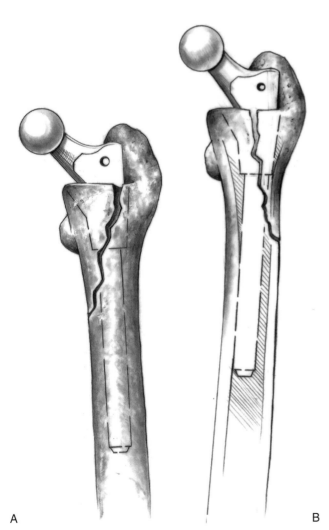

A   B

FIG. 3. A: Distal extent of the fracture exits medial femoral cortex at about the level of the mid stem. **B:** Distal extent of the fracture exits the lateral femoral cortex in the region of the mid stem. Implant stability is compromised.

Complex Metaphyseal Fractures

A metaphyseal split fracture (Fig. 3) with near complete separation of the metaphyseal fragments presents a more difficult problem. This type of fracture is more likely to occur in revision surgery where the bone is compromised. In particular, this fracture pattern must be kept in mind during placement of modular femoral components such as the S-ROM (Joint Medical Corporation, Stamford, CT). The technique of insertion permits separate placement of the metaphyseal module and the long-stem femoral implant. If the axes of both components do not match, significant torsional stresses will be delivered to the femoral metaphysis and this fracture pattern may occur.

This type of split fracture can also be seen during insertion of curved long-stem components, as the femoral shaft begins to make the turn in the canal. It is especially likely if proximal femoral remodeling into varus has occurred. If, during preoperative templating, the proximal metaphyseal varus bow is noted to be significant, consideration should be given to corrective osteotomy. Cerclage wiring with multiple wires alone, or with the addition of wire mesh, is an option in cases where the femoral prosthesis retains significant diaphyseal stability.

If implant stability is questionable, the component is removed and the fracture is fixed as above, or with the addition of an onlay cortical allograft. Further metaphyseal reaming (typically deep to the greater trochanter) may be required. Diaphyseal stabilization of the prosthesis is then achieved by the placement of a long-stem, press-fit, uncemented implant (preferably with enhanced rotational stability) or a cemented device. Postoperative weight bearing will probably be restricted in most cases if an uncemented implant is used. Prophylactic wiring before broaching and implant insertion may prevent these fractures, particularly in cases where proximal filling prostheses are utilized.

Greater Trochanteric Fractures

Care must be taken to observe possible unstable fractures of the greater trochanter. This is especially true during revision surgery and in primary THA when severe osteoporosis is present. It is unusual to cause a displaced intraoperative fracture of the greater trochanter. However, it is, unfortunately, not unusual to note a gradually migrating greater trochanteric fragment during the postoperative period, although at the time of surgery only a minor crack was thought to have been present. This may not result in persistent pain, but the resultant limp may be quite severe and will likely require the indefinite use of a support. Therefore, if trochanteric stability is in question, appropriate fixation should be utilized. If in doubt, err on the side of fixation. Wires or a cable-grip-type system may be utilized. However, the bulkier the system, the greater the likelihood of a bothersome trochanteric bursitis, and the need for removal of the device.

INTRAOPERATIVE DIA-METAPHYSEAL FRACTURES

Simple Fractures

This fracture pattern (Fig. 4) may occur during the course of uncemented THA while attempting to maximize the degree of interference fit in the presence of dense cortical bone, or during the course of revision or primary surgery using a straight or bowed long-stem implant. In the case of a straight stem (longer than 180 cm), fracture may occur as the stem engages the bow of the femur. A more distal, diaphyseal fracture is likely to occur if preparation for a bowed stem is inadequate (e.g. under-reaming).

Hoop stresses and complex torsional stresses extend further distally than in the simple intraoperative metaphyseal fracture. There is typically some degree of displacement. It is essential to differentiate this from the simple, short metaphyseal fracture. If this distinction is

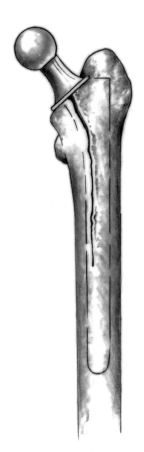

FIG. 4. Intraoperative dia-metaphyseal fracture, simple. This fracture represents a more extensive split than the isolated metaphyseal fracture. It can be stabilized with minimal internal fixation.

not made, fixation may be inadequate. Treatment begins by exposing the entire extent of the fracture. Wire or cable fixation is usually adequate unless bone density is compromised. If the bone is weak, an onlay cortical strut may be added to supplement fixation.

Complex Fractures

The bone may be predisposed to this extensive type of fracture by osteoporosis, osteolysis associated with a previous implant (Fig. 5A), or periprosthetic infection. This fracture is also the type seen in association with the removal of a well-fixed prosthesis (Fig. 6A), either cemented or uncemented. Component removal may be required because of infection, malposition, or, in the case of an uncemented prosthesis, pain thought to be secondary to modulus mismatch, or the relatively new category of impending pathologic fracture secondary to progressive osteolysis (see later). This type of fracture extends over a large area, it is typically displaced and severely comminuted, and implant fixation is clearly compromised. Appropriate management ranges from attempted fracture stabilization, to the use of a proximal femoral allograft using the host bone for onlay autograft.

A unique situation occurs in the presence of both an extensively comminuted dia-metaphyseal fracture and the patulous femoral canal (more than 22 mm in diameter). Rather than place a massive, long-stem femoral implant in the 58-year-old, 6-foot-4-inch-tall man in Figure 5, an intramedullary femoral allograft was used. The long diaphyseal segment was fashioned to achieve a press-fit into the host femur and a femoral component was cemented proximally. Comminuted proximal host bone was wired to the graft (see Fig. 5B,C). Although an excellent clinical result was present at the 7.5-year follow-up (6), the use of impaction grafting with cement should be considered today.

The severely comminuted, extensive dia-metaphyseal fracture is generally considered to be an indication for the use of a proximal femoral allograft/prosthesis composite replacement. Although fracture can be quite challenging in the presence of such severe comminution, there are occasions when an attempt at proximal reconstruction with host bone may be desirable. One approach that the author has found helpful involves the use of an intramedullary PMMA–antibiotic stent (see Fig. 6B). This stent not only assists in fracture stabilization and antibiotic delivery, but it also maintains a minimum canal diameter and a neutral canal axis. In this case, the diaphyseal diameter was minimally prepared to 13 mm using cylindrical reamers. Flexible reamers may also be utilized, but the femoral bow will persist.

The stent shown in Figure 6B was fashioned out of PMMA–tobramycin–vancomycin wrapped around a 9/64th-inch threaded Steinmann pin. The Steinmann pin serves two purposes. First, it allows the creation of a rel-

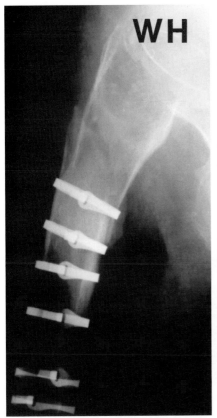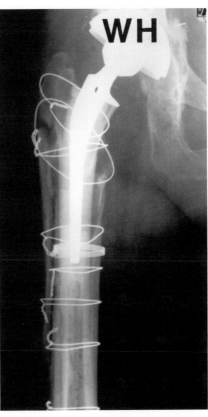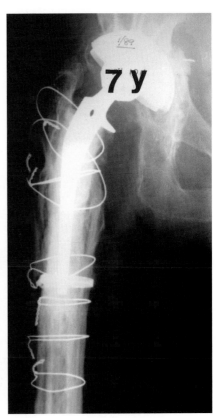

A,B   C

FIG. 5. A: Extensive intraoperative dia-metaphyseal fracture occurred during the course of removal of a loose femoral component associated with marked osteolysis. Multiple fracture lines extended from the upper metaphysis into the upper diaphysis. **B:** This patient's problem was compounded by the fact that he had a patulous medullary canal measuring approximately 22 mm in diameter. An intramedullary femoral allograft was fashioned to achieve a press-fit within the patient's diaphysis. Precoat femoral prosthesis was placed proximally. Fragments of upper dia-metaphyseal bone were wired onto the allograft. **C:** Remodeling is visible in this 7-year follow-up radiograph. The patient continues to function extremely well. He ambulates without support and experiences no pain in this hip. There is minimal intramedullary allograft bone resorption.

atively straight stent of constant diameter. Second, removal is facilitated by the ability to rethread the Steinmann pin and attach to it some type of gripping device (e.g., grip pliers, slap hammer through a Jacobs chuck). The device was initially molded by hand (much as a child molds modeling clay) and as it began to set, it was passed into the diaphysis for final molding. It was then press-fit into the medullary canal, leaving the proximal end proud, approximately to the level of the tip of the greater trochanter. The main fracture fragments were then reduced around the stent and held in place with wires. Defects in this case were packed with calcium sulfate tablets (ORTHOSET/WMT). Additional PMMA—antibiotic beads were placed in the acetabulum to aid in treating the periprosthetic infection.

At re-operation, approximately 7 weeks later, the stent was removed. Femoral continuity was reestablished and revision arthroplasty was carried out using the Ling technique (6). The new component and morselized allograft were placed entirely within the clearly viable, intact,

native femur. Onlay allograft struts were placed prophylactically (Fig. 6C,D).

INTRAOPERATIVE DIAPHYSEAL FRACTURES

Simple Fractures

These diaphyseal fractures may take different forms (Fig. 7). They are typically seen during placement of press-fit porous-coated femoral components. This may appear radiographically as a longitudinal split (Fig. 8), or as a more transversely oriented, short, oblique fracture (Fig. 9A) or more extensive cortical elevation, with or without a transverse fracture component (Fig. 10).

Unless you are performing this operation on a regular basis and have mastered the subtleties of bone preparation and component insertion, it is advisable to obtain anteroposterior (AP) and lateral intraoperative radiographs. It is clearly preferable to extend the incision,

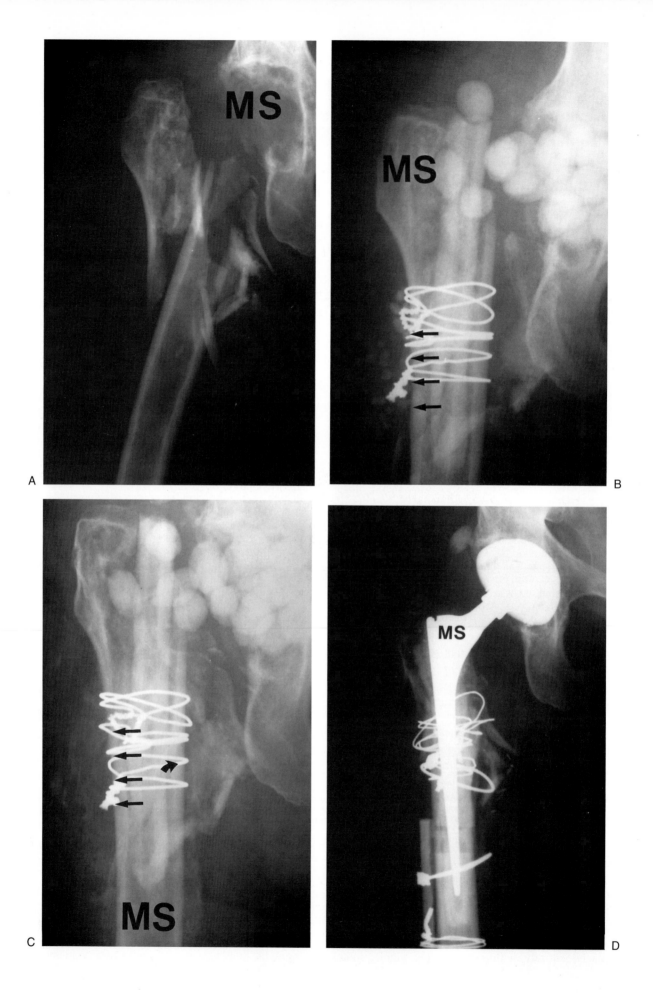

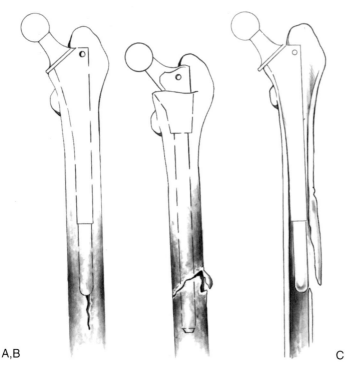

A,B   C

FIG. 7. A: Intraoperative diaphyseal fracture, simple. "Stable" longitudinal split. **B:** Short oblique simple diaphyseal fracture with comminution. **C:** Simple diaphyseal cortical fracture. Cortical "elevation" is noted.

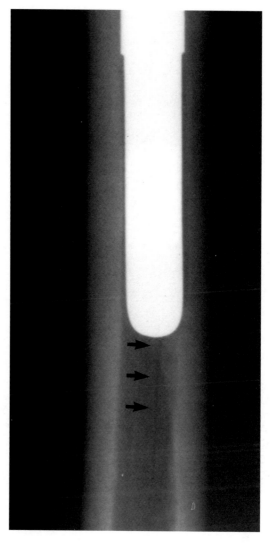

FIG. 8. Approximately 1½- to 2-inch longitudinal split is seen.

assess the nature and type of fracture, and treat appropriately, than to present the patient with the news of a fracture and the necessity of a return to the operating room in the immediate postoperative period.

If a small cortical split is identified, the most prudent treatment would be the placement of one or more cerclage wires to stabilize the fracture and prevent displacement or distal propagation. The degree of protection (e.g., 40 lb, weight of leg, or 50% of body weight) and duration (approximately 6 weeks) will vary depending on the surgeon's interpretation of relative fracture stability and the patient's ability to heal.

The potentially unstable transverse or oblique fracture and the more extensive "cortical elevation" type

FIG. 6. A: This 71-year-old patient suffered an extensively comminuted intraoperative dia-metaphyseal fracture during the course of removal of a Precoat femoral component that had become infected. **B:** One week after initial resection arthroplasty, the patient was treated with open reduction and internal fixation around an intramedullary PMMA-—antibiotic stent. Calcium sulfate pellets (ORTHOSET, Wright Medical, Memphis, TN) are visible adjacent to the lateral cortex. **C:** At 7 weeks after fracture stabilization, debridement, and placement of PMMA-—antibiotic, consolidation of fracture fragments is seen proximally and medially (*solid curved arrow*). In the region of the previously placed calcium sulfate pellets, we see amorphous calcific density. At the time of surgery, this proved to be a mass of new, woven bone. **D:** Final reconstruction is shown here with placement of CPT prosthesis in association with impacted intramedullary allograft [Ling technique (6)].

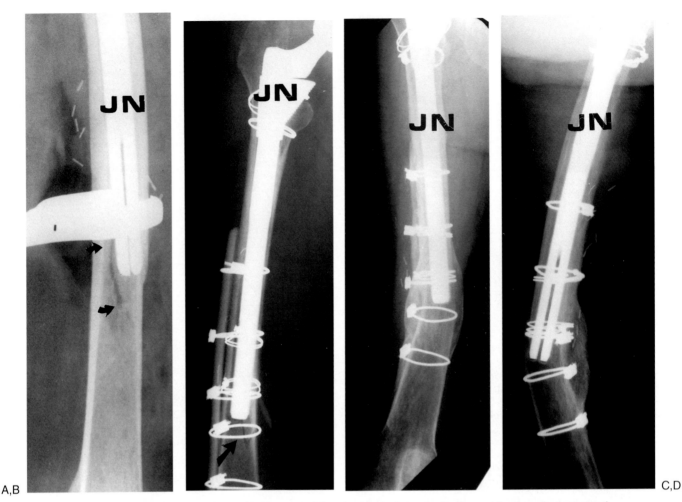

A,B

C,D

FIG. 9. A: This lateral radiograph shows an obliquely oriented simple diaphyseal fracture that occurred during placement of a long-stem uncemented implant. **B:** The fracture was identified at the time of surgery. Single allograft strut was placed along the lateral femoral cortex. **C:** AP radiograph, 3 years postoperative. AP fracture fixation was inadequate. Fracture healed with 15° of valgus angulation. It is also likely that more extensive comminution was present than was initially appreciated. Addition of medial and anterior struts would likely have avoided fracture mal-union. Placement of a DCS or long blade plate alone or in conjunction with medial allograft strut could also have been used (see Fig. 12). The fracture ultimately healed with combined valgus and flexion deformity. The patient currently ambulates with the aid of a cane. **D:** Lateral radiograph 3 years postoperatively. An approximately 22-degree flexion deformity occurred.

require more aggressive treatment. The fracture site is widely exposed (as discussed later). Bone allograft plates, either stainless steel plates alone or combined with cortical allograft plates, are the most desirable treatment options. A single allograft strut (see Fig. 9B) may not be adequate alone in the distal diaphysis when the fracture is distal to the implant. Strut fracture can occur (Fig. 9C), resulting in the loss of fixation and in fracture angulation (see Fig. 9C,D). Although this fracture eventually healed, the preferable fixation technique would have been the placement of two or three struts or a 95-degree DCS type or blade plate anchored in the supracondylar bone (Fig. 11).

Occasionally, after cementing the femoral component in revision arthroplasty in the presence of compromised cortical bone, cement extrusion is identified. If the amount of cement is small, the defect is likely to be small, and, in many cases, it requires no treatment. On the other hand, if the amount of extruded cement is large (greater than 3 cm in the largest dimension), the area should be explored, the cement carefully removed, and the defect assessed. If this is not felt to represent a significant stress riser, autograft or allograft bone chips or paste may be placed over the area. If, on the other hand, a large split or displaced fragment is found, structural integrity must be restored. Onlay cortical allograft struts

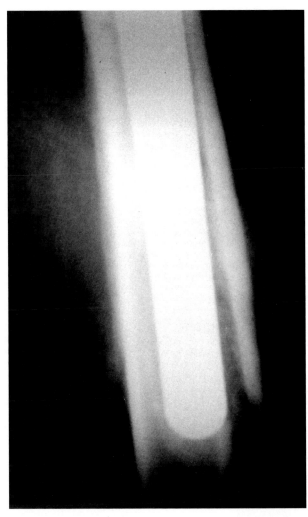

FIG. 10. This cortical-elevation-type fracture occurred at the time of revision surgery using curved long-stem prosthesis.

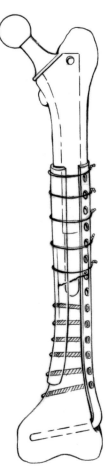

FIG. 11. Distal diaphyseal fractures may be amenable to treatment with DCS or blade-plate device with extended side-plate. Medial onlay allograft strut provides excellent adjunct fixation. Distally, the screws can be positioned so that they aid in securing the allograft. Proximally, cerclage wires secure both the metallic and allograft plates.

(see later section on surgical technique) are an excellent means of treating this type of fracture.

Complex Fractures

This is a typical fracture pattern seen during the course of revision surgery using long-stem femoral implants, and, unlike the simple fracture type, it threatens implant fixation. The fracture may occur in association with a cortical window, osteolysis, or the use of power burrs (Fig. 12). Unstable intraoperative diaphyseal fractures are usually recognized when they occur. A crack may be heard, but, most often, the person holding the leg becomes aware of motion in the previously intact femoral shaft. Occasionally, this type of fracture does not significantly displace during the course of the revi-

sion surgery. Unless a radiograph is taken, the fracture may not be recognized until after surgery. In all such high risk situations, intraoperative radiographs should be a standard part of the procedure.

Management of these potentially difficult fractures has been greatly simplified by the use of onlay allograft struts (see later section on surgical technique) and uncemented long-stem implants that function as intramuscular rods (Fig. 13). An additional level of complexity is present if bone loss is severe and a segmental diaphyseal or dia-metaphyseal defect is also present (see Fig. 14A). This variation is usually seen in association with the use of power equipment for clearing bone cement. It is treated with placement of interpositional segmental allograft and press-fit or cemented femoral component. In the presence of infection, where an interval resection

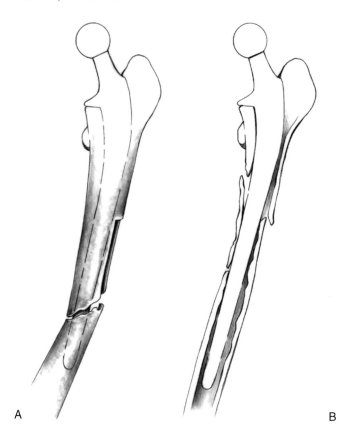

A

B

FIG. 12. A: Angulated distal diaphyseal fracture, which can occur through the lower edge of a cortical window. This fracture may extend proximal enough to compromise implant fixation. **B:** Upper diaphyseal fracture with severe loss of bone may occur in association with the use of high-speed burrs during the course of component or cement removal.

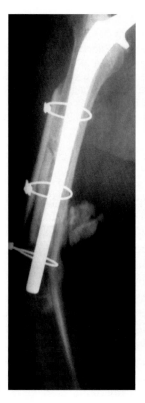
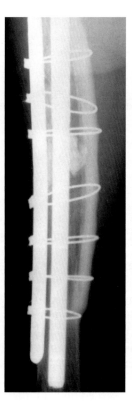
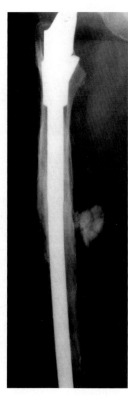

A–C

FIG. 13. A: This diaphyseal spiral fracture occurred through a cortical window. It was recognized at the time of surgery and an unsatisfactory attempt was made to stabilize the fracture using a longer prosthesis in association with an onlay cortical allograft strut. **B:** If this fracture had been recognized during the time of surgery, a more viable stabilization could have been attempted with the use of an uncemented long-stem prosthesis that acts as an intramedullary rod. In this case, a long-stem S-ROM prosthesis was used. A stainless steel plate was placed along the lateral femoral cortex and cortical allograft strut was placed medially. **C:** The patient developed persistent complaint of discomfort along lateral femoral cortex. This was felt to be the result of cable grip sleeves. Symptoms resolved after removal of cables and metallic plate. Previous fracture line is no longer visible. Patient ambulates without assistive devices.

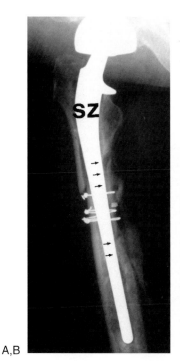
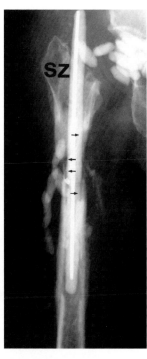
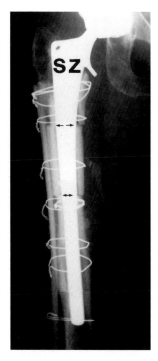
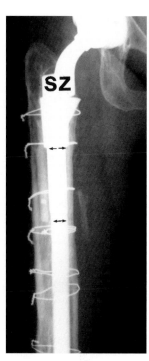

A,B   C,D

FIG. 14. A: Complex proximal diaphyseal fracture. This is associated with approximately 2 inches of moderate segmental diaphyseal bone loss (*arrows*). Long-stem implant was loose and infected. **B:** Resection arthoplasty has been carried out. In an effort to achieve some degree of fracture stability, an internal stent of PMMA-—antibiotic around a Steinmann pin was placed. Additional antibiotic beads were placed within the soft-tissue envelope. **C:** Approximately 8 weeks postoperatively, definitive reconstruction was performed. Upper diaphyseal segmental allograft was placed. Long-stem BIAS femoral prosthesis was used. Additional rotational control was conferred by placement of anteromedial and lateral onlay strut grafts. The patient developed thigh pain approximately 2 years postoperatively. This was felt to be a result of a loose femoral component. Revision was required. **D:** BIAS prosthesis was easily removed. Minimal fibrous tissue fixation was present. As seen by the radiograph (C), segmental interposition allograft union occurred. Revision was then performed with placement of a long-stem S-ROM femoral component. Thigh pain was relieved.

arthroplasty may be required and definitive fixation deferred, temporary limited internal fixation may be desirable. One method of achieving this is the placement of the "customized" internal stent (described previously in the section on complex, dia-metaphyseal fractures) made from PMMA-—antibiotic. An attempt is made to achieve some degree of press-fit by lightly reaming the diaphysis and determining the approximate diameter of the stent (Fig. 14A,B). After the appropriate duration, interval resection arthroplasty reconstruction is carried out using a segmental cortical allograft in association with onlay allograft struts (see Fig. 14C,D).

POSTOPERATIVE METAPHYSEAL FRACTURES

Simple Fractures

As noted, this fracture (Fig. 15) is most likely to be associated with placement of press-fit femoral compo-

nents. Although there is generally minimal displacement, treatment will depend on the surgeon s assessment of component stability. Treatment can be operative if implant fixation is in question (e.g., with proximally coated compared to more extensively porous-coated implants, or for a short stem compared to a long stem), or it can be non-operative if the fracture is not felt to compromise implant fixation. An extended period of protected weight bearing may be helpful if non-operative treatment is chosen.

Another type of metaphyseal fracture is seen in Figure 16. This patient began to experience severe groin pain and an acute, lesser trochanteric fracture was identified. In the presence of osteolysis associated with both cemented and cementless femoral components, metaphyseal compromise can be severe enough to result in spontaneous or pathologic fracture in the absence of trauma. In this case, the femoral component was stable. Associated acetabular-component osteolysis was present, and the acetabular component was revised. All lytic areas,

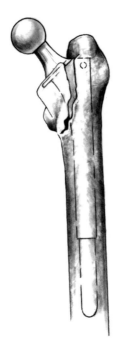

FIG. 15. Postoperative metaphyseal fracture, simple. Implant stability is not compromised. Fracture may heal with some displacement.

including the proximal femoral metaphysis, were treated with curettage and packed with morselized allograft bone.

POSTOPERATIVE COMBINED (OR DIA-METAPHYSEAL) FRACTURES

By definition, these fractures are classified as complex. The fracture extends around the body of the prosthesis, and implant stability is compromised. They may present as relatively uncomplicated two-part fractures (Fig. 17) and they are treated in the manner of postoperative diaphyseal fractures. However, implant-induced osteolysis in association with other patient-related factors such as systemic osteopenia, prior fracture, or periprosthetic infection may lead to more extensive fractures (Figs. 18A,19A). Complex reconstruction is often necessary in these cases.

In general, if less than 50% of the femoral tube is viable, proximal femoral allograft reconstruction must be considered. In elderly or low-demand patients, it may be more prudent to proceed directly to proximal femoral allografting if the reconstruction is likely to be prolonged or tedious (see Fig. 18).

A dia-metaphyseal fracture in cases of moderate to severe proximal bone loss in a younger patient presents a unique reconstructive challenge. A combination of wire mesh (Zimmer, Warsaw, IN) onlay struts, with or without the addition of metallic plates and morselized bone, has

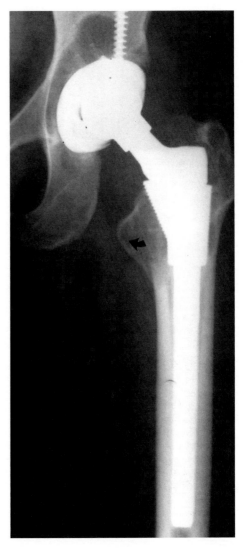

FIG. 16. Lesser trochanteric fracture is visible *(curved solid arrow)*. This occurred in association with severe acetabular and proximal femoral osteolysis.

been used in salvage situations in younger, generally healthy patients (see Fig. 19).

POSTOPERATIVE DIAPHYSEAL FRACTURES

Simple Fractures

This is perhaps the most common type of periprosthetic fracture. The orientation may be transverse (Fig. 20B) or in varying degrees of obliquity (Fig. 21A). In the author's experience, these fractures are often the result of a significant traumatic event, such as a fall, a severe twisting injury, or a motor vehicle accident. However, there may be a cortical lytic defect that predisposes to a type of stress fracture associated with minimal activity. For example, the

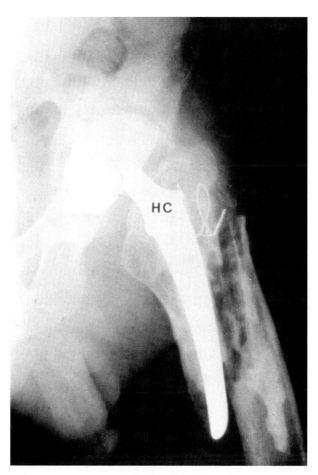

FIG. 17. Dia-metaphyseal fracture, complex. Although some osteolysis is present, cortical tube can be reconstituted by reducing and stabilizing this fracture.

patient whose radiograph is shown in Fig. 20A was sitting in a swimming pool when he felt the fracture occur.

Management of simple postoperative diaphyseal fractures typically requires only fixation of the fracture and not component revision. It is the author's preference to treat these fractures with dual onlay, cortical allograft struts (3) (see later section on surgical technique) (see Fig. 20B,C,D, Fig. 21). Not only does this technique offer superb fracture fixation, but it also eliminates the distal stress riser potential of a metal plate (Fig. 22), as well as the stress shielding that occurs under a metal plate. If apposition is adequate, these grafts will unite (Fig. 23) and potentially offer long-term bone augmentation. Subsequent surgery is not required for device removal as is often recommended with metal plates. After removal of metal plates, the stress risers caused by the remaining screw holes, combined with stress shielding, present yet another risk of periprosthetic fracture. Remodeling of the onlay grafts appears to occur over time. The grafts do appear to thin, thereby reducing the stress riser potential (Fig. 24).

Complex Diaphyseal Fractures

Although rare, diaphyseal fracture in the presence of severe osteopenia, well-fixed femoral components, and failure of a previous attempt at internal fixation with bone struts, has been encountered by the author on three occasions. Bone compromise is usually so severe that whole proximal femoral allograft reconstruction is the only realistic option for restoring function (Fig. 25).

SURGICAL TECHNIQUE

Exposure

To begin, the proximal and distal extent of the fracture must be clearly identified. Conventional wisdom for fracture fixation associated with THA components dictates that two cortical diameters (4) or four to six cortices are appropriate distances for bypassing cortical defects or fractures. Soft-tissue dissection should extend to just below and just above the anticipated extent of the fixation plate (bone or metal). A mid-lateral skin incision is made and the fascia overlying the vastus lateralis is incised along the posterior edge (Fig. 26A), leaving approximately a 1- to 2-cm fascial cuff for repair. Muscle is then elevated from within the posterior fascial sleeve using sharp dissection and moving from distal to proximal. A broad periosteal elevator is used to maintain tension on the muscle just anterior and proximal to the leading edge of the dissection, which progresses medially and proximally toward the linea aspera and then on to the periosteum. The perforating vessels are encountered just before reaching the periosteum (see Fig. 26B), at approximately 1- to 1fi-inch intervals. This can be a relatively bloodless and expeditious dissection if these vessels are patiently identified, isolated under a tonsil (Schnid) clamp, secured using hemoclips (doubly clipped posteriorly and singly clipped anteriorly), and cut well anterior to their point of emergence through the linea aspera.

Allograft Preparation

Beginning with a dia-metaphyseal segment approximately 20 to 25 cm long, the allograft tube is cut longitudinally in thirds, generally centering around the linea aspera (Fig. 27A,B). This may take 10 to 15 minutes and is best accomplished using a thin oscillating saw blade with in-line teeth (see Fig. 27C). Typically, each 2- to 2.5-cm-wide strut will match the corresponding surface of the host femur (e.g., the lateral strut will approximate the contour of the lateral cortex) (see Fig. 27D). Occasionally, in the presence of irregular contours (e.g., heterotopic bone, abundant callus, or mild mal-union from a

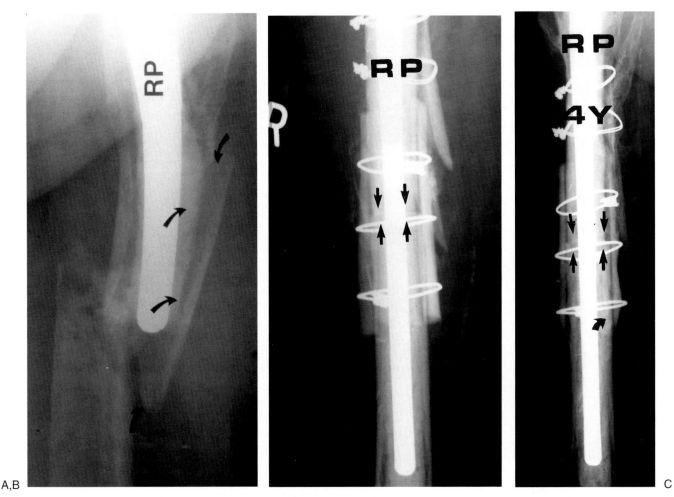

FIG. 18. A: Severely comminuted proximal dia-metaphyseal fracture in the presence of severe osteopenia. **B:** In view of the patient's age (79 years) and relatively limited lifestyle because of moderate obesity and pulmonary disease, treatment of choice was felt to be proximal femoral allograft reconstruction using cemented, long-stem implant. Construct was further stabilized by placing onlay cortical allograft struts as shown. **C:** By 4 years postoperatively, fracture junction has united. Allograft strut remodeling is noted.

previous fracture), the concavity of the anterior cortical strut can be utilized for more precise fit without excess thinning of the strut. A more accurate estimation of length is then made, and the struts are shortened. The grafts likely to provide the best apposition with minimal trimming are then chosen. The medullary trough is then eliminated by running the Midas Rex AM-15 burr over the endosteal surface of the strut graft (Fig. 28). To maximize surface contact, graft contouring is also carried out at this point as the graft is repeatedly trimmed, the contact checked, and the graft trimmed again as necessary. Care must be taken not to thin the graft excessively (i.e., less than 6 mm)! Graft contouring is complete when the struts can be placed directly medially and directly laterally, with minimal tendency to rock or slide as they are compressed. Graft contact does not have to be 100%, because some flexing will occur as the wires are tight-

ened. However, if large gaps are present, the strut may fracture on tightening the wires.

It is safest to place the cerclage wires prior to placement of the strut grafts (Fig. 29). They are arrayed at approximately 2.5-cm intervals and a spare two or three may be added in case of over-tightening and breakage of the primary wire. Tightening usually begins with the middle wire, as this is less likely to toggle the grafts. Particular attention must be paid to the medial strut, as it tends to slide anteriorly as the cerclage wires are tightened. If this occurs, the medial soft-tissue envelope may have to be further developed to accommodate the graft, or the graft may require additional contouring to improve surface contact or remove some of its width. As each subsequent wire is tightened, one of the previously tightened wires may loosen as the graft is further compressed. It is for this reason that final cutting and bending of the wires

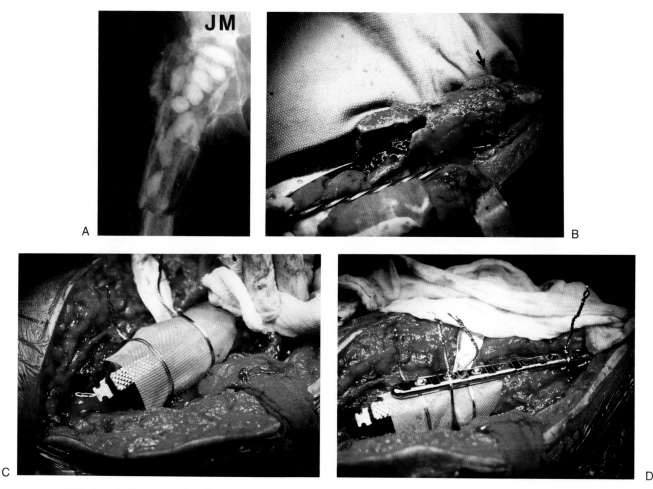

FIG. 19. A: Postoperative dia-metaphyseal fracture occurred during the course of treatment of periprosthetic infection. The patient was treated with resection arthroplasty, and then, approximately 1 week prior to anticipated reimplantation, the patient fell and suffered this fracture. **B:** At the time of reconstruction, severe proximal metaphyseal bone loss was noted. Diaphyseal fracture is seen at the far right of this photograph. **C:** Reconstruction was carried out in a stepwise fashion. Proximal cortical tube was closed initially using stainless steel mesh wired into place. Approximate level of femoral head and shoulder of the prosthesis was determined by placement of broach. **D:** The fracture was then fixed laterally using stainless steel Howmedica plate (East Rutherford, NJ).

is not carried out until all wires have been maximally tightened (Fig. 30).

Author's Note

Although onlay allograft struts appear to offer an excellent method of managing these fractures, certain essential rules for their use warrant emphasis. As stated above, the strength of fixation of these grafts derives from maximizing the surface area in contact with the underlying bone. When cerclage wires or cables are applied, the grafts are compressed onto the host bone and a very strong and stable construct is created. It is essential that the grafts remain arrayed around the femur and do not make contact with each other as the cerclage device (cable or wire) is

tightened. If each of the two or three strut grafts is making edge contact with the other, the cerclage wire tension is being taken up in the compression of one strut against the other and not in the compression of the strut against host bone (Fig. 31). Fracture fixation is significantly compromised and failure is likely if this occurs. To minimize this risk, it is critical that the entire length of each of the struts be checked, either visually or by palpation, for edge-to-edge contact along 30% or more of the length of the strut. If this occurs, the wires or cables should be removed and the struts repositioned. Struts may have to be narrowed or the medial soft-tissue envelope may have to be developed further to permit the medial strut to rest along the medial cortex rather than the anteromedial femur. Ideally, fixation is not finalized if the array is not satisfactory.

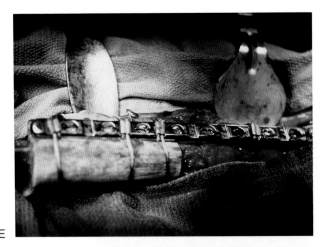

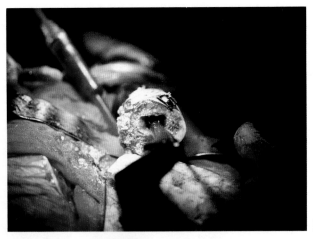

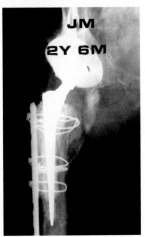

FIG. 19 *Continued.* **E:** Proximal tube was further reinforced by placement of onlay cortical allograft strut. **F:** Reconstruction was then carried out using impaction grafting technique. Looking down from the top, impacted bone is noted. The cast of the bone tamp is seen. **G:** Final orientation of the tamp within impacted bone and reconstituted upper femoral tube. **H:** At 2.5 years postoperatively, component position has been maintained, and the fracture appears healed. The patient is now working on his feet approximately 8 hours per day and experiences no pain.

Impending Fracture

When inserting an uncemented implant in the presence of thin calcar bone, it is advisable to place at least one cerclage wire prior to seating the prosthesis. In the presence of cortical thinning, secondary to either osteolysis or eccentric reaming, consideration should be given to some type of prophylactic fixation (see Fig. 20A). Placement of an onlay strut graft should be considered if the defect is at or below the distal third of the femoral component. If such a lesion is encountered during routine follow-up of an asymptomatic patient (Fig. 32) and is believed to be progressive, an attempt should be made to understand the etiology prior to assessing treatment options. Infection should be ruled out, and if the lesion is felt to be the result of osteolysis without loosening, revision arthroplasty will likely be the treatment of choice.

The impaction bone grafting technique (6) for femoral reconstruction during revision THA has become quite popular. The technique employs the use of a cemented, collarless, polished, conventional-length femoral implant in association with an intramedullary allograft bone mantle. This has led to postoperative fracture in the upper diaphysis. At present, the technique does not call for the use of a long-stem implant. It is now recommended that, in the presence of dia-metaphyseal osteolysis, onlay cortical strut graft(s) be utilized prophylactically (Fig. 33).

Prophylactic Extended Trochanteric Osteotomy

This is an essential technique for minimizing risk of fracture during revision THA. Extended trochanteric osteotomy permits liberal access to bone cement and prosthesis. In the presence of an uncemented femoral

A,B

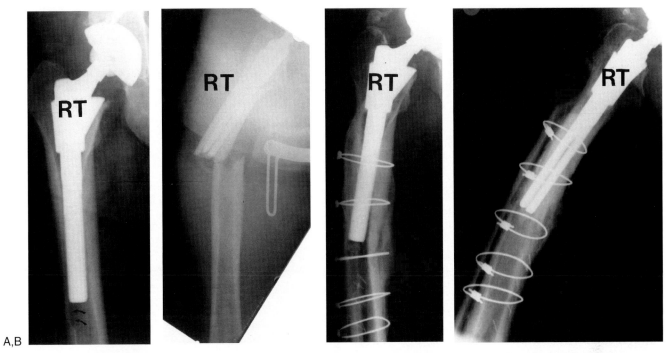

C,D

FIG. 20. A: Postoperative radiograph of 57-year-old man who underwent recent placement of S-ROM prosthesis. Prosthesis is in varus. Deep distal lateral femoral cortical "scalloping" is present. **B:** At 2.5 months postoperatively, acute transverse diaphyseal fracture occurred through the weakened lateral femoral cortex. **C:** Fracture was treated with onlay cortical allograft struts. At 4 years after ORIF of this periprosthetic fracture, the patient remained asymptomatic in spite of persistent angulation. **D:** Lateral views show mild angulation. Remodeling of onlay struts is noted.

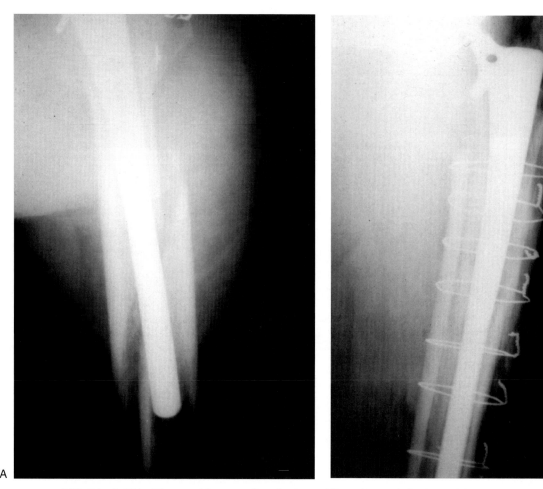

A

B

FIG. 21. A: This 59-year-old man suffered a long oblique femoral diaphyseal fracture approximately 3 weeks after revision of THA with this BIAS prosthesis. **B:** It was felt that proximal implant stability was present in spite of the fracture. The fracture was treated with open reduction internal stabilization using medial and lateral onlay cortical strut allografts. The fracture healed uneventfully.

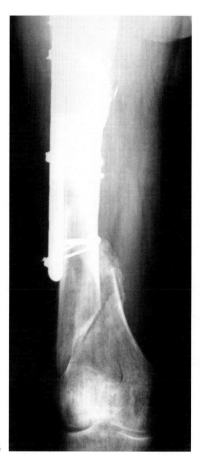 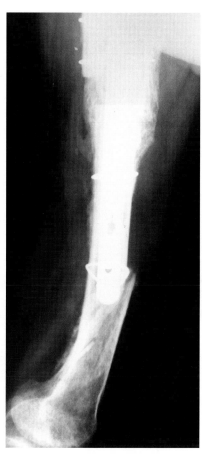

A,B

FIG. 22. A: Although treatment of this patient's proximal periprosthetic fracture was successful, he suffered a fracture through the distal screw hole of this long stainless steel side plate. The patient elected non-operative treatment (i.e., a cast brace). The fracture ultimately healed with some displacement. **B:** Lateral view of distal dia-metaphyseal fracture. Mal-union is noted. The patient is asymptomatic.

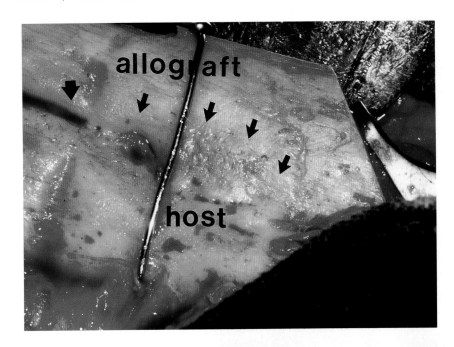

FIG. 23. "Spot welds" are seen between onlay cortical allograft and underlying host bone.

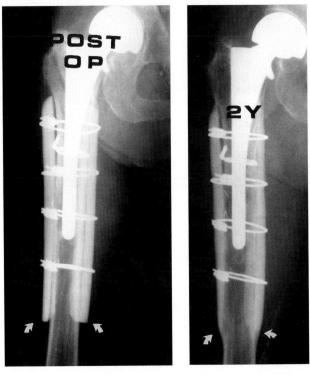

FIG. 24. A: Immediate postoperative radiograph of late diaphyseal fracture treated with onlay cortical strut grafts. **B:** After 2.5 years, proximal and distal allograft bone remodeling is noted.

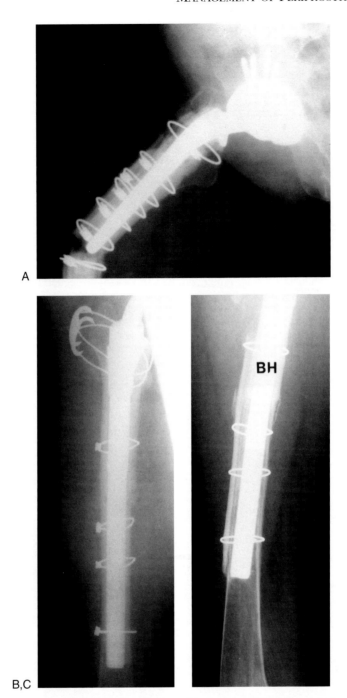

FIG. 25. A: This active, generally healthy, 71-year-old woman suffered the complex diaphyseal fracture within a few weeks of conversion to a cemented Precoat prosthesis. Revision surgery was complicated by upper diaphyseal intraoperative fracture. An attempt was made to treat this with onlay cortical allograft struts. Failure of treatment was felt to be secondary to excessive thinning of onlay struts, as well as edge-to-edge position of strut grafts (see section on pitfalls of management). **B:** Proximal femoral allograft reconstruction has been carried out. **C:** After 4 years, cortical remodeling has occurred.

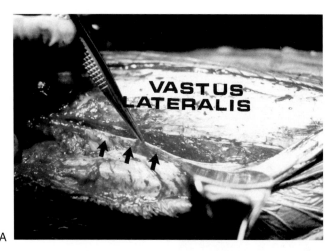
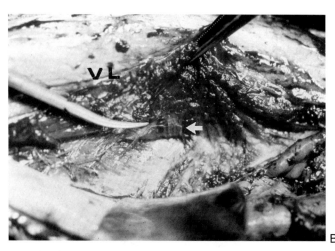

A

B

FIG. 26. A: An incision is made along the posterior edge of the vastus lateralis fascia, leaving an approximately 1- to 2-cm fascial cuff for repair *(arrows).* **B:** Patient dissection allows clear identification of the perforating vessels. They are at approximately 1- to 1¹/₂-inch intervals. These can be isolated and sectioned sequentially, making this a relatively bloodless approach, allowing wide exposure with little, if any, additional blood loss. Vessel clips are quite helpful in securing these vessels. Typically, two clips would be placed posteriorly and one anteriorly. Leaving a few millimeters of vessel length anterior to emergence from the septum allows easy access if a clip becomes dislodged. (VL, vastus lateralis.)

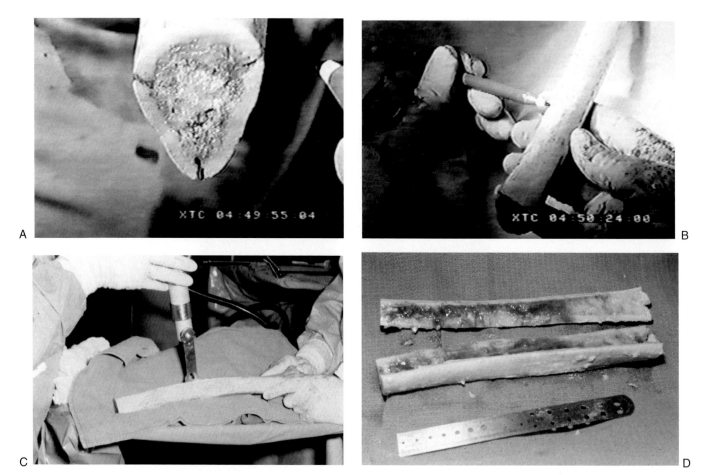

A

B

C

D

FIG. 27. A: Femoral diaphysis is seen end-on. The circumference is divided into thirds, centering over the linea aspera. Marking pen is used to identify each segment. **B:** These lines are then projected along the surface of the diaphysis. **C:** Oscillating saw blade with in-line teeth is used for initial allograft preparation. **D:** Anterior strut prior to final preparation.

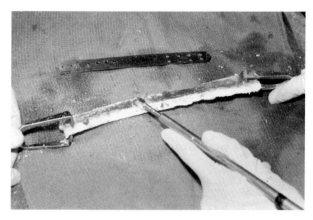

FIG. 28. A barrel burr is used to eliminate the medullary trough. AM-15 burr (Midas Rex, Dallas, TX, not shown) allows creation of a flat surface in a single plane.

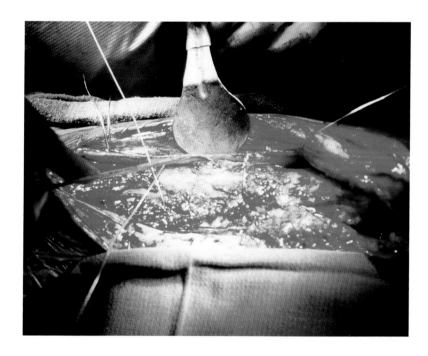

FIG. 29. Cerclage wires are placed prior to laying in the strut grafts.

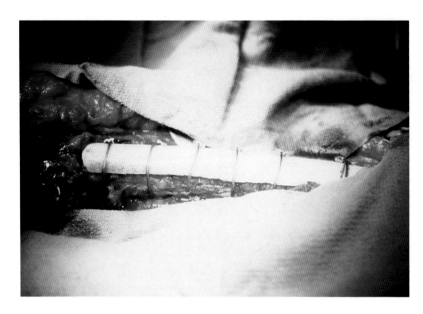

FIG. 30. Wires are generally spaced 1 to 1¹⁄₂ inches apart, depending on relative fracture stability.

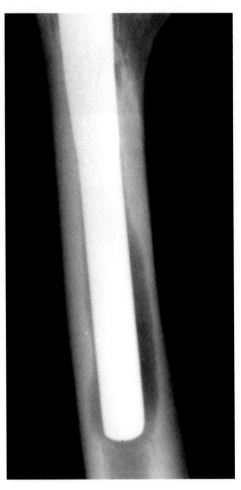

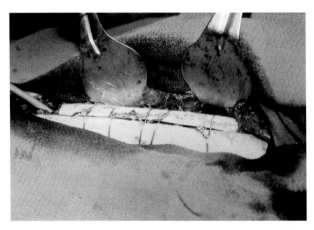

FIG. 31. Edge-to-edge contact of the strut grafts significantly reduces fracture fixation by reducing relative compression of the struts against the underlying cortical bone. Every effort must be made to array the grafts so that when final tension is applied, there is no contact of one against the other.

FIG. 32. Extensive endosteal erosion is noted. Patient is at increased risk of fracture. Revision surgery is anticipated within the near future.

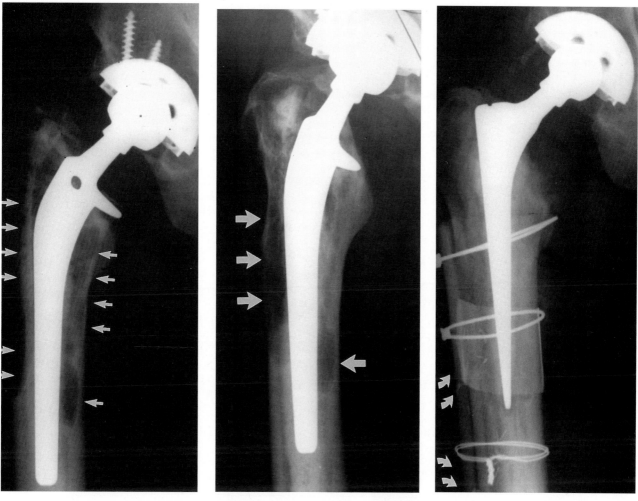

A,B   C

FIG. 33. A: Marked endosteal cortical osteolysis is noted. Full-thickness lysis is noted proximally and laterally. **B:** Lateral radiograph confirms the extent of osteolysis. **C:** At the time of surgery, all soft tissue was removed from these lytic defects. Full-thickness defect proximally and laterally was treated with onlay cortical mesh. Surgery was carried out using the Ling technique, as described previously. Onlay cortical allograft strut is visible *(curved arrows)*. It is felt that placement of the strut significantly reduces stress-riser potential.

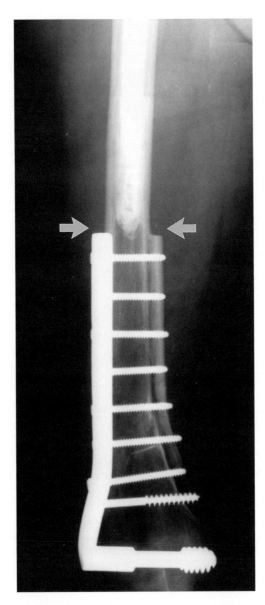

FIG. 34. When using allograft struts and metallic plates, it should be kept in mind that a significant stress riser can be created between the end of a femoral component or associated cement mantel and the adjacent end of a metallic plate or onlay cortical strut graft. Ideally, this would be recognized and fixation device extended to reduce the potential for fracture at such a junction.

component requiring removal for malposition, infection, or pain, the implant is almost always well fixed. Significant fracture is likely unless extensive controlled exposure is carried out.

Pitfalls in Management

Avoid creating a new stress riser when fixing a diaphyseal or proximal dia-metaphyseal fracture in the presence of a total knee arthroplasty with a stemmed femoral component. The problem can be avoided by extending the fixation an appropriate distance distal to the upper end of the stem. Conversely, when fixing a supracondylar femur fracture in the presence of a total hip prosthesis, similar care should be taken to extend the fixation device an appropriate distance proximal to the end of the femoral component of the THA (Fig. 34).

Occasionally, a supracondylar plate is encountered along the lateral femoral shaft. In this case, a medial strut, or both medial and anterior struts, are placed an appropriate distance distal to the plate to eliminate the significant stress riser.

The end of a metal plate, such as the Howmedica (Rutherford, NJ) device designed for these fractures, also sets up a potential stress riser. In most instances, this cannot be avoided. The surgeon and the patient must both be aware that a fracture can occur in the supracondylar area of the distal femur after the use of this device. Should such a fracture occur, treatment options include the removal of the plate and placement of a long blade plate or the use of a cast brace (see Fig. 22). If the underlying bone is very osteoporotic and there is stiffness at the hip, the risk of fracture at the end of this device is high. In this setting, consideration should be given to the use of a long blade or DCS plate as primary fixation for a periprosthetic fracture. If wires are required at the level of the femoral prosthesis, they may be stabilized over the plate by eyelets now provided by Synthes. These eyelets permit anchoring of the wires, keeping them from sliding distally along the conical femur and loosening once they have been tightened.

CONCLUSION

A clear understanding of the nature and extent of these fractures is essential prior to considering treatment. An appreciation for certain patient-specific factors will lead to different treatment techniques for similar fractures. Familiarity with conventional and somewhat unique fixation techniques can lead to successful management of even the most complex periprosthetic fractures.

Each orthopedic surgeon, however, must assess his or her own level of experience and expertise as it relates to the problem being considered. Some of the treatment options discussed will be more appropriate for those surgeons involved in joint replacement surgery on a regular basis.

REFERENCES

1. Bethea J, Andrade J, Fleming L, Lindenbaum S, Welch R. Proximal femoral fractures following total hip arthroplasty. *Clin Orthop* 1982; 170:95–105.
2. Chandler H, Clark J, Murphy S, et al. Reconstruction of major segmental loss of the proximal femur in revision total hip arthroplasty. *Clin Orthop* 1994;298:67–74.
3. Chandler HP, Penenberg BL, eds. *Bone stock deficiency in total hip replacement. Classification and management.* Thorofare, NJ: Slack, 1989.
4. Duncan CP, Masri BA. Fractures of the femur after hip replacement. *Instr Course Lect* 1995;44:293–304.
5. Emerson R, Head W, Berklacich F, Malinin T. Noncemented acetabular revision arthroplasty using allograft bone. *Clin Orthop* 1989;249: 30–43.
6. Gie GA, Linder L, Ling RS, Simon JP, Slooff TJ, Timperley AJ. Impacted cancellous allografts and cement for revision total hip arthroplasty. *J Bone Joint Surg* 1993;75B:14–21.
7. Head W, Wagner R, Emerson R, Malinin T. Revision total hip arthroplasty in the deficient femur with a proximal load-bearing prosthesis. *Clin Orthop* 1994;298:119–126.
8. Johannsson J, McBroom R, Barrington T, Hunter G. Fracture of the ipsilateral femur in patients with total hip replacement. *J Bone Joint Surg* 1981;63(A):1435–1442.
9. Kelley SS, Periprosthetic femoral fractures. *J Am Academy Othop Surg* 1994;2:164–172.
10. Makely J. The use of allografts to reconstruct intercalary defects of long bones. *Clin Orthop* 1985;197:58–75.
11. Malinin T, Latta L, Wagner J, Brown M. Healing of fractures with freeze-dried cortical bone plates. Comparison with compression plating. *Clin Orthop* 1984;190:281–286.
12. Pak J, Paprosky W, Jablonsky W, Lawrence J. Femoral strut allografts in cementless revision total hip arthroplasty. *Clin Orthop* 1993;295: 172–178.
13. Roffman M, Mendes D. Fracture of the femur after total hip arthroplasty. *Orthopedics* 1989;12:1067–1070.
14. Serocki J, Chandler R, Dorr L. Treatment of fractures about hip prostheses with compression plating. *J Arthroplasty* 1992;7:129–135.
15. Stiehl J. Femoral allograft reconstruction in revision total hip arthroplasty. *Orthop Rev* 1992;21:1057–1063.
16. Zehntner M, Ganz R. Midterm results (5.5-10 years) of acetabular allograft reconstruction with the acetabular reinforcement ring during total hip revision. *J Arthroplasty* 1994;9:469–479.

The Adult Hip, edited by J. J. Callaghan,
A. G. Rosenberg, and H. E. Rubash.
Lippincott–Raven Publishers, Philadelphia © 1998.

CHAPTER 78

Management of the Trochanter

Craig D. Silverton and Aaron G. Rosenberg

Osteotomy of the trochanter has long been recognized as the most effective method of obtaining wide exposure of the hip joint. Particularly in cases of periarticular scar, ankylosis, or deformity, osteotomy of the trochanter provides relatively easy circumferential exposure of the joint, minimizing surgical time and soft-tissue trauma where other approaches may prove more tedious. Although initial use of the transtrochanteric approach was recommended for all total hip arthroplasty (THA), most contemporary arthroplasty surgeons prefer to use other approaches in the routine primary case. Nonetheless, osteotomy of the trochanter remains a viable option for exposure of the difficult primary cases of ankylosis, protrusio acetabuli, deformities of the proximal femur, congenital dysplasia of the hip (CDH), and revision surgery. The decision to utilize a trochanteric osteotomy for exposure of the hip involves factors such as the amount of exposure necessary, available bone stock, previous surgical approach, and the type of reconstruction planned.

The number of osteotomy configurations and techniques reported in the literature is superseded only by the volume of reports available on various fixation techniques. Multiple reports of combinations of wires, screws, plates, cables, springs, and bolts holds testimony to the fact that fixation of the trochanter remains the "Achilles

tendon" of the trochanteric osteotomy. This chapter will review (a) indications and contraindications for osteotomy, (b) techniques for osteotomy, (c) techniques for fixation, (d) management of chronic nonunion, trochanteric bursitis, and trochanteric loss, and (e) complications associated with trochanteric fixation.

INDICATIONS AND CONTRAINDICATIONS

Preoperative planning involves not only determining the size and type of components to be utilized in the arthroplasty, but the type and amount of surgical exposure necessary. According to Sir John Charnley, who was taught the method of trochanteric osteotomy by Sir Harry Platt, "If it could be guaranteed that the greater trochanter would unite within three weeks when reattached, and without imposing restrictions which would impede rehabilitation, few surgeons would fail to avail themselves of the easy and beautiful access to the hip joint provided by the lateral [transtrochanteric] approach" (16,17). Indeed, Charnley repeatedly emphasized the importance of utilizing a technique that would provide appropriate exposure to prepare the bone, and the importance of implanting the components in a way that could be easily accomplished by other surgeons. Few would argue that trochanteric osteotomy still provides the most thorough access to the hips in those patients with primary hip disease or in the revision setting where an extensile exposure is required to perform the surgery.

   A. G. Rosenberg: Department of Orthopaedic Surgery, Arthritis and Orthopaedic Institute, Rush Medical College, Chicago, Illinois 60612.
   C. D. Silverton: Department of Orthopaedic Surgery, Rush-Presbyterian–St. Luke's Medical Center, Chicago, Illinois 60614.

Contemporary primary THA is usually approached through a posterior exposure or a modification of the direct lateral (Hardinge) (38). However, certain conditions necessitate a different approach. In the patient with an ankylosed hip, severe protrusio acetabuli, massive periarticular scar, or heterotopic ossification, internal or external rotation may not be possible and access to the hip capsule or pericapsular scar tissue may be impossible. Attempting to force rotation often results in a catastrophic spiral fracture of the femur. Trochanteric osteotomy in these cases will give the surgeon adequate exposure of the hip joint, so that a complete capsulectomy can be performed, and aid in exposure of the proximal femur. Many times, the femoral neck cut must be made prior to dislocation, as intra-articular adhesions or protrusion prevents any motion despite a complete capsulectomy. This is also the case with fusion of the hip.

Patients with congenital dislocation of the hip and acetabular dysplasia may require trochanteric osteotomy for a complete exposure and lengthening of the shortened femur. The size and shape of the trochanteric osteotomy is important in these cases, because trochanteric reattachment becomes difficult after the femoral lengthening.

Deformities of the proximal femur and trochanter may be congenital, developmental, posttraumatic or secondary to primary bone diseases such as Paget's disease or fibrous dysplasia. Previous intertrochanteric or subtrochanteric hip fractures with malunion and a rotatory deformity may make a standard exposure difficult, as can a previous arthrodesis or limited motion of the ipsilateral knee. Trochanteric osteotomy in these cases facilitates exposure and assists in proper orientation of the femoral component.

Inadequate soft-tissue tension after THA can result in chronic dislocations that can be managed with distal transfer of the greater trochanter. It should be noted, however, that nonunion rates increase once the trochanter is shifted more than 1 cm distal to its original bed (36).

The primary indication for trochanteric osteotomy remains revision hip arthroplasty, where adequate exposure of the acetabulum and proximal femur frequently cannot be adequately achieved with standard approaches. Performing total hip revision without adequate exposure risks injury to the sciatic nerve, iatrogenic fractures of the femur and acetabulum, avulsion of the abductors, malposition of both acetabular and femoral components, inadequate preparation of the bone beds, and prolonged surgical exposure.

Although the advantages of trochanteric osteotomy in difficult primary THA and in revision cases are numerous, poor healing of the trochanter remains an unavoidable complication. Inability to reapproximate the trochanter to an adequate bone bed may thus be a relative contraindication to the standard type of trochanteric osteotomy. Cementless ingrowth prostheses that require large metaphyseal filling leave only a thin shell of bone in the trochanteric area after broaching of the canal, and a standard trochanteric osteotomy may be relatively contraindicated in these cases.

TECHNIQUES FOR OSTEOTOMY

The classic trochanteric osteotomy, as initially recommended by Charnley, created a flat cut across the trochanter. The trochanteric fragment was then lateralized and placed distal to its original bed (17). This distal transplantation of the greater trochanter had several advantages according to Charnley: (a) it allowed the use of a short-necked prosthesis that decreased the lever arm of the femoral neck and transmitted forces to the upper shaft of the femur, (b) correction of a fixed lateral (posterior) rotation of the trochanter is moved to the center of the hip joint on the lateral projection, increasing the effective length of the lever arm, and (c) the abductors can be properly tensioned, which reduces the incidence of postoperative dislocation. As the use of modular femoral components along with offset options became available in the 1980s, the advantages of transplantation of the greater trochanter became outdated. Surgeons who continued to use trochanteric osteotomy reapproximated the flat trochanteric fragment to its original bed. Techniques to improve fixation of the trochanteric fragment and lower the rate of nonunion began to appear.

Chevron Osteotomy

As other surgeons recognized the inherent instability of a flat-cut trochanteric osteotomy, an alternative chevron, or biplane, osteotomy was developed. Although probably first used by French surgeons Debeyre and Duliveux in 1954 (24), the Swiss popularized this "dihedral self-stabilizing" trochanteric osteotomy (84,85). The advantages of this osteotomy are obvious: not only is rotation resisted but anatomic replacement of the trochanter is made easier and the surface area of the osteotomy is increased. Weber compared a group of 138 patients, of whom 69 had conventional flat osteotomies and 69 had the biplane osteotomy; he found a pseudoarthrosis rate of 11% in the conventional group and 1.5% in the biplane group (84). Berry and Müller, reporting on 53 primary total hip arthroplasties and 74 revisions, utilized this chevron osteotomy with single-wire fixation and noted 98% and 97% rates of trochanteric union, respectively (11). Wroblewski and Shelley reported equally excellent results in both primary and revision cases: 98% union in 222 arthroplasties, of which half were revisions (Table 1) (86).

The technique of biplane osteotomy is quite simple, and reproducible results should be easily attained. The osteotomy is planned 4 to 5 cm distal to the proximal tip of the greater trochanter. The anterior and posterior limbs

TABLE 1. *Trochanteric fixation with wire*

Author (ref.)	Amstutz and Maki (3)	Eftekhar (26)	Eftekhar (26) (Comparison)			Harris (44) 1986	Berry (11) and Müller	Nutton and Checketts (65) (Comparison)		Wroblewski and Shelley (86) (Comparison)		
Osteotomy type	Flat cut	Chevron	Flat	Chevron	Chevron	Flat cut	Chevron	Chevron	Chevron	Chevron	Chevron	Chevron
Total patients	728	1158	100	100	110	804	127	101	66	66	139	226
Primary/revision	728/0	842/316	100/0	100/1	110/0	725/79	53/74	N/A	N/A	45/21	94/45	77/149
Fixation	2-wire cruciate	3-wire	Single wire, double vertical	Cruciate, 2-wire interlock and double wire	Single wire with spring	3 wires, 2 vertical 1 horizontal (mesh as needed)	Single wire	1 transverse, 1 double (Charnley)	2 double vertical, 1 transverse	Cruciate wire	Double and single wire	Double wire and compression spring
Nonunion: primary/revision	35 (5%)	3 (0.4%)/ 2 (0.5%)	5 (5%)	3 (3%)	4 (4%)	8 (1%)/0	1 (2%)/ 1 (2%)	21 (21%)	8 (12%)	3 (4.5%)	9 (6.5%)	3 (1.3%)
Fibrous union		29 (3.5%)/ 28(8.9%)	2 (2%)	2 (2%)	4 (4%)							
Migration with union		17 (2%)/ 11(3.5%)	6 (6%)	3 (3%)	7 (7%)					2 (3%)	2 (1.5%)	1 (0.5%)
Delayed union—total primary/revision						17 (2.3%)/ 6(7.6%)		32 (32%)	15 (23%)		6 (4%)	4 (1.8%)
Reoperation	8 (1%)		0	0	2 (2%)	6 (<1%)						
Breakage	153 (21%)	3 (0.4%)/ 2 (0.3%)	17 (17%)	8 (8%)	7 (7%)	215 (28%)				3 (4.5%)	11 (8%)	8 (3.5%)
Wire migration												

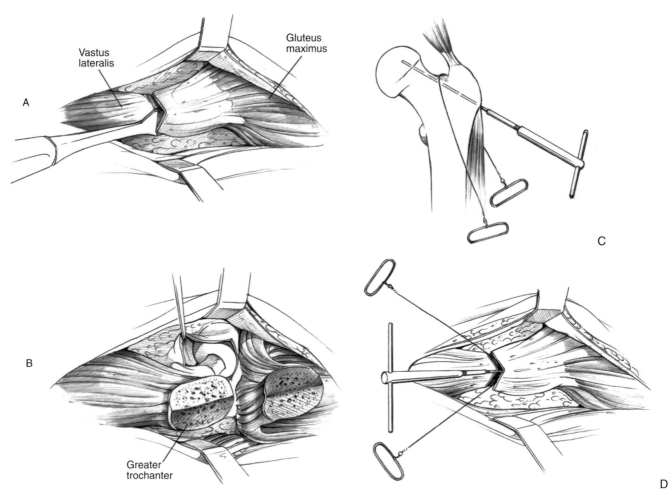

FIG. 1. A: The chevron osteotomy performed with an osteotome. **B:** The dihedral cut provides for stable approximation of the cut surfaces. **C:** The chevron osteotomy performed with a Gigli saw over a smooth Steinmann pin. **D:** The Gigli saw is directed distally, cutting anteriorly and posteriorly and creating a dihedral osteotomy.

of the osteotomy are equal in size and are cut at an angle of about 30° from the parasagital plane, forming a biplanar surface that is convex laterally (like the roof a Swiss chalet). This cut can be made with an oscillating saw or a straight osteotome (Fig. 1A,B). Special chevron-shaped osteotomes are popular with surgeons who routinely use this approach (26,76). Another option is the method used at Wrightington, whereby Wroblewski passes a 4-mm smooth Steinmann pin into the center of the trochanter, starting just below the vastus ridge, directing it at about 45° to the shaft of the femur (86). A Gigli saw is then passed into the notch between the superior aspect of the femoral neck and the trochanter (see Fig. 1C). The saw lies proximal to the Steinmann pin and is directed distally, cutting anteriorly and posteriorly, creating a two-plane osteotomy (see Fig. 1D). Reattachment is performed with a one-, two-, or three-wire technique. Wroblewski and Shelley found their two-wire technique with the compression spring to offer the best union rate,

but other authors have noted equally good results with standard techniques. Although the type of wire fixation may be important, it appears that the self-stabilizing effect of this dihedral osteotomy is the key to its success. This self-stabilizing effect, however, may be negated in the revision situation in the presence of a poor trochanteric bed or substantial bone loss. Additional or alternative fixation techniques may then be required.

Trochanteric Slide

The technique now known as the trochanteric slide was first described by English in 1975 (27). Dissatisfied with the classic techniques of trochanteric detachment used by Ollier and Charnley, English et al. developed a new method of trochanter detachment in an attempt to convert the tensile forces placed across the detached fragment of bone to compressive forces (Fig. 2C)(28,29). McFarland and Osborne (1954) were the first to describe keeping the

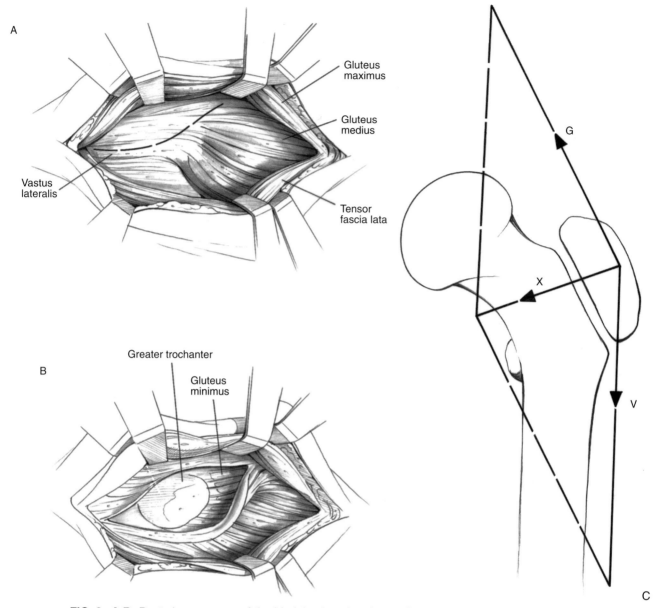

FIG. 2. A,B: Posterior exposure of the hip joint, keeping the tendinous portions of the gluteus medius and vastus lateralis intact (McFarland). **C:** Leaving the gluteal (G) and vastus (V) muscles attached produces a medial component (X) that exerts a compressive force on the plane of osteotomy (English).

tendinous portions of the gluteus medius and vastus lateralis intact during a posterior exposure of the hip. They did not osteotomize the trochanter, instead peeling the insertions of the gluteus medius and vastus lateralis off with a sharp chisel or knife (see Fig. 2A,B) (55). English modified McFarland's technique so that a part of the origin of the vastus lateralis muscle remained attached to the trochanteric fragment. Leaving the gluteal and vastus muscle attachments in combination with the short external rotators, English felt this musculotendinous sleeve would create a compressive force on the osteotomy site, preventing migration and encouraging rapid union (see Fig. 2C). After the osteotomy, the detached fragment is

turned on edge and held forward, and the hip is dislocated in a posterior direction. Reporting on 222 primary arthroplasties, of which 120 involved standard wire techniques for reattachment of the trochanter and 102 involved a bolt and bone graft, the rates of nonunion were 4.3% and 2.5%, respectively (27).

Fulkerson et al. modified this technique slightly by reflecting the gluteus medius and minimis laterally while developing a plane between these two muscles and the anterior head of the origin of the vastus lateralis (33). The osteotomy is then made from this anterior approach, keeping the gluteal and vastus muscles attached to the trochanter along with the short external rotators. They felt that by retracting the trochanteric fragment and its attached muscles posteriorly instead of anteriorly as described by English, the femoral canal might be more easily and accurately approached.

The need for greater exposure during revision hip surgery became evident in the 1980s, and techniques for facilitating this began to emerge. Glassman et al. described the sliding trochanteric osteotomy or anterior trochanteric slide (35). This technique is similar to the original description by English, but the external rotators are divided close to their insertion and preserved for reattachment after reapproximation of the trochanter. Glassman et al. originally reported on 90 hip arthroplasties (of which 88 were revision cases) and noted a 10% nonunion rate. Of the nine patients with trochanteric nonunions, cephalad trochanteric migration was seen in seven (mean, 7.1 mm; range, 2 to 26 mm). Seven additional hips had wire breakage. In no patient was the presence of a nonunion thought to be a significant source of pain and none required trochanteric reattachment. An abductor lurch was seen in 28% of the patients (23 hips). There were no early or late dislocations after a mean follow-up of 21 months (range, 1 to 3 years). A more recent report by Glassman et al. (34), of 129 revision procedures in which a sliding trochanteric osteotomy was utilized, demonstrated a nonunion rate of 13.9% (18 patients): in three, there was more than 2 cm trochanteric migration. There was also a 20.9% incidence of broken wires and a 4.6% rate of postoperative dislocations. Persistent abductor lurches were seen in 18.6%.

Lindgen and Svenson, using the same technique in 189 total hip arthroplasties (of which 39 were revision cases), noted a 2.1% incidence of nonunion and only one case of a postoperative dislocation (52).

Advantages of this technique include the wide exposure of the proximal femur and acetabulum, and its relative simplicity. The continuity of the vastus lateralis with the gluteus medius offers an added margin of safety against trochanteric migration should nonunion occur.

Technique

A standard posterior approach is utilized, centered over the greater trochanter. The fascia lata is divided into anterior and posterior flaps, and the approach follows the course of the gluteus maximus fibers proximally. The interval between the gluteus medius and the tensor fascia is developed anteriorly, exposing the joint capsule that is incised. Internally rotating the femur, the gluteus minimus and medius are identified just above the piriformis tendon, and the entire muscle mass of the gluteus medius is isolated bluntly from the underlying hip capsule working from posteriorly to anteriorly. The

external rotators are now isolated, tagged, and divided; then they are retracted in a posterior direction. The vastus lateralis is incised at a point 10 to 15 cm distal to the vastus ridge and 1 cm anterior to the lateral intermuscular septum. This muscle is now elevated subperiosteally from the anterior and lateral shaft of the femur and held forward with a retractor. The osteotomy is performed with an oscillating saw beginning just posterolateral to the insertion of the gluteus medius, so a that 1-cm-thick piece of the trochanter is removed proximally, and this tapers to about 0.5 cm just distal to the vastus ridge (Fig. 3A). The gluteus minimis should remain attached to the proximal femur. Should the gluteus minimis remain connected to the osteotomized trochanter, this may tend to tether the fragment anteriorly. After repair of the trochanter, this tethering effect may be a problem during external rotation of the femur, but its tendinous insertion can easily be released should this occur. The trochanter, in continuity with the gluteus medius and vastus lateralis, can now be retracted anteriorly, exposing the joint capsule (see Fig. 3B). Repair of the sliding osteotomy is accomplished with two 16- or 18-gauge wires passed through a single drill hole in the lesser trochanter. Two corresponding holes (one superior and one inferior) are drilled in the anterior and posterior cortex of the proximal femur and trochanteric bed. In revision situations or when the trochanteric bed is of poor quality, bone graft and the use of cables and a cable grip device may be necessary. Should significant lengthening occur, reattachment of the trochanter proximal to its original bed may be necessary. If this is not possible, subperiosteal elevation of the gluteus off the ilium may provide some lengthening, but this risks injury to the neurovascular pedicle. An alternative technique of shelling out the trochanteric fragment while preserving the myofascial sleeve of the gluteus medius and vastus lateralis is possible but not ideal. This sleeve is reinforced by suturing it to the undersurface of the posterior flap of the fascia lata and the insertion of the gluteus maximus tendon. No special precautions are necessary postoperatively; weight bearing as tolerated is allowed based on the stability of the prosthetic components and method of fixation.

Partial Trochanteric Osteotomy

Anterior trochanteric osteotomy has the advantage of preserving the continuity of the gluteus medius and vastus lateralis attachments anteriorly with a portion of the trochanter and leaving the posterior part of the gluteus medius intact. This transgluteal approach is a modification of the technique described by Hardinge (38). Dall reported on this technique in 69 primary total hip arthroplasties and noted no cases of nonunion, bursitis, or abductor lurches (22). Because the Hardinge direct lateral

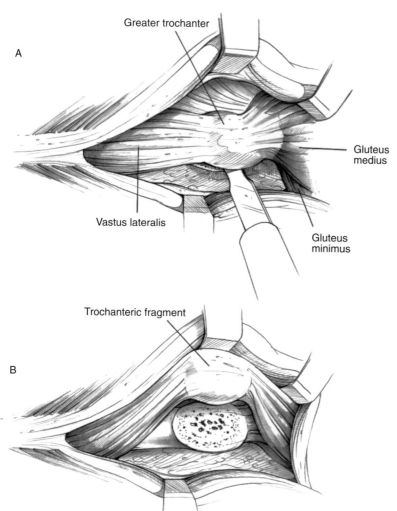

A

Greater trochanter

Gluteus
medius

Vastus lateralis

Gluteus
minimus

B

Trochanteric fragment

FIG. 3. A: The sliding trochanteric osteotomy performed with an oscillating saw, keeping the insertions of the vastus lateralis and gluteus medius in continuity (Glassman). **B:** The trochanteric fragment can now be retracted anteriorly, exposing the hip joint.

approach utilizes soft-tissue intervals only, Dall questioned the integrity and strength of this tendinous reattachment. He felt that a bone-on-bone repair was superior, with minimal risk of nonunion.

Technique (Dall)

In Dall's technique, the cutting diathermy is used to divide the insertion of the gluteus medius and vastus lateralis midway between the anterior and posterior margins of the greater trochanter, extending not more than 2 cm above the tip of the trochanter. The anterior margin of the gluteus medius is identified, and curved forceps are passed behind the gluteus medius and minimis and over the anterior capsule, exiting the original incision in the gluteus medius tendon. A Gigli saw is now passed deep to the vastus lateralis and gluteus medius and minimis with both ends exiting the original incision (Fig. 4A). Partial trochanteric osteotomy is now performed with the hip adducted, slightly flexed, and internally rotated (see

Fig. 4B). The tendency to take a very small fragment of bone is avoided by starting the saw cut in as posterior a direction as possible. A roughly triangular part of the anterior half of the greater trochanter is obtained, which carries with it the continuity of the anterior half of the gluteus medius with vastus lateralis, as well as the insertion of the gluteus minimus. The hip is now dislocated anteriorly (see Fig. 4C). Should there be concern about instability, Dall recommends this osteotomy be performed intracapsularly, passing the Gigli saw deep within the capsule and sawing in a more lateral direction to include the capsular insertion and to avoid taking an excessively large piece of bone. The trochanteric fragment can then be reattached with cerclage monofilament wires or cables. Harris et al. recently reported on a similar technique that they described as an oblique trochanteric osteotomy. The short external rotators are left attached to the femur and the posterior cut is superficial to the intertrochanteric ridge, whereas the anterior cut is wider and contains the insertion of both the gluteus medius and minimis (56).

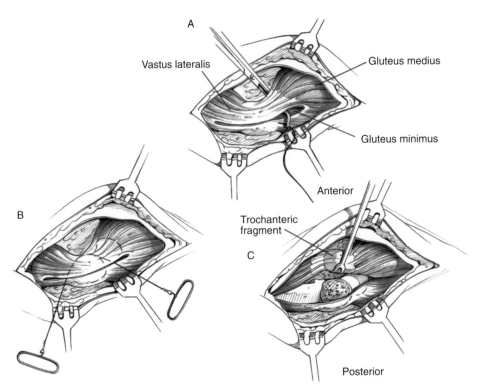

FIG. 4. A: The Gigli saw is passed deep to the gluteus medius and vastus lateralis insertions (Dall). **B:** The hip is adducted, flexed, and internally rotated prior to cutting the fragment. **C:** The trochanteric fragment is retracted anteriorly prior to dislocation.

Technique (Stracathro)

Another modification of the original technique described by McFarland and Osborne (55) is the Stracathro approach, in which exposure is obtained by elevating anterior and posterior slices of the greater trochanter with attachments of the gluteus medius and vastus lateralis proximally and distally and the external rotators posteriorly (Fig. 5) (57). The gluteus minimis is split or detached from the greater trochanter and the hip is dislocated anteriorly. Closure is a simple matter, with the trochanteric slices falling back into position and then being anchored with sutures into the soft tissues. In over 2000 total hip replacements at Stracathro Hospital in Scotland, McLauchlan noted trochanteric bursitis in under 1% of patients (57).

Although both of the above techniques keep the continuity of the gluteus medius and vastus lateralis tendons intact, their usefulness in revision settings is limited. Although there may be a place for these techniques in the occasional difficult primary hip arthroplasty that requires additional but not extensive exposure, they cannot be recommended to routinely obtain the wide exposure generally necessary during revision hip arthroplasty. Once there is a commitment to a partial trochanteric osteotomy, conversion to a trochanteric slide or standard osteotomy may be extremely difficult or impossible.

Myofascial Flap

A further modification of the McFarland approach was described by McMinn et al. of Birmingham, England, in 1991 (58). In this approach, a V-shaped flap with the apex distally, consisting of the belly and tendon of gluteus medius and minimis and part of the vastus lateralis with overlying fascia, is reflected proximally off the greater trochanter (Fig. 6A). The authors note that this approach rivals that which can be obtained with a standard trochanteric osteotomy without the complications of nonunion and migration. In their report on 100 revision THAs, 25 of the most difficult cases required this approach. Routine hip revisions are carried out through a posterior approach. Excellent exposure was noted in all cases and a sound reattachment was possible in all but one case. If the leg was lengthened by the revision procedure, the flap can be repaired as a V-Y plasty (see Fig. 6B). Postoperatively, the patient is kept in bed for 3 weeks with the leg in abduction. There were two cases of dislocation (8%), of which one was caused by component malposition. Functional assessment (measured clinically by grading of abductor power from 1 to 5) after 6 months noted that no patient had a decrease in abductor power or function using this approach.

Repair of myofascial flaps of the quadriceps mechanism, as well as the Achilles tendon, have generally been

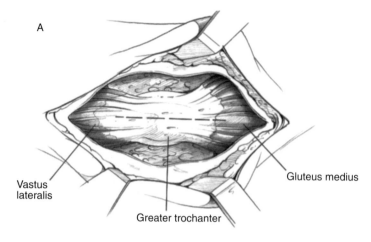

Vastus lateralis

Greater trochanter

Gluteus medius

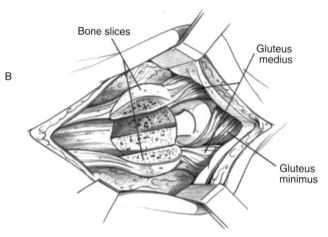

Bone slices

Gluteus medius

Gluteus minimus

FIG. 5. A,B: Elevating anterior and posterior slices of the trochanter with the insertions of the gluteus medius and vastus lateralis provides easy access to the hip joint (Stracathro).

because of the anatomy of the proximal femur. In these cases, a horizontal or short oblique osteotomy is performed as far proximal as possible, preserving the insertions of the abductors (Fig. 7A). The fragment should be of sufficient size, because reattachment may be possible only farther distal to the lateral femoral cortex. Because this type of osteotomy is cut at a greater angle (90° versus 45°), the frictional contact between the two surfaces is decreased, and greater stresses are placed on the fixation system. Bal et al. recently reported on 28 revision trochanteric osteotomies utilizing this technique and noted an 89% union rate (6). Fixation consisted of two horizontal and two vertical monofilament wires, adding mesh to distribute forces evenly on the trochanteric fragment.

In Charnley's original technique, the trochanteric fragment was advanced to the lateral femoral cortex (17). This technique is now only rarely used for tensioning of

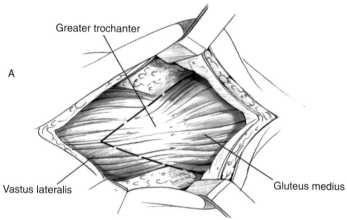

Greater trochanter

A

Vastus lateralis

Gluteus medius

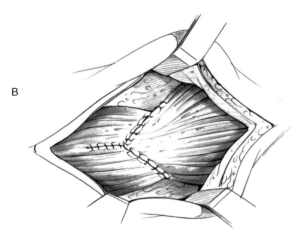

B

FIG. 6. A: Incision used to create the myofascial flap consists of the tendons of the gluteus medius, minimus, and part of the vastus lateralis (McMinn). **B:** V-Y plasty of the flap when the leg has been lengthened.

favorable. Although the hip abductors are an order of magnitude stronger than musculotendinous units that cross the knee and ankle joints, primary tendinous repair as recommended by McMinn et al. may be feasible. However, the abductor forces in a vertical plane are at least twice the body weight with normal walking (67). As the anteroposterior shearing forces can be up to 4 times body weight, any tendinous repair will be subject to a large amount of stress (16). The cancellous nature of osteotomy surfaces provides frictional resistance that is not obtained with this soft-tissue technique. However, there may be a place for this technique in the patient in whom a wide exposure is needed and trochanteric osteotomy is not feasible or possible.

Horizontal and Vertical Trochanteric Osteotomy

In certain revision situations, the use of a chevron-type osteotomy or trochanteric slide may not be possible

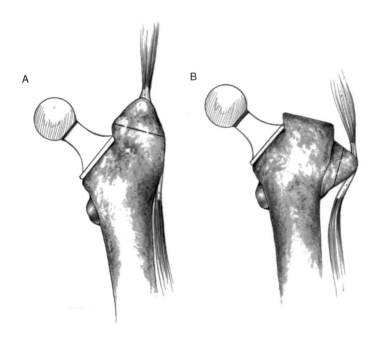

FIG. 7. A: A horizontal osteotomy may be necessary in cases where an adequate cancellous bed is not available. **B:** A vertical osteotomy is indicated in revision cases where the trochanter has previously been advanced to the lateral femoral cortex.

the abductors, as in the case of retention of a monoblock femoral component with an acetabular revision, or during femoral shortening. A compromised trochanteric bed may also necessitate distal transfer of the fragment. Once this fragment has healed to the lateral femoral cortex, a vertical trochanteric osteotomy is indicated parallel to the shaft of the femur. The vertical cut is 3 to 5 mm lateral to the femoral shaft, leaving an adequate bed of cancellous bone for reattachment (see Fig. 7B). Three horizontal wires or cables are used for reattachment. In the study by Bal et al., 10 of 10 osteotomies healed utilizing this technique (6). They found no statistical difference between the healing rates of union for vertical osteotomy, horizontal osteotomy, and standard osteotomy in the revision setting.

Extended Trochanteric Femoral Osteotomy

The surgeon faced with removal of well-fixed femoral implants during revision THA can find this to be an extremely difficult, time-consuming, and occasionally disastrous undertaking. The exposure afforded by a standard trochanteric osteotomy gives minimal access to ingrowth surfaces of cementless implants or the bone–cement interface of a standard cemented stem. In addition, cement remaining distal to the tip of a prosthesis usually requires removal prior to reimplantation. Attempts at removal of these implants and distal cement plugs with flexible osteotomes, high-speed burrs, and cement removal guides may cause damage to existing bone stock, with uncontrolled perforations of the femoral cortex, eccentric reaming, and an occasional total loss in continuity of the trochanteric portion of the femur to the remaining proximal femoral tube. Of equal concern in many revi-

sions is that reattachment of a standard trochanteric osteotomy may be adversely compromised because of the poor quality of the remaining trochanteric bed.

The use of a trochanteric osteotomy with distal extension was described by Cameron in 1991 for use in removal of a square-shouldered Moore cementless implant that had subsided and drifted laterally (14). He felt that removal of the prosthesis in this situation would result in avulsion of the greater trochanter, and the use of a classic trochanteric osteotomy would leave an unacceptable bed for trochanteric reattachment. The technique begins from a posterior or anterolateral exposure and consists of an osteotomy that extends from the tip of the trochanter to a variable point distal to the vastus tubercle where the horizontal osteotomy is made. The trochanteric fragment then includes one quarter to one third of the circumference of the femur, while retaining the gluteus medius and minimis attachments. After completion of the revision, the trochanteric fragment is held in place with cerclage wires and reinforced if necessary with a cortical allograft strut. Emerson and Head reported on the same technique, but their indications were for revision of cemented femoral components (68). They reported on 21 extended trochanteric osteotomies with no cases of trochanteric migration or broken wires. Four of the osteotomies had delayed healing but had united by 6 months.

Wagner also described in detail the extended trochanteric osteotomy with complete anatomic drawings (83). No published results could be found.

Taking advantage of the original technique by McFarland and Osborne, and modifying the technique described by Cameron, Paprosky et al. described a technique in which an intact muscle–osseous sleeve composed of a portion of the anterolateral proximal femur is removed with the greater trochanter, gluteus medius, and vastus lateralis (87). This technique combines the advantages of an extremely wide exposure of component fixation surfaces while preserving the soft-tissue attachments. The proximal femur is addressed via direct visualization, facilitating accurate and safe removal of cement as well as direct access to the bone–prosthesis interface of a well-fixed cementless implant. After component exchange, the osteotomy is replaced into its original bed and secured with several monofilament wires or cables.

The indications for the use of this extended proximal femoral osteotomy include the removal of any well-fixed cemented or cementless implant where access to the bone–cement or bone–prosthesis interface is necessary. Another indication would be in the patient with a failed femoral component that has subsided and standard techniques may risk a fracture of the greater trochanter. Performance of this osteotomy requires careful preoperative planning to determine the appropriate distal extent of the osteotomy so that all work can be adequately completed without unnecessarily compromising host bone. Paprosky et al. recommend that a fully coated cementless revision stem be used to bypass the osteotomy defect, and in this setting it is important to have at least 4 to 5 cm of diaphyseal fixation surface available distal to the extent of this osteotomy. Thus, there are occasions when this osteotomy cannot be extended further distally, because preoperative templating would preclude adequate distal fixation surface. Another option available is to cement a standard stem into the proximal femur. After replacement and securing of the trochanteric segment, the femoral canal is plugged distal to the osteotomy site and third-generation cementing techniques are employed. To prevent extravasation of the cement, Gelfoam can be packed into the gaps of the osteotomy site. Harris et al. recommend that a felt and lead shield be temporarily held in place over the osteotomy site with 0.5-inch hose clamps to facilitate cement pressurization and prevent cement extravasation (56). The hose clamps are then replaced with doubled monofilament wire. Although there are no published results of this option, several centers are currently employing this technique. Another technique available is the use of this osteotomy combined with an allograft bone-packing technique and a standard-length straight stem cemented in place. We have performed this procedure on cadaveric femurs, testing their rotational stability in 70° of flexion, and we noted no difference between these and models in whom no osteotomy was performed. There are now reports of surgeons using this option after an extended trochanteric osteotomy. Currently, only limited experience with these options is available, and the technique of bypassing the defect with a fully coated cementless device appears most reasonable until further studies demonstrate short-term survival of this

technique with cement or bone-impacting techniques used for reconstruction.

Technique

A standard posterior approach is utilized, followed by release of the external rotators off the trochanter and release of the gluteus maximus insertion. It is easier to perform this osteotomy after dislocation of the hip and maximal internal rotation of the femur. The vastus lateralis is elevated off the femur over the length of the proposed osteotomy and held forward with a Bennet retractor (Fig. 8A). Preoperative templating will assist the surgeon in determining the extent of the osteotomy distally, as measured from the tip of the greater trochanter or the vastus ridge. In the unlikely event that the femoral prosthesis is loose and can be removed prior to osteotomy, this can also be utilized as a guide. The osteotomy begins at the base of the greater trochanter proximally and extends distally, staying just anterior to the linea aspera to a predetermined point distal on the femoral shaft. A high-speed pencil burr is used to make multiple holes along the posterior osteotomy line extending through the femur to the anterolateral cortex, which is perforated (see Fig. 8B). A portion of bone representing approximately one third of the circumference of the femur is necessary. The posterior and distal drill holes are connected with either the burr or an oscillating saw. Wide osteotomes are now passed from posterior to anterior and used to crack open the previously perforated anterolateral cortex, hinging on the soft tissues (see Fig. 8C). The gluteus medius and minimis and the vastus lateralis remain attached to the trochanter and lateral femoral osteotomy segment that is retracted anteriorly as a single unit (see Fig. 8D). Direct access to the femoral canal is now possible.

After insertion of the revision prosthesis, the osteotomy fragment is shaped with a high-speed burr to remove any retained cement and to fit along the lateral shoulder of the implant. Multiple cables or monofilament wires are used to secure the fragment to the proximal femur. Should soft-tissue tensioning be necessary, the distal portion of the osteotomy fragment may be trimmed so that the entire musculo-osseous sleeve can be advanced distally. Finally, cancellous bone graft can be placed along the posterior and distal osteotomy junction. Should additional support be necessary in areas of weak bone, allograft strut grafts may be added to the lateral aspect of the construct and secured with wires or cables. After a standard closure, patients are allowed partial weight bearing as tolerated, based on fixation characteristics of the revision components. Although this osteotomy was designed for a posterior approach, a similar technique can be performed from an anterolateral plane as well, but protection of the sciatic nerve must be taken into consideration.

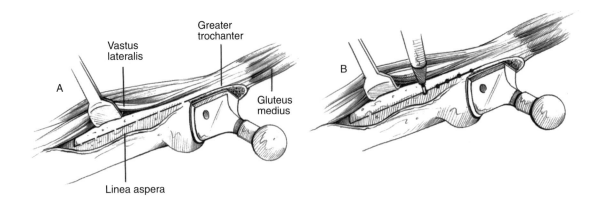

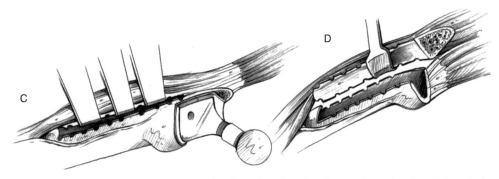

FIG. 8. A: The extended trochanteric osteotomy begins with elevating the vastus lateralis off the shaft of the femur (Paprosky). **B:** A high-speed burr is used to make multiple perforations from the base of the trochanter distally, staying just anterior to the linea aspera and perforating the anterolateral cortex. **C:** Wide osteotomes are now passed from posterior to anterior, cracking the perforated anterior cortex. **D:** The gluteus medius, minimis, and vastus lateralis remain attached to the trochanter and osteotomy segment, which is retracted anteriorly as a single unit.

Paprosky's group reported on 31 revision procedures, with an average follow-up period of 16 months (range, 9 to 24 months), in which this proximal femoral osteotomy was utilized (87). There were no complications relating to the procedure: no change in femoral component position, no breakage of cables or wires, and no change in preoperative Trendelenburg gait status. The osteotomy resulted in predictable clinical and/or radiographic union by 3 months, with callous formation present in most cases.

This type of extended trochanteric osteotomy may be indispensable for allowing access to the proximal femur for the removal of well-fixed cementless fully coated implants or retained distal cement. It is important, however, to realize that in performing this osteotomy, the tube of the proximal femur is disrupted, and thus its inherent stability to support a standard-length femoral component is affected. It is necessary to bypass this defect, which can be done by obtaining stability distally with a fully coated cementless implant. This usually means a 6-inch or an 8-inch stem, but on occasion a 10-inch curved stem is required. Should this stem fail in the future, revision may

be extremely difficult and an allograft prosthetic composite may be the only available reconstructive option. Other potential problems with the use of this osteotomy include the possibility of nonunion of the trochanteric fragment, fracture or fragmentation of the fragment, loss of fixation, poor bone contact apposition of the fragment because of the placement of a large femoral revision stem, and the necessity for multiple wires and/or cables to secure the fragment.

FIXATION TECHNIQUES

The likelihood of union after trochanteric osteotomy is influenced by several factors, including the type of fixation. The vast number of fixation devices and techniques to repair trochanteric osteotomies that have been introduced over the past 30 years is evidence of the inherent problems in trochanteric fixation, nonunion, and migration of the trochanteric fragment. Prior to adopting a particular technique, it is essential to understand the forces acting on the trochanteric fragment. It is a common misconception that the gluteus medius and minimis (which insert along the superior and anterior margins of the trochanter) exert their forces only in a near vertical plane, when actually the forces most likely to detach the trochanter are in an anteroposterior plane, creating rotational forces when the knee and hip are in a flexed position (16). These forces can be up to 4 times body weight, compared to those acting in a vertical plane, which are at least 2 times body weight. For any fixation system to be effective, it must resist the forces in these planes while providing compression across the cancellous surfaces to increase frictional resistance. The type of osteotomy utilized may assist in controlling these forces; for example, in those osteotomies that maintain continuity of the vastus lateralis, the muscles retained on the trochanteric fragment may help prevent superior trochanteric migration and subsequent displacement. The chevron type of trochanteric osteotomy provides additional frictional resistance and rotational control by its geometric configuration. The extended trochanteric osteotomy has a portion of the lateral cortex of the femoral shaft to provide additional bone surface for union and fixation stability. The trochanteric size, shape, bone quality, soft-tissue attachments, and trochanteric bed all play integral roles in fixation and subsequent healing of this fragment. Should any of these factors be compromised, healing rates may be adversely affected. It is therefore important to understand that for any successful fixation system to work properly, the bone surfaces must be in continuity with one another and ideally should be compressed. Bone ischemia from impaired blood supply at the osteotomy site may also be associated with delayed healing and slow revascularization (63). As with any fracture fixation device, the race between bone union and device failure begins at the time of fixation.

Charnley was insistent about obtaining exposure for THA through the transtrochanteric approach. Recognizing the disadvantages of a nonunited trochanter, he felt that trochanteric reattachment tests a surgeon's natural mechanical instincts (16). In his very early days of hip arthroplasty at Wrightington (1958 to 1962), the trochanteric fragment was completely displaced and reattached to the lateral aspect of the femur with one wire (19). Patients were placed in hip spica casts and there were no cases of nonunion. It was not until early rehabilitation was introduced that nonunion became an issue, according to Charnley (16).

Charnley studied the rotational forces acting on the trochanteric fragment and displacing it anteriorly, and his wiring technique was based on his findings. He felt that failure of trochanteric union was caused by failure to achieve and maintain perfect fixation during a critical 3-week period postoperatively (18). This occurred in two phases: the first phase begins when the pull of the abductors separates the osteotomy by the thickness of the necrosed soft tissue beneath the loops of wire, and the second occurs when the direction of the pull of the abductors changes. This pull is initially in line with the axis of the femur in extension, and then a shearing force is created by flexion of the hip and pull of the abductors in an anterior direction. Cyclic anteroposterior movement of the trochanter both abrades the cancellous surface of the osteotomy and results in fatigue fracture of the wires. Despite the thousands of trochanteric osteotomies performed by Charnley (with his superb surgical and mechanical skills), a 5% radiographic nonunion rate persisted. Those surgeons with less technical abilities reported nonunion rates 2 to 3 times higher (16).

An experimental test apparatus to examine various fixation techniques was soon developed by Charnley, and his cruciate wiring technique became the recommended choice for trochanteric reattachment (16). This system consists of two separate wires, one medial (superior) that acts as a pulley, and one lateral (inferior) that pulls down on the pulley. This is combined with a vertical double loop of wire that anchors the trochanter in position while the cruciate system is being woven through the fibers of the abductor muscles close to the surface of the trochanter. The special feature of this cruciate system is that, because the pulley system is being incorporated into the lateral (inferior) wire, tightening of this last wire distributes the forces to all four limbs of the cross simultaneously. In addition, the pulley system tends to multiply the force and compensate for force lost in frictional resistance. The wire of the vertical double loop is not considered part of the cruciate system, even though it contributes two more arms, giving the final cross a total of six radial arms. This method of fixation appears simple, secure, and reliable, but practicing on a plastic model would be advantageous for the hip surgeon with limited trochanteric osteotomy experience.

Monofilament wire has been the mainstay of trochanteric fixation. Multiple variations of techniques, using two, three, or four wires, are reported (Fig. 9) (8,12,20, 44,74,86). The Charnley two-wire and three-wire techniques are probably the most widely used. In reviewing the abundant literature on the various wire fixation techniques, attempting to determine the best wiring configuration is difficult. All of the variables in each study (patient population, primary or revision procedure, the use of mesh, bone union versus fibrous union, trochanteric migration, distal advancement of the trochanter, functional significance, and postoperative protocol) make comparisons difficult. Nonunion rates are reported from 1% to 25% based on these variables (see Table 1). Reports comparing different wiring techniques have been performed *in vivo* and *in vitro*, but all suffer from the large number of variables present. Testing several different wiring techniques on fresh cadaver specimens, Markoff et al. found all of the trochanters displaced when a 27-kg load was applied (59). The Harris and Charnley

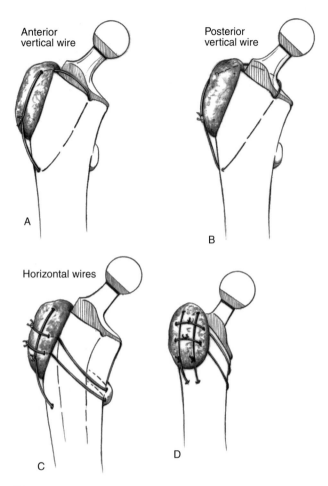

FIG. 9. A–D: The four-wire technique of trochanteric reattachment is simple and reproducible, and it yields a 97% union rate (Harris).

configurations (three wires and four wires, respectively) displaced least (0.7 mm) when repeated loadings (0 to 27 kg) were performed from the previous rest position. Other authors have shown that the type of wiring configuration has little influence on the rate of union or amount of superior migration (86).

Monofilament stainless steel wire (16 or 18 gauge) continues to be the most popular cerclage material, based on its strength, availability, and low cost. Cobalt-chrome-molybdenum (CoCrMo) takes advantage of an increased yield strength and mechanical properties superior to stainless steel. Titanium wires are advocated by some because of their biocompatability and low modulus of elasticity. In comparing these three materials for the use in a monofilament cerclage wire application, CoCr has the advantage of being stronger, although it is stiffer and thus more difficult to work with. In addition, while twisting the CoCr wire, it has more of a tendency to break than to stretch as the more elastic stainless steel and titanium do (37). Titanium wire seems to be the least suitable for cerclage application, based on its notch sensitivity and its

low-modulus of elasticity that leads to lack of an end point in tightening, resulting in overstretching and weakening of the wire.

Charnley originally stated that "wire breakage is never due to tension except at the moment of tightening by the surgeon" (18). The ability to keep sufficient tension on the wire and secure this adequately has created a niche in the instrument market for various wire tighteners. The use of a Kirschner traction bow for wire tightening has the disadvantage of causing difficulty in releasing tension while pulling and twisting the wire. If tension is not released while twisting a wire, then it is overstretched and weakened and will usually break at the first twist. Those materials with a lower modulus of elasticity (stainless steel and titanium) have a lesser tendency to fracture, and thus are more forgiving. However, if too much tension is released prior to twisting, then the cerclage loop becomes loose and loss of fixation may result. The perfect twist should be a symmetrical spiraling of both wires through two to three full twists while maintaining tension across the osteotomy site.

The use of a square knot has been advocated by some authors, and in laboratory testing it appears that this knot is superior to twisting (922 newtons versus 516 N) (Fig. 10) (37). However, the ability to maintain tension on the wire while tying a square knot is both difficult and inconsistent. Even with the use of specialized wire tighteners, the ability to maintain tension after the first throw requires the use of fine needle-nose pliers that can easily notch the wire. Oh has demonstrated that a nick in the wire as small as 1% of its diameter can result in a 63% reduction in its fatigue life (66).

Liu and O'Conner (53) found a stainless steel hose clamp superior to monofilament wire and the Dall-Miles cable system (23) for generating and maintaining com-

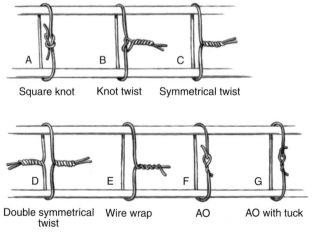

FIG. 10. Although the use of a square knot appears to be superior to twisting, maintaining tension is extremely difficult. Twisting remains the most consistent method of fastening monofilament wire.

pressive forces on a bone model. They recommend the use of a 0.5-inch stainless steel hose clamp to apply the compression during fixation of an extended osteotomy or allograft plates, followed by doubled monofilament wire. The hose clamps are then removed (53,56).

Wroblewski and Shelley , unhappy with the standard monofilament wire and the inherent problem of loss of compression across the osteotomy site, designed a self-tightening wire system that incorporated a compression spring (Fig. 11A) (86). A double cross-over wire is passed first and secured, followed by two 18-gauge wires with end crimps that are passed through the spring in opposite directions, compressing the spring fully, and then secured over the mid portion of the trochanter (see Fig. 11B). The spring lies on the anterior portion of the femoral neck (see Fig. 11C). With an amplitude of 0.75 cm, and when fully closed, the device delivers a compression force of about 25 lb (111 N) of constant pressure across the osteotomy site.

Evaluating 431 hip arthroplasties (half revisions), Wroblewski and Shelley compared this compression spring system to the standard Charnley cruciate wire method and the double- and single-wire method of Boardman et al. (12) and found a 98.2% union rate with the use of the compression spring system (86). Unfortunately, other authors have found no advantage to the use of the spring system compared to other techniques (26,64,79).

Retaining the versatility of wire without the tendency for kinking, Dall and Miles designed a multifilament cable system that had mechanical properties that were far superior to monofilament wire (23). With a better resistance to fatigue and a higher yield and breaking strength (78), the CoCr cable was combined with a trochanteric

grip to provide secure fixation of the trochanteric fragment. This system allowed the cable to be crimped in place while maintaining equal force on each end of the cable strands with a specially designed tensioning device. A series of bench tests were conducted to compare this system to the two-wire, three-wire, and Charnley staple clamp (which was combined with the three-wire system). Vertical deflection and anteroposterior deflection were highest with the two- and three-wire systems and considerably lower with the cable-grip system (23). Similar findings were noted by Hersh et al. comparing three methods of trochanteric fixation in a cadaver model. Utilizing 16-gauge monofilament wire, 2.0-mm cable, and the Dall-Miles cable-grip system, they noted that the forces needed to displace the trochanter 1 cm were significantly greater for the cable-grip system than for the cable and wire group (1397 N, 757 N, and 771 N, respectively) (40).

In a series of 321 osteotomies using this cable-grip system, cable breakage of 6% with a 1.6-mm cable and a nonunion rate of 4% were reported (23). In a subset of 130 patients followed for 4 years using a 2.0-mm cable, the incidence of breakage was 3% and the nonunion rate, 2%. Unfortunately, the report did not differentiate between primary and revision cases. Turner et al. reported on the results of the Dall-Miles system, noting a 2% nonunion rate in 251 trochanteric osteotomies, of which 43% (109 patients) had undergone a previous osteotomy (80).

Unfortunately, other studies have not shown such encouraging results. Ritter et al., using the same system with stainless steel cables, reported on 40 hips (of which 16 were revisions and 24 primary arthroplasties) and noted a nonunion rate of 38% and cable breakage in 33% (70). Johnston et al. reported a retrospective review of

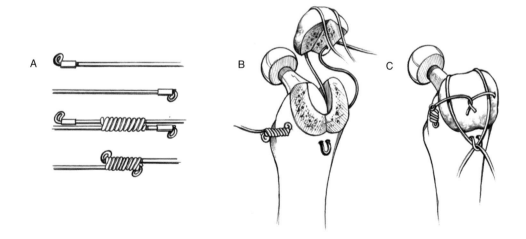

FIG. 11. A: A self-tightening wire system that incorporates a compression spring (Wroblewski). **B:** The compression spring places continuous pressure (25 lb) across the osteotomy site, theoretically facilitating union. **C:** The spring lies anterior on the base of the femoral neck.

322 transtrochanteric osteotomies comparing two methods of fixation in primary cases only: 162 repaired with stainless steel monofilament wire and 160 with 1.5-mm CoCr cable (Zimmer, Warsaw, IN) (47). Trochanteric nonunion rates were 25% for the wire group and 21% for the cable group. Wire breakage was seen in 43% (68 patients), and cable breakage was seen in 12% (20 patients). Our recent review of 68 osteotomies (7 primary and 59 revision arthroplasties) that were repaired with the Dall-Miles system showed a nonunion rate of 25% (17 patients) and a cable breakage rate of 22% (15 patients) (75). Comparing two similar groups of primary Charnley hip replacements, one group fixed with the Dall-Miles cable grip system and the other group fixed with the Wroblewski spring wire technique, Teanby et al. found an astonishing 29% nonunion rate in each group (79).

Galline and Soria utilized a plate and cable system for trochanteric fixation in which the plate is fixed to the lateral shaft of the femur and the two vertical cables secure the trochanteric fragment (Fig. 12). They reported only one case of nonunion in the 61 patients in whom this device was utilized (1.6%) (72).

Although the idea of a multifilament cable system is attractive, the overall nonunion rate and cable breakage rate in studies other than Dall and Miles' series is of concern. Larger and stronger fixation devices do not necessarily translate into higher rates of union and lower rates of trochanteric migration. Similar findings have been noted in nonunions of long bones where bigger and stronger plates have not led to an increase in the rate of healing. The bone biology at the fracture site has more of an influence on healing than the fixation device. This certainly holds true as well in trochanteric fixation. As for the strength of a particular cable or wire, it is interesting to note that a recent report showed that the compression force generated by a doubled monofilament 18-gauge wire was similar to that generated by a 1.6-mm and 2.0-mm cable (53). In another study, cable fastened with a standard CoCr crimping sleeve decreased the tensile strength of the cerclage cable system by 25% compared to cable fastened with a square knot; however, there was elongation of the system fastened with a square knot (30). Cable and cable-grip devices will continue to outperform monofilament wire in bench tests and quasistatic loading tests (23,40,78). However, this is not representative of the *in vivo* situation, as evidenced by the multiple reports of unacceptable cable breakage and nonunion rates (Table 2).

Recognizing the mechanical limitations of monofilament wire, Volz et al. designed a bolt assembly for mechanical fixation of the osteotomized trochanter (81,82). The system consisted of four parts: an angulated intramedullary bolt that is seated in the cemented lateral portion of the proximal femur, an interface shear washer, an outer compressive washer, and a self-locking nut (Fig. 13). Evaluating 229 trochanters after primary THA, Volz and Turner (82) had three trochanteric nonunions (1.3%). They credited the high yield strength of the bolt compared to 16-gauge monofilament wire (340 kg versus 41

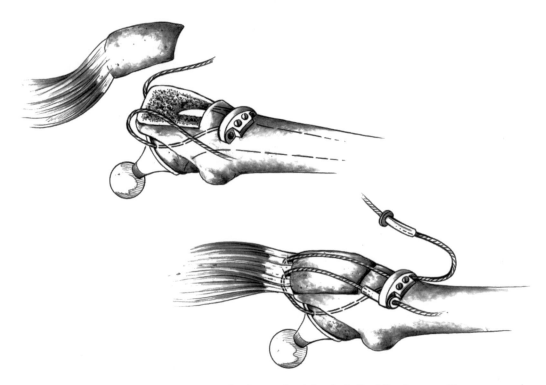

FIG. 12. A cable device providing secure fixation to the lateral shaft of the femur with screws and a cephalad-directed blade (Galline and Soria).

TABLE 2. *Trochanteric fixation with cable devices*

Author (ref.)	Dall and Miles (23)		Ritter et al. (70)	Turner et al. (80)		Johnson and Kelley (45)	Silverton et al. (75)	Soria et al. (72)
Osteotomy type	Flat	Flat	Flat	Flat	Dome	Dome	Flat	Flat
Total patients	62	130	40	272	160	162	68	61
Primary/revision	N/A	N/A24/16	21/251	160/0	162/0	7/59		
Fixation	CoCr 1.6-mm cable-grip	CoCr 2.0-mm cable-grip	Stainless steel 1.6-mm cable-grip	CoCr 2.0-mm cable-grip	CoCr 1.5-mm cable, square knot	Stainless steel 3-wire (two vertical; one horizontal)	CoCr 1.6-mm and 2.0-mm cable-grip	Plate with cable
Nonunion	3 (4.8%)	2 (1.5%)	15 (38%)	0/5 (2%)	13 (8%)	21 (13%)	14 (21%)	1 (1.5%)
Fibrous union	2 (3.2%)	1 (<1%)	N/A	N/A	21 (13%)	19 (12%)	3 (4%)	
Migration with union	N/A	N/A	N/A	N/A				7 (11.5%)
Delayed union	N/A	N/A	N/A	N/A	4 (2.5%)			
Reoperation	N/A	N/A	N/A	5 (2%)	20 (12%)	0	11 (16%)	6 (9.8%)
Breakage	5 (8%)	4 (3.1%)	13 (33%)	22 (8%)	90 (56%)	68 (43%)	15 (22%)	N/A
Fraying/fragmentation	N/A	N/A	N/A	41 (15%)		0	30 (44%)	3 (4.7%)
Calcar lysis and lesser trochanter			N/A		42 (26%)	15 (9%)	7 (10%)	
Debris migration to inferior acetabulum			N/A		25 (16%)	13 (8%)	8 (12%)	

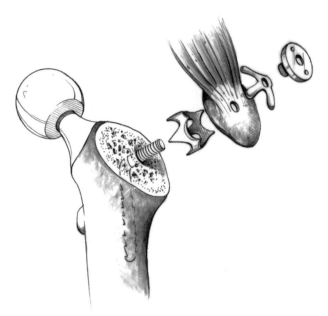

FIG. 13. An angulated bolt is seated in the cemented proximal femur and the trochanteric fragment is secured with a shear washer, outer washer, and nut (Volz).

kg) as a factor in their high success rate. Gottschalk et al. also designed a mechanical system for reattachment of the trochanter (36). Their system consisted of a U-bolt through the shoulder of the femoral prosthesis, along with a toothed clamp and two nuts to obtain firm fixation of the trochanter (Fig. 14). In using this system and comparing various positions of trochanteric reattachment,

they found any superomedial tilt of the trochanter leads to a delay in healing and is associated with a high incidence of nonunion. They concluded that stable fixation alone cannot prevent nonunion of the trochanteric osteotomy (36).

Scher et. al. designed a new method of fixation for trochanteric stabilization to be used in difficult revision hip arthroplasties (73). The fixator is secured to the metaphysis of the femur with two or three screws, and its two malleable prongs encompass the trochanter fragment and stabilize it using the tension-band principle (Fig. 15). In reviewing 49 revisions after a mean follow-up of 40 months, there was bony union in 46 of the 49 hips, the remaining three developing stable fibrous union. There were no cases of migration of the trochanter. Courpied and Postel reported on the use of a similar device, securing it to the femur with horizontal wires rather than screws (Fig. 16). They reported a success of 19 established nonunions treated with this device (21). We have no experience with these devices, but, because the fixator rests over the lateral aspect of the femur and trochanter, one would be concerned about a high incidence of trochanteric bursitis (Table 3).

Regardless of which device is stronger, the question that remains is how much strength is actually necessary to maintain position of the trochanter until healing

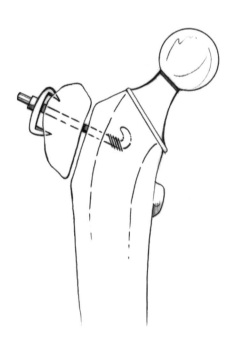

FIG. 14. The use of a U-bolt for fixation of the trochanteric fragment (Gottschalk).

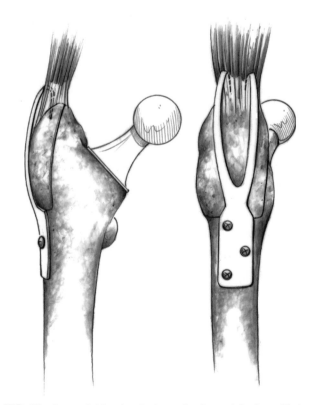

FIG. 15. A special trochanteric reattachment device with two malleable prongs that encompass the trochanter and stabilize it using the tension band principle (Scher).

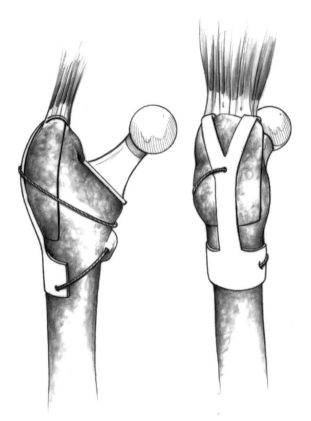

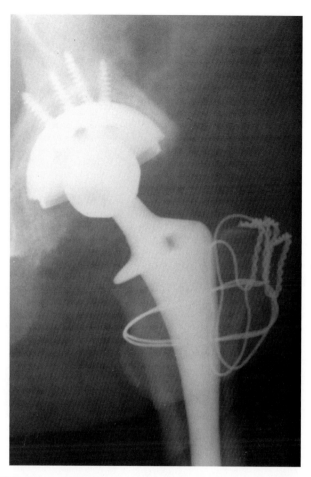

FIG. 16. A similar reattachment device (see Fig. 13) for holding the trochanter with cerclage wires (Courpied and Postel).

FIG. 17. A well-healed trochanteric osteotomy with a three-wire technique (two vertical and one double horizontal). Although the use of multiple twists in the wire appears very elegant on the radiograph, adding more than two full twists does not provide any additional strength and probably only contributes to trochanteric bursitis.

occurs. All fixation cables, wires, screws, and bolts may eventually work harden and break, with or without union of the trochanter. Based on a review of all studies concerning reattachment of the trochanter, it is reasonable to use 16-gauge or 18-gauge monofilament wire (stainless steel or CoCr) with a minimum of three and preferably four wires for fixation (two vertical and two horizontal) (Fig. 17). It is beyond the scope of this chapter to describe in detail the various wiring configurations available. The use of mesh to supplement wire fixation has been advocated by some authors and appears to be a reasonable alternative in selected cases where a weakened, small, or osteoporotic trochanter may be cut by the tensioning of

the monofilament wires (Fig. 18) (74). Additional fixation will be needed with cases of extended trochanteric osteotomies. Cables should be used only in those cases where an obvious delayed union will occur and the additional strength of this system will be of benefit (Fig. 19). The routine use of cables with their inherent problems of fraying, fretting, and fragmentation should be limited

TABLE 3. *Trochanteric fixation with other devices*

Author (ref.)	Courpied and Postel (21)	Scher and Jakim (73)	Volz and Turner (82)	Gottshalk et al. (36)
Total patients	100	49	229	85
(primary/revision)	(84/16)	(0/49)		(85/0)
Osteotomy type	Flat	Flat	Flat	Flat
Fixation	Plate—Stainless steel	Malleable plate	Bolt U-bolt	
Nonunion	3 (3%)	0	3 (1.3%)	9 (10.6%)
Fibrous union			3 (6%)	
Breakage of device			N/A	7 (8%)
Reoperations	N/A	N/A	2 (1%)	

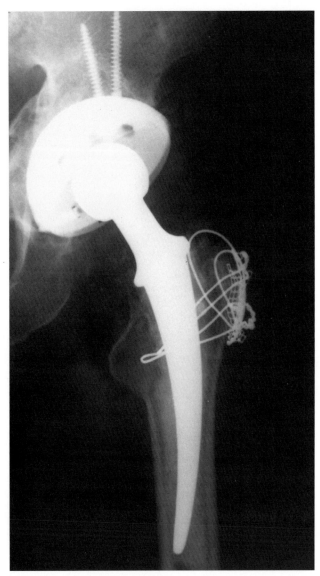

FIG. 18. Mesh is used successfully to provide support and prevent the wires from cutting through the trochanter in the osteoporotic bones of this patient.

(75). Attention to detail in applying the cable-grip system is essential to prevent early failure of the device (Fig. 20).

BONE GRAFTING

In an attempt to facilitate union of the greater trochanter, Stefanich et al. reported on 286 hip arthroplasty procedures performed with a transtrochanteric approach (77). All trochanters were advanced 1 to 2 cm distally and reattached using a three-wire technique. In 111 procedures (of which 26 were revisions), cancellous bone grafting was performed, and in the remaining 175 procedures, no bone grafting was performed. Although there was no statistically significant difference in the

overall incidence of trochanteric nonunion between the two groups, a lower incidence of trochanteric nonunion was found in the grafted group (2.7%) than in the nongrafted group (5.7%) which included the patients undergoing revision arthroplasty.

Although this study does not specifically support the concept of bone grafting the trochanter to increase the likelihood of and reduce time to bony union, we recommend bone grafting in the face of a questionable trochanteric bed. Even based on these results, there may be a partial beneficial effect of cancellous bone grafting after trochanteric osteotomy.

COMPLICATIONS

Management of Trochanteric Nonunion, Bursitis, and Trochanteric Loss

The two major problems relating to trochanteric osteotomy are nonunion of the trochanter and peritrochanteric bursitis. Trochanteric nonunion may lead to pain, a limp, and postoperative dislocations, whereas bursitis is usually an annoying complication secondary to implanted fixation devices.

If nonunion is present radiographically, complaints of trochanteric pain may or may not be related to the nonunion. Several studies have compared healed trochanters

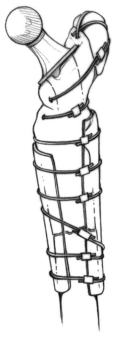

FIG. 19. The routine use of cables should be avoided because of subsequent fraying, fretting, and fragmentation. However, in cases of allograft fixation or in cases where delayed union may be expected, the added strength may be of benefit.

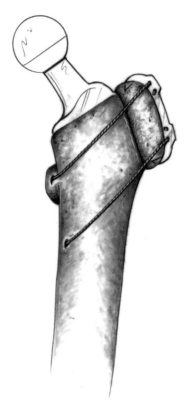

FIG. 20. To prevent a bucket handle effect on the trochanter, cables should be separated by at least 3 cm and placed through predrilled holes (Dall-Miles Cable-Grip System).

to those with nonunion and have found no difference in pain distribution (10,17,51,71). Because most patients with trochanteric nonunions have a stable fibrous union, it is not reasonable to attribute a patient's complaint of pain to a radiographic finding of trochanteric nonunion without further confirmatory findings such as tenderness over the trochanter and gross motion of the ununited segment associated with pain. Other sources of the pain should be ruled out (17).

The prominence of fixation devices over the trochanteric region (including cables, bolts, clamps, screws, and wires) may be responsible for many patients' complaints. It is easy to understand how these mechanical devices would cause local irritation. However, even after removal of these devices, pain relief is inconsistent. In a series by Bernard and Brooks, 36 patients with trochanteric bursitis underwent removal of trochanteric fixation wires and successful relief of pain was obtained in less than half the cases (10). Additionally, they found no difference in pain relief after the removal of intact wires versus broken wires, or trochanters with union versus nonunion. They concluded that pain in the region of the trochanter may well arise from sources other than the radiographically obvious coexisting abnormality of trochanteric fixation, which is frequently revised with poor results. In a patient with peritrochanteric pain complaints, a trial injection of

local anesthetic should be attempted prior to any operative intervention. Patients should also be aware that removal of the device will not guarantee pain relief.

Trochanteric nonunion has been cited as a causative factor in postoperative dislocations. This loss or decrease of the abductor tension across the hip after nonunion would appear to be a plausible explanation for dislocations (4). Several authors have reported dislocation rates to be higher with trochanteric nonunions (15). However, other authors have found no association between dislocation and trochanteric nonunion. Woo and Morrey found a higher rate of dislocation with the posterior approach as compared to the trochanteric approach (60,88). One explanation for this may be that the exposure afforded by removal of the trochanter lessens the likelihood of component malposition, which still remains the most common cause of early dislocations (48,50). The ability to advance the trochanter and increase myofascial tension has been cited as an advantage in minimizing postoperative dislocations, but with the use of prostheses with increased offset and modular heads to adjust neck lengths, this may not play as important a role as in the past with the Charnley-type prosthesis. In the report by Woo and Morrey on 10,500 total hip arthroplasties, of which 8944 underwent a lateral transtrochanteric osteotomy (60,88), nonunion developed in 194 and dislocations occurred only in those patients whose trochanter migrated proximally greater than 2 cm [34 patients (17.6%)]. Those patients with a fibrous nonunion and migration less than 2 cm did not have an increase in the rate of dislocation. They concluded that migration of the trochanter (farther than 2 cm) increased the frequency of postoperative instability sixfold. It is thus reasonable to assume that nonunion of the trochanter will occur in about 5% of cases and, of those, approximately 15% will be unstable.

Instability after THA is a complex, multifactorial phenomenon. When evaluating patients who have presented with postoperative dislocations, nonunion of the trochanter must be considered along with other possible causes, which include malposition of components, soft-tissue impingement, traumatic episodes, sepsis, stretching of the pseudocapsule, and muscle imbalance. Once these other causes are ruled out, advancement and reattachment of the trochanter may be indicated. Kaplan et al. reported on 21 hips with recurrent dislocation and no identifiable cause other than presumed abductor weakness (46). All of the hips underwent trochanteric advancement and recurrent dislocation was eliminated in 17 patients. In two of the four failures, there was trochanteric nonunion and migration farther than 1 cm.

The persistence of a limp after trochanteric nonunion is not unexpected. The degree of trochanteric migration probably represents the primary factor responsible for the limp rather than the radiographic finding of a nonunion (71). Nutton and Checketts showed that displacement of the trochanter of 1 cm or less will almost invariably leave the power of the hip abductor muscles unimpaired (65). However, displacement of more than 1 cm is likely to cause abductor weakness, whether bony union occurs or not. The greater the displacement, the greater the likelihood of an unsatisfactory lurching gait and of a generally poorer clinical result. Amstutz and Maki, in a report on 728 hips of which 5% developed nonunions, found abductor weakness in 50% of patients. With nonunions, weakness was most profound when trochanteric migration was greater than 2 cm (2). It is clear from these reports that the degree of proximal migration of the trochanter is of greater importance than radiographic nonunion in the overall function of the replaced hip. Results of advancement and reattachment of the trochanter in the absence of instability may not improve the clinical result. Unless there is clear reason that the patient originally developed a trochanteric nonunion, the likelihood of a second procedure succeeding is doubtful.

Baker and Coventry reported on 40 patients with nonunion of the trochanter who presented with pain, instability, or weakness; they were able to achieve a 66% union rate (5). Reoperations for trochanteric nonunion and bursitis are not to be taken lightly. Unless one is reasonably sure of the cause for the pain, limp, or instability, results have been less than satisfying. Those surgeons confronted with reattachment of a migrated trochanter should use all possible means to achieve a stable fixation, including cables and a cable-grip device, being fully aware that these additional fixation devices frequently cause trochanteric bursitis by themselves. Should the cancellous bone bed be compromised, iliac bone grafting may be indicated. After replacement of the trochanter, if it is necessary to abduct the hip to oppose the trochanter against the shaft of the femur, the hip may need to be kept in this abducted position for at least 6 weeks in a cast or brace, with delayed weight bearing for 3 to 6 months until healing is complete.

Surgical Technique

Release of the abductors off the iliac crest and/or Z-lengthening of the tendinous portion of the abductors can be attempted to gain additional length. Injury to the superior gluteal nerve (located less than 5 cm proximal to the tip of the greater trochanter) may occur when attempting subperiosteal dissection of the abductors off the ilium (1,43,62). To slide this muscle mass distal, sharp dissection can be used to remove the proximal attachment of the abductors off the iliac crest. This may require a separate incision. Immobilization in a hip spica cast or brace for at least 6 to 8 weeks is recommended to allow the muscle to scar down to its new bed. If this salvage technique is utilized, it is imperative to pay attention to the superior gluteal neurovascular bundle as it exits the sciatic notch to prevent inadvertent injury. Although the complete

mobilization of the abductor mass is utilized occasionally in complex acetabular fractures (e.g., the Rheinhart approach) (69), and these patients regain function of their abductors, the revision patient with scarred periprosthetic tissue and bone loss creates a less-than-ideal environment for healing of the trochanter and soft tissues.

Recent studies have shown that combining a trochanteric slide with proximal dissection of the soft tissues (gluteus medius and minimis) will cause almost complete arrest of blood supply to the greater trochanter (63). Although we have limited experience with this technique, it seems reasonable to caution against its use except in the occasional case where reattachment of the trochanter cannot be accomplished without this mobilization.

Trochanteric loss or avulsion of the abductors off the trochanter creates a special situation. Often, stability of the hip is compromised and a constrained component must be utilized. Attempting to reattach a small fragment of bone or the remnants of the abductors to a trochanteric bed is futile. Shortening of the femur, rotation of the anterior portion of the gluteus medius, subperiosteal elevation of the abductors off the ilium, and reattachment of the remaining abductors to the posterior tensor fascia may all be tried. Occasionally, after shortening of the femur, the abductors can be directly attached to the vastus lateralis insertion. Regardless of the method utilized in these difficult situations, coverage of the prosthesis with a muscular sleeve is imperative. Immobilization in a hip spica for 3 months is usually required.

Wires and Cables

Monofilament wire has been the standard fixation device for reapproximation of the trochanter since the late 1950s. Reports of complications secondary to the wire have been rare. Proper placement of the wires is important, as inadvertent soft-tissue entrapment may have devastating consequences (Fig. 21) (54). Migrating wire fragments have been reported occasionally in the past, but their significance has yet to be determined (13). Radiographic evaluations of hip arthroplasty have, however, shown a significant number of wire fractures even in the presence of healed trochanters (see Table 1). Several authors have reported wire breakage rates of up to 33%, but the significance of this number relates to those wires that fracture early and are associated with subsequent loss of trochanteric position (3,9,25,32). Clark et al., in evaluating 92 patients with trochanteric osteotomy fixed by wires, noted that 50% had early wire fracture (less than 6 weeks) along with trochanteric migration. Their conclusion, and that of multiple other authors, was that wires and other fixation devices probably have only a minor role after the first 6 weeks (9,20,25,32). Although this may be true in the uncomplicated, primary hip arthroplasty, in the revision setting the race between trochanteric fixation device failure and trochanteric union

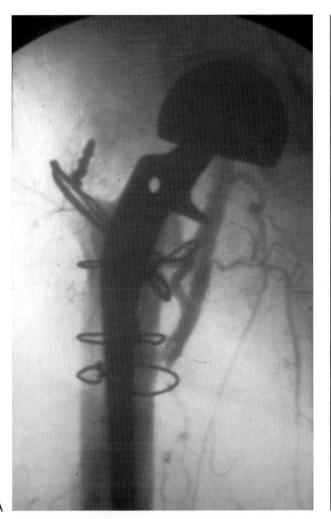
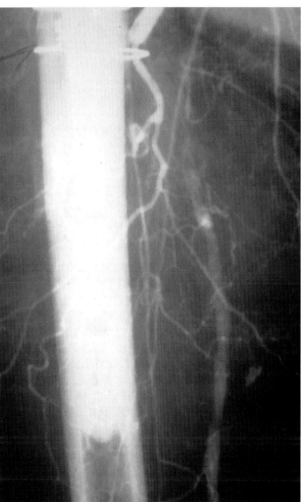

A   B

FIG. 21. A,B: Inappropriate placement of a cable or wire can have catastrophic consequences, as shown by this cerclage wire compromising the femoral artery.

remains competitive. The need for stronger fixation devices prompted the development of cable-grip systems.

Complications unique to cables revolves around the issues of fretting, cable fragmentation, and debris migration. Although there is no question that a multistrand cable is significantly stronger in both fatigue and static tensile strength than monofilament wire, no one has demonstrated that the use of monofilament wire is inferior to a cable system in a prospective randomized study.

Although Dall and Miles reported union rates of 97% using a cable grip, only a few were in the revision setting (23). Harris et al. have reported union rates of 97% with monofilament wire in the revision setting (44,74). If equally good results can be obtained with monofilament wire or cable fixation, then the complications of these fixation systems should be addressed. Johnson et al. compared two groups of patients who were undergoing primary THA via a transtrochanteric approach (47). Of 643 hips, 322 were reattached with stainless steel monofilament wire and 322 with CoCr cable using a three-wire/cable technique (two vertical and one horizontal). Trochanteric union rates were 75% (122 patients) for the wire group and 79% (126 patients) for the cable. Wires broke in 43% of cases (68 hips) and cables in 12% (20 hips). However, migration of wire and cable fragments or debris to the acetabular notch was seen in 8% of the wire cases (13 hips) and 16% of the cable cases (25 hips). They found an increased incidence of acetabular loosening secondary to the cable debris (47). In another study of 68 trochanteric osteotomies of which 59 were revisions, the authors found fraying and fragmentation of the cable in the majority of patients with nonunions (88%), and in 35% of those with healed trochanters (18 patients). Large deposits of metallic debris at the inferior border of the acetabulum were seen in 12% of hips (eight patients) (see Table 2) (Fig. 22). Reports of abrasive three-body wear of polyethylene caused by cable debris have recently been published (7,41).

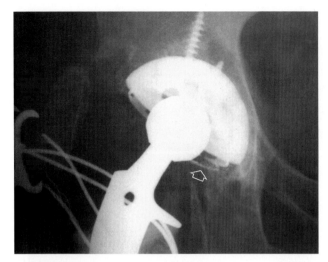

FIG. 22. Nonunion and migration of the trochanter, with broken cables and a large collection of metallic debris at the inferior aspect of the acetabular component.

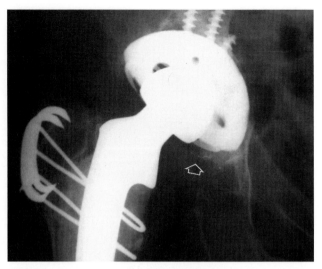

FIG. 24. A well-healed trochanter with evidence of metallic debris at the inferior edge of the acetabulum in the absence of cable breakage.

In evaluating these data, it becomes clear that although the multistrand cable system has mechanical properties far superior to those of monofilament wire, it still breaks. It will not prevent a nonunion. It will not prevent trochanteric migration. However, it can act rather in the manner of

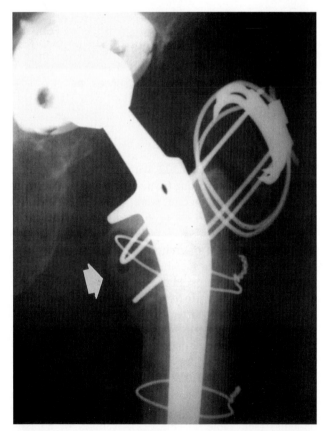

FIG. 23. Nonunion of the trochanter, with an intact cable-grip device and lysis of the lesser trochanter secondary to the Gigli-saw effect from the cables.

a Gigli saw and can abrade the area of the lesser trochanter (Fig. 23). Even with trochanteric union, free ends of the cut cable may be abraded by the soft tissues, resulting in fraying and fragmenting, sending tiny particles of CoCr wires into the joint (Fig. 24). The likelihood that these particles will contribute to three-body wear is of concern. Bauer et al. recently reported three cases of abrasive wear of the acetabular liner and femoral head after fraying of multifilament cables (7). They found multiple fragments of the CoCr cables embedded in the weight-bearing portion of the acetabular liner. As the femoral head is roughened and abraded with each step, the amount of polyethylene debris generated by this surface is of concern and potentially may cause problems of early loosening.

The need to decrease any potential source of particle debris within or around the hip is of prime concern in joint arthroplasty. Although intra-articular interposition of wire fragments has been reported in the past (13), these findings of metallic debris adjacent to the acetabulum and embedded in the polyethylene liner are alarming. Although there may be a role for the use of cables in the repair of an extended trochanteric osteotomy or fixation of allograft plates, removal after radiographic union should be considered to decrease the likelihood of cable fraying and fragmentation.

Heterotopic Ossification

The development of heterotopic ossification after THA is most common in those high-risk patients with a diagnosis of hypertrophic osteoarthritis or ankylosing spondylitis, or a history of ipsilateral or contralateral ectopic bone formation, with reported rates up to 80%. Although there are several studies in the literature suggesting that the use of a trochanteric osteotomy may increase the risk of heterotopic ossification (31), Morrey et al. found that in primary THA, there was no statistically significant difference among the three approaches (anterolateral, transtrochanteric, and posterior) in the development of heterotopic ossification (61). Eftekhar noted a 7% incidence of heterotopic ossification after routine transtrochanteric approach in his first 1500 low-friction arthroplasties (26). However, when a transtrochanteric approach is used only for selected, difficult primary THAs and revision procedures, the incidence may be as high as 90% in some cases if prophylactic measures are not taken (49). For this reason, prophylactic treatment measures are recommended in those high-risk groups regardless of the approach. In summary, the surgeon should select the approach that will give the best exposure for a given situation regardless of concerns for the development of heterotopic ossification.

SUMMARY

As we enter the twenty-first century, removal of the greater trochanter is still a viable option for access to the hip joint. The decision to remove part of the trochanter, the entire trochanter, or the trochanter along with the lateral shaft of the femur becomes the surgeon's choice based on the amount of exposure necessary, the quality of the bone, and the reconstructive options available. Although not useful in all cases of revisions or difficult primary hip arthroplasties, competence in trochanteric osteotomies and fixation techniques will add to a surgeon's armamentarium. Complications relating to the fixation devices should not be a deterrent to the utilization of this technique in the appropriate setting.

REFERENCES

1. Abitbol JJ, Gendron MD, Laurin CA, et al. Gluteal nerve damage following total hip arthroplasty: a prospective analysis. *J Arthroplasty* 1990;5:4.
2. Amstutz HC, Mai LL. Results of interlocking wire trochanteric reattachment and technique refinements to prevent complications following total hip arthroplasty. *Clin Orthop* 1983;183:82.
3. Amstutz HC, Maki S. Complications of trochanteric osteotomy in total hip replacements. *J Bone Joint Surg* 1978;60A:214.
4. Baker AS, Bitounis VC. Abductor function after total hip replacement: an electromyelographic and clinical review. *J Bone Joint Surg* 1985;71B:47.
5. Baker SA, Fitzgerald RH, Coventry MB. Treatment of non-union of greater trochanter of the hip. In: *The hip: proceedings of the scientific meeting of the Hip Society.* St. Louis, MO: Mosby Year Book, 1981.
6. Bal BS, Maurer BT, Harris WH. Trochanteric union following revision total hip arthroplasty. *J Arthroplasty* 1997 *(in press).*
7. Bauer TW, Ming J, D'Antonio JA, Morawa LG. Abrasive three-body wear of polyethylene caused by broken multifilament cables of a total hip prosthesis. A report of three cases. *J Bone Joint Surg* 1996;78A:1244–1247.
8. Bechtol CO, Crickenberger DP, O'Rourke FM. An alternate method of trochanteric reattachment in total hip replacement. *J Bone Joint Surg* 1977;59A:426.
9. Bergström B, Lindberg L, Persson BM, Önnerfält R. Complications after total hip arthroplasty according to Charnley in a Swedish series of cases. *Clin Orthop* 1973;95:91–95.
10. Bernard AA, Brooks S. The role of trochanteric wire revision after total hip replacement. *J Bone Joint Surg* 1987;69B:352–354.
11. Berry DJ, Müller ME. Chevron osteotomy and single wire reattachment of the greater trochanter in primary and revision total hip arthroplasty. *Clin Orthop* 1993;294:155–161.
12. Boardman KP, Bocco F, Charnley J. An evaluation of a method of trochanteric fixation using three wires in the Charnley low-friction arthroplasty. *Clin Orthop* 1978;132:31.
13. Bronson JL. Articular interposition of trochanteric wires in a failed total hip replacement. *Clin Orthop* 1976;121:50–52.
14. Cameron HU. Use of a distal trochanteric osteotomy in hip revision. *Contemp Orthop* 1991;23:235.
15. Carlsson AS, Gentz CF. Postoperative dislocation in the Charnley and Brunswick total hip arthroplasty. *Clin Orthop* 1977;125:177–182.
16. Charnley J. *Low friction arthroplasty of the hip: theory and practice.* Berlin: Springer-Verlag, 1979.
17. Charnley J. The long-term results of low-friction arthroplasty of the hip performed as a primary intervention. *J Bone Joint Surg* 1972;54B:61–76.
18. Charnley J. Total hip replacement by low friction arthroplasty. *Clin Orthop* 1970;72:7.
19. Charnley J, Ferreira A. de SD. Transplantation of the greater trochanter in arthroplasty of the hip. *J Bone Joint Surg* 1954;46B:191.
20. Clarke RP Jr, Shea WD, Bierbaum BE. Trochanteric osteotomy. Analysis of pattern of wire fixation failure and complications. *Clin Orthop* 1979;141:102–110.
21. Courpied JP, Postel M. Pseudarthroses trochantériennes après arthroplastie totale de hanche: leur fixation par une nouvelle plaque-griffe. *Rev Chir Orthop* 1986;72:583–586.
22. Dall D. Exposure of the hip by anterior osteotomy of the greater trochanter: a modified anterolateral approach. *J Bone Joint Surg* 1986;68B:382–386.
23. Dall DM, Miles AW. Re-attachment of the greater trochanter. The use of the trochanter cable-grip system. *J Bone Joint Surg* 1983;65B:55–59.
24. Debeyre J, Duliveux P. *Les arthroplasties de la hanche: étude critique à propos de 200 cas opérés.* Paris: Editions Medicales Flammarion, 1954.
25. Eftekhar NS. Significance of wire breakage. In: Eftekhar NS, ed. *Principles of total hip arthroplasty.* St. Louis, MO: CV Mosby, 1978; 634–637.
26. Eftekhar NS, ed. *Total hip arthroplasty.* St. Louis, MO: CV Mosby, 1993;16–61.
27. English TA. The trochanteric approach to the hip for prosthetic replacement. *J Bone Joint Surg* 1975;57A:1128–1132.
28. English TA, Dowson D. An introduction to biomechanics of joints and joint replacement. In: Dowson D, Wright V, eds. New York: Elsevier, 1975.
29. English TA, Dowson D, Jobbins B. The effect of trochanteric displacement on forces acting at the hip joint. In: *Proceedings of the 15th international conference of the Biological Engineering Society,* Edinburgh, 1975.
30. Ernberg JJ, Bostrom MPG, Asnis SE, Wright TM. Cobalt chrome cerclage: mechanical strength and mechanisms of failure. *Presented at the meeting of the American Academy of Orthopaedic Surgeons,* Orlando, FL, 1995.
31. Errico TJ, Fetto JF, Waugh TR. Heterotopic ossification. Incidence and relation to trochanteric osteotomy in 100 total hip arthroplasties. *Clin Orthop* 1984;190:138.
32. Evanski PM, Waugh TR, Orofino CF. Total hip replacement with the Charnley prosthesis. *Clin Orthop* 1973;95:69–72.
33. Fulkerson JP, Crelin ES, Keggi KJ. Anatomy and osteotomy of the greater trochanter. *Arch Surg* 1979;114:19–21.
34. Glassman AH. Complications of trochanteric osteotomy. *Orthop Clin North Am* 1992;23:321–333.
35. Glassman A, Engh C, Bobyn J. A technique of extensile exposure for total hip arthroplasty. *J Arthroplasty* 1987;2:11–21.
36. Gottschalk FA, Morein G, Weber F. Effect of the position of the greater trochanter on the rate of union after trochanteric osteotomy for total hip arthroplasty. *J Arthroplasty* 1988;3:235–240.
37. Guadagni JR, Drummond DS. Strength of surgical wire fixation. *Clin Orthop* 1986;209:176–181.
38. Hardinge K. The direct lateral approach to the hip. *J Bone Joint Surg* 1982;64B:17.
39. Harris WH. Presented at: *Total hip replacement: back into the future.* Cambridge, MA. 25th Annual Harvard Hip Course, 1995: September 20–23.

40. Hersh CK, Williams RP, Trick LW, Lanctot D, Athanasiou K. Comparison of the mechanical performance of trochanteric fixation devices. *Clin Orthop* 1996;329:317–325.

41. Hop JD, Callaghan JJ, Olejniczak JP, Pedersen DR, Brown TD, Johnston RC. An in vivo model of third body wear contribution of cable debris generation to accelerated polyethylene wear and acetabular component loosening. *The Hip Society and AAHKS*. February 16, 1997.

42. Hunter SG. Component alignment and trochanteric detachment in total hip arthroplasty. *Clin Orthop* 1982;168:53–58.

43. Jacobs LGH, Buxton RA. The course of the superior gluteal nerve in the lateral approach to the hip. *J Bone Joint Surg* 1989;71A:1235.

44. Jensen NF, Harris WH. A system for trochanteric osteotomy and reattachment for total hip arthroplasty with a ninety-nine percent union rate. *Clin Orthop* 1986;208:174–181.

45. Johnston RC, Kelly SS. Debris from cobalt-chrome cable may cause acetabular loosening. *Clin Orthop* 1992;285:140.

46. Kaplan SJ, Thomas WH, Poss R. Trochanteric advancement for recurrent dislocation after total hip arthroplasty. *J Arthroplasty* 1987;2:119–124.

47. Kelley S, Johnston RC. Debris from cobalt-chrome cable may cause acetabular loosening. *Clin Orthop* 1992;285:140–146.

48. Khan MA, Brakenbury PH, Reynolds ISR. Dislocation following total hip replacement. *J Bone Joint Surg* 1981;63B:214–218.

49. Kjaersgaard-Andersen P, Hougaard K, Linde F, Christiansen SE, Jensen J. Heterotopic bone formation after total hip arthroplasty in patients with primary or secondary coxarthrosis. *Orthopedics* 1990;13:1211–1217.

50. Kristiansen B, Jorgensen L, Holmich P. Dislocation following total hip arthroplasty. *Arch Orthop Trauma Surg* 1985;103:375–377.

51. Lazansky MG. Complications in total hip replacement with the Charnley technic. *Clin Orthop* 1970;72:40–45.

52. Lindgren U, Svenson O. A new transtrochanteric approach to the hip. *Int Orthop* 1988;12:37–41.

53. Liu A, O'Connor DO. The comparison of cerclage techniques using a hose clamp versus monofilament cerclage wire or cable. Presented at *Total Hip Replacement; Back Into the Future*, 25th Annual Harvard Hip Course, September 20–23, 1995.

54. Mallory TH. Sciatic nerve entrapment secondary to trochanteric wiring following total hip arthroplasty: a case report. *Clin Orthop* 1983;180:198.

55. McFarland B, Osborne G. Approach to the hip: a suggested improvement on Kocher's method. *J Bone Joint Surg* 1954;36B:364.

56. McGrory BJ, Bal BS, Harris WH. Trochanteric osteotomy for total hip arthroplasty: six variations and indications for their use. *J Am Acad Orthop Surg* 1996;4:258–267.

57. McLauchlan J. The Stracathro approach to the hip. *J Bone Joint Surg* 1984;66B:30–31.

58. McMinn DJ, Roberts P, Forward GR. A new approach to the hip for revision surgery. *J Bone Joint Surg* 1991;73B:899–901.

59. Markoff KL, Hirschowitz DL, Amstutz HC. Mechanical stability of the greater trochanter following osteotomy and reattachment by wiring. *Clin Orthop* 1979;141:111–121.

60. Morrey BF. Instability after total hip arthroplasty. *Orthop Clin North Am* 1992;23:237–248.

61. Morrey BF, Adams RA, Cabanela ME. Comparison of heterotopic bone after anterolateral, transtrochanteric, and posterior approaches for total hip arthroplasty. *Clin Orthop* 1984;188:160–167.

62. Nazarian S, Tisserand PH, Brunet CH, et al. Anatomic basis of the transgluteal approach to the hip. *Surg Radiol Anat* 1987;9:27.

63. Naito M, Ogata K, Emoto G. The blood supply to the greater trochanter. *Clin Orthop* 1996;323:294–297.

64. Nercessian O, Sheikh B, Eftekhar N. Comparison of trochanteric osteotomy by a biplane osteotomy and spring-loaded wire with conventional three-wire fixation. *Presented at the twenty-third annual meeting of the Hip Society*, New York, NY, 1991.

65. Nutton RW, Checketts RG. The effects of trochanteric osteotomy on abductor power. *J Bone Joint Surg* 1984;66B:180.

66. Oh I. Effect of iatrogenic defects on the fatigue resistance of orthopedic wire. *Scientific exhibit, 50th meeting of the American Association of Orthopaedic Surgeons*, Anaheim, CA, February, 1983.

67. Paul JP. Load actions on the human femur in walking and some resultant stresses. *Exp Mech* 1971;11:121–125.

68. Peters PC, Head WC, Emerson RH. An extended trochanteric osteotomy for revision total hip replacement. *J Bone Joint Surg* 1993;75B:158.

69. Reinert CM, Bosse MJ, Poka A, Schacherer T, Brumback RJ, Burgess AR. A modified extensile exposure for the treatment of complex or malunited acetabular fractures. *J Bone Joint Surg* 1988;70A:329–337.

70. Ritter MA, Eizember LE, Keating EM, Faris PM. Trochanteric fixation by cable grip in hip replacement. *J Bone Joint Surg* 1991;73B:580–581.

71. Ritter MA, Gioe JJ, Stringer EA. Functional significance of nonunion of the greater trochanter. *Clin Orthop* 1981;159:177–182.

72. Sabbagh MA, Galline Y, Soria C. Osteosynthèse du grand trochanter par plaque et cables dans les arthroplasties totales de hanche. *J Chir (Paris)* 1990;127(4):230–234.

73. Scher MA, Jakim I. Trochanter reattachment in revision hip arthroplasty. *J Bone Joint Surg* 1990;72B:435.

74. Schutzer SF, Harris WH. Trochanteric osteotomy for revision total hip arthroplasty: 97% union rate using a comprehensive approach. *Clin Orthop* 1988;227:172.

75. Silverton CD, Joshua JJ, Rosenberg AG, Kull L, Conley A, Galante JO. Complications of a cable grip system. *J Arthroplasty* 1996;11:400–404.

76. Sochart DH, Paul AS, Kurdy WM. A new osteotome for performing chevron trochanteric osteotomy. *Acta Orthop Scand* 1995;66(5):445–446.

77. Stefanich RJ, Jabbur MT. Autogenic cancellous bone grafting following transtrochanteric hip arthroplasty. An attempt to facilitate union of the greater trochanter. *Clin Orthop* 1988;228:141–149.

78. Taylor JK, Hayes DEE Jr, Bargar WL, Paul HA. Cerclage systems in total hip replacement: static tension and mechanics of failure. *Presented at the 37th annual meeting of the Orthopaedic Research Society*, Anaheim, CA, March 1991.

79. Teanby DN, Monsell, FP, Goel R, Faux JC, Hardy SK. Failure of trochanteric osteotomy in total hip replacement: a comparison of two methods of reattachment. *Ann R Coll Surg Engl* 1996;78:43–44.

80. Turner RH, McCarthy JC, Kremchek T, Renten JJ. Reattachment of the greater trochanter after total hip replacement: using the Dall-Miles cable grip system. *Presented at the ninth combined meeting of the Orthopaedic Associations of the English Speaking World*, Toronto, Canada, June 1992.

81. Volz RG, Brown FW. The painful migrated ununited greater trochanter in total hip replacement. *J Bone Joint Surg* 1977;59A:1091–1093.

82. Volz RG, Turner RH. Reattachment of the greater trochanter in total hip arthroplasty by use of a bolt. *J Bone Joint Surg* 1975;57A:129–130.

83. Wagner H. *Atlas of hip surgery*. New York: Thieme, 1996.

84. Weber BG. Osteotomy of the greater trochanter total hip replacement. Conventional versus dihedral technique. *Orthopäde* 1989;18:540–544.

85. Weber BG Stühmer G. Improvements in total hip prosthesis implantation technique: a cement-proof seal for the lower medullary cavity and a dihedral self-stabilizing trochanteric osteotomy. *Arch Orthop Traumat Surg* 1979;93:185–189.

86. Wroblewski BM, Shelley P. Reattachment of the greater trochanter after hip replacement. *J Bone Joint Surg* 1985;67B:736–740.

87. Younger TI, Bradford MS, Magnus RE, Paprosky WG. Extended proximal femoral osteotomy. A new technique for femoral revision arthroplasty. *J Arthroplasty* 1995;10:329–338

88. Woo RYG, Morrey BF. Dislocation of THA. *J Bone Joint Surg* 1992;64A(9):1295–1306.

The Adult Hip, edited by J. J. Callaghan,
A. G. Rosenberg, and H. E. Rubash.
Lippincott–Raven Publishers, Philadelphia © 1998.

CHAPTER 79

Sepsis: Etiology, Prophylaxis, and Diagnosis

James P. McAuley and Guy Moreau

ETIOLOGY OF PERIPROSTHETIC INFECTIONS

Sepsis after total hip arthroplasty remains a potentially devastating complication, resulting in major morbidity for the patient and adversely affecting the prosthetic outcome. Further operations are usually required to control the sepsis and, despite the best efforts, can ultimately end in a dysfunctional or disfiguring result, even amputation. The overall incidence of periprosthetic infection is about 1% (12,13,16). This represents approximately 1000 new cases of infection per year, as over 100,000 total hip arthroplasties are performed yearly in the United States. Many factors have contributed to the dramatic decrease in the rate of infection since the early experience of Charnley. His 9% rate of deep infection (6) would be, by current standards, unacceptable. The advent of antibiotic prophylaxis, improved patient selection (including the elimination of remote infections), and operating room measures such as clean-air surgery, body-exhaust suits, and minimized activity in the operating room have all contributed to the lower rate of deep wound infection after total hip arthroplasty.

Patient Factors

Orthopedic patients undergoing hip arthroplasty are often elderly and have secondary illnesses that adversely

J. P. McAuley and G. Moreau: Division of Orthopaedic Surgery, Department of Surgery, University of Ottawa, Ottawa, Ontario K1H 8L6, Canada.

affect their ability to resist the development of infection after bacterial contamination. Age has a known effect on normal immune responses (36), affecting both B-cell and T-cell responses. Age results in decreased mitogen-induced proliferative responses and diminished primary and secondary antibody formation (B-cell, humoral immunity). The decrease in T-cell (cell-mediated) immune response includes depressed, delayed-type hypersensitivity (DTH) responses, decreased proliferative response, and an altered ratio of helper to suppressor cell activity. The aging population has a rate of infection double that of other patients.

Local and regional immunity are the first line of protection against environmental pathogens. Chronic diseases are associated with an acquired reduction of immunoresponsiveness (36). Patients with diabetes mellitus demonstrate deficiencies of neutrophil chemotaxis and phagocytosis and depressed T-cell responses to mitogenic stimulation. Rheumatoid arthritis also results in decreased chemotaxis and phagocytosis. These patients are also often corticosteroid dependent, which also affects their ability to respond to outside pathogens.

Malnutrition is a known factor that may contribute to the development of surgical sepsis. It is estimated that nearly 30% of patients undergoing surgery have some degree of malnutrition. Malnutrition states have an adverse effect on all the components of immunologic activity, from local to systemic immunity (11,36). A quick way of assessing malnutrition is the index validated by Rainey-McDonald et al. (44). The calculation is as follows: [(1.2 × serum albumin) + (0.0013 × serum transferrin)] - 6.43. If the result is 0 or a negative number, the patient is nutritionally depleted and is at high risk of sepsis. These patients should be supplemented prior to undergoing elective surgery.

Preoperative assessment is important to decrease the overall risks of postoperative sepsis. Optimization of chronic illnesses, thorough physical examination to rule out other foci of infection (such as pneumonia, urinary tract, skin folds in obese patient, and other skin conditions) are important to help avoid sepsis. The incidence of postoperative sepsis can be 3 times higher in patients with remote foci of infection, so they must be treated prior to surgery.

Microbiology

The reported incidence of sepsis in total hip arthroplasty varies from series to series. The advent of antibiotic prophylaxis, improved surgical techniques, and clean-air operating rooms have contributed to a decrease in incidence from 9% to as low as 0.27% (16). However, the pathogens have not changed markedly during the last few decades of hip arthroplasty. Gram-positive cocci still dominate the list of pathogens in total hip sepsis, but many different causative organisms are reported. For example, in a combined study from the Mayo Clinic and the Hospital for Special Surgery (17), 97 pathogens were isolated in 76 patients. *Staphylococcus epidermidis* was present in 36 and *Staphylococcus aureus* in 18, accounting for more than 50% of the periprosthetic infections. Other pathogens involved, in decreasing order of frequency, were *Streptococcus viridans*, Group-D streptococci or enterococci, and β-hemolytic streptococci. Seventy-six percent were gram-positive and the rest gram-negative organisms such as *Escherichia coli*, *Proteus mirabilis*, *Pseudomonas aeruginosa*, *Salmonella choleraesuis*, and *Campylobacter intestinalis*. Anaerobic bacteria, accounting for 12%, included *Propionibacterium acnes*, *Peptococcus asaccharolyticus*, *Peptostreptococcus magnus*, *Peptostreptococcus micros*, and *Clostridium bifermentans*. Many other bacteria appear in other series, including *Klebsiella*, *Serratia*, and *Mycobacteria*.

Pathogens can produce an infection by direct contact with the wound at the time of the operation or by hematogenous spread. The source can be the patient's skin, the operating room environment, the operating room personnel, or pathogens in the patient's circulation. It is not well understood why some infections develop in certain patients and not in others, but age, immunologic status, concomitant diseases, active infection, and nutritional status all can contribute to sepsis.

However, even in an optimal patient with no risk factors, periprosthetic infections occur. Work done by Gristina et al. (20–24) described the effects of biomaterials or prostheses on the development of infection in hip arthroplasty. They elucidated the concept of the race for colonization of the biomaterial surface. This is a competition between host tissue and pathogens for the biomaterial surface, devitalized tissue (necrotic bone, traumatized tissue), or acellular tissue (articular cartilage, foreign body). By its nature, normal viable tissue is resistant to infection, but devitalized tissues and biomaterials can provide surfaces for adhesion of particles by various mechanisms.

Three classes of interaction have been described. Class 1 involves Van der Walls forces (physical forces) and hydrophobic interactions constituting the initial mechanism for particle adhesion to the biomaterial. Class 2 is nonspecific chemical binding to exposed biomaterial or tissue substratum surfaces by means of covalent polar or hydrogen-bonding interactions not involving receptor ligand configurations. An example is the glue-like adhesion of the polysaccharide slime to a prosthesis. Finally, class 3 is specific bacterial receptor-to-biomaterial surface protein ligand interactions caused by bacterial receptor surface molecules and their respective protein ligand or lectin molecules (e.g., *Staphylococcus aureus* to collagen fibrils in osteomyelitis).

Once the interaction between inert substratum surface and the pathogens occurs, a microclimate is established that protects bacteria and allows proliferation. *In vitro* and *in vivo* studies have shown that certain organisms have preferential attraction to biomaterials (20–24). *Staphylococcus aureus* has an affinity for metallic implants, and *Staphylococcus epidermidis* to the presence of polymers [polyethylene liners, polymethylmethacrylate PMMA] (46). *Pseudomonas aeruginosa* also has a predilection for polymers, being a frequent cause of bacterial keratitis with extended corneal lens wear.

This affinity for different biomaterials may be explained by the exopolysaccharide glycocalyx slime produced by different bacteria. It consists of an outside moiety related to the cell wall of the bacteria. The polysaccharide slime confers resistance to host defense mechanisms of phagocytes, surfactants, antibodies, and antibiotics (11). This provides an inherent protection for bacterial growth. Once the bacteria grow within the inert substratum, the increased production of polysaccharides allows better fixation and creates a biofilm. This protective layer creates the prefect environment for bacterial proliferation. It effectively seals it from host defense mechanisms such as antibodies, viable tissue integration, and antibiotics. It interferes with phagocytosis and impedes antibiotic penetration. Accumulated biofilm may fragment and detach as inocula, secondary to hemodynamic forces. Inocula of pathogens may be a source of and explanation for hematogenous septic emboli, distant seeding, and secondary infection. The biofilm can also prevent proper isolation of the causative pathogen because of the protective effect of this microenvironment.

Fitzgerald (13) has shown that in 105 patients with an infected total joint arthroplasty, 52% of the isolates of *Staphylococcus epidermidis* and 28% of those of *Staphylococcus aureus* elaborated glycocalyx. In such situations, it is essential to remove all the infected material, and it would seem appropriate to avoid a one-stage procedure because some of the biofilm will undoubtedly remain in the site of excision. It is felt that glycocalyx may contribute to the reported incidence of recurrence after one-stage reconstruction. It is essential for the surgeon to obtain microbiologic specimens not only to identify the pathogen but also to determine if the organism is producing glycocalyx.

The diagnostic test for glycocalyx is based on the procedure of Christensen et al. (13) and is performed in the microbiology laboratory. Several colonies of the organism to be tested are inoculated into 5 mL of trypticase soy broth, and the culture is incubated at 35°C for 48 hours without shaking. The contents of the test tube are then aspirated and replaced with safranin stain for 2 minutes. The safranin solution is aspirated, and the inside of the test tube is examined for the presence of the stain, which indicates the elaboration of glycocalyx by the microorganism (13).

Other factors inherent to different biomaterials and tissues can influence the establishment of infection around an implant. Metals and alloys form an outside layer of oxidation of 20 to 30 nm, and biomolecules interact with this oxide layer. As mentioned, *Staphylococcus aureus* has an affinity for metals and alloys. It seems that titanium and its alloys have less fibrous reaction around the implant, which may be a protective property against colonization. Polymers such as PMMA have a noncrystalline, porous structure that provides large surface areas for diffusion and molecular interaction. Studies by Gristina et al. (20–24) have shown an increased adhesion of *Staphylococcus epidermidis* to polymers, with resultant increased resistance to antibiotics. Traumatized bone exposes collagenous proteins that act as ligands for bacterial adhesion (class 3 interaction). Allografts are obviously devitalized bone and provide a surface for colonization by bacteria with the appropriate receptors.

The fate of the biomaterial surface thus depends on the outcome of the race for the surface by macromolecules, bacteria, and tissue cells as conceptualized by Gristina et al. If viable cells get the initial access to the biomaterial surface and a secure bond is established, local bacteria are confronted by living, integrated cells resistant to bacterial colonization through intact cell membranes, extracellular polysaccharides, and functioning host defense mechanisms. However, bacteria, being prevalent in biologic environments, may colonize the biomaterial first, producing infection and preventing tissue integration. The potential for infection theoretically could be diminished by accelerating the integration of the material surfaces with tissue cells, but clear evidence of this benefit remains to be seen.

Classification

Postoperative periprosthetic infections can occur early or late after implantation. The mode of contamination with bacteria can vary from direct contact at the time of surgery, from a contiguous source, or by hematologic seeding. The pathogens involved can be quite variable, even though more than 50% of the time gram-positive cocci are the culprits. All these variables can affect treatment and outcome, so an appropriate classification system is essential to deal with this complication and allow meaningful analysis of results.

The most widely accepted classification of postoperative wound infection in hip arthroplasty was presented by Coventry in 1975 (8). It divides postoperative infections into three different stages.

Stage I, or acute postoperative infection, is usually not a diagnostic problem. It may be accompanied by persistent discharge of purulent material or serous drainage. Fever is common and is associated with inordinate pain, findings of restricted range of motion, and a red, swollen extremity. Immediate wound debridement and irrigation is warranted. Therefore, stage I infection includes fulminant postoperative infection, the infected hematoma, and the superficial infection with deep extension.

Stage II, or indolent, delayed deep infection, occurs from 6 months to 2 years after the arthroplasty. The patient presents with a painful arthroplasty, often after an uneventful initial postoperative course. Aseptic loosening may be the cause of pain, but deep infection has to be excluded because the treatment and outcomes are markedly different. The investigation and treatment of stage II deep infection will be the subject of later sections in this chapter.

Stage III infections, or late hematogenous infections, usually pose little diagnostic difficulty. The patient may have a had recent surgical procedure, dental manipulation, upper respiratory tract infection, or remote infection. The patient presents in a febrile state with a painful joint. Aspiration and the usual laboratory tests will confirm the diagnosis.

A criticism of this classification is that its division of infections is based on an arbitrary temporal standard. To address this, Schmalzried et al. (48) proposed a pathophysiologic classification system based on clinical history and laboratory findings. It is divided into four modes: mode 1 is considered surgical contamination; mode 2 is defined as hematogenous spread from another source; mode 3 is recurrent sepsis from a previously infected joint; and mode 4 is contiguous spread from a local source.

A newer approach to the classification of periprosthetic infections and recommendations for the proposed management of these patients was developed by Tsukyama et al. (52). This classification has four categories: (a) Positive intraoperative cultures: The infection is diagnosed after two or more specimens, obtained intraoperatively, have been cultured and found to be positive for the same organism. The infection should be treated with 6 weeks of intravenous antibiotics and may not require operative intervention. (b) Early postoperative infection: Apparent within 1 month after implantation of the prosthesis, the infection can be treated with debridement, exchange of polyethylene liner, retention of the components, and intravenous antibiotics for 4 weeks. (c) Late chronic infection: Occurs more than 1 month after implantation. It is of insidious onset. It should be treated with a two-stage procedure. (d) Acute hematogenous infection: Acute onset in a previously well-functioning hip. If the prosthesis is well fixed, it should be treated in the same manner as for early postoperative infection. If the prosthesis is loose, it should be treated as a late chronic infection.

Classification of periprosthetic infections is evolving with the emergence of new knowledge in the pathophysiology of infection in the presence of biomaterials. Newer classifications should take into consideration the timing and the source of infection, the type of organism, glycocalyx production, and the biomaterial used. A consensus on classification is needed for meaningful comparisons of results of various therapies, and for true progress to be made in this very difficult area.

PROPHYLAXIS OF SEPSIS IN TOTAL HIP ARTHROPLASTY

Patient Preparation

The patient's own skin and airborne particles containing bacteria are the major sources of the wound contamination that can lead to sepsis. Preoperatively, the patient should be questioned and examined to rule out any source of infection on the skin, leg, or foot (e.g., ingrown toenail). The patient's medical and nutritional condition should be optimized to maximize their resistance to infection. Dental and urologic surgery should be completed prior to the hip arthroplasty. Preoperative lab results may suggest distant infection such as leukocytosis, white cells or bacteria in the urinalysis, or an unexplained elevation of the erythrocyte sedimentation rate (ESR).

Some recommend that patients shower using an antimicrobial soap prior to their surgery, but no data are available to demonstrate any benefit (39). Hair removal should be done immediately before the surgery, ideally with a depilatory agent to avoid skin laceration. Shaving the night before is not recommended because of the risk of folliculitis and dermatitis, and shaving of the local area should be done as closely as possible to the procedure (39,40).

Operating Room Environment

Total hip arthroplasty is performed by the surgical team in an operating theater environment. Many factors can be addressed in an attempt to lower the potential for contamination of the wound by pathogens. Airborne bacteria concentration varies with the type of air filtration and air exchange. Airborne bacteria usually reside on particles of at least 2 µm in size (39–41). They are almost exclusively gram positive and originate from the circulating personnel in the operating room. The skin and hair are the main sources of airborne bacteria, hence the importance of operating room garment and head piece quality to reduce potential air contamination. As many as 5000 to 55,000 particles are shed per minute by the surgeon (40), the exact number depending on how recently the person has showered and on the type of clothing worn. Interestingly, a person sheds the most particles immediately after a shower.

Attempts have been made to decrease the number of airborne bacteria in operating rooms by improving the quality of air circulation with the clean-air room concept developed in Britain. Nelson (41) showed that in a regular (conventional) operating room the average count of airborne bacteria was 5.4 per cubic foot. In the clean-air room, it was about 0.45. When the clean-air room was combined with body-exhaust system, the count was significantly reduced to 0.1 per cubic foot. In 1974, the Medical Research Council of Great Britain initiated a prospective study (33) of the use of clean-air rooms compared to conventional operating rooms. The results showed an incidence of 1.5% of deep wound infection in conventional rooms as opposed to 0.6% for clean-air rooms. Fitzgerald's (12) appropriate criticism of this study was that the use of prophylactic antibiotics was not controlled. When prophylactic antibiotics were taken into account, the difference between the two operating room environments was no longer statistically significant. To substantiate this criticism, Fitzgerald initiated a prospective study to verify his hypothesis about clean-air rooms and conventional rooms with control of antibiotic prophylaxis. The findings after over 7000 arthroplasties did not show any significant difference between the two systems.

The dress of the surgical team is important to control the amount of airborne particles from desquamation. Because the outermost layer of epithelial cells is shed every 24 hours (1 million cells a day), clothing should haves pores that prevent or decrease transudation of skin bacteria (31). Regular cotton fabric has pores of 80 µm, whereas the size of particles carrying bacteria average 14 μm. Gortex performs much better than cotton. Ultraviolet lights have also proven to decrease bacteria-containing air particles but are not widely used because of the exposure of the surgical team.

Limiting personnel access to the operating theater as well as limiting circulation can help diminish airborne particle generation within the operating room. Knowing that the number of pathogens required to initiate sepsis is much less in the presence of a biomaterial, it is important to do everything possible to limit the amount of wound contamination in total hip arthroplasty.

Surgical Measures

Surface bacteria are easily removed using any of the common disinfectants (31), the choice of which is governed largely by surgeon preference. However, is impossible to completely remove bacteria from skin follicles and subcutaneous glands despite careful preparation (40). Preparation of the skin after standard operating room protocols usually includes a two-step technique of washing the entire limb with an iodophor soap, followed by an iodophor paint. One-step prepping may be as effective as traditional methods in reducing bacterial counts taken both preoperatively and at the completion of the procedure (18).

The limb should be completely covered with a stockinet and waterproof draping. A consistent draping routine is important to complete patient preparation and decrease the potential for contamination.

The millions of bacteria normally present on the surgeon's hands can be decreased by 80% with a disinfectant scrub, and the addition of alcohol can produce a further reduction to 95% (31). Gloves are often punctured during orthopedic procedures, so double gloving is recommended (26,31).

Meticulous surgical techniques are essential for diminishing complications. The principles of gentle handling and retraction of tissues, maintenance of hemostasis and tissue moisture, repetitive irrigation, and careful closure with avoidance of dead space all deserve reinforcement. One should presume that contamination is likely inevitable in these cases of major dissection and long operative times, and the implications of the implanted foreign material are obvious. Avoidance of reaming to cortical bone can avoid the devascularization that occurs when PMMA directly contacts it (40).

When an adhesive barrier dressing is removed from the wound, a layer of epidermis is stripped off, and positive cultures are always obtainable (31). If removed during closure, it should be trimmed away, the skin edges washed with an appropriate antiseptic solution, and outer gloves changed (31).

Antibiotic Prophylaxis

It is widely recognized that antibiotic prophylaxis has been a major factor in the reduction of total joint sepsis (12,16,31,39,40,46). A prospective, placebo-controlled study in 1981 described a reduction in infection rate from 3.3% to 0.9% with prophylactic cephazolin (27), but there was little effect of the addition of ultraclean operating rooms. In a review of 7305 arthroplasties, factors related to infection, including operating room type, antibiotic prophylaxis was felt to be the most important (12).

The ideal prophylactic agent should be rapidly bacteriocidal, have a wide therapeutic index against common pathogens, have an appropriate half-life, and be inexpensive, leading to a virtually universal recommendation for first-generation cephalosporins. Giving the antibiotic 1 or more days preoperatively alters the patient's flora and provides no additional protection (12). The medication should be given just before the surgery to allow the 15 to 60 minutes needed for adequate levels to be obtained during the procedure (39). If intraoperative material will be obtained for culture, antibiotics should be held until the culture specimens are obtained.

The optimal duration of prophylaxis remains unclear (14,16,39,40,54). A study in 1979 (43) compared an extreme duration (2 weeks) with a perioperative regimen and revealed no difference. Another study comparing 7-day, 3-day, and 24-hour courses in 466 total joints showed similarly no difference (40). In a review article (16), no benefit was found in continuing antibiotics for over 24 hours. Taking it further, a randomized study of 2651 arthroplasties showed no statistical difference between one and three postoperative doses (0.83% and 0.45%), but for confirmation the authors felt more patients were required (54).

The option of antibiotic-impregnated cement instead of systemic antibiotics for prophylaxis in primary hip arthroplasty was evaluated in a prospective, randomized, consecutive series of 1688 hips with 10-year follow-up (29) with no difference seen. It seems reasonable to avoid the potential detrimental effects of the antibiotics on mechanical properties of the cement unless its use is clearly beneficial.

The choice of prophylactic antibiotic may well evolve as we are confronted with different organisms and new patterns of resistance. One report questions the continued use of cephalosporins for prophylaxis (28). Their prospective study of skin swabs of 100 consecutive patients admitted for total hip arthroplasty showed cephalosporin-resistant Staphylococcus epidermidis in 25. The prevalence of resistant organisms may well require reassessment of this cornerstone of prevention of postoperative sepsis.

DIAGNOSIS OF THE INFECTED TOTAL HIP ARTHROPLASTY

The presence of infection in a failed total hip arthroplasty is of major clinical significance, affecting the treatment planning, the reconstruction options, and certainly the clinical outcome. The diagnosis of a flagrant infection with systemic symptoms, local erythema, and drainage is straightforward, but the reliable detection of low-grade sepsis in a failed total hip arthroplasty remains a challenge.

After the appropriate history and physical evaluations, there are many options for investigation, including blood work, radiographic studies, joint aspiration, biopsy, and scintigraphic studies. The literature is unfortunately confusing and seemingly contradictory, largely because of differing (a) patient populations, (b) criteria for establishing the presence of infection, and (c) interpretation of what constitute pathogenic versus contaminant organisms. The question to be addressed is, how can a surgeon, presented with a failed total hip arthroplasty, best determine that sepsis is not contributing to the failure?

For example, Figure 1 is a plain radiograph of a 73-year-old woman with a failed cemented revision total hip

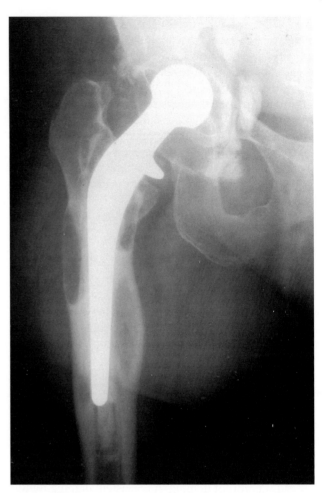

FIG. 2. AP radiograph showing the 7-year follow-up of an all-titanium femoral component.

revision done 5 years previously. Figure 2 illustrates the 7-year follow-up of a failed primary total hip arthroplasty done with an all-titanium femoral component. Neither patient had any postoperative complications or systemic or local findings to suggest sepsis. Is septic loosening a factor in one or both, and how can this be investigated?

Blood Work

The white blood cell count and differential in the absence of flagrant sepsis are universally recognized as being of little diagnostic value (10). Experimental work has been described looking at differential T-cell responses and interleukin levels in patients with septic or aseptic loosening, but clinical indications and applications remain to be clarified (13).

As a result, attention has been directed toward other options, including ESR and C-reactive protein determinations for detection of subclinical sepsis in arthroplasty patients.

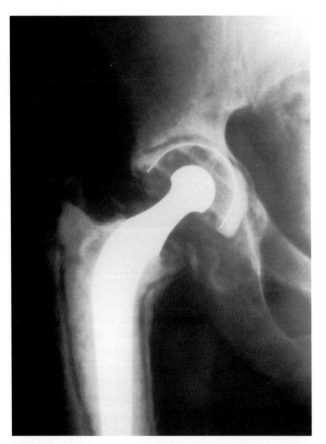

FIG. 1. Anteroposterior (AP) radiograph of 73-year-old woman with a failed cemented revision.

Erythrocyte Sedimentation Rate

The presence of a statistically significant elevation of the ESR in patients with infected arthroplasties compared with aseptic failures is often reported, but its lack of specificity limits its predictive value (9,13,32,47). As expected, numerous conditions other than sepsis can result in an elevated value (10). The level of ESR used as a discriminator varies with the series, making comparisons difficult, but on average a sensitivity of 83% and an accuracy of 80% are reported (9,10).

C-reactive Protein

Considerable interest has been directed at the acute-phase C-reactive protein evaluation as a noninvasive index of the potential for sepsis in total hip arthroplasty. To provide normal values for comparison in each patient, C-reactive protein levels have been shown to return to baseline levels in 3 to 8 weeks after primary and revision hip surgery (1,7,49,55).

One study (47) evaluated the diagnostic value of this test and the ESR, comparing 23 patients with proven deep hip infections with 33 control patients with aseptic loosening. All controls and five of the infected group had C-reactive protein levels below 20 mg/mL. Both the ESR and C-reactive protein level were normal in every control patient and only one of the infected group, suggesting that a combination of the two tests is more useful. The C-reactive protein test has also been used as a factor in deciding whether to proceed to aspiration of the joint (13).

Radiographic Evaluation

Several radiographic options are available to evaluate a failed arthroplasty, including plain film, ultrasonographic, and arthrographic studies.

Plain Radiographic Studies

Just as in examination for aseptic loosening, radiographs should be reviewed for potential signs of sepsis. Plain x-ray findings including endosteal erosions are seldom diagnostic for septic loosening, and their usefulness is controversial, sometimes adding little (9,10,25,32,46) and sometimes being integral to the decision-making process for further investigation (3). Periosteal new bone formation particularly is described as a warning sign for the presence of prosthetic infection (3,13,35) (Fig. 3).

Ultrasonography

Ultrasonography has only recently been described as a tool in the evaluation of failed total hip arthroplasties. It is used to evaluate capsular morphology and fluid collections in the hip region. One series reviewed 15 asymptomatic and 33 patients with a loose, painful arthroplasty who subsequently had arthrography with aspiration (53). Six of the symptomatic patients were shown to be infected, and the results of the three groups were compared. Measurements of the distances from anterior capsule to proximal femoral bone showed normal values (under 3.2 mm), and no hip with a value less than this was infected.

Infected hips showed significantly higher values (mean, 10.2 mm), with marked intra-articular effusions. All patients with intra-articular effusions and extra-articular fluid extension were found to be infected. The reproducibility of these results still needs to be clarified with other studies, before proposing the routine use of ultrasonography in hip evaluations.

Hip Arthrography

Hip arthrography is often described in association with aspiration, but the evaluation of the fluid and radiographic images are related but separate issues. The injection of dye into the hip confirms intra-articular location at the time of needle sampling of fluid or tissue, and it can detect abnormal bursae and sinuses, but, independently, arthrography is of limited predictive value (9,13,37,46) and certainly should be combined with aspiration if performed.

The indications for arthrography/aspiration vary between series: for example, (a) all symptomatic hip failures (9,25,30,32,37,50,51), (b) painful total hip in noninflammatory arthritis with elevated C-reactive protein or ESR (13), (c) history of infection or plain radiographic findings of periosteal new bone and focal or nonfocal aggressive osteolysis (3).

Joint Aspirates

The role and reliability of joint aspiration for detection of sepsis in total hip failure is a very controversial and confusing area with marked variations between reported series and their recommendations. Fluid obtained can be analyzed as in other joint aspirations, including cell count and differential, and glucose and protein levels, with a white cell count over 25,000, a differential count of over 25% polymorphonuclear leukocytes, and low glucose and high protein levels being suggestive of infection (46).

Several cultures should be taken to diminish the inaccuracy caused by contamination, keeping in mind that growth on plated cultures as opposed to in broths and on subcultures is less likely to be a contaminant (46). The emergence of *S. epidermidis* as a common pathogen (13,46), and its potential to be a contaminant can make the distinction difficult. If any material is to

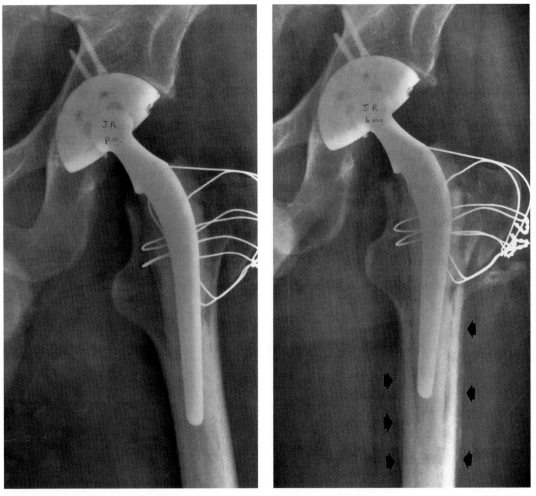

A   B

FIG. 3. AP radiographs of failed infected total hip arthroplasty, immediately postoperative **(A)** and 6 months postoperative **(B)**. Note periosteal reaction and cortical changes (*arrows*) in **(B)**.

be cultured, the patient should be off antibiotics, and preoperative antibiotics should be held until the material is obtained.

The reliability of cultures of aspirated fluid is also very controversial. High degrees of sensitivity, specificity, and accuracy (93%, 96%, and 95%, respectively) were reported in a series of 90 consecutive painful hips (50). Another series of 147 cases showed a sensitivity of 92.8%, a specificity of 91.7%, and a negative predictive value of 99.2% compared with operative cultures (51). Further reports of 178 cases showed no false-positive results and 96% accuracy (37). Several series have shown less dramatic results (5,9,30,32,34). False-positive results are reported as high as 12% and 13% (3,5,10). The largest series with long-term follow-up of 270 patients does not recommend routine aspiration before revision surgery (3), an opinion echoed by others (13). However, many authors feel that aspiration, even with its limitations, is still the most reliable test in their respective institutions, and they continue to advocate its routine use, usually in

association with other investigations (5,9,10,25,30,32,34, 37,46,50,51).

Adjunctive laboratory data can been used to improve the reliability of the aspiration. The presence of more than 10,000 white blood cells in the fluid, or the presence of a fistula on arthrogram, increased the sensitivity from 79% to 91% in one series of 143 revisions with only one false negative (34). Aspiration and fine-needle biopsy of capsular tissues, with the material obtained undergoing radiometric culture technique with carbon-14-impregnated substrate, has been proposed, with 94% of the aspirates proving correct with a specificity of 95% (45).

Polymerase chain reaction technology is an extremely sensitive and powerful tool for reliably detecting the presence of bacterial DNA remnants. The role of this technology remains to be seen. It will likely be helpful when a negative result is obtained, but since most if not all wounds have the potential for bacterial contamination, the significance of a positive result may be unclear (13).

Tissue Biopsy

There remains the option of using tissue obtained at surgery to help in the evaluation of the failed arthroplasty. Unfortunately, there is inconsistency as to what should constitute a positive histologic result, from an average of one or more polymorphonuclear leukocytes or plasma cell per high power field (2) to five polymorphonuclear leukocytes per high power field (46). Even using the more stringent criteria in 106 revisions, excellent results were obtained (sensitivity, 90%; specificity, 96%; accuracy, 95%). Conversely, sending tissue for Gram stain is of dubious value (3,30). Utilizing the material obtained for tissue cultures is more likely to supply valuable information.

Scintigraphic Evaluation

The role of nuclear medicine in the detection of sepsis in a failed hip arthroplasty continues to evolve as the technology expands. Again, the literature can be perplexing with seemingly contradictory results, but patterns do become manifest.

Routine three-phase technetium bone scans alone have generally not proven useful for predicting sepsis (4,9,19,30,32,38), largely because of inadequate specificity. The presence of a negative scan, however, is strongly predictive of the absence of infection (9,46).

The addition of gallium scans to the technetium scan has largely been disappointing (10,30,38), but the addition of indium scanning has improved the predictive capability of nuclear scans (10,12,13). Indium-labeled leukocyte scans were compared to the combination of technetium and gallium in a prospective study of 42 patients with suspected sepsis (38), demonstrating superior results (88% versus 62% correct) with the indium scans. The enthusiasm for indium scans has not been universal, even when combined with technetium studies (9,16,19). In one particular study of 54 patients with operative biopsy correlation, indium scans had a sensitivity of 37% when used alone and 44% combined with technetium; of interest was the time dependency of the results (19). The infections detected by positive scans averaged 1.1 years postoperatively, compared with the false-negative scans, which averaged 6.1 years, suggesting that the usefulness of scintigraphy may diminish with time.

The technology continues to evolve. Technetium-99m nanocolloid scintigraphy has shown promising results, with a sensitivity of 94%, a specificity of 84%, and an accuracy of 87% (15). Another study evaluating indium scans combined with technetium sulfur colloid scans produced a 100% sensitivity, a 97% specificity, and a 98% accuracy (42). Immunoscintigraphy is another evolving area. For example, in one study evaluating antigranulocyte monoclonal antibody scans in 78 prostheses, the authors were able to exclude infection in 36% of the cases with positive bone scans (4). The role of these and other advances in scintigraphy, and their cost effectiveness in routine evaluation of failed prostheses, is still to be determined.

It is clear that there are significant institutional variations in approaches and results, and no regime for evaluation of the failed hip for sepsis has been universally accepted. The optimal protocol for any surgeon should consist of the combinations of tests most reliable in that center. One study (9) found that the combination of ESR, indium, and positive aspirate gave 100% concordance with infection, but this still provided only 80% accuracy.

Our experience in 32 suspected arthroplasties showed white cell count, differential, and blood cultures to be of little diagnostic value. An elevated ESR was found in all infected cases but also in 30% of aseptic failures. In our center, scintigraphic studies have not helped in the discrimination between septic and aseptic failures, and the aspirate continues to be the most useful investigation. If a dry tap is obtained, the joint is rinsed with sterile saline and the recovered fluid sent for culture. It has been our experience, and that of others (34,45), that true infections can be present in the presence of a dry tap. We routinely aspirate all revisions, having detected four cases of true infections in otherwise unsuspected prosthetic failures. Our current protocol includes ESR and C-reactive protein, aspiration with arthrographic confirmation, and plain radiographs. Fluid is sent for analysis and cell count in addition to cultures. In the presence of an equivocal culture result, or if there is concern about the possibility of contamination, the aspirate is repeated. Sequential scintigraphic studies are used only to follow patients with painful arthroplasties in the absence of loosening.

Clearly, there is no perfect screening or evaluation test to determine the presence or absence of infection in a failed total hip arthroplasty. Although we favor the use of hip aspiration, we recognize it is not a 100% sensitive or specific test and it is very important to keep in mind other available information and to maintain a high index of suspicion for the presence of sepsis.

For example, a 68-year-old woman underwent a total hip arthroplasty after developing a painful nonunion of a previous femoral neck fracture. Within 1 year of her total hip arthroplasty, she had developed symptomatic loosening of her hip with obvious radiographic signs of femoral component failure (see Fig. 3). Her referring surgeon had performed a hip aspirate that had failed to grow organisms and a technetium bone scan (Fig. 4) that had showed marked periprosthetic uptake.

Even in the absence of bacterial growth on the initial arthrogram, a very premature failure with such a radiographic and scintigraphic picture should appropriately raise the index of suspicion. Investigations included a C-reactive protein determination, which was elevated, and

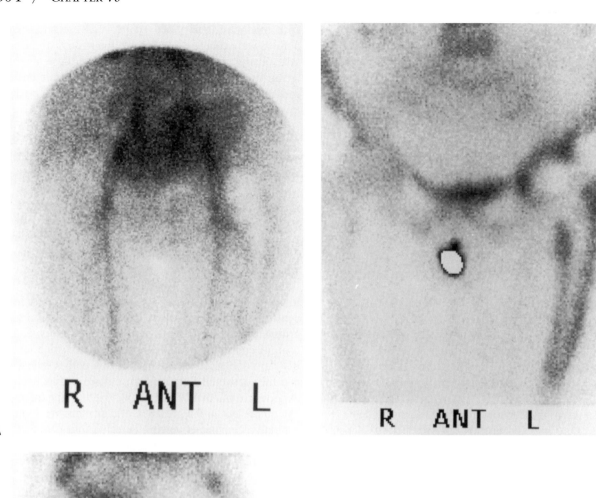

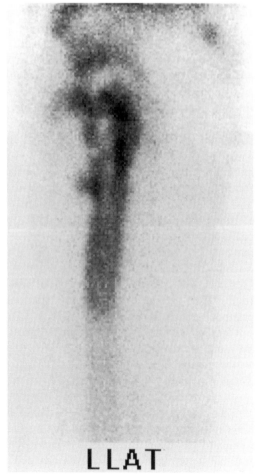

FIG. 4. A: Blood pool portion of technetium bone scan. **B:** Anterior view of technetium bone scan of the hip. **C:** Lateral view of technetium bone scan of the hip.

ESR, which was 35 mm. Repeat aspiration again failed to grow an organism.

Because of the overall picture, we had concerns about the potential for infection contributing to the failure of this arthroplasty and explained to the patient the possibility that we would proceed with a two-stage operation if our concerns continued intraoperatively. At the time of surgery, there was no frank pus present in the joint, but the proximal femur was markedly abnormal with significant granulation tissue present. Intraoperative frozen sections revealed eight polymorphonuclear leukocytes per high power field. Because of the abnormal clinical appearance and the positive frozen section, we elected to leave her initially as an excision arthroplasty with insertion of gentamicin beads. Tissue specimens were sent for culture from the time of surgery and definitively grew a *Streptococcus* species. Such a case typically illustrates that even the most reliable investigation in a particular institution has its limitations, and it is essential to carefully review all aspects and information available in trying to obtain a reasonable index of suspicion for the presence of sepsis in a failed arthroplasty.

SUMMARY

The devastating complication of an infected total hip arthoplasty has tremendous ramifications for the patient, the health care system, and the surgeon's ability to successfully revise the components. Avoidance of the complication is clearly the best defense against it, and this requires a clear understanding of all relevant issues and variables. Recognizing, and where possible decreasing, patient risk factors, and understanding the pathophysiology of the sepsis and its offending organisms will help diminish the incidence of this dreaded complication. Knowing how best to detect the presence of sepsis in a failed arthroplasty and understanding its significance for revision options and techniques is essential to optimize care and outcome of the revision procedure. The potential for sepsis should always be considered, and the patient should be carefully evaluated for it in every revision situation. Constant awareness of avoiding this complication during the preoperative, operative, and postoperative care is paramount, and a high index of suspicion of sepsis in all symptomatic arthroplasties must be maintained.

REFERENCES

1. Aalto K, Osterman K, Peltola H, Rasanen J. Changes in erythrocyte sedimentation rate and C-reactive protein after total hip arthroplasty. *Clin Orthop* 1984;184:118–120.
2. Athanasou NA, Pandey R, De Steiger R, Crook D, Smith PM. Diagnosis of infection by frozen section during revision arthroplasty. *J Bone Joint Surg* 1995;77B(1):28–33.
3. Barrack RL, Harris WH. The value of aspiration of the hip joint before revision total hip arthroplasty. *J Bone Joint Surg* 1993;75A(1);66–76.
4. Boubaker A, Delaloye AB, Dutoit M, Leyvraz PF, Delaloye B. Immunoscintigraphy with antigranulocyte monoclonal antibodies for the diagnosis of septic loosening of hip prostheses. *Eur J Nucl Med* 1995;22(2):139–147.
5. Buchholz HW, Elson RA, Englebrecht E, Lodenkamper H, Rottger J, Siegel A. Management of deep infection of total hip replacement. *J Bone Joint Surg* 1981;63B(3):342–353.
6. Charnley J. Postoperative infection after total hip replacement with special reference to air contamination in the operating room. *Clin Orthop* 1972;87:167–187.
7. Choudhry RR, Rice RP, Triffitt PD, Harper WM, Gregg PJ. Plasma viscosity and C-reactive protein after total hip and knee arthroplasty. *J Bone Joint Surg* 1992;74B(4):523–524.
8. Coventry MB. Treatment of infections occurring in total hip surgery. *Orthop Clin North Am* 1975;6:991–1003.
9. Cuckler JM, Star AM, Alavi A, Noto RB. Diagnosis and management of the infected total joint arthroplasty. *Orthop Clin North Am* 1991; 22(3):523–530.
10. Evans BG, Cuckler JM. Evaluation of the painful total hip arthroplasty. *Orthop Clin North Am* 1992;23(2):303–311.
11. Evans RP, Nelson CL, Lange TA. Pathophysiology of osteomyelitis. In: Evarts CM, ed. *Evarts' surgery of the musculoskeletal system*, New York: Churchill Livingston, 1990;4301–4312.
12. Fitzgerald RH. Total hip arthroplasty sepsis, prevention and diagnosis. *Orthop Clin North Am* 1992;23(2):259–264.
13. Fitzgerald RH Jr. Infected total hip arthroplasty: diagnosis and treatment. J Am Acad Orthop Surg 1995;3(5):249–262.
14. Fitzgerald RH Jr, Thompson RL. Cephalosporin antibiotics in the prevention and treatment of musculoskeletal sepsis. *J Bone Joint Surg* 1983;65A:1201–1205.
15. Flivik G, Sloth M, Rydholm U, Herrlin K, Lidgren L. Technetium 99m nanocolloid scintigraphy in orthopedic infections: a comparison with indium 111 labelled leukocytes. *J Nucl Med* 1993;34(10):1646–1650.
16. Garvin KL, Hanssen AD. Infection after total hip arthroplasty. *J Bone Joint Surg* 1995;77A(10):1576–1588.
17. Garvin KL, Fitzgerald RH, Salvati EA, Brause BD, Nercessian OA, Wallrichs SL, Ilstrup DM. Reconstruction of the infected total hip and knee arthroplasty with gentamycin-impregnated Palacos bone cement. *Instr Course Lect* 1993;42:293–302.
18. Gilliam DL, Nelson CL. Comparison of a one step iodophor skin preparation versus traditional preparation in total joint surgery. *Clin Orthop* 1990;250:258–260.
19. Glithero PR, Grigoris P, Harding LK, Hesslewood SR, McMinn DJ. White cell scans and infected joint replacements. Failure to detect chronic infection. *J Bone Joint Surg* 1993;75B(3):371–374.
20. Gristina AG, Barth E, Webb LX. Microbial adhesion and the pathogenesis of biomaterial-centered infections. In: Gustillo RB, ed. *Orthopaedic Infection: diagnosis and treatment*. Philadelohia: WB Saunders, 1989;3–25.
21. Gristina AG, Barth E, Webb LX. Microbes, metals, and other nonbiological substrata in man. In: Gustillo RB, ed. *Orthopaedic infection: diagnosis and treatment*. Philadelphia: Saunders; 1989;26–36.
22. Gristina AG, Naylor PT, Myrvik QN. Molecular mechanisms of musculoskeletal sepsis. In: Esterhai JL Jr, Gristina AG, Poss R, eds. *Musculoskeletal infection. American Academy of Orthopaedic Surgeons Symposium* 1990;13–28.
23. Gristina AG, Naylor PT, Webb LX. Molecular mechanisms in musculoskeletal sepsis: the race for the surface. *Instr Course Lect* 1990; 471–482.
24. Gristina AG, Shibata Y, Giridhar G, Kreger A, Myrvik QN. The glycocalyx, biofilm, microbes, and resistant infection. *Sem Arthroplasty* 1994;5(4);160–170.
25. Hamblen DL. Diagnosis of infection and the role of permanent excision arthroplasty. *Orthop Clin North Am* 1993;24(4):743–749.
26. Hester RA, Nelson CA, Harrison S. Control of contamination of the operative team in total joint arthroplasty. *J Arthroplasty* 1992;7(3): 267–269.
27. Hill C, Flamant R, Mazas F, Evrard J. Prophylactic cephazolin versus placebo in total hip replacement. *Lancet* 1981;1:795–796.
28. James PJ, Butcher IA, Gardner ER, Hamblin DL. Methicillin resistant *Staphylococcus epidermidis* in infection of hip arthroplasties. *J Bone Joint Surg* 1994;76B(5):725–727.
29. Josefsson G, Kolmert L. Prophylaxis with systemic antibiotics versus gentamicin bone cement in total hip arthroplasty. A ten year survey of 1,688 hips. *Clin Orthop* 1993;292:210–214.
30. Kraemer WJ, Saplys R, Waddell JP, Morton J. Bone scan, gallium scan and hip aspiration in the diagnosis of infected total hip arthroplasty. *J Arthroplasty* 1993;8(6):611–616.

31. Learmonth ID. Prevention of infection in the 1990s. *Orthop Clin North Am* 1993;24(4):735–741.
32. Levitksy KA, Hozack WJ, Balderston RA, Rothman RH, Gluckman SJ, Maslack MM, Booth RE Jr. Evaluation of the painful prosthetic joint. Relative value of bone scan, sedimentation rate, and joint aspiration. *J Arthroplasty* 1991;6(3):237–244.
33. Lidwill OM, Lowbury EJ, White W, Blowers R, Stanley SJ, Lowe D. Effect of ultraclean air in operating rooms on deep sepsis in the joint after total hip or knee replacement, a randomized study. *Br Med J* 1982;285:10–14.
34. Lopitaux R, Levai JP, Raux P, Hermet R, Grenier-Gaudin A, Sirot J. Interet de la ponction-arthrographie de hanche dans le diagnostic d'infection sur prothese totale. *Rev Chir Orthop Reparatrice Appar Mot* 1992;78(1):34–37.
35. Lyons CW, Berquist TH, Lyons JC. Evaluation of radiographic findings in painful hip arthroplasties. *Clin Orthop* 1985;195:239.
36. Marshall JC, Meakins JL. Immune responses and musculoskeletal disease. In: Evarts MC, ed. *Surgery of the musculoskeletal system*. New York: Churchill Livingston, 1990;4381–4397.
37. Maus TP, Berquist TH, Bender CE. Arthrographic study of painful total hip arthroplasty: refined criteria. *Radiology* 1987;162:171.
38. Merkel KD, Brown ML, Dewangee MK. Comparison of indium-labelled leukocyte imaging with sequential technetium-gallium scanning in the diagnosis of low-grade musculoskeletal sepsis, a prospective study. *J Bone Joint Surg* 1985;67A:465–476.
39. Nasser S. Prevention and treatment of sepsis in total hip replacement surgery. *Orthop Clin North Am* 1992;23(2):265–277.
40. Nelson C. Prevention of infection. In: Evarts CM, ed. *Surgery of the musculoskeletal system*. New York: Churchill Livingston, 1990; 4313–4321.
41. Nelson JP. Prevention of postoperative infection by airborne bacteria. In: Gustilo RB. *Orthopaedic infection: diagnosis and treatment*. Philadelphia: WB Saunders, 1989;75–80.
42. Palestro CJ, Kim CK, Swyer AJ. Total hip arthroplasty: periprosthetic indium-111-labelled leukocyte activity and complimentary technetium-99-sulfur colloid imaging in suspected infection. *J Nucl Med* 1990;31:1950.
43. Pollard JP, Hughes SPF, Scott JE. Antibiotic prophylaxis in total joint replacement. *Br Med J* 1979;1:707–709.
44. Rainey-McDonald CG, Holliday RL, Wells GA, Donner AP. Validity of a two-variable nutritional index for use in electing candidates for nutritional support. *J Parenter Enter Nutr* 1983;7(1):15.
45. Roberts P, Walters AJ, McMinn DJ. Diagnosing infection in hip replacements. The use of fine needle aspiration and radiometric culture. *J Bone Joint Surg* 1992;74B(2):265–269.
46. Salvati EA. The infected total hip replacement. In: Evarts CM, ed. *Surgery of the musculoskeletal system*. New York: Churchill Livingston, 1990;4475–4493.
47. Sanzen L, Carlsson A. The diagnostic value of C-reactive protein in infected total hip arthroplasties. *J Bone Joint Surg* 1989;71B:638–641.
48. Schmalzried TP, Amstutz HC, Au MK, Dorey FJ. Etiology of deep sepsis in total hip arthroplasty: the significance of hematogenous and recurrent infections. *Clin Orthop* 1992;280:200–207.
49. Shih LY, Wu JJ, Yang DJ. Erythrocyte sedimentation rate and C-reactive protein values in patients with total hip arthroplasty. *Clin Orthop* 1989;225:238–246.
50. Taylor T, Beggs I. Fine needle aspirates in infected hip replacements. *Clin Radiol* 1995;50(3):149–152.
51. Tigges S, Stiles RG, Meli RJ, Roberson JR. Hip aspiration; a cost effective and accurate method of evaluating the potentially infected hip prosthesis. *Radiology* 1993;189(2):485–488.
52. Tsukayama DT, Estrada R, Gustilo RB. Infection after total hip arthroplasty. A study of the treatment of 106 infections. *J Bone Joint Surg* 1996;78A:512–523.
53. van Holsbeek MT, Eyler WR, Sherman LS, Lombardi TJ, Mezger E, Verner JJ, Schurman JR, Jonnson K. Detection of infection in loosened hip prostheses: efficacy of sonography. *AJR* 1994;163(2):381–384.
54. Wymenga A, van Horn J, Theeuwes A, Muytjens H, Sloof T. Cefuroxime for prevention of postoperative coxitis. One versus three doses tested in a randomized multicenter study of 2651 arthroplasties. *Acta Orthop Scand* 1992;63(1):19–24.
55. Yoon SI, Lim SS, Rha JD, Kim YH, Kang JS, Baek GH, Yang KH. The C-reactive protein in patients with long bone fractures and after arthroplasty. *Int Orthop* 1993;17(3):198–201.

The Adult Hip, edited by J. J. Callaghan,
A. G. Rosenberg, and H. E. Rubash.
Lippincott–Raven Publishers, Philadelphia © 1998.

CHAPTER 80

Sepsis: One-Stage Exchange

Reginald A. Elson

The principles of management of the infected hip arthroplasty (or any other joint arthroplasty) are now clearly understood:

1. Obtain an accurate microbiologic diagnosis and an antibiogram.
2. Excise infected tissue and remove contaminated implant.
3. Institute antibiotic therapy, local and systemic.
4. Reimplant a prosthesis: direct or delayed; cemented or uncemented; if cement, with or without antibiotic; with or without bone graft.
5. Indefinite follow-up.

It is the choice and refinement of these principles that confronts the thinking and responsible practitioner. There are no absolute answers to the many aspects concerned and, in particular, to whether a one- or two-stage exchange for the infection disaster should be advised.

The danger is that a writer should presume to be an advocate for a specific method of treatment. There must be no element of competition in the matter. Everything should depend on experience and a correctly audited evaluation of personal results in comparison with those of other researchers. Undoubtedly, the choice of method of management is likely to be influenced by previous mentors. Certainly, for me this was John Charnley, for whom I worked in 1966, and then Hans Buchholz in Hamburg in 1976. In those days, the advent of a deep infection was confused with so-called sterile inflammation, which Charnley suspected was associated with some ill-understood reaction to acrylic cement. He had to contend with a lot of occult criticisms from colleagues at this time, and the Teflon outcome was still much in mind. So many of the infections seemed to be without bacterial identity. The milestones in our understanding are the contributions of William Petty et al. (16) and Hans Buchholz et al. (3), our small contribution in the identification the multiple strains of the coagulase-negative staphylococci (CNS), and the self-isolation from defense mechanisms and antibiotics by slime formation (glycocalyx) described by Gristina and Kolkin (12).

The incidence of deep infection has declined during the last 20 years; however, infections from one source or another will continue to occur and they will have to be treated. In general, infections should be managed in consultation with or referral to centers dealing with significant numbers, which have the experience and equipment necessary for optimal management. The choice of one- or two-stage management is of secondary importance because the experienced practitioner will know what can be achieved using the chosen methods. The majority of infections treated in special centers nowadays will be from referral.

With these remarks in mind, the following account outlines the principles followed by the Department of Orthopaedics at the Northern General Hospital in Sheffield, United Kingdom. These have been largely influenced by my relationship with the EndoKlinik in Hamburg, but they are modified by local facilities that are not as extensive as those in Germany. Nevertheless, our performance can be regarded as average to good, the result of attempts to optimize the ideals of best management within the framework of a British National Health hospital.

R. A. Elson: Department of Orthopaedics, Northern General Hospital, Sheffield S5 7AU, United Kingdom.

DIAGNOSIS

Crucial to successful management are diagnosis and assessment of bone stock. Apart from obvious signs of infection (pyrexia, raised erythrocyte sedimentation rate, abscess formation, or sinus) diagnosis is mainly from radiologic and microbiologic studies; when a one-stage procedure is envisaged, it is mandatory that the workup should include an accurate bacteriologic identification. When infection is suspected, the suspect joint should be immediately aspirated, with or without tissue biopsy. It is remarkable that in many studies, great emphasis is placed on special investigations before basic microbiologic considerations have been addressed. Even when there is no evidence of infection, the joint should be aspirated if an exchange is contemplated. It is best to obtain a culture and an antibiogram, together with hematologic studies, for both one- and two-stage procedures.

We continue to aspirate and take a tissue sample by a closed cannular technique under a brief anesthetic although the practice is under current review (unfortunately not yet completed). The procedure is performed in a clean-air environment.

Microbiologic processing includes immediate transfer of fluid and tissue fragments in brain–heart and Robertson's cooked-meat media for aerobic and anaerobic culture, as well as Gram staining. Subculturing is performed on the 5th and 12th days. This process takes a minimum of 2 weeks, and the cooperation of a dedicated microbiologist is essential for accuracy.

Using this protocol, assessment of accuracy in 1991 was as follows:

Sensitivity	84%
Specificity	87%
False-positives	13%
False-negatives	16%
Overall accuracy	86%

The reason for laboring the uncertainties of bacteriologic care is that several studies have suggested that such an expensive procedure is unnecessary and that comparable accuracy can be had from simpler methods. Thus, Roberts et al. (18), using a simple fine-needle aspiration performed under radiographic control with local anesthesia, achieved overall accuracy of 94% in a series of 78 cases. Sixty-three (81%) of these proved sterile. In contrast, 56% of our series were definitely infected, and in a further 11% there was strong evidence for suspecting infection.

Barrack and Harris (2) went so far as to state that routine aspiration is unnecessary before exchanging a loose prosthesis. This conclusion was based on a large series of 270 aspirations performed by the radiologist: only 2% of their cases had proven infections, and there was a 13% false-positive rate. It is possible that the latter resulted from aspiration outside a clean-air enclosure (the incidence is similar to ours performed in full aseptic circumstances during the latter part of our series). The small number of infected cases in the preceding series is in contrast to our material, which includes many infected cases referred to us because of our interest in the subject.

Despite the debate, all authors advocate that whenever there is doubt, aspiration, at least, is mandatory. Personal experience will influence the threshold of such doubt.

Our limited experience indicates that radionuclide scans are of uncertain value. Opinions range from agreement with this view to the belief that such investigations are more specific than bacteriologic proof, a very difficult attitude to justify. Nevertheless, there are patients in whom there is pain or some other nonspecific problem for which every scrap of diagnostic evidence must be sought; unexplained pain is a source of anxiety, with the fear of smoldering infection.

Finally, histologic assessment may have a place. Certainly, when a microbiologically "blind" revision is performed and the expert facilities are available, it is worthwhile to be mindful of the impressive results described by Athanasou et al. (1): using the criterion of more than one neutrophil per high power field, a diagnostic accuracy of 95% was achieved with histologic methods. However, the inevitable conclusion is that, in the event of an infection being detected at the time of revision, the execution of a one-stage exchange cannot be entertained, as no antibiogram is available. The benefit of a nonspecific on-the-spot diagnosis of infection cannot be compared with conclusive information from preoperative assessments.

For the present, at least, our unit continues the expensive drill-biopsy routine for most exchanges, and we continue to study the results. Even when a delayed program is envisaged, bacteriologic accuracy is optimal for appropriate systemic antibiotic therapy because of the possible use of antibiotic-loaded acrylic pellets, a valuable means of controlling the infected or contaminated field.

Efforts to classify infection into early, intermediate, or late are of interest, but in individual cases they are without practical value. Violent acute infection can occur late (i.e., more than 1 year postoperatively), and some patients are seen in whom a smoldering low-grade manifestation has presented from the immediate postoperative phase; therefore, every suspected deep infection should be assessed individually. A previous history of revision or infection is immaterial except in respect to loss of bone stock; a new and accurate diagnosis is always necessary. Even when a past history of infection is known, a fresh bacteriologic diagnosis is essential.

Particular care must be devoted to the assessment of infections by the CNS. In our series, between 1974 and 1980, 28% of clinical infections were regarded as sterile; some even presented with a discharging sinus. Between 1980 and 1986, inability to culture organisms fell to 7% as a result of our awareness that the CNS was not an

TABLE 1. *Antibiograms of eight treacherous strains of CNS isolated from one culture from an infected cemented hip arthroplasty (without antibiotic)*

	Biopsy			Excision arthroplasty (~3 mo later)					
Penicillin	S	R	R	R	S	R	R	R	R
Cloxacillin	S	R	S	S	S	R	S	R	S
Erythromycin	R	R	S	R	S	R	R	S	S
Gentamicin	S	S	S	S	S	S	S	R	S
Cefuroxime	M	M	S	M	S	R	S	S	S
Cephalothin	S	S	S	S	M	R	M	S	S

CNS, coagulase-negative staphylococci; S, sensitive; R, resistant; M, moderately sensitive.
Pellets subsequently used to disinfect were Palacos with 3.5 g gentamicin and 2 g cephalothin. At reimplantation (~3 mo after excision arthroplasty), the site was sterile.

organism of "no significance." In contrast, it is now one of our most serious problems, and since 1983 we recognize that within one culture of this treacherous organism, more than one strain can exist, each with a different antibiogram (13). This was a new problem, especially for one-stage exchange procedures, and it explained some former failures.

Table 1 shows the antibiograms of three strains taken at biopsy and five strains taken at the arthroplastic surgery. One of the latter strains was resistant to gentamicin, an antibiotic added to cement for control of the organisms thought to be the main infective agents. In fact, this particular case remains controlled, probably because other antibiotics were incorporated in the cement used for final implantation. As stated, Petty et al. (16) mentioned the significance of the ability of the CNS to colonize pre-polymerized polymethylmethacrylate (PMMA). Later studies (6) confirmed the increased likelihood of contamination on metal implants, in addition to the particular susceptibilities of PMMA in this respect.

Infections associated with CNS need to be treated with particular care, especially when considering one-stage exchange. Fungal infections (e.g., *Candida* species) are fortunately rare. Gram-negative infections are often associated with extensive soft-tissue involvement, which makes excision especially difficult. Nevertheless, the same principles for management apply, and because of the availability of appropriate antibiotic powders and the surety of sensitivity, one-stage procedures can be considered.

ANTIBIOTIC-LOADED ACRYLIC CEMENT

Buchholz and Engelbrecht (5) described the apparently naïve concept of adding antibiotic to acrylic cement. Their claims have been substantiated (8,24); large concentrations of antibiotics can elute from PMMA if powders are incorporated prior to curing. Stable antibiotics such as aminoglycosides elute for longer periods, and other antibiotics elute for brief but nevertheless useful periods. Gentamicin was the agent chosen in Europe, but in the United States, because of Food and Drug Adminis-

tration (FDA) restrictions, other materials had to be used (e.g., tobramycin). Even now, there is some doubt as to the therapeutic place of these composites, and there is justified concern about the potential dangers from denaturing the mechanical properties of PMMA needed for fixation of a new implant.

All acrylic cements afford elution properties, but, because of the nature of the filler agent, the Palacos R brand allows higher amounts to escape for longer periods. It was by chance that Buchholz and Engelbrecht (5) were using this cement at the time they were developing their product, Refobacin Palacos. The higher elution property applies to other antibiotics generally. The stable amino-glycosides are most effective. Wahlig and Dingeldein (24) examined many antibiotics with Palacos R, and some of the elution comparisons are summarized in Table 2. To these can be added vancomycin (for resistant CNS) and fluconazole (for some yeasts).

Antibiotic-loaded acrylic cements (ALAC) can be used in direct or delayed reimplantation for the fixation of a new implant, but the deleterious effect of crudely mixing powder with polymer in the operating room prior to adding monomer is disturbing. As much as 4 g of powder has been added on many occasions, and the resultant texture of the cured cement is alarming (Fig. 1). Nevertheless, the control of infection has been undoubted and the evidence of failure from cement abuse not evident. Comparison of the survival of reimplantations using amounts of antibiotic less or greater

TABLE 2. *Release of antibiotics from Palacos-R in vitro over 10 days*

Antibiotic	Average µg/mL per day
Gentamicin	14.31
Colistin	5.04
Bacitracin	0.43 (IU)
Fucidinic acid	0.11
Erythromycin	2.36
Lincomycin	10.96
Cefazedone	11.77

Multiple strains of coagulase-negative staphylococcus species isolated from one culture. Strains are identified by antibiogram.

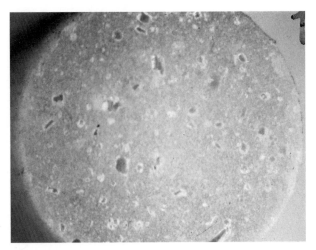

FIG. 1. Appearance of Palacos R cement containing 3.5 g antibiotic powder per 40 g polymer powder, before curing.

than 2 g has not revealed any significant differences; as in all other studies, failures have taken place at a bone–cement interface as a result of the unsuitable surface available for intrusion. It must be recognized that the more recent exploitation of cemented, impacted, morselized bone grafting, which, in effect, provides a new surface for cement attachment, has introduced an additional factor into the equation concerning the advisability of direct exchange. Usually, delayed exchange is advised (whether it be cemented or uncemented) for infected cases when bone grafting is necessary. When cement is removed before the loosening (caused by infective tissue reaction) has progressed to involve the whole bone–cement interface, a surface often remains that is appropriate for recementing. Unfortunately, many cases are referred to us after unnecessarily extensive destruction has occurred, so grafting is necessary.

Antibiotic-loaded acrylic cements can also be used in pellet form during the interval phase of a two-stage

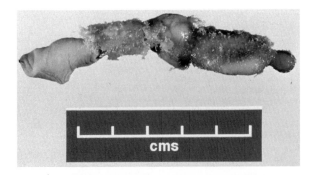

FIG. 2. "Home-made" pellets after removal from femoral medullary cavity 7 weeks after insertion during a two-stage program. Note flattened shape pressed onto braided wire, and the coarsely textured woven bone that has formed within the interstices of the pellets.

exchange. We have been so confident in its effectiveness that we have not seen fit to biopsy the field before conducting the reimplantation. (Regretfully, this confidence was disturbed by one example in November 1995, in which a resistant CNS was not controlled, and reimplantation occurred in a contaminated field; the future for this hip is uncertain.) In pellet form, large amounts of appropriate antibiotic powder can be added because there is no concern for the mechanical function. As an aid to removal, beads can be threaded on braided wire. The only caution is to ensure that the conglomerate of beads should be housed in bone and not allowed to massage the mobile soft tissues. We have had several examples of formation of a seroma of considerable volume (sterile, red, and almost transparent fluid) caused, we believe, by acrylic particles generated by friction with soft tissues. There is no need for pellets to be confined to the commercially available items, although these are convenient; Seligson et al. (21) have shown that the elution from "home-made" beads that can be prepared before or at the time of surgery is similar to that from commercial products. In fact, by squeezing the pellets into flat plates, there is a larger surface area available for elution for a given volume than with spherical beads.

An interesting phenomenon is the presence of woven bone that generates in the interstices of the beads during the interval phase. This is not a specific property of the beads but part of the roughening regeneration of the endosteal bone surface that occurs during the period; this may be another advantage of allowing a two-stage interval (Fig. 2) rather than performing a one-stage procedure, which is the primary scope of this chapter.

TECHNIQUE

Exposure

The trochanteric osteotomy allows the best exposure for excision of the infected field, but in the non-obese subject without tough scarred soft tissues or some complex bony configuration, anterolateral, transgluteal, or dorsal approaches can avoid the inevitable complications of the trochanteric re-attachment especially when the upper femoral bone stock is impoverished; this is especially the case when femoral impaction bone grafting is necessary. A roof or chevron type of osteotomy (Fig. 3) affords marked stability, but there are cases in which the trochanter is eroded to a fragile shell (7).

Excision

The necessity for complete soft-tissue and cement excision is well established and needs no emphasis. It can on occasion be alarmingly hemorrhagic, but it must be

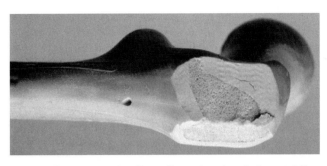

FIG. 3. Chevron or "roof" configuration that helps stabilize the osteosynthesis of the trochanter osteotomy.

complete. A sinus track should be excised in continuity with its source, the infective focus, and all its ramifications. A discharging sinus is not a contraindication to direct exchange. This has been recognized on many occasions: in our series of infected cases, open sinuses were present in 54% of patients at the time of surgery, and in a further 14% there was a past history of a wound discharge. Although cultures were taken routinely, that from a sinus track does not reflect accurately the bacteriology of the source of the deep infection (17). A sinus is related to a source that the body cannot discharge; if the source is removed, the sinus will close. If the track is too dangerous to excise because of nearby structures, when the

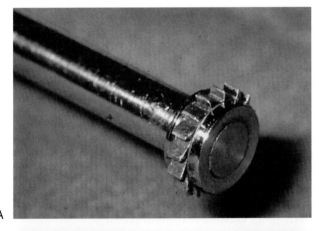

A

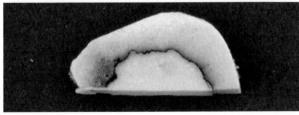

B

FIG. 4. A: Femoral reaming saw. **B:** Configuration of the macrointerlock afforded for cement intrusion. This is vastly coarser than that afforded by the corticocancellous bone, which is often lost.

source has been removed, a chain of ALAC beads can be threaded to the surface and then withdrawn progressively, allowing the sinus to close behind them. In this role, commercially available spherical pellets on a wire, slide more easily than the rough home-made ones.

Cement fragments must be evacuated; sometimes there is a question of whether this has been complete, especially inside the femoral shaft. Perhaps *thin* lamellae that remain firmly attached can be sterilized, but it is preferable to remove them completely. A periscope, headlight, or 90-degree arthroscope can aid inspection. Intraoperative radiographs should be considered if there is concern about cement retention.

In the choice between one- and two-stage procedures, the matter of bone stock becomes crucial. In principle, if excision is performed early (more common in the cemented case), the process of chipping away the cement leaves a rough surface still amenable for intrusion. If, on the other hand, general loosening from the infective process has been allowed to occur, a smooth featureless endosteal surface remains that is entirely unsuited for recementing. Earlier, we attempted to make the best of this poor situation by painstaking attempts to key the cortical bone; whether this contributed to the relatively good survival of our cemented exchanges (usually without grafting) is uncertain, because there is no way of proving the contention. Keying, which provides a macrointerlock, can be done radially in the femur with a femoral reaming saw (Fig. 4), and vertically with an orbital saw with copious irrigation (Fig. 5). Cementing was with routine compression. In both the femur and the acetabulum, the need for grafting precludes one-stage reimplantation.

The amount of bone to be excised can be difficult to define. In general, even when there is vascular soft-tissue attachment and if ALAC is used, areas of necrotic bone can be sterilized by diffusion of the high concentration of local antibiotic. Avascular bone will have to be sacrificed, and in these circumstances a temporary spacer may be helpful. We have on occasion resorted to a temporary one-stage method, loosely cementing a socket and a femoral component, the shank of which has been coated with ALAC. However, this is done at the risk of seroma formation, which in one instance led to enormous swelling of the thigh.

PERSONAL EXPERIENCE

Experience must be interpreted from two viewpoints: control of the infection, and survival of the reimplanted prosthesis. The quality of the function attained is another aspect that relates to any type of revision. Our last comprehensive review of patient material was completed in 1991 and since that time, there have been a few additional failures from re-infection and a more significant

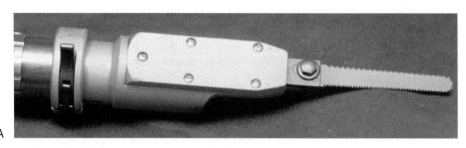

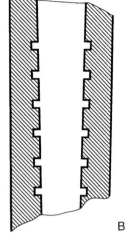

FIG. 5. A: Orbital saw. **B:** Section of femoral shaft showing vertical configuration of stabilizing channels in the cortical bone surface. **B**

number of mechanical failures of the cemented exchanges, which occurred in both infected and noninfected cases. The following is a summary of data published by Scott and Elson (20):

Period of study	1978–1990
Total number of hip and knee exchanges	503
Excluded from study	
Cases left as pseudarthrosis	19
Uncemented revisions	
Saddle arthroplasties	
Included in study	
Patients lost to follow-up	14*
Patients who died	73*
Cemented exchange arthroplasties (total)	440
Definitely infected	247
Possibly infected	49
(Total "probably" infected	296**)
Not infected	144

* No recurrence of infection at time of loss.

** The concept of "probably" infected relates to a variety of uncertainties, sometimes amounting to a discharging sinus from which no positive bacteriologic culture was obtained, or cases in which cultures were not obtained from a minimum of three tissue sample cultures at the time of primary excision.

An analysis of the number of previous operations and exchanges, the bacteriologic species isolated, and the details of antibiotic therapy employed introduce so many variables that this relatively large series becomes fragmented to a degree that really scientific evaluation is impossible. Each center must select its own method of management and exploit it to the full. Only relatively crude comparisons can be made with other series published.

Our results with regard to control of infection apparent at the time of follow-up in 1991 (and with slight deterio-

ration of about 5%) from both one- and two-stage procedures were as follows:

	One stage		Two stage	
	N	Failure rate (%)	N	Failure rate (%)
All infected exchanges	239	10.5–15.0	67	4.5–7.5
Noninfected exchanges	131	5.3–9.2	7	0.0

The range of failure encompasses the definite failures and cases in which there was strong, or some suspicion of, evidence of a reinfection.

There is a significant, fourfold-higher failure rate for one-stage procedures. These results emanate from a period when, undoubtedly, our experience was deficient and our facilities were less comprehensive than at present. The following information has been gathered from the 33 definite failures from re-infection.

Preliminary biopsy inaccurate	8
Inaccuracy from CNS underestimation	12
New infections	
(i.e., with a different bacteriologic species)	4
Inadequate treatment	
(e.g., poor excision or retained cement)	3
Unexplained failures	6

It is also important to note that there was a 6% incidence of deep infection in patients in whom no previous infection had been detected.

These comments are not made to justify the failures or to suggest that they can be avoided; however, by refining the indications for a direct exchange, the risks of re-infection may influence the balance between that risk and the advantages of one operative procedure.

From the point of view of control of infection, in the bacteriologically straightforward case, a one-stage exchange can, in experienced hands, be successfully managed in about 80% of cases irrespective of past history. Control of the infection is the primary aim, and failure caused by recrudescence is a sporadic event: it is most likely to be recognized within 1 year, but much more delayed failures occur. Nevertheless, because failure from reinfection is not inevitable, the result is not appropriate for assessment in actuarial survival.

The advantage of one-stage exchange is the avoidance of the second operative procedure. Almost certainly, there is an enhanced risk of re-infection, but this must be weighed against subjecting the patient to two large operative interventions. If the organism is straightforward, such as *Staphylococcus aureus*, *Corynebacterium*, *Peptococcus*, most streptococci, and sensitive CNS, one-stage exchange can be performed after very careful study. Colleagues at the EndoKlinik in Hamburg remain very definite in their one-stage practice, and, except in cases of bone grafting (17,23,26), they confirm the safety in selected cases. My preferences have modified because of the CNS problem outlined and the increasing need for grafting in the types of patients referred to us, but whenever considered prudent I will resort to a one-stage cemented exchange procedure.

MECHANICAL SURVIVAL

Although in the absence of infection control, all other considerations pale, the survival of a cemented revision is always suspect; this applies especially to the late or repeatedly revised joint when there is serious loss of bone stock. Further, following guidance from the EndoKlinik in Hamburg, one of the most serious concerns is the knowledge that by adding antibiotic powder to acrylic cement in the crude fashion employed in the operating room, there must be serious impairment of mechanical properties of the resulting cement composite. Large voids are apparent, and in screening tests performed by Lee in the Exeter University Department of Mechanical Engineering (personal communications, 1984), it was shown that the effect of adding 2.5 g antibiotic powder to 40 g polymer was a reduction of 12% of the compressive strength compared with plain Palacos R. The addition of 3.5 g caused a decrement of 18%. Both figures were accompanied by very significant scatter. (The texture of the adulterated cement has been noted in Fig. 1.) These facts are labored because when debating the advantages and disadvantages of any particular method, a frank appraisal of the risks is essential. Surprisingly, although there is a progressive mechanical survival failure of our cemented revisions, in both infected and uninfected cases, there is no statistical difference between survival in the cases using cement with less than 2.5 g and those using more than 2.5 g antibiotic powder (weights of antibiotic powder relate to base salt load).

Survival results were assessed in 1991. Knee arthroplasties are included in the results relating to control of infection because the principles are precisely the same as those concerned with hip replacements. The survival statistics of the hip exchanges, on the other hand, concern a subset of 369 hips that were assessed for mechanical or radiologic failure. The assumption was that if an infected case were deemed cured, it could reasonably be included in the group assessed for mechanical or radiologic failure. Mechanical failure was defined as the need for a further exchange (whether performed or not), and possibly impending mechanical failure accounts for the larger figure shown in the range of failures noted. The following table shows the conventional percentages of failure rates, with ranges based on a follow-up period of 2 to 20 years; 389 patients had a follow-up of more than 1 year and 194 had a minimum follow-up period of 5 years.

	One-stage exchange		Two-stage exchange	
	N	Failure rate (%)	N	Failure rate (%)
Infected	200	8.5–12.0	61	3.3–8.2
Not infected	102	2.9–8.8	6	0.0

The range of failure rates occurs because there were still specific instances in which it was impossible to be sure whether failure was going to occur. There *appears* to be a difference in mechanical survivals comparing one- and two-stage procedures; however, comparison of survival (actuarial) curves indicate that there was no statistical difference in this respect. Figure 6 demonstrates the overall survivorship related to mechanical failure.

Radiologic failure is defined as progressive loosening and migration of components. The appearance of a radiolucent line is regarded as impending radiologic failure; many of these cases had radiolucencies from the start. Radiologic failure heralds mechanical failure, but this result is not inevitable (Fig. 7). The curves of survival become uncertain at 14 years because of the few patients followed to that point.

A higher failure rate was exhibited in the age group under 40 years (Fig. 8), but no difference was found between different antibiotic loadings, nor between sterile and infected cases.

The inevitable question is posed: By comparison of published series or by meta-analysis, can we identify a place for one-stage exchange in cases of deep infection? In my view, we cannot. The preponderance of opinion favors two-stage exchange. I have highlighted some salient factors to be used in the decision-making process, such as the CNS, bone grafting, and the much less common, difficult organisms (*Klebsiella*, *Pseudomonas*, group D streptococci, and *Bacteroides* species), but the main influence on choice depends on personal experience.

The results outlined are similar to those of others who use one-stage cemented exchange in preference to other

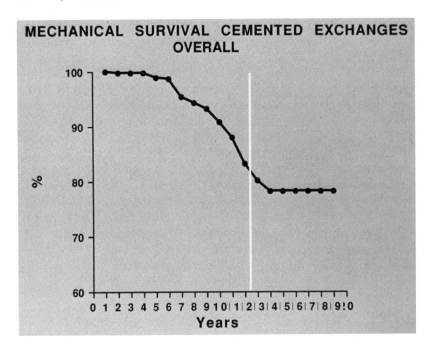

FIG. 6. Survivorship to mechanical failure. After 12 years, the tail of the curve becomes uncertain. All cases included.

methods, but as is often the case, varying criteria and length of follow-up and the enormous number of variables concerned make meaningful comparison difficult.

Buchholz et al. (4) reviewed again the series in an earlier report that contained the original description of the one-stage procedure (Buchholz et al., 1978). Other workers have considered their own methods to be efficacious, but the numbers of their cases have been relatively small and their criteria of assessment vary. Furthermore, the survivals are not always identified in mechanical and radiologic terms. In the United States, Nasser et al. (1989) described 30 septic one-stage exchanges without recurrence; Garvin et al. (9) described slightly better results from two-stage procedures than from one-stage. In

Europe, Raut et al. (17) described 57 cases with discharging sinuses (referred to previously) with good results in 86% of these, and Sanzén et al. (19) referred to 76% success in 72 hips. In an excellent article on infection management, Garvin and Hanssen (10) summarized:

> The complexity of the operative procedure and the many factors involved . . . have discouraged investigators from performing prospective, randomized trials to evaluate the timing (one-stage or two-stage procedure).

I am forced to agree and I have no solution. The relatively recent expansion in bone grafting has required surgeons to resort more to two-stage management. Whether morselized bone could be used as a vehicle for

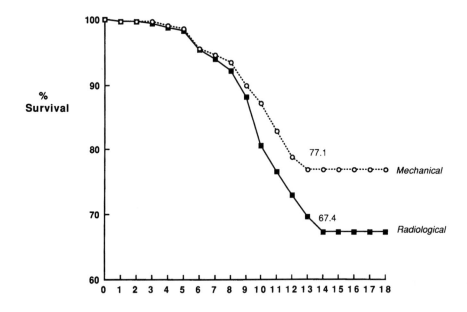

FIG. 7. Comparison of survival curves for hips in patients of over and under 40 years.

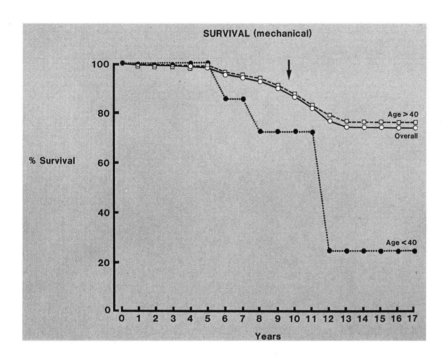

FIG. 8. Comparison of mechanical and radiologic survivals for all cases.

incorporation of antibiotic in clinical practice remains doubtful, although it has been described in animal studies (15).

In summary, the one-stage management of the infected joint arthroplasty has a definite place, but it should not be regarded as a routine policy. In these days of cost constraints, it should be considered in the appropriate situation. It requires the use of ALAC and should be restricted to cases with an early intervention, which allows preservation of bone stock, and to cases that afford an endosteal surface adequate for cement intrusion. Accurate bacterial diagnosis is essential. One-stage management is inappropriate when bone grafting is required. Whenever in doubt, recourse to a two-stage operation is wise. Finally, it should be noted that although most failures from reinfection are apparent within 18 months from the time of exchange, whether direct or delayed, failure can occur at any time in the future. Therefore, signs of radiologic and mechanical failure should be sought at regular examination for an indefinite period.

REFERENCES

1. Athanasou NA, Pandy R, de Steiger R, Crook D, McLardy Smith P. Diagnosis of infection by frozen section during revision arthroplasty. *J Bone Joint Surg* 1995;77B:28–33.
2. Barrack RL, Harris WH. The value of aspiration of the hip joint before revision total hip arthroplasty. *J Bone Joint Surg* 1993;75A:66–76.
3. Buchholz HW, Elson RA, Engelbrecht E, Lodenkämper H, Röttger J, Siegel A. Management of deep infection in total hip replacement. *J Bone Joint Surg* 1981;63B:342–353.
4. Buchholz HW, Elson RA, Heinert K. Antibiotic-loaded acrylic cement: current concepts. *Clin Orthop* 1984;190:96–108.
5. Buchholz HW, Engelbrecht H. Über die Depotwirkung einiger Antibiotica bei Vermischung mit dem Kunstharz Palacos. *Chirurg* 1970;40:511.
6. Cordero J, Manuera L, Folgueira MD. Influence of metal implants on infection. *J Bone Joint Surg* 1994;76B:717–720.
7. Dall DM, Miles AW. Re-attachment of the greater trochanter. *J Bone Joint Surg* 1983;65B:55–59.
8. Elson RA, Jephcott AE, McGechie DB, Verettas D. Antibiotic-loaded acrylic cement. *J Bone Joint Surg* 1977;59B:200–205.
9. Garvin KL, Evans BG, Salvati EA, Brause BD. Palacos gentamicin for the treatment of deep periprosthetic hip infections. *Clin Orthop* 1994; 298:97–105.
10. Garvin KL, Hanssen AD. Infection after total hip arthroplasty *J Bone Joint Surg* 1995;77A:1576–1588.
11. Gie G, Templey J, Ling RSM. Impaction cancellous grafting in cemented revision hip arthroplasty. In: J Older, ed. *Bone implant grafting*. Berlin: Springer-Verlag, 1992.
12. Gristina AG, Kolkin J. Current concepts review. Total joint replacement and sepsis. *J Bone Joint Surg* 1983;65A:128–134.
13. Hope PG, Kristinsson KG, Norman P, Elson RA. Deep infection of total hip arthroplasties caused by coagulase-negative staphylococci. *J Bone Joint Surg* 1989;71B:851–855.
14. Izquierdo RJ, Northmore-Ball MD. Long-term results of revision hip arthroplasty. *J Bone Joint Surg* 1994;76B:34–39.
15. Lindsey RW, Probe R, Miclau T, Alexander JW, Perren SM. The effects of antibiotic-impregnated autogeneic cancellous bone graft on bone healing. *Clin Orthop* 1993;291:303–311.
16. Petty W, Spanier S, Shuster JJ, Silverthorne C. The influence of skeletal implants on incidence of infection. *J Bone Joint Surg* 1985;67A: 1236–1244.
17. Raut VV, Siney PD, Wroblewski BM. One-stage revision of infected total hip replacements with discharging sinuses. *J Bone Joint Surg* 1995;76B:721–724.
18. Roberts P, Walters AJ, McMinn DJW. Diagnosing infection in hip replacements. *J Bone Joint Surg* 1992;74B:264–269.
19. Sanzén L, Carlsson AS, Josefsson G, Lindberg LT. Revision operations on infected total hip arthroplasties. *Clin Orthop* 1988;229:165–172.
20. Scott IR, Elson RA. Cemented exchange hip arthroplasties—a 17 year experience. *J Bone Joint Surg* 1991;73B(suppl 2):165.
21. Seligson D, Popham GH, Voos K, Henry SL, Faghri M. Antibiotic-leaching from polymethylmethacrylate beads. *J Bone Joint Surg* 1993; 75A:514–720.
22. Sloof TJJF. Acetabular augmentation in cemented arthroplasty: preoperative assessment and surgical technique. In: J Older, ed. *Bone implant grafting*. Berlin: Springer-Verlag, 1992.
23. Steinbrink K. The case for revision arthroplasty using antibiotic-loaded acrylic cement. *Clin Orthop* 1990;261:19–22.
24. Wahlig H, Dingeldein E. Antibiotics and bone cements. *Acta Orthop Scand* 1980;51:49–56.
25. Went P, Krismer M, Frischhut B. Recurrence of infection after revision of infected hip arthroplasties. *J Bone Joint Surg* 1995;77B: 307–309.
26. Wroblewski BM. One-stage revision of infected cemented total hip arthroplasty. *Clin Orthop* 1986;211:103–107.

The Adult Hip, edited by J. J. Callaghan,
A. G. Rosenberg, and H. E. Rubash.
Lippincott–Raven Publishers, Philadelphia © 1998.

CHAPTER 81

Sepsis: Two-Stage Exchange

Bassam A. Masri and Eduardo A. Salvati

Infection continues to be one of the most feared complications of total hip arthroplasty, second only to fatal pulmonary embolism in its devastating effect. Despite many advances over the past three decades, this complication continues to be a blemish on the face of an otherwise very successful and highly predictable procedure. In 1982, the late Sir John Charnley wrote, "Postoperative infection after total hip replacement is the saddest of all complications: it is sad because it seriously limits the success of any subsequent operations undertaken to revise a poor result following a first intervention" (15). Nelson, in 1977, expressed an equally pessimistic view when he reported the death of 10 of 16 patients with infected total hip arthroplasties (68). Fortunately, today the picture is not as bleak. With contemporary aseptic techniques and prophylaxis, the incidence of infection should be less than 1%. Furthermore, with the philosophy and treatment protocol outlined in the following pages, if deep infection should occur, it should be possible to achieve a cure and a well-functioning reimplantation in over 90% of these patients.

Although excision arthroplasty (Fig. 1) has been the accepted treatment of infection in total hip arthroplasty in the past, this method of treatment has fallen out of favor because of its poor functional outcome (5,6,17,39).

Obviously, it is ideal to retain a well-functioning total hip replacement after infection. Unfortunately, in most cases with longstanding implant sepsis, this is not possible, for a variety of reasons. These include the biologic behavior of microorganisms, such as their production of glycocalyx (40,41) in the presence of antibiotics. The relatively avascular environment around an infected total hip replacement also precludes effective treatment with antimicrobial agents alone. Goulet et al. (38) reported a 52.6% failure in 19 patients treated with suppressive antibiotics after an average follow-up of 4 years. They defined the limited indications for antibiotic suppression, including those cases in which there is a contraindication to removal of the implant, and those in which the patient refuses surgical treatment. The patient should have no systemic symptoms of infection, and the prosthetic components should be well fixed. Otherwise, this treatment may lead to progressive bone loss. The infecting organism must be sensitive to oral antibiotics, and the antibiotics must be well tolerated by the patient. All these requisites are rarely encountered. Accordingly, removal of the implant is mandatory for the treatment and cure of implant sepsis in the great majority of cases. Once the implants are removed, the surgeon has the option of either reimplanting a new hip replacement prosthesis immediately, as in the so-called one-stage exchange arthroplasty, or delaying the reimplantation for a few weeks or months, as in two-stage exchange arthroplasty. One-stage exchange arthroplasty was the subject of Chapter 80. In this chapter, the indications, contraindications, technique, and results of two-stage exchange arthroplasty will be discussed. The role of two-stage

   B. A. Masri: Division of Reconstructive Orthopaedics, University of British Columbia, and Vancouver Hospital and Health Sciences Center, Vancouver, British Columbia V5Z 4E1, Canada.
   E. A. Salvati: The Hospital for Special Surgery, Cornell University College of Medicine, New York, New York 10021.

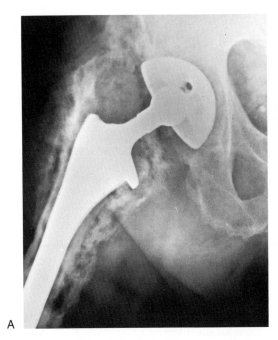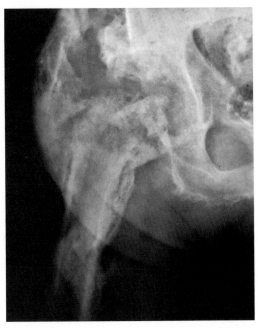

A

B

FIG. 1. A: Severe infection after a cementless total hip replacement. At the time of surgery, there was a severe infection of the periprosthetic tissues with marked periostitis and osteomyelitis. The septic process involved the proximal two-thirds of the femur. In view of the severity of the infection, this patient was not considered a candidate for reimplantation. **B:** A follow-up radiograph, obtained 3 years after surgery, revealed severe ectopic ossification. The patient has mild pain and a stable hip with limited range of motion resulting from ectopic ossification, and two crutches are required for ambulation.

exchange arthroplasty in the management of the chronically infected total hip arthroplasty is summarized in Figure 2.

SOURCES OF PERIPROSTHETIC INFECTIONS

Over the past three decades, it has become clear that the infecting organisms in a deep periprosthetic infection may be acquired by three mechanisms. The first, bacterial contamination at the time of surgery, has been well documented as a source of early deep postoperative infection. Charnley's pioneering work on ultra-clean-air operating rooms with laminar flow and body exhaust suits has shown that with these practices, the infection rate was dramatically reduced from 9.5% to about 0.5%, with no perioperative antibiotic prophylaxis. This decrease in the rate of infection corresponded to a significant reduction of bacterial counts in the air around the wound, by using ultra-clean air and total-body exhaust suits by the surgical team (13,14). This association between infection and bacterial counts in the operating room air has been demonstrated by others (57,58,77). Not all infections that are acquired in the operating room manifest themselves early. Some infections, caused by organisms of low virulence that are acquired at the time of surgery, can become symptomatic months or years after hip replacement.

However, the longer the postoperative period before the infection is manifested, the less likely the intraoperative origin (34).

The second mechanism of infection is contiguous spread (76). This is a more significant problem with joints that are close to the surface, such as the knee or the elbow, where a wound-healing complication, such as slough, can predispose to a deep prosthetic infection. In the hip, superficial wound infections have been associated with a higher incidence of deep sepsis (59,81). The organisms migrate to the deeper tissues by contiguous spread.

The third pathway by which organisms can reach the prosthesis is through the hematogenous route (31,63). Any remote infection in the body may seed and cause a deep infection in total hip arthroplasty (81). The most common sites of remote infection that may lead to an infected total hip replacement are skin and soft-tissue infections and psoriasis (46%), dental infections or manipulation (15%) (79,80), and urinary infections (13%) (63). Urinary catheterization in the perioperative period has not been shown to be a definite source of infection (74).

Deep infections of total hip arthroplasties may be categorized as acute postoperative infections, chronic infections, or acute but delayed infections secondary to hematogenous spread from other sources.

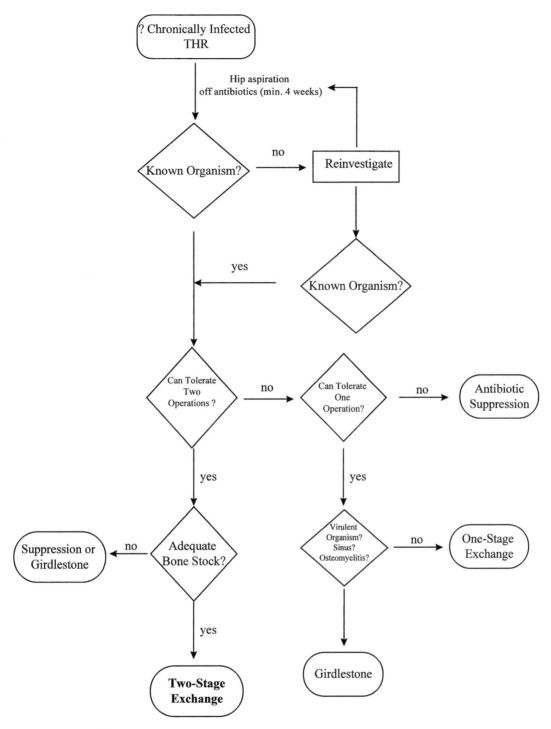

FIG. 2. The role of two-stage exchange arthroplasty in the management of the infected total hip replacement is outlined.

INDICATIONS FOR TWO-STAGE EXCHANGE ARTHROPLASTY

Two-stage exchange is often the treatment of choice for chronic periprosthetic infections. In addition, after the failure of radical debridement and antibiotic therapy in early postoperative or acute hematogenous infections, two-stage exchange arthroplasty becomes indicated (34).

Because of the prolonged course of two major operative procedures, separated by a few weeks' course of intravenous antibiotics, the patient has to be medically fit to withstand the rigors of such treatment. The frail, elderly, or medically unwell patient is best treated using other techniques (38,87).

For any treatment of infection, and particularly for exchange arthroplasty, preoperative intimate knowledge

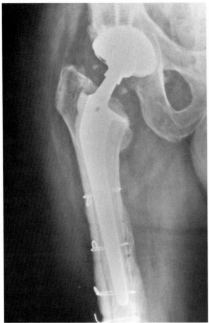
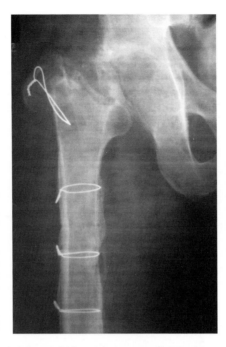
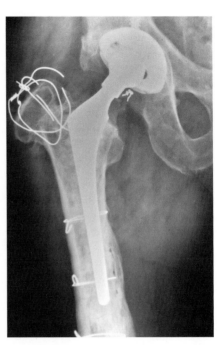

A,B   C

FIG. 3. A: Loose and infected right total hip replacement. Original surgery of a cementless stem was complicated by an intraoperative fracture, requiring cerclage wiring 2 weeks later. The stem loosened, requiring revision to a cemented stem, 15 months after the original surgery. The patient was referred to our institution with these radiographic findings. He underwent removal of the prosthetic components, acrylic cement, and all necrotic and devitalized tissue through a transtrochanteric approach. **B:** Resection of the hip performed through a transtrochanteric approach. All foreign body was removed, except the cerclage wires. The patient was kept at bed rest with tibial skeletal traction for 2 weeks and then progressed in ambulation with a walker and two Canadian crutches. **C:** Postoperative radiograph obtained 3½ years after reimplantation. Patient has no pain, ambulates without a limp and without external support, and has resumed a normal life.

of the identity and antimicrobial susceptibility of the infecting organism is optimal. Without proper antibiotic therapy, exchange arthroplasty has a high risk of recurrence of infection. Effective antibiotic treatment is discussed further in Chapter 83.

Adequate bone stock, or bone stock deficiency that can be properly reconstructed, is a requirement for a biomechanically successful two-stage exchange arthroplasty. In most cases, there is adequate bone stock, and it is feasible to perform a two-stage exchange arthroplasty as outlined in this chapter. Figure 3 is an example of a patient who underwent removal of the infected implant. After 6 weeks of antibiotic therapy, another hip replacement was implanted, with a successful long-term result.

TECHNIQUE OF TWO-STAGE EXCHANGE ARTHROPLASTY

The technique of two-stage exchange arthroplasty (Figs. 3,4) involves the removal of the infected prosthesis, with all associated foreign material and inflamed and necrotic tissue. This includes the complete excision of all

sinus tracts, abscess cavity walls, scarred avascular tissue, necrotic tissue, trochanteric and other cerclage wires, and loose and solidly fixed cement. A careful search for abscesses is performed, particularly along the tendon of iliopsoas, to rule intrapelvic abscesses. All abscesses should be drained and debrided. After this step, the joint is thoroughly and profusely irrigated. In the traditional two-stage exchange arthroplasty, the wound is then closed over suction drains, and the patient is treated in tibial skeletal traction for about 2 weeks to allow early scarring about the hip to occur. Thereafter, ambulation is started with a walker, partial weight-bearing is allowed on the affected lower extremity, and the patient progresses to crutches as tolerated.

During the interval between stages, the patient is treated with intravenous antibiotics for a minimum of 4 to 6 weeks. The antibiotics are started at the time of surgery as soon as all the intraoperative cultures are obtained. If the clinical evolution, wound healing, and the effectiveness of the antibiotic therapy assessed by minimal serum bactericidal titers are favorable, the patient undergoes reimplantation of another hip prosthesis, thus completing the two-stage exchange protocol.

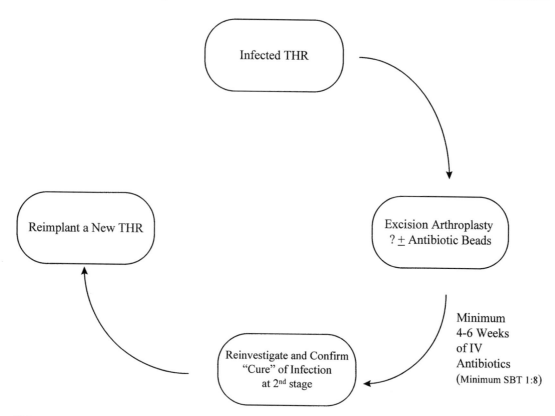

FIG. 4. A two-stage exchange arthroplasty involves a complete excision arthroplasty at the first stage. Antibiotic beads may or may not be used to fill the resulting cavity. After a minimum of 6 weeks of intravenous antibiotic therapy, a definitive total hip replacement prosthesis is reimplanted.

First Stage

Removal of the Cemented Femoral Component

One of the main principles of the current management of the infected hip replacement is the complete removal of all foreign material and devitalized tissue. Early infections do not result in loosening of cemented implants, but late infections do produce septic loosening. The removal of a solidly fixed cemented implant, particularly on the femoral side, can be a very challenging undertaking. In general, a wider exposure than normal is required to remove these solidly fixed stems. It is easy to remove a smooth stem from the cement mantle. Removal of a solidly fixed cement mantle requires special instrumentation, experience, and meticulous technique to avoid compromising the upper end of the femur. The cemented stem that is precoated with methylmethacrylate, such as the Zimmer Precoat or Centralign stem (Zimmer, Warsaw, IN), poses a major challenge. The stem bonds thoroughly to the underlying cement mantle, and, when solidly fixed, it is almost impossible to remove without bivalving the femur. For this reason, an extended trochanteric osteotomy is recommended. Unlike the case of the smooth stem, the osteotomy is more difficult to perform because

the stem is in the way. A few anterior perforations through the vastus lateralis are often required, so that the far medial cortex is weakened and allowed to crack at the proper location when the osteotomy is completed. The extended trochanteric osteotomy, as popularized by Paprosky (84), is useful. The posterior aspect of the hip joint is exposed in a routine manner. A small portion of the vastus lateralis is elevated off the posterolateral portion of the femur to maintain the blood supply to the extended trochanteric fragment (Fig. 5). Especially in the infected situation, it is optimal to avoid devascularization of the femur. Continuity of the vastus lateralis distally prevents proximal migration and avulsion of the osteotomized fragment. A trochanteric osteotomy is then performed from posterior to anterior, and extended distally so that one third of the cortex of the femur is removed in continuity with the greater trochanter. The osteotomy is extended as far distally as necessary to remove the entire cement mantle. If the stem is easy to remove after posterior dislocation of the hip, this should be done first, because the osteotomy is technically easier to perform with the stem out of the way. The osteotomy is performed across the intact cement mantle, and, once the femur is opened, it is easy to remove the cement mantle, now under direct vision, using conventional techniques. At the end of the procedure, the

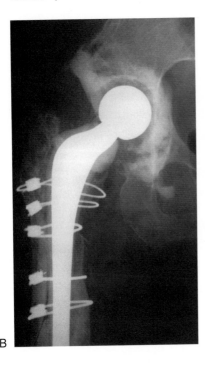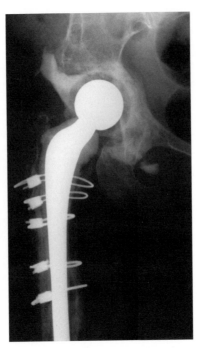

A,B

FIG. 5. A: An extended trochanteric osteotomy was used to remove the cement mantle. In this early postoperative radiograph, the osteotomy line is still visible. The rounded corners at the distal end of the osteotomy minimize the stress-riser effect. B: Two months later, the osteotomy is healed, and a second-stage procedure may be performed without having to violate the femur again. The prosthesis is a temporary antibiotic-loaded facsimile of a true hip replacement prosthesis, known as the PROSTALAC (discussed in Chapter 82). It is a modification of the two-stage exchange technique described in this chapter.

osteotomy is fixed with cerclage wires. Cables have an increased risk of fraying and are not recommended. Luque wires are particularly useful because of their strength, ease of application, and low cost.

Protracted infections lead to progressive prosthetic loosening. Generally, removal of a loose cemented femoral stem is not difficult. The loose cement can be removed without the need for a trochanteric osteotomy. A solidly fixed cement plug can pose a challenge, and several techniques are available to remove it, including the use of manual instruments, power instruments, and ultrasonic devices (9,32). Techniques that require a distal window are not recommended, as they require longer stems to bypass the defect. Manual techniques include drilling a hole in the distal cement column and plug, followed by insertion of a large tap with an attached handle for a slap hammer. The plug is then removed in a retrograde fashion. Another technique involves the use of a high-speed burr with special attachments designed to capture the plug, so that it can be pulled in a retrograde fashion. A similar technique can be used with ultrasonic devices (9,32).

In some cases, the distal plug is rigidly fixed, or the femur is deformed proximally, making it impossible to remove the plug in a retrograde manner. For these cases, a carefully planned osteotomy of the anterior cortex of the femur at the site of the distal plug can be performed. This technique has been described as the pencil-box osteotomy by Duncan. (Duncan CP, personal communication). This osteotomy is performed with rounded corners through the anterior cortex of the femur, while maintaining the attachment of the vastus lateralis to the cortical fragment. At the completion of the procedure, the osteotomy is fixed with cerclage wires.

Every effort should be made to remove all bone cement because of the increased risk of recurrence of infection when contaminated bone cement is left behind (28,29, 50,62). However, Lieberman et al. (59) have shown that small amounts of retained cement had no detrimental effect on the treatment outcome in their series.

Removal of the Cementless Femoral Component

Early infections may delay or prevent bone ingrowth in cementless stems, making it easier to remove them. However, late infections have been observed with solidly fixed cementless stems and their removal is also challenging. Three types of cementless stems are encountered. The first type is the press-fit stem, with or without hydroxylapatite coating. The noncoated stems are generally easy to remove without specialized techniques. The coated stems require techniques similar to the porous-coated stems, which will be described later. The other two types of stems are the proximally and extensively porous-coated cementless stems. The proximally coated stem can be removed using flexible osteotomes to break the bony bond between the porous coating and the bone. Fine-tipped attachments for high-speed burrs have been developed for this purpose. Where the greater trochanter obstructs adequate access to the medullary canal and proximal stem, a trochanteric or extended osteotomy may be required for exposure.

Extensively porous-coated implants are more difficult to remove, and a variety of techniques are available. Whereas flexible osteotomes may be used from the top, this technique is generally inadequate for freeing the middle and distal thirds of the stem. If a large collar is present, such as in the Anatomic Medullary Locking prosthesis (AML, DePuy, Warsaw, IN), the medial portion of the proximal one third of the implant cannot be accessed until after the collar is removed with a metal-cutting high-speed burr. After loosening of the implant proximally, an anterior window may be made in the femur at the junction of the metaphyseal proximal portion of the prosthesis and the straight diaphyseal portion of the implant. A metal-cutting high-speed burr is then used to cut the prosthesis at that level (36). The proximal portion is then removed without difficulty, and the distal portion is removed using a special trephine (Moreland Instruments, DePuy, Warsaw, IN). Alternatively, an extended trochanteric osteotomy may be performed and the stem sectioned as described above. A Gigli saw is then used to debond the proximal portion of the prosthesis, and the distal portion of the stem is removed using the Moreland trephines.

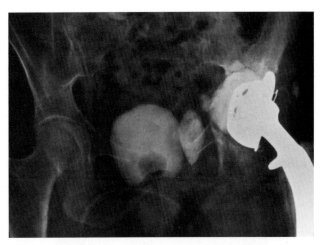

FIG. 6. Cytogram of a patient with an infected hip and intrapelvic cement. Note the medial cement adjacent to the contrast dye in the bladder.

Removal of the Acetabular Cup

The acetabular component is generally easier to remove. Cemented components can be removed by freeing the prosthesis from the underlying cement using curved gouges and osteotomes. Once the cup is removed, the underlying cement is carefully removed piece-meal by creating controlled fractures of the cement mantle under direct vision. Drilling holes in selected locations can weaken and guide the breakage of the cement. The cement within the anchoring holes should also be carefully removed. The main difficulty arises when intra-pelvic cement is present, or when the acetabular component has migrated into the pelvis. Extreme care should be exercised during maneuvers of removal to avoid rupture of intrapelvic structures. Frequently, the intrapelvic cement is larger than the acetabular perforation that allowed the intrusion. Although in aseptic revisions, leaving intrapelvic cement may obviate the risk of removal, in the presence of infection it may contribute to the risk of persistence of infection, and every effort to remove it is indicated. Minimal enlargement of the acetabular defect through which cement has protruded may allow removal of the cement. Preoperative Foley catheterization of the bladder, which is routine for most revision total hip arthroplasty, will prevent bladder perforation as well as any displacement of vital structures by an enlarged bladder towards the pelvic wall (Fig. 6).

Al-Salman et al. (2) described a technique by which intrapelvic components may be removed using a re-troperitoneal approach. Because of the proximity of the major vascular structures within the pelvis, it is best to perform these procedures with the help of an experienced vascular surgeon. Porous-coated cementless acetabular components may be removed with the help of specialized curved acetabular gouges. It is important to be meticu-lous and patient with these instruments, so that bone loss can be kept to a minimum. Another technique for the removal of solidly fixed porous-coated acetabular components is the use of pneumatic impactors that apply a rotational torque and allow loosening of the solidly fixed implant (53). Occasionally, these metal cups need to be sectioned to prevent excessive bone loss.

After removal of the prosthetic components and cement, and after thorough debridement, it has been the current trend to insert antibiotic-loaded cement beads (Fig. 7) (1,44) within the acetabulum, joint space, and femoral canal. Some authors recommend an intraopera-tive radiograph after debridement for assurance that all cement is removed. Others are using endoscopic fiberop-tics to examine the femoral canal for retained cement. Sensitivity of the infecting organism to the antibiotics in the beads is essential. If the organism is resistant, the beads will act as a foreign body, with persistence of the infection. Tobramycin in the dose of 1.2 g per package of bone cement is most commonly used. The beads are strung on a suture, and they should be counted and their number carefully recorded in the operative report, to enssure complete removal at the time of reimplantation. There is no definitive literature to suggest whether this is superior to leaving the joint space empty. These beads and other antibiotic-loaded cement spacers will be covered in more detail in Chapter 82.

Suction–irrigation between stages has been used in the past. However, this is a technique that requires meticu-lous care and balance of inflow and outflow, and it is fre-quently fraught with complications, such as accumulation of fluid within the soft tissues, blockage of the suction tubes, and superinfection. Moreover, if antibiotic-loaded cement beads are used between stages, the antibiotic-rich periprosthetic milieu is disturbed by the suction irriga-tion. Finally, there is no evidence in the literature to sug-

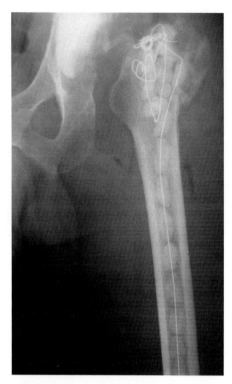

FIG. 7. Home-made antibiotic-loaded cement beads were used in this case after excision arthroplasty. A cement spacer filled the acetabular fossa, and beads filled the joint space and medullary canal of the femur.

gest that suction–irrigation adds to the efficacy of two-stage exchange arthroplasty in the management of the infected total hip arthroplasty. For these reasons, we no longer use this technique.

Interval Period

Between stages, the patient is treated in skeletal traction for about 2 weeks, until a manual push–pull test of the lower extremity reveals stability and minor discomfort. The period of skeletal traction allows the formation of scar tissue and stabilization of the pseudarthrosis. Thereafter, the patient is allowed partial weight-bearing ambulation with the support of a walker, progressing to crutches as tolerated.

During this interval, intravenous antibiotics under the supervision of an infectious disease consultant should be administered. Excellent results, with infection cure rates of 90.6% (10,59) and 95% (33), have been reported, with a protocol using a minimum of 6 weeks of intravenous antibiotics achieving a minimal serum bactericidal titer of 1:8 against the infecting bacteria identified in the individual periprosthetic infection (52). This has been the routine at The Hospital for Special Surgery since 1975, and it is still the recommended antibiotic treatment pro-

tocol. This concept of serum bactericidal titers will be elaborated upon in Chapter 83.

The exact duration of the interval between stages continues to be controversial. In the absence of antibiotic-loaded bone cement, the administration of systemic antibiotics for less than 28 days was associated with a higher recurrence rate (62). Because of pain, persistent shortening, and poor function after an excision arthroplasty (5,6,17,39), most patients are eager to proceed with the definitive reimplantation as soon as indicated.

During the last two decades, we have delayed the second stage for 6 weeks, provided the clinical evolution, wound healing, and antibiotic treatment were satisfactory. Otherwise, the reimplantation has been delayed further, and in 30% of cases it was elected not to proceed with reimplantation. Main factors dictating this approach included extensive periostitis and osteomyelitis (see Fig. 1), poor bone stock, antibiotic-resistant organisms, mixed flora, recurrent local infection, poor wound healing with prolonged wound drainage, limited interval antibiotic therapy because of poor patient tolerance, inadequate serum bactericidal titers (less than 1:8), femoral shaft fracture, decubitus ulcers, or limited rehabilitation potential (59).

In some cases, when the patient is a good candidate for reimplantation but there are some concerns regarding infection control (e.g., if the erythrocyte sedimentation rate remains high or continues to climb), reimplantation can be delayed for an additional few weeks. Infection eradication may be confirmed by an aspiration biopsy performed at least 4 weeks after cessation of all antibiotic therapy. An earlier culture may yield false-negative results because of antibiotic therapy. If the results of the aspiration biopsy are negative, a new hip prosthesis may be reimplanted. If the joint continues to be infected, despite an adequate course of intravenous antibiotics, a second incision and debridement may be indicated to re-excise retained foreign body and devitalized infected tissues.

Intervals ranging from a few weeks to at least 1 year have been recommended in the literature. Fitzgerald (30) recommends at least 3 months for less virulent organisms, and 1 year for more virulent organisms. In our experience, a failed debridement is generally a result of retained foreign body, an inadequate debridement, or inadequate antibiotic therapy. Waiting for a longer period of time will not remedy the problem, unless the cause of persistence of infection is treated. Therefore, a delay of 1 year between stages is not necessary when the debridement and antibiotic therapy are adequate. The best results for two-stage exchange arthroplasty have been reported with an interval of at least 6 weeks between stages (10,59).

There is only one series in which the interval between stages was deliberately shortened to under 6 weeks: Colyer and Capello (18) attempted to perform the second stage within 4 weeks of the first stage. In a series of 41 consecutive patients with infected hip implants, only 37 were entered into this protocol, and of these 37 patients, only 13 were able to have both stages within a 4-week period. The overall success rate in this series was 83%, and the success rate for the 13 patients in whom reimplantation was done within 4 weeks of the initial debridement was 86%. Because of the small numbers in this series, and the selection bias with respect to the patients who were able to complete the proposed protocol, it is difficult to draw firm conclusions from this experience.

Second Stage

At the second stage, numerous intraoperative samples are obtained for Gram stain, cultures, and frozen section, looking for an acute inflammatory tissue response. The procedure should be abandoned if the intraoperative macroscopic findings or the results of the Gram stain or frozen section suggest ongoing infection. It is safer to repeat the debridement and irrigation and, depending on the results of intraoperative cultures, to administer another course of intravenous antibiotics, than to subject the patient to reimplantation with a higher risk of recurrence of infection. If the above intraoperative findings are benign, we proceed with reimplantation. Intravenous antibiotics are continued until the results of the intraoperative cultures are negative. If positive, intravenous antibiotics should be continued, followed by suppressive oral antibiotics depending on the sensitivity of the bacteria. The duration will be dictated by the overall clinical picture and infectious disease consultation (38).

The surgical exposure for the second stage is generally easy if the interval between stages was only a few weeks. The longer the interval, the more complex the exposure (because of scarring and limb shortening), and adequate and generous soft-tissue release is generally required. If antibiotic-loaded cement beads were used at the first stage, they should be removed. The beads tend to be scarred in the soft tissues and the longer the interval between the first and second stages, the more the scarring. It is often quite difficult to find all these beads, and for this reason, we recommend that the beads be counted at the time of their insertion, and their exact number clearly documented in the operative report (Fig. 8). The addition of a small amount of methylene blue (0.5 to 1 mL) to the bone cement at the time of mixture, makes it easier to visualize the beads at the time of their removal. Palacos cement, which has better leaching characteristics for antibiotic delivery, stains green because of its chlorophyll content, and this aids in its removal, thus obviating the need for addition of other dyes. Prior to proceeding with the definitive reimplantation, any retained cement from the first stage should also be removed and cultured.

On the acetabular side, cementless fixation is preferred, as long as there is adequate bone stock. If bone is deficient, and bulk bone graft will represent more than half of the surface for fixation, a cemented cup is preferred, perhaps with a reinforcement ring. Antibiotics are mixed with the cement. Careful mixture to assure even distribution is most important. Palacos R (Smith and Nephew Richards, Memphis, Tennessee) is preferred because of its superior antibiotic elution properties (25,42,64,85). Fixation on the femoral side has been controversial in revision total hip arthroplasty. We favor the use of antibiotic-impregnated cement for the fixation of

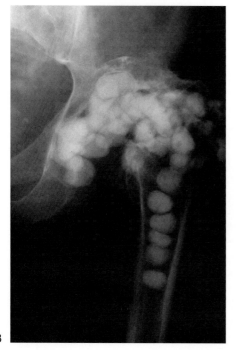 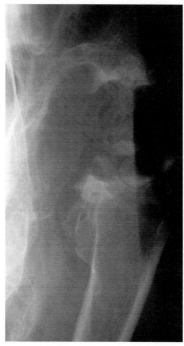

A,B

FIG. 8. A: Antibiotic-loaded beads were inserted elsewhere, and their number was not recorded. **B:** An intraoperative radiograph revealed a few retained beads, which were removed prior to the insertion of the final components.

femoral stems and for the reimplantation of infected hip prostheses. Nestor et al. (69) showed an 18% recurrence of infection and 18% loosening rate with cementless fixation. We believe that this risk of recurrence of infection is significantly higher than when antibiotic-loaded cement is used (less than 10% in the latter case), and we therefore caution the reader against the use of cementless implants for reimplantation after infection, until further studies are available. We use antibiotic-loaded Simplex P bone cement (Howmedica, Rutherford, NJ), or a cement with a similar viscosity. The higher molecular weight of Palacos cement makes it more viscous and more difficult to inject with a cement gun. Furthermore, premixed antibiotic-loaded Palacos cement is not available in the United States, as it has not been approved by the U.S. Food and Drug Administration. The use of less than 2 g of antibiotic powder does not seem to weaken the bone cement significantly (19,55). However, the use of more than 4.5 g has deleterious biomechanical effects (54).

Severe Bone Loss

For the hip with severe bone loss, Fitzgerald (29,30) developed a new technique of bone stock reconstruction

known as the three-stage technique. The first stage is similar. The second stage involves bone grafting of the deficient bone stock in the femur and acetabulum, using a combination of autogenous iliac crest bone graft and morselized allograft; this is done 3 to 12 months after the first stage. At least 9 months later, the third stage is performed, at which time a cementless revision total hip arthroplasty is performed. This technique has been performed at only one center, with no published results. Because of the prolonged interval between the stages, most patients would not consent to such a treatment protocol. Furthermore, the cost of such a protocol in the current climate of cost containment may be prohibitive.

In some cases, however, because of severe bone loss, it is difficult to apply the principles outlined in this chapter. For example, consider the patient with the infected proximal femoral prosthetic replacement or the infected proximal femoral allograft (Fig. 9). This patient will have poor control of such a flail limb after removal of the components. An antibiotic-loaded temporary implant may be required to maintain soft-tissue tension and stability of the limb (20,21,90). This technique is discussed further in Chapter 82.

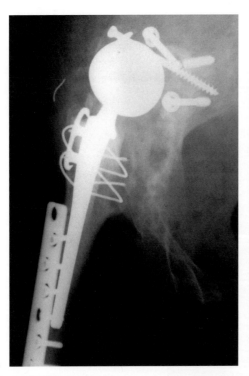 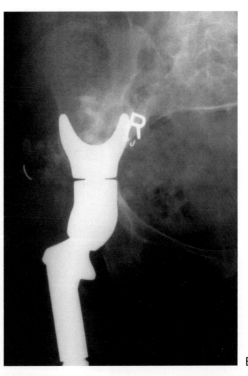

A   B

FIG. 9. A: This patient had an infected proximal femoral allograft replacement with an infected and collapsed allograft reconstruction of the acetabulum. Excision arthroplasty would have left a massive defect with severe functional disability. A standard two-stage exchange arthroplasty is impractical and a spacer that maintains the limb length and stability is preferred. An intramedullary nail coated with antibiotic-loaded bone cement was fashioned to resemble a femoral component. **B:** At the second stage, the spacer was removed and replaced by a Saddle prosthesis. A case of this magnitude should only be treated at tertiary care centers that specialize in the management of severe periprosthetic infections.

RESULTS OF TWO-STAGE EXCHANGE ARTHROPLASTY

For many decades, the insertion of prosthetic devices in the presence of infection has contradicted all classic orthopedic teaching. The pioneering work of Buchholz and Engelbrecht at the Endo-Klinik in Hamburg (8) paved the way to successful reimplantation of infected hip replacements. They championed direct exchange of the infected implant with antibiotic-loaded Palacos R bone cement. Since then, many reports of reimplantation in the treatment of the infected total hip prostheses have been published (1,7,12,16,20,21,26,37,44,47,48,65,67, 76,78,86–89). Despite some early negative reports (48,71), exchange arthroplasty has become the standard of care in most periprosthetic infections. Although one-stage exchange is still popular at some European centers, two-stage exchange arthroplasty has dominated in the United States and Canada.

The results of two-stage exchange arthroplasty, with (1,20,21,44,78,89) or without (26,45,62,67) antibiotic-loaded cement spacers, have been clearly outlined in the literature. Despite acceptable salvage rates for one-stage exchange arthroplasty, equivalent or better results have been reported using two-stage exchange arthroplasty (Table 1). In a multicenter study from Sweden, Carlsson et al. (12) attempted to reproduce Buchholz's results. Seventy-seven patients with infected total hip arthroplas-

ties were treated with the single-stage exchange arthroplasty (59 hips) or with two-stage exchange arthroplasty (18 hips) with antibiotic-loaded Palacos bone cement. Out of 77 patients, 60 had a good result, whereas eight remained infected, and nine hips, despite the lack of obvious evidence of infection, continued to be painful. The authors considered these cases "doubtful" results. For the sake of this discussion, they will be considered treatment failures. This gave a success rate of 78%, which is slightly higher than Buchholz's original success rate of 73%. Carlsson et al. (12) used systemic antibiotics for 6 months, unlike Buchholz who did not use any systemic antibiotics. The success rates of the single-stage and two-stage exchange procedures were identical (78%). The authors concluded that they were unable to detect a difference between the single- and the two-stage exchange arthroplasties, and they recommended the use of single-stage exchange in the presence of infection, because of its expediency.

In a review of their 12-year experience with reimplantation without the use of antibiotic-loaded bone cement, Salvati et al. (76) divided their patients into three groups, the third being the most recently treated. Their trend, over the years, was towards performing more two-stage exchange arthroplasties. The recurrence rate with single-stage exchange was between 10% and 15%. In the third group, where the predominant procedure was a two-stage exchange arthroplasty, the recurrence rate was 6%. The

TABLE 1. *Comparison between one- and two-stage exchange arthroplasty, with and without antibiotic-impregnated cement*

Author (ref.)	One-Stage		Two-Stage	
	Hips (N)	Success (%)	Hips (N)	Success (%)
Cement with antibiotics				
Buchholz et al. (7)	667	77.0	—	—
Lindberg (60)	59	90.0	18	78.0
Murray (66)	13	38.5	22	95.5
Turner et al. (84)	101	86.0	—	—
Wroblewski (88)	102	91.0	—	—
Hope et al. (43)	72	87.5	19	100.0
Elson (23)	235	87.5	61	96.5
Garvin et al. (33)	21	90.5	55	92.7
Johnston et al. (49)	24	91.7	—	—
Tsukayama et al. (83)	—	—	34	85.3
Total	1294	82.0	209	92.3
Cement without antibiotics				
Hunter (46)	55	18.0	10	60.0
Talbott et al. (82)	—	—	25	80.0
Cherney and Amstutz (16)	5	80.0	28	64.0
Fitzgerald (27)	—	—	111	90.0
Jupiter et al. (50)	18	78.1	—	—
Salvati et al. (76)	31	91.0	28	89.0
Salvati et al. (75)	14	86.0	18	94.5
McDonald et al. (62)	—	—	82	86.6
Lieberman et al. (59)	—	—	32	91.0
Total	123	55.5	334	85.6

These studies show the superiority of two-stage exchange arthroplasty with antibiotic-loaded cement.

authors recommended that parenteral antibiotics be continued for at least 6 weeks prior to reimplanting the new prosthesis, and they emphasized the importance of identifying the infecting organism preoperatively to select the appropriate antibiotic treatment. They also stressed the importance of removal of all infected bone cement, foreign body, and devitalized tissue, to minimize the recurrence rate. Their contraindications for a one-stage exchange arthroplasty were gram-negative infections, mixed flora, open wounds and draining sinuses, and intraoperative findings of severe inflammation and suppuration. They also reviewed the literature and compared the results obtained with and without antibiotic-loaded bone cement, as well as the results obtained with one-stage and with two-stage exchange arthroplasties. Salvati et al. (76) concluded that two-stage exchange arthroplasty with antibiotic-impregnated bone cement was the most effective method of treatment, with a cure rate of 87.5%. One-stage exchange without antibiotic-loaded bone cement was the least effective treatment with a cure rate of 57%.

The early experience with one-stage reimplantation has been poor. In a large review of 1112 hip arthroplasties performed between 1971 and 1976, Murray (67) reviewed 151 infected total hip arthroplasties. The salvage rate for one-stage exchange using antibiotic-loaded bone cement was only 46.7%, compared with 92% when the two-stage exchange method (with antibiotic-loaded bone cement) was used. More recently, Hope et al. (43) reported an infection recurrence rate of 13% with the single-stage method. They concluded that the role for a one-stage exchange arthroplasty should be highly selective, and they recommended two-stage exchange. Furthermore, Elson et al. (24) reported a 12.4% failure rate with the one-stage method, compared with a 3.5% failure rate with the two-stage method. Based on the information thus presented, it seems that the success rate of two-stage exchange with antibiotic-loaded bone cement is higher and more predictable, despite the obvious disadvantages.

Recent studies questioned the need for antibiotic-loaded bone cement (62,87). In a series of 82 hips treated with two-stage exchange arthroplasty for hip sepsis, the success rate was 87% without the use of any antibiotic-loaded bone cement (62). Once again, there was a high correlation between the presence of retained cement at the time of the initial excision and the rate of recurrence of infection. Moreover, it was noted that reimplantation less than 1 year after resection arthroplasty was associated with a higher recurrence rate (27%) than that performed later than 1 year after the resection arthroplasty (7%). The administration of parenteral antibiotics for less than 28 days was associated with a higher recurrence rate. Other poor prognostic factors included the presence of a virulent organism (gram-negative rods and group D streptococci) and retention of cement at the time of first stage debridement. Therefore, for a two-stage exchange arthroplasty without antibiotic-loaded bone cement to be

successful, a prolonged period (over 1 year) of disability and poor function with prolonged antibiotic therapy are necessary, according to this study (62). By comparing this study to others where antibiotic-loaded bone cement is used, it becomes clear that antibiotic-loaded bone cement allows more predictable results. Moreover, Cherney and Amstutz (16) reported only a 63% salvage of infected total hip arthroplasties when treated with one- or two-stage exchange arthroplasty without the use of antibiotic-loaded bone cement. Based on these data, they recommended the use of antibiotic-loaded cement in the hope of improving their results. In a phase II FDA-approved trial, Garvin et al. (33,35) showed that the use of a commercial preparation of gentamicin-loaded Palacos bone cement (0.5 g per 40 g cement) improved the outcome of infected total hip and knee replacements. A total of 211 patients, some of whom were at risk for infection, some of whom were suspected of having an infected implant, or others of whom had definite prosthetic infections, were studied. The infection recurrence rates were 10.1% and 5.6% for one- and two-stage exchange, respectively. The higher success in the two-stage exchange group occurred despite the careful selection of patients undergoing single-stage exchange (i.e., these patients had less severe infections). This compares favorably with a recurrence rate of 13% when antibiotic-loaded bone cement was not used (62). This improved infection rate was in spite of the shorter interval prior to reimplantation in the antibiotic-loaded cement group (27 weeks versus 52 weeks). The infection recurrence rate after exchange arthroplasty with gentamicin-loaded bone cement was 13% if the organism was resistant to gentamicin, and 3.9% if the organism was sensitive to gentamicin (35). These studies provided further support for the efficacy of antibiotic-loaded bone cement in the treatment of infected total hip arthroplasties.

Based on the information available, it is clear that the use of antibiotic-loaded bone cement can improve the salvage rate in the infected total hip arthroplasty, regardless of the treatment philosophy that is adopted. Carlsson et al. (11) examined the radiographic loosening seen in hip arthroplasties implanted with antibiotic-loaded bone cement for the treatment of sepsis. They concluded that the addition of 0.5 g of gentamicin to bone cement does not lead to worse radiographic loosening than is seen in revision arthroplasties performed with plain bone cement.

Although their study was not designed to specifically study the effect of antibiotic-loaded bone cement on the rate of aseptic loosening, Garvin et al. (35) showed that there was no mechanical loosening in any of 211 total hip and knee prostheses implanted with gentamicin-loaded Palacos cement, at a minimum 2 year follow-up. Furthermore, Elson (23) showed that the use of antibiotic-loaded bone cement did not increase the rate of prosthetic loosening.

CONCLUSION

Despite the lack of properly controlled, randomized, and prospective trials, the results of two-stage exchange arthroplasty with antibiotic-loaded bone cement are superior and more predictable to those of one-stage exchange arthroplasty, particularly for the severe, chronic, and extensive infections, especially if caused by virulent organisms. According to our work at The Hospital for Special Surgery, the most important predictor of a good outcome is patient selection, with good potential for rehabilitation and adequate bone stock and soft tissues to achieve a sound biomechanical reconstruction. In addition, meticulous surgical technique and intravenous antibiotics achieving minimal serum bactericidal titers of 1:8 against the patient's infecting bacteria for a minimum period of 6 weeks (59), followed by reimplantation with antibiotic-impregnated cement, are also of paramount importance. Cure rates of about 90% can be achieved, regardless of whether antibiotic-loaded cement beads or spacers are used. Over the past three decades, the outlook for a successful outcome for the treatment of an infected total hip replacement has improved significantly, and with further refinements in patient selection, surgical techniques, and medical management, these results should improve even further.

AKNOWLEDGMENTS

This chapter was supported in part by Ms. Emma A. Daniels, president of the May Ellen and Gerald Ritter Foundation, and by Dr. and Mrs. Gianbattista Foglio.

REFERENCES

1. Abendschein W. Arthroplasty rounds. Salvage of infected total hip replacement: use of antibiotic/PMMA spacer. *Orthopedics* 1992;15: 228–229.
2. Al-Salman A, Taylor DC, Beauchamp CP, Duncan CP. Prevention of vascular injuries in revision total hip replacement. *Can J Surg* 1992; 35:261–264.
3. Amstutz HC, Ma SM, Jinnah RH, et al. Revision of aseptic loose total hip arthroplasties. *Clin Orthop* 1982;170:21–33.
4. Barrack RL, Folgueras AJ. Revision total hip arthroplasty: the femoral side. *J Am Acad Orthop Surg* 1995;3:79–85.
5. Bittar ES, Petty W. Girdlestone arthroplasty for infected total hip arthroplasty. *Clin Orthop* 1982;170:83–87.
6. Bosquet M, Duncan CP, Mulier J, Patterson FP. Girdlestone excision arthroplasty of the hip. A review of 49 patients. *Orthop Trans* 1982;6: 336.
7. Buchholz HW, Elson RA, Engelbrecht E, Lodenkämper H, Röttger J, Siegel A. Management of deep infection of total hip arthroplasty. *J Bone Joint Surg Br* 1981;63:342–353.
8. Buchholz HW, Engelbrecht H. Über die Depotwwirkung einiger Antibiotica bei Vermischung mit dem Kunstharz Palacos. *Chirurg* 1970;41:11–515.
9. Caillouette JT, Gorab RS, Klapper RC, Anzel SH. Revision arthroplasty facilitated by ultrasonic tool cement removal. Part II: Histologic analysis of endosteal bone after cement removal. *Orthop Rev* 1991; 20:435–440.
10. Callaghan JJ, Salvati EA, Brause BD, Rimnac CM, Wright TM. Reim-

11. plantation for salvage of the infected hip: rationale for the use of gentamicin-impregnated cement and beads. In: Fitzgerald RH Jr, ed. *The hip: proceedings of the thirteenth open scientific meeting of the Hip Society.* St. Louis: CV Mosby, 1985;65–94.
12. Carlsson AS, Engund A, Gentz C, Hussenius A, Josefsson G, Lindberg L. Radiographic loosening after revision with gentamicin-containing cement for deep infection in total hip arthroplasties. *Clin Orthop* 1985; 194:271–279.
13. Carlsson AS, Joseffson G, Lindberg L. Revision with gentamicin-impregnated cement for deep infections in total hip arthroplasty. *J Bone Joint Surg Am* 1978;60:1059–1064.
14. Charnley J. A clean-air operating enclosure. *Br J Surg* 1964;52: 202–205.
15. Charnley J. *Low friction arthroplasty of the hip. Theory and practice.* New York: Springer-Verlag, 1979.
16. Charnley J. The future of total hip arthroplasty. In: Nelson JP, ed. *The hip.* St. Louis: CV Mosby, 1982;198–210.
17. Cherney DL, Amstutz HC. Total hip replacement in the previously septic hip. *J Bone Joint Surg Am* 1983;65:1256–1265.
18. Clegg J. The results of the pseudarthrosis after removal of an infected total hip prosthesis. *J Bone Joint Surg Br* 1978;59:298–301.
19. Colyer RA, Capello WN. Surgical treatment of the infected hip implant: two-stage reimplantation with a one-month interval. *Clin Orthop* 1994;298:75–79.
20. Davies JP, O'Connor DO, Burke DW, Harris WH. Influence of antibiotic impregnation on the fatigue life of Simplex P and Palacos R acrylic bone cements, with and without centrifugation. *J Biomed Mater Res* 1989;23:379–397.
21. Duncan CP, Beauchamp CP. The antibiotic-loaded hip replacement: a valuable tool in the management of the complex infected total hip arthroplasty. *J Bone Joint Surg Br* 1991;73(suppl 2):115.
22. Duncan CP, Beauchamp CP. Total hip replacement for the management of chronic infection. *J Bone Joint Surg Br* 1992;74(suppl 3):275.
23. Elson RA. Exchange arthroplasty for infection. Perspectives from the United Kingdom. *Orthop Clin North Am* 1993;24:761–767.
24. Elson R. Results of primary exchange in infected total hip replacement. *Combined meeting of the Orthopaedic Associations of the English-Speaking World,* Toronto, June 1992.
25. Elson R, Norman P, Scott I, Stockley I. Exchange cemented joint arthroplasties for deep infection. *J Bone Joint Surg Br* 1992;74(suppl 3):295.
26. Elson RA, Jephcott AE, McGechie DB, Verettas D. Antibiotic-loaded acrylic cement. *J Bone Joint Surg Br* 1977;59:200–205.
27. Evans RP, Nelson CL. Staged reimplantation of a total hip prosthesis after infection with *Candida albicans:* a report of two cases. *J Bone Joint Surg Am* 1990;72:1551–1553.
28. Fitzgerald RH. Indirect exchange of the infected hip implant. *Orthop Trans* 1981;5:372.
29. Fitzgerald RH Jr. The infected total hip arthroplasty: current concepts in treatment. In: Welch RB, ed. *The hip. Proceedings of the twelfth open scientific meeting of the Hip Society.* St. Louis: CV Mosby, 1984.
30. Fitzgerald RH Jr. Problems associated with the infected total hip arthroplasty. *Clin Rheum Dis* 1986;12:537–553.
31. Fitzgerald RH Jr. Infected total hip arthroplasty: diagnosis and treatment. *J Am Acad Orthop Surg* 1995;3:249–262.
32. Fitzgerald RH Jr, Nolan DR, Ilstrup DM, Van Scoy RE, Washington JA, Coventry MB. Deep wound sepsis following total hip arthroplasty. *J Bone Joint Surg Am* 1977;59:847–855.
33. Gardiner R, Hozack WJ, Nelson C, Keating EM. Revision total hip arthroplasty using ultrasonically driven tools. A clinical evaluation. *J Arthroplasty* 1993;8:517–521.
34. Garvin KL, Evans BG, Salvati EA, Brause BD. Palacos gentamicin for the treatment of deep periprosthetic hip infections. *Clin Orthop* 1994; 298:97–105.
35. Garvin KL, Hanssen AD. Current concepts review: infection after total hip arthroplasty. Past, present, and future. *J Bone Joint Surg Am* 1995; 77:1576–1588.
36. Garvin KL, Fitzgerald RH Jr, Salvati EA, Brause BD, Nercessian OA, Wallrichs SL, Ilstrup DM. Reconstruction of the infected total hip and knee arthroplasty with gentamicin-impregnated Palacos bone cement. *Instr Course Lect* 1993;42:293–302.
37. Glassman AH, Engh CA. Removal of porous-coated femoral hip stems. *Clin Orthop* 1992;285:164–180.
38. Goodman SB, Schurman DJ. Outcome of infected total hip arthro-

plasty: an inclusive and consecutive series. *J Arthroplasty* 1988;3: 97–102.

38. Goulet JA, Pellicci PM, Brause BD, Salvati EM. Prolonged suppression of infection in total hip arthroplasty. *J Arthroplasty* 1988;3: 109–116.

39. Grauer JD, Amstutz HC, O'Caroll PF, Dorey FJ. Resection arthroplasty of the hip. *J Bone Joint Surg Am* 1989;71:669–678.

40. Gristina AG. Biomaterial-centered infection: microbial adhesion versus tissue integration. *Science* 1987;237:1588–1595.

41. Gristina AG, Costerton JW. Bacterial adherence to biomaterial and tissue: the significance of its role in clinical sepsis. *J Bone Joint Surg Am* 1985;67:264–273.

42. Hoff SF, Fitzgerald RH Jr, Kelly PJ. The depot administration of penicillin G and gentamicin in acrylic bone cement. *J Bone Joint Surg Am* 1981;63:798–804.

43. Hope P, Kristinsson KG, Norman P, Elson RA. Deep infection of cemented total hip arthroplasties caused by coagulase-negative staphylococci. *J Bone Joint Surg Br* 1989;71:851–855.

44. Hovelius L, Josefsson G. An alternative method for exchange operation of infected arthroplasty. *Acta Orthop Scand* 1979;50:93–96.

45. Hughes PW, Salvati EA, Wilson PD, Blumenfeld EL. Treatment of subacute sepsis of the hip by antibiotics and joint replacement: criteria for diagnosis and evaluation of twenty-six cases. *Clin Orthop* 1979;141: 143–157.

46. Hunter GA. The results of reinsertion of a total hip prosthesis after sepsis. *J Bone Joint Surg Br* 1979;61:422–423.

47. Hunter G, Dandy D. The natural history of the patient with an infected total hip replacement. *J Bone Joint Surg Br* 1977;59:293–297.

48. James ETR, Hunter GA, Cameron HU. Total hip revision arthroplasty: does sepsis influence the results? *Clin Orthop* 1982;170:88–94.

49. Johnston RC, Katz RP, Callaghan JJ, Sullivan PM. One stage reimplantation of the infected total hip arthroplasty: a minimum 10 year study. *Proceedings of the meeting* of the American Academy of Orthopaedic Surgeons, New Orleans, February 1994.

50. Jupiter JB, Karchmer AW, Lowell JD, Harris WH. Total hip arthroplasty in the treatment of adult hips with current or quiescent sepsis. *J Bone Joint Surg Am* 1981;63:194–200.

51. Kavanagh BF, Ilstrup DM, Fitzgerald RH Jr. Revision total hip arthroplasty. *J Bone Joint Surg Am* 1985;67:517–526.

52. Kaye D, ed. *Infective endocarditis.* Baltimore: University Park Press, 1976.

53. Lachiewicz PF, Anspach WE 3d. Removal of a well fixed acetabular component. A brief technical note of a new method. *J Bone Joint Surg Am* 1991;73:1355–1356.

54. Lautenschlager EP, Jacobs JJ, Marshall GW, Meyer PR. Mechanical properties of bone cements containing large doses of antibiotic powder. *J Biomed Mater Res* 1976;10:929–938.

55. Lautenschlager EP, Marshall GW, Marks KE, Schwartz J, Nelson CL. Mechanical strength of acrylic bone cements impregnated with antibiotics. *J Biomed Mater Res* 1976;10:837–845.

56. Lawrence JM, Engh CA, Macalino GE. Revision total hip arthroplasty: long-term results without cement. *Orthop Clin North Am* 1993;24: 635–644.

57. Lidwell OM. Clean air at operation and subsequent sepsis in the joint. *Clin Orthop* 1986;211:91–102.

58. Lidwell OM, Elson RA, Lowbury EJL, Whyte W, Blowers R, Stanley S, Lowe D. Ultraclean air and antibiotics for prevention of postoperative infection. *Acta Orthop Scand* 1987;58:4–13.

59. Lieberman JR, Callaway GH, Salvati EA, Pellicci PM, Brause BD. Treatment of the infected total hip arthroplasty with a two-stage reimplantation protocol. *Clin Orthop* 1994;301:205–212.

60. Lindberg LT. The experience with antibiotic cement in Sweden. Read at the *second American Orthopaedic Association Symposium*. Boston, 1981.

61. McCarthy JC, Mattingly D, Turner RH, et al. Revision of the deficient femur with a modular femoral component. *Orthop Trans* 1993;17: 966.

62. McDonald DJ, Fitzgerald RH Jr, Ilstrup DM. Two-stage reconstruction of a total hip arthroplasty because of infection. *J Bone Joint Surg Am* 1989;71:828–834.

63. Maderazo EG, Judson S, Pasternak H. Late infection of total joint prostheses: a review and recommendation for prevention. *Clin Orthop* 1988;229:131–142.

64. Marks KE, Nelson CL, Lautenschlager EP. Antibiotic-impregnated acrylic bone cement. *J Bone Joint Surg Am* 1976;58:358–364.

65. Miley GB, Scheller AD, Turner RH. Medical and surgical treatment of the septic hip with one-stage revision arthroplasty. *Clin Orthop* 1982;170:76–82.

66. Murray WR. Treatment of established deep wound infection after hip arthroplasty: a report of 65 cases. In: Leach RE, Hoaglund FT, Riseborough EJ, eds. *Controversies in orthopaedic surgery.* Philadelphia: WB Saunders, 1982:382–398.

67. Murray WR. Use of antibiotic-containing bone cement. *Clin Orthop* 1984;190:89–95.

68. Nelson JP. Deep infection following total hip arthroplasty. *J Bone Joint Surg Am* 1977;59:1042–1044.

69. Nestor BJ, Hanssen AD, Ferrer-Gonzalez R, Fitzgerald RH Jr. The use of porous prostheses in delayed reconstruction of total hip replacements that have failed because of infection. *J Bone Joint Surg Am* 1994;76: 349–359.

70. Paprosky WG, Jablosky W, Magnus RE. Cementless femoral revision in the presence of severe proximal bone loss using diaphyseal fixation. *Orthop Trans* 1993;17:965–966.

71. Patterson FP, Brown CS. The McKee-Farrar total hip replacement. *J Bone Joint Surg Am* 1972;53:257–275.

72. Pellicci PM, Wilson PD Jr, Sledge CB, et al. Revision total hip arthroplasty. *Clin Orthop* 1982;170:34–41.

73. Pellicci PM, Wilson PD Jr, Sledge CB, et al. Long-term results of revision total hip replacement: a follow-up report. *J Bone Joint Surg Am* 1985;67:513–516.

74. Redfern TR, Machin DG, Parsons KF, Owen R. Urinary retention in men after total hip arthroplasty. *J Bone Joint Surg Am* 1986;68: 1435–1438.

75. Salvati EA, Callaghan JJ, Brause BD. Prosthetic reimplantation for salvage of the infected hip. *Instr Course Lect* 1986;35:234–241.

76. Salvati EA, Chekofsky KM, Brause BD, Wilson PD. Reimplantation in infection: a 12-year experience. *Clin Orthop* 1982;170:62–75.

77. Salvati EA, Robinson RP, Zeno SM, Koslin BL, Brause BD, Wilson PD. Infection rates after 3175 total hip and total knee replacements performed with and without a horizontal unidirectional filtered air-flow system. *J Bone Joint Surg Am* 1982;64:525–535.

78. Sanzén L, Carlsson AS, Josefsson G, Lindberg LT. Revision operations on infected total hip arthroplasties: two to nine year follow-up study. *Clin Orthop* 1988;229:187–172.

79. Strazzeri JC, Anzel S. Infected total hip arthroplasty due to *Actinomyces israelii* after dental extraction: a case report. *Clin Orthop* 1986; 210:128–131.

80. Sullivan PM, Johnston RC, Kelley SS. Late infection after total hip replacement caused by an oral organism: a case report. *J Bone Joint Surg Am* 1990;72:121–123.

81. Surin VV, Sundholm K, Bäckman L. Infection after total hip replacement, with special reference to a discharge from the wound. *J Bone Joint Surg Br* 1983;65:412–418.

82. Talbot RD, Glassburn AR, Nelson JP, et al. Implantation of total hip arthroplasty after known deep infection. *Orthop Trans* 1980;4:97.

83. Tsukayama DT, Estrada R, Gustilo R. Infection after total hip arthroplasty. A study of the treatment of one hundred and six infections. *J Bone Joint Surg Am* 1996;78:512–523.

84. Turner RH, Miley GB, Fremont-Smith P. Septic hip replacement and revision arthroplasty. In: Turner RH, Scheller AS, eds. *Revision total hip arthroplasty.* New York: Grune and Stratton, 1982:291–314.

85. Younger TI, Bradford MS, Magnus RE, Paprosky WG. Extended proximal femoral osteotomy. A new technique for femoral revision arthroplasty. *J Arthroplasty* 1995;10:329–338.

86. Wahlig H, Dingeldein E. Antibiotics and bone cement. *Acta Orthop Scand* 1980;5:49–56.

87. Wilson MG, Dorr LD. Reimplantation of infected total hip arthroplasties in the absence of antibiotic cement. *J Arthroplasty* 1989;4: 263–269.

88. Wroblewski BM. One-stage revision of infected cemented total hip arthroplasty. *Clin Orthop* 1986;211:103–107.

89. Wroblewski BM. Revision of infected hip arthroplasty. *J Bone Joint Surg Br* 1983;65:224.

90. Zilkens K-W, Casser H-R, Ohnsorge J. Treatment of an old infection in a total hip replacement with an interim spacer prosthesis. *Arch Orthop Trauma Surg* 1990;109:94–96.

The Adult Hip, edited by J. J. Callaghan,
A. G. Rosenberg, and H. E. Rubash.
Lippincott–Raven Publishers, Philadelphia © 1998.

CHAPTER 82

Sepsis: Antibiotic-Loaded Implants

Bassam A. Masri and Clive P. Duncan

Since the introduction of the modern total hip replacement by Sir John Charnley, excellent results have been reported, with excellent clinical outcomes in up to 85% of patients at 15-year follow-up (53). These excellent results are severely tarnished if deep infection occurs. In addition to the increased morbidity, infection has a marked economic impact. Sculco (50) reviewed the incidence and economic impact, based on U.S. Medicare data, of infected total hip and knee arthroplasty. In 1989, 80,647 total knee replacements were performed on Medicare patients in the United States. During the same year, 1795 implants were removed for infection, for an estimated incidence of total knee sepsis of 2.23%. Sculco also estimated the cost of treatment of each infection at $50,000 to $60,000. The overall annual cost for the treatment of infected total knee replacements would therefore be between $90 million and $110 million per year. Most of the cost of treatment is the expense of the prolonged hospitalization that is often required. Any treatment method that allows earlier discharge from the hospital and effective control of infection would be welcomed. Economic issues, however, should not be the orthopedic surgeon's foremost concern. Nothing is accomplished if a lower-cost treatment protocol is less effective.

In this chapter, a method of treating the infected total hip replacement will be outlined. This method is a modification of the well-accepted two-stage exchange arthro-

plasty outlined in Chapter 83, in which the implant is removed and the hip is debrided at the first stage, and after a period of at least 6 weeks, a permanent prosthesis is reimplanted. The modification of this method includes the insertion of an antibiotic-loaded facsimile of a total hip arthroplasty between stages. In addition to the elution of high levels of antibiotics into the joint, this prosthesis allows ambulation, rehabilitation, and earlier discharge from hospital between stages. The patient is readmitted for the second stage on an elective basis. This temporary functional spacer is currently known as the prosthesis of antibiotic-loaded acrylic cement, or the PROSTALAC (30).

BASIC SCIENCE CONSIDERATIONS

Deep periprosthetic infections are difficult if not impossible to eradicate predictably using antibiotic therapy alone. This difficulty is related to a variety of host, as well as pathogen, factors. For this reason, an aggressive approach to the management of these infections is often required. For the most part, a chronic deep periprosthetic infection cannot be controlled without removing the infected implants. With the poor results of excision arthroplasty, it is often desirable to reimplant another prosthesis, despite the presence of infection. Prior to the early 1970s, this was thought to be impossible. With the advent of antibiotic-impregnated bone cement, this has not only become a reality but even the standard of care in the management of infected total hip arthroplasties. An

B. A. Masri and C. P. Duncan: Department of Orthopaedics, Vancouver Hospital and Health Sciences Center, University of British Columbia, Vancouver, British Columbia V5Z 4E1, Canada.

understanding of the biology of prosthetic infections, as well as the basic science of antibiotic-loaded bone cement, is important for the proper application of the principles of this reimplantation technique.

SPECIAL CONSIDERATIONS IN PROSTHETIC INFECTION

The difficulty in eradicating postoperative infection (Fig. 1) is not unique to total joint replacements. The same phenomenon is seen with any prosthetic material, whether it is in the form of vascular bypass grafts, implantable pacemakers, total artificial hearts, or even intravenous cannulas. This is directly related to the interaction between the host, the infecting organism, and the prosthetic device.

Ninety percent of bacteria exist in nature in a layer of adherent, protective biofilm (19). The periprosthetic space in a total hip replacement is not unlike many natural ecosystems. When bacteria are present within this environment, they tend to adhere to biomaterials by a variety of mechanisms. This bacterial adherence is a major factor in the pathogenesis of total joint infections. The necrotic debris from the mechanical trauma of bone

reaming and the thermal trauma from cement polymerization is bound to act as a culture medium for bacteria if they are present in the wound or migrate to the wound from remote sources. Another major factor in the pathogenesis of prosthetic joint infection is the effect of the various biomaterials on host defense mechanisms (22). These factors are unique to prosthetic infections and will be discussed in more detail.

Bacterial Adherence

It has been shown that almost all bacteria growing in natural, industrial, or aquatic systems tend to produce a network of fibrous polysaccharides, glycoproteins, or both. This has been referred to by Gristina and Costerton (20) as glycocalyx. A similar phenomenon is seen in biomaterials when they become colonized with bacterial cells: they become coated with a biofilm that is an aggregate of bacterial colonies with their surrounding glycocalyx (19). Within this new ecosystem, one or more bacterial species may live in relative isolation from the host defense mechanism and from antibiotics. If more than one bacterial species survive in this biofilm, a symbiotic relationship develops and a polyclonal infection results.

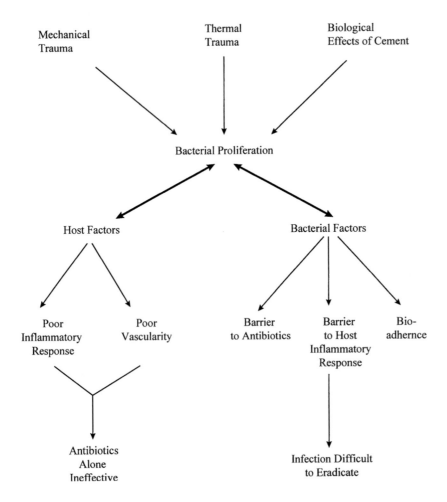

FIG. 1. Flow chart illustrating the interaction between the various factors that contribute to the difficulty in eradicating periprosthetic sepsis. The mechanical and thermal trauma of the preparation of the femoral canal and the cementing of implants, as well as the potential biologic effects of the bone cement monomer on the host's inflammatory response, make joint replacements particularly susceptible to periprosthetic sepsis. The protected periprosthetic milieu, with its relatively poor blood supply, insulates the bacteria from the effects of the host's inflammatory response as well as the effect of systemically administered antibiotics. Moreover, glycocalyx acts not only as a means of bioadherence of microorganisms, but also as a barrier against the host's inflammatory response and the antibiotics administered. For these reasons, deep periprosthetic infections are difficult to eradicate.

Glycocalyx not only isolates the infecting organism from the host's endogenous and exogenous defense mechanisms, but it also makes it difficult to detect certain bacteria in aspirated fluid from the infected joint (21). The importance of glycocalyx in mediating bacterial adherence to metal surfaces in industrial and natural ecosystems has been well demonstrated (11). A similar function has been proposed (20) in biomaterial infections. In fact, the primary role of glycocalyx is to allow adhesion of bacteria to biomaterial surfaces.

Glycocalyx can act as a barrier to the diagnosis and treatment of difficult total-implant-associated infections. Not every orthopedic implant infection, however, is accompanied by glycocalyx formation. Gristina and Costerton (21) demonstrated the presence of glycocalyx in 59% of 17 infected orthopedic implants. It then follows that not every bacterial organism is capable of producing glycocalyx to the same degree, and, in fact, different bacterial species are capable of responding differently to different biomaterial surfaces. *Staphylococcus epidermidis* is able to adhere better to polymers, whereas *S. aureus* is able to adhere better to metal surfaces (19). Certain therapeutic interventions may change the bacterial response and glycocalyx production. Dall et al. (12) showed that the use of clindamycin can inhibit glycocalyx production in an experimental streptococcal endocarditis. Whether such an interaction is applicable in the case of orthopedic implant infections remains to be seen.

Integration of biomaterials by the ongrowth or ingrowth of host tissue can be desirable. Once the prosthesis is stable and covered with living tissue, the biomaterial surface is less vulnerable to bacterial adherence. It becomes difficult for a clinical infection to become established, because the lack of adherence allows the host defenses to reach and destroy the infecting organisms (19). Gristina has elegantly summarized this concept as the "race for the surface" (19).

Effect of Biomaterials on Host Defense Mechanisms

Polymethylmethacrylate is thought to be particularly prone to infection. In monomeric forms, methylmethacrylate can inhibit phagocytic, lymphocytic, and complement function *in vitro*. Gristina and Kolkin (22) summarized some of the changes that occur in macrophages when they are exposed to bone cement. Macrophages tend to remain spherical when they come in contact with polymethylmethacrylate, whereas they spread when they come in contact with Vitallium (Howmedica, Rutherford, NJ), glass, or stainless steel. The spreading of macrophages is necessary for their phagocytic ability. The polymerization process itself has also been shown to enhance the likelihood of infection in the dog model (7). All of these properties have been

shown only in *in vitro* experiments or in animal models. There has been no convincing evidence, however, that implants inserted with bone cement are at a higher risk of infection than those inserted without bone cement.

Host responses to bone cement may also contribute to infection in total joint arthroplasties. Fibronectin has been shown to enhance the binding of *S. aureus* to biomaterials (7,45). Trauma to tissues is also a predisposing factor in the development of *S. aureus* infection by similar mechanisms (45). These mechanisms involve the attachment of *S. aureus* cells to the N-terminal portion of fibronectin. Invasive strains of this organism tend to have better adherence characteristics than less invasive strains. In addition to glycocalyx formation, this is another important mechanism by which bacteria adhere to bioimplants.

Failed cemented (48) and cementless (47) total hip prostheses have been associated with aggressive granulomatous lesions that can cause significant bone destruction and debris generation. This changes the balance of power in Gristina's "race for the surface" (19), and in the presence of microorganisms, it may predispose to infection.

PROPERTIES OF ANTIBIOTIC-LOADED CEMENT

The properties of antibiotic-loaded bone cement have been thoroughly investigated over the past two decades. It is now known, through *in vitro* (2,5,6,10,14,17,18,25, 26,31,32,35,49,51) and *in vivo* (2,5,6,8–10,17,37,43, 51,52) studies that many commonly used antibiotics are released from bone cement is such a way that the local antibiotic levels vastly exceed the minimal inhibitory concentration that is effective against most susceptible pathogens, and that these levels are much higher than those achieved with parenteral therapy (8,46). In our own patients, tobramycin levels as high as 232 mg/L and vancomycin levels as high as 54 mg/L were measured in the suction drainage fluid within 24 hours after insertion of an antibiotic-loaded cement spacer containing these two antibiotics. These values represent highly therapeutic levels. Different antibiotics have different elution characteristics. For example, when tobramycin is compared to vancomycin (Fig. 2), it becomes clear that tobramycin elutes in much higher concentrations early on. The elution of both antibiotics decays with time, but tobramycin elution decays at a much faster rate than that of vancomycin (39). Only a few studies have addressed the long-term elution of antibiotics from bone cement (9,10,25,38,51).

In an *in vitro* assay, clindamycin was found to elute for up to 56 days (25). In rabbits, antibiotic-loaded cement pellets can elute antibiotics for up to 37 days (10). In a series of three sheep with gentamicin-loaded bone

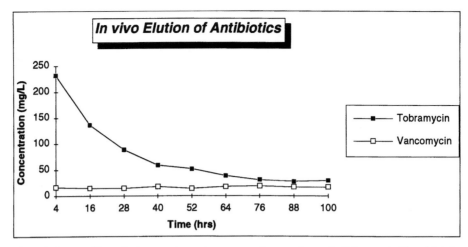

FIG. 2. The elution profiles of tobramycin and vancomycin are shown in this graph. Very high levels are obtained early, with a rapid decline to steady-state levels. Tobramycin elutes in consistently higher levels than vancomycin.

cement within the femur, gentamicin levels in bone at 18 months after insertion of the antibiotic-loaded cement was 7 to 36 mg/kg (9).

The *in vivo* long-term elution of antibiotics in humans has been reported in two series (38,51). In one study (51), therapeutic levels of gentamicin were measured in the periprosthetic connective tissue, and in cancellous or cortical bone in 17 patients several months after total hip arthroplasty with gentamicin-loaded bone cement. In one patient, 5.75 years following surgery, gentamicin concentrations of 5.4 to 6.6 mg/kg of tissue (wet weight) and 6.6 mg/kg were measured from periprosthetic connective tissue and cancellous bone, respectively. Joint fluid, in this study, was not assayed for gentamicin levels. In an investigation by Masri et al. (38), long-term antibiotic elution from the PROSTALAC hip (15,30) and knee (41) systems was studied in 49 patients. Based on these investigations, the recommended dose of tobramycin and vancomycin in antibiotic-loaded spacers in two-stage exchange arthroplasty of the hip are 3.6 g of tobramycin and 1.0 g of vancomycin in each 40-g package of bone cement (Table 1).

Not only does antibiotic-loaded bone cement allow the elution of high levels of antibiotics into the periprosthetic milieu, but it has been shown that antibiotics in bone cement implanted within the medullary cavity of a cadaver femur are able to permeate through dead cortical bone (17). This finding has obvious therapeutic advantages in the case of the severely infected total hip arthroplasty with devascularization and osteomyelitis.

The safety of this antibiotic depot has also been clearly established. In our own patients treated with antibiotic-loaded bone cement for infected hip and knee arthroplasties, we have never been able to detect tobramycin or vancomycin serum levels higher than 3 mg/L. This has also

been shown by other investigators in humans and in animal models (1,10,17,26,37,51,52).

Baker and Greenham (5), using *in vivo* and *in vitro* studies with scanning electron microscopy, described the mechanism of elution of antibiotics from bone cement. The release of antibiotics occurs from the surface only through voids and cracks in the bone cement. They concluded that increasing the concentration of antibiotics within the bone cement would improve the elution characteristics of the antibiotics. This was confirmed in human studies by Wahlig and Dingeldein (52), who showed that doubling the concentration of

TABLE 1. *Levels* of antibiotics, eluted from the bone cement of the PROSTALAC, in the fluid of the prosthetic space*

Antibiotic added to bone cement (g)	Tobramycin (mg/L)		Vancomycin (mg/L)	
	Mean	CI	Mean	CI
Vancomycin, 1 g				
Tobramycin ≤ 2.4 g	2.23	1.72–2.74	0.77	0.56–0.98
Tobramycin ≥ 3.6 g	9.43	4.24–14.6	2.02	0.83–3.21
Vancomycin, ≥ 1.5 g				
Tobramycin ≤ 2.4 g	3.3	NA	1.40	NA
Tobramycin ≥ 3.6 g	5.93	4.05–7.82	2.49	1.97–3.01

* Antibiotic levels were measured in 34 consecutive hips, after a mean interval of 118 days from implantation.

CI, 95% confidence interval; NA, not applicable.

From Masri BA, Duncan CP, Beauchamp CP. Long-term elution of antibiotics from bone cement: an *in vivo* study using the PROSTALAC system. *J Bone Joint Surg Br* 1995; 77(suppl 3):308.

gentamicin from 0.5 g to 1.0 g per 40 g of cement allowed doubling of the concentration of gentamicin in wound secretions. Baker and Greenham (5) also concluded that bone cements with a higher porosity would be expected to allow higher antibiotic release than those with a lower porosity. It is then no surprise that Palacos-R bone cement, which has a higher surface pore size (37) than other cements, has the best *in vitro* elution characteristics (17,26,37,51). Moreover, they also concluded that methods of cement preparation that are designed to minimize porosity (such as vacuum mixing or centrifugation) could have a deleterious effect on antibiotic elution.

The change in mechanical strength of antibiotic-loaded bone cement, when compared with plain cement, has also been studied (4,13,33,34). In some studies, the addition of small amounts of antibiotics in the powder form did not seem to significantly weaken bone cement (13,34), whereas the addition of antibiotics in liquid form to the bone cement caused significant weakening (34). Other studies have shown that the addition of any amount of antibiotic powder will cause some weakening of the antibiotic–bone cement composite, regardless of the amount of antibiotic added to the cement (4). The degree of weakening depends on the proportional weight of antibiotics added to the bone cement (33). Lautenschlager et al. (33) showed that mixing more than 4.5 g of gentamicin sulfate can significantly weaken bone cement to the point that its compressive strength is decreased to below the minimum acceptable standards. This was only when samples were tested in compression. Fatigue testing of the cement is difficult to perform because physiologic cycling would require a very prolonged period of time. Based on the literature, a limit of about 2 g of antibiotic powder per 40 g of bone cement appears to be a safe estimate for the maximum allowable concentration of antibiotics in bone cement, particularly when the bone cement is used for the fixation of a permanent revision hip prosthesis. These limits do not necessarily apply when antibiotics are added to bone cement in temporary spacers, which are removed a few weeks or months after insertion in two-stage exchange arthroplasty.

Another possible advantage to the use of antibiotic-loaded bone cement is its potential role in decreasing bacterial bioadherence. In one study (42), the adherence of *S. epidermidis* was reduced when tobramycin was added to bone cement. Another study (12) showed that the use of clindamycin can inhibit glycocalyx production in an experimental streptococcal endocarditis model. Whether such an interaction is applicable in the case of orthopedic implant infections remains to be seen. Also, whether these interactions are as applicable *in vivo* as they are *in vitro* is not well documented.

With an understanding of the basic properties of antibiotic-loaded bone cement, the surgeon can take better advantage of this material in the treatment of infected total hip replacements.

INDICATIONS AND APPLICATIONS OF ANTIBIOTIC-LOADED IMPLANTS

With the advantages of antibiotic-loaded bone cement, it is at least theoretically advantageous to utilize this material in the treatment of the infected total hip arthroplasty. Buchholz introduced antibiotic-loaded bone cement in the prophylaxis and one-stage exchange treatment of the infected hip replacement. With the introduction of two-stage exchange arthroplasty, the role of antibiotic-loaded cement at the time of the second stage became obvious. It was not until Hovelius and Joseffson (27) introduced antibiotic-loaded cement beads as a spacer between stages that antibiotic-loaded implants became popular between stages. These beads have also been used in the management of open fractures, and soft-tissue and bone infections (23,24,36,44). Because of the advantages of antibiotic-loaded bone cement, particularly in its capacity as an antibiotic depot (16), it has become very popular to insert such beads within the hip joint between stages in two-stage exchange arthroplasty of the hip. The use of these beads, however, does not change the functional status of the patient between stages.

In addition to having to perform two surgical procedures, the other disadvantages of two stage exchange arthroplasty include (a) a period of poor function and relatively increased morbidity between stages, (b) soft-tissue contractures and difficulty with reimplantation, and (c) the inability to stabilize a limb where major bone deficit exists.

To address these difficulties, antibiotic-loaded implants may be inserted between stages to allow the patient some function, and also to maintain the soft tissues out to length and decrease scarring within the periprosthetic tissues. Since 1987, we have abandoned the standard two-stage exchange arthroplasty in favor of the PROSTALAC system, in which a facsimile of a total hip replacement prosthesis is inserted between stages. This technique, as well as the results in the first 60 patients treated with the latest design, will be described.

THE PROSTALAC SYSTEM

Overview and Rationale

Not unlike a routine modern total hip replacement, the PROSTALAC system consists of a modular femoral component with an acetabular component. The difference between this system and a standard hip replacement is that in the former, the components are deliberately inserted loose, and no attempts are made to achieve permanent fixation of either the acetabular or the femoral components.

The rationale for this is that these components are routinely removed at about 3 months after insertion. Rigid fixation of the implants would defeat this purpose, and would render this method of treatment no different from one-stage exchange arthroplasty, and therefore the potential advantage of the second operation is lost. It was our belief, when this system was being developed, that adding new foreign material in the presence of an infected implant is safe, provided that some basic principles are strictly adhered to. These include the following.

1. An attempt should be made to remove all infected foreign material, including prosthetic implants, devitalized tissue, wires, and cement. If retained cement is noted after surgery, every effort should be made to remove it at the time of the second stage, in order to remove any

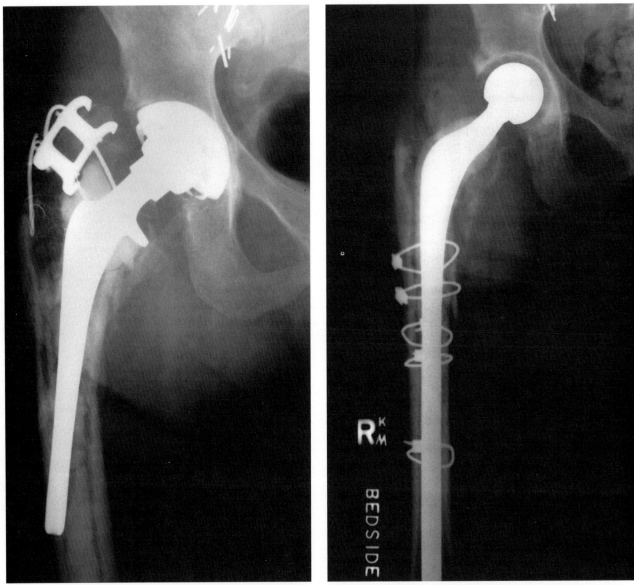

A   B

FIG. 3. A: Despite excellent cementing technique at the time of implantation 18 months prior to presentation, this femoral prosthesis failed with a pathologic periprosthetic fracture of the proximal femur. Infection was diagnosed and the implants were removed. Intraoperatively, bone loss was marked with loss of the posterior and medial cortices proximally. There were multiple perforations of the femoral cortex laterally and anteriorly. It would have been impossible to stabilize the femur after excision arthroplasty without a solid spacer. B: Excellent stability was achieved with a 250-mm PROSTALAC femoral prosthesis after open reduction and internal fixation of the fractured femur. This example illustrates the versatility and utility of antibiotic-loaded implants in the management of the infected hip replacement with marked bone loss.

potentially adherent microorganisms that are protected by glycocalyx.

2. A high-concentration-antibiotic-loaded reservoir is implanted to increase the periprosthetic antibiotic levels, above and beyond what may be achieved by parenteral therapy alone.

3. The dose of antibiotics included within this reservoir should be high enough that adequate antibiotic levels remain at the time of removal of the temporary implant, so that at no point is the hip left with an implant without the protective effect of antibiotic therapy.

4. Every effort is made to maintain an adequate blood supply to the bones, and unnecessary stripping of soft tissues is minimized.

5. A stable reconstruction is achieved so that mobilization is possible, thus justifying the potential disadvantages of adding more foreign material.

The PROSTALAC system was designed to address all of these principles. A meticulous dissection with an extensile exposure is critical, so that the prosthesis along with the entire cement mantle is removed. A retroperitoneal approach for the removal of retained intrapelvic cement is performed if necessary (3). At times, the intrapelvic cement can be removed by minimally widening a previous pilot hole. On the femoral side, osteotomies and windows of the femur are performed in such a way that the osteotomized fragment or cortical window is never deprived of its muscular attachment and blood supply. After removal of the components, a thorough debridement with copious irrigation is performed so that the appearance of the tissues prior to the insertion of the PROSTALAC components is no different from the appearance of the wound at the time of revision surgery for aseptic reasons. The dose of antibiotics used in the cement is large enough that very high antibiotic levels within the joint cavity are present immediately, and some antibiotics remain at the time of the second stage procedure. In fact, our most commonly used antibiotic combination is 3.6 g of tobramycin and 1.0 g of vancomycin per package of bone cement. This is in contrast to the doses of Wahlig et al. (52), who used 0.5 g of gentamicin per package of bone cement. Our dose is based on *in vivo* measurements of antibiotic levels early following the insertion of the PROSTALAC implants, as well as at the time of the second stage (an average of 4 months after the first stage) (38,40). Finally, the PROSTALAC system is designed with sufficient versatility so that most cases, regardless of the degree of severity of bone loss (Fig. 3), may be handled. Subsequently, a stable reconstruction can be obtained in most patients.

Surgical Technique

After a thorough debridement and irrigation of the wound, the acetabulum is reconstructed using the PROSTALAC acetabular component. A single size is available (42-mm outer diameter, 32-mm inner diameter) (Fig. 4), and there is a simple snap-fit design to reduce the risk of dislocation. There is a thin (5-mm) ultra-high-molecular-weight polyethylene shell, which is cemented to the remaining acetabular bone stock using antibiotic-loaded bone cement. The degree of acetabular bone loss is noted at this time, so that the second-stage procedure can be planned. Bone deficiency is built up using antibiotic-loaded bone cement at the first stage (Fig. 5). The ultra-high-molecular-weight polyethylene component is inserted at a late stage of cement polymerization, so that marked cement intrusion into the remaining bone stock does not occur. This facilitates the removal of the acetabular component at the second-stage procedure.

The femur is then prepared by adequate reaming and broaching with one of five broaches. A trial reduction is performed and the appropriate femoral offset and neck length are determined. The choice of PROSTALAC femoral component is not limited only to prosthetic size, but also to femoral offset, neck length, and stem length. For the standard-length implants, two femoral offsets, five stem sizes, and five neck lengths are available for each stem size. A mid-stem and a long-stem femoral component are also available. These may be used in cases of segmental femoral deficiency or in the case of a weak proximal femur that needs to be bypassed. The technique for manufacturing the femoral component is the same regardless of the size or length of the stem. A stainless steel endoskeleton is inserted within a metal mold (Fig. 6), which was previously filled with antibiotic-loaded bone cement. A total of six endoskeletons are available. There are standard-offset

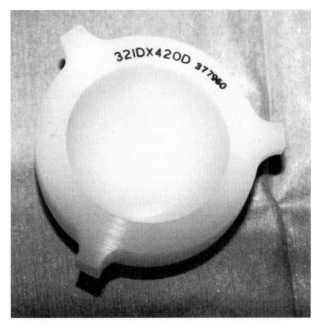

FIG. 4. The PROSTALAC acetabular component.

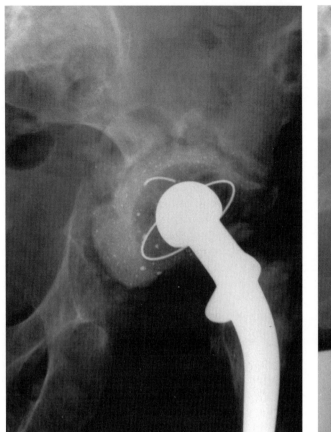 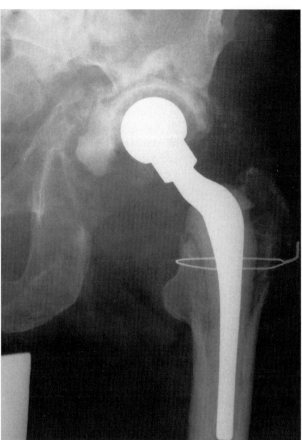

A   B

FIG. 5. Despite significant distortion and deficiency of the acetabular bone stock **(A)**, a PROSTALAC acetabular component was inserted **(B)**, and antibiotic-loaded bone cement was used to fill in the bone defects. The cement is not pressurized, to allow easy removal at the time of the second stage.

and increased-offset endoskeletons that may be used for any of the five standard-length molds. In addition, a mid-stem and a long-stem endoskeleton are available (Fig. 7) for use with the long-stem mold. Because of the bowed nature of these stems, right- and left-sided endoskeletons are available. After determination of the appropriate size and length of the stem, the PROSTA-LAC femoral stem is manufactured on the back table, and the antibiotics within the cement are customized based on the identity and antibiotic sensitivity profile of the infecting organism. The femoral neck of the endoskeleton is also coated with antibiotic-loaded bone cement to minimize the amount of exposed metal. With experience, the acetabular component and femoral component may be manufactured simultaneously, thus minimizing the surgical time. The final neck length is determined after the final seating of the stem. For added joint stability, the articulation is designed with a 32-mm head diameter, and a prosthetic design with an acetabular component rim that projects beyond the equator, so that a snap-fit configuration is achieved.

After insertion of the implants, the wound is closed in an appropriate manner. If possible, a suction drain is avoided so that an accumulation of antibiotic-rich fluid is allowed to collect. This bathes the implant and helps control the infection. After surgery, the patient is allowed up to 50% partial weight bearing, depending on the stability of the reconstruction. Under no circumstances should the patient be left in traction or on bed rest after surgery. Intravenous antibiotics are administered for a period of 3 weeks, and oral antibiotics are given for another 3 weeks. Two to 3 weeks later, a repeat aspiration biopsy is performed, in preparation for the second stage. If the wound has healed uneventfully with no evidence of ongoing sepsis, and if the aspiration biopsy results are negative, the second stage is planned for 3 months after the first stage.

At the second stage, the femoral component is removed without difficulty using a stem extractor. The acetabular component easily debonds from the cement mantle, and the underlying cement mantle is fragmented and removed piece-meal, without sacrificing acetabular bone stock. Appropriate implants are then reimplanted. At the second stage, we have used either cemented or cementless components, as well as allograft if necessary.

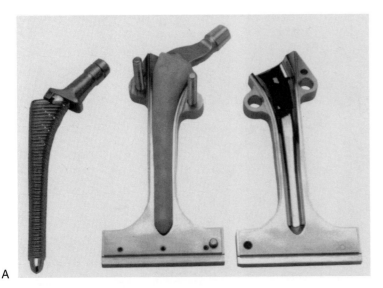

A

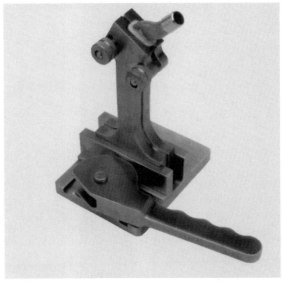

B

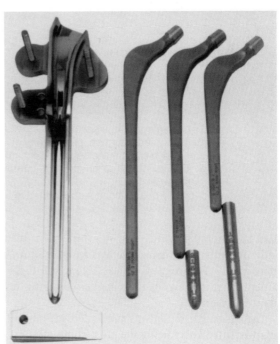

C

FIG. 6. A: The PROSTALAC short-stem mold, trial broach, and completed PROSTALAC implant. **B:** The PROSTALAC short-stem mold with the implant within the mold, prior to hardening of the cement. **C:** Long-stem molds. Antibiotic-loaded cement is packed into the mold, followed by the endoskeleton. Plugs of different lengths are inserted within the long-stem mold to obtain stems of varying lengths.

Results of the PROSTALAC System

To date, minimum 2-year follow-up results are available for the first 60 hip PROSTALAC two-stage exchange arthroplasties that were performed at our center between March 1991 and January 1994. The two-stage protocol was completed successfully in all but four patients. In one patient, the function with the PROSTALAC temporary implant was so good that the patient refused to undergo a second procedure. In another, drainage continued, and a Girdlestone arthroplasty was performed. Multiple cultures were attempted, and to the best of our knowledge, no organisms were ever isolated, suggesting that this was a sterile synovial fistula. The patient refused reimplantation because of good function. Another patient developed complications of chronic renal failure and hemodialysis after his first stage, and a second stage was never performed. He later died of complications related to chronic renal failure, and the hip became infected with a different organism prior to his death. The final patient presented with systemic sepsis secondary to an infected total hip arthroplasty. A first-stage PROSTALAC procedure was performed, and after recovery, it became apparent that his mental status was not compatible with reimplantation, and he underwent a definitive excision arthroplasty. He

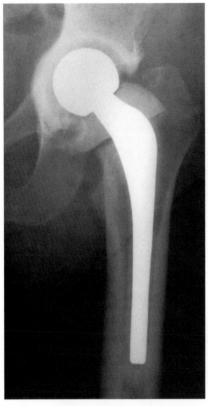
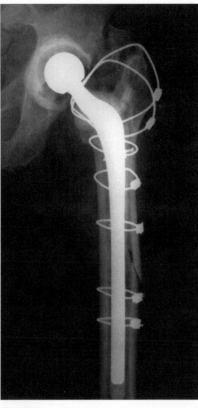
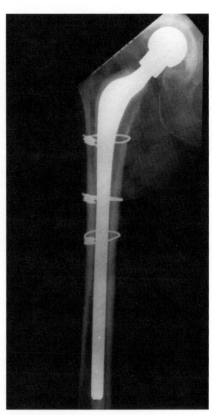

A,B

C

FIG. 7. Radiographs showing PROSTALAC implants of various lengths. **A:** A standard PROSTALAC stem was used because of adequate bone stock distally. **B:** A mid-length PROSTALAC stem was required to bypass the extended trochanteric osteotomy and the weak proximal femur. **C:** Because a very long extended trochanteric osteotomy was required for the removal of an infected long-stem cemented prosthesis, a 250-mm long PROSTALAC stem was required for fixation and stability. Antibiotic-loaded beads alone would not have been sufficient for stability after excision arthroplasty.

died at a nursing home, with his hip still infected. In addition to these patients, one was lost to follow-up and three died of unrelated causes. None of these three patients had any evidence to suggest ongoing sepsis at the time of death.

The causative organisms are listed in Table 2, with gram-positive cocci being the most common.

TABLE 2. *Bacteria identified as agents of infection in 60 hips prior to undergoing PROSTALAC two-stage exchange arthroplasty*

Number	Organism
22	*Staphylococcus epidermidis* (coagulase-negative)
7	*Staphylococcus aureus*
6	*Streptococcus* species
3	*Enterococcus* species
1	*Propionibacterium* species
4	Gram-negative (1 *Escherichia coli*, 1 *Yersinia*, 1 *Pseudomonas*)
1	*Mycobacterium tuberculosis*
2	More than 1 organism: one hip with 2 *Staph.* types, one hip with *Strep.* and *Staph.*
1	Negative culture, but pus present at two surgeries.

At the first stage, there was only one complication: an intrapelvic hemorrhage controlled with retroperitoneal dissection with the assistance of a vascular surgeon.

The mean delay between stages was 91 days. One patient, however, underwent a repeat debridement and revision of the first stage because of suspected ongoing sepsis; however, all cultures at that time remained negative. In most patients, a cementless acetabular component and a cemented femoral component were used at the second stage. Notable exceptions are four patients in whom a cementless stem was used, and two patients in whom a proximal femoral allograft was used for the reconstruction of a very deficient femur.

The overall complications following the second stage included one dislocation in five patients, two of whom dislocated their hip a second time. Two patients had a late periprosthetic fracture, both of which united uneventfully.

Of the patients who completed the two stages, clinical outcome was excellent in 27, good in 10, fair in 5, and poor in 2. The mean Harris Hip Score at presentation was 33.5 points, improving to a mean of 55.2 after the first stage, and to 75.2 at final review. The mean length of stay at the hospital, after the first stage, is currently 12 days, and after the second stage it is 9 days.

Recurrent infection was seen in only two patients of the 46 in whom the two stages were completed, for an infection cure rate of 96%. If the entire group is considered with no exclusion, the recurrent infection rate was 4 out of 60, for a cure rate of 93%.

CONCLUSION

The techniques described in this chapter allow the surgeon to reconstruct even the most deficient femur safely and effectively using a modified two-stage exchange arthroplasty technique. Similar deficiencies on the acetabular side can be handled after removal of the implants. Because of the improved function even in the more straight-forward case, this technique is recommended so that the patient may mobilize and may be discharged from the hospital.

This is but one technique in the management of the difficult problem of the infected total hip arthroplasty. Other techniques utilizing the same principles outlined in this chapter are possible. One such technique, involving a large bone-cement spacer that is shaped like a large hemiarthroplasty femoral component, has been described by Ivarsson et al. (28), although their experience was limited to only five cases. In another technique reported by Kane et al. (29), the prosthesis was removed at the first stage, and after autoclaving, a temporary spacer was fashioned using the removed prosthesis. Initial experience with the first 18 patients was encouraging. This approach, however, lacks the versatility of the PROSTALAC system.

Despite the versatility of the approach outlined in this chapter, there are still certain clinical situations in which other treatment strategies, such as a standard two-stage exchange arthroplasty, a one-stage exchange arthroplasty, suppressive antibiotic therapy, an excision arthroplasty, or even an amputation, would be preferable.

REFERENCES

1. Abendschein W. Arthroplasty rounds. Salvage of infected total hip replacement: use of antibiotic/PMMA spacer. *Orthopedics* 1992;15: 228–229.
2. Adams KA, Couch L, Cierny G, Calhoun J, Mader MT. *in vitro* and *in vivo* evaluation of antibiotic diffusion from antibiotic-impregnated polymethylmethacrylate beads. *Clin Orthop* 1992;278:244–252.
3. Al-Salman A, Taylor DC, Beauchamp CP, Duncan CP. Prevention of vascular injuries in revision total hip replacement. *Can J Surg* 1992;35: 261–264.
4. Bargar WL, Martin RB, deJesus R, Madison MTI. The addition of tobramycin to contrast bone cement. *J Arthroplasty* 1986;1:165–168.
5. Baker AS, Greenham LW. Release of gentamicin from acrylic bone cement. *J Bone Joint Surg Am* 1988;70:1551–1557.
6. Bayston R, Milner RDG. The sustained release of antimicrobial drugs from bone cement. *J Bone Joint Surg Br* 1982;64:460–464.
7. Brause BD. Infections associated with prosthetic joints. *Clin Rheum Dis* 1986;12:523–536.
8. Brien WW, Salvati EA, Klein R, Brause B, Stern S. Antibiotic impregnated bone cement in total hip arthroplasty. An *in vivo* comparison of the elution properties of tobramycin and vancomycin. *Clin Orthop* 1993;296:242–248.
9. Bunetel L, Segui A, Langlais F, Cormier M. Osseous concentrations of

10. gentamicin after implantation of acrylic bone cement in sheep femora. *Eur J Drug Metab Pharmacokinet* 1994;19:99–105.
11. Chapman MW, Hadley WK. The effect of polymethylmethacrylate and antibiotic combinations on bacterial viability: an *in vitro* and preliminary *in vivo* study. *J Bone Joint Surg Am* 1976;58:76–81.
12. Costerton JW, Geesey GG, Cheng K-J. How bacteria stick. *Sci Am* 1978;238:86–95.
13. Dall L, Keilhofner M, Herndon B, Barnes W, Lane J. Clindamycin effect on glycocalyx production in experimental viridans streptococcal endocarditis. *J Inf Dis* 1990;161:1221–1224.
14. Davies JP, O'Connor DO, Burke DW, Harris WH. Influence of antibiotic impregnation on the fatigue life of Simplex P and Palacos R acrylic bone cements, with and without centrifugation. *J Biomed Mater Res* 1989;23:379–397.
15. DiMaio FR, O'Halloran JJ, Quale JM. *in vitro* elution of ciprofloxacin from polymethylmethacrylate cement beads. *J Orthop Res* 1994;12: 79–82.
16. Duncan CP, Beauchamp CP. A temporary antibiotic-loaded joint replacement system for management of complex infections involving the hip. *Orthop Clin North Am* 1993;24:751–759.
17. Duncan CP, Masri B. Antibiotic depots. *J Bone Joint Surg Br* 1993;75: 349–350.
18. Elson RA, Jephcott AE, McGechie DB, Verettas D. Antibiotic-loaded acrylic cement. *J Bone Joint Surg Br* 1977;59:200–205.
19. Goodell JA, Flick AB, Herbert JC, Howe JG. Preparation and release characteristics of tobramycin-impregnated polymethylmethacrylate beads. *Am J Hosp Pharm* 1986;43:1454–1461.
20. Gristina AG. Biomaterial-centered infection: microbial adhesion versus tissue integration. *Science* 1987;237:1588–1595.
21. Gristina AG, Costerton JW. Bacterial adherence and the glycocalyx and their role in musculoskeletal infection. *Orthop Clin North Am* 1984;15: 517–535.
22. Gristina AG, Costerton JW. Bacterial adherence to biomaterial and tissue: the significance of its role in clinical sepsis. *J Bone Joint Surg Am* 1985;67:264–273.
23. Gristina AG, Kolkin J. Current concepts review: total joint replacement and sepsis. *J Bone Joint Surg Am* 1983;65:128–134.
24. Hedstrom S-A, Lidgren L, Torholm C, Onnerfalt R. Antibiotic containing bone cement beads in the treatment of deep muscle and skeletal infections. *Acta Orthop Scand* 1980;51:863–869.
25. Henry SL, Seligson D, Mangino P, Popham GJ. Antibiotic-impregnated beads. Part I: Bead implantation versus systemic therapy. *Orthop Rev* 1991;20:242–247.
26. Hill J, Klenerman L, Trustey S, Blowers R. Diffusion of antibiotics from acrylic bone-cement *in vitro*. *J Bone Joint Surg Br* 1977;59: 197–199.
27. Hoff SF, Fitzgerald RH Jr, Kelly PJ. The depot administration of penicillin G and gentamicin in acrylic bone cement. *J Bone Joint Surg Am* 1981;63:798–804.
28. Hovelius L, Josefsson G. An alternative method for exchange operation of infected arthroplasty. *Acta Orthop Scand* 1979;50:93–96.
29. Ivarsson I, Wahlstrom O, Djerf K, Jacobsson S-A. Revision of infected hip replacement. Two-stage procedure with a temporary gentamicin spacer. *Acta Orthop Scand* 1994;65:7–8.
30. Kane KR, Plaster RL, Tkach TK, Kennedy EJ, Hofmann AA. Treatment of infected total hip arthroplasty using an articulating spacer. Read at the *62nd annual meeting of the American Academy of Orthopaedic Surgeons*, Orlando, FL, 1995.
31. Kendall RW, Masri BA, Duncan CP, Beauchamp CP, McGraw RW, Bora B. Temporary antibiotic loaded acrylic hip replacement: a novel method for management of the infected THA. *Sem Arthroplasty* 1994;5: 171–177.
32. Kirkpatrick DK, Trachenberg LS, Mangino PD, Von Fraunhofer JA, Seligson D. *in vitro* characteristics of tobramycin-PMMA beads, compressive strength and leaching. *Orthopedics* 1985;8:1130–1133.
33. Kuechle DK, Landon GC, Musher DM, Noble PC. Elution of vancomycin, daptomycin, and amikacin from acrylic bone cement. *Clin Orthop* 1991;264:302–308.
34. Lautenschlager EP, Jacobs JJ, Marshall GW, Meyer PR Jr. Mechanical properties of bone cements containing large doses of antibiotic powder. *J Biomed Mater Res* 1976;10:929–938.
35. Lautenschlager EP, Marshall GW, Marks KE, Schwartz J, Nelson CL. Mechanical strength of acrylic bone cements impregnated with antibiotics. *J Biomed Mater Res* 1976;10:837–845.
36. Lawson KJ, Marks KE, Brems J, Rehm S. Vancomycin and tobramycin

elution from polymethylmethacrylate: an *in vitro* study. *Orthopedics* 1990;13:521–523.

36. Majid SA, Lindberg LT, Gunterberg B, Siddiki MS. Gentamicin-PMMA beads in the treatment of chronic osteomyelitis. *Acta Orthop Scand* 1985;56:265–268.

37. Marks KE, Nelson CL, Lautenschlager EP. Antibiotic-impregnated acrylic bone cement. *J Bone Joint Surg Am* 1976;58:358–364.

38. Masri BA, Duncan CP, Beauchamp CP. Long-term elution of antibiotics from bone cement: an *in vivo* study using the PROSTALAC system. *J Bone Joint Surg Br* 1995;77(suppl 3):308.

39. Masri BA, Duncan CP, Beauchamp CP, Paris NJ, Arntorp J. Tobramycin and vancomycin elution from bone cement. An *in vitro* and *in vivo* study. *Orthop Trans* 1994;18:130.

40. Masri BA, Kendall RW, Duncan CP, Beauchamp CP, Bora B. The PROSTALAC System—a microbiological analysis. *J Bone Joint Surg Br* 1995;77(suppl 1):74.

41. Masri BA, Kendall RW, Duncan CP, Beauchamp CP, McGraw RW. Two-stage exchange arthroplasty using a functional antibiotic-loaded spacer in the treatment of the infected knee replacement: the Vancouver experience. *Sem Arthroplasty* 1994;5:122–136.

42. Oga M, Arizono T, Sugioka Y. Inhibition of bacterial adhesion by tobramycin-impregnated PMMA bone cement. *Acta Orthop Scand* 1992;63:301–304.

43. Penner MJ, Masri BA, Duncan CP. Elution characteristics of vancomycin and tobramycin combined in acrylic bone cement. *J Arthroplasty* 1996;8(11):939–944.

44. Popham GJ, Mangino P, Seligson D, Henry SL. Antibiotic-impregnated beads. Part II: Factors in antibiotic selection. *Orthop Rev* 1991;20: 331–337.

45. Proctor RA, Hamill RJ, Mosher DF, Textor JA, Olbrantz PJ. Effects of subinhibitory concentration of antibiotics on *Staphylococcus aureus* interactions with fibronectin. *J Antimicrob Ther* 1983;12(suppl C):85–95.

46. Salvati EA, Callaghan JJ, Brause BD, Klein RF, Small RD. Reimplantation in infection: elution of gentamicin from cement and beads. *Clin Orthop* 1986;207:83–93.

47. Santavirta S, Hoikka V, Eskola A, Konttinen YT, Paavilainen T, Tallroth K. Aggressive granulomatous lesions in cementless total hip arthroplasty. *J Bone Joint Surg Br* 1990;72B:980–984.

48. Santavirta S, Konttinen YT, Bergroth V, Eskola A, Tallroth K, Lindholm S. Aggressive granulomatous lesions associated with hip arthroplasty: immunopathological studies. *J Bone Joint Surg Am* 1990;72:252–258.

49. Seyral P, Zannier A, Argenson JN, Raoult D. The release *in vitro* of vancomycin and tobramycin from acrylic bone cement. *J Antimicrob Chemother* 1994;33:337–339.

50. Sculco TP. The economic impact of infected total joint arthroplasty. *Instr Course Lect* 1993;42:349–351.

51. Wahlig H, Dingeldein E. Antibiotics and bone cement. *Acta Orthop Scand* 1980;5:49–56.

52. Wahlig H, Dingeldein E, Buchholz HW, Buchholz M, Bachmann F. Pharmacokinetic study of gentamiciloaded cement in total hip replacements: comparative effects of varying dosage. *J Bone Joint Surg Br* 1984;66:175–179.

53. Wroblewski BM. 15–21 year results of the Charnley low-friction arthroplasty. *Clin Orthop* 1986;211:30–35.

The Adult Hip, edited by J. J. Callaghan,
A. G. Rosenberg, and H. E. Rubash.
Lippincott–Raven Publishers, Philadelphia © 1998.

CHAPTER 83

Sepsis: The Rational Use of Antimicrobials

Barry D. Brause

The popularity of the total hip arthroplasty procedure is a proper testament to its magnificent success in restoring function to disabled arthritic individuals. However, 1% to 5% of indwelling joint prostheses develop infection, associated with significant morbidity and occasionally death. This chapter discusses the pathogenesis of these infections as it relates to the current spectrum of pathogens, the difficulties encountered in designing effective antimicrobial therapy in the present era of emerging multidrug resistance, and specific approaches to sepsis prevention.

BACTERIOLOGY OF PROSTHETIC HIP INFECTION

Infection of prosthetic joints occurs by either the introduced/contiguous or hematogenous route. The relative frequencies of these pathogenetic mechanisms observed at The Hospital for Special Surgery is 51% introduced/contiguous and 34% hematogenous, with the remainder being cryptogenic (Table 1) (5).

The introduced/contiguous form of joint sepsis results from wound infection overlying the prosthesis, or from operative contamination. Any factor or event that delays wound healing increases the risk of infection. Ischemic necrosis, infected wound hematomas, superficial wound infection, and suture abscesses are common events preceding joint replacement sepsis. During the early postoperative period when these infections develop, the fascial tissue layers are not yet healed, and the deep, periprosthetic tissue is unprotected by the

usual physical barriers. Rarely, latent foci of chronic, quiescent osteomyelitis are reactivated by the disruption of tissue that accompanies implantation surgery. Although operative cultures at the time of joint replacement are sterile, *Staphylococcus aureus* and *Mycobacterium tuberculosis* infections have recrudesced in this setting.

Introduced/contiguous-type infections are usually caused by a single pathogen, whereas polymicrobial sepsis with as many as three to five different organisms is seen in 24% of patients (Table 2) (5). Two thirds of introduced/contiguous infections are caused by gram-positive aerobes. Coagulase-negative staphylococci (*Staphylococcus epidermidis* and other species), the principal constituents of skin microflora, are the predominant etiologic agents, isolated in 37% of cases, followed by *Staphylococcus aureus* in 16% and Group D streptococci (enterococcal and nonenterococcal) in 10%. Gram-negative aerobes are found in 22% and anaerobes in 10% of patients.

Any bacteremia can cause infection of a total joint replacement by the hematogenous route. Sepsis usually becomes established at the interface of the bone with the foreign body (cement or prosthesis), and the pathogens reflect the resident microflora at the source of the bacteremia. Table 3 describes the attributed pathogenetic events in 36 patients with hematogenous prosthetic joint

B. D. Brause: New York, New York 10021.

TABLE 1. *Routes of infection for joint prostheses (The Hospital for Special Surgery)*

Route	Patients	Percent
Introduced/contiguous	54/105	51
Hematogenous	36/105	34
Unknown	15/105	14

TABLE 2. *Introduced/contiguous type prosthetic joint infection bacteriology (The Hospital for Special Surgery)*

Pathogen	Frequency in patients (%)
Gram-positive aerobes	67
Staphylococcus epidermidis	37
Staphylococcus aureus	16
Group D streptococci	10
Group B streptococci	1
Corynebacteria	3
Gram-negative aerobes	22
Proteus	6
Enterobacter	6
Pseudomonas aeruginosa	4
Serratia	4
E. coli	1
Klebsiella	1
Anaerobes	10
Propionibacteria	3
Clostridia	3
Peptococcus	1
Peptostreptococcus	1
Bacteroides	1
Arachnia	1
Polymicrobial infections	24

TABLE 3. *Pathogenesis of hematogenous prosthetic joint infection*

Clinical event	Organisms involved (N)
Dental	
Manipulation with extensive gingival bleeding, abscesses, root canal	Viridans streptococci (4)
Infected wisdom tooth	*Peptostreptococcus* (1)
Capping	*Peptococcus* (1)
Urinary tract	
Infection	*P. mirabilis* (6)
	E. coli (4)
Skin	
Abscesses, infected cyst, infected dermatitis, cellulitis, infected IV site	*Staphylococcus aureus* (9)
Cellulitis	Group G streptococci (2)
Desquamative dermatitis	*Staphylococcus epidermidis* (1)
Bowel	
Tumor, radiation colitis, diverticulitis, multiple enemas for obstipation	Viridans streptococci (4)
Proctitis	*Peptococcus* (1)
Diverticulitis	*E. coli* (1)
Enteritis	*Salmonella* (1)
Genital tract	
Cervical polypectomy	*Lactobacillus* (1)

TABLE 4. *Microbiology of prosthetic joint infection (all routes)*

Pathogens	Frequency (%)
Staphylococci	44
S. aureus	22
S. epidermidis	22
Streptococci	21
Viridans streptococci	9
Groups A, B, G	5
Group D (enterococci)	7
Gram-negative aerobic bacilli	25
Anaerobes	10
Fungi	<1
Mycobacteria	<1

infections evaluated at The Hospital for Special Surgery over a 3-year period (5). Dentogingival infections and manipulations are known causes of viridans streptococcal and anaerobic (peptococci and peptostreptococci) infections around prostheses (35,36). Pyogenic skin processes can cause staphylococcal (*Staphylococcus aureus* and *Staphylococcus epidermidis*) and streptococcal (Group A, B, C, and G streptococci) infections of prosthetic joint arthroplasties. Genitourinary and gastrointestinal tract procedures and infections are associated with gram-negative bacillary, enterococcal, and anaerobic infections of total joint replacements (2,27).

A general view of the microbial spectrum observed among joint implants infected by all routes is described in Table 4 (5). Staphylococci are the principal causative agents (44%), evenly divided between *Staphylococcus epidermidis* and *Staphylococcus aureus* in frequency. Aerobic streptococci are responsible for more than 20% of infections. Gram-negative aerobic bacilli are identified in 25% of patients, and anaerobes represent 10% of culture-proven pathogens. Anaerobes may not be isolated by routine culture techniques because of their fastidious growth requirements and their rapid demise upon exposure to air. Therefore, the frequency of anaerobic involvement in prosthetic joint infections is likely understated and several studies report no incidence of anaerobic organisms (13). Recovery of anaerobes from infected tissues and fluids can be substantially increased by placing the specimen directly and immediately into a pre-reduced incubation medium, such as thioglycollate broth. Supplies of this inexpensive medium can be made available in the operating room and at the bedside to encourage its use. The frequency of culture-negative cases should be reduced with this approach to delineating the microbiological diagnosis. In those difficult clinical situations in which antibiotic therapy is designed empirically because there is a high suspicion of infection in the absence of positive cultures, strong consideration should be given to include an antianaerobic agent in the therapeutic regimen.

FUNGAL INFECTIONS

Although these pathogens have been isolated in less than 1% of infected total joint arthroplasties, they represent significant problems for both diagnosis and treatment. All four principal species of *Candida* (*C. albicans*, *C. parapsilosis*, *C. tropicalis*, and *C. glabrata*) are capable of infecting joint prostheses (12,19,31,33,34). Because of the rarity of mycotic infection in this setting, initial cultures revealing *Candida* species may be interpreted as contaminants, thereby delaying appropriate therapy. Usually, fungal infections are found in patients with underlying conditions, including immunosuppression, prolonged antibiotic therapy, or intravenous drug abuse, but this is not true for patients with *Candida* infection of prosthetic articulations. The majority of patients described have had no identifiable predisposing conditions, have not had *Candida* infections elsewhere in their body, and have not had evidence of disseminated candidiasis. These infections present within 5 years of joint replacement, and symptom evolution follows an indolent course with an average of 10 months (range, 2 weeks to 4 years) between the onset of joint pain and diagnosis. Clinical presentations are the same as seen in bacterial infections of prosthetic joints. The periarticular fluid and tissues examined reveal purulent material with polymorphonuclear leukocytes. The individualized therapeutic approaches have varied from resection arthroplasties with intravenous amphotericin B to suppressive oral therapy with an imidazole (Brause, unpublished observations).

TUBERCULOUS INFECTIONS

Bacillemia during the earliest stage of tuberculous infection (*Mycobacterium tuberculosis*) can seed osseous tissue without causing systemic or local symptoms. Then, many years later, these foci of old, quiescent tuberculosis can reactivate in bones receiving prosthesis implantation (3,17,18,30,32,44). The risk of recrudescent infection is very low (in the 1% range) in patients with inactive tuberculosis for more than 10 years, but it can be as high as 43% in patients with active tuberculosis within the previous 10 years (28). It appears that perioperative antituberculous therapy is an appropriate consideration, especially if the initial tuberculous infection had been inadequately treated and if the patient is likely to tolerate antituberculous medication (6). The possibility of a mycobacterial infection should be considered in patients with otherwise unexplained recurrent joint prosthesis failure.

Optimally, patients with active tuberculosis should be treated prior to undertaking prosthesis implantation. Occasionally, *M. tuberculosis* infection is discovered at the time of joint replacement arthroplasty on the basis of subsequently available histopathology or culture results. In this clinical situation, successful treatment can be accomplished with triple-drug antituberculous chemotherapy given for 18 months postoperatively (29). It is noteworthy that almost all of these tuberculous infections were effectively controlled by antimicrobial therapy without removal of the prosthesis. However, the recent emergence of multidrug-resistant tuberculosis makes the efficacy of future treatments uncertain (4).

ESTABLISHING THE DEFINITIVE MICROBIOLOGIC DIAGNOSIS

The diagnosis of joint replacement infection is dependent, in large part, on isolation of the pathogen. Usually, the clinical history, physical examination, radiographs, and radioisotopic scans have inadequate specificity. Therefore, the single observation that delineates the presence of implant infection is isolation of the pathogen by arthrocentesis or surgical debridement. Moreover, microbiologic evaluations (e.g., susceptibility studies) of the etiologic microorganism are essential to design optimal antibiotic therapy.

Prosthetic joint fluid aspirates demonstrate the pathogen in 85% to 98% of cases (16,40). Fluoroscopic guidance and arthrography are useful, and in many cases necessary, to confirm accurate needle placement. When difficulty is encountered in obtaining intra-articicular fluid, irrigation with sterile normal saline (without antiseptic preservative additives) can be used to provide fluid for culture. If initial cultures reveal a relatively avirulent organism (coagulase-negative staphylococci, corynebacteria, propionibacteria, or *Bacillus* species), a second aspirate should be considered to confirm that the isolate is the pathogen and not a contaminant artifact. Early isolation of the infecting organism is important in establishing the correct cause of the patient's painful prosthesis, and it is essential for optimal selection of the surgical and medicinal therapeutic approaches. Availability of antibiotic susceptibility studies preoperatively permits proper selection of the appropriate antimicrobial agent for incorporation into the antibiotic-loaded cement spacer. Preoperative knowledge of the pathogen's quantitative sensitivity (minimum bactericidal concentration) should be extremely valuable in determining whether a single-stage or a two-stage (prosthesis removal and re-implantation) procedure is the best alternative in individual cases. Because the success of the single-stage exchange procedure is largely dependent on the efficacy of the antibiotic selected for mixing with cement during reimplantation, the choice of antimicrobial agent should be based on the quantitative susceptibility of the specific pathogen being treated. Most often tobramycin or gentamicin is used in the antibiotic–cement admixture, because it is known that these agents leach from polymethylmethacrylate cement in predictably therapeutic concentrations (46). With the recent emergence of aminoglycoside (tobramycin, gentamicin)-resistant staphylococci and streptococci, a successful clinical outcome may be related to how sensitive the pathogen is to these drugs. Most of these resistant gram-positive cocci remain sensitive to vancomycin, but vancomycin leaches from cement in only very low concentrations (8). Recent *in vivo* data have demonstrated significantly higher release of vancomycin when it is combined with tobramycin in the cement admixture (37). Anaerobes are not susceptible to aminoglycosides but are usually sensitive to clindamycin. As more information is obtained regarding the usefulness (pharmacokinetics and patient tolerance) of clindamycin–cement admixtures, clindamycin may become the agent of choice for local depot therapy of anaerobic prosthesis infections.

Operative cultures are definitively diagnostic. Therefore, in the absence of acute illness, the patient should not receive any antibiotic therapy for several weeks before the procedure. Multiple specimens (five to seven) of tissue and fluid should be submitted for culture. Samples of purulence, abnormal tissue, and fluid are preferable to swabs for cultivation. Cultures should be obtained by the surgeon with no intermediary handling, to avoid contamination. Specific cultures for anaerobes using pre-reduced medium (e.g., thioglycollate broth) should be inoculated in the operating room, if possible. Fungal and mycobacterial cultures should be arranged, if appropriate. After culturing has been completed, intraoperative antibiotic therapy can be commenced.

Once the specific microbiologic diagnosis has been delineated, quantitative sensitivity studies (optimally, minimum bactericidal concentrations) can be utilized to design the best antimicrobial regimen for each individual patient. Selection of specific antibiotic agents and their route of administration (intravenous or oral) are facilitated by the availability of this data. Decisions regarding the utility of combinations of antibiotics can also be made more easily with these studies, to provide additive or synergistic therapy. The isolated pathogen can then be used to determine the potency of the therapeutic regimen by incubating it with a sample of the patient's blood in the serum bactericidal test (SBT). This test has been very useful for confirming the efficacy of antibiotic therapy for prosthetic joint infection. For this purpose, the SBT blood is drawn at the post-peak period, 25% into the interval between doses. When this post-peak SBT titer is equal to or greater than 1:8, cure rates are 90% to 95% for prosthetic hip arthroplasties and 97% for prosthetic knee arthroplasties (9,43,49).

For all of these reasons, it is essential to isolate the pathogen in total joint replacement infections. However, there will always be clinical situations in which the etiologic microorganism is not isolated. In these uncommon circumstances, empiric antibiotic therapy should be designed on the basis of the likely pathogen(s), with special attention to the possible involvement of anaerobes in the infection.

ANTIMICROBIAL RESISTANCE

In the presence of prosthetic devices, many bacteria (especially strains of staphylococci and *Pseudomonas*) elaborate a fibrous exopolysaccharide material often termed glycocalyx. Organisms can grow within this matrix, forming thick biofilms. The glycocalyx modifies the local tissue environment in favor of the pathogen by concentrating microbial nutrients and by protecting the organism from surfactants, opsonic antibodies, phagocytes, and antimicrobial agents. These conditions increase the density of colonization on the surface of foreign materials *in vivo* and may predispose toward tissue invasion (6,11,23). These protective biofilms may also result in persistence of infection despite treatment with systemic antibiotic therapy (especially in the absence of extensive and meticulous debridement). Infections associated with biofilms and biomaterials may require special studies to determine the efficacy of specific antimicrobial agents (14,20,42). The routine tests for minimum inhibitory and minimum bactericidal concentrations are performed on suspensions of microorganisms in the logarithmic phase of growth. When the same bacteria are studied while they are adhering to foreign-body substrates or in the stationary phase of growth, their resistance to antibiotics increases markedly (24). By this mechanism, all microorganisms that induce biofilms in association with prosthetic device infection are more resistant to the effects of antimicrobial agents.

Resistance of bacteria in general to specific antibiotics continues to increase as a consequence of microbial genetic responses to antimicrobial agents. Certain microorganisms, important in prosthetic joint infections, have developed particularly troublesome patterns of resistance. Methicillin-resistant *S. aureus* (MRSA) and *S. epidermidis* (MRSE) have become common nosocomial pathogens often requiring multidrug, substantially toxic antibiotic regimens for effective treatment (21). Vancomycin, associated with frequent chemical phlebitis and potential nephrotoxicity, is usually the drug of choice in combatting these pathogens. Recently, vancomycin-resistant strains of *Enterococcus faecalis* (VREF) and *E. faecium* have been isolated in hospital settings, representing potentially untreatable microorganisms (45,47). These vancomycin-resistant organisms are able to transfer vancomycin resistance to staphylococci *in vitro*, thereby producing MRSA (and potentially MRSE) strains that would also be untreatable with presently available antimicrobial agents. Because staphylococci together with enterococci account for 63% of introduced-type prosthetic joint infection, the potential emergence of this degree of antibiotic resistance would be a clinical problem of immense proportions. Aminoglycoside (gentamicin, tobramycin, amikacin, streptomycin) resistance is also being observed among staphylococci and streptococci (38). This eliminates our ability to utilize these antibiotics in combination with cell-wall-active agents in synergistic, multidrug, systemic therapeutic regimens. Even more important, the emergence of this resistance will substantially interfere with the efficacy of antibiotic-impregnated cement for local therapy, because tobramycin and gentamicin are the most commonly employed antibiotics in these admixtures, worldwide.

Antibiotic resistance among gram-negative bacilli continues to outpace the development of new antibiotics. Treatment of these bacteria has been problematic and often ineffective. As a result of this experience, patients with gram-negative infections of their joint prostheses have often been refused reimplantation, or reimplantation has been delayed for many months, because insufficient confidence could be established regarding the eradication of this type of infection. Because this resistance pattern is strain specific, decisions concerning therapeutic approaches, including the timing of reimplantation, should be made on the basis of the quantitative sensitivity (minimum bactericidal concentration and serum bactericidal testing) of the particular microbe isolated (5,43,49). Treatment choices should not be based on the Gram stain characteristics of the organism or the genus and species involved. Instead, each cultured strain should be evaluated for our ability to eradicate it from the infected tissue with currently available antimicrobial strategies (including the variety of systemic agents as well as local therapy with aminoglycoside-loaded polymeric cement). At the present time, we encounter gram-negative bacilli that are far more readily eradicated than specific strains of gram-positive cocci (such as MRSA, MRSE, and VREF).

Our ability to control and eliminate specific pathogens is uncertain as antibiotic resistance continues to increase. The present problems we encounter with routine and nosocomial bacteria may be dwarfed by the recent reemergence of multidrug-resistant *M. tuberculosis* (4). Infection has often plagued the development of novel biotechnological advances, including total joint arthroplasty. Innovative solutions to these clinical problems will require continued collaboration between clinicians and researchers from the different disciplines of orthopedics, bioengineering, and infectious disease.

Although the treatment of infected total hip arthroplasty with debridement and suppressive antibiotics has not been markedly successful, the use of combination antibiotic therapy to include Ofloxacin or Ciprofloxacin and rifampin has recently yielded encouraging results. Encouraging results have also been demonstrated using the 1-to-8 bacteriocidal concentration protocol for 6 weeks, followed by long-term suppression (15,22,48).

PROPHYLACTIC USE OF ANTIBIOTICS

Perioperative antibiotic prophylaxis has been shown to reduce deep wound infection effectively in total joint replacement surgery (39). Oxacillin and cefazolin are commonly administered as antistaphylococcal agents immediately before implantation and for 24 hours thereafter. Vancomycin is an appropriate antimicrobial in those patients allergic to penicillins and cephalosporins. The duration of prophylactic antibiotic administration postoperatively has steadily decreased over the past two decades. Presently, prophylaxis is justifiable for 24 hours after surgery, but, as more data accumulates, even shorter courses may become standard (26,41).

In patients with indwelling joint prostheses, early recognition and treatment of infection in any location is critical to decrease the risk of seeding the implant hematogenously. Circumstances likely to cause bacteremia should be avoided. Prophylactic antibiotic administration in anticipation of bacteremic events (i.e., dental surgery, cystoscopy, colonoscopic biopsy, surgical procedures on infected or contaminated tissues) has been suggested on the same empiric basis upon which endocarditis prophylaxis is recommended (6,7,10,36). This approach to prevention is controversial, and no data are available with which to determine the adequacy or cost effectiveness of such measures.

The rationale for recommending prophylactic antibiotics for procedures associated with substantial bacteremias is based on the following:

1. Prosthetic joint infection is accompanied by significant morbidity, and occasionally death. Prosthesis removal, which is usually necessary to treat these infections, produces large skeletal defects, shortening of the extremity, and severe functional impairment.

2. The patient population at risk is identifiable. All patients with prosthetic articulations are predisposed to infection at that site. It is likely that certain populations of these patients have increased vulnerability to joint sepsis (i.e., patients during the initial 2 years after implantation), and perhaps these individuals should be particularly targeted (25).

3. The pathogenic organisms are identifiable. Although the spectrum of microorganisms in prosthetic joint infection is very broad, the probable pathogens have been delineated and are susceptible to many available antimicrobial agents.

4. The procedures associated with bacteremia are identifiable.

5. There is widespread belief that bacteremic procedures can cause prosthetic joint infection. Animal models have proved that bacteremia can induce these infections, and hematogenous seeding of human prostheses has been reported.

The prophylactic use of antibiotics for expectant bacteremias is not universal. The frequently stated arguments against recommending prophylaxis are as follows:

1. Only a minority of prosthetic joint infections are hematogenous in origin, and most of them are not associ-

ated with medical or dental procedures. Therefore the risk of prosthesis infection represented by dental procedures, for example, is too low to justify the use of prophylactic antibiotics.

2. The potential toxicity of widespread antibiotic use in prophylaxis may outweigh the potential benefit.

3. The financial cost of widespread antibiotic prophylaxis is not justifiable.

4. Recommendations for or against prophylaxis could create difficult medicolegal problems for the medical or dental practitioner.

The wording of a recent consensus recommendation published in *The Medical Letter* is as follows:

> Patients with indwelling prosthetic joints generally do not require antimicrobial prophylaxis when undergoing dental, gastrointestinal or genitourinary procedures; for long procedures, surgery in an infected area (including periodontal disease) or other procedures with a high risk of bacteremia, prophylaxis may be advisable. (1)

Clinical decisions regarding prophylactic antibiotics for expected bacteremias in patients with prosthetic joints should be made on an individual basis.

REFERENCES

1. Abramowicz M. Antimicrobial prophylaxis in surgery. *The Medical Letter* 1995;79–82.
2. Ahlberg A, Carlsson AS, Lindberg L. Hematogenous infection in total joint replacement. *Clin Orthop* 1978;137:69–75.
3. Baldini N, Toni A, Gregg I, Giunta A. Deep sepsis from *Mycobacterium tuberculosis* after total hip replacement. *Arch Orthop Trauma Surg* 1988;107:186–188.
4. Barnes PF, Barrows SA. Tuberculosis in the 1990s. *Ann Intern Med* 1993;119:400–410.
5. Brause BD. Infected orthopedic prostheses. In: Bisno AL, Waldvogel FA, eds. *Infections associated with indwelling medical devices.* Washington, DC: American Society for Microbiology, 1989;111–127.
6. Brause BD. Prosthetic joint infections. *Curr Opinion Rheum* 1989;1:194–198.
7. Brause BD. Infectious disease perspectives on musculoskeletal sepsis. In: Esterhai JL Jr, Gristina AG, Poss R, eds. *Musculoskeletal infection.* Park Ridge: American Academy of Orthopaedic Surgeons, 1992;35–48.
8. Brien WW, Salvati EA, Klein R, Brause BD, Stern S. Antibiotic impregnated bone cement in total hip arthroplasty, an in vivo comparison of the elution properties of tobramycin and vancomycin. *Clin Orthop* 1993;296:242–248.
9. Callaghan JJ, Salvati EA, Brause BD, Rimnac CM, Wright TM. Reimplantation for salvage of the infected hip: rationale for the use of gentamicin-impregnated cement and beads. In: *The hip: proceedings of the 13th open scientific meetings of The Hip Society.* St. Louis: CV Mosby, 1986;65–94.
10. Cioffi GA, Terezhalmy GT, Taybos GM. Total joint replacement: a consideration for antimicrobial prophylaxis. *Oral Surg Oral Med Oral Pathol* 1988;66:124–129.
11. Costerton JW, Irvin RT, Cheng K-J. The bacterial glycocalyx in nature and disease. *Annu Rev Microbiol* 1981;35:299–324.
12. Darouiche RO, Hamill RJ, Musher DM, Young EJ, Harris RL. Periprosthetic candidal infections following arthroplasty. *Rev Infect Dis* 1989;11:89–96.
13. Davies IM, Leak AM, Dave J. Infection of a prosthetic knee joint with *Peptococcus magnus.* *Ann Rheum Dis* 1988;47:866–868.
14. Dix BA, Cohen PS, Laux DC, et al. Radiochemical method for evaluating the effect of antibiotics on *Escherichia coli* biofilms. *Antimicrob Agents Chemother* 1988;32:770–772.
15. Drancourt M, Stein A, Argenson JN, Zannier A, Curvale G, Raoult D. Oral rifampin plus ofloxacin for treatment of staphylococcus-infected orthopedic implants. *Antimicrob Agents Chemother* 1993;37:1214–1218.
16. Eftehar NS. Wound infection complicating total hip joint arthroplasty. *Orthop Rev* 1979;8:49–64.
17. Eskola A, Santavirta S, Konttinen YT, Tallroth K, Hoikka V, Lindholm ST. Cementless total replacement for old tuberculosis of the hip. *J Bone Joint Surg* 1988;70B:603–606.
18. Eskola A, Santavirta S, Konttinen YT, Tallroth K, Lindholm ST. Arthroplasty for old tuberculosis of the knee. *J Bone Joint Surg* 1988;70B:767–769.
19. Evans RP, Nelson CL. Staged reimplantation of a total hip prosthesis after infection with *Candida albicans*: a report of two cases. *J Bone Joint Surg* 1990;72A:1551–1553.
20. Farber BF, Kaplan MH, Clogston AG. *Staphylococcus epidermidis* extracted slime inhibits the antimicrobial action of glycopeptide antibiotics. *J Infect Dis* 1990;161:37–40.
21. Goetz MB, Mulligan ME, Kwok R, O'Brien H, Caballes C, Garcia JP. Management and epidemiologic analyses of an outbreak due to methicillin-resistant *Staphylococcus aureus.* *Am J Med* 1992;92:607–614.
22. Goulet JA, Pellicci PM, Brause BD, Salvati EM. Prolonged suppression of infection in total hip arthroplasty. *J Arthroplasty* 1988;3:110–116.
23. Gristina AG, Kolkin J. Total joint replacement and sepsis. *J Bone Joint Surg* 1983;65A:128–134.
24. Gristina AG, Jennings RA, Naylor PT, et al. Comparative in vitro antibiotic resistance of surface-colonizing coagulase-negative staphylococci. *Antimicrob Agents Chemother* 1989;33:813–816.
25. Hanssen AD, Osmon DR, Nelson CL. Prevention of deep periprosthetic joint infection. *J Bone Joint Surg* 1996;78A:458–471.
26. Heydemann JS, Nelson CL. Short-term preventive antibiotics. *Clin Orthop* 1986;205:184–187.
27. Inman JN, Gallegos KV, Brause BD, Redecha PB, Christian CL. Clinical and microbial features of prosthetic joint infection. *Am J Med* 1984;77:47–53.
28. Kim YH, Han DY, Park BM. Total hip arthroplasty for tuberculous coxarthrosis. *J Bone Joint Surg* 1987;69A:718–727.
29. Kim YH. Total knee arthroplasty for tuberculous arthritis. *J Bone Joint Surg* 1988;70A:1322–1330.
30. Kim YY, Ko CU, Ahn JY, Yoon YS, Kwak BM. Charnley low friction arthroplasty in tuberculosis of the hip—an 8 year to 13 year follow-up. *J Bone Joint Surg* 1988;70B:756–760.
31. Koch AE. *Candida albicans* infection of a prosthetic knee replacement. *J Rheumatol* 1988;15:362–365.
32. Laforgia R, Murphy JCM, Redfern TR. Low friction arthroplasty for old quiescent (Tb) infection of the hip. *J Bone Joint Surg* 1988;70B:373–376.
33. Lambertus M, Throdarson D, Goetz MB. Fungal prosthetic arthritis: presentation of two cases and review of the literature. *Rev Infect Dis* 1988;10:1038–1043.
34. Levine M, Rehm SJ, Wilde AH. Infection with *Candida albicans* of a total knee arthroplasty: a case report and review of the literature. *Clin Orthop* 1988;226:235–239.
35. Lindqvist C, Slatis P. Dental bacteremia-a neglected cause of arthroplasty infections? *Acta Orthop Scand* 1985;56:506–508.
36. Maderazo EG, Judson S, Pasternak H. Late infections of total joint prostheses: a review and recommendations for prevention. *Clin Orthop* 1988;229:131–142.
37. Masri BA, Duncan CP, Beauchamp CP. Long-term elution of antibiotics from bone cement: an in vivo study using the prostalac system (abstr). *J Bone Joint Surg* 1995;77B(suppl 3):308.
38. Montecalvo MA, Horowitz H, Gedris C, et al. Outbreak of vancomycin-, ampicillin-, aminoglycoside-resistant *Enterococcus faecium* bacteremia in an adult oncology unit. *Antimicrob Agents Chemother* 1994;38:1363–1367.
39. Norden C. A critical review of antibiotic prophylaxis in orthopedic surgery. *Rev Infect Dis* 1983;5:928–932.
40. O'Neill DA, Harris WH. Failed total hip replacement: assessment by plain radiographs, arthrograms and aspiration of the hip joint. *J Bone Joint Surg* 1984;66A:540–546.
41. Page CP, Bohnen JMA, Fletcher JR, McManus AT, Solomkin JS, Wittmann DH. Antimicrobial prophylaxis for surgical wounds: guidelines for clinical care. *Arch Surg* 1993;128:79–88.
42. Prosser BL, Taylor D, Dix BA, et al. Method of evaluating effects of antibiotics on bacterial biofilm. *Antimicrob Agents Chemother* 1987;31:1502–1506.

43. Salvati EA, Chekofsky KM, Brause BD, Wilson PD Jr. Reimplantation in infection: a 12 year experience. *Clin Orthop* 1982;170:62–75.
44. Santavirta S, Eskola A, Konttinen YT, Tallroth K, Lindholm ST. Total hip replacement in old tuberculosis: a report of 14 cases. *Acta Orthop Scand* 1988;59:391–395.
45. Shales DM, Bouvet A, Shales JH, Devine D, Al-Obeid S, Williamson R. Inducible, transferable resistance to vancomycin in *Enterococcus faecalis* A256. *Antimicrob Agents Chemother* 1989;33:198–203.
46. Trippel SB. Antibiotic impregnated cement in total joint arthroplasty. *J Bone Joint Surg* 1986;68A:1297–1302.
47. Whitman MS, Pitsakis PG, Zausner A, Livornese LL, Osborne AJ, Johnson CC, Levison ME. Antibiotic treatment of experimental endocarditis due to vancomycin- and ampicillin-resistant *Enterococcus faecium. Antimicrob Agents Chemother* 193;37:2069–2073.
48. Widmer AF, Gaechter A, Ochsner PE, Zimmerli W. Antimicrobial treatment of orthopedic implant-related infections with rifampin combinations. *Clin Infect Dis* 1992:13:1251–1253.
49. Windsor RE, Insall JN, Urs WK, Miller DV, Brause BD. Two- stage reimplantation for the salvage of total knee arthroplasty complicated by infection. *J Bone Joint Surg* 1990;72A:272–278.

SECTION VII

Revision of Total Hip Arthroplasty

The Adult Hip, edited by J. J. Callaghan,
A. G. Rosenberg, and H. E. Rubash.
Lippincott–Raven Publishers, Philadelphia © 1998.

CHAPTER 84

Preoperative Planning for Revision Total Hip Arthroplasty

Michael A. Catino, Janet E. Whirlow, Nicholas G. Sotereanos, Lawrence S. Crossett, and Harry E. Rubash

Preoperative planning for primary total hip arthroplasty (THA) has been discussed extensively in the literature. Unfortunately, little has been written with regard to revision THA. Preoperative planning is invaluable in revision THA, and, as shown for primary THAs, considerable attention to detail is required to provide the most beneficial results (37).

Preoperative planning for revision THA consists of a thorough history and physical examination, proper radiograph evaluation, bone deficiency classification, and selection of one or a variety of prosthetic possibilities as judged by preoperative templating. The initial evaluation should focus on the need for surgical reconstruction. Proper planning will identify any special needs for a given case, help avoid intraoperative complications, reduce operating room time, and optimize clinical results. The inclusion of alternative plans is also prudent (7,17, 19,37).

HISTORY AND PHYSICAL EXAMINATION

Assessment of the patient's need for reconstructive surgery begins with the history and physical exam. Absolute indications for revision THA include progressive disabling pain, sepsis, and limitation of function. In addition, the patient's current quality of life and expected outcome should be considered (15). The patient should be asked to describe the location and onset of pain. Patients with hip disease will typically report having groin or thigh pain, generally indicating acetabular or femoral component dysfunction, respectively. Pain associated with supine straight-leg raising can be an indicator of a loose acetabular component. However, referred pain may be the only symptom, manifesting as generalized knee discomfort without specific physical signs (11). Pain associated with the onset of activity is often characteristic of a loosened component. An infected component is commonly associated with extreme or generalized pain during periods of rest. Patients with an infection may have a history of a postoperative hematoma or delayed wound healing after the primary THA. Extensive pelvic or femoral osteolysis, secondary to excessive polyethylene or metallic wear, is often silent and may surprisingly result in only minimal hip discomfort.

Although infection and prosthetic loosening are common causes of intrinsic hip pain, such pain also can result from periarticular problems or disease extrinsic to the hip (25). For example, spinal stenosis or a herniated vertebral disk can cause hip pain. Methylmethacrylate or wire migration from primary THA can produce peripheral nerve symptoms by impinging on the sciatic or obturator nerve. Intermittent claudication secondary to lower extremity ischemia after THA also can produce symptoms perceived as joint pain, as can a fracture of the pubic rami or femur after relatively minor trauma in an elderly patient. Heterotopic ossification after THA is rarely the

M. A. Catino, N. G. Sotereanos, L. S. Crossett, and H. E. Rubash: Department of Orthopaedic Surgery, University of Pittsburgh Medical Center, Pittsburgh, Pennsylvania 15213-3221.

J. E. Whirlow: Arizona Center for Joint Replacement, Phoenix, Arizona 85018-3424.

source of significant pain. When groin pain is the patient's predominant complaint, a thorough physical exam will reveal the occasional femoral or inguinal hernia in the postarthroplasty patient.

The initial evaluation also should identify factors that may lead to operative or postoperative complications. The patient's cardiac and pulmonary status is of primary importance. Thromboembolic disease and endocrine abnormalities should be addressed and stabilized before surgery. Estimating the patient's risk for postoperative infection is extremely important. Several studies have shown that the rate of postoperative deep sepsis is influenced by obesity, advanced age, metabolic diseases, concurrent remote infections, prolonged preoperative hospitalization, steroid therapy, prophylactic antimicrobial agents, and suppressed immune status (20,21,40,49). Patients with rheumatoid arthritis or previous hip surgery have also been shown to be at increased risk for deep sepsis (20).

The physical examination both confirms impressions gained from the patient's history and provides a baseline for postoperative evaluation (31). It begins with gait analysis as the patient arrives for examination. The use of a walking aid, a limp, or a deformity of the lower extremity should be documented. Antalgic gait resulting from pain in all phases of weight bearing is characterized by a short stance phase and is commonly seen with hip-joint disease. Neuromuscular weakness also can be identified by recognizing characteristic gait patterns. The abduction lurch, also known as the gluteal or Trendelenburg gait, results from a weak gluteus medius (L5 nerve root). When ambulating, the patient's center of gravity is shifted over the affected hip. A weak gluteus maximus (S1 nerve root) forces the thorax posteriorly during hip extension, creating the characteristic extensor lurch. Weakness of the quadriceps (L2, L3, and L4 nerve roots) prevents full extension of the knee at heel strike. A foot drop is seen with a weak tibialis anterior (L4 nerve root).

Previous incisions in the hip and pelvis should be examined for proper healing or evidence of infection. Although skin flap necrosis is less common in hip as opposed to knee surgery, incisions should be planned to maximize distance and angles between incisions. Discrepancies in leg length must be identified to allow surgical correction during revision. True leg-length discrepancies are easily appreciated by comparing measurements from the anterior superior iliac spine to the medial malleolus on each extremity of the supine patient. If one leg appears shorter than the other but the measurements taken as described are equal, a false leg-length discrepancy likely exists. This is confirmed by differing measurements taken from the umbilicus of the supine patient to each medial malleolus. Recognition of pelvic obliquity and fixed flexion contractures of the lower extremity is crucial since these are sources of false leg-length discrepancies that should be thoroughly evaluated prior to

revision THA, and these may not require correction. The anterior and posterior superior iliac spines will not be horizontal in a standing patient, allowing identification of an oblique pelvis. Foot blocks of increasing incremental sizes can confirm objective measurements and give patients the ability to determine the "feel" of various leg lengths. The patient should be informed that stability is the primary focus of the procedure and will be favored over leg-length equality. Therefore, an orthosis to equalize leg lengths may be necessary on the non-operative extremity. The gluteus medius and minimus are the primary muscles involved in maintaining a level pelvis when upright. The strength of the gluteus medius can be assessed by asking the patient to stand on one leg. A positive Trendelenburg sign exists when the pelvis tilts toward the unaffected hip when weight is placed on the affected hip. Neural disruption or approximation of the origin and insertion of the muscle results in weakness and pelvic obliquity. This is often seen in patients with advanced degenerative changes of the spine resulting in lumbosacral scoliosis, previous spinal surgery, coxa vara, or fracture of the greater trochanter. A fixed flexion contracture of the hip can be concealed by increased lumbar lordosis. The Thomas test is useful for detecting flexion contractures of the hip because it eliminates lumbar lordosis by flexing the normal hip of the supine patient, preventing full extension of the involved extremity.

The strength and range of motion of the hip girdle musculature is then evaluated by functional groups. The primary hip extensor is the gluteus maximus (inferior gluteal nerve, S1 nerve root). Along with the lateral biceps femoris and medial semitendinosus and semimembranosus muscles, approximately 30° of hip extension is attainable. Flexion is mediated primarily by the iliopsoas (femoral nerve, L1, L2, and L3 nerve roots) in addition to the rectus femoris and sartorius muscles. A normal hip allows 135° of flexion. The adductor longus muscle (obturator nerve, L2, L3, and L4 nerve roots), along with the gracilis, pectineus, adductor brevis, and adductor magnus muscles, provides 20° to 30° of hip adduction. Forty-five degrees to 50° of abduction is provided mainly from the gluteus medius with less contribution by the gluteus minimus (superior gluteal nerve, L5 nerve root). Normal values for internal and external rotation are 35° and 45°, respectively.

The neural and vascular status of the involved extremity is evaluated next. The hip musculature is supplied by nerve roots from the lower thoracic, lumbar, and sacral spine. Damage of these nerve roots can be identified by assessing their cutaneous sensory distributions. Vascular exam begins with palpation of the abdomen to exclude the presence of an aortic aneurysm. The strength and character of the femoral, popliteal, dorsalis pedis, and posterior tibial pulses should then be evaluated. Patients with a history of peripheral vascular disease require appropriate preoperative arterial or venous vascular studies.

If the history and physical examination to this point show the need for revision arthroplasty, further studies and tests are indicated. Our standard laboratory studies include a white blood cell (WBC) count, erythrocyte sedimentation rate (ESR), and C-reactive protein (CRP). Although the WBC count has proven to be of little value in the absence of fulminant sepsis, ESR and CRP are useful in discriminating between septically and aseptically loosened implants (18). Technetium diphosphonate- and indium-labeled leukocyte scans do not clearly differentiate loosening from infection in a cemented hip prosthesis, but they are useful as negative tests (24). If there is a discrepancy between the technetium- and indium-labeled scans, further elucidation is mandatory to rule out the possibility of sepsis. The long-term bone remodeling associated with noncemented hip implants may limit the value of radionuclide scanning in these cases unless marked uptake of the isotope is noted in the periprosthetic regions. However, dynamic computed tomography (CT) scanning is a useful technique for diagnosing a loosened uncemented femoral stem (4). We routinely obtain an aspiration prior to most revisions. Because aspiration has been shown to be associated with a significant number of false positives, we also incorporate clinical, radiographic, and laboratory information increasing our ability to detect infection (25).

RADIOGRAPHIC EVALUATION

The preliminary radiographic evaluation includes plain roentgenograms of the pelvis and involved hip. Extensive bony defects may require additional radiographs. The required roentgenograms are an anteroposterior (AP) view of the pelvis (Fig. 1A) and both AP and lateral views of the involved hip (see Fig. 1B,C). Judet views (obturator and iliac obliques) and CT scans are useful in assessing extensive acetabular and pelvic defects. The proximal half of the involved femur should be rotated internally 15° to 25° for the AP view, to eliminate the normal hip anteversion and thus allow true measurement of the neck–shaft angle and offset. If a patient presents with bilateral hip disease preventing internal rotation of either femur, a posteroanterior radiograph, taken as shown in Figure 2, also can eliminate the natural femoral neck anteversion. The AP view of the hip should include as much of the femur as possible so that the tip of the prosthesis or the cement column is visible. Problems with cement fixation or extraction thus can be anticipated.

The lateral hip roentgenogram can be attained by a variety of methods. The Lowenstein lateral (Fig. 3) or "table down lateral" roentgenogram is taken with the patient's hip, knee, and ankle on the table; the x-ray beam is directed over the lesser trochanter at a 90-degree angle to the proximal femur (2) minimizing distortion of the intramedullary canal. Although this technique does

not produce the optimal femoral rotation for lateral templates, it does show the maximal anterior femoral bow and it is reproducible, making it the radiographic view of choice (17). Alternatively, for the modified surgical lateral roentgenogram, the involved leg is extended and internally rotated while the contralateral leg is suspended. The x-ray beam is directed perpendicular to the femoral neck. This view is good for determining acetabular version, but it is often difficult to obtain, especially if a patient has bilateral hip prostheses. A third, less commonly used, and often difficult technique is the unilateral frog-leg lateral. This view requires flexion of the involved hip and knee while abducting the same hip. The x-ray beam is directed through the femoral neck, perpendicular to the table. Regardless of the radiographic technique used, examination of serial roentgenograms will allow identification of component loosening and osteolysis.

Three categories of radiographic signs of cemented femoral component loosening have been identified (27). Definite loosening is defined by evidence of migration of the component or cement column (Fig. 4). This includes subsidence of the component or cement–component complex (28,41). Other findings include progressive varus positioning, fracture or fragmentation of the cement, and, rarely, fracture or deformation of the femoral component. Probable loosening requires a complete radiolucent zone around the cement–bone interface on at least one radiograph. Possible loosening requires a radiolucent zone occupying more than 50% but less than 100% of the cement–bone interface. Scalloping of the endosteal surface and a lacy periosteal reaction is suggestive of infection.

The radiographic signs of instability in uncemented femoral components differ from those in cemented components. In the former, stability can be gauged by the formation of new bone between the porous coating and the endosteal surface (i.e., osseointegration). The major signs of osseointegration include the absence of motion-induced reactive lines around the porous coating, the absence of pedestal formation at the tip of the implant, and the presence of spot welds (14). Stress shielding is an absolute indicator of osseous integration. On these components, a radiation beam tangential to the porous coating, necessary for evaluation, may be difficult to achieve. Proximally coated implants are designed for proximal fixation; therefore, radiolucencies and reactive lines around the smooth distal portion of the component do not indicate absence of bone ingrowth into the proximally coated areas (16). Identification of reactive lines and spot welds is less difficult when viewing radiographs of fully coated femoral components, because a tangential radiation beam is more likely to be attained. Specific signs of uncemented femoral component instability are calcar hypertrophy, an intramedullary weight-bearing pedestal at the tip of the prosthesis,

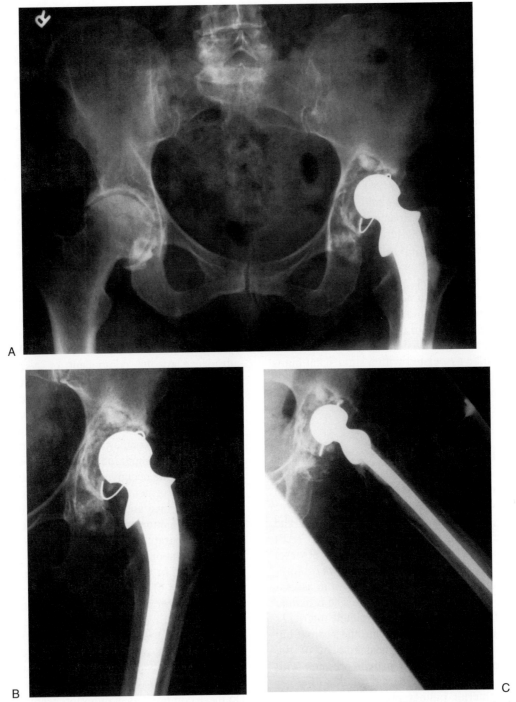

FIG. 1. The requisite preoperative roentgenograms are AP views of the pelvis **(A)** and hip **(B)** and a lateral view of the hip **(C)**. The femur is internally rotated approximately 15° for the AP views to eliminate the normal hip anteversion.

and the absence of proximal resorptive remodeling secondary to stress shielding, as seen in fully porous-coated implants (16) (Fig. 5).

Cemented acetabular components, unlike the femoral components, rarely loosen at the implant–cement interface. Signs of a loose cemented acetabular component include a radiolucent zone more than 2 mm wide surrounding the entire component (30,52), medial migration of the cup and cement (socket break-in), fracture of the acetabular bone stock, and changes in the degree of inclination or version of the component seen on serial roentgenograms (socket break-out) (Fig. 6).

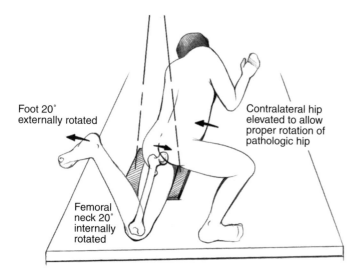

FIG. 2. When bilateral hip disease prevents internal rotation of a femur, the natural femoral neck anteversion can be avoided with a posteroanterior radiograph, as shown here. (From Engh CA. Recent advances in cementless total hip arthroplasty using the AML prosthesis. *Techniques Orthop* 1991;6(3):59–72.)

A comparison of acetabular-component fixation at 5 to 7 years found that bone ingrowth may provide superior fixation to that of cement (46). Furthermore, the rate of cemented acetabular loosening increases significantly after the first 10 years. A loose uncemented acetabulum commonly is associated with socket migration, screw breakage, defoliation of the porous surface, and fracture of the metal shell (Fig. 7). The importance of radiolucent lines surrounding the implant, which correlates with cemented acetabular component instability (30), is unclear in regard to the uncemented component.

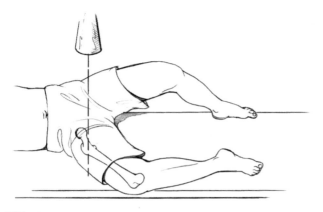

FIG. 3. The Lowenstein lateral roentgenogram taken as shown here is easily reproducible and shows the maximum anterior femoral bow; thus, it is the lateral view of choice. (Engh CA, Engh CA Jr, Cadambi A, Lauro G, Piston RW. Cementless revision of failed total hip arthroplasty: preoperative planning, surgical technique, and postoperative rehabilitation. *Techniques Orthop* 1993;7(4):9–26.)

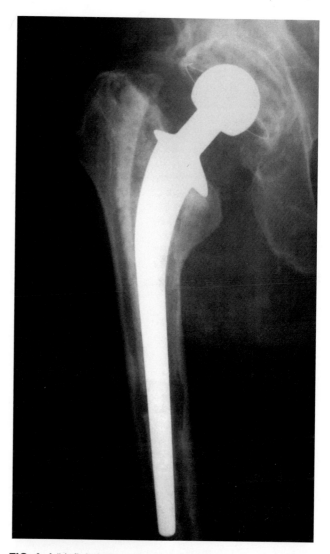

FIG. 4. A "definitely loose" cemented femoral component with component subsidence, cement fragmentation, varus positioning, and radiolucency at the implant–cement interface.

Osteolysis, the process of progressive destruction of periprosthetic bony tissue, is characterized on serial roentgenograms as a progressive radiolucent line or cavity at the implant–bone or cement–bone interface. Although occasionally a result of infection, this process typically results from a granulomatous reaction to polyethylene and metallic wear particles shed by the implant. This process was initially referred to as cement disease because it was thought to be caused by particles of fragmented cement (32,34,55). However, osteolysis is also associated with acetabular polyethylene wear, as was seen in the initial surface replacement arthroplasties (3). More recently, excessive rates of polyethylene wear, noted radiographically by changes in the position of the femoral head within the acetabular shell, have been shown to lead to excessive femoral and pelvic osteolysis (1) (Fig. 8).

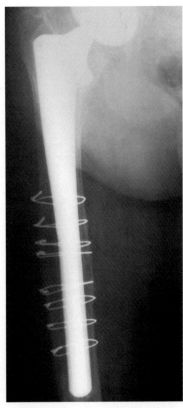

FIG. 5. A loose uncemented femoral component with an intramedullary weight-bearing pedestal and radiolucent lines at the smooth and porous portions of the implant.

Early osteolysis commonly manifests as component loosening associated with subjective pain, but if gone unrecognized, will ultimately lead to a significant bone stock deficiency. When rapidly progressive, osteolysis is an absolute indication for surgical reconstruction.

Femoral osteolysis occurs most commonly at the proximal medial femoral neck or calcar region and greater trochanteric bed (23) (Fig. 9), but it may extend along the entire length of the component. Although originally thought to be limited to cemented femoral components, femoral osteolysis has been associated with radiographically stable and unstable uncemented femoral components (Figs. 8,10). In fact, the rate of femoral osteolysis for both cemented and uncemented implants has been shown to be approximately 7% to 24% (29,32,51,56). Metallic and polymeric wear debris from uncemented implants may play a synergistic role in the development of osteolysis and implant loosening (36,38).

Acetabular osteolysis is also associated with both cemented and uncemented acetabular components. Particulate debris, consisting predominantly of polyethylene, appears to enter the effective joint space, initiating a granulomatous foreign body reaction that results in aggressive bone loss. The effective joint space refers to the area in the periprosthetic region that is contiguous with the articulating surfaces (45).

The pelvic osteolysis associated with uncemented cups is more localized and expansive than that associated with

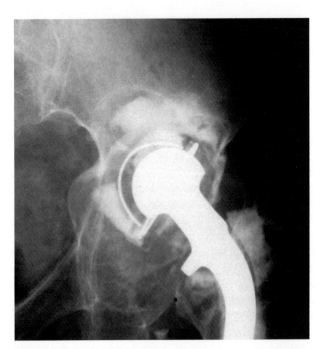

FIG. 6. The radiograph of this loose cemented acetabular component shows medial migration, circumferential radiolucency around the entire cement column, and cement fragmentation.

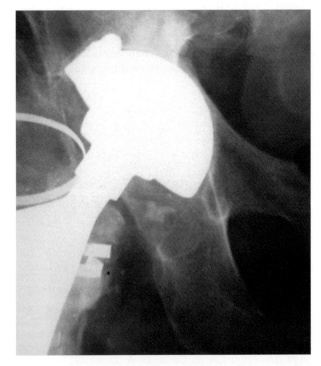

FIG. 7. A loose uncemented acetabular component with implant migration and circumferential implant–bone radiolucencies.

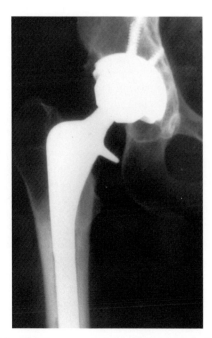

FIG. 8. Polyethylene wear, noted radiographically by changes in the position of the femoral head within the acetabulum, can lead to femoral osteolysis as shown in the greater trochanter region as well as pelvic osteolysis.

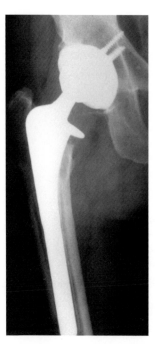

FIG. 10. Osteolysis, initially thought to be limited to cemented components, increasingly has been found in patients with first-generation uncemented femoral components.

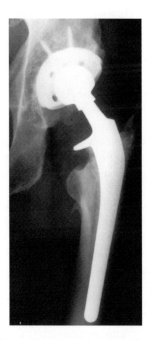

FIG. 9. Femoral osteolysis occurs most often at the proximal medial neck, or calcar, as in this patient with a hybrid total hip prosthesis and accelerated polyethylene wear.

cemented components, and it results in greater pelvic bone loss. The fibrous layer that forms between the cement and bone in cemented acetabular components may limit the migration of wear particles, resulting a more linear pattern of pelvic osteolysis (30,34,47,48). Interestingly, component loosening is more commonly seen with cemented acetabular components with concur-

rent osteolysis. In some studies, pelvic osteolysis has been seen in as many as 37% of cemented and 18% of uncemented acetabular components (57). Because uncemented acetabular components are associated with significant pelvic osteolysis while remaining well fixed, regularly scheduled radiographic evaluations are very important to prevent progressive pelvic bone loss. Therefore, the use of 26-mm to 28-mm femoral heads, a polyethylene thickness of at least 8 mm, precise liner shell contact, rigid fixation of the acetabular metal shell, and intimate bone–acetabular shell contact will decrease the amount of, and migration potential of, polyethylene debris, resulting in less significant pelvic osteolysis (5).

CLASSIFICATION OF BONY DEFICIENCIES

Along with the patient's age, activity level, and current medical problems, recognition of bony changes in the acetabulum and femur since the primary arthroplasty is also very important when selecting the appropriate prosthesis and method of fixation. After the radiographs have been examined, any bony deficiencies present should be documented and classified according to the system developed by the American Academy of Orthopaedic Surgeons Committee on the Hip (Table 1) (9,10). Most acetabular deficiencies are segmental or cavitary. By definition, segmental defects include deficiencies in the supporting rim or medial wall of the acetabulum; cavitary defects occur within the acetabular substance. These two types of defects, which can present alone or in combination, are further described by location, as shown in the table.

TABLE 1. *AAOS Committee on the Hip Classification system for bony deficiencies*

A. Classification of acetabular deficiencies

Type I: Segmental deficiencies
  Peripheral
    Superior
    Anterior
    Posterior
  Central (medial wall absent)
Type II: Cavitary deficiencies
  Peripheral
    Superior
    Anterior
    Posterior
  Central (medial wall intact)
Type III: Combined deficiencies
Type IV: Pelvic discontinuity
Type V: Arthrodesis

B. Classification of femoral deficiencies

Type I: Segmental deficiencies
  Proximal
    Partial
    Complete
    Intercalary
  Greater trochanter
Type II: Cavitary deficiencies
  Cancellous
  Cortical
  Ectasia
Type III: Combined deficiencies
Type IV: Malalignment
  Rotational
  Angular
Type V: Femoral stenosis
Type VI: Femoral discontinuity

From D'Antonio JA, et al. Classification of femoral abnormalities in total hip arthroplasty. *Clin Orthop* 1993;296:133–139; and D'Antonio JA. Periprosthetic bone loss of the acetabulum. Classification and management. *Orthop Clin North Am* 1992;23(2):279–290.

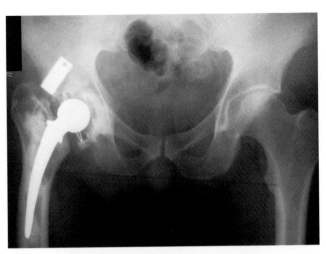

FIG. 11. Templating begins with drawing a line across the inferior aspect of the ischial tuberosities. By comparing the position of this line with the position of the lesser trochanters, leg-length discrepancies can be identified.

Pelvic discontinuity represents a defect across the anterior and posterior columns, separating the superior and inferior acetabulum. Arthrodesis is considered a deficiency because bone obscures the location of the acetabulum (8).

Femoral deficiencies are similarly classified. Segmental defects are any loss of bone in the outer cortical shell of the femur. A cortical window (intercalary defect) is a segmental defect with intact bone above and below. Cavitary defects here involve an excavation of cancellous and/or cortical bone from within, leaving the outer cortical shell inviolate. Femoral ectasia, a type of cavitary defect, refers to dilation of the outer cortical shell without perforation. Again, cavitary and segmental deficiencies may occur alone or in combination.

TEMPLATING

An accurate fit of the components is essential for firm prosthetic fixation. Templating not only determines the approximate component size and position to use, but it also provides the surgeon with a schematic of the revision procedure before entering the operating room.

Templating begins on the AP pelvic roentgenogram by evaluating leg-length discrepancy. First, a line is drawn across the most inferior aspect of the ischial tuberosities. The distances between each lesser trochanter and this line are then compared (Fig. 11). Any discrepancies in leg length are compared with the clinical measurement. For any discrepancy greater than 2 cm, a scanogram can be performed to localize the source of the discrepancy to the hip center, femur, knee joint, or tibia. Measurements on the scanogram should be relative to a fixed point on the pelvis, such as the sciatic notch, anterior superior iliac spine, or iliac crest if radiographically symmetrical (Fig. 12).

Continuing with the AP pelvic roentgenogram, the general size and more importantly the position and center of the acetabular component is determined. Unless a very large (jumbo) or very small (mini) component is required, establishing the precise size is not crucial at this time because 2-mm increments are generally available. However, the ultimate position of the component and hip center depends on the shape and size of the acetabulum, the degree of damage to the bone stock, and the surgeon's willingness to use bone graft for structural and cavitary defects. If the bony integrity of the acetabulum is relatively well preserved, the appropriate template is that which contacts the lateral aspect of the radiographic teardrop and extends to the lateral acetabular rim (Fig.

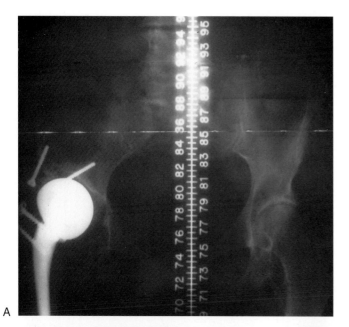

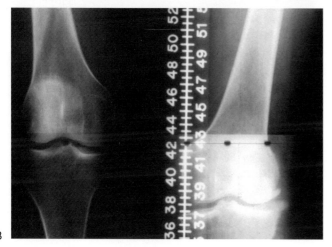

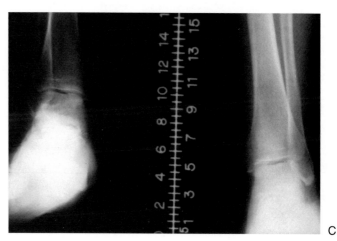

FIG. 12. A,B,C: A scanogram is indicated to localize any leg-length discrepancy greater than 2 cm. In this example, the iliac crest serves as a relative fixed point for measurement. A 6-cm leg-length discrepancy is identified.

13). The orifice of the cup should be as completely contained within the acetabulum as possible (50). An attempt is normally made to place the acetabular component at a 45-degree angle from the inferolateral teardrop to the lateral acetabular rim. In our experience, the most commonly selected implant for revision of the acetabulum is the porous hemispherical acetabular component.

When the acetabular bone stock is significantly compromised, preestablishing a biomechanically correct center of rotation presents a challenge. Placing the cup in a nonanatomic position produces characteristic findings and complications. Component medialization (protrusio acetabuli) is defined by migration of the femoral head medial to Kohler's line, that is, the line from the medial border of the ilium to the medial border of the ischium, also known as the ilioischial line (39). If the medial wall is not violated, this medial position of the acetabular component promotes bony coverage of the porous com-

ponent, contact of the bone with cement, and a close fit at the rim. Although originally advocated by Charnley because of the decreased body-weight lever arm and joint reactive forces, this acetabular location also has many disadvantages when compared to normal anatomic positioning. The most serious of these are decreased offset and hip stability, increased abductor muscle laxity, increased likelihood of femoral impingement on the anterior and posterior columns, and possible weakness or perforation of the medial wall. Protrusio acetabuli is often seen in patients with rheumatoid arthritis who require revision THA.

Treatment of protrusio acetabuli usually requires the use of bone graft to compensate for the medial deficiency and lateralize the component. After reaming the acetabular rim to allow for lateralization of the cup, previously prepared bone graft is placed medially within the acetabulum and a press-fit component is placed at the orifice of

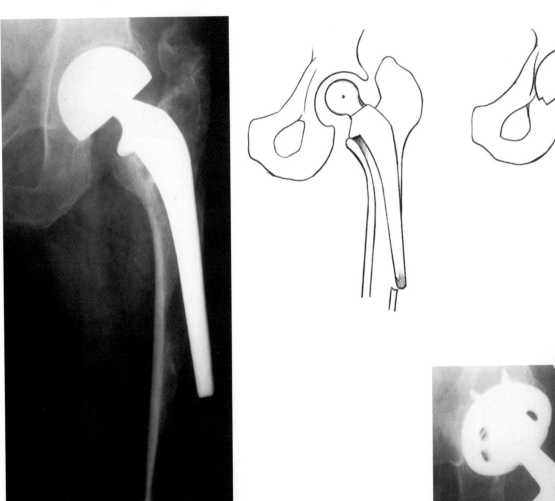

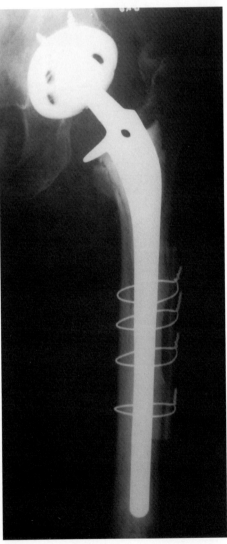

FIG. 13. The preoperative film shows well-preserved bony integrity of the acetabulum **(A)**. Therefore, the appropriate acetabular template should contact the lateral aspect of the teardrop and extend to the lateral acetabular rim **(B)**. Postoperatively, roentgenograms showed an unaltered hip center **(C)** when compared to the preoperative film.

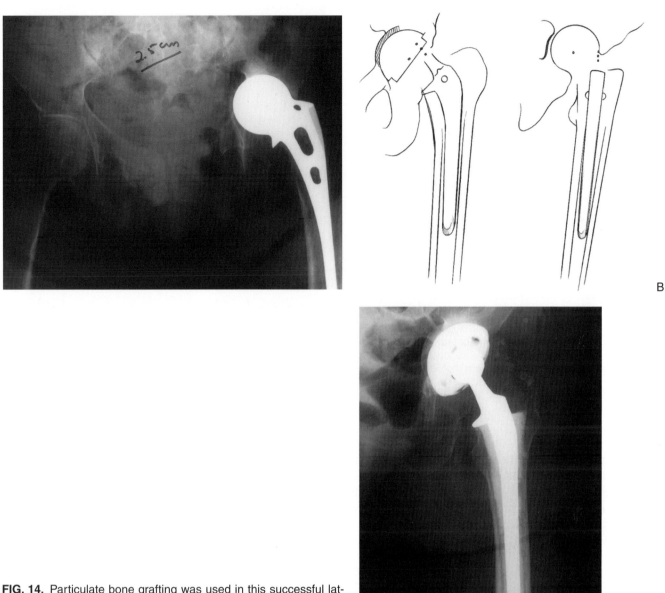

FIG. 14. Particulate bone grafting was used in this successful lateralization of a medially migrated endoprosthesis. **A:** Preoperative radiograph. **B:** Preoperative template with the *hatched area* representing bone graft. **C:** Postoperative radiograph.

the rim (Fig. 14). A deficient acetabular rim may require the use of metal protrusio rings or a special cup such as the anti-protrusio cage (6) (Fig. 15). If extensive bone has been lost from the acetabulum, the use of bulk structural allograft may be indicated (Fig. 16). In such cases, cement may be used to affix the component into the allograft. For a failed cemented cup that has entered the pelvis where no medial acetabular bone exists, an arteriogram should be obtained to define the relationship between the component, the fragmented cement, and the iliac vessels. If the cement or component is close to these vessels, a vascular surgeon may be required to dissect and mobilize the vessels to prevent intraoperative traumatic

injury during replacement of the acetabular component (42) (Fig. 17). Templating on the non-operative side facilitates reproduction of normal hip positioning and biomechanical properties. However, tightness of the soft tissue on the operative hip often prevents placing the acetabular component in an exact anatomic lateral position.

Lateralization of the normal center of rotation often results from inadequate reaming of the bony acetabulum, which prevents approximation of the implant with the medial quadrilateral plate. Associated complications may include suboptimal bony ingrowth secondary to insufficient contact with the host bone, poor cup stability, excessive abductor lever arm and offset, and high joint reactive forces.

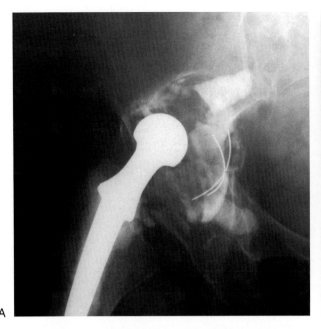 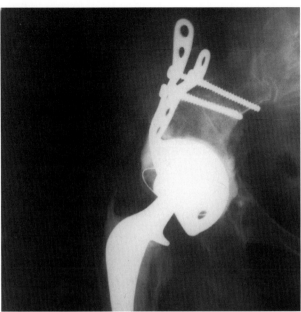

FIG. 15. A: Medial and superior migration of the acetabular component is a potential problem when reconstructing an acetabulum with a deficient rim. **B:** The anti-protrusio cage provides a useful treatment alternative for the reconstruction of this defect, providing protection of the medial femoral head allograft until it has been incorporated.

In contrast to lateralization of the cup, superior placement of the acetabular component without lateralization does not adversely affect the biomechanics of the hip (12,44) (Fig. 18). In one study, the hip center was placed an average of 43 mm (range, 35 to 61 mm) proximal to the interteardrop line (44). Furthermore, this position is recommended over the use of structural bone grafting for patients with acetabular deficiencies, because it is generally an area of good bone quality, and bulk structural weight-bearing acetabular bone grafts have a high late failure rate (26). However, failure to compensate for the high center of rotation during placement of the femoral component will cause the femur to impinge on the anterior column during flexion, adduction, and internal rotation, and to impinge on the posterior column during extension and external rotation of the hip. Consequently, a limited resection of the anterior column, anterior inferior iliac spine, and ischium may be required. Advancement of the greater trochanter may be required to restore abductor tension. Restoration of leg length can be accomplished by using a long head–neck implant or calcar replacement femoral implant (9).

A cup placed too inferiorly will have poor superior coverage and will be in an area of relatively poor bone quality. Such conditions subject these components to significant instability. Furthermore, the lower hip center of rotation will cause leg lengthening unless the femoral component compensates.

Leg lengthening with lateral displacement of the extremity has been associated with palsies of the sciatic nerve and its divisions (13,33,54). The use of somatosensory evoked potentials (SSEPs) provides a noninvasive method of monitoring the physiologic function of peripheral nerves during THA. Although it has not been shown to be of value when routinely used, it is thought to be a useful tool when used for high-risk patients (53). Included are those undergoing revision THA and those with expected limb lengthening. In one study, no postoperative peripheral nerve complications were reported in 23 revision THAs requiring an average leg lengthening of 18 mm (range, 6 to 43 mm) while using intraoperative sciatic nerve monitoring (35). We currently utilize SSEP on all intraoperative leg lengthenings anticipated to be greater than 2 cm.

The femoral component can be templated utilizing the AP roentgenogram of either the pelvis or the hip, although the latter includes the entire length of the femur and thus is preferred. The femoral templating technique varies depending on the type of implant to be used. For an uncemented fully porous-coated component such as an AML (Depuy Inc., Warsaw, IN), extensive diaphyseal ingrowth is essential (Fig. 19). Place the femoral template over the intramedullary canal on the AP roentgenogram and choose the caliber that contacts the medial and lateral endosteal surfaces of the isthmus over a 4- to 5-cm distance. Make note of the component size and position of

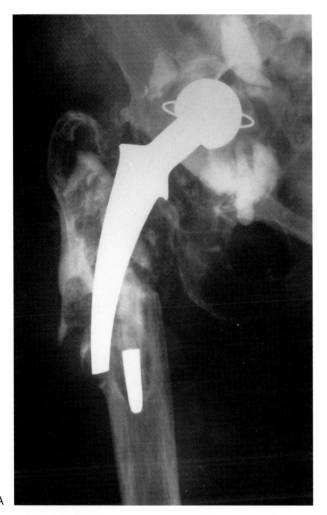

A

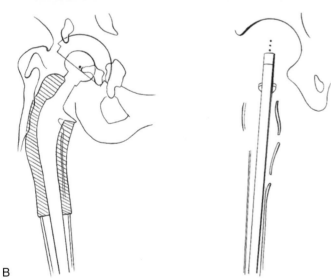

B

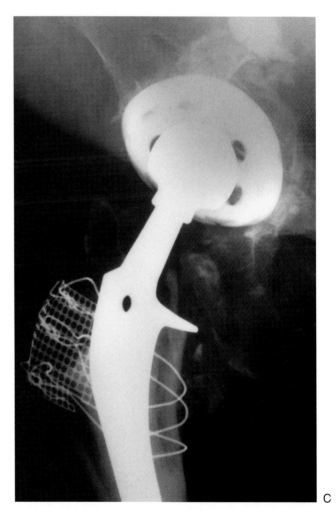

C

FIG. 16. A: Extensive acetabular bone loss is often an indication for the use of extensive allograft. **B:** The preoperative template shows the location of the appropriate hip center. **C:** Fixation of the acetabular prosthesis to the patient's own acetabular rim protects the medial allograft until the bone incorporates.

the pilot hole. Then select the proximal flare (standard or modified medial aspect) that provides the most complete endosteal apposition at the metaphysis.

For proximally porous-coated components such as the MultiLock Hip Prosthesis (Zimmer Inc., Warsaw, IN), it is also important to choose a template that closely approximates the proximal femur (Fig. 20). After selecting a component that fills the medullary canal at the isthmus on the AP roentgenogram, the apposition of the porous surface at the metaphysis is assessed. Ideally, the

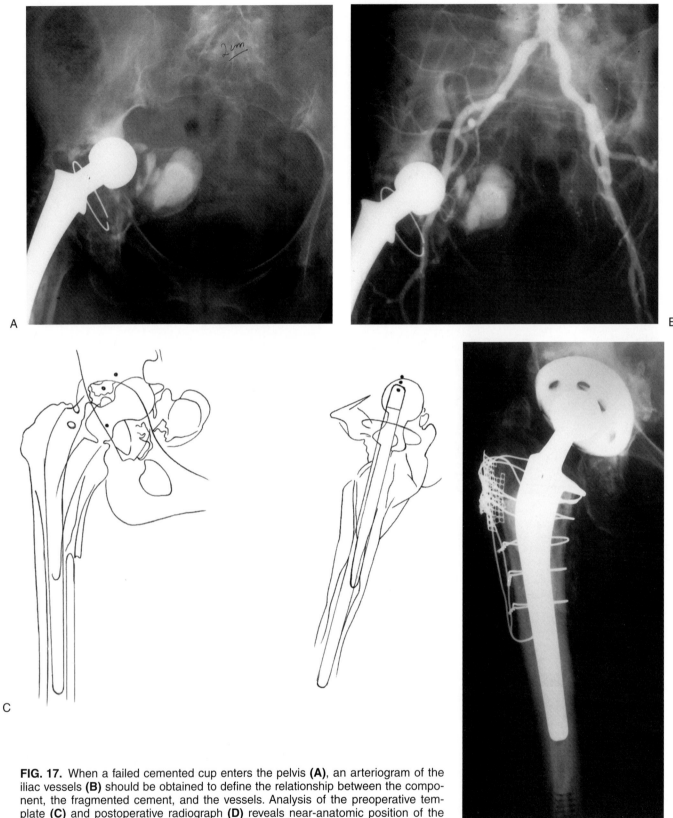

FIG. 17. When a failed cemented cup enters the pelvis **(A)**, an arteriogram of the iliac vessels **(B)** should be obtained to define the relationship between the component, the fragmented cement, and the vessels. Analysis of the preoperative template **(C)** and postoperative radiograph **(D)** reveals near-anatomic position of the acetabulum and the extensive acetabular particulate allograft.

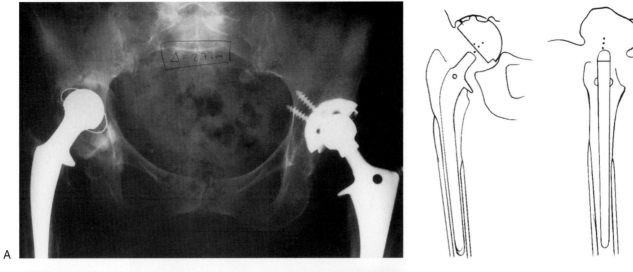

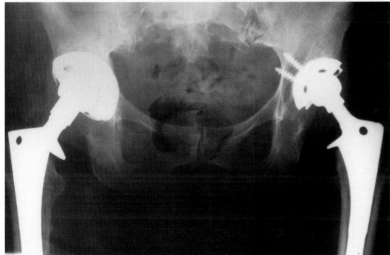

FIG. 18. Superior placement of the acetabular component without lateralization is an alternative to structural bone graft in the reconstruction of superior acetabular deficiencies **(A)**. Note preoperative template **(B)** and postoperative film **(C)**.

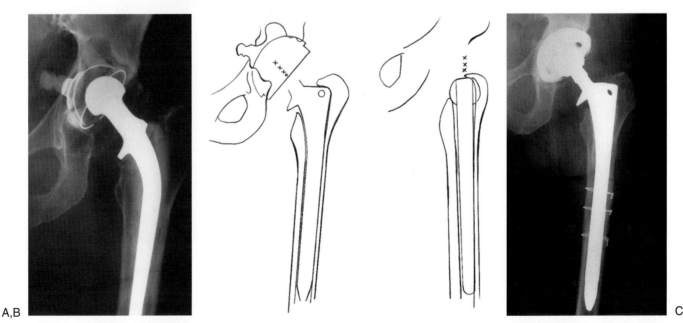

FIG. 19. When revising a failed femoral component **(A)** with an uncemented, fully porous-coated component, the templates **(B)** should closely approximate the endosteal surfaces on the AP and lateral hip films. Postoperative radiographs in this case revealed appropriate endosteal apposition and excellent component alignment **(C)**.

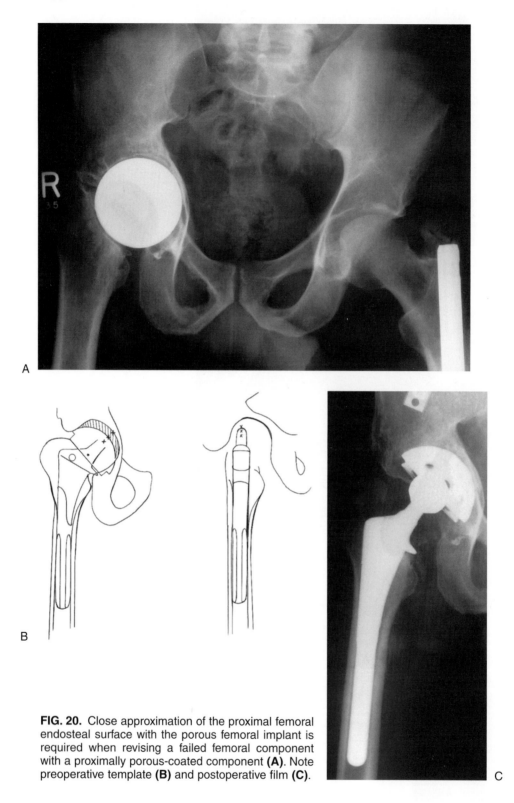

FIG. 20. Close approximation of the proximal femoral endosteal surface with the porous femoral implant is required when revising a failed femoral component with a proximally porous-coated component **(A)**. Note preoperative template **(B)** and postoperative film **(C)**.

body of the prosthesis will be parallel to the proximal medial femoral cortex.

If a cemented femoral component is indicated, an additional 2 mm or more is required circumferentially around the component for cement. This is normally allotted in the template. Intraoperatively, the intramedullary canal will be prepared by removing a majority of the cement and neocortex, attempting to preserve as much cancellous bone as possible. This will often allow a complete 2-mm cement mantle to form between

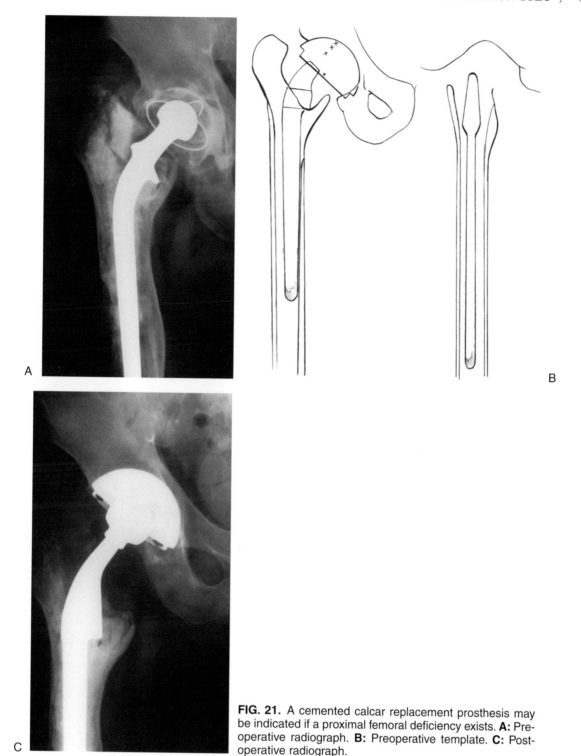

FIG. 21. A cemented calcar replacement prosthesis may be indicated if a proximal femoral deficiency exists. **A:** Preoperative radiograph. **B:** Preoperative template. **C:** Postoperative radiograph.

the endosteal surface and the implant. If a partial calcar deficiency exists, a cemented calcar replacement prosthesis may be indicated (Fig. 21). When confronted with more severe osteolysis or other femoral deficiencies, impaction grafting and use of structural allograft are reasonable alternatives.

Because the cortex of the proximal femur transmits load, a cortical segmental allograft is a rarely used option in the treatment of extensive proximal femoral bone deficiencies (Fig. 22). This technique requires that a long-stemmed femoral component be fixed within the allograft. Cement generally should also be used for fixation

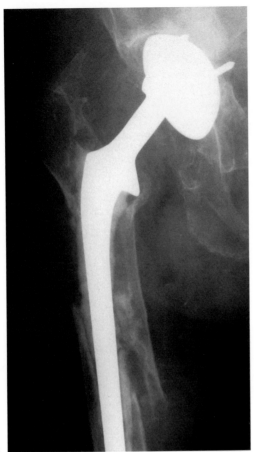

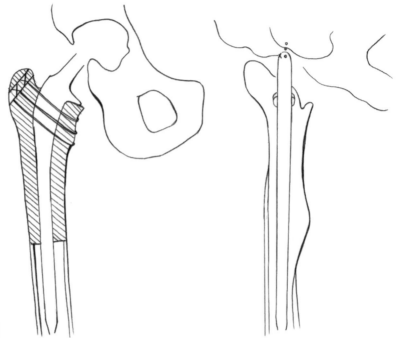

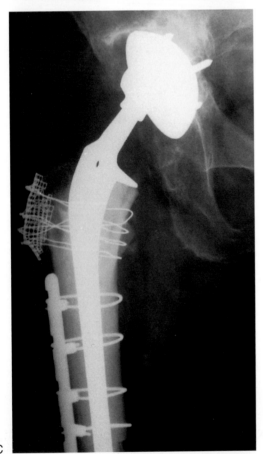

FIG. 22. For extensive proximal femoral bone deficiencies, a cortical segmental allograft is a less commonly used reconstructive option. Preoperative radiograph **(A)** and the template **(B)** illustrate the planned femoral allograft *(hatched area)*. Note the postoperative radiograph **(C)**. The acetabular component was stable when inspected during the operative procedure.

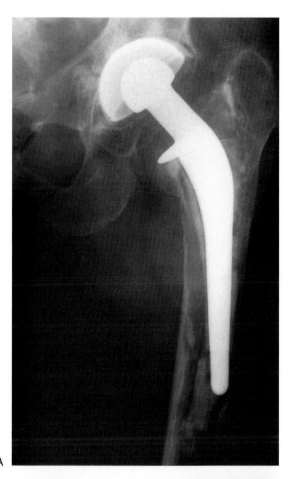

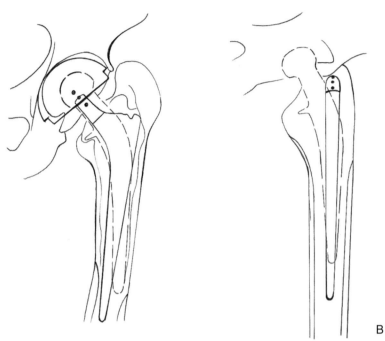

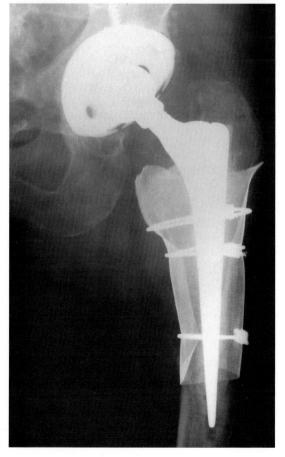

FIG. 23. The new technique of impaction grafting is an alternative for treating proximal femoral deficiencies. Cancellous allograft is used to compensate for the bony deficiency, and then a tapered femoral component is cemented in place. **A:** Preoperative radiograph. **B:** Preoperative template. **C:** Postoperative radiograph.

between the implant and the host bone (43). The placement of autograft at the host–allograft interface also is recommended to ensure fixation. The preoperative plan must include determining the level of the host femoral resection, the length of the femoral allograft, and the need for additional types of fixation.

An alternative for treating proximal femoral deficiencies is the recently introduced technique of impaction grafting (Fig. 23). This method uses impacted cancellous allograft and cement to compensate for the loss of bone stock. Defects in the femoral cortex initially are covered with a fine wire mesh supported by cerclage wires. Cancellous allograft bone chips are then placed into the prepared femoral canal and tamped with a trial femoral component two sizes larger than the size estimated by preoperative templating. This process is repeated until the intramedullary canal is filled with impacted chips and a "neomedullary" canal exits within the allograft bone chips. Reduced-viscosity cement is pressurized into the newly formed canal, and a tapered femoral component is inserted (22). Less severe cortical defects in the distal femur are filled with bone graft and bypassed with the implant by at least two bone diameters.

After the acetabular and femoral components have been selected, the neck length and the position of the femoral component within the femur are determined. At this point, it is critical to restore the normal anatomic offset between the femur and pelvis as closely as possible. Doing this helps to preestablish the normal biomechanical properties of the hip and eliminate the need for additional procedures such as trochanteric advancement. Failure to restore Shenton's line (15), which depends on the femoral–pelvic offset, results in characteristic abnormalities. A reduction in offset leads to instability and limp, increased joint reactive forces, a decreased abductor lever arm (which increases the energy required for walking), instability secondary to bony impingement, soft-tissue laxity, and hastened component failure. Increased offset has the opposite effect: an increased abductor lever arm (which decreases the energy required for walking), decreased joint-reactive forces, decreased bony impingement, and taut soft tissues.

If the pelvis and the femur have a normal anatomic relationship, templating on the operative side will reproduce the desired offset. The centers of rotation of the femoral head and acetabulum are superimposed, and the neck resection level is noted relative to the superior aspect of the lesser trochanter or any other prominent bony landmark. The appropriate modular neck length is then selected.

Unfortunately, this pelvic-femoral relationship is rarely maintained on the operative hip, in which case templating should be performed on the non-operative hip to more accurately determine the position for the femoral component. This method equalizes the offset of the diseased hip from the contralateral hip, producing near-nor-

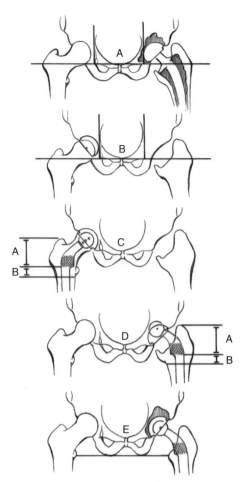

FIG. 24. When the pelvic–femoral relationship is distorted on the operative side, preoperative templating can be performed on the non-operative side. The prosthetic acetabular center of rotation is first transferred from the operative side (A) to the normal side (B). The height of the femoral component is selected next by superimposing the center of rotation of the femoral component upon that of the acetabular component (C). The position of the femoral component is measured relative to a bony landmark such as the greater trochanter (a) or lesser trochanter (b). The component templates then are transferred to the operative side while maintaining their relative positions (D). Components placed in this manner will equalize the offset of the diseased and contralateral hips (E). (Modified from Engh CA, Engh CA Jr, Cadambi A, Lauro G, Piston RW. Cementless revision of failed total hip arthroplasty: preoperative planning, surgical technique, and postoperative rehabilitation. *Techniques Orthop* 1993;7(4):9–26.)

mal biomechanical properties in the hip postoperatively. Contralateral templating requires the prosthetic acetabular center of rotation to be transferred from the operative side to the normal side (Fig. 24). This position is measured relative to horizontal and vertical lines drawn through the inferolateral teardrop. Having selected the appropriate femoral component size, the height of the component placement is determined next. This is per-

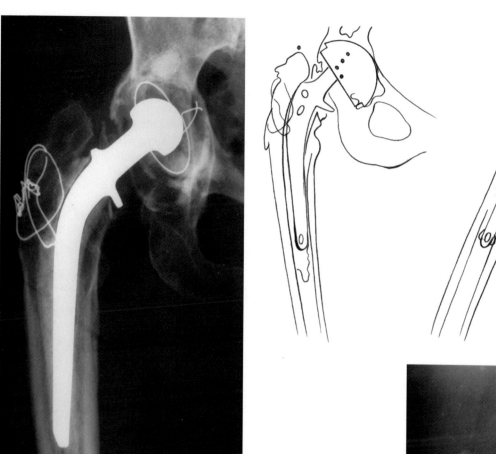

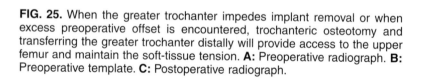

A

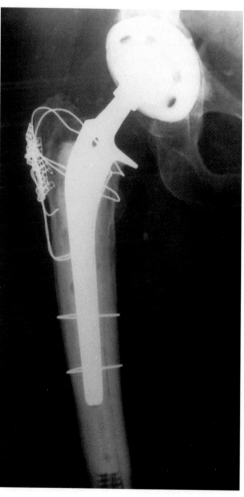

B

C

FIG. 25. When the greater trochanter impedes implant removal or when excess preoperative offset is encountered, trochanteric osteotomy and transferring the greater trochanter distally will provide access to the upper femur and maintain the soft-tissue tension. **A:** Preoperative radiograph. **B:** Preoperative template. **C:** Postoperative radiograph.

formed by raising and lowering the template within the intramedullary canal until one of the centers of rotation of the femoral heads superimposes on the center of the acetabular cup. Once the placement height of the component has been determined, the position of the component relative to a bony landmark, such as the lesser trochanter, is measured. The component templates are then transferred to the operative side while maintaining their relative positions. Occasionally, the anatomic offset is noted to be greater than the prosthetic offset. This is best corrected using a prosthesis capable of greater offset. Other options include using a longer prosthetic neck and transferring the greater trochanter distally to maintain soft-tissue tension (Fig. 25).

The final aspect of templating is performed on the lateral hip roentgenogram. Initially, the amount of anterior bow and presence of deficiencies in the femur should be determined. Deficiencies in the distal femur, distal to the implant, also must be recognized as they can contribute to postoperative morbidity. Next, the stem length and diameter selected on the AP roentgenogram are confirmed to be appropriate for the intraosseous shape. When utilizing a noncemented prosthesis such as the AML or MultiLock femoral implants, precise endosteal apposition is much more important than when using cemented implants. If the AP diameter of the intramedullary canal (noted on the lateral radiograph) is found to be greater than the mediolateral diameter, selection of a larger implant should be considered if the femoral cortex is dense enough to permit intramedullary reaming. Lateral templating also can avoid intraoperative perforation of the femoral cortex by the anterior bow (19).

SUMMARY

Preoperative planning should be the first step performed when preparing a patient for revision surgery of the hip. This process consists of a complete history and physical examination, proper radiographs, classification of bone deficiencies, and the selection of the proper prosthesis based on preoperative templating. The history and physical should focus on the patient's need for revision surgery, the location and source of pain, risk factors for infection, the neuromuscular and vascular status of the involved extremity, and identification of any leg-length discrepancy. The standard radiographs are an AP view of the pelvis and both AP and lateral views of the involved extremity. Arteriography, computed tomography, Judet views, and other advanced radiographic studies are indicated for more complicated cases. These modalities enable the assessment of component loosening and failure, the detection of osteolysis, and the classification of bony deficiencies—information important for selecting the appropriate prosthesis and fixation method during templating. When performed properly, this process pro-

vides the surgeon with a schematic of the revision before entering the operating room. Special requirements, such as the use of allograft or modified implant systems, can be identified. The operating room can be notified in advance, ensuring that the necessary equipment will be available for surgery. Moreover, potential problems can be anticipated, so that alternative plans can be formulated and intraoperative complications avoided. Ultimately, thorough preoperative planning reduces operating room time and promotes the best possible result.

REFERENCES

1. Amstutz HC, Campbell P, Kossovsky N, Clarke IC. Mechanism and clinical significance of wear debris-induced osteolysis. *Clin Orthop* 1992;276:7–18.
2. Ballinger PW. *Merrill's atlas of radiographic positions and radiologic procedures*, 6th ed. St. Louis: CV Mosby, 1986.
3. Bell KS, Schatzker J, Fornasier VL, Goodman SB. A study of implant failure in the Wagner resurfacing arthroplasty. *J Bone Joint Surg* 1985;67A:1165.
4. Berger R, Fletcher F, Donaldson TK, Wasilewski RL, Peterson M, Rubash HE. A dynamic test to diagnose loose uncemented femoral total hip components. *Clin Orthop* 1996;330:115–123.
5. Berman AT, Avolio Jr A, DelGallo W. Acetabular Osteolysis in total hip arthroplasty: prevention and treatment. *Orthopedics* 1994;17:963–965.
6. Berry DJ, Muller ME. Revision arthroplasty using an anti-protrusio cage for massive acetabular bone deficiency. *J Bone Joint Surg Br* 1992;74B:711–715.
7. Capello WN. Preoperative planning of total hip arthroplasty. *Instr Course Lect* 1986;35:249–257.
8. D'Antonio JA, Capello WN, Borden LS, Bargar WL, Bierbaum BF, Boettcher WG, Steinberg ME, Stulberg SD, Wedge JH. Classification and management of acetabular abnormalities in total hip arthroplasty. *Clin Orthop* 1989;243:126–137.
9. D'Antonio JA, McCarthy JC, Bargar WL, et al. Classification of femoral abnormalities in total hip arthroplasty. *Clin Orthop* 1993;296:133–139.
10. D'Antonio JA. Periprosthetic bone loss of the acetabulum. Classification and management. *Orthop Clin North Am* 1992;23(2):279–290.
11. DeOrio JK, Blasser KE. Indications and patient selection. In: Morrey BF, ed. *Joint Replacement Arthroplasty*. New York: Churchill Livingstone, 1991;547–559.
12. Doehring TC, Rubash HE, Shelley FJ, Schwendeman LJ, Donaldson TK, Navalgund YA. Effect of superior and superiolateral relocation of the hip center on hip joint forces: an experimental and analytical analysis. *Journal of Arthroplasty* 1996;11(6):693–703.
13. Edwards BN, Tullos HS, Noble PC. Contributory factors and etiology of sciatic nerve palsy in total hip arthroplasty. *Clin Orthop* 1987;218:136.
14. Engh CA, Bobyn JD. The influence of stem size and extent of porous coating on femoral bone resorption after primary cementless hip arthroplasty. *Clin Orthop* 1988;231:7.
15. Engh CA, Engh CA Jr, Cadambi A, Lauro G, Piston RW. Cementless revision of failed total hip arthroplasty: preoperative planning, surgical technique, and postoperative rehabilitation. *Techniques Orthop* 1993;7(4):9–26.
16. Engh CA, Massin P, Suthers KE. Roentgenographic assessment of the biologic fixation of porous-surfaced femoral components. *Clin Orthop* 1990;257:107.
17. Engh CA. Recent advances in cementless total hip arthroplasty using the AML prosthesis. *Techniques Orthop* 1991;6(3):59–72.
18. Evans BG, Cuckler JM. Evaluation of the painful total hip arthroplasty. *Orthop Clin North Am* 1992;23:303–311.
19. Fitzgerald RH Jr, Brindley GW, Kavanagh BF. The uncemented total hip arthroplasty: intraoperative femoral fractures. *Clin Orthop* 1988;235:61–66.
20. Fitzgerald RH Jr, Nolan DR, Ilstrup DM, Van Scoy RE, Washington JA II, Coventry MB. Deep wound sepsis following total hip arthroplasty. *J Bone Joint Surg* 1977;59A:847–855.

21. Fogelberg EV, Zitzmann EK, Stinchfield FE. Prophylactic penicillin in orthopaedic surgery. *J Bone Joint Surg* 1970;52A:95–98.

22. Gie GA, Linder L, Ling RSM, Simon JP, Slooff TJJH, Timperley AJ. Impacted cancellous allografts and cement for revision total hip arthroplasty. *J Bone Joint Surg Br* 1993;75B:14–21.

23. Gruen TA, McNeice GM, Amstutz HC. "Modes of failure" of cemented stem-type femoral components. A radiologic analysis of loosening. *Clin Orthop* 1979;141:17.

24. Harris WH, Barrack RL. Contemporary algorithms for evaluation of the painful total hip replacement. *Orthop Rev* 1993;22(5):531–539.

25. Harris WH, Barrack RL. Development in diagnosis of the painful total hip replacement: *Orthop Rev* 1993;22(4):439–447.

26. Harris WH. Management of the deficient acetabulum using cementless fixation without bone grafting. *Orthop Clin North Am* 1993;24:663–665.

27. Harris WH, McCarthy Jr JC, O'Neill DA. Femoral component loosening using contemporary techniques of femoral cement fixation. *J Bone Joint Surg* 1982;64A:1063–1067.

28. Harris WH, McGann WA. Loosening of the femoral component after the use of the medullary-plug cementing technique: follow-up note with a minimum five-year follow-up. *J Bone Joint Surg* 1986;68A:1064.

29. Heekin RD, Callaghan JJ, Hopkinson WJ, et al. The porous coated anatomic total hip prosthesis, inserted without cement. *J Bone Joint Surg* 1993;75A:77–91.

30. Hodgkinson JP, Shelley P, Wroblewski BM. The correlation between the roentgenographic appearance and operative findings at the bone-cement junction of the socket in the Charnley low friction arthroplasties. *Clin Orthop* 1988;228:105–109.

31. Hoppenfeld S. *Physical examination of the spine and extremities.* East Norwalk, CT: Appleton and Lange, 1976;133–167.

32. Huddleston HD. Femoral lysis after cemented hip arthroplasty. *J Arthroplasty* 1988;3:285–297.

33. Johanson NA, Pellicci PM, Tsairis P, et al. Nerve injury in total hip arthroplasty. *Clin Orthop* 1983;179:214.

34. Jones LC, Hungerford DS. Cement disease. *Clin Orthop* 1987;225;192–206.

35. Kennedy WF, Byrne TF, Majid HA, Pavlak LL. Sciatic nerve monitoring during revision total hip arthoplasty. *Clin Orthop* 1991;264:223–7.

36. Kim KJ, Rubash HE, Wilson SC, D'Antonio JA, McClain EJ. A histologic and biochemical comparison of the interface tissues in cementless and cemented hip prostheses. *Clin Orthop* 1993;287:142–152.

37. Knight JL, Atwater RD. Preoperative planning for total hip arthroplasty: quantitating its utility and precision. *J Arthroplasty* 1992;7(suppl):403–409.

38. Maloney WJ, Lane Smith R, Castro F, Schurman DJ. Fibroblast response to metallic debris in vitro: enzyme induction, cell proliferation, and toxicity. *J Bone Joint Surg* 1993;75A:835–844.

39. McCollum DE, Nunley JA, Harrelson JM. Bone-grafting in total hip replacement for acetabular protrusion. *J Bone Joint Surg* 1980;62A:1065–1073.

40. Miller WE, Counts GW. Orthopaedic infections: a prospective study of 378 clean procedures. *South Med J* 1975;68:386–391.

41. Moreland JR, Gruen TA, Mai L, Amstutz HC. Aseptic loosening of total hip replacement: incidence and significance. In: Reily LH Jr, ed. *The hip: proceedings of the 8th open scientific meeting of the Hip Society,* St. Louis: CV Mosby, 1980;281.

42. Petrera P, Trakru S, Mehta S, Steed D, Towers J, Rubash H. Revision total hip arthroplasty with a retroperitoneal approach to the iliac vessels. *J Arthroplasty* 1996;11(6):704–708.

43. Rock MG. Allograft. In: Morrey BF, ed. *Joint replacement arthroplasty,* New York: Churchill Livingstone, 1991;810–819.

44. Russotti GM, Harris WH. Proximal placement of the acetabular component in total hip arthroplasty. *J Bone Joint Surg* 1991;73A:587–592.

45. Schmalzried TP, Guttmann D, Grecula M, Amstutz HC. The relationship between the design, position, and articular wear of acetabular components inserted without cement and the development of pelvic osteolysis. *J Bone Joint Surg* 1994;76A:677–688.

46. Schmalzried TP, Harris WH. The Harris-Galante porous-coated acetabular component with screw fixation: radiographic analysis of eighty-three primary hip replacements at a minimum of five years. *J Bone Joint Surg* 1992;74A:1130–1139.

47. Schmalzried TP, Jasty M, Harris WH. Periprosthetic bone loss in total hip arthroplasty. Polyethylene wear debris and the concept of the effective joint space. *J Bone Joint Surg* 1992;74A:849–863.

48. Schmalzried TP, Kwong LM, Jasty M, Sedlacek RC, Haire TC, O'Connor DO, Bragdon CR, Kabo JM, Malcolm AJ, Harris WH. The mechanism of loosening of cemented acetabular components in total hip arthroplasty. Analysis of specimens retrieved at autopsy. *Clin Orthop* 1992;274:60–78.

49. Stevens DB. Postoperative orthopaedic infections. A study of etiological mechanisms. *J Bone Joint Surg* 1964;46A:96–102.

50. Sutherland CJ, Wilde AH, Borden LS, Marks KE. A ten-year follow-up of one hundred consecutive Muller curved-stem total hip-replacement arthroplasties. *J Bone Joint Surg* 1982;64A:970.

51. Tanzer M, Maloney WJ, Jasty M, et al. The progression of femoral cortical osteolysis in association with total hip arthroplasty without cement. *J Bone Joint Surg* 1992;74A:404–410.

52. Tehranzadeh J, Schneider R, Freiberger RH. Radiological evaluation of painful total hip replacement. *Radiology* 1981;141:355.

53. Wasielewski RC, Crossett LS, Rubash HE. Neural and vascular injury in total hip arthroplasty. *Orthop Clin North Am* 1992;23:219–235.

54. Weber ER, Daube JR, Coventry MB. Peripheral neuropathies associated with total hip arthroplasty. *J Bone Joint Surg* 1976;58A:66.

55. Willert HG, Bertram H, Buchhorn GH. Osteolysis in alloarthroplasty of the hip. *Clin Orthop* 1990;258:108–121.

56. Wroblewski BM, Siney PD. Charnley low-friction arthroplasty in the young patient. *Clin Orthop* 1992;285:45–47.

57. Zicat B, Engh CA, Gokcen E. Patterns of osteolysis around total hip components inserted with and without cement. *J Bone Joint Surg* 1995;77A:432–439.

The Adult Hip, edited by J. J. Callaghan,
A. G. Rosenberg, and H. E. Rubash.
Lippincott–Raven Publishers, Philadelphia © 1998.

CHAPTER 85

Evaluation of the Painful Total Hip Arthroplasty

Richard E. White, Jr.

Pain is a very common complaint in patients with a total hip arthroplasty (THA). Kavanagh reported pain in 25% of patients at 1 year and 20% of patients at 5, 10, and 15 years after cemented total hip replacement (26). Patients with cementless total hip replacements also have a significant percentage of pain if carefully questioned (16). Although the pain is not always severe, it can be disabling in many patients to the extent that careful evaluation is required.

INTRINSIC AND EXTRINSIC CAUSES

A painful THA has a differential diagnosis that includes causes that are intrinsic and extrinsic to the arthroplasty. The intrinsic causes that are most commonly considered are mechanical loosening and sepsis. Other intrinsic causes of pain include prosthetic failure, subluxation or impingement, occult fracture, and cementless femoral component thigh pain without loosening. When a patient presents with THA pain, the surgeon must also consider causes that are extrinsic to the arthroplasty. These causes may be periarticular problems or extrinsic to the hip area itself. Because the pain may be multifactorial, these extrinsic causes must be ruled out even if there is an obvious diagnosis of loosening or sepsis. These extrinsic causes include lumbar spine disease such as spinal stenosis (5) or disc disease (29), trochanteric

bursitis, trochanteric nonunion (36), claudication, abdominal aortic aneurysm, sciatic (24) or obturator nerve (40) impingement, abductor or iliopsoas tendinitis, stress fractures of the pubic ramus (34), and heterotopic bone, especially that in the process of maturation (32). In addition to the history and physical examination, a thorough evaluation of the painful THA may include laboratory tests, plain radiographs, aspiration, arthrography, and nuclear medicine evaluations. A careful history and physical examination often contribute the most important information to the diagnosis of the pain, being especially critical in ruling out extrinsic causes of the pain.

HISTORY

The history gives valuable clues to the source of pain in a THA. The location, time of onset, severity, and character of the pain all contribute to the investigation. Groin pain or deep buttock pain is associated with acetabular or capsular sources of pain. But groin pain can also be caused by iliopsoas tendinitis or proximal femoral problems. Buttock pain can also be caused by arthritic changes of the lumbar spine or sacroiliac joint. Femoral-component problems usually present with anterior proximal thigh pain. Posterior buttock and thigh pain, especially when associated with calf pain, is usually related to lumbar spine disease. Pain over the greater trochanter implicates trochanteric bursitis, trochanteric nonunion, or painful trochanteric hardware.

Temporal relationships may aid in the difficult diagnosis. If there has been a pain-free period after the THA, the

R. E. White, Jr.: Department of Orthopaedic Surgery and Rehabilitation, University of New Mexico School of Medicine, Albuquerque, New Mexico 87131.

late onset of pain suggests loosening or sepsis (27). Failure to achieve resolution of the preoperative symptoms after surgery suggests that an extrinsic cause was the cause of the pain. The most common example is a patient with obvious mechanical loosening. The mechanical loosening may cause few symptoms, because the majority of the hip pain is caused by lumbar spine disease. After revision of the loose component, the patient still experiences the majority of the preoperative pain.

If pain increases in severity with increased walking or standing and is relieved by rest, it is usually associated with loosening, but loosening is rarely associated with rest pain alone. Night pain, rest pain, or constant pain can be associated with sepsis (11,13). Knowledge of the postoperative clinical course may assist in making the diagnosis. Delayed wound healing, prolonged febrile course, and constant pain after surgery are raise suspicion for sepsis.

Start-up pain, produced when starting to walk after having been seated or resting, has been linked to loosening or significant micromotion in cementless THA, but it can also be caused by iliopsoas tendinitis or quadriceps weakness (if the pain is anterior) or lumbar spine disease (if the pain is posterior).

The severity and character of the pain may contribute to determination of the diagnosis. Pain secondary to loosening may be severe but is always improved by rest. It rarely has a constant nature. Constant pain points to sepsis or a neurologic cause. The lumbar spine should be investigated if the pain has neurologic features such as radiation below the knee, numbness, paresthesias, or dysesthesias. Lumbar spine diseases to be considered include spinal stenosis, mechanical low back pain, radiculopathy, and neuropathy. Spinal stenosis may become symptomatic after total hip replacement: the symptoms may not have been evident before the surgery because walking was so limited (5). The contribution of the lumbar spine to the pain syndrome is the most difficult to quantify and the most easily missed diagnosis.

PHYSICAL EXAMINATION

A thorough physical examination of the hip frequently reveals abnormalities and reproduces the patient's pain. The gait should be carefully evaluated. Limp and abductor weakness are common with the intrinsic causes of pain. The presence of a normal gait and a negative Trendelenburg test suggest that the source of pain is other than the THA. Neurologic abnormalities and leg-length discrepancies cause or contribute to a gait abnormality. A leg-length discrepancy may be a true discrepancy or an apparent discrepancy related to abduction or adduction contracture, or to scoliosis of the lumbar spine.

Range of motion of the hip can be revealing. Pain throughout a passive range of motion suggests sepsis. Pain at extremes of motion suggests loosening. Pain in certain reproducible positions suggests instability or impingement. The patient cannot always perceive subluxation itself but will guard against motions that cause pain from impingement against inflamed capsule or soft-tissue structures. Trochanteric bursitis and tendinitis can often be diagnosed by direct palpation and resistive muscle testing. Careful muscle testing can clearly diagnose abductor or iliopsoas tendinitis. Firm compression or palpation of the pelvis, especially the pubic ramus, can detect sacroiliac disease or raise the possibility of pubic ramus stress fracture.

The physical examination should evaluate two important extrinsic causes of pain—the lumbar spine and the vascularity of the lower extremity. Neurologic sources of pain include the femoral, sciatic (24), and obturator nerves (40). Evaluation of peripheral pulses and skin temperature can usually adequately evaluate vascularity; imaging studies can give additional objective information in equivocal cases.

LOOSENING AND SEPSIS

Periarticular and extrinsic causes of the painful THA are best eliminated by the history and physical examination. After these causes are excluded, loosening and sepsis must be evaluated. The diagnosis of loosening or sepsis is often obvious. It is important to preoperatively predict the fixation status of both components, especially if only one is obviously loose. This may dramatically change the preoperative planning and the revision prosthesis requirements. In painful cases where sepsis is not clinically obvious, controversy exists concerning the necessity for preoperative aspiration and the value of laboratory tests to rule out sepsis. Revision total hip replacement in the face of undiagnosed, occult sepsis has a potentially disastrous result.

The diagnostic tools for evaluation of mechanical loosening include plain radiographs, arthrography, and nuclear medicine studies. The diagnostic tools available to evaluate the presence or absence of sepsis include laboratory tests, aspiration and nuclear medicine studies.

The widespread use of cementless THA has added additional complexity to evaluation of mechanical loosening. Although there are some similarities, the diagnostic criteria for loosening of cemented and cementless THAs have important differences that justify a separate discussion of each type of evaluation.

Loosening

Plain Radiographs—Cemented

In evaluation of a painful cemented THA, critical examination of serial plain radiographs is the most accurate method of predicting the status of implant fixation.

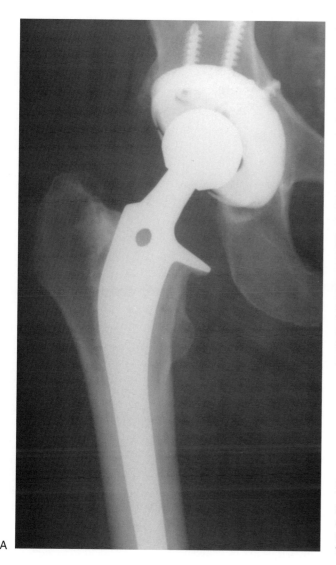

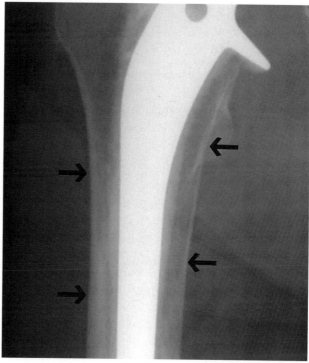

FIG. 1. A: Postoperative radiograph of right hybrid THA in 71-year-old woman with osteoarthritis. **B:** The 7-year follow-up radiograph reveals significant intense bone remodeling of femoral cortex in zones 1, 2, 6, and 7. This may be misinterpreted as a radiolucency at the bone–cement interface.

The reliability of plain radiographs and other diagnostic tools is difficult to determine because standard criteria for loosening have not been accepted by all investigators (14,15,28,35). The most widely accepted criteria have been proposed by O'Neill and Harris (35). This classification includes definite, probable, and possible loosening. Definite component loosening is determined by migration, cement fracture, or component fracture.

Two other commonly accepted criteria are the prosthesis–cement radiolucent line, if not present on the immediate postoperative radiographs, and a continuous cement–bone radiolucent line with some aspects of the radiolucent line greater than 2 mm. Recent studies question the accuracy of the last two criteria. Callaghan et al. (7) reported that the development of a prosthesis–cement radiolucency may be nonprogressive and not necessarily an indication of impending failure. This finding may be prosthesis or design specific. Radiolucent lines at the bone–cement interface around cemented total hip replacements may actually represent internal bone

remodeling and not necessarily any weakness of the bone–cement interface (21,22) (Fig. 1). Therefore, it seems most logical to report a component as either loose or not loose. The diagnosis of loosening on plain radiographs should be based on (a) migration or subsidence and (b) cement or component fracture.

Our evaluation of 65 failed cemented total hip replacements found plain radiographs to be the most accurate tool for the evaluation of loosening for both the femoral and acetabular component (25). The sensitivity was high, at 91% for the femoral component and 92% for the acetabular component. Specificity was even higher, at 93% and 94%, respectively, for the two components. The positive predictive values were 86% and 90% for the femoral and acetabular components. False positives could cause the surgeon to perform unnecessary surgery. There were only two false positives of the femoral component and one false positive for the acetabular component.

Most authors report that plain radiographs are more accurate for the femoral component than for the acetabular component (18,28,35). The accuracy of evaluation of acetabular fixation can be improved by using obturator and iliac oblique views in questionable cases. Our investigation contradicts these reports as the accuracy of plain radiographs was equal for both components.

Hodgkinson et al. made an important contribution to understanding the plain radiographic evaluation of the cemented acetabular component (19). In 200 cemented Charnley acetabular components, they reported that surgically identifiable loosening was found in 94% of components that had a complete radiolucent line regardless of width. If the radiolucent line involved two thirds of the interface, 74% of the components were loose. Therefore, the extent of the radiolucency around the acetabular bone–cement interface does in fact have a predictive value for loosening.

Plain Radiographs—Cementless

Evaluation of fixation of cementless components by plain radiographs involves different criteria. Migration or subsidence is the only reliable criterion for loosening of either component. The classification of Engh et al. for femoral component stability has been widely accepted (9). Major signs of osseointegration are absence of reactive, radiodense lines around the porous portion of the implant and endosteal spot welds. Minor signs include calcar atrophy, stable distal stem, and the absence of a pedestal (Fig. 2). Unfortunately, these signs are prosthesis dependent. Proximally porous-coated stems have a different picture of osseointegration than extensively coated stems.

Radiodense, reactive lines are common around the smooth distal portion of the stem in proximally porous-coated implants (41). The stem has bone ingrowth stability proximally, but the more flexible femur will flex over the more stiff distal stem. The radiodense, reactive lines are more common the more distant from the point of proximal fixation. Extensively coated stems have a more distal point of fixation and, therefore, will have fewer radiodense reactive lines than in a proximally porous-coated implant (9). Radiodense lines around a porous implant and radiolucent lines around a cemented implant have different causes and significances.

The two reliable criteria for loosening of a cementless femoral component are migration and a radiodense, reactive line around the entire porous-coated portion of the implant (Fig. 3). Less reliable criteria are usually prosthesis dependent. Migration is the only accurate criterion for loosening of the cementless acetabular component. The determination of migration is critical to make the diagnosis of loosening in both cemented and cementless femoral and acetabular components. This requires meticulous comparison of sequential radiographs. Standardization of radiographic views makes this determination more

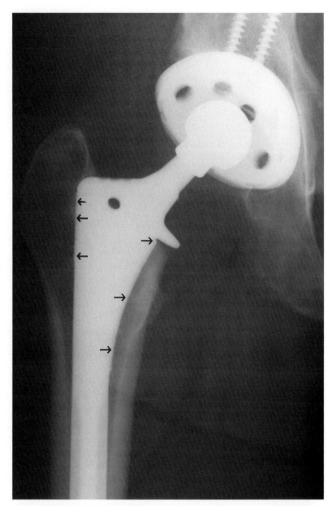

FIG. 2. The 5-year follow-up radiograph of a cementless femoral component in a 64-year-old man with osteoarthritis reveals signs of osseointegration, including endosteal spot welds, condensation of cancellous bone in the proximal medial metaphysis and femoral neck, calcar rounding or atrophy, and the absence of a pedestal.

accurate. The use of reproducible anatomic or prosthetic landmarks is also helpful. The careful radiographic evaluation can usually determine the fixation status of each component.

Arthrography

Contrast and radionuclide arthrography have been supported as an adjunct to the evaluation of loosening in the painful THA. Determination of the accuracy of this diagnostic tool has been clouded by two problems. First, the lack of standardization of diagnostic criteria makes it very difficult to compare studies. Second, arthrography is very technique dependent. Because many techniques have been suggested to improve the accuracy of this test, the variability of the performance of the arthrography

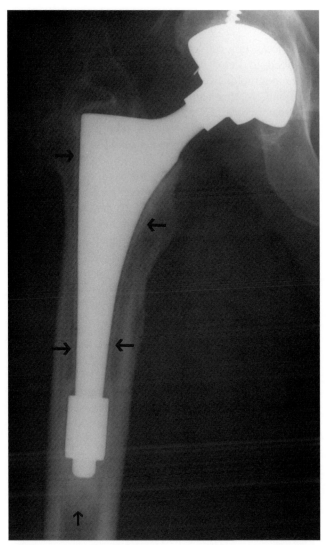

FIG. 3. The 5-year follow-up radiograph of a cementless femoral component in a 55-year-old man with osteoarthritis. The complete radiodense, reactive line is indicative of a loose femoral component. The large distal pedestal confirms stress transfer at the tip of the prosthesis and suggests inadequate proximal fixation of the femoral stem.

questions its accuracy. If contrast arthrography is to be of value, meticulous technique should include high injection pressure, postambulation films, and subtraction techniques (3,35,38).

Cemented

The sensitivity and specificity of contrast arthrography have been reported to be from 60% to 100% for both the femoral and the acetabular components in the evaluation of the painful cemented THA (10). Most reports have found contrast arthrography to be more valuable for the acetabular component than the femoral component (14,18,35).

Our study revealed contrast arthrography to be less accurate than plain radiographs for both femoral and acetabular components (25). The sensitivities were 66% and 87%, and the specificities were 93% and 73% for the femoral and acetabular components, respectively. Positive predictive values were 62% and 80% for the two components. We no longer use contrast arthrography in the evaluation of the painful cemented total hip replacement. The unpredictable accuracy cannot justify the additional cost or potential patient discomfort.

Cementless

Contrast arthrography has not been frequently studied in the evaluation of the painful cementless THA. The concept of the effective joint space in cementless THA explains the access routes of joint fluid to aspects of the prosthesis–bone interface even in components that are bone ingrown and well fixed (30). This explains the reports of significant numbers of false positive arthrograms (2). There are not yet substantial data to support the routine use of contrast arthrography in evaluation of the painful cementless THA.

Radionuclide Arthrography

This technique uses a medium that is less viscous and has a longer half-life than contrast dye. As a result, more uniform penetration may be achieved. In contrast arthrography, it is sometimes difficult to distinguish a thin line of contrast from either cement or a reactive radiodense line. This difficulty does not exist in radionuclide arthrography. Welman et al. (43) and Maxon et al. (31) have reported improved accuracy but only on the femoral component. More investigation is necessary to define the accuracy of radionuclide arthrography.

Nuclear Medicine Images—Cemented

Technetium-99m methylene diphosphonate (MDP) bone images are frequently suggested to assess the fixation of cemented components. MDP bone images are very sensitive indicators of bone turnover and activity, but they are not very specific. Increased radionuclide uptake can be caused by infection, loosening, heterotopic ossification, stress fracture, Paget's disease, tumor, or reflex sympathetic dystrophy (20).

Our evaluation of loosening in painful cemented THA revealed that MDP bone images have the highest sensitivity, at 97% and 98%, for the femoral and acetabular components, respectively. However, the specificities were low, at 67% and 79%, for the two components. This inaccuracy was manifest by the frequent presence of false-positive bone images (25).

The MDP bone images are of greatest value in cases where loosening is uncertain from the plain radiographs. A negative or normal MDP bone image strongly supports the diagnosis of no loosening. Observation should be recommended in these cases (42). The diagnosis of loosening should not be based solely on the presence of a positive MDP bone image (23). If the plain radiographs do not reveal loosening, the MDP bone image should be considered a false positive.

Nuclear Medicine Images—Cementless

The interpretation of MDP bone images after cementless THA is very different from that of cemented THA. Bone remodeling occurs after cementless THA, but its characteristics are dependent on bone quality and prosthetic design. The sensitivity of MDP bone images makes this diagnostic tool seem attractive in evaluation of the cementless THA.

Forty primary cementless total hip arthroplasties and 16 revision cementless THAs were evaluated at routine follow-up examinations through 5 years by MDP bone images. The grading system for the MDP bone images was as follows: 0, less than normal uptake; I, normal uptake; II, slight or moderate increased uptake; and III, intense increased uptake. The natural history of the MDP bone images after cementless THA followed a very consistent chronologic evolution of the radionuclide uptake. Between 2 and 6 weeks postoperatively, there was uniform increased tracer activity of either grade II or intense grade III activity around both components. This increased radionuclide uptake began to decrease towards normal, or to a stable state, between 6 and 12 months after surgery. Further resolution of increased tracer activity continued from 12 to 24 months after surgery. At 2 years, 66% of acetabular components but only 21% of femoral components had returned to a normal bone image (44).

Thigh pain is a common complaint after cementless THA. If the thigh pain is of prosthetic origin, two characteristic bone image sequences were noted that are different from the normal chronologic evolution of radionuclide uptake. Increased radionuclide uptake after initial resolution suggested prosthetic origin of the thigh pain. An intense grade III activity that never resolved also suggested a prosthetic cause of the thigh pain. An MDP bone image that followed the anticipated normal chronologic sequence suggested nonprosthetic causes of thigh pain (44).

A single MDP bone image may not be helpful in the diagnosis of loosening of cementless THA unless it is negative or normal and associated with normal plain radiographs. An abnormal MDP bone image associated with normal radiographs should not encourage operative intervention. This initial MDP bone image can be used as a baseline to compare further studies if symptoms persist and the cause is not determined.

Dynamic Computed Tomographic Scan

A new, innovative technique has recently been described to help in the diagnosis of loosening in a roentgenographically stable uncemented femoral stem with pain. In this technique, a computed tomographic (CT) scan is obtained in the proximal and distal femur of the affected hip. Posterior femoral condyles are used as a reference point, and the affected extremity is internally and externally rotated and held in position as a CT scan is made at the level of the component collar. Two lines are drawn on the CT image, one between the posterior aspects of the condyles and the second drawn parallel through the center of the femoral component. The angle between these two lines is measured, and if the change in angle between the two positions of internal and external rotation is greater than 2°, the result has been shown to strongly correlate with intraoperative stem loosening (37).

Evaluation of Sepsis

Plain Radiographs

Plain radiographs often do not reveal signs of sepsis. They may be indistinguishable from those showing a loose THA, because many septic THAs develop loosening. Several radiographic findings are highly suggestive of infection (1,28). Periostitis or periosteal new bone formation, endosteal scalloping, and extensive generalized lysis and osteopenia suggest sepsis. Within the first year, rapid development of a continuous wide radiolucency greater than 2 mm is highly suggestive of sepsis (4).

Laboratory Tests

White blood cell count (WBC), erythrocyte sedimentation rate (ESR), and C-reactive protein (CRP) are available to assist in the identification of the septic THA. As an isolated test, the WBC is felt to be of little value (6,8). It is frequently normal in septic cases and abnormal in aseptic cases, as there are many conditions that affect its value.

The ESR may be of value not as an isolated test but as support for the diagnosis of sepsis. It may be beneficial in patients without a known reason for ESR elevation (8). The ESR can be elevated for 6 months after THA. It has been found to have a sensitivity of 73% to 100%, a specificity of 69% to 94%, and an accuracy of 73% to 88% (10).

C-reactive protein has gained support as a tool to assist in the diagnosis of the septic arthroplasty. Sanzer and Carlsson studied patients with asymptomatic THA, loose aseptic THA, and septic THA (39). Their results showed CRP to be similar to ESR in sensitivity and specificity when considered as an isolated test. The combination, however, of both ESR and CRP increases the accuracy of the preoperative evaluation of sepsis. This concept was also supported by Garvin, who reported that the combination of ESR and CRP yielded 100% sensitivity and 100% specificity in the preoperative detection of a septic THA (12). When CRP was used as an isolated test, the sensitivity was 100% but the specificity was only 79%. Additional studies will more accurately determine the role of CRP.

Aspiration

Preoperative aspiration of the painful THA is recommended by most authors (10). The aspiration can rule out sepsis as the source of pain in the initial evaluation or in most patients with obvious mechanical loosening that requires revision. Discovery of a previously undiagnosed infection in the postoperative period is usually a catastrophe. Removing a recently implanted prosthesis, especially cemented, can be a difficult procedure with a high rate of complication. If the infection can be diagnosed preoperatively, the surgical plan changes dramatically and an organism can be identified preoperatively.

Therefore, it seems routine aspirations should be advocated. Unfortunately, the reliability of aspiration is not reproducibly good (1,10,16,28,30,33,35). The sensitivity has been reported to be from 40% to 91%, and the specificity varies from 60% to 100%. False-negative and false-positive results are common. If the aspiration is performed by the radiologist, the surgeon does not know the sterility and technique of the procedure. Aspiration should always be performed by the surgeon. The surgeon then knows whether the aspiration was adequate, a dry tap, a traumatic or bloody tap, or whether saline was injected and then aspirated. It is also controversial whether "light growth" or "liquid media growth only" should be interpreted as pathologic or as a contaminant. Although the concept of aspiration is ideal, these factors give an unpredictable accuracy. Therefore, Barrack (1) does not recommend routine aspiration in the evaluation of the failed THA.

After 12 years of obtaining routine preoperative aspirations, I now use aspiration in selected cases. In a significant number of cases, diagnosis of sepsis is obvious, because there is a draining sinus or dramatic radiographic finding of longstanding sepsis. In other cases, history and physical examination, or plain radiographic findings such as periostitis or endosteal scalloping suggest sepsis. In these cases, ESR, CRP, and aspiration are performed. In patients requiring revision for mechanical loosening, aspiration is not performed unless there is clinical evidence to suspect sepsis.

Aspiration is also performed in cases where significant pain is present but an obvious diagnosis cannot be found. History and physical examination are not diagnostic. Plain radiographs do not reveal loosening or sepsis. MDP bone image is negative. ESR and CRP are normal.

Extrinsic causes of pain have been eliminated. Aspiration is therefore used to exhaust all diagnostic options in these problem cases.

Nuclear Medicine Imaging

Numerous studies have documented the sensitivity and specificity of both gallium-67 citrate images and indium-111-labeled leukocyte images (10,17). Unfortunately, the results have been quite variable. The sensitivity of both types of images has been reported as low as 50% and the specificity as low as 45%. This lack of predictability and the cost do not appear to justify their routine use. They may be used in difficult diagnostic problems. We do not routinely use gallium and indium scans in the evaluation of the painful THA.

CONCLUSION

A logical and careful evaluation of the painful THA can be performed at a reasonable cost and make the correct diagnosis to a high degree of accuracy (Fig. 4). The evaluation should depend on those examinations that have predictable accuracy: history, physical examination, and plain radiographs. Narrow indications should be followed for tests such as MDP bone images and aspirations, to minimize their inaccuracies but to take advantage of their contribution to the evaluation. Costly tests with unpredictable accuracy, such as arthrography and gallium and Indium nuclear images, are rarely necessary to make the diagnosis.

A complete history and physical examination can usually eliminate extrinsic causes of pain. In addition, plain radiographs are the most accurate diagnostic tool for mechanical loosening. A negative MDP bone image supports the diagnosis of no loosening in equivocal cases. Arthrography is very technique dependent and expensive, and it has variable results. For these reasons, arthrography is not routinely used in the evaluation of loosening of the painful THA.

The diagnosis of sepsis is often obvious. If not obvious, history and physical examination, plain radiographs, ESR, and CRP can define cases in which aspiration should be performed. Routine aspiration is technique dependent, adds expense, and has frequent false positives, false negatives, and contaminants. Gallium or indium images add expense, have variable results, and are rarely required to make the diagnosis of sepsis.

Surgical exploration should be performed only when there is clear evidence of loosening or sepsis. Exploratory procedures without documentation of loosening or sepsis are rarely productive. In aseptic cases with no evidence of loosening, observation is prudent and not harmful. Early or occult loosening or sepsis will eventually become clinically obvious.

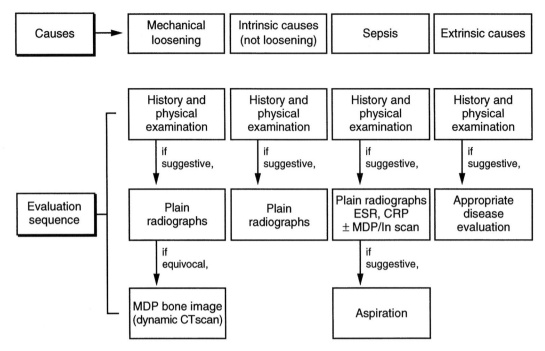

FIG. 4. Algorithm for evaluation of painful THA.

REFERENCES

1. Barrack RI, Harris WH. The value of aspiration of the hip joint before revision total hip arthroplasty. *J Bone Joint Surg* 1993;75A:66–76.
2. Barrack RI. *Presented at the annual meeting of the American Academy of Orthopaedic Surgeons*, February, 1992.
3. Bassett LW, Loftus AA, Mankovich NJ. Computer-processed subtraction arthrography. *Radiology* 1985;157:821.
4. Bergstrom B, Lindgren L, Lindberg L. Radiographic abnormalities caused by postoperative infection following total hip arthroplasty. *Clin Orthop* 1974;99:95–102.
5. Bohl WR, Steffee AD. Lumbar spinal stenosis: a cause of continued pain and disability in patients after total hip arthroplasty. *Spine* 1979;4:168–173.
6. Callaghan JJ, Salvati EA, Pellicci PM, et al. Results of revision for mechanical failure after cemented total hip replacement: 1979–1982. *J Bone Joint Surg* 1985;67A:1074.
7. Callaghan JJ, Mohler CG, Collis DK, Johnson RC. Early loosening of the femoral component at the cement-prosthesis interface after total hip replacement. *J Bone Joint Surg* 1995;77A:1315.
8. Cuckler JM, Star AM, Alivi A, et al. Diagnosis and management of the infected total joint arthroplasty. *Orthop Clin North Am* 1991;22:523.
9. Engh CA, Bobyn JD, Glassman AH. Porous-coated hip replacement: the factors governing bone ingrowth, stress shielding, and clinical results. *J Bone Joint Surg* 1987;69B:45–55.
10. Evans BG, Cuckler JM. Evaluation of the painful total hip arthroplasty. *Orthop Clin North Am* 1992;23:303.
11. Fitzgerald R. The infected total hip arthroplasty: current concepts of treatment. In: Welch RB, ed. *Proceedings of the twelfth open scientific meeting of the Hip Society.* St. Louis, MO: CV Mosby, 1984.
12. Garvin KL. *Presented at the annual meeting of the American Academy of Orthopaedic Surgeons*, February, 1996.
13. Gristina AG, Kolkin J. Current concepts review: total joint replacement and sepsis. *J Bone Joint Surg* 1983;65A:128–134.
14. Harris WH, McCarthy JC, O'Neill DA. Femoral component loosening using contemporary techniques of femoral cement fixation. *J Bone Joint Surg* 1982;64A:1063.
15. Harris WH, Peneberg BL. Further follow-up on socket fixation using a metal-backed acetabular component for total hip replacement. *J Bone Joint Surg* 1986;69A:1140.
16. Harris WH, Barrack RL. Developments in diagnosis of the painful total hip replacement. *Orthop Rev* 1993;April:439.
17. Harris WH, Barrack RL. Contemporary algorithms for evaluation of the painful total hip replacement. *Orthop Rev* 1993;May:531.
18. Hendrix RW, Wixson RL, Raina NA, et al. Arthrography after total hip arthroplasty: a modified technique used in the diagnosis of pain. *Radiology* 1983;148:647.
19. Hodgkinson JP, Shelley P, Wroblewski BM. The correlation between the roentgenographic appearance and operative findings at the bone-cement junction of the socket in Charnley low friction arthroplasties. *Clin Orthop* 1988;228:105.
20. Holder LE. Radionuclide bone imaging in the evaluation of bone pain. *J Bone Joint Surg* 1982;64A:1391–1396.
21. Jacobs ME, Koeweiden EM, Slooff TJ, et al. Plain radiographs inadequate for evaluation of the cement-bone interface in the hip prosthesis: a cadaver study of femoral stems. *Acta Orthop Scand* 1989;60:541–543.
22. Jasty M, Maloney WJ, Bragdon CR, et al. Histomorphological studies of the long-term skeletal responses to well fixed cemented femoral components. *J Bone Joint Surg* 1990;72A:1220–1225.
23. Jensen JS, Madsen JL. Tc-99m-MDP scintigraphy not informative in painful total hip arthroplasty. *J Arthroplasty* 1990;5(suppl):S11–S13.
24. Johanson NA, Pellicci PM, Tsairis P, et al. Nerve injury in total hip arthroplasty. *Clin Orthop* 1983;179:214.
25. Johnson RA. *Presented at the annual meeting of the American Academy of Orthopaedic Surgeons*, February, 1986.
26. Kavanagh BF, DeWitz MA, Ilstrup DM, et al. Fifteen year results of cemented Charnley total hip arthroplasty. *J Bone Joint Surg* 1989;71A:1496.
27. Kavanagh BF. Evaluation of the painful total hip arthroplasty. In: Morrey BE, ed. *Joint replacement arthroplasty.* Philadelphia: Churchill Livingstone, 1991;779–788.
28. Lyons CW, Berquist TH, Lyons JC, et al. Evaluation of radiographic findings in painful hip arthroplasties. *Clin Orthop* 1985;195:239.
29. Mallory TH, Halley D. Posterior buttock pain following total hip replacement: a case report. *Clin Orthop* 1973;90:104–106.
30. Maus TP, Berquist TH, Bender CE, Rand JA. Arthrographic study of painful total hip arthroplasty: refined criteria. *Radiology* 1987;162:721–727.
31. Maxon HR, Schneider HJ, Hopson CN, et al. A comparative study of indium-111 DTPA radionuclide and iothalamate meglumine roentgeno-

graphic arthrography in the evaluation of painful total hip arthroplasty. *Clin Orthop* 1989;245:156–159.

32. Morrey BF, Adams RA, Cabanela ME. Comparison of heterotopic bone after anterolateral, transtrochanteric, and posterior approaches for total hip arthroplasty. *Clin Orthop* 1984;188:160–167.

33. Mulcahy DM, Fenelon GC, McInerney DP. Aspiration arthrography of the hip joint: its uses and limitations in revision hip surgery. *J Arthroplasty* 1996;11:64–67.

34. Oh I, Hardacre JA. Fatigue fracture of the inferior pubic ramus following total hip replacement for congenital hip dislocation. *Clin Orthop* 1980;147:154–156.

35. O'Neill, DA, Harris WH. Failed total hip replacement: assessment by plain radiographs, arthrograms, and aspiration of the hip joint. *J Bone Joint Surg* 1984;66A:540–546.

36. Ritter MA, Gioe TJ, Stringer EA. Functional significance of nonunion of the greater trochanter. *Clin Orthop* 1981;159:177–182.

37. Rubash, Donaldson, Wasielewski, et al. 1997; accepted.

38. Salvati EA, Ghelman B, McLaren T, Wilson PDJ. Subtraction technique in arthrography for loosening of total hip replacement fixed with radiopaque cement. *Clin Orthop* 1974;101:105–109.

39. Sanzen L, Carlsson AS. The diagnostic value of C-reactive protein in infected total hip arthroplasties. *J Bone Joint Surg* 1989;71B: 638.

40. Siliski JM, Scott RD. Obturator nerve palsy resulting from intrapelvic extrusion of cement during total hip replacement: report of four cases. *J Bone Joint Surg* 1985;67A:1225.

41. Teter K. *Presented at the annual meeting of the Western Orthopaedic Association*, October, 1991.

42. Weiss PE, Mall JC, Hoffer PB, et al. ^{99m}Tc-methylene diphosphonate bone imaging in the evaluation of total hip prostheses. *Radiology* 1979;133:727–729.

43. Wellman HN, Schauwecker DS, Capello WN. Evaluation of metallic osseous implants with nuclear medicine. *Semin Nucl Med* 1988;18: 126–136.

44. White RE. *Presented at the annual meeting of the American Academy of Orthopaedic Surgeons*, February, 1988.

The Adult Hip, edited by J. J. Callaghan,
A. G. Rosenberg, and H. E. Rubash.
Lippincott–Raven Publishers, Philadelphia © 1998.

CHAPTER 86

Removal of Components and Cement

William J. Hozack

Revision total hip arthroplasty as a procedure can be divided conveniently into three phases: exposure and closure, cement and component removal, and reconstruction with new components. Each phase is critically important and deserves equal focus and attention. The trick to total hip revision, therefore, is to minimize the time needed for each phase in case one particular phase creates a special challenge deserving of extra time and attention. The goal of this chapter is to provide a framework for the time-efficient yet atraumatic and high-quality removal of components and cement. In this chapter, a potpourri of tools and techniques will be discussed, and it is important for the revision total hip surgeon to be familiar with all of them. But it is equally important that each surgeon develop a degree of comfort with the tools and techniques that best suit the individual skills and aptitudes of that surgeon. Similar tools and similar techniques used by different surgeons do not necessarily work in a similarly efficient and effective fashion. Finally, nothing beats proper preparation and having the right tool for the job.

TOOLS OF THE TRADE

The following figures and descriptions represent most of the tools necessary for removal of components and cement. The specific application of each tool is described briefly in this section, but more detailed explanations are to be found in the sections dealing with acetabular component removal, femoral component removal, and cement removal.

Hand Tools

With a few additions, the hand tools on the Moreland cemented and cementless revision sets (DePuy, Warsaw, IN) suffice for most revision situations. However, alternative tools similarly designed can be used with equal efficacy.

  W. J. Hozack: Department of Orthopaedic Surgery, The Rothman Institute, Thomas Jefferson University Hospital, Philadelphia, Pennsylvania 19107.

Tool	Function	Figure
Curved acetabular osteotomes	Disrupt cement–prosthesis, cement–bone, and prosthesis–bone interface of acetabular component	1
Pointed osteotome	Fragments acetabular cement	2
Large cup grasper	Grabs acetabular component for removal	3
Polyethylene implant extractor	Attaches to cemented acetabular components to facilitate removal	4
Polyethylene insert extractor	Attaches to modular polyethylene inserts in cementless cups to facilitate removal	5
Cup lever	Levers cementless cup out of acetabular bed	6
Screw trephine	Removes broken acetabular screws	7
Universal femoral extractor (a)	Attaches to nonmodular femoral components	8
Universal femoral extractor (b)	Removes modular femoral components	9
Carbide punch	Femoral component removal, removal of fractured stems, perforates distal bony pedestal	10
Disimpactor	Femoral component removal if collared or nonmodular; used with mallet	11
Flexible osteotomes	Disrupt prosthesis–bone interface of cementless stems	12
Trephine reamers	Disrupt prosthesis–bone interface of cementless stems	13
Cement tap	Engages cement column for removal of cement with weak cement-bone interface	14
Pituitary rongeur	Grasps loose cement fragments, grasps distal plastic cement restrictor	15
Cement splitters (T, V)	Create longitudinal fissures in cement column	16
Curved cement osteotomes	Separate cement from bone at the cement-bone interface	17
Reverse hook curettes	Extracts distal cement plug, removes residual cement in canal, flattens distal bony pedestal	18
x osteotome	Perforates distal bony pedestal	19

Power Tools

Tool	Function	Figure
Drill bits, centering cone	Cannulate distal cement plug	—
High speed tools		
Carbide burr	Metal cutting bit	20
Pencil bit	Loosens cement–prosthesis interface and cement–bone interface	21
Round-ended burrs	Cortical windows	22
Flat-ended burrs	Cannulate distal cement plug	23

High speed instrumentation is available from two manufacturers—Midas Rex (Fort Worth, TX) and Anspach (Lake Park, FL). Both provide similar high speed, low torque tools for special situations in revision total hip arthroplasty. Both systems have similar tools with equal efficacy. The choice of system should be based on preference, experience, and practicality. Special training courses are offered and are recommended.

Ultrasonic Tools

Ultrasonic powered tools have been developed in an attempt to mimic the function of hand tools while avoiding the impact needed for effective function. The ultrasonic console converts electrical energy to mechanical energy with specially designed tool tips that shape and concentrate this mechanical energy. Basic science studies have shown ultrasonic tools to be relatively safe, in that they provide both tactile and auditory feedback when cortical bone is contacted instead of to cement (3). Furthermore, ultrasonic tools require considerable force to perforate cortical bone, a force much higher than that required to remove cement (2). Clinical experience has been favorable (8,9,17), but some concern exists regarding possible systemic effects during the surgery (29). As with all power instrumentation, experience with the ultrasonic system reveals its true potential.

Tool	Function	Figure
Power console	Converts electrical energy into a synchronized waveform	—
Hand piece	Converts electrical to mechanical energy	24
Tool tips	Shape and concentrate the mechanical energy	
Osteotome	Creates longitudinal splits in the cement mantle	25
Plug puller	Distal plug removal, removal of cement columns with poor cement–bone interface	26
Disc drills	Cannulates distal cement plugs, reshapes intact cement column to fit new femoral component	27

Component-Specific Tools

Component-specific tools are available from the manufacturer for a variety of different tasks. Awareness of their availability can reduce operative time and inconvenience significantly. The following is a list of the variety of available component-specific tools:

1. Stem extractors (Fig. 28)
2. Polyethylene liner extractors
3. Cup extractors
4. Screwdrivers (some have a special end designed specifically for a particular screw)
5. Modular head/neck detachment devices

Other Tools

Several other devices are available and are potentially useful in specific situations that will be discussed in the appropriate sections of the chapter. These include the Bohn modular stem extractors (Biomet, Warsaw, IN) (Fig. 29) and the Segces cement extraction system (Zimmer, Warsaw, IN) (see Fig. 61).

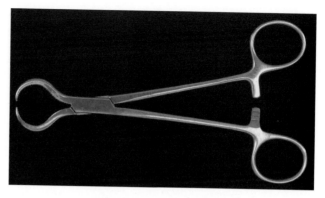

FIG. 3. Large cup grasper.

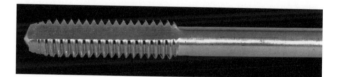

FIG. 4. Polyethylene implant extractor.

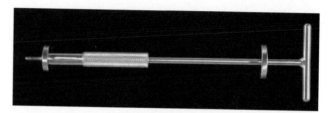

FIG. 5. Polyethylene insert extractor.

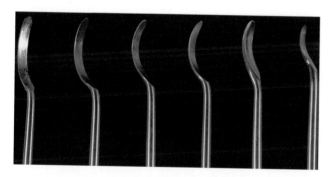

FIG. 1. Curved acetabular osteotomes.

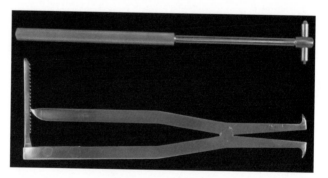

FIG. 6. Cup levers.

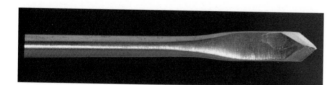

FIG. 2. Pointed osteotome.

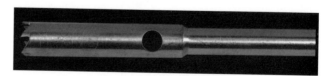

FIG. 7. Screw trephine.

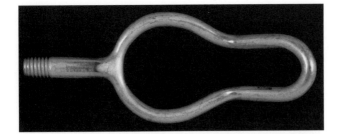

FIG. 8. Universal femoral extractor for nonmodular components.

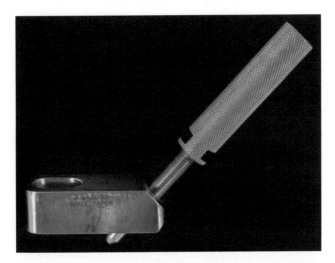

FIG. 9. Universal femoral extractor for modular components.

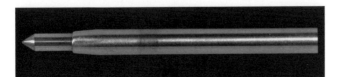

FIG. 10. Carbide punch.

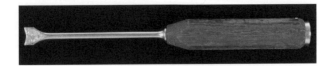

FIG. 11. Component disimpactor.

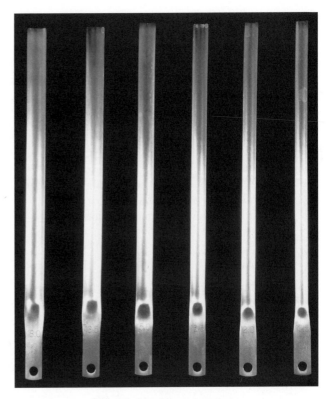

FIG. 12. Flexible osteotomes.

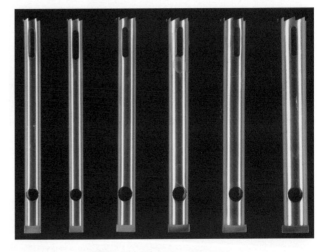

FIG. 13. Trephine reamers.

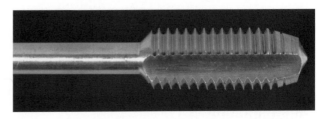

FIG. 14. Cement tap.

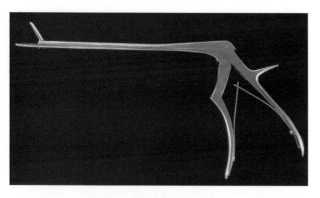

FIG. 15. Pituitary rongeur.

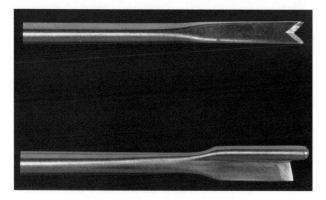

FIG. 16. T and V cement splitters.

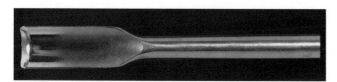

FIG. 17. Curved cement osteotomes.

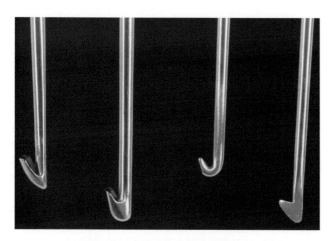

FIG. 18. Reverse hook curettes.

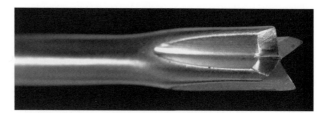

FIG. 19. X osteotome.

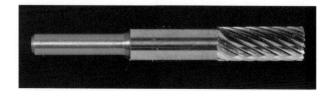

FIG. 20. High speed carbide burr.

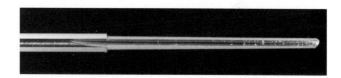

FIG. 21. High speed pencil bit.

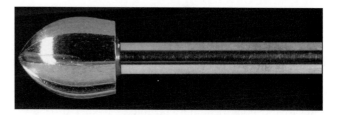

FIG. 22. High speed round-ended burr.

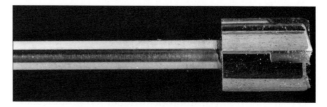

FIG. 23. High speed flat-ended burr.

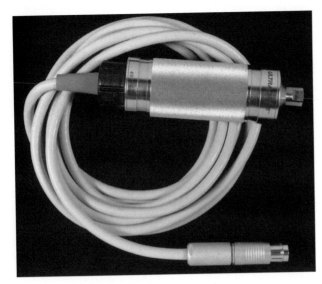

FIG. 24. Ultrasonic hand piece.

FIG. 25. Ultrasonic osteotome.

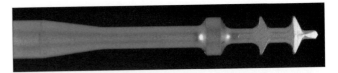

FIG. 26. Ultrasonic plug puller.

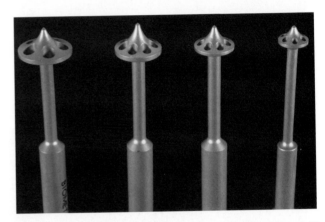

FIG. 27. Ultrasonic disc drills. There are four disc drills of different sizes ranging from 7 mm to 13 mm in diameter.

ACETABULAR COMPONENT REMOVAL

While generally felt to be relatively straightforward and simple, acetabular component removal can be tricky, especially if the surgeon is attempting to preserve bone stock while removing a well-fixed bone-ingrown cementless component. In these situations, the relative osteopenia of the bone near the cup makes it very difficult to remove the component with minimal bone damage. Therefore, it should be questioned whether acetabular component revision is necessary at all in every situation. Although there is some debate about the need to remove both components if there is a problem in only one side (i.e., the femoral side), the following represent the indications for acetabular component revision:

1. Mechanical loosening at any interface, either cement–bone, cement–prosthesis, or prosthesis–bone.

2. Malposition or improper orientation of the acetabular component.

3. Significant polyethylene wear or damage. This is a rather ill-defined endpoint, as all components will have some wear, albeit microscopic. However, if wear or scratching is actually visible intraoperatively, then revision of the acetabular component is warranted.

4. Instability of the hip after femoral component revision. This situation can occur if the acetabular component has a small internal polyethylene diameter (22 mm or 26 mm), in which neck-length choices for the femoral component are limited.

Liner Exchange

The simplest form of acetabular component revision is the polyethylene linear exchange—an alternative available only for cementless components. Although it is an attractive alternative, liner exchange must be used judiciously. For example, some of the older cementless cup designs were marginal at best (inadequate locking mechanism, poor liner–cup articulation with multiple areas of unsupported polyethylene, or nonuniform polyethylene thickness with the hexagonal polyethylene inserts), and to replace an older inadequate design with a new polyethylene insert of the same inadequate design would be unwise. In addition, as time passes, some of these older polyethylene designs may no longer be available. It is important to check the operative report for the type of liner in place, and with the manufacturer for the availability of a replacement.

Polyethylene thickness is a critical concern for the modular liners. A minimum thickness of 8 mm is ideal, although a 6-mm thickness may be acceptable in special situations (e.g., for older, minimally active patients with a short life expectancy). If the replacement liner will be under the acceptable thickness limit, then complete revision of the acetabular component is indicated.

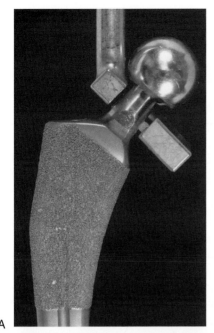

A

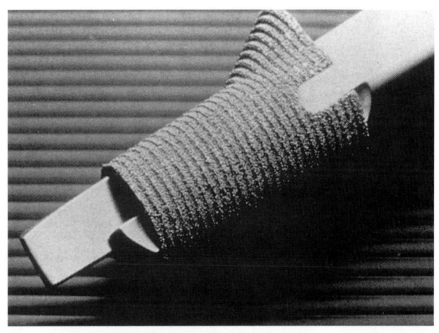

B

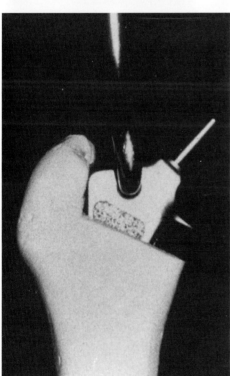

C

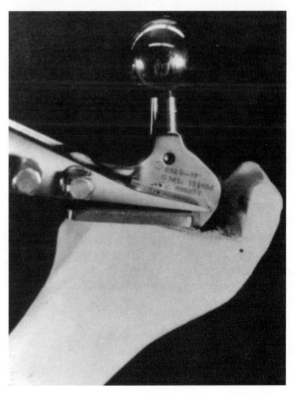

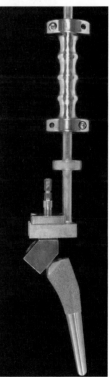

D,E

FIG. 28. A: Custom stem extractor for Biomet femoral components. The extraction mechanism locks around a specially designed area on the femoral neck. **B:** Custom extractor for proximal modular component of S-ROM cementless femoral stem. (Reprinted with permission from Pierson JL, Jasty M, Harris WH. Techniques of extraction of well-fixed cemented and cementless implants in revision total hip arthroplasty. *Orthop Rev* 1993;22:904–916. **C:** Special hook for extraction of Zimmer femoral component with an extraction hole. (Reprinted with permission from Rubash et al. *Instr Course Lect.*) **D:** Wedge platform technique to remove a collared femoral component without extraction hole. (Reprinted with permission from *Instr Course Lect.*) **E:** Special femoral component extractor for porous-coated arthroplasty.

overgrowth. Once the liner is removed, re-assess the true orientation of the acetabular component. A high wall liner may have been inserted to compensate for a malpositioned acetabular component. If the acetabular component truly is malpositioned, then the surgeon must strongly consider full acetabular component revision rather than simple liner exchange.

The locking mechanism may be damaged by liner extractors; certainly, the locking strength is compromised. As shown by Greenwald (12), repeated removal and re-insertion of liners leads to gradual decrements in liner–cup locking strength. Some components have locking mechanisms that can be replaced (Fig. 31) and these need to be ordered from the manufacturer. Removal of cup screws at the time of liner exchange is controversial. Screws provide conduits for polyethylene debris to filter up into the acetabular bone, and they may also be sources of metal debris from fretting against the cup–metal interface. In addition, screws generally are used to provide

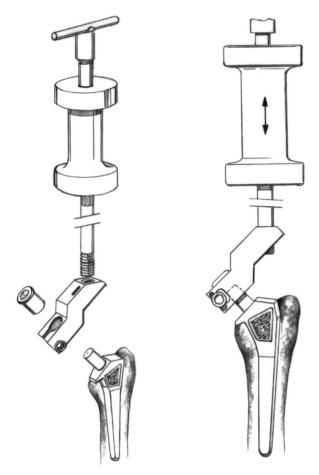

FIG. 29. Bohn modular stem extractor, which can be used to fit a variety of different modular femoral neck tapers.

Once it has been determined that liner exchange is a viable option, the surgeon must review the operative report for the type and size of the acetabular component in place. Occasionally, operative reports are inaccurate (through either dictation or transcription), so it is wise to review the patient chart from the previous surgery in which stickers listing component size and manufacturer are placed at the time of surgery.

Locking mechanisms for the polyethylene liner are different for each component. Review the specific mechanism for the liner to be exchanged. Although wedging a curved osteotome between the liner and cup, and then levering the liner out, generally suffices for removal of most liners, a special gadget may be available that will minimize the damage to the locking mechanism. An alternative technique to remove the polyethylene liner is to use a special threaded extractor device (see Fig. 5). After drilling a hole through the polyethylene liner, the extractor is treaded into the polyethylene. After it emerges through the back of the polyethylene liner and abuts against metal shell, the liner is forced out (Fig. 30).

Prior to attempting liner removal, fully expose the liner so that removal is not inhibited by soft tissue or bony

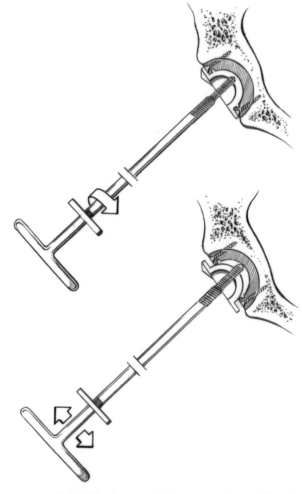

FIG. 30. Polyethylene insert extractor. A ¼-inch drill hole is placed through the center of the insert down to the medal, and then a threaded polyethylene extractor is inserted into the hole. After inserting it through the polyethylene, it abuts against the metal shell, forcing the liner out.

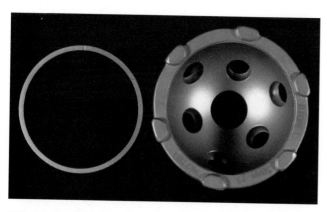

FIG. 31. Acetabular component ring lock device, which can be replaced if damaged but must be ordered from the manufacturer prior to surgery.

only initial stability to the cup, with long-term stability coming from bony ingrowth. Therefore, their presence is likely to be vestigial in nature at the time of liner exchange. For these reasons, screw removal appears warranted. However, there may be instances in which cup stability comes to depend, at least partially, on the screws. In these situations, screw removal will compromise component stability.

Cemented Acetabular Component Removal

Cemented component removal can be divided conveniently into three stages:

1. Exposure
2. Disruption of the cement–prosthesis interface
3. Component extraction

Although extensile exposure of the hip provides adequate access to the acetabular area, addition exposure of the acetabular component may be necessary. Specifically,

migration and micromotion of the acetabular component may lead to a situation in which the cup is hidden within the acetabular bed. In these situations, the entrance/exit aperture of the bony acetabular margin may extensively obscure the acetabular component, thereby restricting access to the cup and cement. In these situations, judicious and careful expansion of the acetabular bony rim with rongeurs and high speed burrs should be undertaken to simplify the subsequent extraction procedure.

Disrupting the cement–prosthesis interface is the safest means of removing the acetabular component, as it prevents inadvertent damage to the bone of the acetabular bed. The superior aspect of the acetabular component needs to be exposed and some lateral cement removed with a narrow osteotome. Then a curved osteotome (see Fig. 1) is introduced into the cement–prosthesis interface and gradually insinuated around the acetabular component. With gentle twists of the handle, the acetabular component can be separated from the cement (Fig. 32). A special ultrasonically driven, curved osteotome is available that can be used in a fashion similar to this hand tool.

Although disrupting the cement–prosthesis interface is the safest means of acetabular component removal, newer cup designs with enhanced cement–prosthesis bonding (precoating, porous coating, textured coating) may stymie the best attempts to access that interface. In these situations, the cement–bone interface is often loosened, and the use of the curved osteotome in this interface is generally successful. The surgeon must be careful not to damage the bony rims of the acetabulum, thereby compromising the subsequent reconstruction. In addition, the radiographs must be scrutinized: any anchoring holes or intrapelvic cement must be separated from the cement mantle prior to extracting the component.

Once the component is separated from the cement, the acetabular component is grasped with a large cup grasper (see Fig. 3) and the acetabular component gently maneuvered from the acetabular bed. Gentle twists of the

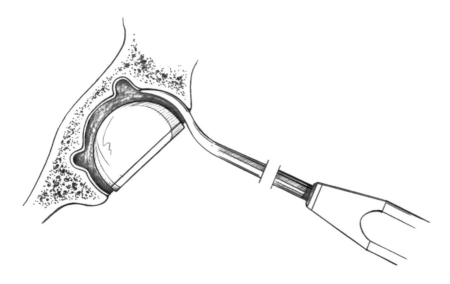

FIG. 32. The acetabular gouge can be inserted between the polyethylene and the cement, or between the cement and the bone. Gentle placement of this around the edges of the component and cement can loosen them from the underlying bone, allowing removal of the component or cement or both.

curved osteotome facilitate this maneuver. If this is not successful, a firmer grasp on the acetabular component can be obtained using a special Moreland tool that can be threaded into a hole drilled into the polyethylene. After proper attachment of the device, the acetabular component can be removed with a gentle rocking of the acetabular component and a gentle extraction force (Figs. 4,33).

Two other techniques of the acetabular component removal are available. Using high speed burrs, a cemented acetabular component can be cut into sections, then imploded upon itself, with subsequent removal. A special power instrument has recently been designed to remove the well-fixed acetabular component (19). Designed as a pneumatic impact wrench, it can deliver repetitive rotatory loads to the acetabular component that create shear stresses at the cement–prosthesis or cement–bone interface, thereby loosening the component. (see Fig. 36). Grooves are created in the polyethylene or the metal component itself to allow attachment of the device to the component. Clinical experience with this device has not been reported extensively.

Cementless Acetabular Component Removal

The three phases of component removal are the following:

1. Polyethylene liner removal
2. Screw removal
3. Metal shell removal

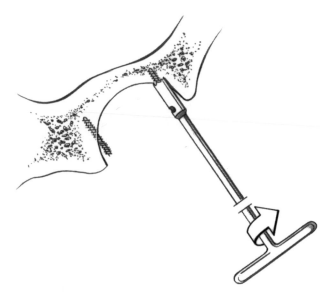

FIG. 34. After removal of the acetabular component, all broken screws can be extracted using the screw trephine reamer.

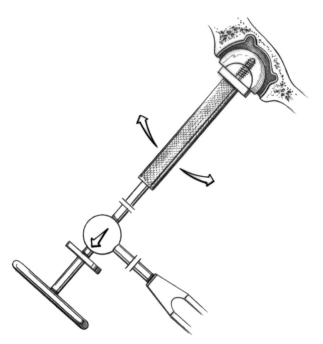

FIG. 33. Attaching the acetabular component extractor can be accomplished by pre-drilling with a ¼-inch drill bit and then tapping the threaded portion into the acetabular component. A gentle rocking motion with a gentle extraction force can then extract the acetabular component from the acetabular bed.

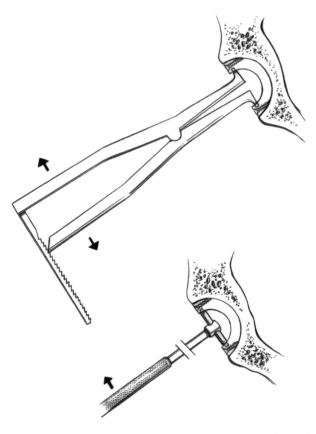

FIG. 35. The cementless-cup extractors/levers can lock into the metal portion of the cementless acetabular component. A gentle rocking motion will allow extraction of the component. Prior to levering with these tools, it is important to loosen the bone–prosthesis interface with the curved acetabular osteotomes.

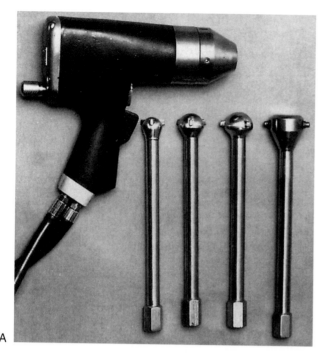

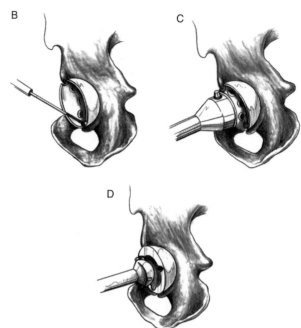

FIG. 36. A: Pneumatic impact wrench with drivers of various sizes available for different-sized acetabular components. **B:** A metal-cutting burr is used to create holes in the edge of the component. **C:** A driver of the correct size is introduced to sit within the acetabular component, the impact wrench is attached, and torch is applied to loosen the acetabular component. **D:** Nonmodular polyethylene components can be removed through the use of three grooves instead of two. (Reprinted from Lachiewicz PF, Anspach WE. Removal of a well-fixed acetabular component: a brief technical note of new method. *J Bone Joint Surg* 1991;73A:1355–1356.)

Removal of the polyethylene liner was discussed previously. Although liner removal is not absolutely necessary in all situations (e.g., nonmodular cementless components or cementless components inserted without screws), it is often useful to do so anyway. Removal of the liner can provide the surgeon with better visualization of the metal shell margins, thus allowing easier extraction.

Screw removal seems almost too mundane a topic to discuss. However, nothing is more embarrassing than discovering that the acetabular component screw heads require a special screwdriver that is not available in your operating room. Preoperative evaluation of the operative record and conversation with the appropriate manufacturer will identify any special screwdriver needs that might be necessary. Flexible screwdrivers are helpful. If the screw becomed stripped or cannot be removed for some reason, then the screw head must be cut off with a high speed carbide bit. Once the acetabular component is removed, these screws and any other broken screw tips can be removed with a special trephine (Figs. 7,34).

Removal of the cementless acetabular component itself can be relatively easy if the component is mechanically loose, but it can also be very difficult if the acetabular component is well fixed by bony ingrowth. In this situation, think long and hard about the absolute need for component removal, as attempts at extraction of the well-fixed acetabular component can lead to extensive bone destruction despite the most meticulous technique.

The first step in cementless acetabular component removal is to fully expose the margins of the metal shell. It is important to remember that the porous coating may extend beyond the margins of the outer metal shell, and proper exposure of the outer confines of this porous coating is essential. A high speed burr can be used to remove the rim of bone that generally overhangs the acetabular component and its porous coating.

A series of narrow, curved osteotomes are available in the Moreland cementless revision set (see Fig. 1), which must be introduced around the edge of the cup. The surgeon should aim circumferentially around the cup, starting with the shortest osteotome, and gradually progress to longer ones. It is important to stay as close as possible to the bone–prosthesis interface and resist the urge to lever with the tools. Patience is necessary! Areas of the cup where the bone is thickest—the ilium, ischium, and pubic ramus—should be accessed while avoiding the anterior and posterior rim areas. Once the component is loosened, it can be removed with a large cup grasper (see Fig. 3). In addition, two special tools are available that can also extract the acetabular component (Figs. 7,35). One final alternative may be a Cup-Out device, used as described by Lachiewicz and Anspach (Fig. 36).

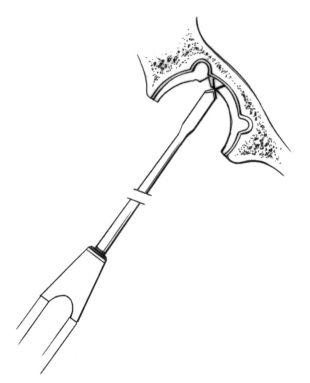

FIG. 37. Fragmentation of the cement within the acetabular bed can be achieved using the pointed osteotome. After fragmentation, the cement can be curetted free.

ACETABULAR CEMENT REMOVAL

Residual cement within the acetabular bed is often poorly fixed to the bone and can be removed with curettage. If it is well fixed, fragmentation with a narrow osteotome (the pointed Moreland osteotome can be used) generally disrupts the cement–bone bond, allowing easy extraction (Figs. 2,37).

Anchoring-hole cement can create problems with extraction. Gentle twisting of the cement with a curette is often successful. If it is not, then a narrow osteotome can fragment the cement prior to extraction with a curette. Alternatively, a high speed burr can debulk the cement within the anchoring hole, and the residual cement can be extracted with hand tools. Occasionally, larger anchoring-hole cement plugs have been removed with the ultrasonic plug-puller tools (Fig. 38). In these situations, the plug puller is inserted and locked into the anchoring-hole cement. A gentle disimpaction force is then applied, effecting removal of the anchoring-hole cement.

Intrapelvic Cement and Components

Components or cement that have passed the ilio-pectineal line can be considered intrapelvic in location. In the majority of cases, extraction is still possible through the standard extensile hip incision. With the addition of an extended trochanteric osteotomy, the problem of femoral component removal is minimized. This allows subsequent access to the acetabular component and cement.

A thick layer of fibrous pericapsular tissue is generally found around the loose components and cement. By identifying the plane between the component or cement and this fibrous layer, careful dissection can free up the components and the cement to allow for extraction. The urge to remove the intrapelvic component or cement by a direct forceful extraction should be resisted, because this could seriously damage intrapelvic vital structures. Using gentle traction, and a curette to separate the components and cement from the fibrous layer, gradual extraction of the intrapelvic components and cement is possible, leaving the fibrous layer intact.

There are occasional situations in which removal of intrapelvic cement or components is not possible through the standard hip approach. One example is intrapelvic cement that has penetrated through a small hole in the bone only to expand in size behind the hole, making it

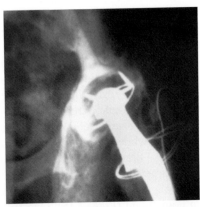

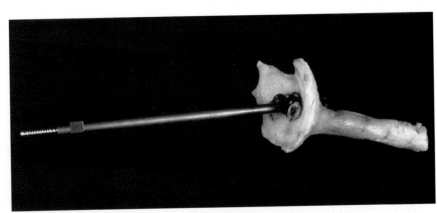

A   B

FIG. 38. Use of the ultrasonic tools can facilitate removal of anchoring-hole cement plugs. In this case, a large anchoring-hole cement plug was removed using a plug-puller device.

impossible to remove from the exterior of the acetabulum. Furthermore, this cement may have coiled around or become adherent to iliac vessels that could be damaged if attempts at extraction of the cement are too vigorous. One alternative course is not to remove all the intrapelvic cement. This is an option only in aseptic cases.

If removal of the cement and components is necessary in these situations, a retroperitoneal approach to the interior wall of the acetabulum can be undertaken. As described by several authors (4,13,16,25), it is a variation of the ilioinguinal approach used for acetabular fracture exposure (Fig. 39). During this exposure, the surgeon is usually impressed by the degree of intrapelvic scarring present, often affecting the bladder, ureter, nerves, and iliac vessels. The assistance of a general surgeon is useful for those unfamiliar or uncomfortable with this exposure. The exact indications for this intrapelvic retroperitoneal exposure are not well defined—Eftekar and Nercessian (4) employed it in only four cases, and Grigoris et al. (13) in nine. Fehring et al. (7) suggested preoperative evaluation with enhanced computed tomography (CT) scanning of all patients with intrapelvic cement or screws. When intimate contact with a major pelvic structure is found,

then the retroperitoneal approach is indicated. However, what "intimate contact" actually means was not well defined. Grigoris et al. stated that MRI might be equally useful at evaluating the relationships of intrapelvic structures to cement and components.

FEMORAL COMPONENT REMOVAL

Removal of the femoral component and cement can be accomplished using the standard exposure of the hip with which the surgeon is most familiar and comfortable. However, because of the intricacies of component removal, cement removal, and the ultimate reconstruction, the surgeon must be familiar with more extensile exposures which can be added to the standard exposure. Specifically, the surgeon must be able to perform a trochanteric osteotomy, which provides undeniably the best hip exposure. Although a standard trochanteric osteotomy may be sufficient, the poor trochanteric bone stock that is often present in the revision situation compromises the reattachment procedure. Use of a cable-grip system may be useful in these situations.

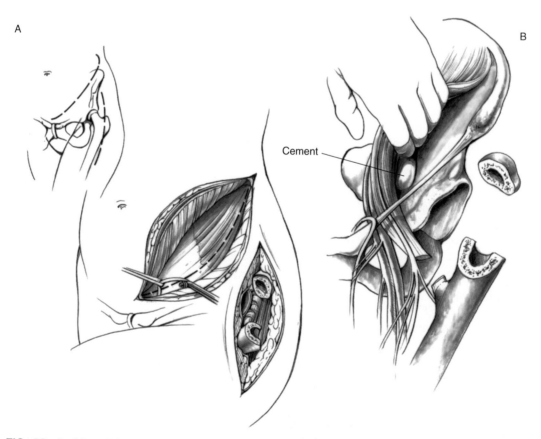

FIG. 39. A: After determining that removal of the acetabular component or cement is impossible through the standard hip incision, a separate ilioinguinal incision is made for exposure. **B:** Reflection of the iliac muscle off the iliac wing allows direct access to the intrapelvic cement or components. (Reprinted with permission from Eftekhar NS, Nercessian O. Intrapelvic migration of total hip prosthesis. *J Bone Joint Surg* 1989;71A:1480–1486.)

A sliding trochanteric osteotomy as described by Glassman et al. (11) may be a better alternative. In this approach, both the proximal and distal muscular attachments of the greater trochanter are preserved, thus preventing proximal migration of the trochanteric fragment should a nonunion occur. An extended trochanteric osteotomy technique provides the best alternative for extensile exposure, greatly facilitating cement and component removal. In this technique, which can be used to extend both anterior and posterior approaches to the hip (24,30), the lateral third of the femur for 3 to 10 cm is osteomized in continuity with the greater trochanter. Careful elevation of this segment with its attached muscles provides unparalleled exposure of the femur. Reattachment is provided via cerclage wires or cables.

Unlike acetabular component revision, femoral component revision is more complicated, and accordingly the surgeon is faced with many choices of tools and techniques. In addition, the extent of this femoral revision can vary considerably.

Isolated Head/Neck Exchange

In cases where revision is being undertaken only because of acetabular component failure, the option of head/neck exchange exists only if the femoral component has a Morse-taper modular head/neck. Indications for removal of the modular head/neck include the need for adequate surgical exposure, the need for change in neck length to equalize leg length or improve hip stability, or the need for change in head size to maximize polyethylene thickness. It is important to identify the component type and manufacturer prior to revision, as many component-specific tools are available to extract the head/neck from the stem taper. A useful technique is to tap the femoral head lightly with a ½-inch osteotome (thereby disrupting the lock between the head/neck and the taper), and then to use a mallet and disimpaction tool (see Fig. 11) to sharply disimpact the head/neck from the taper. This simple technique has been effective in all but one of my revisions over the past 5 years.

Cemented Stem Removal

Two steps make up this chore: (a) disruption of the cement–prosthesis interface, and (b) extraction of the component.

Disruption of the cement–prosthesis interface can be relatively straightforward in components with no special surface treatments such as precoating or porous coating to enhance the interface. In general, disimpaction of the component with a retrograde force is sufficient to disrupt the cement–prosthesis bond. However, before this force is applied, it is critical to remove any bone or cement over-hanging the proximal aspect of the femoral component (Fig. 40). Most components curve gently in the proximal lateral area, and if overlying cement or bone in this area is not removed, disimpaction can be impeded or fracture of the greater trochanter can occur. Similarly, a component that has subsided as a result of mechanical loosening may have bone overgrowing the collar. This must be removed prior to component disimpaction.

In cemented prostheses with enhanced cement–prosthesis interface bonding (precoating, porous coating, textured), disruption of this interface can be more difficult. Although the hand-held osteotomes are able to disrupt the interface, they run the risk of bone fracture or perforation. In general, the most effective means of solving this dilemma is to use the thin, high speed, pencil-bit burrs (see Fig. 21) to remove a thin layer of cement at the cement–prosthesis interface. If a collar obstructs access to the medial interface, it may be necessary to remove it with a high speed carbide drill (see Fig. 20).

Prior to the surgery, it is important to have an accurate idea of the extent of the cement–prosthesis enhancement. If the enhanced interface extends distally past the meta-

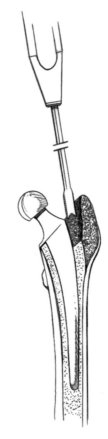

FIG. 40. Removal of proximal/lateral bone and cement is important to facilitate stem removal without fracture of the trochanteric region.

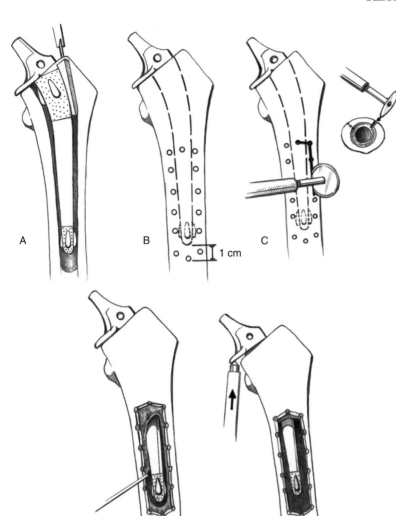

FIG. 41. A: Disruption of the proximal cement–prosthesis interface can be accomplished using a high speed pencil bit. **B:** Outlining the anterior femoral cortical window with drill holes is useful. This window should extend past the tip of the prosthesis by approximately 1 cm. **C:** A high speed drill can be used to create the actual window. Beveling of the cuts is helpful for subsequent replacement of the fragment after removal of the components and cement. **D:** Again, a high speed pencil bit is used to disrupt the distal cement–prosthesis interface. **E:** Once the proximal and distal cement–prosthesis interface bonding has been disrupted, a carbide bit can be used to extract the prosthesis. (Reprinted with permission from Pierson JL, Jasty M, Harris WH. Techniques of extraction of well-fixed cemented and cementless implants in revision total hip arthroplasty. *Orthop Rev* 1993;22:904–916.)

physeal flare of the femur, access is restricted with a standard hip approach. In these situations, an extended trochanteric osteotomy greatly facilitates the exposure to the distal cement–prosthesis interface. A more radical technique would be to transect both femur and femoral component, and then to extract the distal prosthesis with a combination of high speed burrs and trephines. A femoral window technique has also been described (18,26) that can provide access to this area (Fig. 41).

Extraction of the femoral component is relatively straightforward once the cement–prosthesis interface is disrupted. If the component is nonmodular, an extraction force can be applied to the femoral head with a punch or a special component-extraction device (Figs. 8,42). If the component has a collar, then the punch can be used to apply an extraction force at that location. Some components have custom devices designed specifically for extraction, which can be used if ordered from the manufacturer prior to surgery (see Fig. 28). Components with modular heads can create special problems, especially if

no collar is present. In these situations, the Moreland universal extraction device can be employed (Figs. 9,43). Special notches on the component must be created with a high speed carbide burr to allow the universal extraction device to attach securely. Alternatively, the carbide burr can be used to create a divot on the component, into which the carbide punch can be inserted to provide an extraction device. The Bohn-Modular stem extractor (see Fig. 29) is a specially designed instrument that can be fitted to a variety of head/neck tapers, allowing for easier extraction of the femoral component. (It is not usually necessary to purchase this device, as there are multiple alternative techniques for component extraction.)

Cementless Stem Removal

The scope and extent of the removal of cementless femoral components depend on two factors: (a) fixation status of the component, and (b) extent of the porous coating.

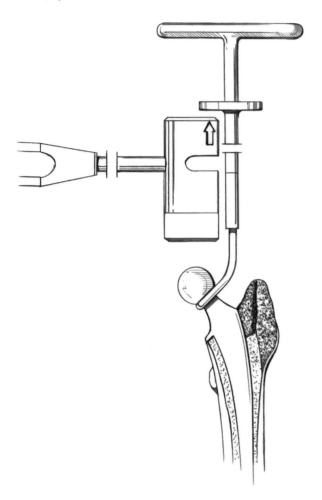

FIG. 42. Looping the nonmodular femoral component extractor over the stem can allow for extraction.

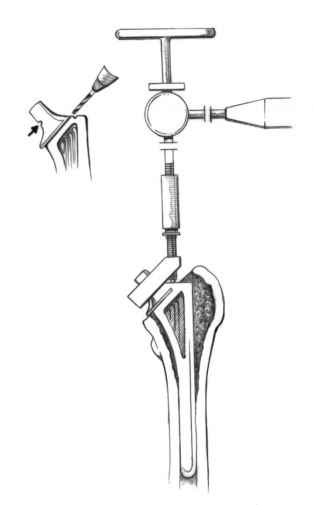

FIG. 43. A Universal extraction device can be used for nonmodular femoral components. If not already present, special notches must be made on the femoral component using a carbide bit, and attachment of the device to the femoral component allows extraction.

It is important to evaluate the preoperative radiographs to determine whether or not the femoral component is loose or well fixed. The Engh classification (6) of stable—bone ingrown, stable—fibrous ingrown, or unstable, is extremely useful. If the femoral component is mechanically loose, as judged radiographically, extraction requires merely clearance of the proximal bone overhang and a firm disimpaction force using any one of the techniques described for removal of cemented femoral components. In this situation, a manual disimpaction force should be applied only four or five times, and then abandoned if unsuccessful. Persistence in disimpaction after this can lead to fracture of the femur. If the four or five disimpaction blows are unsuccessful, then the component is reclassified as intraoperatively stable and should be approached as if bone ingrown. If the femoral component is bone ingrown, then special instruments and special approaches must be employed to remove the implant. The extent of the porous coating also influences the approach to the extraction procedure. If the well-ingrown porous surface is only proximal in extent, then disruption of the prosthesis–bone interface can be achieved with standard approaches, with or without trochanteric osteotomy. On the other hand, if extended porous coating is present and bone ingrowth has occurred distally, then special approaches such as cortical windows or extended trochanteric osteotomies must be utilized.

There are two techniques that can successfully remove a well-ingrown cementless component. The first technique involves a graduated exposure that depends on the level of fixation of the porous coat (10). The proximal porous coat (primarily metaphyseal in extent) can be interrupted with thin, flexible osteotomes (Figs. 12,44). Alternatively, a thin, high speed, pencil-bit burr can be employed (see Fig. 21). Access to the medial portion of the prosthesis is the most difficult and can be hampered by

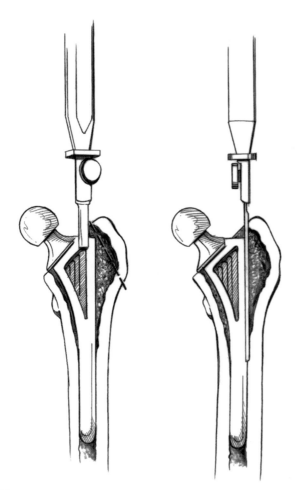

FIG. 44. Insertion of thin flexible osteotomes between the prosthesis and the bone can disrupt the prosthesis–bone interface. Start with shorter osteotomes and proceed to the longer ones. However, as the osteotomes reach into the diaphyseal area, they may cause perforations or fracture unless there is space between the prosthesis and the endosteal cortical bone.

a collar. Removal of the collar can be undertaken with a metal-cutting high speed bit. Once the prosthesis–cement interface is disrupted, disimpaction of the femoral component is undertaken.

If the porous coating extends distally into the diaphysis, use of the flexible osteotomes is limited and potentially dangerous (Fig. 45). In this situation, a cortical window is created in the femur at the level where the proximal tapered and distal cortical portions of the stem intersect (Fig. 46). Through this cortical window, the stem is transected with a high speed metal-cutting bit. Then the proximal portion of the femoral component is removed using the standard technique described for the proximally porous-coated stem. The remaining distal stem is removed using trephines (see Fig. 13), which can overdrill the distal stem, thereby disrupting the prosthesis–bone interface (Fig. 47). An extraction device can then be attached to the trephine, thus effecting femoral component removal.

An alternative approach to remove porous-coated implants involves the use of an extended trochanteric osteotomy. As described by Younger et al. (31), the distal extent of the osteotomy is placed at the junction of the tapered and cylindrical portions of the femoral component. It can be extended even more distally, but care must be given to the subsequent reconstruction—at least 4 to 6 cm of longitudinal endosteal contact must be available for the revision femoral component. Once the osteotomy exposes the femoral component, a Gigli saw is used to disrupt the proximal prosthesis–bone interface. If the stem is still secure, the prosthesis is transected and removed as described previously (Fig. 48).

Some cementless femoral components are modular in nature, in addition to having the modular head/neck. Removal of the distal modular segment can create slight dilemmas (26). Fortunately, most components of this type have special extraction equipment. It is imperative to

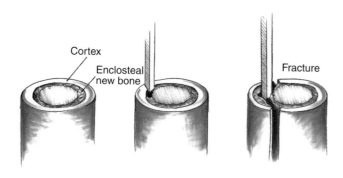

FIG. 45. Using flexible osteotomes in cementless components where there is little space between the component and the endosteal bone risks fracture of the femur. (Reprinted with permission from Glassman AH, Engh CA. The removal of porous-coated femoral hip stems. *Clin Orthop* 1992;285:164–180.)

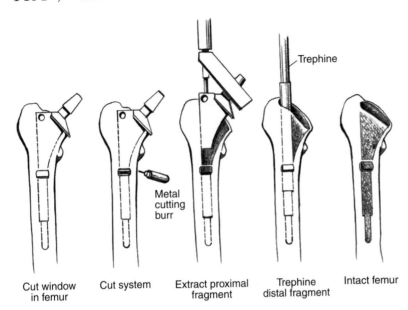

FIG. 46. Step-by-step technique for removal of distally fixed porous coated femoral component. (Reprinted with permission of *Clin Orthop.*)

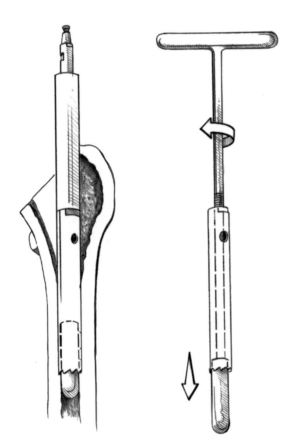

FIG. 47. After removal of the proximal uncemented femoral component, the distal conical section can be removed using the hollow trephines. The trephine of the proper size over-drills the distal segment and then, because the reamer generally entraps the femoral component, a T-bar attachment and mallet can be used to extract the femoral stem from the canal.

assess the need for this equipment preoperatively and to have it available (Fig. 49).

Fractured Stems

Stems fracture as a result of a combination of good distal fixation (either cement or cementless) and inadequate proximal fixation. Ultimately, cantilever-bending fatigue-fracture occurs. Although increasingly uncommon, stem fracture presents a special technical challenge to the removal of the well-fixed distal segment. Removal can be achieved by creating a hole in the proximal end of the distal fragment using high speed instrumentation (15), but this approach is less satisfying than two alternatives.

Moreland et al. (23) described the window technique for removal of fractured distal stems (Fig. 50). An anterior cortical bone window is created just below the proximal end of the fracture. A small divot in the component is then created, either with a sharp carbide steel punch or with a high speed metal-cutting burr. Then the punch is used to drive the stem out of the canal. The two steps are repeated as necessary until the distal segment is removed. This technique may not be applicable to cementless stems that fracture, as the distal fragment can be well fixed by bone ingrowth. However, extraction is possible using the technique described in the section on cementless femoral component removal (see Fig. 48).

An alternative approach to creating a femoral window is to use an extended trochanteric osteotomy, with the distal aspect of the osteotomy based just below the level of the femoral component fracture. After exposure, the distal stem can be removed in the same stepwise fashion as that described by Moreland et al. (23).

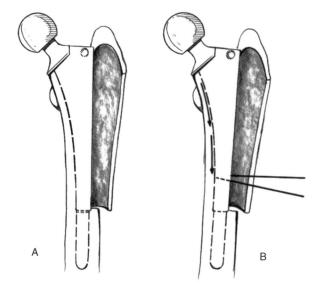

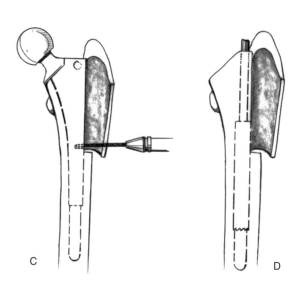

FIG. 48. A: An extended trochanteric osteotomy is used to expose the proximal aspect of the femoral component. **B:** A Gigli saw is used to disrupt the bone–prosthesis interface. Multiple Gigli saws may be necessary. **C:** If distal bony ingrowth prevents removal of the stem, then a metal-cutting high speed burr is used to transect the stem with subsequent removal of the proximal segment. **D:** Trephining the distal stem will allow for extraction of that segment. (Reprinted with permission from Younger TI, Bradford MS, Paprosky WG. Removal of a well-fixed cementless femoral component with an extended proximal femoral osteotomy. *Contemp Orthop* 1995;30:375–380.)

FEMORAL CEMENT REMOVAL

Cement to Cement

Prior to attacking the potentially formidable task of cement removal, it is important to decide if it is necessary at all. One alternative is to recement a femoral component into the preexisting cement mantle. This technique has been utilized by several authors (1,21,22) with excellent results. Recementing of a femoral component into a retained mantle should be considered only in instances where the cement–bone interface and the cement mantle are close to ideal. However, when they are less than ideal, exceptions might be made if removal of the cement mantle might seriously jeopardize the existing bone stock, which is particularly a problem with very osteopenic thin bone (Fig. 51). Situations in which the cement-to-cement approach should receive serious consideration include revisions for instability or leg-length inequality, in which the femoral cement is adequate. In addition, an isolated acetabular revision in association with a nonmodular femoral component may require femoral component revision to adjust leg length, stability, or femoral head size. Furthermore, the need for increased exposure may make femoral component removal necessary (without femoral cement mantle removal). This technique also may be useful for fractured femoral components with satisfactory cement mantles or for isolated debonding at the cement–prosthesis interface.

Although the original prosthesis can be used (1), surface modification of the cement mantle usually is necessary to fit a new femoral component into the old cement mantle. After adequate exposure of the proximal femur, tap out the original prosthesis. Inspect the cement mantle to confirm maintenance of an excellent cement-to-bone bond. Small proximal deficiencies in the cement mantle may be acceptable, but they require further preparation to ensure an adequate cement–bone interface. The proximal cement is modified using a high speed burr to remodel the cement mantle to fit the metaphyseal flare of the new prosthesis. The distal cement mantle can be enlarged or lengthened as necessary to fit the new component. Although high speed burrs can be used, the perforation rate may be unacceptable (21). An alternative technique is to prepare the distal cement mantle using ultrasonic tools. Small circular tool bits (disc drills) are used to widen or lengthen the preserved cement mantle for a larger or longer prosthesis. Sequentially larger disc drills are used, thus enlarging the canal for the new femoral implant. Care should be taken to stay as central as possible within the canal. Preoperative radiographs should be scrutinized to determine where the stem is located within the canal and cement mantle. Adjustments can then be made to keep the new canal centered within the bony tube.

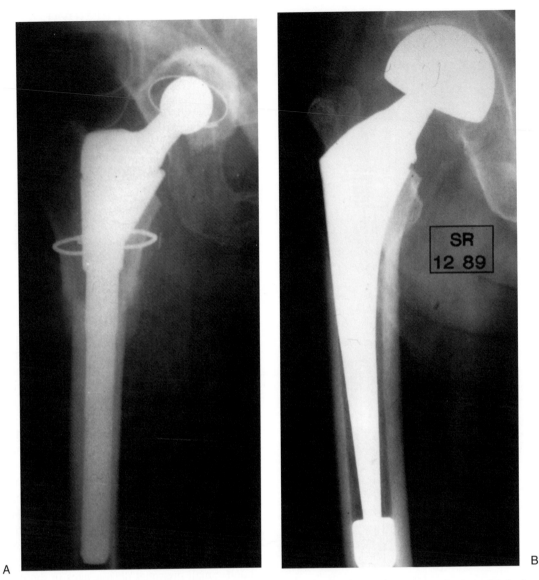

FIG. 49. A: For extraction of the proximal segment of this modular femoral component, a special device is required, which must be ordered from the manufacturer. **B:** Extraction of the distal bullet of this femoral component often requires a special attachment.

Cement Removal Techniques

If the cement needs to be removed, it is best approached in three stages:

Stage 1. Metaphyseal cement, above the lesser trochanter.

Stage 2. Diaphyseal cement, below the lesser trochanter but proximal to the cement plug.

Stage 3. Distal plug cement.

It must be understood that femoral component removal is a prerequisite to cement removal. The workhorses of femoral cement removal are the hand tools. A variety of other tools and techniques are available, but they should be viewed as complementary to the hand instrumentation, not as replacements for them. These include the high speed drills, ultrasonic tools, and the segmental extraction technique of cement removal.

Occasionally, the entire cement mantle is loose within the canal. In this situation, a tool can be anchored into the cement mantle and then the entire cement mantle removed with a single disimpaction force. A metal tap can be threaded into the cement (Fig. 14,52) or the ultrasonic plug puller can be similarly anchored. If only some of the cement is removed with the first disimpaction, the steps can be repeated as needed. The success of this technique depends on a greater mechanical bond between the instrument and cement than between the cement and the

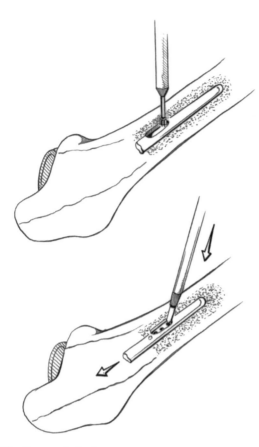

FIG. 50. Removal of a fractured femoral component requires creation of a distal cortical window just below the level of the fracture. A small divot is created in the component using a burr or carbide punch. Then the fragment is disimpacted with the carbide bit. Multiple divots may be required.

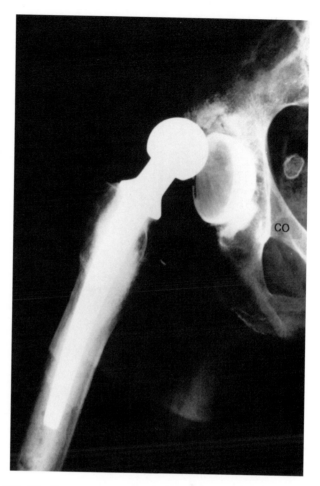

FIG. 51. Removal of cement by attacking the cement–bone interface may be hazardous in this patient with extreme osteopenia and thin cortical bone. In these situations, the cement-to-cement technique may be a better alternative.

bone. When preoperative radiographs show a radiolucent line at the cement–bone interface comprising 100% of the interface, then this technique can be successful. It is important in this situation to clear away any bone overhanging the proximal cement mantle so as to avoid bone fracture. Unfortunately, this technique is rarely an option.

Adequate visualization of the femoral canal is essential to avoid bone perforation and fracture. Aiming an operating room light over the shoulder of the surgeon may be adequate, but a fiberoptic head-light is the best way to illuminate the femoral canal. In addition, both hands of the surgeon are free to use cement removal tools. Hand-held lights can also be used but can obscure access to the canal for the hand tools. Extended trochanteric osteotomy is another way of fully exposing the femoral canal cement.

Metaphyseal Cement

Cement in the metaphyseal area tends to be bulky and the bone tends to be thin and weak. Although hand instru-

ments are needed in this stage of cement removal, initial debulking of the cement using a high speed burr is helpful. The cement should then be split longitudinally into three or four segments using either a /-inch osteotome or the special T or V osteotomes from the Moreland set (Figs. 16,53). Sharp taps are necessary to split the cement, but care must be taken to avoid splitting the metaphyseal bone as well. An ultrasonically driven osteotome (Figs. 27,54) can be used to create the longitudinal splits, avoiding the force needed to crack the cement manually. A curette is then used to separate the cement from the bone, with the cement fragments being retrieved by a pituitary rongeur. A fibrous membrane is generally apposed to the bone and should be curetted away before progressing to the next stage. At this time, it is critical to remove cement and bone from the trochanteric bed to allow direct longitudinal access to the diaphyseal part of the femur. Failure to do so could lead to subsequent perforation of the lateral cortex of the femur during attempts to remove the distal cement.

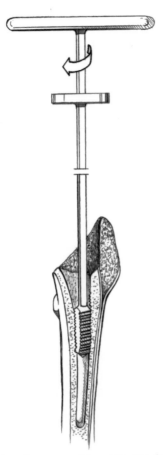

FIG. 52. Tapping the cement tap into the femoral cement mantle may allow extraction of the femoral cement if the cement bone interface is weak.

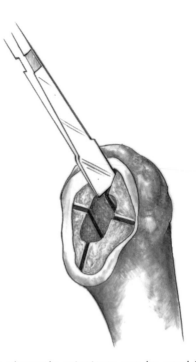

FIG. 54. An ultrasonic osteotome can be used to split the metaphyseal cement without the forceful impaction needed with the hand tools.

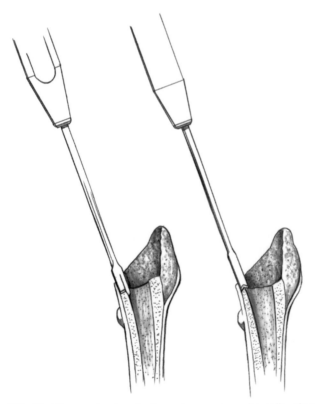

FIG. 53. The proximal metaphyseal cement can be split using special T or V osteotomes. Sharp taps are necessary, but care must be taken to avoid splitting the metaphyseal bone as well.

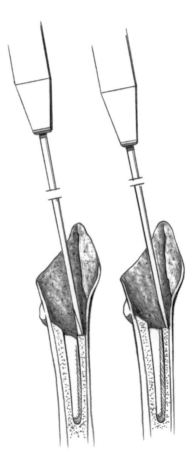

FIG. 55. Sharp curved cement osteotomes introduced at the cement–bone interface can chip away the diaphyseal cement after splitting of the cement mantle using the T or V shaped osteotomes.

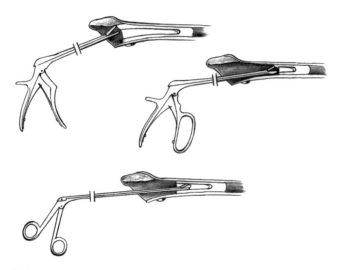

FIG. 56. A pituitary rongeur can be used to remove loose cement after the osteotomes have been employed.

Diaphyseal Cement

The following sequence of steps should be repeated in this stage of cement removal:

1. Split the cement mantle circumferentially with the T or the V osteotome.

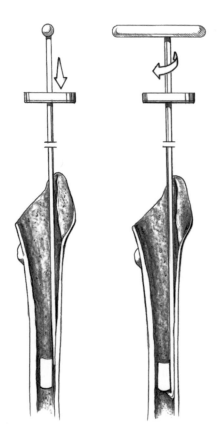

FIG. 57. If there is a space between the distal cement plug and the bone, a thin hook curette can be used to slip by the cement plug and then disimpact it.

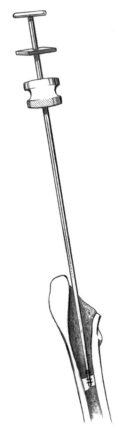

FIG. 58. An ultrasonic plug puller can be inserted in the cement plug, and then the cement plug can be disimpacted using a small 1-lb weight. This technique works only if the cement–bone interface is weak. In addition, this should not be used if the cement plug expands past the isthmus of the femoral canal.

2. Chip the cement away from the bone using a sharp curved osteotome. Keep the curved osteotome at the cement–bone interface for best efficacy (Figs. 17,55).
3. Use a curette or pituitary rongeur to remove the loose cement and fibrous membrane (Figs. 15,56).
4. Irrigate the canal and then dry it with an E-tape to restore proper visualization.

Advancing in 1- to 2-cm increments while repeating this series of steps allows for efficient and safe removal of all cement from the diaphyseal area.

Distal Plug Cement

Removal of distal plug cement can be a tedious and frustrating chore. Hand tools can be used successfully but often seem less than adequate. It is important to evaluate the preoperative radiographs to determine the extent and nature of the cement plug: How long is it? Does it pass the isthmus of the femur and then expand? Is it well bonded to bone, or is the cement–bone interface loose?

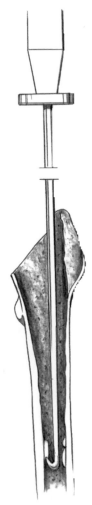

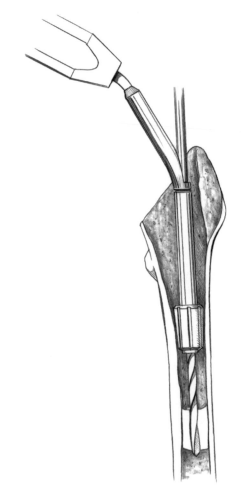

FIG. 59. After removal of most of the cement plug, the reverse hook curettes can be used to remove all residual cement.

FIG. 60. Using graduated centering cones to guide a drill, the distal cement plug can be cannulated.

Can an instrument be passed between the plug and the endosteal bone, or does the cement plug completely obliterate the canal?

If a space exists between the distal plug and the endosteal bone (Figs. 18,57), then a thin hook curette can be insinuated past the plug and rotated 90°. An extraction force can then remove the plug. If no space exists for the hook curette, but the cement–bone interface is weak, the plug can be removed in one of two ways. First, a sharp osteotome can work the bone–cement interface and with gentle twists fully free up the plug. The plug can then be grasped by pituitary forceps. Alternatively, the ultrasonic plug puller can be employed as described previously to engage and then disimpact the loose cement plug (Figs. 28,58).

The most difficulty occurs when the distal cement plug is well fixed and fills the canal completely. In this situation, hand tools alone are insufficient and power instrumentation is necessary to remove the distal cement plug. The general principle is to drill a hole through the distal plug, thus converting it to a cement mantle similar to that in the proximal diaphyseal area. The remainder of the cement can then be excised in the fashion previously described for the diaphyseal cement removal stage. In addition, the reverse hook curettes should be employed to remove all residual cement (Fig. 59).

Drilling through the cement can be accomplished in several ways, with standard drills, high speed burrs, or ultrasonic drills. The standard drills are used through graduated centering cones (Fig. 60) to guide the drill through the approximate center of the distal plug. Unfortunately, the femoral curvature makes the drilling much more precarious than can be shown diagrammatically. In these situations, an extended exposure of the femur should be undertaken and controlled perforation of the femoral bone should be performed to ensure proper orientation of the drills within the canal (31). Controlled perforation involves subperiosteal stripping of the vastus lateralis off the femur and the creation of 9-mm round holes in the shaft of the femur using a high speed burr (see Fig. 22). This portal should be placed just proximal to the distal plug, which allows the surgeon direct visualization of the drill as it enters into the distal plug. Illumi-

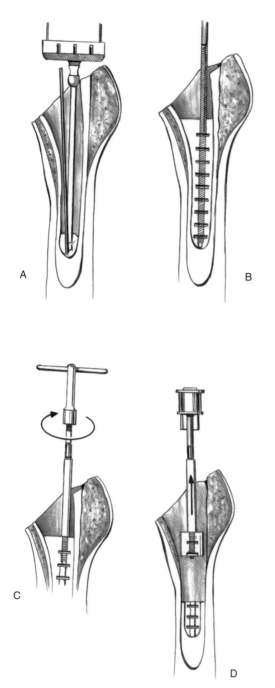

FIG. 61. A: After removing the prosthesis, new cement is injected into the old cement. **B:** A thread-forming rod with nuts is placed into the liquid cement and the cement is allowed to harden. **C:** Extraction rods are then inserted into the threaded canal and attached to a slap hammer. **D:** The old cement, now bonded to the new, is removed in segments.

nation and irrigation of the canal can also be accomplished through the portal. Additional controlled perforations can be created, each 5 cm apart, as needed. During the reconstruction phase of the revision procedure, these defects must be bypassed by the new femoral component (20). High speed burrs can also be used for the drilling of

the distal cement plug. They tend to be more efficient at cement removal than the standard drills and are relatively safe if guided by the controlled perforation technique (14). However, if improperly guided, high speed burrs can preferentially remove bone rather than cement with no tactile feedback to the surgeon using the tool. Facility with the high speed instrumentation is definitely experiential. Fluoroscopic control of the drilling process has been employed, but it is cumbersome, time consuming, and less safe than the controlled perforation technique.

Ultrasonically driven tools can also be used to drill through the distal cement plug. The main advantage of this approach is that tactile and auditory feedback is provided by the instrumentation, allowing the experienced surgeon to differentiate between bone and cement. Thus the ultrasonic tool can be guided gently through the distal plug, avoiding damage to the surrounding bone. Four disc drills (with diameters of 7, 9, 11, and 13 mm) are available to perforate the distal plug (see Fig. 28). They are used sequentially, with copious irrigation, to push through the distal plug, enlarging the hole as the disc drills increase in size. After using the largest disc drill possible, the residual cement is removed with the hand tools as previously described.

Distal cement plugs that extend past the isthmus and around the curvature of the femur pose special problems of removal. Complete removal of the cement plug may not be necessary. If a new cemented component is to be implanted, the distal cement can act as a cement restrictor. If a new cementless component is to be implanted, removal of cement need be undertaken only to the level of the tip of the new stem. Drilling through an extended distal cement plug from the proximal end of the femur is likely to result in either perforation or eccentric cement removal (which will encourage bone perforation during insertion of the new femoral stem). In these situations, the extended trochanteric osteotomy exposure with the distal aspect of the osteotomy near the apex of the curvature of the femur is the best approach. Drilling of the cement mantle can then be performed in a more controlled fashion.

After the cement is removed, there are two additional obstacles that need to be overcome prior to reconstruction. First, a plastic cement restrictor may be in place and must be excised. Often, this plastic plug does not come out with the cement mantle and must be retrieved with a pituitary rongeur. Occasionally, the plastic plug is not free enough in the canal for the pituitary rongeur to remove it, but gentle use of the curved osteotomes around the outer margins of the plastic plug will loosen it up for subsequent removal. Finally, there is often a reactive bony pedestal below loose prostheses, which must be removed prior to reconstruction. The first step is to perforate through the bony pedestal, and the X osteotome (see Fig. 19) is most beneficial in these situations. The remainder of the pedestal is removed with the reverse hook curettes.

Segmental Cement Extraction

Segmental cement extraction using the Segces cement extraction system (Zimmer, Warsaw, IN) is a novel, albeit counterintuitive, approach to the removal of femoral canal cement (5,27). Although initially advocated for removal of all cement within the femoral canal, currently it is best utilized for the diaphyseal cement removal stage and the distal cement plug removal stage. Prior to utilizing this technique, it is important to review in detail the step-by-step technique recommended by the manufacturer (Fig. 61). New cement is inserted into the femoral canal over a special threaded rod. After setting, this cement is then removed in steps with a special extraction system. A special plug-removal device is also available. The segmental extraction system is based on two principles: first, the new cement injected into the femoral canal will bond firmly with the preexisting cement; second, the bond between the new and old cement will be stronger than the bond between the old cement and bone. Contraindications for the use of the segmental extraction system include a distal cement mantle that expands past the isthmus such that the cement mantle diameter distally is greater than proximally, and situations in which cement has extruded through defects in the femoral bone. Clinical experience with this technique continues to accumulate, as do specific indications and contraindications.

REFERENCES

1. Archibald DA, Protheroe K, Stother IG, Campbell A. A simple technique for acetabular revision. *J Bone Joint Surg* 1988;70B:838.
2. Brooks AT, Nelson CL, Hofmann DE. Minimal femoral cortical thickness necessary to prevent perforation by ultrasonic tools in joint revision surgery. *J Arthroplasty* 1995;10:359–362.
3. Callaghan JJ, Elden SH, Stranne SK, Fulghum CF, Seaker AV, Myers BS. Revision arthroplasty facilitated by ultrasonic tool cement removal. *J Arthroplasty* 1992;7:495–500.
4. Eftekhar NS, Nercessian O. Intrapelvic migration of total hip prosthesis. *J Bone Joint Surg* 1989;71A:1480–1486.
5. Ekelund AL. Cement removal in revision hip arthroplasty, *Acta Orthop Scand* 1992;63:549–551.
6. Engh CA, Bobyn JD. Biological fixation in total hip arthroplasty. Thorfare, NJ: Slack, 1985;89–107.
7. Fehring TK, Guilford WB, Baron J. Assessment of intrapelvic cement and scores in revision total hip arthroplasty. *J Arthroplasty* 1992;7:509–518.
8. Frankel A, Hozack WJ. Ultrasound for revision hip arthroplasty. *Curr Opin Orthop* 1993;4:43–45.
9. Gardiner R, Hozack WJ, Nelson CL, Keating EM. Revision total hip arthroplasty using ultrasonically driven tools. *J Arthroplasty* 1993;8:517–521.
10. Glassman AH, Engh CA. The removal of porous-coated femoral hip stems. *Clin Orthop* 1992;285:164–180.
11. Glassman AH, Engh CA, Bobyn JD. A technique of extensile exposure for total hip arthroplasty. *J Arthroplasty* 1987;2:11–21.
12. Greenwald AS. A comparison of the dissociation strength of modular acetabular components. *Clin Orthop* 1993;296:154–160.
13. Grigoris P, Roberts P, McMinn DJW, Villar RN. A technique for removing an intrapelvic acetabular cup. *J Bone Joint Surg* 1993;75B:25–27.
14. Harris WH, Oh I. A new power tool for removal of methylmethacrylate from the femur. *Clin Orthop* 1978;132:53–54.
15. Harris WH, White RE, Mitchel S, Barber F. A new technique for removal of broken femoral stems in total hip replacement. *J Bone Joint Surg* 1981;63A:843–845.
16. Head WC. Prevention of intraoperative vascular complications in revision total hip replacement arthroplasty. *J Bone Joint Surg* 1984;66A:458–459.
17. Klapper RC, Caillouette JT, Callaghan JJ, Hozack WJ. Ultrasonic technology in revision joint arthroplasty, *Clin Orthop* 1992;285:147–154.
18. Klein AH, Rubash HE. Femoral windows in revision total hip arthroplasty. *Clin Orthop* 1993;291:164–170.
19. Lachiewicz PF, Anspach WE. Removal of a well fixed acetabular component: a brief technical note of new method. *J Bone Joint Surg* 1991;73A:1355–1356.
20. Larson JE, Chao EYS, Fitzgerald RH. Bypassing femoral cortical defects with cemented intrameduely stems. *J Orthop Res* 1991;9:414–421.
21. Lieberman JR, Moeckel BH, Evans BG, Salvati EA, Ranawat CS. Cement-within-cement revision hip arthroplasty. *J Bone Joint Surg* 1993;75B:869–871.
22. McCallum JD, Hozack WJ. Recementing a femoral component into a stable cement mantle using ultrasonic tools. *Clin Orthop* 1995;319:232–237.
23. Moreland JR, Marder R, Anspach WE. The window technique for the removal of broken femoral stems in total hip replacement. *Clin Orthop* 1986;212:245–249.
24. Peters PC, Head WC, Emerson RH. An extended trochanteric osteotomy for revision hip replacement. *J Bone Joint Surg* 1993;75B:158–159.
25. Petrera P, Trakru S, Mehta S, Steed D, Towers JD, Rubash HE. Revision total hip arthroplasty with a retroperitoneal approach to the iliac vessels. *J Arthroplasty* 1996;11:704–708.
26. Pierson JL, Jasty M, Harris WH. Techniques of extraction of well-fixed cemented and cementless implants in revision total hip arthroplasty. *Orthop Rev* 1993;22:904–916.
27. Schurman DJ, Maloney WJ. Segmental cement extraction at revision total hip arthroplasty. *Clin Orthop* 1992;285:158–163.
28. Sydney SV, Mallory TH. Controlled perforation: a safe method of cement removal from the femoral canal. *Clin Orthop* 1990;253:168–172.
29. Woo R, Minster GJ, Fitzgerald RH, Mason LD, Lucas DR, Smith FE. Pulmonary fat embolism in revision hip arthroplasty. *Clin Orthop* 1995;319:41–53.
30. Younger TI, Bradford MS, Magnus RE, Paprosky WG. Extended proximal femoral osteotomy: a new technique for femoral revision arthroplasty. *J Arthroplasty* 1995;10:329–338
31. Younger TI, Bradford MS, Paprosky, WG. Removal of a well-fixed cementless femoral component with an extended proximal femoral osteotomy. *Contemp Orthop* 1995;30:375–380.

The Adult Hip, edited by J. J. Callaghan,
A. G. Rosenberg, and H. E. Rubash.
Lippincott–Raven Publishers, Philadelphia © 1998.

CHAPTER 87

Cementless Acetabular Reconstruction

Douglas E. Padgett

Revision acetabular surgery presents one of the most difficult challenges to any orthopedic surgeon (40,66,87). Failure of a prior acetabular component, whether caused by aseptic loosening, sepsis, or in the setting of osteolysis, often results in a pelvis with distorted anatomy because of deformity, volumetric bone loss, or inferior bone quality, often sclerotic (3,14,16). The challenge to the surgeon is to obtain acetabular implant stability while at the same time restoring loss of bone and maintaining hip mechanics (44,70,92).

It is becoming increasingly apparent that the use of porous, noncemented acetabular components in revision acetabular surgery yields predictably good results (21,33, 34,61,76,81,82). Although there was some initial success employing cemented acetabular components in the setting of revision surgery, longer-term follow-up has shown that component loosening rates, as well as revision rates, were not acceptable (11,13,19,23,36,42). Amstutz et al. (1) reported that 61% of cemented revision sockets had evidence of progressive radiolucent lines and 10% had already failed by the 2-year follow-up. Pellicci et al. (66, 67) demonstrated 9% progressive loosening and a 5% revision rate at 3 years. Finally, Kavanaugh et al. (46) reported that 70% of their cemented acetabular revisions showed evidence of progressive radiolucent zones, with 2% already revised at the 5-year follow-up. Even with the development of devices such as anti-protrusio rings as

described by Müller, clinical results at intermediate-term follow-up have not yielded predictable results, with aseptic failure rates of 12% (5,23,71,93). Unfortunately, alternative techniques for reconstruction utilizing threaded screw-in rings, as well as the use of bipolar implants in conjunction with bone graft, have not been uniformly successful (2,10,37,56,58,75,89–91). With the advent of porous cementless components, especially those being used in acetabular reconstruction, short-term and longer-term follow-ups have shown this method of reconstruction to be far superior to those using acrylic cement for the same degree of deficiency (7,21,24,61,76,82). It appears, therefore, that porous noncemented acetabular components are the treatment of choice for the vast majority of acetabular revisions.

In this chapter, we will attempt to define the indications for cementless acetabular reconstruction, to evaluate defects that are amenable to this type of reconstruction, to outline preoperative planning including type of bone graft when needed, to describe surgical technique for reconstruction, to review the results employing this technique, and, finally, to discuss future directions using cementless acetabular reconstruction.

INDICATIONS FOR CEMENTLESS ACETABULAR RECONSTRUCTION

The use of porous noncemented acetabular components in revision hip arthroplasty relies on the ability to achieve biologic fixation of the component to the underlying host

D. E. Padgett: Department of Orthopaedic Surgery, Hospital for Special Surgery, New York, New York 10021.

bone. For biologic fixation to be achieved, an implant must have appropriate porous structure (in the range of 150 to 400 μm), intimate host bone contact avoiding gaps, and rigid implant stability (7,24,32,49,79,83). The basic object of reconstruction using cementless acetabular components is to maximize host bone apposition to achieve stabilization. Therefore, any situation that can satisfy these requisites is amenable to cementless acetabular reconstruction.

The most common indication for the use of a cementless acetabular component is in the setting of revision for aseptic failure of either a cemented or a cementless component. Unfortunately, the ever-increasing rate of periprosthetic bone loss caused especially by osteolysis, whether combined with implant loosening or in isolation, can also be an indication for the use of a cementless acetabular component. Although component malposition leading to recurrent instability and eventual revision is not common, certainly revision of the acetabular component to improve orientation can be successfully performed using a cementless implant. Finally, although some authors have questioned the use of porous cementless femoral components during reimplantation after sepsis because of an alarmingly high rate of recurrence of infection (59), the use of cementless acetabular components during reimplantation has led to predictable fixation and has not been shown to be associated with increased rates of recurrent sepsis (34,61) (Table 1.)

There are only two instances in which reconstruction utilizing a porous, noncemented acetabular component should not be employed. Because cementless reconstruction relies on the process of biologic fixation, the use of these components in situations with suspect bone biology is questioned. This would include revision in the setting of tumor, metabolic bone disease such as Paget's disease, and pelvic osteonecrosis such as that after pelvic irradiation (41).

Second, although the use of hemispherical acetabular components is successful for most classes of pelvic deficiency, the sole use of a hemispherical noncemented component in the setting of pelvic discontinuity (pelvic diastasis) should be avoided. It is felt that this degree of pelvic compromise should be managed by restoration of pelvic ring structure with plating (usually of the posterior column), followed by the use of cementless acetabular techniques for reconstruction. Attempts to use the component itself to serve this function has not been uniformly successful (61,81).

PREOPERATIVE EVALUATION

A systematic preoperative approach to revision acetabular surgery is essential to produce predictably successful results. The initial operative note is a source of valuable information, including type of component, details of fixation, and any noteworthy defects that were encountered at the time of surgery. Plain radiographs are probably the most useful piece of information the surgeon has at hand

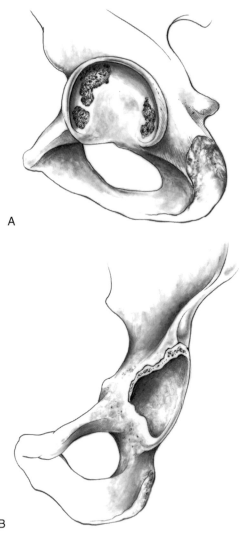

FIG. 1. A: Schematic of isolated cavitary defects in the acetabular vault. These defects, which represent volumetric loss of bone with an intact underlying bed of often sclerotic bone, are amenable to particulate grafting. **B:** Segmental defects are those that involve the supporting columnar support of the acetabulum. In this case of an anterior segmental defect, there is a noncontained deficiency of the anterior column extending to the anterosuperior acetabular dome.

TABLE 1. *Indications for cementless acetabular reconstruction*

Aseptic loosening of either a cemented or cementless component
Periprosthetic bone loss associated with osteolysis
Component malposition
Reimplantation after treatment for sepsis

(14,17,26,45,62,63,65,80). Anteroposterior (AP) projections of the pelvis provides an excellent sense of the integrity of the pelvic ring, and the intactness of the medial wall and the superior dome. Contained defects (Fig. 1A) can often be identified on the plain radiographs, but major segmental or columnar defects (see Fig. 1B) are often detectable only on oblique radiographs (Judet views). The role of computerized tomography (CT), acetabular version analysis, and studies such as arteriograms and contrast pyelography should be used on an individual basis and are not routinely necessary. Details of the preoperative evaluation are described in Chapter 88.

The ultimate goal of the preoperative evaluation is the determination of the extent of pelvic deficiency one can anticipate at the time of revision. Stratification of defects as described by the American Academy of Orthopaedic Surgeons Committee on the Hip is useful (17). Preoperative planning for acetabular revision is simplified by determining the status of the supporting columns (segmental defects), the presence of contained defects that represent volumetric loss of bone without loss of structural integrity, and the overall integrity of the pelvic ring.

PREOPERATIVE TEMPLATING FOR CEMENTLESS ACETABULAR RECONSTRUCTION

Preoperative templating with acetabular overlays is an important part of the preoperative planning for acetabular revision surgery. The technique for templating involves the initial marking of the interteardrop line on the AP radiograph. The acetabular inclination line is then drawn from a point 5 mm lateral to the teardrop, along the interteardrop line superolaterally at an angle of 40°, which represents the desired acetabular abduction. Delineation of acetabular defects is noted, including integrity of medial wall and superolateral rim. Ideal acetabular placement is at the level of the teardrop, but in the revision setting, our primary goal is to maximize host bone coverage of implant and therefore some proximal placement of the component is accepted. This is commonly referred to as the high hip center (48,72,85). Variables encountered include the ability to obtain rim fit of the implant, the ability to maximize host contact (which may result in proximal placement of implant), bone loss encountered (which may require bone grafting, either

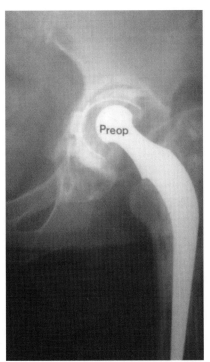
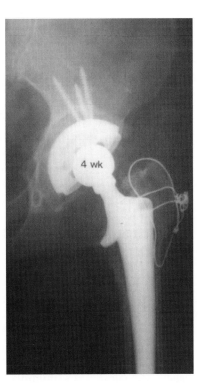
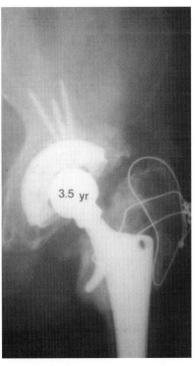

A,B   C

FIG. 2. A: A preoperative AP radiograph demonstrating cavitary defects of the medial wall and superior dome. Note that although there is thinning of the medial wall, there remains continuity with a thin sclerotic rim of bone. **B:** Reconstruction has been accomplished with particulate graft both medially and superiorly. Note that the implant is now lateral to Kohler's liner. Supplemental screw fixation into the wing of the ilium has ensured implant stability in the early postoperative period while awaiting bone graft consolidation and host bone–implant fixation. **C:** At 3.5 years, acetabular bone stock has been restored and the implant has stabilized without evidence of migration.

structural or particulate), and the effect of implant placement on offset and leg lengths. The anticipated position of the component is now marked either directly on the radiograph or on templating paper.

The stability of the acetabular component relies on the ability to obtain a press-fit between ischium, pubis, and ilium. Despite the inevitable bone loss encountered during revision acetabular surgery, accepting some degrees of proximal implant placement to maximize implant–bone contact obviates the need for any type of bulk structural bone graft in the majority of cases. However, in situations such as advanced degrees of dysplasia or in acetabular "break-out," where the superolateral acetabular defect results in component uncovering by host bone of more than 30% to 40%, consideration of using bulk structural graft with either a cementless or a cemented component should be given (4,6,9,15,18,20,22,25,28,29,31,39,43,52, 57,60,64,73). This situation should be anticipated preoperatively by appropriate preoperative planning.

The most difficult of acetabular revisions are those associated with advanced degrees of bone loss or pelvic deformity. In situations with global bone loss manifested by expansile loss of superior dome, lack of medial wall integrity, and advanced ischial osteolysis, large-segment allograft may be necessary. In these situations, where extensive allograft bone is used to reconstruct major defects with or without pelvic discontinuity, cementless acetabular reconstruction may be inappropriate because of the unpredictable nature of biologic fixation from cadaveric bone. It is in these rare instances that acetabular reconstruction utilizing acrylic cement fixation is recommended (5,9,15,27,35,38,54,65,69,74,77,78,84,94).

For the vast majority of acetabular revisions, the use of particulate graft is sufficient to graft contained defects as well as noncontained medial defects (Fig. 2). Graft sources include (a) autograft, either from local host bone reaming, trochanter, or iliac crest; (b) freeze-dried allograft; (c) fresh-frozen allograft; or (d) a combination of these. Because the graft is not structural and weight bearing in function, the type of graft used is of little significance (13,27,39,51).

SURGICAL TECHNIQUE OF CEMENTLESS ACETABULAR RECONSTRUCTION

Exposure

Regardless of the surgical approach used, extensile exposure is mandatory during acetabular revision (30, 65,87). The decision to use previous incisions and previous tissue planes, or to employ new approaches is often determined by the status of the trochanter, whether femoral revision is being performed at the same time, the presence of modular femoral components in situations when the component is not being revised, and,

most important, the surgeon's familiarity. The ability to completely visualize both anterior and posterior columns, as well as to displace the femur out of the field, is essential to corroborate acetabular defects anticipated preoperatively, to quantitate bone loss, to assess the ability to perform cementless acetabular reconstruction, and to successfully complete the reconstruction. This author prefers to avoid trochanteric osteotomies and favors either an extended posterolateral approach or a combined anterolateral and posterior approach with anterior displacement of the femur or femoral component in situations where it is not being revised. Removal of pseudocapsule around the entire acetabular orifice is essential to enable identification not only of the periphery of the implant but also of the bony rim. Identification of the inferior extent of the acetabulum to the level of the obturator foramina, and visualization of the ischium and pubis provide complete acetabular anatomy. At this point, intraoperative Gram staining and frozen sections as indicated are sent for appropriate laboratory analysis.

In certain instances, a second separate incision and exposure may be required during revision acetabular surgery. The use of the retroperitoneal approach in combination with standard hip exposure has been described by Petrera et al. (68). These authors have used the retroperitoneal exposure in patients whose pelvic vasculature is felt to be at risk. This includes patients with medial-wall bone loss with resultant intrapelvic component protrusion, those with large masses of intrapelvic cement, or those with osseous deformity that may place pelvic vascular structures at risk during acetabular reconstruction. Preoperative CT is useful in detailing the local pelvic anatomy and in determining the need for the retroperitoneal approach. This approach should be performed either by or in consultation with a vascular surgeon who is familiar with this anatomic region. Identification and isolation of the iliac vessels prior to embarking on acetabular reconstruction appears to minimize the risk of major bleeding in this selected group of patients.

Implant Removal and Debridement

The ability to remove the previously placed implant is dependent on method of fixation, integrity of fixation, and association with periprosthetic bone loss. The key is to minimize bone loss and avoid iatrogenic bone destruction. To accomplish this, the surgeon requires the proper exposure, the proper tools, and, above all, patience. Although removal of a loose implant proceeds without difficulty, extraction of a well-fixed implant, whether cemented or cementless, is more challenging, and it should never be forcibly levered out, a sure way to fracture the supporting acetabular rim or to remove a sizable piece of acetabular bone stock with the implant. The use of curved osteotomes or pneumatic-driven gouges can break the interface between implant and bone with little bone destruction. When removing a well-fixed cementless acetabular component, care should be taken to circumferentially free-up the implant, especially inferiorly where biologic fixation can be extensive but access with curved osteotomes difficult.

With the component removed, the surgeon should begin the tedious task of thorough debridement of the acetabular vault. In the case of previously cemented implant, attempts should be made to remove all retained portions of acrylic, especially in the regions of fixation holes. Acrylic cement that is intrapelvic and not readily accessible should be left *in situ*. Large boluses of cement that extravasated during insertion through small defects in the acetabular cavity prior to polymerization may not be removable without making major perforations in the remaining acetabular bone (73). In the setting of aseptic loosening, discretion would dictate leaving the acrylic in place. Granulomatous tissue often accompanies acrylic cement fixation holes, and these regions and should be curetted out as well. Regions of periprosthetic osteolysis that were suspected on the preoperative radiographs should be investigated and debrided as well.

Bone Stock Assessment

Perhaps the most crucial time during acetabular reconstruction is the confirmation of acetabular deficiency previously suspected during preoperative evaluation. Identification of defects is undertaken by inspection and palpation. The size and location of contained defects previously debrided are noted. More important is the status of supporting rim: anterior, medial, superior (dome), and, most important, the posterior supporting column. Partly because of the posteriorly directed vector of forces across the hip joint during activities of daily living, the posterior supporting column is the key to acetabular reconstruction. The lack of an intact posterior supporting rim makes cementless acetabular reconstruction tenuous at best. If there is no intact posterior rim, reconstruction of pelvic integrity using pelvic reconstruction plates with allograft bone as needed is mandatory. The acetabular component alone cannot be relied on to span major osseous defects with resultant implant stability. Fortunately, the most common defects encountered are medial wall defects, isolated superior dome defects, and defects in the anterior column.

Loss of superior bone in the region of the acetabular dome is frequently encountered during revision acetabular surgery. Bone loss at this level may be caused by migration of a prior implant, osteolysis with or without migration, or placement at a superior level at the time of index surgery. When superior bone loss is encountered, the surgeon needs to decide whether to accept some degree of proximal placement of the implant or to employ bulk graft in order to lower the acetabular center of rotation to its normal (anatomic) level (70). Proximal placement of 20 to 25 mm is usually acceptable and obviates the need for bulk graft. The decision to employ a high hip center or to strive to place the implant in its anatomic location will influence subsequent reaming (81). My personal preference is to avoid the use of bulk grafts and accept varying degrees of proximal implant placement (61,76).

Finally, in addition to the integrity of the rim, the quality of the bone is important to note, although a sclerotic bed of host bone with varying degrees of cancellous bone is usually present.

Hemispherical Reaming

At this point, hemispherical reaming of the acetabular vault is begun. The purpose of reaming is to initially debride the sclerotic bone to a smooth hemispherical surface. Smaller-diameter reamers (in the range of 44 to 50 mm) are used with little force. There is little rationale for attempts at forceful reaming. Reaming down to, but not through, the medial wall is one method to improve host bone coverage of implant. Reaming into the anterior column will also provide some degree of improved host bone contact and has little consequence. However, reaming of the posterior column should be avoided. Sequentially larger hemispherical reamers are then utilized until the reamer makes three-point contact between the ischium, pubis, and ilium (55). Reaming should be performed in the desired direction of implant insertion, usually 40° of abduction and 20° of anteversion. The last-used reamer shell can be used as a trial to assess contact throughout the acetabulum. The decision to use a component or trial shell 1 to 2 mm larger to obtain an improved press-fit should be based on bone quality or presence of osseous defects. However, impaction of the trial reamer shell should be performed gently: sclerotic bone may not be compliant and the risk of fracture is real (50). This author currently favors line-to-line reaming for most acetabular revisions and to enhance initial component stability with the use of adjuvant screw fixation.

Bone Graft

With the trial shell in desired position, the degree of uncovering should be noted. An implant that is more than 30% uncovered may be difficult to stabilize despite using adjuvant screw fixation, and therefore structural bone graft may be indicated. Although the long-term success of structural grafts in cemented acetabular sock-

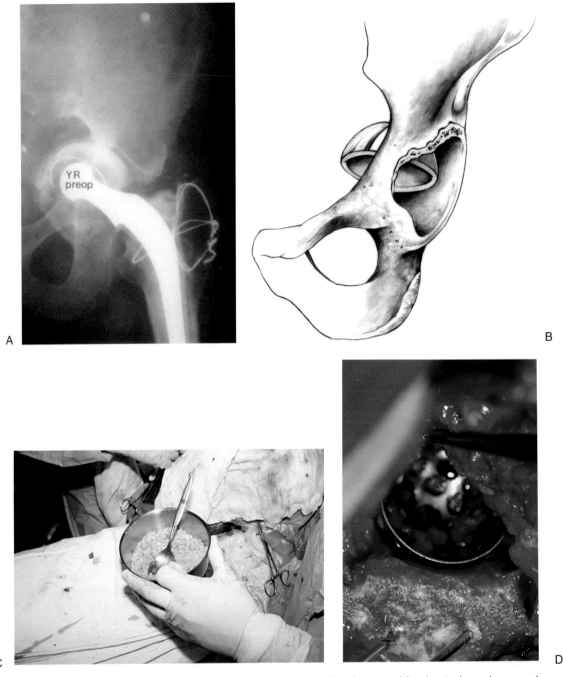

FIG. 3. A: A failed cemented acetabular reconstruction resulting in a combined anterior column and medial wall defect. The posterior supporting column is intact, making this defect amenable to cementless acetabular reconstruction. **B:** Schematic representation of the defect. **C:** Particulate allograft bone that is mixed with local autograft bone and bone marrow aspirate. The graft can be "spooned" into the defect and then compressed using hemispherical reamers on reverse. **D:** Acetabular reamer shell has been used to compress and shape the particulate graft into the medial and anterior defects. Using the shell as a provisional "trial," the surgeon can check for component orientation in addition to amount of host bone contact.

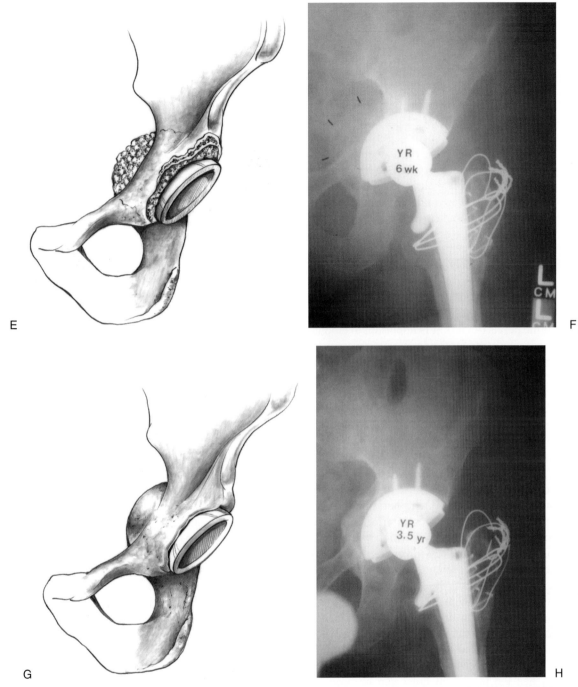

FIG. 3. (*cont.*) **E:** Particulate graft has been gently packed into the noncontained medial defect. **F:** With the particulate graft placed medially, acetabular component obtains three-point fixation between ischium, pubis, and ilium. Note that the component is at the level of the radiographic teardrop. Adjuvant cancellous screw fixation provides implant stability. **G,H:** By 3.5 years, the medial bone graft has consolidated to a firm sclerotic rim of bone, effectively reconstituting the medial wall defect. There has been no evidence of implant migration.

ets has been questioned, its use in cementless acetabular reconstruction to provide initial implant stability while awaiting for the process of biologic fixation to occur has been demonstrated (6,20,31,38,51,57,61).

Particulate bone graft of either cancellous autograft, allograft, or both should be placed into all contained defects. In addition, noncontained medial defects can be successfully grafted using particulate graft laid directly onto the fascial surface of the obturator internus muscle. Gentle compression of the particulate graft into position can be accomplished by using the hemispherical reamer on reverse (Fig. 3).

Implant Insertion

Implant insertion is often facilitated with a commercial holder, which aids in proper component orientation. In general, the implant is placed in approximately 40° of cup abduction and 20° of anteversion. The final orientation may be influenced by surgical approach utilized, amount of host bone available, and hip joint stability. Implant stability is dependent on factors such as remaining host bone, effect of bone graft whether particulate or bulk, and whether reaming was performed in a line-to-line manner (final reamer size equals implant size) or whether under-reaming to obtain a press-fit was utilized. As stated previously, under-reaming and impaction may be associated with fracture, especially in cases of sclerotic, noncompliant bone (50).

The use of adjuvant screw fixation when utilizing cementless porous hemispherical implants improves initial fixation and is associated with enhanced biologic fixation. Screw placement should be directed into the "safe quadrants" of the pelvis (47,85). It is important to emphasize that the safe quadrants for screw insertion were originally described for an anatomically located component (i.e., at the level of the teardrop). In revision surgery, varying degrees of bone loss will result in the acetabular component being more proximal (cranial) than in primary arthroplasty. Acetabular bone stock for screw fixation will change as the implant is placed more proximal (Fig. 4). Wasielewski et al. (86) recently described safe zones for adjuvant screw fixation in association with an acetabular component placed at a high hip center. It is apparent from their work that the peripheral one half of the posterior superior and posterior inferior quadrants contain the optimal bone for screw fixation while minimizing the risk of injury to the pelvic vessels. In general, anterior quadrant screw placement should be used only with extreme caution.

Unfortunately, placing adjuvant screws through the implant at its periphery can often cause the implant to shift position, especially when the initial impaction fit is tenuous. Placement of a relatively short adjuvant screw in the central or polar hole can effectively secure implant position, and then the peripheral holes can be used for longer screw insertion and improved mechanical stability. The polar screw, although often short in length, very often obtains secure cortical purchase. Once adequate peripheral screw placement has been completed, usually with two to three screws, the polar screw may be either removed or left in place to provide additional fixation. It is at this time that cup stability should be assessed. This can be performed by using a Kocher clamp or hemostat to check for gross implant motion. The component should also be checked for host bone contact, ensuring that there are no significant gaps between implant and bone. Implant orientation as well as implant location is next evaluated.

Localization of the acetabular implant relies on bony landmarks when available. The degree of craniocaudad component placement is best assessed by identifying the most inferior aspect of the acetabular vault: the entrance into the obturator foramina. In primary hip arthroplasty, identification of the transverse acetabular ligament is a useful guide to the most caudad aspect of the acetabulum. In the setting of revision surgery, this landmark is often absent and palpation of the osseous floor of the acetabulum with an instrument, such as a pair of forceps, must be relied on, proceeding inferior until the forceps fall into the obturator foramina. This level corresponds to the radiographic teardrop. Determination of cup position relative to this level can aid in determining the extent of any cranial or caudad implant placement. It is important to remember that acetabular component placement will influence leg lengths, as will the femoral reconstruction.

In addition to determining cup position relative to the inferior aspect of the acetabulum, the degree of component coverage by the superolateral ilium is important. Excessive implant coverage or lack of coverage may indicate too much or too little implant lateral opening (abduction). Preoperative planning and drawing on the AP radiograph will give some indication of expected degree of cup coverage, which should be confirmed at this time (53).

After acetabular component shell insertion, a modular polyethylene liner is inserted. The decision to employ high wall or elevated liners is controversial. Although there is literature to support their use to reduce the incidence of hip instability in primary total hip arthroplasty (12), there are also concerns about early neck impingement leading to hip instability. Thus, routine use does not appear warranted and the use of high wall or even constrained types of liners should be reserved for those cases in which hip joint stability is not satisfactory to the surgeon.

The postoperative management of patients undergoing cementless porous acetabular revision surgery is dependent on several factors. Weight-bearing status can be influenced by factors, such as stability of the construct as measured by the quality of interference fit of the cementless socket or by the quality of purchase of adjuvant screw fixation. In addition, bone grafting of either contained or noncontained defects may require protected weight bearing until incorporation has occurred. Finally, the type of femoral reconstruction as well as the status of the trochanter/abductor mechanism will influence the surgeon's decision about what degree of weight bearing to permit. Our current recommendations are to permit 50% weight bearing with crutches or a walker for the first 6 to 8 weeks, and then progressive weight bearing as tolerated. As cementless fixation relies on an ordered process of inflammation ultimately leading to the formation of mature osseous fixation, the use of medications that may inhibit the inflammatory response during the initial 2-month postoperative period is discouraged.

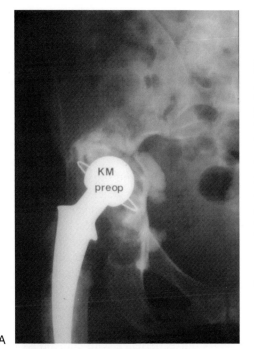

A

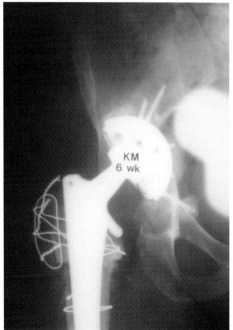

B

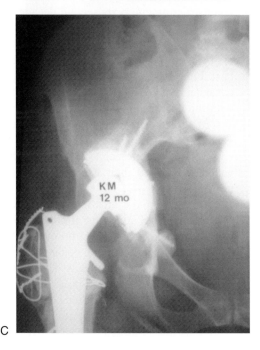

C

FIG. 4. A: Failed cemented acetabular component with a noncontained defect medially and cavitary defects superiorly in the dome. **B:** Reconstruction has been accomplished with a cementless hemispherical component, utilizing particulate bone graft in the medial and cavitary dome defects. Supplemental screw fixation has been used to enhance initial component stability. Component position is above the level of the teardrop, but this proximal placement has maximized host bone contact and obviated the need for bulk graft. **C:** At 1 year, component position has been maintained and implant interfaces appear stable. Note that extravasated intrapelvic cement has been left in place. The decision to remove intrapelvic cement must be balanced with the associated risks, such as great vessel injury.

RESULTS OF CEMENTLESS ACETABULAR RECONSTRUCTION

Reconstruction of a failed acetabular component presents the surgeon with a formidable task. Periacetabular bone loss coupled with a sclerotic bone bed limits reconstructive options. Revision of failed acetabular components employing acrylic cement have been shown by numerous authors not to be successful (1,46,66). The ability to obtain acrylic interdigitation into sclerotic bone has yielded high rates of progressive radiolucent zones and unacceptably high migration rates at relatively short

follow-up. Techniques using bipolar hemiarthroplasties (10,75,91), protrusio rings (5,93), and threaded acetabular components (2,37) unfortunately did not lead to predictable rates of success. It was the failures of these techniques that gave impetus to the development and refinement of cementless, porous acetabular reconstruction.

The early results of cementless acetabular reconstruction using a porous component have been uniformly successful. In two separate studies performed at the Massachusetts General Hospital and the Rush-Presbyterian Medical Center, authors were able to demonstrate predictable implant fixation in the majority of patients (33,61,76,81). The majority of patients in both these studies presented with either cavitary or combined cavitary and columnar defects. Using the technique of cementless reconstruction as described was successful for all classes of acetabular deficiency. The incidence of migration as detected by serial radiographs was less than 2%, and, in the study by Padgett et al. (61), there were no revisions for loosening without infection. Pelvic osteolysis was not identified in this series. However, it is apparent that the use of modular acetabular components with adjuvant screw fixation may lend itself to eventual osteolytic reactions. In a follow-up of these patients at 9 to 12 years, Silverton et al. reported peripheral osteolysis observed in 4% of patients, but none required surgical intervention (76). The low incidence of osteolysis observed may be related to the relatively short duration of follow-up, as well as to the relatively low demand of many patients undergoing acetabular reconstruction.

Initial stability of the implant is aided by adjuvant screw fixation, and many authors have demonstrated success in obtaining secure mechanical fixation at the time of insertion with low rates of complications resulting from inadvertent screw placement. Familiarity with the safe zones of the pelvis for screw placement has been outlined by several authors and is recommended reading for all surgeons employing this technique (47,85,86).

In addition, these studies have demonstrated that the use of particulate bone grafting was successful in restoring bone stock for both cavitary defects and noncontained medial defects. Medial wall reconstruction can be performed using bulk structural allograft. However, as described by White and Cook (88), graft resorption to a sclerotic rim of bone was common. We have found that the use of particulate graft can accomplish the same goal of medial wall restoration with a technique that is much less complex.

Failures of cementless acetabular reconstruction did occur in hips with a greater degree of pelvic deficiency. As has been pointed out, the use of a hemispherical component to span defects across a pelvic diastasis is associated with loss of fixation, implant migration, and failure. These severe degrees of pelvic deficiency are best served by the use of pelvic reconstructive plating and reestablishment of the pelvic ring (76).

Perhaps it should be noted that not all cementless acetabular components have yielded uniform success. Although the short- and intermediate-term results of cementless acetabular revision surgery are excellent, concerns about the generation of wear debris and osteolysis have been raised. Although the incidence of pelvic osteolysis after cementless revision acetabular surgery is low (range, 0% to 10%) (34,61,76,82), the long-term consequence of this phenomenon is worrisome. Design characteristics of some components, which resulted in liners with unacceptably thin polyethylene, exhibited rapid wear of some polyethylene liners and are associated with early failures (8). In addition, material failures of some types of polyethylene that were affected by gamma irradiation, heat pressing, or other types of treatment may predispose certain acetabular components to premature wear and failure. With these concerns in mind, it is recommended that all patients undergoing cementless revision surgery be followed on an annual basis radiographically. The presence of osteolysis as well as progression should be noted. Large expansile lesions of pelvis may necessitate debridement and grafting. Although the exact mechanism is unknown, (a) the generation of particulate debris at the articulating surface or at the junction between implant and liner shell; (b) corrosion between screws and implant shell; or (c) motion at other modular sites may be the source of particulate debris that can evoke the tissue response that then initiates the osteolytic cascade.

FUTURE DIRECTIONS

As our experience with cementless porous acetabular reconstruction enters its second decade, identifiable successes as well as problems can be seen. Specifically, fixation of implant to bone has been predictable for the vast majority of revision cases. The principles of maximizing host bone–implant contact and implant stability have consistently been successful. Aims at improving fixation with the use of adjuvants applied to the implant such as any of the bioactive ceramics or recombinant morphogenetic proteins are exciting and could complement the currently used approach (49). Whether cost of such adjuvants will justify their use is still an unanswered economic issue.

Clearly, the major area for improvement in all implant systems is combating the problems of osteolysis and wear-generated bone lysis. Improvements in hemispherical shell and liner locking mechanism, reduction in screw holes that may be a pathway for debris to access the pelvis, and the use of one-piece liner-shell components may eliminate potential sources of particle debris.

The most important focus of current research has been on the bearing surface, specifically the polyethylene. Improvements in quality of polyethylene leading to improved wear characteristics as well as searching for alternative bearing surfaces will hopefully eliminate the major problem of particle-driven osteolysis. It is hoped that elimination of particle-driven osteolysis will enhance the longevity of all arthroplasties.

SUMMARY

The reconstruction of a failed acetabular component present one of the most difficult challenges to any orthopedic surgeon. The use of cementless porous acetabular components supplemented with bone graft has led to predictable, reproducible results. The ability to use bone graft to restore bone stock and obtain stable fixation of the socket, with either interference fit or adjuvant screw fixation, has been successful for most classes of acetabular deficiencies. This method of reconstruction appears to be the treatment of choice for the majority of hips requiring revision acetabular surgery.

REFERENCES

1. Amstutz HC, Ma SM, Jinnah RH, Mai L. Revision of aseptic loose total hip arthroplasties. *Clin Orthop* 1982;170:21–33.
2. Ayerza M, Pierson RH III, Sheinkop M, Rosenberg AG, Landon G, Galante JO. A clinical review of a conical screw-in acetabular design. *Orthop Trans* 1988;12:662.
3. Berman AT, Iorio R, Marine JM. Classification and staging system for revision total hip arthroplasty. *Scientific exhibit presented at the annual meeting of the American Academy of Orthopaedic Surgeons*, New Orleans, LA, February 1990.
4. Berry DJ, Chandler HP, Reilley DT. The use of bone allografts in two stage reconstruction after failure of hip replacement due to infection. *J Bone Joint Surg* 1991;73A:1460.
5. Berry DJ, Muller ME. Revision arthroplasty using an anti-protrusio cage for massive acetabular bone deficiency. *J Bone Joint Surg* 1992;74B:711.
6. Berrey BH, Lord FC, Gebhardt MC, Mankin HS. Fracture of allografts. *J Bone Joint Surg* 1990;72A:825.
7. Bobyn JD, Pilliar RM, Cameron HU, Weatherly GC, Dent GM. The effect of porous surface configuration on the tensile strength of fixation of implants by bone ingrowth. *Clin Orthop* 1980;149:291.
8. Bono JV, Sanford L, Toussaint JT. Severe polyethylene wear in total hip arthroplasty. *J Arthroplasty*, 1994;9(2):119–125.
9. Borja FJ, Mnaymeh W. Bone allografts in salvage of difficult hip arthroplasties. *Clin Orthop* 1984;197:123.
10. Brien WW, Bruce WJ, Salvati EA, Wilson PD Jr, Pellicci PM. Acetabular reconstruction with a bipolar prosthesis and morseled bone grafts. *J Bone Joint Surg* 1990;72A:1230–1235.
11. Callaghan JJ, Salvati EA, Pellicci PM, Wilson PD Jr, Ranawat CS. Results of revision for mechanical failure after cemented total hip replacement, 1979 to 1982. *J Bone Joint Surg* 1985;67A:1074–1085.
12. Cobb TK, Morrey BF. The elevated-rim acetabular liner in total hip arthroplasty: relationship to postoperative dislocations. *J Bone Joint Surg* 1996;78A:80–86.
13. Conn RA, Peterson LFA, Stauffer RN, Ilstrup D. Management of acetabular deficiency; long-term results of bone grafting the acetabulum in total hip arthroplasty. *Orthop Trans* 1985;9:451–452.
14. Chandler HP, Penenberg BI. Bone stock deficiency in total hip replacement. Classification and management. Thorofare, NJ: Slack; 1989.
15. Chandler HP. Use of allografts and prostheses in the reconstruction of failed total hip replacements. *Orthopedics* 1992;15:1207.
16. D'Antonio JA. Periprosthetic bone loss of the acetabulum. *Orthop Clin North Am* 1992;23:279.
17. D'Antonio JA, Capello WN, Borden LS, Bargar WL, Bierbaum BF, Boettcher WG, Steinberg ME, Stulberg SD, Wedge JH. Classification and management of acetabular abnormalities in total hip arthroplasty. *Clin Orthop* 1989;243:126–131.
18. Dartee DA, Huij J, Tonino AJ. Bank bone grafts in revision hip arthroplasty for acetabular protrusion. *Acta Orthop Scand* 1988;59:513.
19. DeLee DG, Charnley J. Radiological demarcation of cemented sockets in total hip replacement. *Clin Orthop* 1976;121:20–32.
20. Emerson RH Jr, Head WC, Berklacich FM, Malinin TI. Non-cemented acetabular revision arthroplasty using allograft bone. *Clin Orthop* 1989;249:30–43.
21. Engh CA, Glassman AH, Griffin WL, Mayer JG. Results of cementless revision for failed total hip arthroplasty. *Clin Orthop* 1988;235:91–110.
22. Frick S, Tsahakis PJ, Barr S, Peindl R, Brick GW. Distal femoral allografts for the reconstruction of structural acetabular defects in revision total hip arthroplasty: a clinical study with biomechanical correlation. *Presented at the American Academy of Orthopaedic Surgeons annual scientific meeting*, New Orleans, Feb. 24–March 1, 1994.
23. Fuchs MD, Salvati EA, Wilson PD Jr, Sculco TP, Pellicci PM. Results of

acetabular revisions with newer cement techniques. *Orthop Clin North Am* 1988;19:649–655.
24. Galante JO, Rostoker W, Luick R, Ray RD. Sintered fiber composites as a basis for attachment of implants to bone. *J Bone Joint Surg* 1971;53A:101.
25. Gates HS III, McCollum DE, Poletti SC, Nunley JA. Bone grafting in total hip arthroplasty for protrusio acetabuli: a follow-up note. *J Bone Joint Surg* 1990;72A:248.
26. Goodman SB, Adler SJ, Fyhrie DP, Schurman DJ. The acetabular teardrop and its relevance to acetabular migration. *Clin Orthop* 1988;236:199–204.
27. Gordon SL, Binkert BL, Rashoff ES, Britt AR, Esser PD, Stinchfield FE. Assessment of bone grafts used for acetabular augmentation in total hip arthroplasty. *Clin Orthop* 1985;201:18.
28. Gross AE, Allan DG, Catre M, et al. Bone grafts in hip replacement surgery: the pelvic side (review). *Orthop Clin North Am* 1993;24:679.
29. Gross AE, Lavoie MV, McDermott P, Marks P. The use of allograft bone in revision of total hip arthroplasty. *Clin Orthop* 1985;197:115.
30. Hardinge K. The direct lateral approach to the hip. *J Bone Joint Surg* 1982;64B:17.
31. Harris WH. Allografting in total hip arthroplasty: in adults with severe acetabular deficiency—including a surgical technique for bolting and grafting to the ilium. *Clin Orthop* 1982;162:150–164.
32. Harris WH, Jasty M. Bone ingrowth into porous coated canine acetabular replacements: the effect of pore size, apposition, and dislocation. In: Fitzgerald RH, ed. *The hip. Proceedings of the thirteenth open scientific meeting of The Hip Society*, St. Louis, MO: CV Mosby, 1987:214–234.
33. Harris WH, Krushell RJ, Galante JO. Results of cementless revisions of total hip arthroplasties using the Harris-Galante prosthesis. *Clin Orthop* 1988;235:120–127.
34. Hedley AK, Gruen TA, Ruoff DP. Revision of failed total hip arthroplasties with uncemented porous-coated anatomic components. *Clin Orthop* 1988;235:75–90.
35. Henry JD, Brick GW, Reilly DT. Whole acetabular allograft reconstruction during revision total hip arthroplasty. *Presented at the American Academy of Orthopaedic Surgeons annual scientific meeting*, San Francisco, Feb 18–23, 1993.
36. Hodgkinson JP, Shelley P, Wroblewski BM. The correlation between the roentgenographic appearance and operative findings at the bone-cement junction of the socket in Charnley low friction arthroplasties. *Clin Orthop* 1988;228:105–109.
37. Hoikka V, Schlenzka D, Wirta J, et al. Failures after revision hip arthroplasties with threaded cups and structural bone allografts: loosening of 13/18 cases after 1-4 years. *Acta Orthop Scand* 1993;34:403.
38. Hooten JP, Engh CA Jr, Engh CA. Failure of structural acetabular allografts in cementless revision hip arthroplasty. *J Bone Joint Surg* 1994;76B:419.
39. Huo MH, Friedlander GE, Salvati EA. Bone graft and total hip arthroplasty; a review. *J Arthroplasty* 1992;7:109.
40. Hunter GA, Welsh RP, Cameron HU, Bailey WH. The results of revision total hip arthroplasty. *J Bone Joint Surg* 1979;61B(4):419–421.
41. Jacobs JJ, Kull LR, Frey GA, Gitelis S, Sheinkop MB, Kramer T, Rosenberg AG. Early failure of acetabular components inserted without cement after previous pelvic irradiation. *J Bone Joint Surg* 1995;77A:1829–1835.
42. Jasty M, Harris WH. Results of total hip reconstruction using acetabular mesh in patients with central acetabular deficiency. *Clin Orthop* 1988;237:142–149.
43. Jasty MJ, Harris WH. Salvage total hip reconstruction in patients with major acetabular deficiency using structural femoral head allografts. *J Bone Joint Surg* 1990;72B:63–67.
44. Johnston RC, Brand RA, Crowninshield RD. Reconstruction of the hip: a mathematical approach to determine optimum geometric relationship. *J Bone Joint Surg* 1979;61A:639.
45. Johnston RC, Fitzgerald RH, Harris WH, Poss R, Muller ME, Sledge CB. Clinical and radiographic evaluation of total hip replacement. *J Bone Joint Surg* 1990;72A:161–168.
46. Kavanagh BF, Ilstrup DM, Fitzgerald RH Jr. Revision total hip arthroplasty. *J Bone Joint Surg* 1985;67A:517–526.
47. Keating EM, Ritter MA, Faris PM. Structures at risk from medially placed acetabular screws. *J Bone Joint Surg* 1990;72A:509–511.
48. Kelley SS. High hip center in revision arthroplasty. *J Arthroplasty* 1994;9:503.
49. Kienapfel H, Sumner DR, Turner TM, Urban RM, McLeod BC, Skipor

AK, Yang A, Galante JO. Efficacy of autograft, freeze dried allograft and fibrin glue to enhance fixation of porous coated implants in the presence of interface gaps. *Trans ORS* 1990;15:432.

50. Kim YS, Callaghan JJ, Ahn PB, Brown TD. Fracture of the acetabulum during insertion of an oversized hemispherical component. *J Bone Joint Surg* 1995;77A:111–117.

51. Kwong LM, Jasty M, Harris WH. High failure rate of bulk femoral head allografts in total hip acetabular reconstructions at 10 years. *J Arthroplasty* 1993;8:341.

52. Madsen-Cummings N, Brick GW, Reilly DT, Poss R. Acetabular reconstruction with allograft and fixed uncemented cups in revision total hip arthroplasty. *Presented at the American Academy of Orthopaedic Surgeons annual scientific meeting*, New Orleans, Feb. 8–13, 1990.

53. Massin P, Schmidt L, Engh CA. Evaluation of cementless acetabular component migration. *J Arthroplasty* 1989;4:245.

54. McGann WA, Mankin HJ, Harris WH. Massive allografting for severe failed total hip replacement. *J Bone Joint Surg* 1986;68A:4.

55. McGann WA, Welch RB, Picetti GD. Acetabular preparation in cementless revision total hip arthroplasty. *Clin Orthop* 1988;235:35–46.

56. Muldoon MP, Padgett DE, Rothen R, Cady GW, Melillo AS. Failure of a non-porous coated acetabular component inserted without cement in primary total hip arthroplasty. *J Bone Joint Surg* 1996;78A:1486–1491.

57. Mulroy RD, Harris WH. Failure of acetabular autogenous grafts in total hip arthroplasty. *J Bone Joint Surg* 1990;72A:1536–1540.

58. Murray WR. Salvage of acetabular insufficiency with bipolar prostheses. In: Welch RB, ed. *Proceedings of the twelfth open scientific meeting of the Hip Society*. St. Louis: CV Mosby, 1984;296.

59. Nestor BJ, Hanssen AD, Ferrer-Gonzalez R, Fitzgerald RH. The use of porous prostheses in delayed reconstruction of total hip replacements that have failed because of infection. *J Bone Joint Surg* 1994;76A: 349–359.

60. Oakeshott RD, Morgan DAF, Zuker DJ, Rudan JF, Brooks PJ, Gross AE. Revision total hip arthroplasty with osseous allograft reconstruction. *Clin Orthop* 1987;225:37.

61. Padgett DE, Kull L, Rosenberg AG, Sumner DR, Galante JO. Revision of the acetabular component without cement after total hip arthroplasty. *J Bone Joint Surg* 1993;75A:663–673.

62. Paprosky WG, Lawrence J, Cameron HU. Acetabular defect classification: clinical application. *Orthop Rev* 1990;19(suppl):23–35.

63. Paprosky WG, Lawrence JM, Cameron HU. Classification and treatment of failed acetabulum: a systematic approach. *Contemp Orthop* 1991;22:121.

64. Paprosky WG, Magnus RE. Principles of bone grafting in revision total hip arthroplasty: acetabular technique. *Clin Orthop* 1994;298:147.

65. Paprosky WG, Perona PG, Lawrence JM. Acetabular defect classification and surgical reconstruction in revision arthroplasty. *J Arthroplasty* 1994;9:33.

66. Pellicci PM, Wilson PD Jr, Sledge CB, Salvati EA, Ranawat CS, Poss RB. Revision total hip arthroplasty. *Clin Orthop* 1982;170:34–41.

67. Pellicci PM, Wilson PD Jr, Sledge CB, Salvati EA, Ranawat CS, Poss R, Callaghan JJ. Long term results of total hip replacement. *J Bone Joint Surg* 1985;67A:513–516.

68. Petrera P, Trakru S, Mehta S, Steed D, Towers JD, Rubash HE. Revision total hip arthroplasty with a retroperitoneal approach to the iliac vessels. *J Arthroplasty* 1996;11(6):704–708.

69. Pollock FH, Whiteside LA. The fate of massive allografts in total hip acetabulat revision surgery. *J Arthroplasty* 1992;7:271.

70. Ranawat CS, Dorr LD, Inglis AE. Total hip arthroplasty in protrusio acetabula of rheumatoid arthritis. *J Bone Joint Surg* 1980;62A: 1059–1065.

71. Rossen J, Schatzker J. The use of reinforcement rings to reconstruct deficient acetabula. *J Bone Joint Surg* 1992;74B:987.

72. Russotti GM, Harris WH. Proximal placement of the acetabular component in total hip arthroplasty. *J Bone Joint Surg* 1991;73A:587–592.

73. Salvati EA, Bullough P, Wilson Jr PD. Intrapelvic protrusion of the acetabular component following total hip replacement. *Clin Orthop* 1975;111:212–227.

74. Samuelson KM, Freeman MAR, Levak B, et al. Homograft bone in revision acetabular arthroplasty: a clinical and radiographic study. *J Bone Joint Surg* 1988;70B:367.

75. Scott RD. Use of a bipolar prostheses with bone grafting in acetabular reconstruction. *Contemp Orthop* 1984;9:35.

76. Silverton C, Rosenberg AG, Sheinkop MB, Kull LR, Galante JO. Revision of the acetabular component without cement after total hip arthroplasty. A follow-up note regarding results at seven to eleven years. *J Bone Joint Surg* 1996;78A:1366–1370.

77. Sloof TJ, Huiskes R, Van Horn J, Lemmens AJ. Bone grafting in total hip replacements for acetabular protrusion. *Acta Orthop Scand* 1984;55:593.

78. Sloof TJ, Schimmel JW, Buma P. Cemented fixation with bone grafts. *Orthop Clin North Am* 1993;24:667.

79. Sumner DR, Jasty M, Turner TM, Urban R, Galante JO, Bragdon C, Harris WH. Bone ingrowth in porous coated cementless acetabular components retrieved from human patients. *Trans ORS* 1987;12:509.

80. Sutherland CJ. Radiographic evaluation of acetabular bone stock in failed total hip arthroplasty. *J Arthroplasty* 1988;3:73.

81. Sutherland CJ. Treatment of type III acetabular deficiencies in revision total hip arthroplasty without structural bone-graft. *J Arthroplasty* 1996; 11:91–98.

82. Tanzer M, Drucker D, Jasty M, McDonald M, Harris WH. Revision of acetabular component with an uncemented Harris-Galante porous coated prosthesis. *J Bone Joint Surg* 1982;74A:987–994.

83. Tooke SM, Nugent PJ, Chotivichit A, Goodman W, Kabo JM. Comparison of in vivo cementless acetabular fixation. *Clin Orthop* 1988;235: 253–260.

84. Trancik TM, Stulberg BN, Wilde AH, Feiglin DH. Allograft reconstruction of the acetabulum during revision total hip arthroplasty. *J Bone Joint Surg* 1986;68A:527.

85. Wasielewski RC, Britton C, Donaldson T, Rubash HE. Acetabular anatomy and transacetabular screw fixation in acetabular arthroplasty at the high hip center. *J Bone Joint Surg* 1997 *(submitted)*.

86. Wasielewski RC, Cooperstein LA, Kruger MP, Rubash HE. Acetabular anatomy and the transacetabular fixation of screws in total hip arthroplasty. *J Bone Joint Surg* 1990;72A:501–508.

87. Weber BJ. Total hip replacement revision surgery: surgical technique and experience. In: *The hip*. St. Louis: CV Mosby, 1981:3–14.

88. White RE, Cook J. Resorption of large intrapelvic bone grafts for medial acetabular defects in cementless revision total hip replacement. *Presented at the 56th annual meeting of the American Academy of Orthopaedic Surgeons*, Las Vegas, Nevada, Feb. 9, 1989.

89. Wilson-MacDonald J, Morscher E, Masar Z. Cementless uncoated polyethylene acetabular components in total hip replacement. *J Bone Joint Surg* 1990;72B(3):423–430.

90. Wilson MG, Nikpoor N, Aliabi P, Poss R, Weissman BN. The fate of acetabular allografts after bipolar revision arthroplasty of the hip. A radiographic review. *J Bone Joint Surg* 1989;71A:1469–1479.

91. Wilson MG, Scott RD. Reconstruction of the deficient acetabulum using the bipolar socket. *Clin Orthop* 1990;251:126.

92. Yoder SA, Brand RA, Pedersen DR, O'Gorman TW. Total hip acetabular component position affects component loosening rates. *Clin Orthop* 1988;228:79–87.

93. Zehntner MK, Ganz R. Midterm results (5.5-10 years) of acetabular allograft reconstruction with the acetabular reinforcement ring during total hip revision. *J Arthroplasty* 1994;9:469.

94. Zmolek JC, Dorr LD. Revision total hip arthroplasty: the use of solid allograft. *J Arthroplasty* 1993;8:361.

The Adult Hip, edited by J. J. Callaghan,
A. G. Rosenberg, and H. E. Rubash.
Lippincott–Raven Publishers, Philadelphia © 1998.

CHAPTER 88

Structural Grafting in Acetabular Reconstruction

Hugh P. Chandler and Russell G. Tigges

The longest experience with structural weight-bearing grafts used to reconstruct bone defects has been with the acetabulum. In 1977, Harris et al. reported their experience with structural autogenous femoral head grafts (12). In 1982, Harris described a technique of bolting autologous femoral heads to the deficient ilium and cementing a polyethylene cup in place (11). There are many other reports of good short-term results with autograft and allograft augmentation of the acetabulum combined with cemented sockets (7,8,12,15,19,25–27). However, the mid- and long-term results of structural grafting of the acetabulum have had mixed reviews (4,11,13,14,16,18, 21–24,32–34). Gerber and Harris (8) reported an 8.5% aseptic loosening at 7-year follow-up with structural grafts used with cemented sockets. Mulroy and Harris (23), reviewing the same group of patients, reported a 46% failure at 11.8 years. They no longer recommend the use of bulk acetabular grafts except for extreme deficiencies. However, Gross and Catre (10) had 100% graft union and only a 6% failure rate using an autogenous femoral head grafts, with a follow-up of 99 months. They felt that their better results were related to an older patient population (less active), less graft coverage of the implant (28% versus 42%), and differences in surgical technique.

With the early success of cementless total hip arthroplasties, this method of fixation was also used with bulk acetabular grafts (30,31). Hooten et al. reported a 44% failure rate at an average follow-up of 29 months when femoral head and distal femoral allografts were used with

uncemented components (15). They noted an increased risk of failure of an uncemented acetabular component when less than 50% of the host bone was in contact with the implant. Paprosky and Magnus had a 4% incidence of migration of uncemented acetabular components used against structural grafts at an average of 5.7 years of follow-up (26). In a second series, Paprosky et al. reported a 70% failure rate in porous cups when more than 60% of the surface of the acetabular component was in contact with the allograft (27). These poor results were in contrast to those with cemented acetabular components, used with whole structural acetabular grafts, where there was a 100% survival rate at 5.1 years of follow-up (33).

The purpose of this chapter is to report our experience with structural acetabular grafts and to outline the principles that are important, not only for acetabular grafts, but for all structural weight-bearing grafts.

TREATMENT OPTIONS FOR THE DEFICIENT ACETABULUM

If the rim is capable of providing stability to an uncemented component, intra-acetabular defects, protrusio of the medial wall, and perforation of the medial wall can all be treated with nonstructural morselized bone (2). Allograft morselized bone seems to work as well as autograft bone. Small uncemented components can be used in a high center of rotation (24.30,31). There is a place for very large jumbo cups (above 70 mm) when an intact but expanded rim is present. Oblong cups can be used when only a superior defect is present and there is adequate

    H. P. Chandler and R. G. Tigges: Department of Orthopaedics, Massachusetts General Hospital, Boston, Massachusetts 02114.

anterior and posterior bone stock. Protrusio cages, combined with morselized bone and cemented components, are also helpful with major central perforations. In primary total hip replacement for dysplastic hips with a small superior defect, deliberately creating a controlled central defect with medialized reamers, grafting the defect with morselized bone from the reamers, and press-fitting an uncemented component to the rim is a viable option. With larger superior defects, use of cement to fill the defect, combined with cemented acetabular components, has been shown to be successful, but we have no experience with this technique (21).

INDICATIONS FOR STRUCTURAL GRAFTING OF THE ACETABULUM

With all of these treatment options now available, structural acetabular grafts are rarely necessary. There are only two indications now for structural grafting of the acetabulum. The first is a deficient rim that will not support an uncemented component. This may occur in the primary hip with developmental dysplasia of the hip (DDH) with significant superior rim deficiency and in the revision circumstance with significant segmental loss of the rim. The second indication is major global deficiency of the acetabulum.

RESULTS OF STRUCTURAL ACETABULAR GRAFTS

In 1995, we reviewed 24 patients with 24 grafts that were followed for a minimum of 10 years and an average of 12½ years (2). There are now 29 grafts in 26 patients that have been followed for a minimum of 10 years.

There were nine primary hips and 20 revisions. Five of the nine primary hips had undergone previous surgery, and the 20 patients with revisions each had an average of three previous hip operations.

There are five areas of interest concerning the results of structural acetabular grafts. These are union of the graft, survival of the graft, survival of the acetabular component, function of the patient, and complications related to the procedure.

Union

Radiographic union of the graft to the host was often difficult to determine, as immediate postoperative radiographs frequently showed no lucency between the graft and the host bone, and follow-up radiographs showed no interval changes. If there was an initial gap between the graft and the host, union was assumed to have occurred when this gap had radiographically disappeared. There were two definite nonunions (7%), and both patients had proven sepsis. Union probably occurred in all the remaining patients (93%).

Survival of the Graft

Minor peripheral resorption occurred in virtually all superior rim grafts. This resorption was in the peripheral area of the graft that was not subjected to weight-bearing forces (lateral to the cup). Washers that were used with lag screws in this area commonly migrated proximally up to 5 to 10 mm. This type of peripheral resorption was usually evident by the second year and was not progressive (Figs. 1,2,3,4).

Of the 29 structural grafts, six (20%) failed. Two failed because of sepsis. There were four nonseptic failures (13%). There were technical errors at the time of the index grafting procedure in all the failed aseptic grafts. These errors include a poor choice of bone in two procedures, failure to use cement in one graft, and transverse trabeculae screws in all. Two autografts failed. One femoral head autograft had been previously used beneath a cup arthroplasty. The cemented acetabular component required revision because of loosening at 18 years. Further grafting was not necessary, but the majority of the graft had resorbed. A second femoral head autograft had previously been used beneath a surface replacement (Fig.

FIG. 1. A: This 76-year-old woman had degenerative arthritis secondary to DDH. The femoral head is in a false acetabulum. **B:** The head is scuffed with an oscillating saw to remove soft tissues. It is not necessary to remove the cortex. **C:** The acetabulum is curetted to remove soft tissues. **D:** The relationship of the head and the acetabulum is previously marked with the hip in extension, prior to dividing the neck. The head is placed back in the acetabulum, matching these marks, to ensure that the trabeculae are anatomically aligned. The head is temporarily fixed with three smooth wires that are used in the area where the new acetabulum was eventually placed. **E:** After the acetabulum is reamed, a preliminary thin bead of cement is placed at the graft–host junction and allowed to harden to prevent the final cement from intruding between the graft and the host. **F:** The false acetabulum acts as a buttress. The trabeculae of the head are anatomically aligned with weight-bearing forces. Three cancellous screws are placed in the periphery of the head. The screws are parallel and aligned with weight-bearing forces. There should be no threads in the graft so the head can impact against the buttress. The screws bear no weight, but just hold the graft against the buttress. The acetabular component should be cemented. **G:** At 12 years, 4 months, the graft and the patient are doing well.

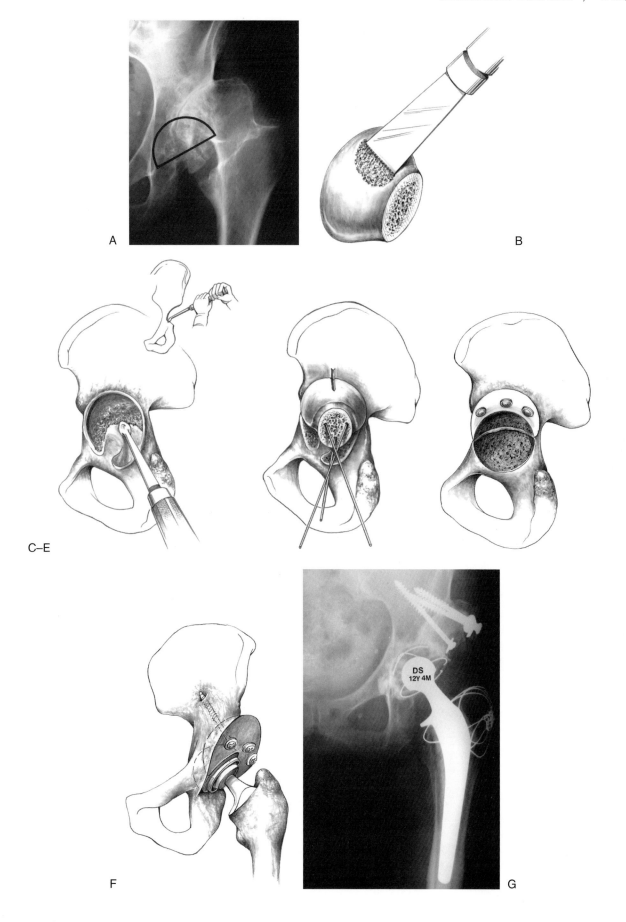

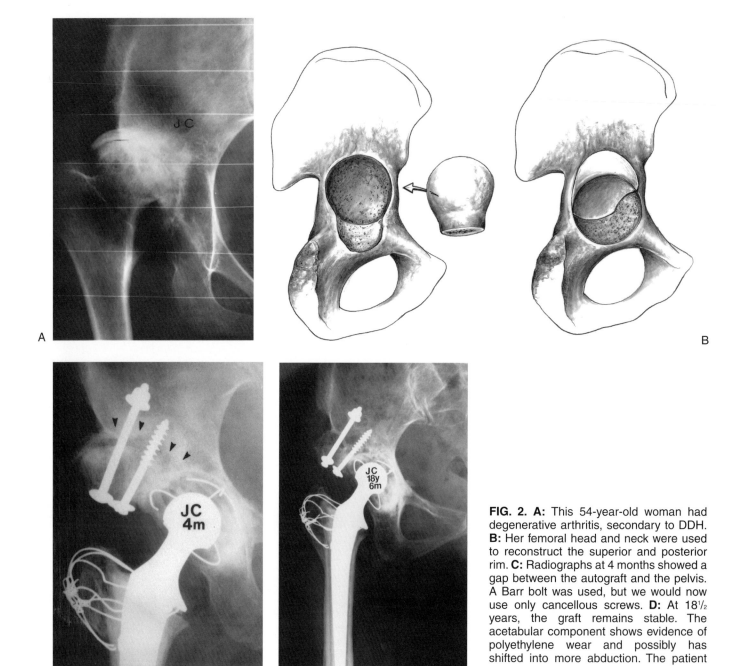

FIG. 2. A: This 54-year-old woman had degenerative arthritis, secondary to DDH. **B:** Her femoral head and neck were used to reconstruct the superior and posterior rim. **C:** Radiographs at 4 months showed a gap between the autograft and the pelvis. A Barr bolt was used, but we would now use only cancellous screws. **D:** At 18½ years, the graft remains stable. The acetabular component shows evidence of polyethylene wear and possibly has shifted into more abduction. The patient has minimal symptoms.

FIG. 3. A: This 60-year-old man had DDH with degenerative arthritis. **B:** His femoral head was used to reconstruct the superior rim. **C:** The junction between the graft and the host is hard to determine in the postoperative radiographs. The screws are more transverse than ideal. **D:** At 19 years, 10 months, the graft and the patient continue to do well.

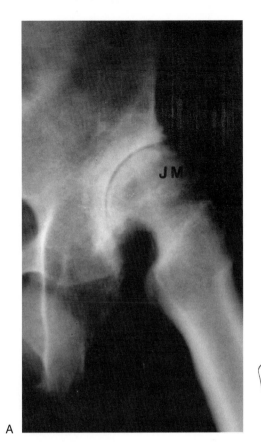

A

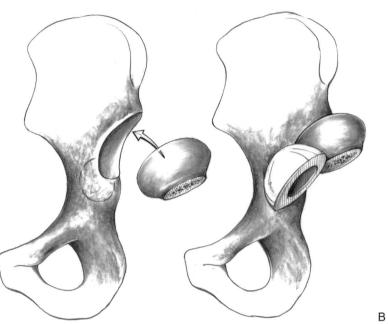

B

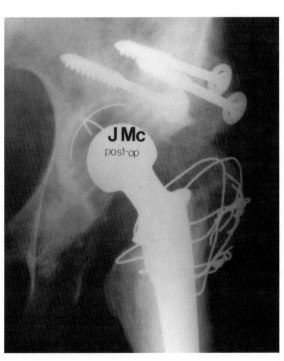

C

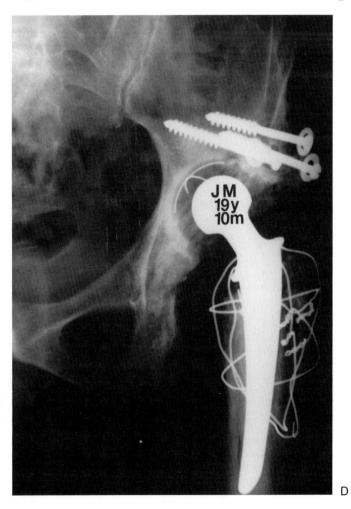

D

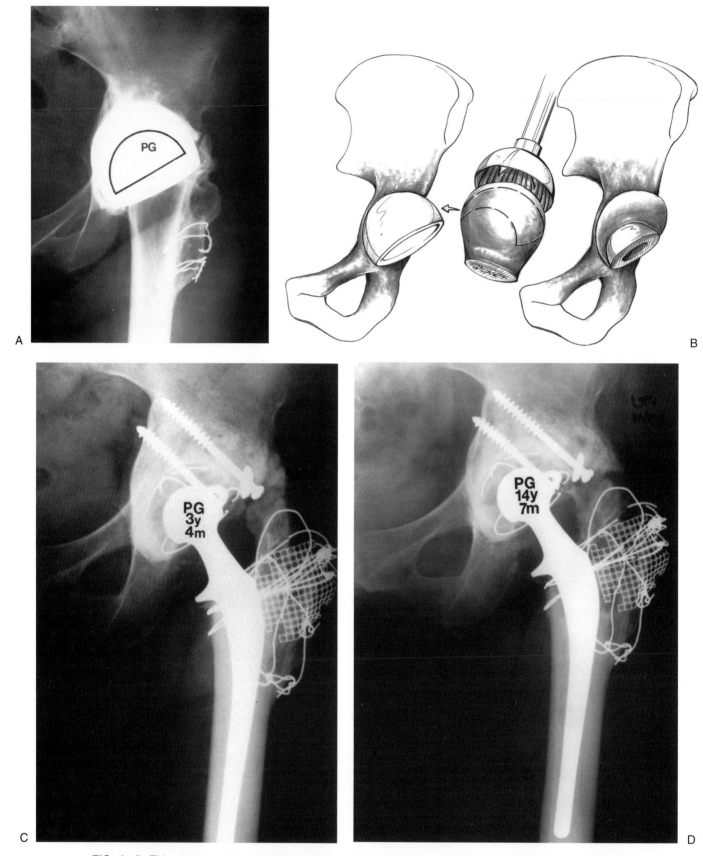

FIG. 4. A: This 40-year-old woman had a painful left hip after two failed mold arthroplasties. **B:** The acetabulum was reamed with a male reamer. A very large allograft femoral head was reamed with a female reamer of the same size. **C:** At 3 years, 4 months, there is mild peripheral resorption of the graft in the area that is not stressed and the washers have migrated medially a bit. **D:** At 14 years, 7 months, the graft and the patient continue to do well. The acetabular component is entirely supported by the graft.

5). Cement was not used and revision was required at $3^{1}/_{2}$ years after surgery. The graft had resorbed significantly and another allograft was necessary. Both of these autograft heads were of poor quality and were probably involved with the repair process of avascular necrosis. Two allografts failed. One patient had major resorption of a distal femoral allograft used in the left hip and required revision 5 years after surgery (Fig. 6). The trabeculae of the graft were inadvertently placed transverse to weight-bearing forces. An identical procedure was performed on the patient's right hip except for the fact that the trabeculae were properly aligned (Fig. 7). The right hip of this patient continues to do well $12^{1}/_{2}$ years after the grafting procedure. A second patient has had major radiographic resorption of a femoral head allograft but still functions well at $14^{1}/_{2}$ years with a Harris rating of 96. The cemented acetabular component does not show radiographic evidence of loosening.

Survival of the Acetabular Component

There were 11 acetabular components that were loose at final follow-up (38%). Two were loose because of sepsis.

There were nine nonseptic acetabular components that were loose (31%). In four patients, the acetabular component failed because the graft failed. In four other patients, loosening of the acetabular component occurred, but the graft was largely intact and further grafting was not required at revision. In one of these patients, a sintered acetabular component was cemented to the graft but was press-fit to viable host bone at the time of the index grafting procedure. This was an obvious error in judgment and the component loosened at $9^{1}/_{2}$ years. One uncemented acetabular component was used in conjunction with an allograft and loosened at 2 years (see Fig. 5G). At rerevision, the graft was largely intact and appeared to be revascularized. A new uncemented acetabular component was used, but, at the 8-year follow-up, the patient is mildly symptomatic and the acetabular component has probably shifted in position as seen on most recent radiographs.

Ten components have been revised. Two of the ten revisions have required a second allograft. The average time of failure for the nonseptic cases was just under 9 years (range, $3^{1}/_{2}$ to 18 years). None of the nonseptic patients had precipitous failure of their acetabular components and most were followed for several years before symptoms required revision.

For the whole series, the average coverage of the acetabular component by the graft was 60% (range, 20% to 100%). We did not find a correlation between the percentage of coverage by the graft and failure of the acetabular component. The average coverage of the acetabular component in the patients that did not loosen was 57%, and in those that had acetabular loosening, it was 64%. These differences are not statistically significant.

Function of the Patient

The average Harris rating preoperatively was 43 and postoperatively was 81, including the failures. If the failures are eliminated, the rating at follow-up of the remaining patients was 93.

Complications Related to the Procedure

Sepsis is clearly a catastrophic complication and there were two patients (6.4%) in this small series with this problem. One of these patients had undergone five previous hip operations, including three total hip replacements, but did not have a previous history of sepsis. *Staphylococcus aureus* infection was identified and resection arthroplasty was performed 5 months after the index graft. This patient subsequently had a second allograft and the new graft is still intact $12^{1}/_{2}$ years after surgery without evidence of sepsis. The second patient with sepsis had undergone ten previous hip operations including seven total hip replacements. He had a recurrence of a previous *Pseudomonas* infection. In the early years of this study, laminar flow operating rooms combined with body exhaust systems were not available, but we now use these techniques in all arthroplasties.

One patient, with four previous hip operations, had a laceration of the iliac artery that was repaired without subsequent vascular problems.

There were four dislocations. All were treated with closed reduction and functional bracing for 6 weeks. None required revision.

CURRENT TECHNIQUES FOR STRUCTURAL BONE GRAFTS FOR THE ACETABULUM

As we have looked back at our long-term experience with structural acetabular grafts, particularly looking at those that have failed and comparing failures to those that have succeeded, it is obvious that the success or failure of such grafts is distinctly related to technique. Factors that affect the results of structural grafts include exposure, choice of graft material, trabecular orientation, fixation of the graft, fixation of the acetabular component, and postoperative management.

Surgical Exposure. It is necessary to have adequate exposure to do difficult reconstructions. Our choice for most easy structural grafts is the transtrochanteric approach, which provides good superior exposure of the acetabulum. The extended iliofemoral approach gives excellent and extensive exposure to the iliac wing, the anterior and posterior columns, and the ischium. The

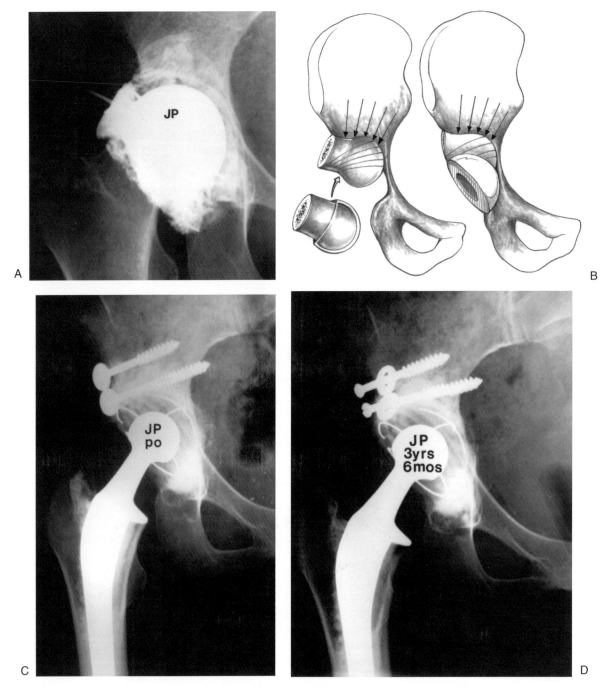

FIG. 5. A: This 40-year-old woman had DDH. The original operation was a surface replacement that failed at 4 years. **B:** The patient's femoral head (beneath the surface replacement) was used as an autograft. The trabeculae were placed transverse to the weight-bearing axis. The head was of poor quality and probably was involved with avascular necrosis. **C:** The screws were placed transversely. **D:** The graft resorbed completely and the acetabular component required revision because of loosening at 3½ years.

ilioinguinal approach provides exposure of the pubic ramus, allowing for the use of anterior column plates. We have used the extended iliofemoral approach, combined with conventional trochanteric osteotomy and with the ilioinguinal approach, in only two patients. This exposure is extraordinary. One of these patients developed a minor breakdown at the junction of the two approaches and required debridement and later secondary closure. If these approaches are combined, it is essential that the skin incision over the pubis intersect the extended iliofemoral incision at 90-degree angles to prevent skin necrosis.

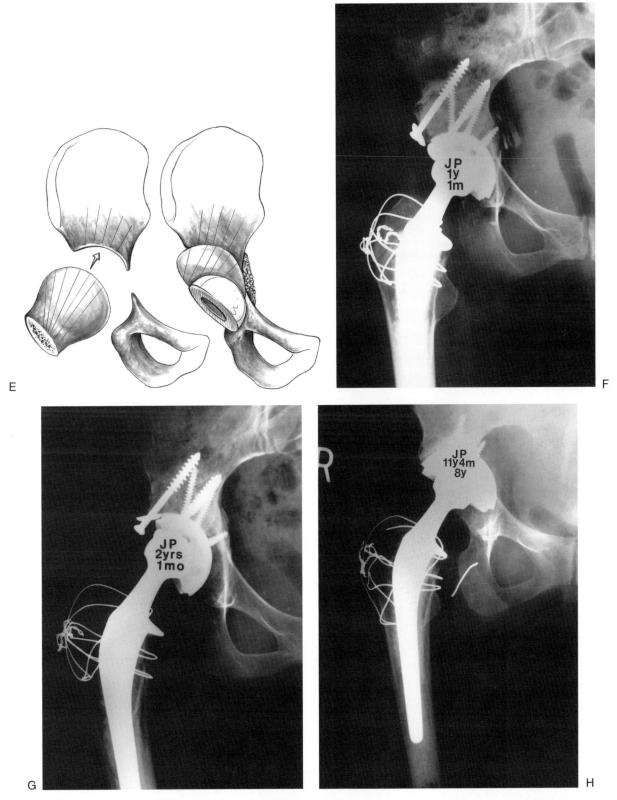

FIG. 5. *Continued.* **E:** A new femoral head allograft was necessary. The trabeculae were properly oriented. **F:** The graft was technically done well but the acetabular component was not cemented. **G:** The acetabular component loosened at 2 years. **H:** A new uncemented component was used because the previous allograft had incorporated and bled well. The graft is intact at 12 years, 4 months. At 8 years after revision, the patient has mild symptoms with a possibly loose acetabular component.

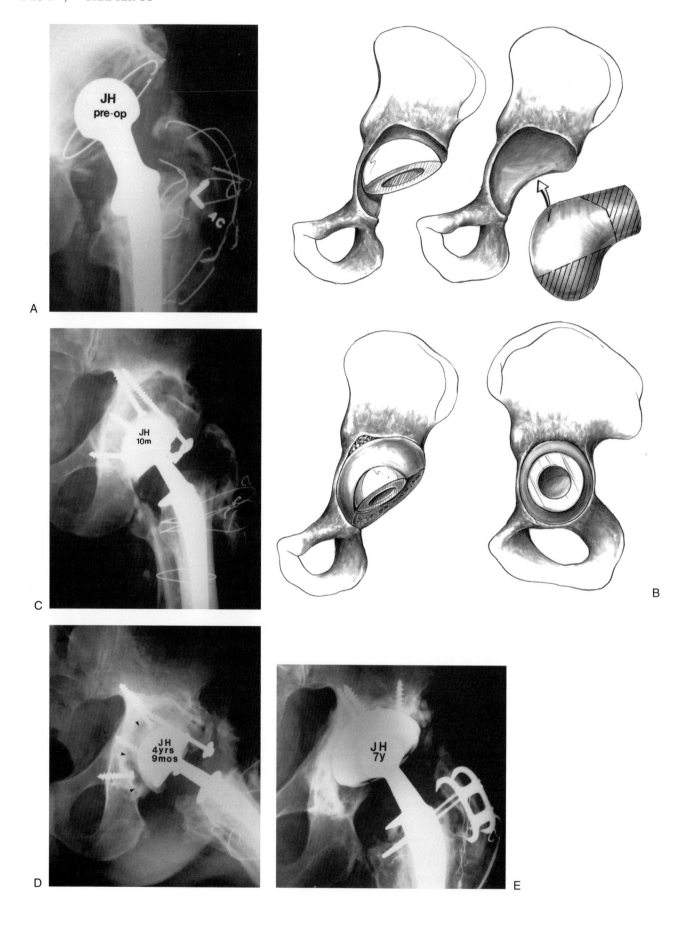

Choice of Graft Material. Autograft heads are ideal sources of bone grafts in patients with subluxed hips who have DDH. Despite the fact that femoral heads beneath mold arthroplasties or surface replacements are potential autografts, they are usually small and are apt to be involved with avascular necrosis (see Fig. 5B,C,D). Large allograft femoral heads from active young patients are inexpensive and easily available. Small heads from elderly osteopenic women are helpful only to provide morselized bone.

Distal femurs and proximal tibias can be used for larger defects. An allograft hemipelvis can be used for major global bone loss. One of the most useful sources of allograft bone is the acetabulum itself (Fig. 8).

Trabecular Orientation. In life, the trabeculae form in response to the stresses that the bone is subjected to. With properly aligned trabeculae, structural grafts are strong enough to bear immediate full weight, and, as incorporation of cancellous bone progresses, new bone is added to the dead trabeculae and the graft becomes even stronger (6,32). However, if the trabeculae of the graft are placed transverse to weight-bearing forces, they will routinely fracture and the graft will always fail (see Fig. 6B,C,D).

Fixation of the Graft. The graft must be placed beneath a buttress of host bone that is capable of bearing weight (see Fig. 1F). The graft must fit the host defect accurately to give optimal chance for bony union. It is often easier to change complex host and graft geometries to simple flat or hemispherical shapes to make an accurate fit easier to achieve (see Fig. 4B). Temporary fixation can be achieved by two or three smooth K-wires, usually placed in the area where the new acetabulum will be placed (see Fig. 1D). Permanent fixation is often satisfactory with three lag screws that are aligned with weight-bearing forces (see Fig. 1F). Screws that are placed perpendicular to the axis of weight bearing, or that have threads in the graft itself, can prevent the graft from impacting against the host buttress (see Fig. 1). Reconstruction plates are occasionally necessary for major deficiencies. If such plates are used, compression lag screws that impact the graft against the buttress should be used first. Fixation devices should never be subjected to weight-bearing loads. Such forces are resisted by the host buttress alone and fixation devices are used only to hold the graft against the buttress.

Choice of Acetabular Components. If the rim is intact, uncemented press-fit acetabular components are very helpful in primary and revision surgery, but ingrowth can never occur in the contact area between sintered surfaces and structural grafts. Grafts combined with uncemented components have not been successful (15,26,27) (see Fig. 3). We now prefer to use all-polyethylene cemented acetabular components (with methacrylate studs to ensure an optimal cement mantle) in all structural grafts if there is more than 10% or 15% contact of the cup with a structural graft that does not have a blood supply. For practical purposes, cement should be used with all structural acetabular grafts. A preliminary bead of cement between the graft and the host bone ensures that the final cement will not intrude between the graft and the host (see Fig. 1E). Bipolar components are absolutely contraindicated with structural acetabular grafts, as they will routinely erode through the graft (6,8,9).

Postoperative Management. If the trabeculae are properly aligned in the graft, and the graft is properly secured beneath the host buttress, it is strong enough to support full weight bearing immediately. Weight-bearing forces impact the graft against the buttress, stimulating union and later remodeling of the graft. Because trochanteric osteotomies are frequently required for exposure, we ask the patient to use partial weight bearing (60 to 80 pounds) for the first 6 weeks to allow healing of the trochanter, and then use full weight bearing as tolerated, regardless of whether the graft has united radiographically. If trochanteric osteotomy is not necessary, immediate full weight bearing is encouraged as comfort allows. An exception might be an entire hemipelvis allograft that is supported by anterior and posterior column plates. We would favor protecting these massive grafts with crutches and 60 pounds of weight bearing for about a year.

CONCLUSION

Structural acetabular grafts are now rarely necessary. However, if other methods are not applicable, structural grafts do work. The success or failure of such grafts is

---

FIG. 6. A: This 43-year-old man had undergone five previous operations on his left hip including a mold arthroplasty that was revised once and a total hip that was also revised once. He presented with a loose polyethylene acetabular component with an outer diameter of 74 mm. **B:** A distal femur, including both condyles, was used to construct the defect. The trabeculae of the graft were inadvertently placed transverse to the weight-bearing axis. We would now have used a jumbo uncemented acetabular component rather than a graft. **C:** At 10 months, the graft appears to have united to the host bone. The inferior screw is transverse to the weight-bearing axis. **D:** At 4 years, 9 months, there is evidence of resorption of the graft. **E:** At 5 years, revision was required. The majority of the graft had resorbed. An uncemented component was used and remains stable at 7 years.

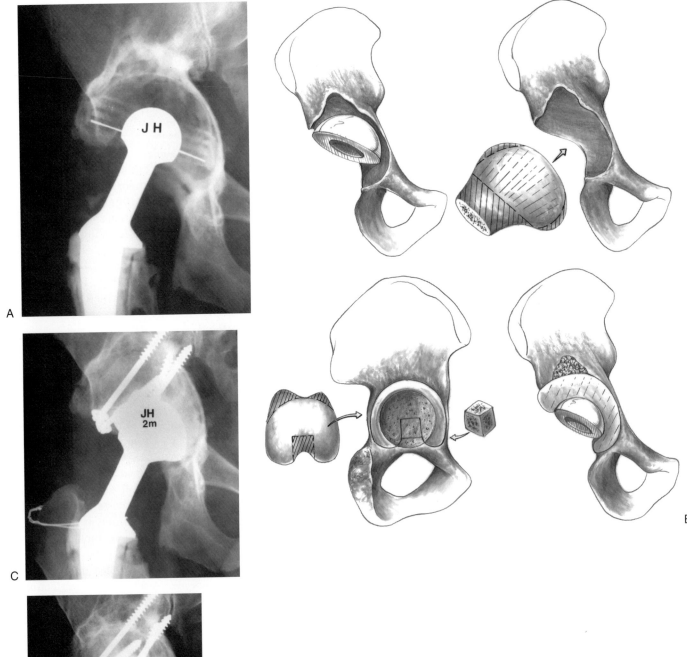

FIG. 7. A: Three years after the left hip was done, the patient required revision of his right hip for an identical acetabular problem. He had undergone nine previous operations on this hip including a Moore prosthesis, an arthrodesis, four cup arthroplasties, and three total hip replacements. **B:** The reconstruction was identical to that performed on the left hip except for the fact that the trabeculae of the femoral allograft on the right side were properly aligned with weight-bearing stresses. **C:** At 2 months, he was doing well and began to use a cane. The screws were in proper alignment. The cemented acetabular component is 100% covered by the graft. **D:** At 12 years, the acetabular component remains well fixed. Note the dramatic difference in the behavior of this graft compared to the graft in the left hip. The only difference is the fact that the trabeculae of the graft were transverse in the left hip and properly aligned in the right.

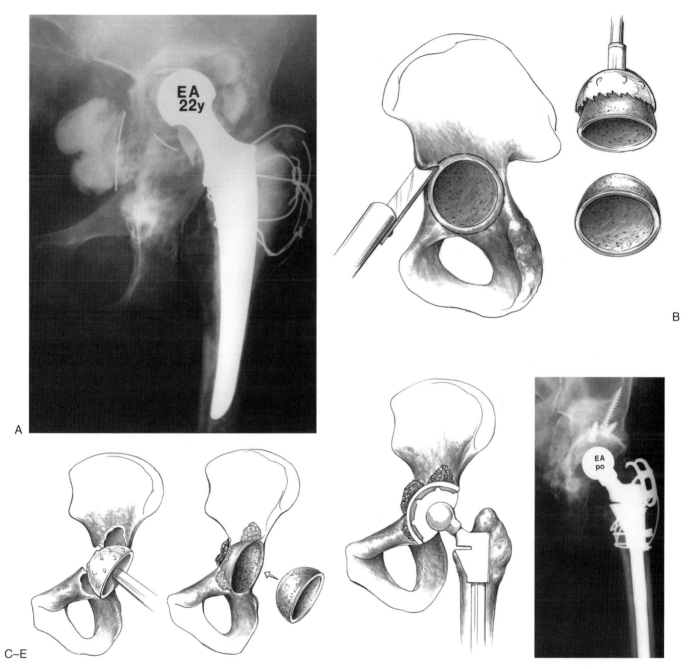

FIG. 8. A: This 60-year-old woman had DDH of both hips. She had pain and loosening 22 years after her index total hip replacement. At revision, the cement was removed through a separate retroperitoneal incision. **B:** The acetabulum from an allograft hemipelvis was removed using a saw. After rough shaping with a saw, the medial side of the allograft acetabulum was shaped with a female hemispherical reamer. **C:** The rim of the acetabular component was touched with a male reamer of the same outer diameter as the inner diameter of the female reamer. Morselized bone was packed within the acetabulum to fill the intra-acetabular defects. It was also used to fill the central defect. **D:** The allograft acetabulum was press-fit to the rim. Three screws were used in zone 1 to compress the graft to the host. A polyethylene acetabular component with methacrylate studs was cemented to the allograft. **E:** Postoperative radiographs show the allograft acetabulum is supported by the rim and by some central bone. This graft is not included in our statistical series, but this technique appears to have promise.

technique related. The principles learned in structural allografting of the acetabulum hold true in proximal femoral allografts, distal femoral grafts, and proximal tibial grafts.

REFERENCES

1. Bradford MS, Paprosky WG. Total acetabular transplant allograft reconstruction of the severely deficient acetabulum. *Semin Arthroplasty* 1995;6(2):86–95.
2. Chandler HP, Lopez C, Murphy S, Van Eenenamm DP. Acetabular reconstruction using structural grafts in total hip replacement: a 12½ year follow-up. Semin Arthroplasty 1995;6(2):118–130.
3. Emerson RH, Head WC. Dealing with the deficient acetabulum in revision hip arthroplasty. Semin Arthroplasty 1995;6(2):96–102.
4. Engh CA, Glassman AH, Griffin WL, Mayer JG. Results of cementless revision for failed cemented total hip arthroplasty. *Clin Orthop* 1989;235:91–110.
5. Engh CA, Griffin WL, Marx CL. Cementless acetabular components. *J Bone Joint Surg* 1990;72B:53–59.
6. Evans FC. Mechanical properties of bone. Springfield, IL: Charles C. Thomas, 1973.
7. Garbuz D, Morsi E, Mohamed N, Gross AE. Classification and reconstruction in revision acetabular arthroplasty with bone stock deficiency. *Clin Orthop* 1996;323:98–107.
8. Gerber SD, Harris WH. Femoral head autografting to augment acetabular deficiency in patients requiring total hip replacement: a minimum five-year and average seven-year follow-up study. *J Bone Joint Surg* 1986;68A:1241–1248.
9. Gross AE, Allan DG, Catre M, Garbuz DS, Stockley I. Bone grafts in hip replacement surgery; the pelvic side. *Orthop Clin North Am* 1993; 24(4):679–695.
10. Gross AE, Catre MG. The use of femoral head autograft shelf reconstruction and cemented acetabular component in the dysplastic hip. *Clin Orthop* 1994;298:60–66.
11. Harris WH. Allografting in total hip arthroplasty in adults with severe acetabular deficiency including a surgical technique for bolting the graft to the ilium. *Clin Orthop* 1982;162:150–164.
12. Harris WH, Crother O, Oh I. Total hip replacement and femoral-head bone grafting for severe acetabular deficiency in adults. *J Bone Joint Surg* 1977;59A:752–759.
13. Harris WH, Penenberg BL. Further follow-up on socket fixation using a metal-backed acetabular component for total hip replacement: a minimum ten-year follow-up study. *J Bone Joint Surg* 1987;69A: 1140.
14. Hasegawa Y, Iwata H, Iwase T, Kawamoto K, Iwasada S. Cementless total hip arthroplasty with autologous bone grafting for hip dysplasia. *Clin Orthop* 1996;324:179.
15. Hooten JP, Engh CA Jr, Engh CA. Failure of structural acetabular allografts in cementless revision hip arthroplasty. *J Bone Joint Surg Br* 1994;76:419–422.
16. Jasty M, Harris WH. Total hip reconstruction using frozen femoral head allografts in patients with acetabular bone loss. *Orthop Clinic North Am* 1987;18(2):291.
17. Kwong LM, Jasty M, Harris WH. High failure rate of bulk femoral head allografts in total hip acetabular reconstructions at ten years. *J Arthroplasty* 1993;8(4):341.
18. Marti RK, Schuller HM, VanSteiger MJA. Superolateral bone grafting for acetabular deficiency in primary total hip replacement and revision. *J Bone Joint Surg* 1994;76B:728.
19. McAllister CM, Border LS. Cementless acetabular reconstruction and the use of allograft in revision hip arthroplasty. *Presented at the 59th meeting of the American Academy of Orthopaedic Surgeons*, Washington, D.C., February, 1992.
20. McFarland EG, Lewellen DG, Cabanela ME. Use of bipolar endoprosthesis and bone grafting for acetabular reconstruction. *Clin Orthop* 1991;268:128.
21. McQuenry FG, Johnston RC. Coxarthrosis after congenital dysplasia: treatment by total hip arthroplasty without acetabular bone-grafting. *J Bone Joint Surg* 1988;70A:1140.
22. Morsi E, Garbuz D. Stockley I, Catre M, Gross AE. Total hip replacement in dysplastic hips using femoral head shelf autografts. *Clin Orthop* 1996;324:164.
23. Mulroy JG, Harris WH. Failure of acetabular autogenous grafts in total hip arthroplasty. Increasing incidence: a follow-up note. *J Bone Joint Surg* 1990;72A:1536.
24. Pagnano MW, Hanssen AD, Lewallen DG, Shaughnessy WJ. The effect of superior placement of the acetabular component on the rate of loosening after total hip arthroplasty. Long term results in patients who have Crowe type II congenital dysplasia of the hip. *J Bone Joint Surg* 1996;78A:1004–1014.
25. Papagelopoulos PJ, Lewellen DG. Cabanela ME, McFarland EG, Wallrichs SL. Acetabular reconstruction using bipolar endoprosthesis and bone grafting in patients with severe bone deficiency. *Clin Orthop* 1995;312:170.
26. Paprosky WG, Magnus RE. Principles of bone grafting in revision total hip arthroplasty: acetabular technique. *Clin Orthop* 1994;298:147–155.
27. Paprosky WG, Perona PG, Lawrence JM. Acetabular defect classification and surgical reconstruction in revision arthroplasty: a six year follow-up evaluation. *J Arthroplasty* 1994;9(1):33.
28. Rant VV, Stone MH, Sineg PD, Wroblewski BM. Bulk autograft for a deficient acetabulum in Charnley low-friction arthroplasty. A two–nine year follow-up study. *J Arthroplasty* 1994;9(4):393.
29. Rodriquez JA, Huk OL, Pellicci PM, Wilson PD. Autogenous bone grafts from the femoral head for the treatment of acetabular deficiency in primary total hip arthroplasty with cement: long-term results. *J Bone Joint Surg* 1995;77A:1227.
30. Russotti GM, Harris WH. Proximal placement of the acetabular component in total hip arthroplasty—A long term follow-up study. *J Bone Joint Surg Am* 1991;73:587–592.
31. Schutzer SF, Harris WH. High placement of porous coated acetabular components in complex total hip arthroplasty. *J Arthroplasty* 1994;9: 359–368.
32. Springfield DS. Massive autogenous bone grafts. *Orthop Clin North Am* 1987;18:249–256.
33. Stiehl JB. Extensive anterior column acetabular reconstruction in revision total hip arthroplasty. *Semin Arthroplasty* 1995;6(2):60–67.
34. Trancik TM, Stulberg BN, Wilde AH, Feiglin DH. Allograft reconstruction of the acetabulum during revision total hip arthroplasty. Clinical, radiographic and scintigraphic assessment of the results. *J Bone Joint Surg* 1986;68A:527.
35. Wilson MD, Nipoor MD, Alibadi P, Poss R, Weisman B. The fate of acetabular allografts after bipolar revision arthroplasty of the hip. A radiographic review. *J Bone Joint Surg* 1989;71A:

The Adult Hip, edited by J. J. Callaghan,
A. G. Rosenberg, and H. E. Rubash.
Lippincott–Raven Publishers, Philadelphia © 1998.

CHAPTER 89

Revision of the Acetabular Component: Use of Cement

William N. Capello, Edward J. Hellman, and Judy R. Feinberg

The hope that a cemented total hip replacement might be a permanent solution to the problem of advanced hip arthritis was short lived. Enthusiasm for this procedure was initially dampened by femoral loosenings (33,34), thought to be a function of deficiencies in prosthetic design and technique, both of which were considered to be solvable problems. To a large extent, this has proven to be correct. Strides made in the design of implants and in the handling of the polymethylmethacrylate have dramatically improved the results of cementing of the femoral component (21,29). Fixation of the acetabular component remains an enigma. Early cemented components remained well fixed to the pelvis for up to 10 years, but then loosening rates dramatically increased (3,11,21,31, 34,37). Unlike the situation on the femoral side, neither changes in prosthetic design nor improved cementing techniques have had a major impact on our ability to keep acetabular components secured to the pelvis with the use of bone cement (21).

CEMENTED CUP IN REVISION HIP ARTHROPLASTY

Once loosening of an acetabular component has occurred, the surgeon is faced with problems that fre-

W. N. Capello, E. J. Hellman, and J. R. Feinberg: Department of Orthopaedic Surgery, Indiana University Medical Center, Indianapolis, Indiana 46202-5111.

quently include multiple cavitary lesions and, at times, significant segmental defects in the rim of the acetabulum. Recementing into this compromised bony bed has proven to be almost universally unsuccessful. Many studies have reported mechanical failure rates between 10% and 20% at less than 10 years of follow-up (13,14,16,27) (Table 1).

Our own experience at Indiana University using cemented acetabular components in the revision setting includes 75 hips with 5-year minimum follow-up (average, 13 years). The majority of patients were women (61%), and the average age at the time of the revision surgery was 64 years (range, 33 to 87). Of these 75 hips, 12 have required re-revision (eight for aseptic loosening, one each for pain, recurrent dislocation, infection, and component failure) (Fig. 1). Therefore the re-revision rate for aseptic loosening in this group of cemented acetabular revisions is 10.7% at the 5-year-minimum follow-up. One case of postradiation necrosis was re-revised at 2 years, with the remaining re-revisions performed between 5 and 16 years after the revision procedure. These data are consistent with other reports in the literature, and they reinforce our thinking that the routine use of cement as a means of managing acetabular revision is unjustified at the present time.

OPTIONS IN ACETABULAR REVISION ARTHROPLASTY

The difficulties in acetabular revision surgery are manifold. First, the surgeon almost invariably has to deal with a

TABLE 1. *Results of cemented cups in revision surgery*

Author (ref.)	Hips (N)	Follow-up (yr)	Hips with three-zone radiolucent lines (%)	Hips with migration (%)	Hips with aseptic revisions (%)	Mechanical failure rate (%)
Kavanaugh et al. (13)	165	4.5	117 (70.9)	15 (9.1)	3 (1.8)	21.8
Marti et al. (16)	60	8.9	7 (11.7)	3 (5.0)	3 (5.0)	10.0
Kershaw et al. (14)	60	6.3	2 (3.3)	5 (8.3)	2 (3.3)	11.6
Raut et al. (27)	387	5.5	38 (9.8)	35 (9.0)	7 (1.8)	20.6

sizable cavity that is often devoid of cancellous bone. In addition, the multiple cavitary lesions that are created by the loosening process of the previously cemented implant make it very difficult for the surgeon to thoroughly cleanse and dry the area, to then fill those cavities with cement, and, finally, to pressurize the cement. Yet another problem is the lack of containment as a function of segmental defects in the acetabular rim. These defects compound the difficulties not only in pressurizing the cement but also in obtaining a substantial interlock between the cement and the existing cancellous bone that remains in the acetabulum.

Because changes in implant designs and cement techniques have had little positive effect on the acetabular side, surgeons have continued to search for alternative methods of managing acetabular loosening. The use of the bipolar prosthesis enjoyed a certain amount of popularity, but this technique proved to be unpredictable, with high rates of migration and subsequent pain (17,36). Threaded rings, which have been used in large numbers in Europe, were tried in this country, but exceedingly high failure rates in very short time periods caused them to fall from favor

rapidly (1,7,26). The cementless acetabular component with a porous ingrowth surface has proven to be the method of choice in managing acetabular failures (6,10,22,32,35). The addition of the larger, or jumbo, sizes has now allowed the orthopedic surgeon to address a variety of acetabular revision problems (12).

Thus, we believe that the use of cement as a means of directly fixing the acetabular component to the pelvis in the revision setting is extremely limited. Certainly, in those situations where the acetabulum is nearly normal relative to the existence of good cancellous bone, and where there are no significant segmental defects, cement may be used effectively. In these limited situations, results of cemented revisions may approach those of a cemented primary acetabulum.

One other indication for the use of cement in the revision setting is its use in conjunction with structural allografting (5,23,30). This approach allows the surgeon to reconstruct cavitary and segmental defects with the use of bulk allograft. It may also allow him to reestablish the mechanics of the hip by placing the hip at its anatomic center as well as to provide the opportunity for restoration of

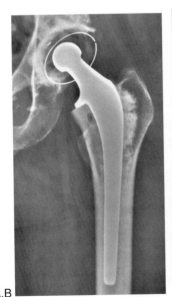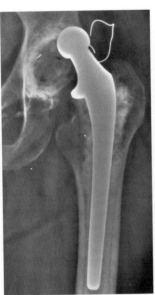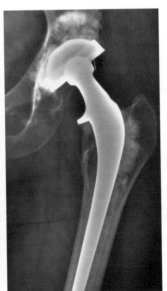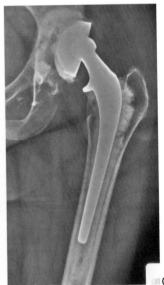

A,B   C,D

FIG. 1. A failed cemented cup. **A:** This 72-year-old woman had a diagnosis of degenerative joint disease and had had a primary cemented total hip arthroplasty. **B:** Failure of primary cemented cup 3.5 years later. **C:** After cemented cup revision. **D:** Failure of revised cemented cup 4.5 years later.

bone stock. Numerous reports in the literature support the use of this technique, but not in conjunction with cementless acetabular components. Patch and Lewallen (24), in their recent presentation to the American Association of Orthopaedic Surgeons (AAOS), summarized current thinking quite well. They were able to demonstrate an increasing mechanical failure rate of cementless acetabular components as a function of the percentage of the component in contact with the bone graft. When prosthesis–bone graft contact exceeded 50%, the mechanical failure rate approached 75%. Cementing into a grafted bed eliminates a number of the problems facing the surgeon who attempts to cement into an ungrafted acetabulum. Bleeding is not an issue with allograft bone. Multiple cavitary defects are addressed by the bone graft, and containment is provided by the graft. Thus, one can achieve excellent interdigitation of the cement into the bone graft. Chapter 94 is devoted to the use of cement in conjunction with packed allograft bone in addressing major acetabular problems.

REINFORCING RINGS IN ACETABULAR REVISION ARTHROPLASTY

We will focus on one other situation in which we believe the use of cement is appropriate in acetabular revision, not to attach the component to bone, but rather to attach modular acetabular components together (e.g., to bond the polyethylene liner into a metal shell). The idea of using a supporting ring in concert with cemented acetabular components is not a new one. Theoretically, it permits the surgeon to fulfill a number of goals of revision surgery. First, it provides a painless, stable, and, hopefully, durable construct. Second, it maintains or augments existing bone stock. And third, it restores hip mechanics to as near as normal as possible.

Mueller (20) in Switzerland and Harris and Jones (9) in this country recognized early the need for ancillary fixation devices to manage unique situations in both primary and revision surgery. Originally designed to handle the medial cavitary or protrusio defect, use of support rings was gradually expanded to handle minor segmental defects also. The introduction of even more substantial devices [e.g., the Ganz ring and the Burch-Schneider anti-protrusio cage (APC), Protek, Berne, Switzerland) (Fig. 2)] now allows the surgeon to address rather substantial segmental and cavitary defects without the need for structural bone graft. Although several designs of reinforcing rings are now available, the primary aims of these various rings are similar. They are all designed to address those cases with major loss of pelvic bone stock through use of cancellous allograft bone. The support ring allows for accurate reconstitution of the hip center of rotation, and the packed allo-

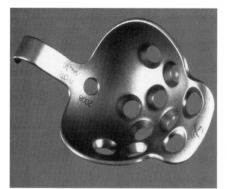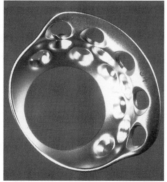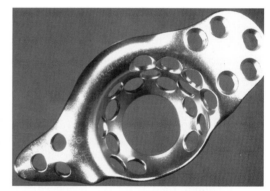
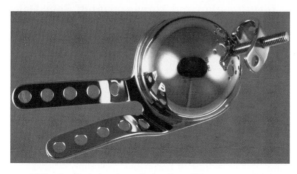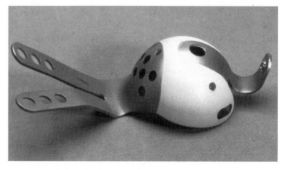

FIG. 2. Reinforcing rings for difficult acetabular reconstruction. *Top left,* Ganz Ring (Protek, Berne, Switzerland). *Top center,* Mueller Ring (Protek, Berne, Switzerland). *Top right,* Burch-Schneider Antiprotrusio Cage (Protek, Berne, Switzerland). *Bottom left,* Link Pelvic Reinforcing Ring (Waldemar Link, Hamburg, Germany). *Bottom right,* Graft Augmentation Prosthesis (GAP) (Osteonics Corporation, Allendale, NJ).

graft behind the ring facilitates restoration of bone stock. Depending on the ring design, screw holes are available not only in the ring itself but also through flanges (e.g., Protek AG, Bern, Switzerland) or malleable superior plates (e.g., Graft Augmentation Prosthesis, Osteonics, Allendale, NJ). An attachable inferior hook is a unique feature of one reinforcing ring (Link Pelvic Reinforcing Ring, Waldemar Link, Hamburg, Germany), although attaching this hook can be a challenge even to the most skilled arthroplasty surgeon. The Graft Augmentation Prosthesis (GAP) (Osteonics, Allendale, NJ) features a crimpable hook inferiorly as part of the ring itself. In all cases, the screw fixation of the reinforcing ring is through host bone, thus bypassing the bony defect. This provides stability of the construct so bone graft incorporation is promoted. These acetabular components have a common characteristic: all require a polyethylene insert to be cemented into the metal ring or shell to complete the acetabular construct.

SURGICAL TECHNIQUE FOR ACETABULAR REINFORCING RINGS

Exposure

Any standard approach to the hip that affords excellent acetabular exposure can be used to place a reinforcing ring. Although neither a trochanteric slide nor a trochanteric osteotomy is necessary for the acetabular procedure, one should not hesitate to use this type of approach if it will facilitate the patient's femoral reconstruction. However, we prefer to use a posterolateral approach.

Several simple techniques to improve acetabular exposure can be employed when using a posterolateral approach to the hip. For instance, the posterolateral approach requires that the femur be displaced far anteriorly to visualize the acetabulum. This displacement is facilitated by a complete release of the bony insertion of the gluteus maximus tendon. The entire anterior capsule must also be cut to permit anterior translation. If one is using an extended reinforcing ring that obtains significant fixation from the ilium, such as the Burch-Schneider ring, a Link pelvic reconstruction cage, or a GAP acetabular reinforcing ring, it is necessary to expose the ilium anterior and superior to the acetabulum itself. This exposure can be achieved by using electrocautery for a short distance onto the outer table of the ilium from the acetabular rim. A periosteal elevator can then be used to elevate the abductor musculature superiorly and anteriorly from the acetabu-

lum. It is important not to dissect posteriorly towards the sciatic notch, as this places the gluteal vessels and nerves at risk. It is not necessary to completely clear the outer table of the ilium, but merely to lift the muscles so that the superior extension of the reinforcing ring can be placed under them, thereby minimizing damage to the abductor musculature. If a reinforcing ring that obtains significant fixation interiorly is being used, such as the Link pelvic reconstruction ring or the GAP acetabular reinforcing ring, it is necessary to obtain excellent exposure inferiorly as well.

It is helpful to identify several landmarks during the course of this dissection. First, the superior pubic ramus is identified by dissecting along the anterior wall in an inferior direction until a finger can be placed over the acetabular rim onto the pubic ramus. It is not necessary to visualize the ramus directly. Then proceed to dissect along the posterior wall until the ischium is easily palpable. The posterior hip capsule can be dissected for a short distance from the posterior wall, allowing a spike retractor to be placed into the ischium, thereby retracting soft tissues while protecting the sciatic nerve from excessive tension caused by this retraction. The next landmark that one must identify is the acetabular teardrop, which marks the inferior-medial extent of the anatomic acetabulum and is located along the medial wall between the pubic ramus anteriorly and the ischium posteriorly. The medial wall is followed inferiorly until the bone is seen to curve medially at the inferior margin of the acetabulum. The obturator foramen is entered by dissecting around this usually stout bone with a curved periosteal elevator. The acetabular branch of the obturator artery is present in this area and usually requires cautery. Devices such as the GAP acetabular reinforcing ring and the Link pelvic reconstruction ring require significant exposure in this area. To adequately position the hook for either of those devices, it is usually necessary to expose the teardrop well enough to place an index finger through the obturator foramen along the medial wall of the acetabulum.

Identification and Management of Bony Defects

Once the acetabulum has been adequately exposed, preexisting components, cement, and any osteolytic membrane present are removed. The remaining bony acetabulum is thoroughly debrided with curettes to remove incompetent bone. Once this debridement has

---

FIG. 3. A: Radiograph of 70-year-old woman with loose total hip arthroplasty and massive acetabular bone loss. **B:** Intraoperative photo of acetabulum showing the extent of bone loss including superior segmental; and superior, medial, and posterior cavitary defects. *Top,* cephalad; *right,* anterior. **C:** The same patient's acetabulum after insertion of the morselized bone to fill defects. **D:** Same patient with acetabular reinforcing ring in place just prior to cementing polyethylene liner. **E:** Radiograph 6 months after reconstruction: there is good positioning of acetabular reinforcing ring. **F:** Close-up of same radiograph (6 months after reconstruction).

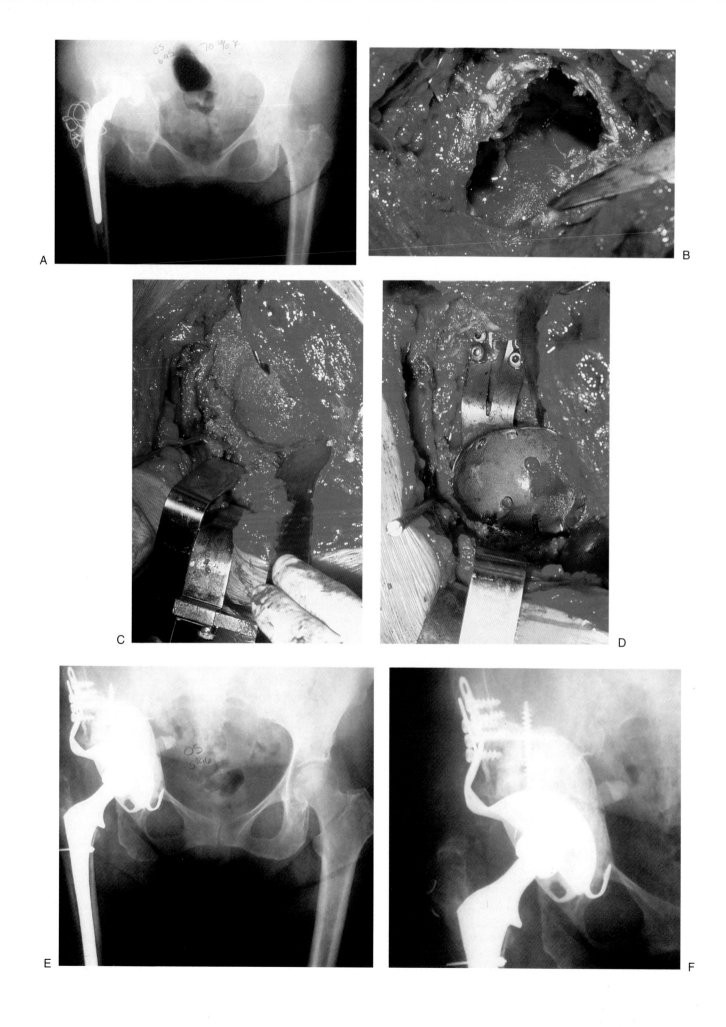

been adequately performed, an assessment of the remaining bone and the bony deficits is made (Fig. 3A,B). We prefer to use the AAOS classification of defects (4). Cavitary defects are those in which the bony rim is intact but the acetabular cavity is significantly expanded. Segmental defects are those in which a portion of the bony rim is completely missing. Combinations of these two general types of defects are very common and are referred to as type III, combined defects. A type IV acetabular defect is a pelvic discontinuity. This classification system is useful to help determine the type of reconstruction necessary.

Once the bony defect has been identified, the acetabulum is reamed lightly with hemispherical reamers to determine the necessary implant size. The bony defects are then addressed with the use of bone graft. In patients with only cavitary defects, the defect is usually managed with morselized bone graft, and a hemispherical porous-coated acetabular component is used. Acetabular reinforcing rings are used primarily in those acetabula that have segmental and combined defects as well as those exhibiting pelvic discontinuity. In cases with medial segmental defects, the membranous tissue and muscle medial to the acetabulum is usually sufficient to contain morselized bone graft. In patients with true rim defects, it is necessary to place some type of containment device if morselized bone graft is to be used and structural allograft is to be avoided. We prefer to use prolene mesh. This material, frequently used by general surgeons for hernia repairs, can easily be cut to fit the size and shape of an existing rim defect and can be stapled to the existing bony rim. Fresh-frozen allograft bone can then be morselized in a bone mill and packed into the defect. The prolene mesh will contain the bone graft in the area of the segmental defect. The bone graft must be tightly packed into the existing defect. Firmly packed bone graft can be achieved by using hemispherical tamps and a mallet (see Fig. 3C).

We currently plate the posterior column with a pelvic reconstruction plate to manage pelvic discontinuity. Next, an acetabular reinforcing ring, such as the Link or GAP device, is used to obtain both inferior and superior fixation. Because these devices do not depend on hoop stress for initial component stability, it is not necessary to plate the anterior column. Once the posterior column has been reconstructed with a plate, remaining bony deficits are addressed as described.

Selection of the Implant

Many different designs of acetabular reinforcing rings are currently available. These range from the Mueller ring, which primarily supports the rim, to rather large devices that allow for significant reconstruction, such as the Link, Burch-Schneider, and GAP devices. It is important to obtain maximal stability on host bone rather than on bone graft. If the patient has an essentially intact acetabular rim or only a small segmental defect, then devices such as the Mueller ring will obtain adequate fixation on host bone. In these situations, a porous-coated hemispherical component can also be used, and it is generally the component of choice in our practice. In patients with significant posterior or superior defects where a hemispherical device will not obtain adequate stability on host bone, a more extensive type of reinforcing ring must be selected. In this situation, fixation on host bone is maximized by obtaining an inferior lock with a hook around the teardrop in addition to fixation superiorly on the ilium by means of plates. The size of the ring should be chosen to maximize contact with host bone, especially superiorly along the acetabular dome.

Placement of the Acetabular Reinforcing Ring

Once the acetabulum has been grafted and the graft has been packed, the construct should appear almost as a normal acetabulum. The appropriate-size acetabular reinforcing ring is then brought into the field. It is very important to place the ring into the patient's acetabulum and to be sure that fit is adequate. If either the Link or GAP reconstruction devices is being used, it will be necessary to pre-bend the plates to fit appropriately against the ilium, with the hemispherical portion of the ring supported by the dome. The acetabular reinforcing ring can then be positioned for final fixation by sliding the plates under the abductor muscles along the ilium and tapping the hemispherical portion into the grafted acetabulum. It is important that the hemispherical portion be tightly inserted against the rim of the acetabulum as well as against the packed morselized bone graft. Inferior fixation can then be obtained by either crimping the hook around the teardrop as for a GAP device, or by attaching the inferior hook by means of a bolt for the Link device. Screws (6.5 mm in diameter) are then placed through the ring into the existing superior bone to further compress the graft. Supplementary fixation can then be obtained by placing the fully threaded 6.5-mm cancellous screws through the holes in the plate and into the ilium. These screws are placed in a bicortical fashion to obtain maximum purchase (see Fig. 3D,E,F). A polyethylene acetabular component is then cemented into the ring. Prior to placement of cement, the screw heads within the ring are filled with bone wax to facilitate their removal should it be necessary in the future. It is often necessary to place acetabular reinforcing rings in an orientation that might not be optimal for joint mechanics to obtain maximal contact with the patient's existing bone. It is possible to orient the polyethylene area of the component independently from the acetabular reinforcing ring if this should be necessary to obtain proper abduction and anteversion for joint stability.

REINFORCING RINGS IN REVISION ARTHROPLASTY

Recent reports of the use of various reinforcing rings indicate encouraging results for the short term (2,8,15,19, 25,28) (Table 2). At follow-up periods between 30 and 60 months, re-revision rates range from 0% to almost 12%, with an average failure rate of 3.3%. It would appear that, at least with these early results, the use of cement to secure the polyethylene liner into these various metal rings is appropriate. Of note is the fact that only two (0.5%) of the 418 reconstructions examined in the literature review had failed at the cement (i.e., polyethylene-reinforcement ring) interface. Osteonics Corporation (Allendale, NJ) recently completed testing on six hybrid cups (polyethylene liner cemented into a GAP metal shell) under simulated *in vitro* 10-million-cycle fatigue loading with a grafted superior defect. The cyclic loading of 60 to 600 lb at 10 Hz was applied through a 32-mm head at 45° from the cup centerline. Results showed no shell, cement, or insert failures (R & D Internal Tech Report #940620).

We have performed 56 acetabular reconstruction procedures in the past 27 months at Indiana University. These include 18 Ganz rings, six Link Pelvic Reconstruction rings, and 32 Graft Augmentation Prostheses. Twenty-four (43%) have 5- to 27-month follow-ups. The majority of these reconstructions (81%) were done for aseptic loosening, and one half had both cavitary and segmental defects (i.e., type III acetabular deficiencies). The most common areas of deficiency were superior and medial. Twelve hips (21%) underwent femoral revision at the time of the acetabular revision. In addition, ten of the acetabular components were constrained and five had polypropylene mesh for additional containment of the bone graft. Complications have been similar to other reports for reconstruction of major bony loss. Component

removal was necessary in two patients with deep joint infection, and a constrained insert was required in three patients who suffered dislocations. There have been three re-revisions (5.4%) for aseptic loosening. In two of the three cases, inadequate bone graft technique had been noted on early postoperative radiographic analysis.

Our current surgical technique for the GAP cup varies with the type and size of the defects present. In all cases, however, it is our goal to integrate the implant into the host bone so that fixation is not solely dependent on the hook and plates. In cases with modest defects in which the implant has greater than 50% contact with host bone, the defects are managed with packed allograft and an implant coated with hydroxyapatite to enhance subsequent integration. In cases where more extensive bone loss exists, whether segmental or cavitary, cementing the implant into the packed cancellous bone is preferred. This technique of cementing through the bone graft and subsequently to the host bone is much like the impaction grafting technique currently used in femoral revision surgery.

Case Example

N. K. is a 65-year-old man who underwent a primary cemented total hip arthroplasty in 1988. He subsequently underwent multiple procedures including at least one revision surgery for treatment of recurrent dislocations and infection. He first presented in our clinic in early 1992 complaining of increasing pain in his left hip. Examination of his radiograph (Fig. 4A) indicated loosening of the acetabular component. At the time of his revision surgery in June, 1992, he was noted to have a large cavitary defect superiorly, combined with a superior segmental defect. These defects were managed with a jumbo hydroxyapatite-coated cup with two AO cancellous screws through a structural allograft (see Fig. 4B). A constrained liner was inserted in October 1992 for recurrent dislocations. By February 1994, this construct had loosened (see Fig. 4C). Re-revision was delayed because

TABLE 2. *Results of reinforcing rings in revision surgery*

Author (ref.)	Component	Hips (N)	Follow-up	Hips with three-zone radiolucent lines	Hips with aseptic loosenings	Hips with re-revisions (%)
Korovessis et al. (15)	Mueller	20P, 10R	30 mo	1	0	0 (0.0%)
Rosson and Schatzker (18)	46 Mueller, 20 B-S	66	5 yr	5	NR	5 (7.6%)
Berry and Muller (2)	B-S	42	5 yr	0	0	5 (11.9%)
Haentjens et al. (8)	Mueller	22P, 21R	40 mo	9	2	3 (7.0%)
Morscher (19)	Ganz Ring	209	<5 yr	NR	NR	1 (0.5%)
Peters et al. (23)	B-S	28	33 mo	0	4	0 (0.0%)

Total N = 418
Total re-revision rate = 14 (3.3%)
Two failures (0.5%) occurred at the polyethylene–metal ring interface

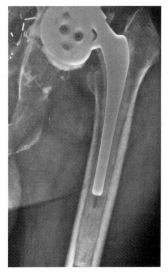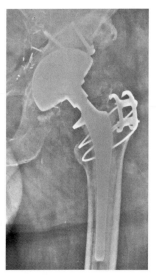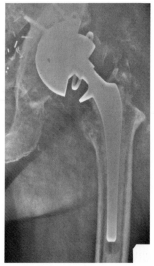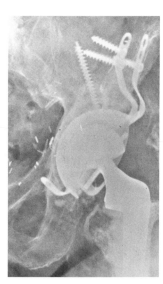

A,B

C,D

FIG. 4. Reinforcing ring in acetabular reconstruction. **A:** Failure of cemented cup 3 years after implantation. **B:** After acetabular revision with jumbo cup and structural allograft. **C:** Failure of that construct 20 months later. **D:** Acetabular revision with reinforcing ring at 15 months after surgery.

of an infection that was effectively treated. In February 1995, he underwent reimplantation using a cemented calcar replacement femoral component and a GAP acetabular reinforcing ring with a constrained liner insert. At his most recent follow-up in May 1996 (15 months after surgery), he was pain free and walking without support except for the use of a cane for long walks (see Fig. 4D).

CONCLUSION

A common concern about the use of acetabular reinforcing rings is the potential for stress shielding of the pelvis and the ultimate reabsorption into the periacetabular bone stock. However, stress shielding is a concern with any metal-backed, hemispheric acetabular component used either in the primary or revision setting. Use of jumbo cups (60 to 80 mm) that increase in thickness so as to accept a common insert are particularly worrisome because of the amount of metal. The GAP reinforcing ring is relatively thin walled and is made of titanium, so, at least theoretically, it should be a better transmitter of stresses than a comparably sized jumbo cup. The validation of this theory will be possible only with continued follow-up and careful roentgenographic assessment.

Dislocation is another concern in revision hip arthroplasty. Dislocation rates for primary total hip arthroplasty average about 2.3%, but it is widely recognized that the incidence significantly increases with subsequent hip surgeries (18). In our series of 56 reinforcing rings, we used a constrained insert in ten cases (17.9%). Six other patients suffered one or more dislocations postoperatively, three of which required reoperation to insert a constrained liner, all within 3 months of the reinforcing ring

implantation. Because the surgeon places the polyethylene insert into the metal shell in what is believed to be the correct alignment independent of the reinforcing ring, dislocation as a function of component malalignment should be minimized. However, dislocation as a function of lack of muscle balance still poses a problem, as it does in any revision situation. In those cases where this imbalance is recognized, a constrained liner may be cemented into the reinforcing ring. Finally, the lack of proper tissue tension is another cause of dislocation. Use of a reinforcing ring allows the surgeon to position the acetabular component at or near the anatomic hip center and thus balance tissue tension more easily than if a high hip placement is accepted. Therefore this cause of dislocation should also be minimized. Our postoperative management with the reinforcing ring does not differ from that of other acetabular revision cases. Patients are instructed in the usual motion restrictions to minimize dislocation. If dislocation occurs, the patient may be casted or provided with a brace for a period of 6 weeks to allow for tissue healing. In cases of recurrent dislocation, reoperation may be necessary.

In summary, management of the pelvis with major bone loss poses a difficult problem for the arthroplasty surgeon. To date, we have not found the perfect solution. No single technique is likely to provide the solution to the full spectrum of acetabular defects. If no or minimal defects exist, one may use a cemented or a cementless cup, but larger defects may require the use of a jumbo cup or reinforcing ring with bone grafting (Fig. 5). With each failure and subsequent revision, the patient is often left with greater bone loss and the surgeon with a more difficult reconstruction. Re-revision rates for reconstruction of severely deficient acetabula will no doubt be greater than those for

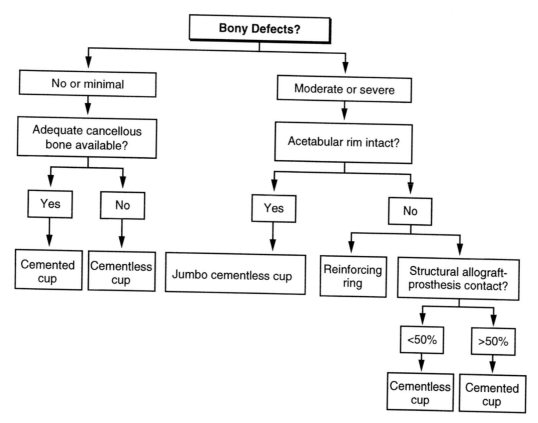

FIG. 5. Decision-making in acetabular revision surgery.

primary or nondeficient bone revisions. Conceptually, the use of a reinforcing ring with morselized allograft appears to be a sound solution for the patient with cavitary and segmental acetabular defects. Short-term failure rates are acceptable; long-term results are unknown. We do know that adequate bone graft technique is critical and that short-term failures at the cement interface have been rare. Long-term follow-up is necessary to determine if this use of cement in revision acetabular surgery will be an effective means of reconstruction of severely deficient acetabula or if the polyethylene–reinforcing ring interface will become a source of osteolysis from either cement or polyethylene debris.

REFERENCES

1. Apel DM, Smith DG, Schwartz CM, Paprosky WG. Threaded cup acetabuloplasty: early clinical experience. *Clin Orthop* 1989; 241: 183–189.
2. Berry DJ, Muller ME. Revision arthroplasty using an anti-protrusio cage for massive acetabular bone deficiency. *J Bone Joint Surg* 1992; 74B:711–715.
3. Callaghan JJ, Kelly SS, Johnston RC. The outcome of Charnley total hip arthroplasty with cement after a minimum twenty-year follow-up. *J Bone Joint Surg* 1993;75A:961–975.
4. D'Antonio JA, Capello WN, Borden LS, Bargar WL, Bierbaum BF, Boettcher WG, Steinberg ME, Stulberg SD, Wedge JH. Classification and management of acetabular abnormalities in total hip arthroplasty. *Clin Orthop* 1989;243:126–137.
5. Emerson RH, Head WC, Berklacich FM, Malinin TI. Noncemented acetabular revision arthroplasty using allograft bone. *Clin Orthop* 1989;249:30–43.
6. Engh CA, Glassman AH, Griffin WL, Mayer JG. Results of cementless revision for failed cemented total hip arthroplasty. *Clin Orthop* 1988; 235:91–110.
7. Fox GM, McBeath AA, Heiner JP. Hip replacement with a threaded acetabular cup. *J Bone Joint Surg* 1994;76A:195–201.
8. Haentjens P, DeBoeck H, Handelberg F, Casteleyn P, Opdecam P. Cemented acetabular reconstruction with the Mueller support ring. *Clin Orthop* 1993;290:225–235.
9. Harris WH, Jones WN. The use of wire mesh in total hip replacement surgery. *Clin Orthop* 1975;106:117–121.
10. Harris WH, Krushall RJ, Galante JO. Results of cementless revision of total hip arthroplasties using the Harris-Galante prosthesis. *Clin Orthop* 1988;235:120–126.
11. Hirose I, Capello WN, Feinberg JR, Shirer RM. Primary cemented total hip arthroplasty: five to twelve year clinical and radiographic follow-up. *Iowa Orthop J* 1995;15:43–47.
12. Jasty M. Jumbo revisions. *Presented at the 22nd annual Hip Course, Massachusetts General Hospital, Boston, MA, September 16–19, 1992.*
13. Kavanaugh BF, Ilstrup DM, Fitzgerald Jr RH. Revision total hip arthroplasty. *J Bone Joint Surg* 1985;67A:517–526.
14. Kershaw, CJ, Atkins RM, Dodd CAF, Bulstrode CJK. Revision total hip arthroplasty for aseptic failure. *J Bone Joint Surg* 1991;73B: 564–568.
15. Korovessis P, Spastris P, Sdougos G, Salonikides P, Christodoulou G, Katsoudas G. Acetabular roof reinforcement rings. *Clin Orthop* 1992; 283:149–155.
16. Marti RK, Schuller HM, Besselaar PP, Haasnoot ELV. Results of revision of hip arthroplasty with cement. *J Bone Joint Surg* 1990;72A: 346–354.
17. McFarland EG, Lewellen DG, Cabanela ME. Use of bipolar endoprosthesis and bone grafting for acetabular reconstruction. *Clin Orthop* 1991;268:128–139.
18. Morrey BF. Instability after total hip arthroplasty. *Orthop Clin North Am* 1992;23:237–248.

19. Morscher EW. Management of the bone-deficient hip: management of acetabular deficiency. *Orthopedics* 1995;18:859–862.

20. Mueller ME. Acetabular revision. In: Salvati EA, ed. *The hip: proceedings of the ninth open scientific meeting of the Hip Society*, St. Louis: CV Mosby, 1981;46.

21. Mulroy Jr RD, Harris WH. The effect of improved cementing technique on component loosening in total hip replacement. *J Bone Joint Surg* 1990;72B:757–760.

22. Padgett DE, Kull L, Rosenberg A, Sumner DR, Galante JO. Revision of the acetabular component without cement after total hip arthroplasty. *J Bone Joint Surg* 1993;75A:663–673.

23. Paprosky WG, Magnus RE. Principles of bone grafting in revision total hip arthroplasty: acetabular technique. *Clin Orthop* 1994;298: 147–155.

24. Patch DA, Lewallen DG. Bone grafting about porous ingrowth acetabular components: a five-year roentgenographic review. *Presented at the 61st annual meeting of the American Academy of Orthopaedic Surgeons*, New Orleans, LA, February 24–March 1, 1994.

25. Peters CL, Curtain M, Samuelson KM. Acetabular revision with the Burch-Schneider antiprotrusio cage and cancellous allograft bone. *J Arthroplasty* 1995;10:307–312.

26. Pupparo F, Engh CA. Comparison of porous-threaded and smooth-threaded acetabular components of identical design. *Clin Orthop* 1991;271:201–205.

27. Raut VV, Siney PD, Wroblewski BM. Cemented revision for aseptic acetabular loosening. *J Bone Joint Surg* 1995;77B:357–361.

28. Rosson J, Schatzker J. The use of reinforcement rings to reconstruct deficient acetabula. *J Bone Joint Surg* 1992;74B:716–720.

29. Russotti GM, Coventry MB, Stauffer RN. Cemented total hip arthroplasty with contemporary techniques. *Clin Orthop* 1988;235: 141–147.

30. Samuelson KM, Freeman MAR, Levack B, Rassmussen GL, Revell PA. Homograft bone in revision acetabular arthroplasty. *J Bone Joint Surg* 1988;70B:367–372.

31. Schulte KR, Callaghan JJ, Kelley SS, Johnston RC. The outcome of Charnley total hip arthroplasty with cement after a minimum twenty-year follow-up. *J Bone Joint Surg* 1993;75A:961–975.

32. Silverton CD, Rosenberg AG, Sheinkop MB, Kull LR, Galante JO. Radiographic evaluation of a cementless acetabular component used for revision total hip arthroplasty at seven to ten-year follow-up. *Presented at the 62nd annual meeting of the American Academy of Orthopaedic Surgeons*, Orlando, FL, February 16–21, 1995.

33. Stauffer RN. Ten-year follow-up study of total hip replacement, with particular reference to roentgenographic loosening of the components. *J Bone Joint Surg* 1982;64A:983–990.

34. Sutherland CJ, Wilde AH, Borden LS, Marks KE. A ten-year follow-up of one hundred consecutive Muller curved-stem total hip replacement arthroplasties. *J Bone Joint Surg* 1982;64A:970–982.

35. Tanzer M, Drucker D, Jasty M, McDonald M, Harris WH. Revision of the acetabular component with an uncemented Harris-Galante porous-coated prosthesis. *J Bone Joint Surg* 1992;74A:987–994.

36. Wilson MG, Nikpoor N, Aliabadi P, Poss R, Neissman BN. The fate of acetabular allografts after bipolar revision arthroplasty of the hip: a radiographic review. *J Bone Joint Surg* 1989;71A:1469–1479.

37. Wroblewski BM. Wear and loosening of the socket in the Charnley low-friction arthroplasty. *Orthop Clin North Am* 1988;19:627–630.

The Adult Hip, edited by J. J. Callaghan,
A. G. Rosenberg, and H. E. Rubash.
Lippincott–Raven Publishers, Philadelphia © 1998.

CHAPTER 90

Revision of the Acetabular Component: Bone Packing

Tom J. J. H. Slooff, Pieter Buma, Jean W. M. Gardeniers, B. Willem Schreurs, Jan W. Schimmel, and Rik Huiskes

Most total hip arthroplasties, cemented and cementless, fail because of aseptic loosening, a slow but progressive process that often results in loss of bone stock. The key problem in revision surgery is how to manage the periprosthetic bone loss. Although controversy still exists about the best treatment for bone stock deficiencies, this chapter presents an excellent biologic method that uses impaction allografting with cement.

This chapter explores the historical development of small-fragment grafts and cement use in revision total hip arthroplasty. It also presents the indications for acetabular reconstruction and describes surgical technique. Finally, the clinical and radiographic results are presented and discussed.

HISTORY

Reconstructive bone surgery is an ancient art. Animal bone tissues were used as transplants in Hippocrates' time. According to Mankin (32), the legend called "the miracle of the black leg" is considered to be the first known allograft procedure in humans. In 1668 Job van Meekeren (35), a Dutch surgeon, reported the first bone-grafting procedure, and Anthony van Leeuwenhoek (29),

a Dutch scientist, first described the microscopic structure of bone.

The popularity of using autogenous grafts and allografts in clinical practice has waxed and waned. During the latter half of the nineteenth century and the early part of the twentieth century, well-known surgeons such as Ollier (39) from France, McEwen (31) from Scotland, Curtis (12) from the United States, and Barth (3), Axhausen (1), and Lexer (30) from Germany popularized these grafting techniques. During this period, bone transplantation was still considered experimental, with an unpredictable outcome. Clinical need spurred its development as a surgical procedure. Between 1947 and 1950, Bush (7) and Wilson (54) developed preservation techniques that enabled storage of allograft bone at minus 20° centigrade. This breakthrough made it possible to use allografts clinically on a larger scale, particularly to replace traumatic or tumor-related bone loss.

In the fifties, Herndon and Chase (25), Burwell and Gowland (6), Campbell (8), and Urist (52) performed extensive laboratory and animal experiments to provide scientific support for the clinical application of bone grafting. Most of these investigations were aimed at the processes of union, incorporation, osteoinduction, and immunogenetic reactions of the grafts.

In the seventies, clinicians began to use bone grafting to repair osseous defects in association with primary and revision hip arthroplasty. The size of the bone grafts used differed among the various surgeons. Currently, some surgeons (26,38) adhere to the use of small-fragment

T. J. J. H. Slooff, P. Buma, J. W. M. Gardeniers, B. W. Schreurs, J. W. Schimmel, and R. Huiskes: Department of Orthopaedics, University Hospital Nijmegen, 6500 HB Nijmegen, The Netherlands.

grafts, while others (19–21) advocate the use of large-fragment grafts with or without cement for revision hip arthroplasty. This chapter deals with the use of morselized grafts (small fragments) with cement.

In 1975, Hastings and Parker (23) described the combination of cemented total hip replacement and autogenous morselized cancellous grafting in intrapelvic protrusio. The graft was not impacted and was subsequently totally covered with a narrow-rimmed, coarse-mesh cup. In 1978, McCollum et al. (34) reported their first experience with autogenous wafers of corticocancellous bone to augment acetabular bone stock in 25 patients with protrusio acetabuli after failed total hip arthroplasty. They utilized gel foam to avoid direct contact between cement and graft material, thereby preventing cement penetration into the graft. They subsequently tucked a fine Vitallium mesh into acetabular anchoring holes to distribute the forces across the acetabulum. They combined a cemented cup with an Eichler ring if the medial wall was absent.

In 1983, Marti and Besselaar (33) introduced a technique for protruded and dysplastic acetabuli. They closed medial segmental defects with a corticocancellous graft and supplemented this with autogenous chips. They compressed intact acetabular host bone to anchor the cement. They also used an Eichler ring. They repaired peripheral segmental defects with segmental plugs from the pelvic crista and fixed these to the iliac wall with screws.

In 1983, Roffman et al. (41) investigated the fate of autogenous chips under a layer of polymethylmethacrylate bone cement in an animal model with intrapelvic protrusio. Their model had a medial segmental defect. Histologic evaluation revealed bone formation from the acetabular wall towards the graft. The graft appeared viable, and new bone formation was induced along the surface adjoining the bone cement. Based on these experimental results in dogs, Mendes and his co-investigators Roffman and Silbermann (36) published the results of a clinical study on primary cemented arthroplasties combined with autogenous bone chips supported with a metal mesh for intrapelvic protrusio. Their follow-up studies of up to 6 years showed clinical success in all patients.

In 1984, Slooff et al. (49) published their experience with a new technique using morselized allografts. Acetabular segmental defects were closed with corticocancellous slices or with flexible metal wire meshes. The contained acetabulum was tightly packed with allograft chips [sized ~1.0 cm³]. The cup was inserted after pressurizing the cement directly onto the graft. The anatomy of the hip was reconstructed by packing as much chip graft material as necessary to build up the socket to the level of the transverse ligament. In the meantime, although it was occasionally modified, other surgeons (26,38) adopted this bone packing and cement technique.

By the mid eighties, animal experiments were performed at the University of Nijmegen (5,46,47,48) to pro-

vide additional scientific support for this reconstruction method. In these experiments, a study in goats was designed to histologically evaluate the processes involved in graft incorporation. The surgical technique was comparable to that used in the human procedures. This experiment demonstrated rapid union of the graft with host

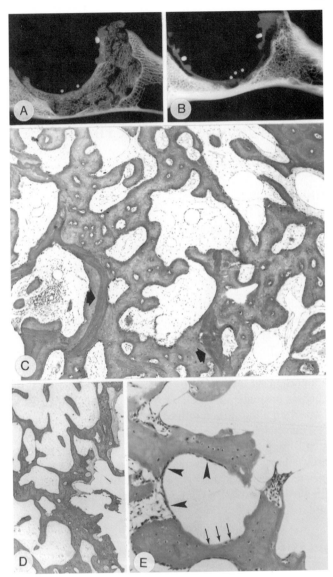

FIG. 1. Histologic analysis of graft incorporation in the goat acetabulum after impaction grafting with morselized allograft bone. **A:** Roentgenogram of thick sections through the acetabulum of the goat taken directly after surgery shows large pieces of graft and the clear transition zone to the host bone-bed. **B:** Complete consolidation with the host bone and incorporation of the graft at 12 weeks postoperatively. **C:** Structure of new trabecular bone after 12 weeks with only scarce remnants of the graft *(arrows)* (× 40). **D:** Interface between cement (C, removed during histotechnical processing) and new bone. **E:** Detail of bone–cement interface showing direct bone cement (C), contact sites *(arrows)*, and locations with a thin-soft tissue interface *(arrowheads)* (× 140).

bone using this method. From 24 weeks onwards, very little of the original graft bone remained, and a new immature trabecular bony structure was formed (Fig. 1). In the course of time, no signs of resorption or collapse of the reconstruction were seen. The results of this study encouraged more extensive clinical use of this biologic reconstruction method.

INDICATIONS

The main indication for revision arthroplasty was the progressive loss of periprosthetic bone, followed by pain and physical disability in otherwise healthy patients. Radiographic signs of loosening often preceded the clinical symptoms of failure. Since the seventies, regular follow-up had been included in the standard postoperative protocol after primary total hip arthroplasty to prevent extensive loss of bone (Fig. 2).

When planning revision arthroplasty, attention should be paid to assessing the diagnosis of loosening and establishing the cause of failure. A thorough physical examination should be followed by laboratory tests and good quality plain radiographs in three views: anteroposterior, axial, and abduction-external. These radiographs could be used to evaluate the severity of anatomic distortion, the location and the extent of bone lysis, the distribution of cement, and any acetabular or femoral deficiencies. Serial radiographs could be compared to monitor changes in the position of the component, cement, and bone stock over the course of time. If loosening is suspected, pre-revision management should include nuclear arthrography combined with an intra-articular needle biopsy and gamma-immunoglobulin scintigraphy to exclude infection.

MATERIALS AND METHODS

Between January 1979 and January 1988, 91 cemented revision hip arthroplasties in 83 patients were done at the University of Nijmegen using the acetabular reconstruction technique with impaction grafting and cement. All patients reported pain and functional disability. Patients were excluded from the follow-up study if the revision procedure was done without bone grafts, or if solid bone grafts or metal acetabular reinforcement rings had been used. In the first half of 1990, all patients eligible to take part in this study were invited for a clinical and radiographic examination. Seven patients (seven hips) had died of causes unrelated to the revision procedure. One patient (one hip) was lost to follow-up. The majority of patients had been to yearly follow-ups, so it was possible to study the records and radiographs of their previous visits. Finally, 88 hips (80 patients) entered the study with an average follow-up of 70 months (range, 24 to 132

months). The average age at the time of revision was 62 years (range, 33 to 89 years). The acetabular defects were classified on the basis of the preoperative and immediate postoperative radiographs and the operation charts. The American Academy of Orthopedic Surgeons (AAOS) classification for acetabular defects (13) was used. In the early period of this series, bone grafts were taken from the iliac crest as autografts, sometimes combined with allografts. Most of the allografts were deep-frozen femoral heads from the hospital bone bank. Allografts were used in 65 hips. The grafts were prepared with a rongeur during surgery. The average chip size was approximately 1 cm^3. The amount of the graft used varied from 1 to 3 femoral heads per patient, depending on the severity of the acetabular defect. The treatment strategy (Fig. 3) to correct structural acetabular integrity loss and impairment of implant mechanical support was aimed to do the following:

1. Repair hip mechanics by positioning the cup at the level of the anatomic acetabulum (tear drop).
2. Close segmental defects with metal wire mesh to achieve containment: a cavitary defect remains.
3. Replace the periprosthetic bone loss by augmenting the cavitary defect with allograft bone chips.
4. Restore stability by impacting the chips and using bone cement.

The X-Change Acetabular Revision Instrumentation System was developed (Howmedica International, Staines, United Kingdom) to achieve these goals.

SURGICAL TECHNIQUE

The posterolateral approach was used in all cases. This enabled extensive exposure of all aspects of the acetabulum and proximal femur. Trochanteric osteotomy was necessary in three cases. Identifying major landmarks was helpful for orientation purposes if the anatomy was disturbed by scarring and distortion. These landmarks included the tip of the greater trochanter, the tendinous part of the gluteus maximus, the lower border of the gluteus medius and minimus, and the sciatic nerve. Aspiration of the hip was repeated at this stage to obtain fluid for Gram staining and frozen sectioning to exclude infection. The proximal part of the femur was exposed and mobilized extensively before the hip was dislocated. Free exposure of the entire socket was achieved by removing all scar tissue, performing circumferential capsulotomy, and dividing the iliopsoas tendon. After removing the components and the cement, the fibrous interface was freed completely from the irregular acetabular wall using sharp spoons and curettes. Special care was taken to locate the transverse ligament on the inferior side of the acetabulum. The socket was reconstructed up to this level. At least

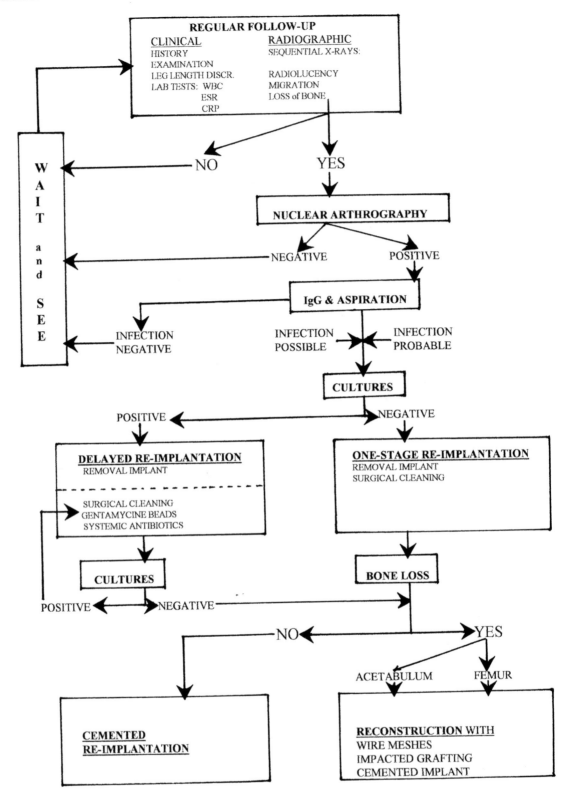

FIG. 2. Flow chart.

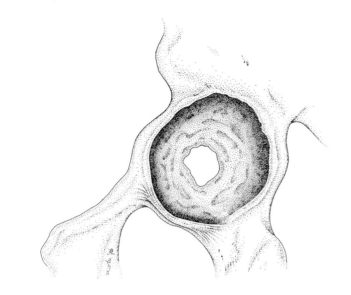

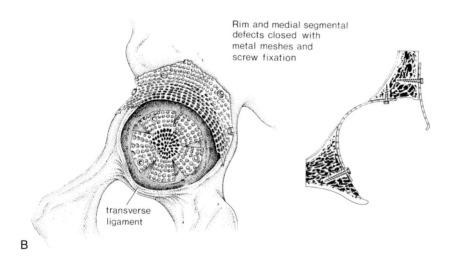

Rim and medial segmental
defects closed with
metal meshes and
screw fixation

transverse
ligament

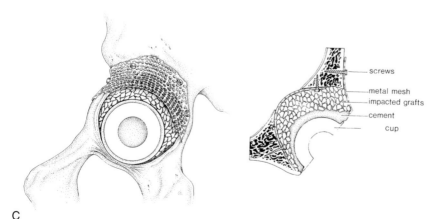

screws

metal mesh

impacted grafts

cement

cup

FIG. 3. A: Schematic view of a combined rim and medial segmental cavitary defect. **B:** Closure of the segmental defects with metal meshes and screw fixation. **C:** Filling of the cavitary defect with packed morselized allografts *(left)*. Transverse section of the reconstruction and the cemented cup *(right)*.

three specimens were taken from the interfacial fibrous membrane for frozen sectioning and bacterial culture. After taking these samples, systemic antibiotic therapy was started. The acetabular floor and wall were examined meticulously for any hidden medial or peripheral segmental defects. Using a pair of scissors, a flexible stainless steel mesh was trimmed and adapted to fit the defects. The mesh was then screwed to three points of the iliac wall to ensure rigid fixation. Any medial segmental defects were closed in a similar manner with a metal mesh. In this way, the acetabulum was contained and transformed into a cavitary defect. Small holes were then drilled into the sclerotic acetabular wall to enhance surface contact and promote vascular invasion into the graft. Deep-frozen femoral heads from the hospital bone bank were divided into four equal parts. Substantial chips were cut with a rongeur or scissors. After cleaning the acetabulum, any small cavities were packed tightly with chips. Next, the entire socket was filled, layer by layer. Impactors hammered the chips *in situ*, starting with the largest-possible-size impactor and ending with the size suitable for a 50-mm-diameter cup. Care was taken to reconstruct the anatomy of the hip until the socket reached the level of the transverse ligament. Consequently, the whole acetabular hemisphere was covered with a layer of impacted allograft chips. It was evident after impaction that this layer was not of uniform thickness. This depended locally on the depth of the acetabular defect. After impaction, the preexisting enlarged acetabular diameter had been reduced to normal size. While the antibiotic-loaded cement was being prepared, pressure on the graft was maintained using a trial socket. After inserting and pressurizing the cement, the cup was placed and held in position with the pusher until the cement had polymerized.

Postoperative management included anticoagulation therapy for 3 months and systemic antibiotics for 24 hours. Indomethacin was administered for 7 days to prevent the development of heterotopic ossification. Mobilization of the patient was individualized according to the different circumstances of the revision arthroplasty. A period of 3 to 6 weeks bed rest was required after major acetabular reconstruction.

All patients were seen in the out-patient department at 6 weeks, 3 months, 6 months, and 1 year, and then yearly after the operation. Harris Hip Scores (HHS) were estimated preoperatively and postoperatively by interview and examination. All pre- and postoperative radiographs were examined and graded on a consensus basis by two surgeons and a radiologist. Acetabular defects were classified as segmental or cavitary according to the AAOS classification scheme (13). Radiographic evaluation was used to examine the process of consolidation, to measure migration of graft incorporation, and to record the occurrence of radiolucencies. Consolidation was defined as the presence of clearly delineated trabecular bone crossing

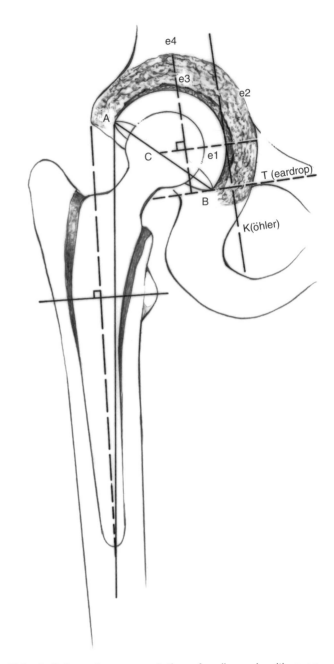

FIG. 4. Schematic representation of radiograph with overprojected coordinate system for measurement of migration. In each radiograph, the magnification factor was determined based on the prosthetic head of 32 mm, which was used in all patients. Köhler's line was chosen as y-axis, K, the line along the medial aspect of ilium and ischium. The line T running perpendicular to the line K and tangential to the inferior aspect of the teardrop was chosen as the x-axis. As a reference point on the acetabular cup, the center of the projected elliptical image of the metallic ring at the periphery of the cup was chosen. This point c, considered as the center of the cup, was determined by bisecting the long axis a-b of the projected ellipse.

the graft–host junction. Graft incorporation was assessed according to the criteria of Conn et al. (11), and graft was considered incorporated when an identical radiodensity of the graft and host bone with a continuous trabecular pattern throughout existed. Migration of the cup was established after digitization of the serial radiographs. Reliable and reproducible measurements were done on the monitor (Fig. 4). The position of the socket was determined by the metal wire, and the cup was measured relative to Köhler's line and the teardrop line. Radiographs were digitized (TEA Image Manager System, DIFA Measuring Systems Ltd., Breda, The Netherlands) with a computer program that was developed for this purpose. This program enabled reproducible measurements based on a coordinate system that was applied in each radiograph. The magnification factor was determined based on the prosthetic head of 32 mm, which was used in all patients. The Köhler line, K, was chosen as the y-axis, a line along the medial aspect of the ilium and ischium. The line T, running perpendicular to the line K and tangential to the inferior aspect of the teardrop, was chosen as the x-axis. The center of the metallic ring's projected elliptical image at the periphery of the acetabular cup was chosen as the reference point for this cup. This point, C, considered the cup's center, was determined by bisecting the long axis a-b of the projected ellipse.

Radiolucency at the graft–cement interface was assessed according to the criteria of DeLee and Charnley (14). Cups with continuous radiolucent lines of thicker than 2 mm in all three segments were considered to be loose.

RESULTS

At the time of the study, four acetabular components had been re-revised because of recurrent infection in two cases and aseptic loosening with migration in two other cases. The postoperative HHS averaged 87 points and, compared with the average preoperative score of 44 points, showed that the clinical results were improved after the reconstruction. Consolidation of the graft (i.e., union of the graft to the host bone) was complete in all 88 hips. Signs of incorporation were difficult to assess because of the irregularities at the graft–cement interface (Fig. 5). Eight acetabula showed incomplete graft incorporation: two cups had remained stable during the follow-up period, five cups had migrated with partial graft resorption but were clinically asymptomatic, and one cup had been re-revised because of progressive loosening (Fig. 6). Migration occurred in the five cups with incomplete graft incorporation. They were considered to be radiographically loose. One cup showed progressive continuous lucency with signs of incomplete graft incorporation. However, migration was not present in this case. Evaluating these results, clinical failures were seen in

four cases, and radiographic symptoms were seen in five cases because of more than 5-mm migration (four cases) or continuous lucency thicker than 2 mm in one case.

DISCUSSION

The process of aseptic loosening results in a widening of the original acetabulum and a weakening of the pelvic bone bed. The implant is progressively unstable and the patient often complains of pain and disabled function. To solve this clinical and biomechanical problem, a choice must be made as to how to reconstruct the loss of bone to restore normal hip mechanics and to achieve stability of the new implant. These goals are essential to guarantee a result that can stand the test of time. Several treatment strategies to achieve these goals have been reported in the literature (9,10,22,27,43,45). The most effective treatment is directed toward replacing the loss of bone, repairing normal hip mechanics, and obtaining stability of the reconstruction. All of these requirements can be fulfilled with the use of impacted morselized grafts, the establishment of containment of the graft, and the use of bone cement. Sotelo-Garza and Charnley (51) and Fuchs et al. (16) reported good results with cement alone to treat the bone loss in acetabular protrusion. In contrast with these findings, Salvati et al. (44), Ranawat et al. (40), and Azuma (2) found high failure rates with cement alone, and they advised the use of bone grafts.

It is evident that in revisions that use only cement, the bone defects remain and excellent cement interlock is not obtained. Also, the addition of rigid metal reinforcements (43) will fail because of the mismatch between the more elastic pelvic bone and the rigid metal shell. When failure of these rigid metal rings occurs, it will cause an additional and larger defect and a challenging surgical problem.

Therefore, the use of these implants requires larger porous-coated implants (22,24,45). Although the hip center can be moved back to the true hip center with jumbo components, the longevity resulting from such a procedure is not yet reported, and the indications are not yet clear.

The preferred treatment is the use of morselized bone grafts. Because of the limited availability of autogenous bone, mainly allografts are recommended in failed total hip reconstruction. The appropriate use of bone grafts requires knowledge of the basic events of bone graft incorporation. It is generally accepted that the early phases of graft incorporation are essentially similar in cortical and cancellous grafts. In cortical grafts, the inflammatory response is followed predominantly by osteoclastic activity. This causes a temporary widening of the haversian canal system and results in a mechanical weakening of the graft. The internal repair takes place very slowly and is confined to the superficial / contact

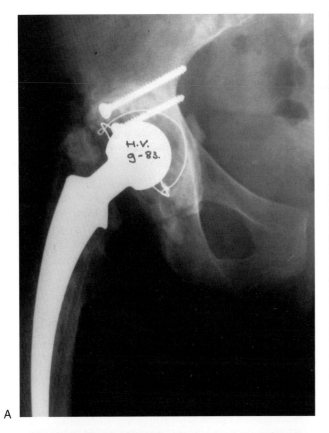

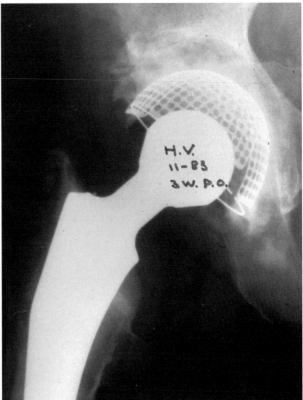

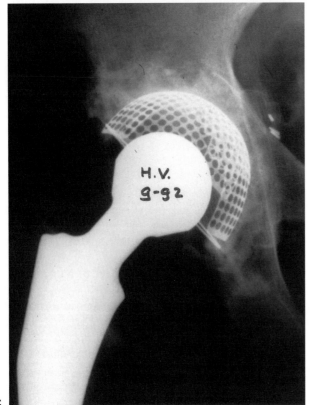

FIG. 5. Radiographic follow-up of a patient with a failed cemented total hip resulting in a combined cavitary and peripheral cemented defect of the right acetabulum. **A:** Preoperative radiograph. **B:** Radiograph 3 weeks after reconstruction with bone packing and cement. **C:** Radiograph 9 years after the reconstruction. There are no signs of lucency or resorption. The homogeneous structure of the periacetabular bone is normal.

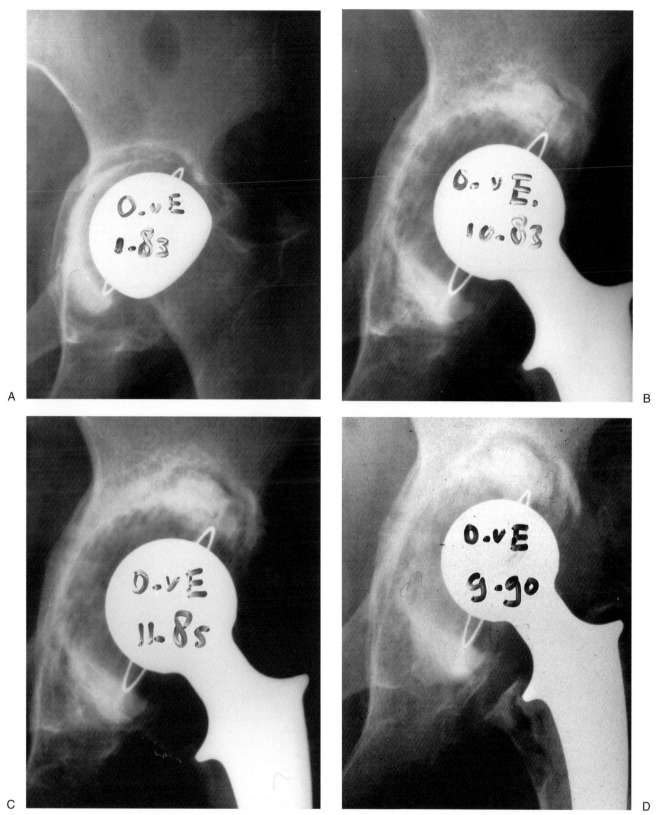

FIG. 6. Radiographic follow-up of a patient with a failed double-cup arthroplasty of the left hip resulting in a combined cavitary and peripheral segmental defect. **A:** Preoperative radiograph. **B:** Radiographs 6 months after reconstruction with bone packing and cement. **C:** Radiograph 1.5 years after surgery: clear signs of bone resorption and reduction of the graft layer. Patient had no clinical symptoms of loosening. **D:** Radiograph 6.5 years after surgery: there has been progressive loosening and migration of the acetabular cup, and there is evidence of graft resorption.

zone only, as reported by Enneking and Mindell (15). Whereas the incorporation of cancellous grafts in general shows rapid vascular invasion, there is subsequent deposition of bone matrix on top of the existing bone trabeculae and finally a more complete incorporation. Again, there is a difference in incorporation between the structural cancellous and the morselized impacted cancellous grafts. Structural cancellous grafts appear to result in unpredictable clinical and radiographic outcomes. Resorption of the graft and failure of stability was reported by Harris and co-workers (20,21,27,28,37). The reasons are not yet completely understood, but it is thought that the size of the transplant is important to the incorporation process. Furthermore, it is also very difficult to achieve a permanent fixation of structural cancellous grafts to host bone because of the existing mismatch of the contact surfaces.

It must be stressed that the containment of the graft in a defect-acetabulum is possible only when these defects in the medial wall and acetabular rim are closed with flexible wire meshes. It is also essential to achieve the stability of the graft by packing it very tightly. Small, 1 × 1 cm morselized chips are a prerequisite, and after impaction a stable and rough surface is obtained that improves the mechanical cement–bone interlock and the easy adaptation of the chips to the irregular surface of the bone bed. This will reduce gap formation between the host and graft and the union process will not be delayed. The stability of the reconstruction is even more improved by pressurizing the cement.

Concern has been expressed about cement being in direct contact with a morselized allograft. Positive results with this combination have been reported by Roffman, Silbermann, and Mendes (36,41,42), and they have been confirmed by the results of histologic studies performed by Schimmel (46) and Schreurs (47,48) with animal models. In these experiments, they also demonstrated that unconstrained grafts in direct contact with cementless implants resulted in resorption of the graft and implant instability.

From 1979 onwards, morselized bone packing with cement has been successfully used in our department as the standardized reconstruction method for protrusio acetabuli and in distorted acetabular anatomy, serious dysplastic acetabula, and column defects. With flexible wire meshes, the medial and peripheral segmental defects were closed and transformed to a cavitary defect. This now-contained defect was completely filled with impacted morselized cancellous grafts starting at the level of the transverse ligament. A new acetabulum at a normal anatomic location is reconstructed in this way.

As previously mentioned, the use of substantially sized chips, approximately 1 cc, is recommended for the acetabulum. Reduction of the chip size may result in early migration of the acetabular cup during the incorporation process, because of the lack of initial stability. Although the various reports (26,36,38,50) of the good

clinical results of this technique are in agreement with each other, the surgical techniques have been improved, and the biology and mechanics in total hip failure are better understood, the performance of this procedure is demanding and needs skillful handling.

This use of the method continues to be recommended, with caution advised, for reconstructing bone defects after failed total hip (17,18) and knee arthroplasty (53). Our clinical and radiographic results are promising and encourage us to promote this technique more intensely in orthopedic practice. The primary requirements of this technique, as expressed in the treatment strategy (Fig. 3), must always be kept in mind to obtain good results.

REFERENCES

1. Axhausen G. Arbeiten aus den Gebiet der Knochenpathologie und Knochenchirurgie. Kritische Bemerkungen und neue Beitrage zur freien Knochentransplantationen. *Arch Klin Chir* 1911;94:241–281.
2. Azuma T. Preparation of the acetabulum to correct severe acetabular deficiency for total hip replacement with special reference to stress distibution of the peri-acetabular region of the operation. *Nippon Seikeigeka Gakkai Zasshi* 1985;59:269–283.
3. Barth A. Ueber histologische Befunde nach Knochenimplantationen. *Arch Klin Chir* 1893;46:409–417.
4. Bayley JC, Christy MJ, Ewald FC, Kelley K. Long term results of total hip arthroplasty in protrusio acetabuli. *J Arthoplasty* 1987;2:275–280.
5. Buma P, Schreurs BW, Versleyen D, Huiskes R, Slooff TJ. Histologic evaluation of allograft incorporation after cemented and non-cemented hip arthroplasty in the goat. In: Older J, ed. *Bone implant grafting*. London: Springer-Verlag, 1992;12–15.
6. Burwell RG, Gowland G. Studies in the transplantation of bone. Assessment of antigenicity. Serological studies. *J Bone Joint Surg* 1962;43B:814–819.
7. Bush LF. The use of homogenous bone grafts. A preliminary report on the bone bank. *J Bone Joint Surg* 1847;29A:620–628.
8. Campbell CJ. Experimental study of the fate of bone grafts. *J Bone Joint Surg* 1953;35A:332–346.
9. Chandler HP, Penenberg BL. *Bone stock deficiency in total hip arthroplasty*. Thorofare, NJ: Slack, 1989.
10. Clarke HJ, Jinnah RH, Lennox D. Osseointegration of bone grafts in porous-coated total hip replacement. *Clin Orthop* 1988;258:160–168.
11. Conn RA, Peterson LFA, Stauffer RN, Ilstrup D. Management of acetabular deficiency: long term results of bone grafting the acetabulum in total hip arthroplasty. *Orthop Trans* 1985;9:451–454.
12. Curtis BF. Cases of bone implantation and transplantation for cyst of tibia, osteomyelitic cavities united fractures. *Am J Med Sci* 1893;106:30–37.
13. D'Antonio JA, Capello WN, Borden LS. Classification and management of acetabular abnormalities in total hip arthroplasty. *Clin Orthop* 1989;243:126–137.
14. DeLee JG, Charnley J. Radiological demarcation of cemented sockets in total hip replacement. *Clin Orthop* 1976;121:20–26.
15. Enneking WF, Mindell ER. Observations on massive retrieved human allografts. *J Bone Joint Surg* 1991;73A:1123–1142.
16. Fuchs MD, Salvati EA, Wilson PD, Senko TD, Pellici PM. Results of acetabular revisions with newer cementing techniques. *Orthop Clin North Am* 1988;19:649–656.
17. Gie GA, Linder L, Ling RSM, Simon JP, Slooff TJ, Timperley AJ. Impacted cancellous allograft and cement for revision total hip arthroplasty. *J Bone Joint Surg* 1993;75B:14–21.
18. Gie GA, Linder L, Ling RSM, Simon JP, Slooff TJ, Timperley AJ. Contained morsellized allograft in revision total hip arthroplasty. *Orthop Clin North Am* 1993;24:717–727.
19. Gross A. Reconstruction of the acetabulum. In: Galante JO, Rosenberg AG, Callaghan JJ, eds *Total hip revision surgery*. New York: Raven Press, 1995;335–346.
20. Harris WH, Crothers O, Oh J. Total hip replacement and femoral head

bone grafting for severe acetabular deficiency in adults. *J Bone Joint Surg* 1977;59A:752–763.

21. Harris WH. Allografts in total hip arthroplasty in adults with severe acetabular deficiency including a surgical technique for bolting the graft to the ilium. *Clin Orthop* 1982;162:150–159.

22. Harris WH. Management of the deficient acetabulum using cementless fixation without bone bone grafting. *Orthop Clin North Am* 1993;24:663–665.

23. Hastings DE, Parker SM. Protrusio acetabuli in rheumatoid arthritis. *Clin Orthop* 1975;108:76–84.

24. Hauwaert van der N, Vandenburghe L, Demuynck M. Reprises par cotyles non cimentés et greffes osseuses. *Acta Orthop Belg* 1995;2:117–121.

25. Herndon CH, Chase SW. The fate of massive autogenous and homogenous bone grafts including articular surfaces. *Surg Gynecol Obstet* 1954;98:273–290.

26. Hirst P, Esser M, Murphy JC, et al. Bone grafting for protrusio acetabula during total hip replacement. *J Bone Joint Surg* 1987;69B:229–236.

27. Jasty M, Harris WH. Total hip reconstruction using frozen femoral head allografts in patients with acetabular bone loss. *Orthop Clin North Am* 1987;18:291–297.

28. Kwong LM, Jasty M, Harris WH. High failure rate of bulk femoral head allografts in total hip acetabular reconstructions at 10 years. *J Arthroplasty* 1993;8:341–347.

29. Leeuwenhoek van A. Microscopical observations about blood, milk, bones, the brain, spittle, cuticula, sweat, fat and tears. *Philes Trans R Soc Lond* 1674;9:121–131.

30. Lexer E. Die Verwendung der freien Knochenplastik nebst Versuchen über Gelenkversteifung und Gelenktransplantation. *Arch Klin Chir* 1908;86:939–954.

31. MacEwen W. Observations concerning transplantation of bones. *Proc Soc Lond* 1881;32:232–247.

32. Mankin HJ, Doppelt S, Tomford W. Clinical experience with allograft implantation. *Clin Orthop* 1983;174:69–87.

33. Marti RK, Besselaar PP. Bone grafts in primary and secondary total hip replacement. In: Marti RK, ed. *Progress in cemented total hip surgery and revision.* Amsterdam: Excerpta Medica 1983:107–129.

34. McCollum DE, Nunley JA, Harrelson JM. Bone grafting in total hip replacement for acetabular protrusion. *J Bone Joint Surg* 1980;72A:248–252.

35. Meekeren van J. *Heel—en geneeskundige aanmerkingen.* Amsterdam L Commelijn, 1668.

36. Mendes DG, Roffman M, Silbermann M. Reconstruction of the acetabular wall with bone graft in arthroplasty of the hip. *Clin Orthop* 1984;186:29–38.

37. Mulroy RD, Harris WH. Failure of acetabular autogenous grafts in total hip arthroplasty. *J Bone Joint Surg* 1990;72A:1536–1543.

38. Olivier H, Sanouiller JL. Acetabular reconstruction with cancellous bone grafts for revision of total hip arthroplasties. *French Orthop Surg* 1991;5:2–9.

39. Ollier L. *Traité experimental et clinique de la regeneration des os et de la production artificièlles dutissue osseux.* Paris: Victor Masson et fils, 1867.

40. Ranawat CS, Dorr LD, Inglis AE. Total hip arthroplasty in protrusion acetabuli of rheumatoid arthritis. *J Bone Joint Surg* 1980;62A:1059–1065.

41. Roffman M, Silbermann M, Mendes D. Incorporation of bone graft covered with methyl-methacrylate onto the acetabular wall. *Acta Orthop Scand* 1983;54:580–586.

42. Roffman M, Silbermann M, Mendes D. Viability and osteogenity of bone coated with methyl-methacrylate cement. *Acta Orthop Scand* 1982;53:513–519.

43. Rosson J, Schatzker J. The use of reinforcement rings to reconstruct deficient acetabular. *J Bone Joint Surg* 1992;74B:716–724.

44. Salvati EA, Bullough P, Wilson PD. Intrapelvic protrusio of the acetabular component following total hip replacement. *Clin Orthop* 1975;111:212–227.

45. Samuelson KM, Freeman MAR, Leval B, et al. Homograft bone in revision acetabular arthroplasty. *J Bone Joint Surg* 1988;70B:367–374.

46. Schimmel JW. *Acetabular reconstruction with impacted morsellized cancellous bone grafts in cemented revision hip arthroplasty.* Thesis, University of Nijmegen.

47. Schreurs BW, Buma P, Huiskes R, Slagter JLM, Slooff TJJH. A technique for using impacted trabecular allografts in revision surgery with cemented stems. *Acta Orthop Scand* 1994;65:267–275.

48. Schreurs BW. *Reconstructive options in revision surgery of failed total hip arthroplasties.* Thesis, University of Nijmegen, 1994.

49. Slooff TJ, van Horn J, Lemmens A, Huiskes R. Bone grafting for total hip replacement in acetabular protrusion. *Acta Orthop Scand* 1984;55:593–597.

50. Slooff TJ, Schimmel JW, Buma P. Cemented fixation with bone grafts. *Orthop Clin North Am* 1993;24:667–677.

51. Sotelo-Garza A, Charnley J. The results of Charnley arthroplasty of the hip performed for protrusio acetabuli. *Clin Orthop* 1978;132:22–24.

52. Urist MR. The physiological basis of bone graft surgery with special references to the theory of induction. *Clin Orthop* 1953;1:207–215.

53. Waal Malefijt de MC, Kampen van A, Slooff TJJH. Bone grafting in cemented knee replacement. *Acta Orthop Scand* 1995;66(4):325–328.

54. Wilson PD. Experience with the use of refrigerated homogenous bone. *J Bone Joint Surg* 1951;33B:301–315.

The Adult Hip, edited by J. J. Callaghan,
A. G. Rosenberg, and H. E. Rubash.
Lippincott–Raven Publishers, Philadelphia © 1998.

CHAPTER 91

Revision of the Acetabular Component: Oblong Cup

David K. DeBoer and Michael J. Christie

Reconstruction of the acetabulum in patients with significant acetabular bone deficiency remains a major challenge in modern joint replacement arthroplasty. Although there are several classification schemes to describe acetabular defects (4,17), the American Academy of Orthopedic Surgeons (AAOS) Committee on the Hip devised a classification scheme that has become the standard for describing acetabular bone loss (Table 1). Type I defects are segmental deficiencies with complete loss of bone in the supporting hemisphere. These defects can be either peripheral rim defects or central defects with an absent medial wall. Type II defects are cavitary deficiencies that represent volumetric loss of bone with an intact acetabular rim. Type III defects represent a combination of segmental (type I) and cavitary (type II) bone loss. Type IV and V defects represent special circumstances where there is either a pelvic discontinuity or hip arthrodesis. Although the AAOS system has shortcomings, it is simple and applicable to both primary and revision cases.

During the 1980s, we began to notice a common pattern of bone loss in patients with failed acetabular components. As the implant loosened, it often migrated superiorly, creating an oblong-shaped defect in the

acetabulum. In other words, the acetabular anatomy was distorted such that the craniocaudal dimension of the acetabular recess was greater than the anteroposterior dimension. This type of defect corresponds to the AAOS type I superior rim defect. Frequently, the superior rim defect is combined with a medial cavitary defect, creating an AAOS type III deficiency.

The optimal method of acetabular reconstruction under these circumstances depends on the severity of the acetabular bone loss. If the degree of superior migration is small, the acetabulum can be reconstructed using an oversized hemispherical cup by simply converting the oblong defect back into a hemisphere (8). However, if the defect is large, reconstruction using an oversized cup is not feasible, because hemispherical reaming will cause obliteration of either the anterior or the posterior columns of the acetabulum, eliminating these structures that are required for implant stability and fixation (Fig. 1).

There are several methods of reconstruction available to the surgeon when a significantly large acetabular defect makes an oversized cup unfeasible. Many authors have advocated using large structural allografts in this situation to restore acetabular bone stock, provide stability for the acetabular implant, and allow restoration of the normal hip center. The initial results of acetabular reconstructions using large structural allografts were encouraging, with excellent initial implant stability and predictable relief of symptoms. As these reconstructions

D. K. DeBoer and M. J. Christie: Arthritis and Joint Replacement Center, Vanderbilt University Medical Center, Nashville, Tennessee 37212.

TABLE 1. *AAOS acetabular defect classification*

I. Segmental
    Peripheral
    Central
II. Cavitary
III. Combined segmental and cavitary
IV. Pelvic discontinuity
V. Arthrodesis

were followed longer, however, the majority of authors reported increasing failure rates, between 30% and 50% at 5- to 10-year follow-up (13,21). Although the variability in the amount of acetabular bone loss, and the location, size, quality, and orientation of the structural allografts have made the clinical studies difficult to compare and interpret, the etiology of the failures appears to be related to graft resorption (3,13).

The reports of long-term failures using structural allografts, combined with the poor early results experienced by many surgeons, led to a resurgence in the use of various anti-protrusio rings and cages to reconstruct these acetabular defects (1,16,18,22). These implants are metal rings with iliac and ischial extensions that are secured to the pelvis with multiple screws. Morselized allograft is commonly used with these devices to fill cavitary defects. Once the flanged component is fixed to the pelvis, a polyethylene cup is cemented in the proper orientation within the center of the cage. In an excellent series, Zehntner and Ganz (22) reported the intermediate-term outcome using the Mueller (Protek AG, Bern, Switzerland) reinforcement ring for patients with AAOS type I, II, and III acetabular defects. Kaplan-Meier survivorship analysis revealed a 79% probability of implant survival at 10 years using revision as the endpoint for failure; however, 44% of the reconstructions had pending failures, with component migration of 2 mm or greater at 7.2 years follow-up. In another series,

Berry and Muller (1) reported a 24% revision rate (12% aseptic loosening, 12% septic loosening) for patients undergoing acetabular revision using the Burch-Schneider cage at an average 5-year follow-up.

Another method of acetabular reconstruction developed to avoid using structural allograft is the technique using the "high hip center" most recently described by Schutzer and Harris (19) and others (11,12). In this method, a standard small hemispherical cup is press-fit high on the ilium to bypass the acetabular defect and gain stability on healthy host bone. This reconstruction technique has yielded good short-term results (19). In a series of 56 hips followed and for an average of 3.5 years, no revisions of the acetabular component were reported. This technique allows reconstruction of the acetabulum without structural allograft. Unfortunately, the femoral component may need to be revised to restore normal limb lengths if the hip center is placed too superiorly. Under these circumstances, replacing the modular femoral head to a femoral head with greater neck length will not adequately reconstitute normal limb lengths and a calcar replacement femoral prosthesis is required. Additionally, the trochanter must be advanced to restore normal soft-tissue tension. Thus, the revision of a well-fixed and positioned femoral component may be required to reconstruct a failed acetabulum.

Another alternative method of reconstruction was derived from our observation of the oblong-shaped defect created by the loosening and migration of the failed acetabular component led to the design of an oblong-shaped prosthesis. This implant replaced the deficient acetabular bone stock with metal, avoiding the need for structural allograft and allowing implant stability directly on host bone. In this chapter, we will outline the design rationale behind the oblong cup, the surgical indications, the surgical technique, and our 3- to 6-year results using this implant.

DESIGN RATIONALE

The oblong cup was designed to have several characteristics that were hoped would provide long-term stability. First, the cup is fully porous-coated and relies on biologic ingrowth for fixation. Mid-term studies using standard porous-coated hemispherical cups in revision patients have demonstrated failure rates of less than 1% (14,15) . Second, the cup is designed to obtain mechanical stability on host bone, thereby avoiding the use of structural allograft. Last, the cup is designed to reestablish the normal anatomic hip center. In addition to decreasing the risk of bony impingement observed with an elevated hip center, cups placed in a nonanatomic, superolateral position have been shown experimentally to significantly increase the hip joint reactive forces (7). Clinical studies have confirmed this experimental find-

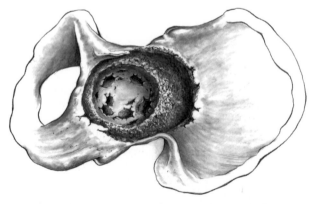

FIG. 1. Combination acetabular defect demonstrating superior rim and medial cavitary bone deficiencies; anterior and posterior columns are intact.

ing with a substantially higher femoral component loosening rate in patients with cemented cups placed in a superolateral position compared to cups that were placed in a nearly anatomic position (20).

ANATOMY

In the mid 1980s, we began to reconstruct large acetabular defects with custom implants because of our dissatisfaction with structural allografts. Solid models of each patient's hemipelvis were made from computerized axial tomographic (CAT) scan data (Fig. 2). Several observations have been made based on these models. Because the defect was created essentially by the linear migration of a hemispherical cup, the geometric shape of the distorted acetabular recess resembled two overlapping hemispheres. Furthermore, the orientation of the pubis, ischium, and ilium relative to the normal acetabulum was noted to be somewhat variable (5). Superior migration of a failed acetabular component results in a defect in the ilium that is also variable in geometric shape and orientation. The larger the defect in the ilium becomes, the greater the degree of retroversion of the acetabular recess. This phenomenon is a result of the fact that the posterior inclination of the ilium increases dramatically at the level of the gluteal ridge (Fig. 3).

To maintain intimate contact between the prosthesis and host bone, an implant that resembled two overlapping hemispheres with a variety of major and minor axis diameters is desirable to completely fill the majority of acetabular defects. In addition, to restore the normal ori-

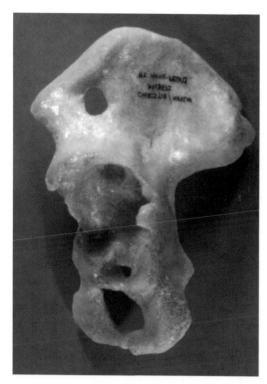

FIG. 2. Hemipelvis model created from CAT scan data of a 41-year-old woman after multiple procedures; CDH was the original diagnosis. Note pattern of bone loss associated with migration of a cemented component placed high.

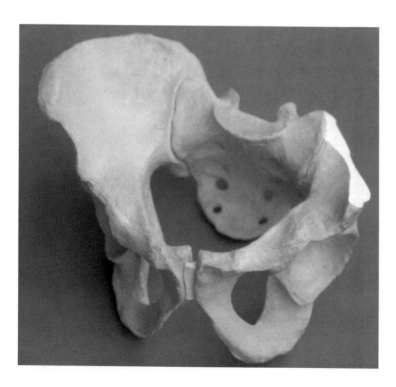

FIG. 3. *Demarcated area* denotes posterior inclination of ilium respective to the gluteal ridge.

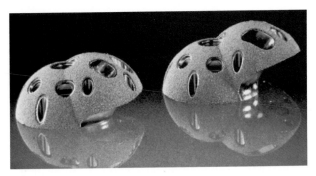

FIG. 4. Acetabular component design consisting of E-15 *(left)* and E-25 *(right)* elongation. (Courtesy of Johnson and Johnson, Inc.; Raynham, Mass.)

entation of the acetabular component, the ability to increase the anteversion and adduction of the component was also deemed necessary.

E-15 AND E-25 CUPS

The oblong cups were named after the amount of elongation of the major cup axis (Fig. 4). The E-15 cup is elongated 15 mm, whereas the E-25 cup is elongated 25 mm. The diameter of the cup hemispheres begins at 51 mm and increases in 3-mm increments to 66-mm for both the E-15 and the E-25 cups. The E-15 cup is designed with neutral anteversion and 10° of adduction. The E-25 cup is larger and designed with 15° of anteversion and 20° of adduction.

The prostheses are made of cobalt–chrome and manufactured with two layers of beads on the outer surface for bone ingrowth. Each prosthesis is secured to the acetabulum with 6.5-mm dome screws and with 5.0-mm peripheral rim screws. The polyethylene liner is locked into position with the rim screws.

SURGICAL INDICATIONS

An indication for using the oblong cup is a large superior rim defects (AAOS type I or III) for which placement of an oversized hemispherical cup would result in reaming away either the anterior or the posterior column. The radiographic assessment of the degree of migration of the hip center is an important indicator for using the oblong cup. In general, approximately 10% to 15% of the patients undergoing revision hip procedures performed at our institution are candidates for the oblong cup. Patients with superior defects demonstrating 1.5-cm or greater vertical migration of the hip center compared to the contralateral hip should strongly be considered candidates for the oblong cup. Our general approach to acetabular revision is to examine the preoperative anteroposterior (AP) pelvis and lateral hip radiographs to determine the location and degree of acetabular bone loss. We refrain from using standard hemispherical cups or oblong cups in patients with massive bone loss, where there is a significant defect involving either the posterior column, a pelvic discontinuity with bone loss in both columns, or a large medial wall defect. We perform salvage acetabular revisions in these patients using custom flanged acetabular components. If the host acetabulum has intact columns, then we plan preoperatively to use either an oversized hemispherical cup or an oblong cup for the reconstruction. The decision whether to use a standard cup or an oblong

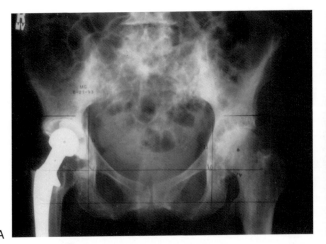
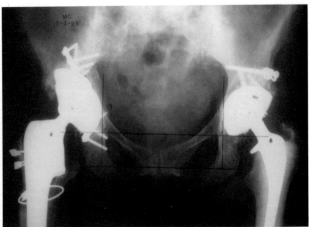

A   B

FIG. 5. Anteroposterior pelvic preoperative **(A)** and postoperative **(B)** radiographs; the patient was a 79-year-old woman who had undergone a cemented arthroplasty in 1983. Both the femoral and acetabular components had migrated significantly, necessitating revision with a calcar replacement stem in addition to the E-15 oblong component. The posterior column plate was created from a curved 3.5-mm reconstruction plate bent to match the bony contours of the acetabulum and fixed with 3.5-mm screws.

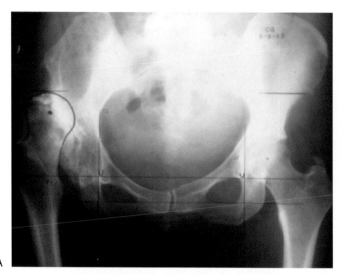
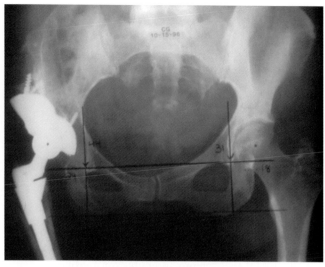

A   B

FIG. 6. Anteroposterior pelvic preoperative **(A)** and postoperative **(B)** radiographs; the patient was a 50-year-old woman with a history of CHD and secondary degenerative arthritis. A pseudoacetabulum and a dysplastic hip were evident preoperatively; primary arthroplasty was performed with an E-25 oblong component and a modular femoral stem.

cup is determined intraoperatively. After reaming to a size where an adequate press-fit is obtained, the degree of coverage of the hemispherical trial acetabular implant is assessed and a decision is made whether to use an oblong cup. Some clinical studies suggest that leaving the acetabular implant uncovered 25% or less is acceptable (10); however, the long-term results using this criterion are unknown. If the amount of uncoverage is greater than 25%, then the decision is to use an oblong cup. In general, we use at least one dome screw and multiple peripheral rim screws for initial implant stability. In addition to providing stability, the peripheral rim screws also provide the locking mechanism for the polyethylene insert with this implant.

We extended our indications for using the oblong cup in one patient with a pelvic diastasis as well as a large superior rim defect. The discontinuity was treated in the usual fashion with a posterior column plate (Fig. 5), and the oblong cup was placed in the standard fashion. The patient healed the discontinuity and the oblong cup has remained stable clinically and radiographically.

We have also used the oblong cup in primary cases. Specifically, patients with congenital dislocation of the hip (CDH) or who have had an acetabular fracture with concurrent avascular necrosis (AVN) of the femoral head (Fig. 6). In this setting, if the femoral head bone stock is not sufficient for structural autograft, then the oblong cup provides a viable alternative for acetabular reconstruction.

SURGICAL TECHNIQUE

A wide exposure of the acetabulum is usually necessary in these cases. We generally use a standard posterior

approach to the hip, although any approach including anterolateral, direct lateral, or transtrochanteric may be used. We identify the sciatic nerve and protect it throughout the procedure. Cobb elevators and large curettes are used to gain circumferential exposure of the bony acetabulum and remove any debris or soft tissue from the acetabular recess down to bleeding bone. The location, size, and geometric shape of the defects are identified. Likewise, the extent of posterior column and anterior column involvement is carefully observed. The transverse acetabular ligament and medial wall of the acetabulum are identified if they are present. These landmarks provide a reference for the normal center of rotation of the acetabulum. If these landmarks are not present, then we determine the

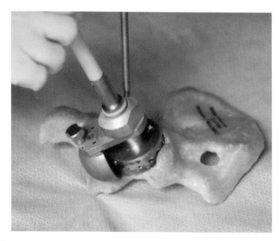

FIG. 7. Reamer assembly (E-25, 51-mm shown); also see Figure 2 for complete view of bone model and Figure 8 for view of trial component.

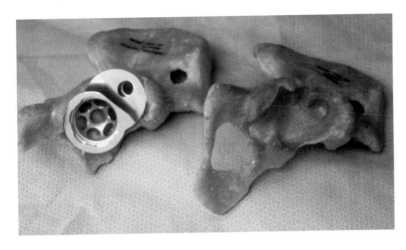

FIG. 8. Bone model with *(left)* and without *(right)* E-25 51-mm trial component.

orientation of the ischium and pubis for a visual estimate of the acetabular center. Standard hemispherical reamers are then used in preparation for the inferior hemisphere of the oblong cup. Attention should be directed toward placing the inferior hemisphere into the correct position to restore the normal hip center, and toward obtaining a press-fit with the anterior and posterior walls of the acetabulum. Next, a special reamer attachment is selected and the superior hemisphere is reamed (Fig. 7). We generally ream the superior hemisphere diameter 1 mm less than the inferior hemisphere to get a press-fit. It is important not to ream the superior hemisphere too far medially because this may cause the cup's orientation to be less anteverted and less abducted than desired. At this point in the procedure, we methodically ream the acetabular defect, removing a minimal amount of bone. A trial implant is inserted to assess the contact and orientation of the cup as well as the stability of the hip after the femoral component has been implanted. We often repeat the reaming, trial reduction, and assessment of orientation and stability several times until the optimal cup position is achieved (Fig. 8). Particulate allograft is used to fill contained medial defects when necessary.

THE 3- TO 6-YEAR RESULTS

Since 1990, we have followed 18 patients who underwent acetabular reconstruction using the Johnson and Johnson oblong acetabular prosthesis (Table 2). The average patient age was 65.5 years, and there were ten men and eight women. There were 15 revision cases and three primary cases. Two of the primary patients had AVN of the femoral head following skeletal trauma. The other primary patient had CDH. All three primary patients had insufficient femoral head bone stock available to be used as autograft. Among the revision patients, there were three with failed bipolar prostheses, nine with failed cemented cups, and three with failed press-fit cups. In revision patients, the average number of previous procedures was 2.2. The acetabular defects were classified as isolated segmental rim defects (AAOS type 1) in five patients, combined segmental rim and medial cavitary defects (AAOS type 3) in 12 patients, and a pelvic discontinuity (AAOS type IV) in one patient. All patients underwent a standard posterior approach to the hip. All cavitary defects were grafted using particulate allograft. The postoperative regimen was identical to the regimen used for hip revision using a standard hemispherical cup. This consists of routine physical therapy for range of motion exercises and non–weight bearing on the affected limb for a 6-week period. We do not use any specialized abduction braces or other orthoses.

Clinical and radiographic results were measured at the initial preoperative visit and at the most recent follow-up visit. The clinical scores were determined using the functional assessment described by Harris et al. (9), the Harris Hip Score (HHS). Radiographic results were determined based on AP pelvis films, and AP and lateral hip films. Radiographs were specifically examined for evidence of pending failures, such as component migration or radiolucent lines at the bone–implant interface. The locations of radiolucent lines were reported for the acetabulum according to a modified method described by DeLee, Ferrari, and Charnley (6).

The location of the hip center was measured using the method described by Callaghan et al. (2). Two measurements were made using a templated AP pelvis film to describe the two-dimensional location of the hip center. A horizontal line was made through the inferior margins of the right and left teardrops, or the superior margins of the right and left obturator foramina if the teardrops were not visible. The center of rotation of the prosthesis was marked and the vertical distance from the interteardrop line was recorded. Likewise, the horizontal distance from the teardrop to the center of rotation was recorded. These two measurements were used to document any change in the location of the hip center. Comparisons were made with the contralateral native hip.

TABLE 2. *A summary of the 18 patients who underwent acetabular reconstruction using the Johnson and Johnson oblong acetabular prosthesis*

Patient ID	Defect type	Previous component
RM	Superior rim	Cemented cup, 1988; uncemented cup, 1991
JK	Superior rim + medial cavitary	Cemented cup
LW	Superior rim + medial cavitary	Bipolar
FM	Superior rim + medial cavitary	Cemented cup
JS	Superior rim + medial cavitary	Cemented cup
CC	Superior rim	Uncemented cup
LO	Superior rim + medial cavitary	Cemented cup
TM	Superior rim + medial cavitary	Uncemented cup
JL	Superior rim + medial cavitary	Bipolar with structural allograft
EN	Superior rim + medial cavitary	Cemented cup
JC	Superior rim + medial cavitary	Cemented cup
MC	Superior rim + medial cavitary	Cemented cup
RR	Superior rim	Primary—DHS with AVN, failed DHS
CG	Superior rim	Primary—CDH with no femoral head for graft
CB	Superior rim + medial cavitary	Cup arthroplasty 1984, bipolar 1987
LG	Superior rim	Primary—acetabular fracture with AVN
TW	Superior rim + medial segmental	cemented cup
TP	Superior rim + medial cavitary	cemented cup

CDH, congenital hip dysplasia; AVN, avascular necrosis.

Clinical Results

The follow-up period for the 18 patients in the study ranged from 3.4 to 6.5 years, with a mean of 4.5 years. The average preoperative HHS was 41.1. The average HHS improved to 91.1 at latest follow-up. No revisions have been performed at latest follow-up. Furthermore, no patients have reported clinical symptoms suggestive of acetabular component loosening.

Radiographic Results

Sequential AP pelvis and lateral hip radiographs demonstrated excellent mechanical stability. There has been no evidence of acetabular component migration, implant dissociation, or prosthetic fracture. Radiolucent lines have been observed in six patients. All radiolucencies were 1 mm or less and nonprogressive. Two patients had radiolucencies in two Charnley zones, and the remaining four patients had radiolucencies in only one Charnley zone. The radiolucencies occurred in an area where particulate allograft was used to fill cavitary defects in four of the six patients. The location of the radiolucencies involved the major cup diameter in five instances and the minor cup diameter in three instances.

Hip Center Analysis

Four patients had a previous hip arthroplasty on the contralateral side and were excluded from the comparison of the prosthetic hip center to the native hip center. The average preoperative vertical migration of the hip center was 45.7 mm (range, 25 to 72 mm) above the interteardrop line. This compared to an average 18.8 mm (range, 13 to 25 mm) for the native contralateral hip. Postoperatively, the reconstructed hip center improved to 20.7 mm (range, 14 to 31 mm) above the interteardrop line (Fig. 9).

Horizontal migration was classified as either medial or lateral based on the comparison with the contralateral hip center. Eight patients had superolateral migration with an average distance of 45.8 mm (range, 41 to 53 mm) from the teardrop. This compared to an average 33.8 mm (range, 25 to 42 mm) for the native contralateral hip. Five of the remaining six patients had less than a 5-mm difference preoperatively between the affected hip and the native hip. These patients were not classified as being medially or laterally migrated. One patient had superomedial (protrusio) migration of 21 mm from the teardrop compared to 34 mm for the native hip. The average postoperative horizontal migration for the reconstructed hip was 35.2 mm (range, 33 to 45 mm). The average postoperative difference between the reconstructed hip center and the native hip center was 5.2 mm for all patients.

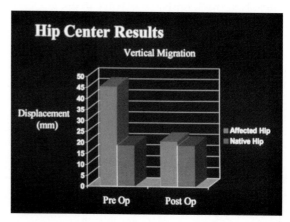

FIG. 9. Graph demonstrating vertical migration of the hip center.

Complications

One patient dislocated 1 year postoperatively after minor trauma. This patient was reduced closed and has not had any subsequent dislocations.

SUMMARY

The oblong cup provides another alternative for acetabular reconstruction. This implant was designed for patients with specific types of acetabular defects, namely large isolated superior rim defects (AAOS type I) or superior rim defects with contained medial cavitary defects (AAOS type III). The inferior hemisphere of the cup relies on the anterior and posterior walls of the acetabulum for a rim-fit similar to that obtained using oversized hemispherical cups. We do not advocate using the oblong cup in patients with massive bone loss where either column is significantly deficient.

There are two areas that need improvement with the oblong cup. A new reamer assembly will be forthcoming to ensure that the orientation of the two hemispheres matches the actual implant with a closer tolerance and reproducibility. Second, the next generation of implants should provide a wider variety of choices for implant anteversion and adduction to provide the proper orientation of the cup face.

Designing an acetabular implant to provide stability on host bone, restore the anatomic hip center, and rely on bone ingrowth for fixation has proven to be successful for standard hemispherical cups. We can hope that the oblong cup will enjoy a similar success rate. Mid-term clinical and radiographic results using the oblong cup to reconstruct the acetabulum in our series of patients with large superior defects have been encouraging.

ACKNOWLEDGMENT

The authors wish to express appreciation to Melanie J. Capps, RN, BSN, for her assistance in the preparation of the manuscript.

REFERENCES

1. Berry DJ, Muller ME. Revision arthroplasty using an anti-protrusio cage for massive acetabular bone deficiency, *J Bone Joint Surg Br* 1992;74-B:711–715.
2. Callaghan JJ, Salvati EA, Pellicci PM, Wilson PD, Ranawat CS. Results of revision for mechanical failure after cemented total hip replacement, 1979 to 1982. *J Bone Joint Surg Am* 1985;67A:1074–1085.
3. D'Antonio JA. Acetabular reconstruction in revision total hip arthroplasty. *Semin Arthroplasty* 1995;6(2):45–59.
4. D'Antonio JA, Capello WN, Borden LS, Bargar WL, Bierbaum BF, Boettcher WG, Steinberg ME, Stulberg SD, Wedge JH. Classification and management of acetabular abnormalities in total hip arthroplasty. *Clin Orthop* 1989;243:126–137.
5. DeBoer DK, Christie MJ. A comparision of acetabular anatomy: computer generated CT scan images versus direct measurements in human cadaver specimens. *Presented at the 8th annual international symposium on technology in arthroplasty*, Puerto Rico, Sept. 27 to Oct. 1, 1995.
6. DeLee J, Ferrari A, Charnley J. Ectopic bone formation following low friction arthroplasty of the hip. *Clin Orthop* 1976;121:53–59.
7. Doehring TC, Rubash HE, Shelley FJ, Schwendeman LJ, Donaldson TK, Navalgund YA. Effect of superior and superolateral relocations of the hip center on hip joint forces. *J Arthroplasty* 1996;11(6):693–703.
8. Emerson RH, Head WC. Dealing with the deficient acetabulum in revision hip arthroplasty: the importance of implant migration and use of the jumbo cup. *Semin Arthroplasty* 1995;4(1):2–8.
9. Harris WH. Traumatic arthritis of the hip after dislocation and acetabular fracture: treatment by mold arthroplasty. *J Bone Joint Surg Am* 1969;51A:737–744.
10. Hozack WJ. Techniques of acetabular reconstruction. *Semin Arthroplasty* 1993;4(2):72–79.
11. Jasty M, Freiberg AA. The use of a high-hip center in revision total hip arthroplasty. *Semin Arthroplasty* 1995;6(2)103–108.
12. Kelley SS. High hip center in revision arthroplasty. *J Arthroplasty* 1994;9(5):503–510.
13. Kwong LM, Jasty M, Harris WH. High failure rate of bulk femoral head allografts in total hip acetabular reconstructions at 10 years. *J Arthroplasty* 1993;8:341–346.
14. Lachiewicz PF, Hussamy OD. Revision of the acetabulum without cement with use of the Harris-Galante porous-coated implant. *J Bone Joint Surg Am* 1994;76A:1834–1939.
15. Padgett DE, Kull M, Rosenberg A, Sumner DR, Galante JO. Revision of the acetabular component without cement after total hip arthroplasty. *J Bone Joint Surg Am* 1993;75A:663–673.
16. Peters CL, Curtain M, Samuelson, KM. Acetabular revision with the Burch-Schneider anti-protrusio cage and cancellous allograft bone. *J Arthroplasty* 1994;10(3):307–312.
17. Paprosky, WG, Perona PG, Lawrence JM. Acetabular defect classification and surgical reconstruction in revision arthroplasty. *J Arthroplasty*, 1994;9(1):33–44.
18. Rosson J, Schatzker J. The use of reinforcement rings to reconstruct deficient acetabula. *J Bone Joint Surg Br* 1992;74B(5):716–720.
19. Schutzer SF, Harris WH. High placement of porous-coated acetabular components in complex total hip arthroplasty. *J Arthroplasty* 1994;9: 359–367.
20. Yoder SA, Brand RA, Pedersen DR, O'Gorman TW. Total hip acetabular position affects component loosening rates. *Clin Orthop* 1988;228: 79–87.
21. Young SK, Dorr LD, Kaufman RL, Gruen TAW. Factors related to failure of structural bone grafts in acetabular reconstruction of total hip arthroplasty. *J Arthroplasty* 1991;6(suppl):S73–S82.
22. Zehntner MK, Ganz R. Midterm results (5.5-10 years) of acetabular allograft reconstruction with the acetabular reinforcement ring during total hip revision. *J Arthroplasty* 1994;9(5):469–479.

The Adult Hip, edited by J. J. Callaghan,
A. G. Rosenberg, and H. E. Rubash.
Lippincott–Raven Publishers, Philadelphia © 1998.

CHAPTER **92**

Revision of the Femoral Component: Extensive Coatings

Wayne G. Paprosky and Anil B. Krishnamurthy

HISTORY OF EXTENSIVELY COATED IMPLANTS

Revision surgery has rapidly become the major focus of total hip arthroplasty. The number of revision hip arthroplasties performed in the United States continues to be on the increase. Although the incidence of revision total hip arthroplasty has been reported at 5% to 9% (1, 21,24,28), these figures may be misleading, as Kavanagh et al. (22) reported a 45% probable radiographic loosening and a 21% symptomatic loosening 4½ years after the revision surgery. Ten-year follow-up studies of both cemented and cementless total hip arthroplasties have reported rates of 1.5% to 19% for revision surgery for aseptic loosening (19,30–32).

The choice of cemented versus cementless total hip arthroplasty continues to be a topic of debate and controversy within the orthopedic community. Early results of cemented revision arthroplasty were less than encouraging. Pellicci and co-workers (29) reported a failure rate of 29% at a mean follow-up of 8.1 years. Kavanagh and Fitzgerald (20) evaluated multiple cemented revisions in 45 patients at an average follow-up of 41 months. The femoral revision rate was 8.3%.

Cementless revision surgery utilizing a porous-coated femoral prosthesis has increasingly gained acceptance

over the last decade (22,25). Varieties of porous-coated devices are currently available. Traditionally, proximally coated femoral components have been used in both primary and revision hip surgery. One of the main problems encountered in revision hip surgery is the presence of bone loss, particularly in the proximal part of the femur. Therefore, fixation of the femoral component becomes increasingly difficult while using a proximally coated device. Although there are few reports in the literature reviewing the results of cementless revision hip surgery, the failure rates reported by various authors utilizing different techniques vary from 5% to 11.5% (8,9,12,15,16, 22,25). Hence, the need for extensively coated stems that afford rigid fixation and eventual ingrowth in the intact diaphyseal portion of the femur was envisaged.

In 1977, Engh began utilizing a modified Austin-Moore straight-stemmed, porous-coated femoral component. The prosthesis was made of cast cobalt–chromium and had a powder-made, sintered, beaded surface of the same material. The initial pore size of 100 μm applied to the entire stem. In 1980, based on animal research, the pore size was increased to a mean of 250 μm. Although this prosthesis was initially used in younger patients, the indications were rapidly expanded. In 1982, the first 100 cases were presented to the Food and Drug Administration and the implant was approved for use without cement in primary hip arthroplasty. In the same year, many stem sizes were made available with porous coating of the proximal 80% of the stem. In 1983, the AML (Anatomic Medullary Locking) stem was made available in distal stem diameters ranging from 9.0 to 21.5 mm, in 1.5-mm

W. G. Paprosky: Department of Orthopaedic Surgery, Rush-Presbyterian–St. Luke's Medical Center, Chicago, Illinois 60190.
A. B. Krishnamurthy: Department of Orthopaedic Surgery, Wright State University, Dayton, Ohio 45409.

increments. Increasing use of the stem led to the recognition of proximal/distal-sizing mismatch in the femur. This, therefore, prompted the development of a second stem with reduced medial to lateral dimension (Modified Medial Aspect). This series of changes allowed for improved canal filling, both proximally and distally. Modular head and neck segments were than added to the system to further refine the prosthesis, allowing for independent leg-length and off-set adjustment. Increasing experience with revision surgery led to the recognition of the fact that, in the presence of significant damage to the proximal femur, fixation of the stem could be reliably achieved at a more distal level. Therefore, longer, extensively coated stems were made available in 205- and 250-mm lengths. Further refinements included the addition of 1.5 mm and 3.0 mm calcar replacement prostheses.

THEORY OF EXTENSIVELY COATED IMPLANTS

Revision of the femur poses a considerable challenge in the presence of significant bone loss in the proximal part of the femur. This problem has been overcome by the use of an allograft–prosthetic composite (2,5,23,33) and bone-packing (4,13,14) in revision surgery utilizing cement. In the setting of revision surgery without cement, this problem has to some extent been addressed by the use of cortical strut grafts (3,17,18,26). To avoid the need for structural allografts, the femoral stem must be supported by the remaining host bone. This stability can reliably be achieved by secured diaphyseal fit, the part of the femur where the best quality of bone is located. Although most implants provide axial stability, rotational control is difficult to achieve. This is particularly true in the revision setting. In revision surgery, a reliable method of achieving bone ingrowth is to gain immediate and rigid fixation of the prosthesis, and to simultaneously allow the porous surface to come in direct contact with well-vascularized and structurally sound host bone with a distal canal filling femoral component. If implanted properly, the extensively porous-coated surface can provide initial stability to both axial and rotational forces. Engh et al. (8,11) reported on a series of 166 cementless revision arthroplasties with a mean follow-up of 4.4 years. They reported a 1% incidence of instability with an extensively porous-coated femoral prosthesis.

Initial stability of the femoral component may be achieved intraoperatively by utilizing an extensively coated prosthesis that is rigidly fixed in the diaphysis of the femur. The current recommendation is to under-ream the femoral canal by 0.5 mm. Fully fluted, rigid reamers that increase in 0.5-mm increments are available. With the currently available refinements, the ability to achieve a press-fit in the femoral isthmus approaches 100%.

Long-term stability of the extensively coated prosthesis is best assessed radiographically. Engh et al. (10), observing the changes that occur between 1 and 3 years postoperatively, have described three basic patterns of radiographic changes: (a) bone-ingrowth fixation, (b) stable fibrous fixation, and (c) unstable fixation. The bone ingrowth pattern is characterized by absence of migration of the implant, absence of radiolucent lines around the porous portion of the stem, absence of endosteal hypertrophy at the distal limit of the porous coating, and no pedestal formation. Also seen in this pattern is a varying degree of bone resorption in the proximal portion of the femur. Such an implant is determined to be bone-ingrown.

The second observed pattern of fibrous ingrowth consisted of either little or no implant migration, and the appearance of a reactive line adjacent to both the porous coating and the smooth portion of the stem. The characteristic feature of this line is that it parallels the contours of the implant, is separated from it by a narrow width (usually 1.0 to 1.5 mm), and is not divergent and does not progress with time. Other changes include a variable pedestal and absence of or minimal proximal bone atrophy. Such an implant is deemed to have a stable fibrous fixation.

The final pattern is characterized by progressive implant migration, rotary instability, and tilting of the component into varus. Progressive, divergent sclerotic lines are seen. Hypertrophy, rather than atrophy, of the proximal portion of the femur is seen. A definite endosteal pedestal is present at the tip of the stem. Such an implant is deemed to be grossly unstable and lacks either fibrous or bone ingrowth.

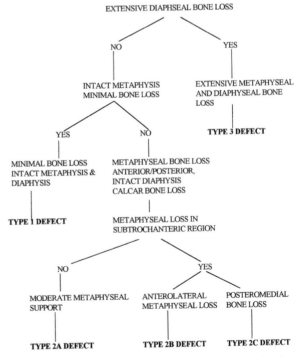

FIG. 1. Algorithm to aid in classification of femoral defects.

INDICATIONS

Indications to use extensively coated implants are varied. The revision surgeon has a variety of implants that are available to suit the needs of individual patients. However, there are certain situations in which only an extensively coated implant is the device of choice. The type of device that is suitable in a given patient depends on a number of factors. The most significant consideration is the amount of bone loss that is present in the femur and the quality of bone that is available. Also of concern is the method chosen to remove existing implants (i.e., the need for trochanteric osteotomy, extended proximal femoral osteotomy, or collapsing osteotomy).

A classification has been developed to assess femoral bone loss, and treatment recommendations are made based on the classification. An algorithmic approach is available to determine the type of bone loss (Fig. 1). The presence of bone loss in the femur is classified into three broad categories. The classification system (27) was discussed in Chapter 57. Briefly, in type 1 defects, the metaphysis is expanded but intact (Fig. 2). In type 2A, the calcar is nonsupportive (Fig. 3); in type 2B, the anterolateral metaphysis is deficient (Fig. 4); and in type 2C, the posteromedial part of the diaphysis is also deficient (Fig. 5). In a type 3 defect, there is complete circumferential bone loss in the metaphysis and it extends into the diaphyseal region (Fig. 6).

Revision of a failed hip is frequently performed in older patients where osteoporosis is frequently encountered. In the presence of Dorr type A or type B bone (7), the choice of implant may be less critical. In the presence of osteopenic type C bone (7) with a wide endosteal canal, the revision surgeon has a number of choices including the utilization of cancellous bone packing with cement discussed in Chapter 97. Although extensively coated stems may be used in type C bone with wide canals, the use of large-diameter stems in such femora is controversial. Engh and Bobyn (10) have shown that there is a strong correlation between cobalt–chrome stem diameters greater than 13.5 mm, extensive porous coating, and pronounced bone resorption. Clinical experience has also shown that in the presence of type C bone (7), utilization of large-diameter stems results in significant proximal bone resorption.

The advances made in revision hip arthroplasty have been not only in the field of biomaterial and implant design, but also in the area of surgical techniques used to remove implants. Notable among them is the technique of the extended proximal femoral osteotomy. This technique may be used to extract ingrown (or stable) fibrous fully coated implants, ingrown proximally coated implants, and loose cemented implants. The osteotomy results in

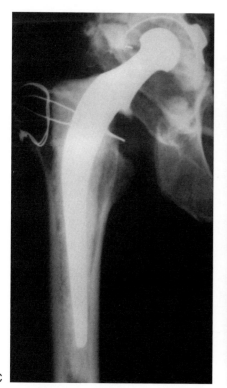
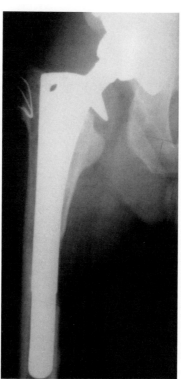
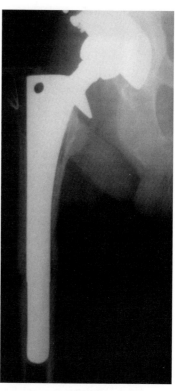

A–C

FIG. 2. A: Preoperative radiograph of the right hip showing a type 1 defect in the proximal femur. Note the expansion of the intact metaphysis. **B:** Immediate postoperative radiograph of the same patient after reconstruction with an extensively coated stem. **C:** Postoperative follow-up radiograph of the same patient at 6 years.

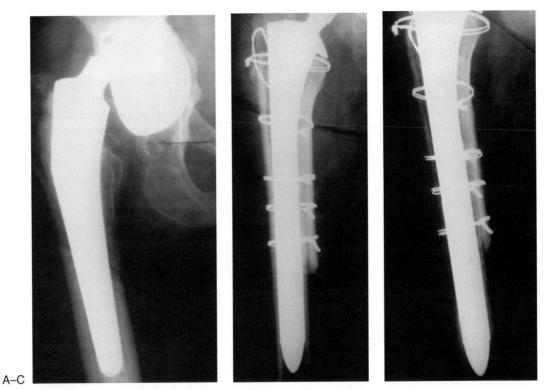

A–C

FIG. 3. A: Preoperative radiograph of a type 2A defect in the proximal femur. The calcar is nonsupportive, the diaphysis is intact. Also note the dissociation of the bipolar hemiarthroplasty prosthesis. **B:** Immediately postoperative radiograph of the same patient after reconstruction. Note the use of strutgraft to fill in the defect on the medial side. **C:** Radiograph of the same patient at 7-year follow-up. Note the incorporation of the strut-graft into the proximal portion of the femur and remodeling of bone.

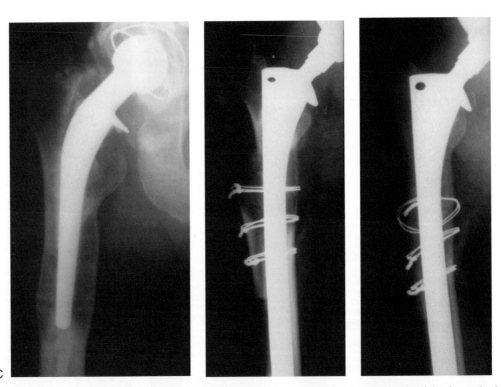

A–C

FIG. 4. A: Preoperative radiograph of a type 2B defect. The anterolateral metaphysis of the femur is deficient. Diaphysis is intact. **B:** Postoperative radiograph after reconstruction of a type 2B defect. An extensively coated stem has been utilized to achieve tight fixation in the diaphysis of the femur, and a strutgraft has been used over the anterolateral defect. **C:** Radiograph of same patient 5 years after reconstruction. There is evidence of bone ingrowth into the prosthesis and incorporation of the strut-graft.

1472

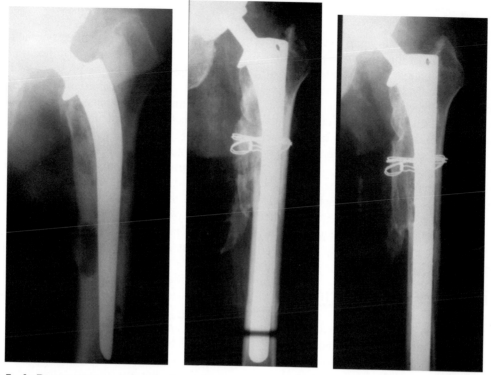

A–C

FIG. 5. A: Preoperative radiograph of a patient demonstrating a type 2C defect. The posteromedial part of the metaphysis is also deficient. Diaphysis is intact. **B:** Radiograph of the same patient after reconstruction. **C:** Radiograph of the same patient at the 11-year follow-up. There is no evidence of loosening, subsidence, or stress-shielding.

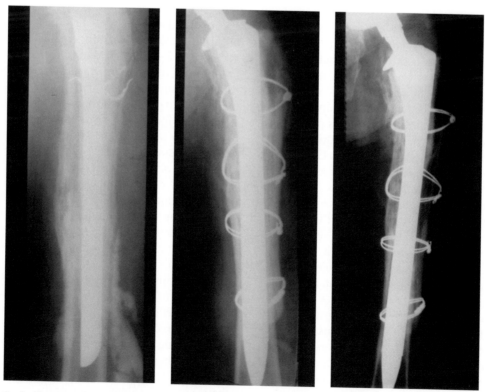

A–C

FIG. 6. A: Preoperative radiograph of the diaphysis of the femur showing complete circumferential bone loss in the metaphysis that extends into the diaphysis. **B:** Immediate postoperative radiograph of the same patient after reconstruction with an extensively coated stem and strut-grafts. **C:** Postreconstruction radiograph at 9-year follow-up. Note evidence of bone-ingrowth and incorporation of the strut-grafts.

1473

the anterolateral third of the femur being opened in the form of a book. As a result of this, the proximal portion of the femur is no longer suitable for the rigid fixation of a proximally coated device. In such a situation, an extensively coated implant will be the prosthesis of choice, being able to provide stable, rigid fixation in the intact diaphyseal portion of the femoral canal. The same is true when a Wagner osteotomy or a transverse femoral osteotomy is utilized (see Chapter 78).

An extensively coated stem may also be the implant of choice in periprosthetic fracture, where, to achieve rotational stability at the fracture site and rigid fixation of the implant, an extensively porous-coated, long-stemmed implant would be the most appropriate choice.

SURGICAL TECHNIQUE FOR INSERTION

Preoperative planning is very essential to achieving a good outcome after revision surgery. Standard, long-length anteroposterior (AP) and lateral radiographs and an AP view of the pelvis with both hips are obtained for preoperative planning. The films must include the entire prosthesis that is to be revised, including the entire cement column in the case of a failed cemented prosthesis. Templates of the extensively coated stems to be used must be available in all the stem sizes and different lengths, including the calcar replacement stems and bowed or curved stems, if their use is contemplated.

The size of the acetabular implant to be used is first determined by placing templates over the AP radiographs of the pelvis with both hips. The center of the hip is marked appropriately, based on the template. The need for bone grafts in the acetabulum is also determined at this stage of the planning. In most hip revisions, the extended proximal femoral osteotomy is performed. The indications and the surgical technique for the extended femoral osteotomy are discussed in Chapter 78. The level of the osteotomy is determined preoperatively based on the AP and lateral radiographs. The distal extent of the osteotomy is based on the length of the prosthesis that is to be revised, the length of the cement column in cemented implants that are being revised, and the level of the cement plug or pedestal. The length of the extensively coated stem is also dependent on the level of the osteotomy and the amount of distal bone that is available for the fixation of the implant. A minimum of 4 cm of distal canal is required for adequate fixation of the extensively coated stem. To achieve this, it may be necessary to use longer (i.e., 8-inch or 10-inch) stems. Based on the bowing of the femoral canal, it may be necessary to utilize the bowed or curved 8- and 10-inch extensively coated femoral stems. By placing the appropriate templates on the AP and lateral radiographs, it is possible to determine the exact type of implant that is best suited for that particular patient. The templates also are a useful guide to the diameter of the implant that may give the best fixation, as determined on both the AP and lateral radiographs. In the presence of bone loss in the proximal femur, particularly on the calcar portion of the neck, it may be necessary to use a calcar replacement prosthesis to restore adequate limb length and soft-tissue tension. Based on the hip center determined by the acetabular implant, it will be possible to make this determination during the planning of the case. The ultimate decision to use a calcar replacement stem and the appropriate length of the neck of the implant is determined intraoperatively based on the soft-tissue tension and stability of the hip joint.

A standard posterolateral approach is used in the majority of patients. The surgical anatomy, approach, and technique of removal of the implants have already been discussed. The technique of proximal femoral osteotomy has also been outlined. After prosthesis removal and after the canal has been cleared of all cement debris, or after removal of the pedestal, reaming of the canal may be commenced. Reaming of the femoral canal for the insertion of extensively coated stems is performed utilizing the AML cylindrical reamers. They are available in 0.5-mm increments starting at 7 mm. The reamers are also marked for different lengths of the implant (i.e., 6 and 10 inches). Reaming of the femoral canal is started with a small-diameter reamer to the appropriate length as determined preoperatively. The canal is reamed progressively by 0.5-mm increments, to beyond cortical chatter. The canal is under-reamed by 0.5 mm after the reamings show cortical bone. This achieves a 2-mm scratch-fit of the component, with 1.5-mm of the fit being provided by the porous beads. Trial stems of all diameters and lengths are available. Trial reduction may be performed with the trial stem in place. The need for calcar replacement stems and the neck-length may be determined after trial reduction. Once the stem diameter and length of the implant have been determined, the actual implant is impacted into the canal. The extensively coated implant is driven into the canal with firm, sustained impactions. Care must be taken to maintain the appropriate anteversion of the stem during the insertion. In the presence of hypertrophic, dense cortical bone in the distal portion of the femur, it may be necessary to prophylactically place a circlage cable over the distal shaft prior to impaction of the implant. During the impaction of the stem, the implant must advance with each impaction: failure to do so may indicate a tight fit and may predispose to fracture of the distal femur. Further reaming of the femur may be necessary to prevent this complication. At the end of the procedure, any osteotomy performed is closed and fixed with two or three cerclage cables. Strut grafts may be used in the presence of bone defects or poor-quality proximal bone, to augment any cables that hold the osteotomy or to supplement more proximal bone loss.

RESULTS

We had the opportunity to review 297 patients [with a mean follow-up of 8.3 years (range, 5 to 14 years)] who underwent revision total hip arthroplasty utilizing the extensively coated AML (De Puy, Warsaw, IN) prosthesis. The proximal femora were classified according to the system proposed by Paprosky et al. (27). There were 45 patients (15%) with type 1 or type 2A defects, 156 patients (52%) were type 2B or type 2C, and 96 patients (33%) were type 3.

All patients were evaluated radiographically and clinically at a minimum of 60 months. Postoperative follow-up radiographs were evaluated using the classification scheme described by Engh and Massin (8) for evaluation of the stability of cementless fixation, and reviewed previously in this chapter. The clinical outcome was assessed using the D'Aubigne and Postel (6) scale for pain and walking.

Definite radiographic instability was noted in seven hips, all of which were type 3 defects. Two of these hips had 3 to 4 mm of subsidence with distal pedestal formation and circumferential radiolucencies. They were, however, not painful, and therefore they were not revised, and the patients were, at the time of follow-up, ambulating with a cane. The remaining five patients demonstrated similar radiographic findings and were all symptomatic, pain being the predominant symptom, and they were therefore revised. At the time of revision, there was no evidence of bone ingrowth but a large amount of fibrous tissue was present. In each of the failures, the stems were undersized and straight. The stems appeared to have a three-point fixation, with the tip of the stem abutting against the anterior femoral cortex. The five revisions were performed with more canal-filling, curved, extensively porous-coated stems. At the time of follow-up, these patients had good clinical function and satisfactory radiographs.

As a group, the seven stem failures showed less than 75% of femoral canal fill as measured from each endosteal surface on postoperative radiographs. The average canal fill in the remaining 290 patients was greater than 88%, and all showed stable fixation. There were no pedestals seen or progressive radiolucencies identified. None of the stems showed subsidence greater than 2 mm. All of the cancellous bone grafts showed evidence of incorporation, and the strut grafts united with the host bone with revascularization of the graft. All of these stable stems had at least 4 cm of intimate diaphyseal contact with the porous coating.

The results of our study were evaluated using the mechanical failure rate. This is defined as the total number of stems showing radiographic evidence of an unstable interface or stems requiring revision surgery, divided by the total number of cases. The mechanical failure rate in our series was a total of seven stems with evidence of loosening out of a total of 297 patients or a rate of 2.4% at a mean follow-up of 8.3 years.

Complications seen in our series were two superficial infections (0.67%) and two sciatic nerve palsies (0.67%) that resolved spontaneously in 5 months. There were no deep infections requiring prosthesis removal or revision. There were eight hip dislocations (2.6%), and six of these patients required only one attempt at closed reduction. Two of the remaining patients had recurrent hip dislocations requiring multiple closed reductions.

Intraoperative complications included the following patterns; fracture of the greater trochanter in 2.1%; proximal femur fractures in 3.1%; fractures at the distal tip of the femoral prosthesis that did not require fixation in 4.4%; and displaced diaphyseal fractures that required fixation in 1.2% of the patients.

Lawrence et al. (22) published the results of revision hip arthroplasty done without cement in 1994. They reported on 83 revision hips that were followed for a minimum of 5 years and a maximum of 13 years, with a mean follow-up of 9 years. All 83 patients underwent revision of the femoral component, and 43 also underwent revision of the acetabular component. The femoral revisions were performed with extensively coated stems in all cases.

At latest follow-up, 23% of the hips that had been revised had had an additional operation. The re-revision rate in the series has been 20%. The rate of re-revision of the femoral component has been 10% and the mechanical failure rate for the femoral implant in this series has been 11%. Early complications included dislocations in three patients and deep vein thrombosis in two patients, with one patient developing a pulmonary embolism. Intraoperative complications included fracture of the calcar in one and nondisplaced fracture of the distal femur in one patient. One patient developed deep infection and had to undergo removal of the implant and reimplantation 8 months later. Patient-defined outcome was satisfactory in 93% of the patients who could be contacted to answer the questionnaire.

Moreland and Bernstein (25) presented their series of 175 patients who underwent revision of the femoral component with extensively coated stems. The patients were followed for a minimum of 2 years and a maximum of 10 years. At a mean follow-up of 5 years, 96% of the revised femoral implants remain in place. They reported a re-revision rate of 4% in their series. Radiographic analysis showed 82.8% to be bone ingrown, 15.5% to be stable fibrous, and 1.7% to be unstable. Severe stress shielding was seen in 7.6% of the femora.

Intraoperative complications included one longitudinal femoral fracture and three perforations of the femoral cortex during removal of cement. One patient developed a partial peroneal nerve palsy. Dislocations occurred in five patients, one patient developed a nonfatal pulmonary embolism and one patient, a fat embolism. Both patients recovered without sequelae. Late infections were reported in three patients.

PITFALLS OF EXTENSIVE COATINGS

Two issues continue to be associated with extensively coated components. The issue of stress shielding seen with the use of extensively coated components seems to be of major concern. The second issue is that of the difficulties encountered during the revision of an extensively coated implant.

Atrophy of the proximal portion of the femur of varying severity has been reported in both cemented and uncemented femoral components. The implantation of a rigid stem in the femoral canal drastically alters the distribution of stress in the femur. The stresses are directly transferred to the distal part of the femur through the stem, thereby shielding the proximal portions of the femur. Therefore, as expressed by Wolfe's law, the decrease in stresses at the level of the proximal femur results in atrophy of that part of the bone. This phenomenon is seen with both cemented and uncemented prostheses.

Various factors appear to be responsible for the phenomenon of stress shielding. Engh and Bobyn (10) have shown that stem sizes greater than 13.5 mm demonstrate a fivefold increase in stress shielding. Also, coating of the stem along its entire length or up to two-thirds its length, results in a two- to fourfold increase in the incidence of stress shielding. Similarly, a canal-filling stem causes a sixfold increase, and age over 50 years results in a threefold increase, in the incidence of stress shielding. Radiographic appearance of bone ingrowth causes a 2.5-fold increase in proximal bone resorption.

Stress shielding has been categorized into four degrees of bone resorption (10). In the first degree, only the most proximal medial edge of cut femoral neck is slightly rounded off. In the second degree, rounding of the proximal medial femoral neck is combined with loss of medial cortical density, as viewed on an AP radiograph. In the third degree, more extensive loss of density is seen extending to the level of the diaphysis but not into it. In the fourth degree, loss of density extends into the diaphyseal portions of the femur.

Although there is a great deal of concern about stress shielding, it must be emphasized that stress-mediated bone loss is only partially attributable to extensively porous-coated femoral implants. Previous publications have demonstrated that a dominant factor influencing bone remodeling is the stiffness of the stem relative to the bone (10). Although titanium alloy has lower modulus compared to that of cobalt–chrome based alloys, the reduction is stem stiffness using titanium are minimized when larger stem diameters are used. Stress shielding has not manifested adverse clinical effects and studies have shown that they have been nonprogressive beyond 2 years (25). To date, no fractures of the femur have been reported that were related directly to stress shielding.

The removal of an extensively coated stem is an arduous task. The indications to remove a well-bone-ingrown, extensively coated stem are few and far between. In the event that removal becomes inevitable, utilizing the technique of performing an extended proximal femoral osteotomy has been very helpful. This allows complete access to the stem. The stem can then be sectioned at the level of the cylindrical portion of the stem and removed in two parts. The distal part may be extracted with the help of trephines that are specially designed for this purpose.

SUMMARY

Strict adherence to important principles is necessary to produce consistent, reliable results. The most important principle in femoral component revision surgery is to be able to achieve immediate and long-term stable fixation of the femoral component. In the presence of bone loss in the proximal femur, which is frequently encountered in revision surgery, this is best achieved in the diaphyseal portion of the femur, where the bone is best suited for this. The use of extensively coated implants, in our opinion, achieves a tight diaphyseal fit and affords rotational stability to the femoral prosthesis.

The results of revision surgery utilizing extensively coated implants have been very encouraging (12,22,25). Results in younger patients and in revisions seem to be better than those performed with cement. Although long-term data are still not available, results to date show that bone-ingrowth does occur and affords long-term stability to the implant, thereby making loosening of the component in the long-run unlikely. In the inevitable event of having to revise such an implant, current techniques, such as the extended proximal femoral osteotomy, have made it easier to do so. Although stress shielding continues to be of concern, the absence of adverse clinical effects to date is encouraging. It is hoped that efforts to design more isoelastic implants with lower-modulus materials will decrease the incidence of stress shielding without compromising the full coating.

REFERENCES

1. Agins HJ, Alcock NW, Bansal M, et al. Metallic wear in failed titanium-alloy total hip replacements: a histological and qualitative analysis. *J Bone Joint Surg* 1988;70A:347–356.
2. Allan DG, Lavoie GJ, MacDonald S, Oakshott R, Gross AE. Proximal femoral allografts in revision hip arthroplasty. *J Bone Joint Surg* 1991; 73(2):235–240.
3. Burchardt H, Jones H, Glowczewski F. Freeze dried allogenic segmental cortical-bone grafts in dogs. J Bone Joint Surg 1978;60A:1082–1090.
4. Capello WN. Impaction grafting plus cement for femoral component fixation in revision hip arthroplasty. *Orthopedics* 1978;17(9):878–879.
5. Chandler HP. The use of allografts and prostheses in the reconstruction of failed total hip replacements. *Orthopedics* 1978;15(10):1207–1218.
6. D'Aubigne RM, Postel M. Functional results of hip arthroplasty with acrylic prosthesis. *J Bone Joint Surg* 1954;39A:451.
7. Dorr LDD. Total hip replacement using APR system. Tech Orthop 1986;1(suppl)3:23–34.
8. Engh CA, Glassman AH. Cementless revision for failed total hip replacement: an update. *Instr Course Lect* 1991;40:189–197.

9. Engh CA, Massin P. Cementless total hip arthroplasty using the anatomic medullary locking stem: results using survivorship analysis. *Clin Orthop* 1954;249:141–158.

10. Engh CA, Bobyn JD, Glassman AH. Porous coated hip replacement: the factors governing bone ingrowth, stress shielding, and clinical results. *J Bone Joint Surg* 1954;69B:45–55.

11. Engh CA, Glassman AH, Suthers KE. The case for porous coated hip implants. *Clin Orthop* 1990;261:63–81.

12. Engh CA, Glassman AH, Griffin WL, Mayer JG. Results of cementless revision for failed cemented total hip arthroplasty. *Clin Orthop* 1988;235:91–110.

13. Gie GA, Linder L, Ling RS, Simon JP, Sloof TJ, Timperley AJ. Contained morselized allograft in revision total hip arthroplasty. Surgical technique. *Orthop Clin North Am* 1988;24(4):717–725.

14. Gie GA, Linder L, Ling RS, Simon JP, Sloof TJ, Timperley AJ. Impacted cancellous allografts and cement for revision total hip arthroplasty. *J Bone and Joint Surg* 1988;75(1):14–21.

15. Harris WH, Krushell RJ, Galante JO. Results of cementless revisions of total hip arthroplasties using the Harris-Galante prosthesis. *Clin Orthop* 1988;235:120–126.

16. Hedley AK, Gruen TA, Rouff OP. Revision of failed total hip arthroplasties with uncemented porous coated anatomic components. *Clin Orthop* 1988;235:75–90.

17. Jablonsky WS, Paprosky WG, Magnus RE, Lawrence JM, Pak JH. Cementless femoral revision arthroplasty: Long-term evaluation of surgical techniques, allografting methods and prosthetic design. *Scientific exhibit at the 59th annual meeting of the American Association of Orthopaedic Surgeons*, Washington, DC, Feb. 20–24, 1992.

18. Johanson NA, Bullough PG, Wilson PD Jr, et al. Microscopic anatomy of the bone-cement interface in failed total hip arthroplasties. *Clin Orthop* 1987;218:123–135.

19. Johnston RC, Crowninshield RD. Roentgenologic results of total hip arthroplasty. A ten year follow-up study. *Clin Orthop* 1983;181:92–98.

20. Kavanagh BF, Fitzgerald RH Jr. Multiple revisions for failed total hip arthroplasty not associated with infection. *J Bone Joint Surg* 1983;69A:1144–1149.

21. Kavanagh BF, Ilstrup DM, Fitzgerald RH Jr. Revision total hip arthroplasty. *J Bone Joint Surg* 1985;67A:517–526.

22. Lawrence JM, Engh CA, Macalino GE, Lauro GR. Outcome of revision hip arthroplasty done without cement. *J Bone Joint Surg* 1994;76A:965–973.

23. Martin WR, Sutherland CJ. Complications of proximal femoral allografts in revision total hip arthroplasty. *Clin Orthop* 1993;295:161–167.

24. McBeath AA, Foltz RN. Femoral component loosening after total hip arthroplasty. *Clin Orthop* 1979;141:66–70.

25. Moreland JR, Bernstein ML. Femoral revision hip arthroplasty with uncemented, porous-coated stems. *Clin Orthop* 1995;319:141–150.

26. Paprosky WG, Lawrence J. Use of femoral strut graft in cementless revision total hip arthroplasty: functional or decorative? Presented at *The 58th annual meeting of the American Academy of Orthopaedic Surgeons*, Anaheim, CA, 1991.

27. Paprosky WG, Lawrence J, Cameron H. Femoral defect classification: clinical application. *Orthop Rev* 1990;Suppl:9–16.

28. Pellicci PM, Wilson PD, Sledge CB, Salvati EA, Ranawat CS, Poss R. Revision total hip arthroplasty. *Clin Orthop* 1982;170:34–41.

29. Pellicci PM, Wilson PD, Sledge CV, Salvatt EA, et al. Long-term results of revision total hip replacement. A follow-up report. *J Bone Joint Surg* 1985;67A:513–516.

30. Salvati EA, Wilson PD Jr, Jolley MN, Vakil F, Aglietti P, Brown GC. A ten year follow-up study of our first one hundred consecutive Charnley total hip replacements. *J Bone Joint Surg* 1981;63A:753–767.

31. Stauffer RN. Ten year follow-up study of total hip replacement. *J Bone Joint Surg* 1982;64A:983–990.

32. Sutherland CJ, Wilde AH, Borden LS, Marks KE. A ten year follow-up of one hundred consecutive Muller curved stem total hip-replacement arthroplasties. *J Bone Joint Surg* 1982;64A:970–982.

33. Zmolek JC, Dorr LD. Revision total hip arthroplasty. The use of solid allograft. *J Arthroplasty* 1993;8(4):361–370.

The Adult Hip, edited by J. J. Callaghan,
A. G. Rosenberg, and H. E. Rubash.
Lippincott–Raven Publishers, Philadelphia © 1998.

CHAPTER 93

Revision of the Femoral Component: Modularity

Hugh U. Cameron

HISTORY

Sixteen years ago, modular head–neck junctions were introduced into North America (8). These junctions enabled orthopedic surgeons to combine different materials for the head and stem (in this case, ceramic and metal) to allow equalization of leg lengths after the final stem had been inserted and to reduce inventory and costs. Other benefits include the ability to remove the head in isolated acetabular revisions to allow visualization, and then to replace it. Incidentally, one trick to protect the trunion from damage during this maneuver is to use an old 22-mm head. If instability was present, a longer neck or a larger head could be substituted. Also, where a high hip center acetabular component was the position of choice, stem extensions could be applied (4), leaving a well-fixed femoral component. The potential disadvantages include problems with the coupling, such as dissociation, fracture, fretting with liberation of wear debris, and corrosion. In general, the realized disadvantages found with head–stem modularity have been minimal.

When initially introduced from Europe, the taper size was 14/16. In North America, small 10/12 tapers were introduced to increase the head–neck diameter difference and, therefore, to increase stability and reduce dislocation by decreasing the possibility of neck–cup impingement. Other 11/13 and 12/14 tapers are also now in common use. These smaller tapers can accommodate the use of 22-mm heads as well as 32-mm heads.

A Morse taper is a tapered male component that fits into a female component. Taper angles generally range from 2° to 12°. The two surfaces lock together because of high contact stresses that develop at the interface during forced assembly. This locking can result in co-integration with some cold welding or transfer of material across the zone of contact (12).

A number of groups have investigated degradation of the taper. Initial observations of corrosion between titanium stems and cobalt–chrome heads suggested that galvanic (mixed alloy) reactions were a potential problem, at least with smaller 10/12 tapers. Some of these tapers initially did not have their tolerances tightly held. Subsequent laboratory investigations and clinical reports of taper corrosion between similar-composition alloys and between metal alloys and nonelectrically conducting ceramics have shown, however, that mixed alloy corrosion was not the cause of the degradation. The corrosion turned out to be mediated by fretting, and directly influ-

H. U. Cameron: Departments of Surgery, Pathology, and Engineering, Orthopaedic and Arthritic Hospital, Toronto M4Y 1H1, Canada.

enced by component tolerance (fit). The poorer the fit, the more the relative movement of one part on the other and, therefore, the greater the degree of liberation of debris into the surrounding environment (12).

Other than seven reported cases of head–neck dissociation during attempted closed reduction of a hip dislocation (14,15) and a few reported cases of aluminum ceramic ball fracture (5), no clinical problems have been noted as a result of the introduction of modular heads. Skirted components should be avoided if possible as they will reduce head–neck diameter difference, thus decreasing the range of movement. It is preferable, therefore, that a hip system have a variation in neck length built into the stem.

Few surgeons would trade the ease and convenience of modular heads for a return to fixed head components. In a recent study of 100 consecutive hips, 19% of the cases reported change in the neck length after insertion of the femoral component. The authors concluded that "the final neck length adjustment needed to maintain hip stability and leg-length equality would have resulted in wastage of $51,300 in these 100 patients. Alternatively, not to change these 19 components would have left the patients with unequal leg lengths or instability" (11).

TYPE OF STEM MODULARITY

Cemented hip stems are not required to accurately reproduce the interior of the femoral canal, as the gap is filled with cement. The introduction of non-cemented hips, primarily porous-coated, changed that requirement. As the femur has an anterior bow beginning at the 200 mm level, any longer stem than that can get at least three-point fixation regardless of the diameter. Animal experiments showed that the closer the porous metal coating came to the endosteal cortical bone, the more rapid and complete the bone ingrowth was. The concept of "fit and fill" thus arose, the objective being to fit the implant to the patient such that it filled the canal. A certain adjustment of canal size and geometry is possible by reaming, but this is limited by the thickness of the cortical bone. The amount of adjustment possible is greater where the cortical bone is thicker than it is in thin osteoporotic bone or in the damaged bone of a revision. This is an everyday experience, as monolithic stems can be fitted quite successfully to a fair percentage of young people with type A bone, but difficulties are experienced in poor quality bone and revision surgery.

There is no consistent relationship between the diameter of the diaphysis and metaphysis. Consequently, to even remotely fill the canal with a monolithic stem, a very large number of implants have to be available with significantly different metaphyseal and diaphyseal diameters, and this does not even begin to address the geometry of the calcar region. One way around the problem is

to ignore the metaphysis completely and ensure diaphyseal fill over a sufficient distance with a fully porous-coated, fully hydroxyapatite (HA)-coated, or grit-blasted titanium stem. Although fixation can be achieved by this method, it does introduce the problem of proximal stress shielding above the most distal fixation point, and it makes implant removal considerably more difficult should revision be required.

Proximal fixation by bone ingrowth is theoretically more attractive, as it limits the length of the stress-shielded segment of bone and makes removal much easier. To achieve proximal fixation, however, initial stability is essential (Fig. 1). The greater the degree of initial proximal stability achieved, the less distal stability is required. With very good initial proximal press-fit, no distal stability may be necessary. In general, however, it is

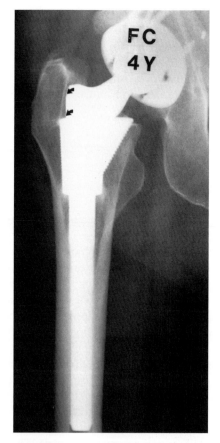

FIG. 1. The expected appearance of a well-fixed proximal ingrowth stem. The main site of ingrowth is always the lowest part of the ingrowth zone, where spot welds can be found. It is uncertain if this is a mechanical effect resulting from a change in stem diameter, or an electrochemical effect, as the sharp change in radius tends to produce a higher free surface energy at that point. The implant makes firm cortical contact distally over more than 5 cm, and the sleeve approaches the lateral cortex proximally. The *arrows* indicate the cavity in the greater trochanter left by the reamer passage and sleeve insertion. If significant wear debris is generated, this area tends to become a magnet for osteolysis.

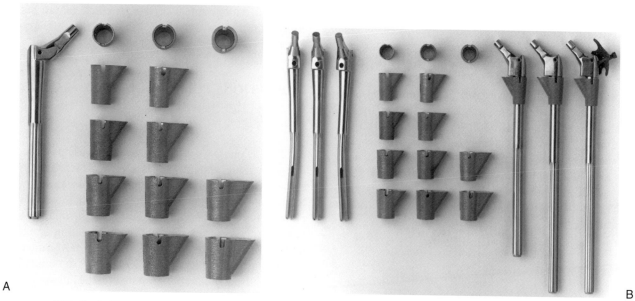

FIG. 2. A: The primary S-ROM system. The stem comes in a variety of neck lengths, from 30 to 42 mm. Various geometries of sleeve can be fitted to the stem. **B:** This is the revision calcar replacement stem. As the proximal femur has a 15° anteversion twist, left and right stems are required. The straight stem should be used only after a diaphyseal osteotomy. One implant shows a trochanteric bolt and washer attached to the prosthesis.

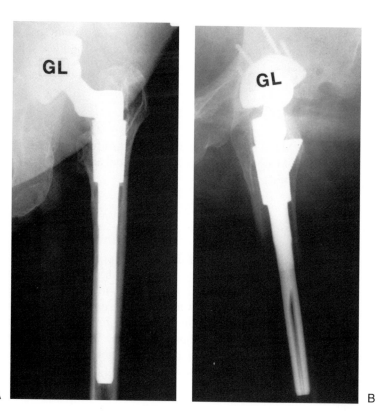

FIG. 3. In this CDH case, the sleeve has been inserted 90° out of phase to allow it to achieve maximum metaphyseal fill. AP **(A)** and lateral **(B)** radiographs.

prudent to obtain some distal stability by using the distal end of the prosthesis even in the best circumstances. This can be done by under-reaming the distal press-fit, using thin, sharp flutes, or using large flutes for filling prepared channels.

In an attempt to produce a monolithic stem that would fit a fair percentage of canals, the sales figures for the size and shape of S-ROM (Joint Medical Corporation, Stamford, CT) sleeves for 1 year were plotted against the stem diameter, hoping to find that a bell curve would result from this study. The figures, however, were scattered, indicating that there is no optimal geometry that fits the majority of canals. In the end, a modular system was preferred.

TYPE OF MODULAR IMPLANT

The description of stem modularity depends on where the coupling occurs in the stem.

Distal Modularity

To achieve distal modularity it is necessary to use a stem that is significantly undersized distally, such as the APR II (Sulzer, Wintertur, Switzerland) and the Omniflex (Osteonics, Allendale, New Jersey). The canal is then filled by a tube or bullet that attaches to the distal end of the stem, usually by means of a Morse taper.

Mid-Stem Modularity

In this design, diaphyseal and metaphyseal segments meet in the mid stem as with Impact and Mallory-Head Modular (Biomet, Warsaw, Indiana). The distal rod fills the diaphyseal canal, and a range of proximal geometries can be attached to it.

Proximal Modularity

In a proximal modular system, the stem fills the diaphysis and is undersized proximally. Canal fill is then achieved by having a series of geometrically different sleeves that can be attached to the stem (Fig. 2). Although wedges have also been used, they leave a gap between the metal and the bone, which is a potential channel for joint fluid and polyethylene debris to gain access to the distal stem.

Version change is one potential advantage of proximal modularity. Because the stem is undersized proximally, it can be inserted in any degree of version with respect to the metaphysis. The sleeve can then be coupled at an angle that allows metaphyseal fill. The ability to change version is particularly important in cases where there is

rotational malalignment of the proximal femur, such as congenital dislocation of the hip or after injury or osteotomy (Fig. 3).

INDICATIONS FOR MODULARITY

General

There is one particular indication for use of a modular non-cemented system: any case in which the use of cement is undesirable for whatever reason and in which templating has shown that a monolithic implant fits poorly. It is important to note that while distal templating is easy and accurate, metaphyseal templating is exceedingly inaccurate. In a patient who has fairly advanced osteoarthritis or congenital dislocation of the hip (CDH), the hip is usually externally rotated on the anteroposterior (AP) radiograph, and there may also be a fixed flexion deformity, resulting in a fore-shortened view. Therefore, with a proximally modular system, the templated size of the sleeve is frequently smaller than the actual size that is employed at the time of surgery. In the lateral radiograph, the position of the proximal end of the implant will vary depending on where the distal end of the implant rests with respect to the femoral bow, making accurate metaphyseal templating even more difficult. Faced with this difficulty, the author has abandoned metaphyseal templating, preferring to use a proximally modular stem in all non-cemented cases.

Specific

Many of the following indications refer only to the S-ROM stem, which has both proximal and distal rotational stability.

Version Change

A modular system that allows version change greatly simplifies the surgery in cases with proximal rotational deformity such as CHD. The ability to insert the sleeve in any version is also very useful in cases with proximal bone destruction, as it allows proximal vertical loading onto the best host bone available. The version of the sleeve with respect to the stem has not been found to produce any clinical or radiologic effect (7).

Femoral Osteotomies

If a proximal–distal osteotomy is performed, rotational and angular stability will be required. Osteotomies can be classified as follows:

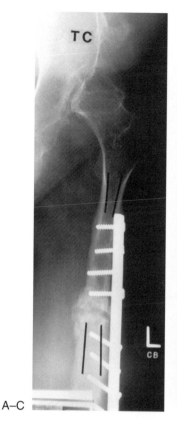
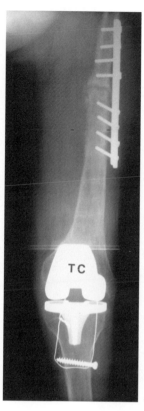
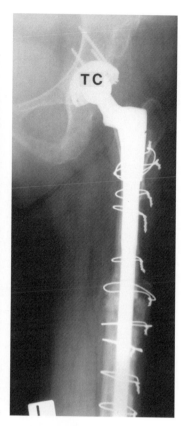

A–C

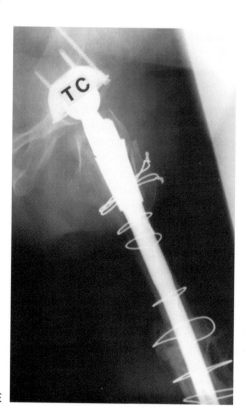
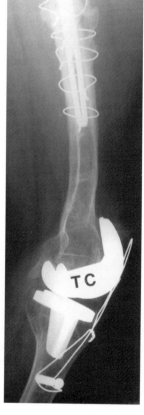

D,E

FIG. 4. This woman with a fibular hemimelia and a high CDH had a total knee replacement. She fractured her femur **(A)**. Attempts at plating and grafting failed, leaving her with a nonunion **(B)**. The proximal femoral canal has a smaller diameter than a distal canal. To pass an adequate-sized stem for distal stability, a vertical osteotomy through the narrowed proximal diameter was carried out to allow reamer passage **(C,D)**. She underwent slight shortening through the nonunion to allow anatomic replacement of the acetabulum. Multiple prophylactic cerclage wires were used **(E)**. Segments of the resected head were wired over the open vertical osteotomy.

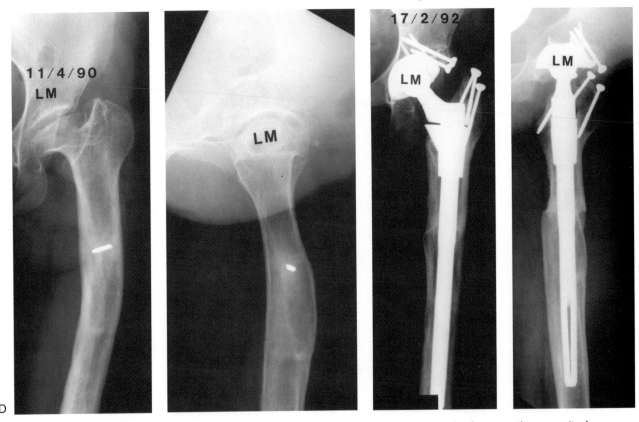

A–D

FIG. 5. This femur was very deformed with a broken screw encased within the femur at the summit of the deformity. AP **(A)** and lateral **(B)** radiographs. A horizontal osteotomy was carried out at the summit of the deformity. The sleeve provides proximal rotational control and the distal fluting distal rotational stability, so that a simple butt joint is all that is required. A crack of the greater trochanter was stabilized by screws **(C)**. Some acetabular bone grafting was required. A straight stem was used in this case **(D)**.

Expansion osteotomy. This is required where there is a narrowing of the bone at some point. A two-thirds horizontal osteotomy with a vertical osteotomy will allow canal expansion for reamer passage (Fig. 4).

Reduction osteotomy. Where the proximal femur is exceedingly patulous, one or more vertical osteotomies can be performed. By serial tightening of cerclage wires, the canal diameter can be reduced.

Angular osteotomy. This should be performed where a change of femoral alignment is required (Fig. 5) (3).

Rotational osteotomy. This should be performed where a change of femoral rotation is required.

Exposure osteotomy. This group includes trochanteric and extended trochanteric osteotomies (2,6) (Fig. 6), and windows where proximal and distal rotational stability is required to prevent a stress fracture at the site of the window (Fig. 7).

Femoral releasing osteotomy. These are vertical osteotomies at the level of the isthmus for primary stems, and at the level of the bow for long-bowed revision stems. When broaching, if the broach becomes stuck and cannot be removed, it is usually jammed in the isthmus or subtrochanteric region. Depending on the implant geometry,

many non-cemented stems also become wedged in the same area. To release those, a vertical cut down to the implant is made on the anterior face of the femur beginning 2 cm below the lesser trochanter and extending distally, usually over a distance of 5 cm. This releases enough hoop tension on the femur to allow withdrawal of the broach or implant, and the osteotomy does not have to be pried open. If a long-bowed stem has been in place for any length of time, a peri-implant bone plate forms around it preventing withdrawal. This is even more so if the stem has a double curve. The releasing osteotomy in this case is a vertical osteotomy through the lateral side of the femur, carried down to the implant, to divide the peri-implant bone plate over the area of bowing. This allows the femur to expand a little to accommodate the bow of the component as the implant is being hammered out. These osteotomies are closed by one or several cerclage wires prior to new stem insertion.

Femoral shortening osteotomies. These include ring shortening, which is excision of a ring of bone in the subtrochanteric or diaphyseal region. Another method of shortening is the calcar episiotomy. This is a vertical osteotomy 3 or 4 cm in length down the calcar or medial

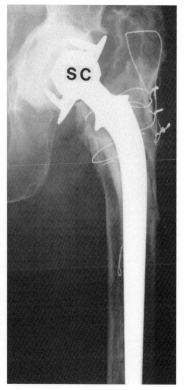

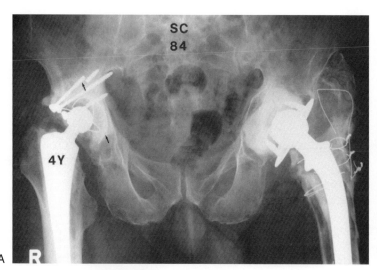

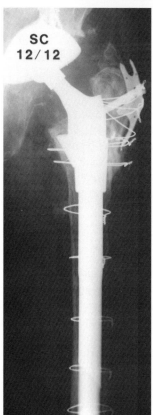

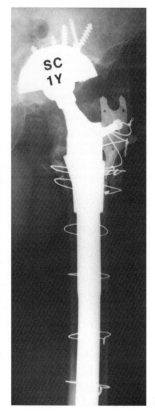

FIG. 6. An 84-year-old man with a loose left femoral component and acetabular protrusion **(A,B)**. An extended trochanteric osteotomy was used for exposure and was reattached by means of a trochanteric bolt and washer. Multiple prophylactic cerclage wires were used because of the poor quality of his osteolytic bone **(C)**. Excellent canal fill was achieved with reconstitution of leg length **(D)**.

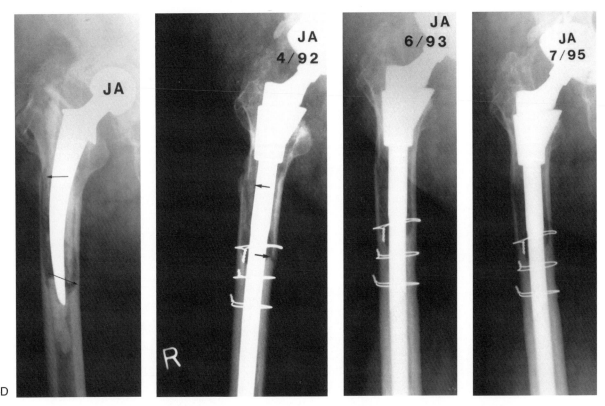

A–D

FIG. 7. A preoperative femoral shaft fracture *(arrows)* can be thought of an exposure auto-osteotomy that greatly simplifies implant and cement removal **(A)**. With proximal and distal canal fill and rotational stability, minimal proximal fixation is required, in this case one cerclage wire. The two distal wires were used to avoid splitting the distal femur **(B)**. The femoral fracture healed rapidly **(C)**. The area of osteolysis that was not grafted has been very slow to recover **(D)**.

face of the femur. As the implant is driven in, the osteotomy gapes open. This allows 10 to 15 mm of shortening. It is mandatory to protect this osteotomy with cerclage wires before implant insertion. The most distal wire is tight, the middle wire is a little loose, and the proximal wire is very loose. As the implant is driven down, the bone expands against the wires, which then become tight. If wires are not used, there is a very real possibility that the osteotomy will extend and break off the anterior or posterior part of the femur.

TECHNIQUE OF INSERTION

Forces to be Resisted in Non-Cemented Stem Fixation

Vertical

The vertical component of load has to be resisted by the wedge shape of the upper end of the femoral stem. Distally, the stem is a round rod in a round hole. No matter how tightly it is inserted, some slippage is likely to occur. The usual method of implant subsidence is that the stem moves into valgus and can then slide down the

inside of the calcar. The shift into valgus is prevented by approaching the lateral femoral endosteal cortex with the implant. Once contact has been made, the only way that further subsidence can occur is by cutting through the calcar, which is very unusual. The geometry, therefore, has to be wedge-shaped with proximal medial/lateral fill.

Angular

Angular forces have to be resisted proximally and distally. This implies reasonable metaphyseal fill in the sagittal plane. The bulk of the angular resistance is probably easiest achieved distally where the medullary canal can be reamed to an exact size over a distance of several centimeters. If the stem is inserted with a press-fit, it is unlikely that significant angular micromotion will occur.

Rotational

On arising from a chair, there is out-of-plane loading of the femoral head, tending to rotate it posteriorly. Proximally, these rotatory forces can be resisted by friction. Consequently, the larger the area of metal–endosteal bone contact, the greater the resistance. The principal area of resistance, however, is the posterior calcar and the anterior femoral cortex. Endosteal cortical contact in these two areas is therefore of some importance.

Distal rotational resistance is required where diaphyseal osteotomies have been performed or where the proximal femur is in poor shape, as it may be in some revision cases. A long-bowed stem in and of itself will provide some resistance to rotation if it reasonably matches the bowing of the femoral canal. Distal fluting with thin sharp flutes inserted with a press-fit have been shown to provide excellent rotational resistance. A heavy press-fit with a rough surface porous coating, a so-called scratch fit, will also provide some distal rotational stability.

Distal Reaming

Distal reaming is generally required in all modular stems. Distal reaming is carried out until firm cortical contact is made over a distance of at least 5 cm. In straight primary stems, rigid reaming can be used over a guide wire if required. The stem is then inserted with a press-fit technique. The definition of a press-fit is the insertion of an oversized implant into an undersized hole. The degree of oversizing will vary depending on the specific implant insertion recommendations. Good quality bone will accept a greater stem-to-canal mismatch. In poor quality bone, there is a risk of fracture, especially if a very rigid implant is used and, therefore, protection with prophylactic cerclage wires may be considered in some instances. In the distally fluted S-ROM, for example, the canal is reamed to the minor diameter (i.e. the diameter of the stem minus the flutes). The flutes are 0.6 mm deep, which gives a 1.2-mm press-fit. In virtually every case, full distal canal fill can be achieved in the AP radiograph. It may not, however, be achieved in the lateral radiograph, as osteoporosis is more active initially in the sagittal plane (10).

Where a revision bowed stem is to be inserted, distal reaming is carried out with a flexible reamer over a guide wire. When flexible reamers are being used, it is unlikely that an exact channel is being created. Furthermore, femurs have different degrees of bowing. This means that the implant is unlikely to be a perfect fit. Reaming should, therefore, be carried out to at least the major diameter of the stem. In nonfluted bowed stems, 1 to 2 mm of over-reaming is usually recommended.

Subsequent insertion techniques will vary with implant type and geometry. The following refers to the S-ROM prosthesis only (7).

Proximal Reaming

Once the canal has been reamed distally to the appropriate size, proximal reaming is carried out with conical reamers. A distal pilot maintains the reamers centrally in the canal. Progressively larger reamers are used until cortical bone is encountered, usually the anterior femoral cortex.

Calcar Preparation

The calcar is then milled with a side-cut drill until cortical bone has been reached.

Trials

Trial reduction is carried out to check sleeve size and neck length, head length, version, and offset, all of which can be varied independently.

Insertion

Where a primary stem is to be inserted, the canal will have been prepared with rigid reamers, producing an exact straight channel. The sleeve is, therefore, inserted first and then the stem is inserted through the sleeve and driven home until the Morse taper has locked.

In the revision situation, because the position of the proximal end of the stem will be controlled by the position of the distal end of the stem and will vary depending on where the stem is with respect to the femoral bow, the sleeve is inserted loosely on the stem. The sleeve should be held inside or distal to the tip of the greater trochanter as the area is usually not completely reamed because the sleeve is flexible enough to bend away from the proximal reamers during canal preparation. The sleeve is orientated to its approximate version a couple of centimeters away from final seating, as by that time the position of the proximal end of the stem will have become fixed. The stem sleeve composite is then driven home.

It must be remembered that it is difficult to change the version of a stem that is pre-bowed. At best, the version can be changed by 5° in either direction. For these reasons, virtually every bowed stem is manufactured with a 15-degree anteversion twist. The stem, therefore, should be inserted in 15° of anteversion.

Once the stem length is greater than 200 mm, it is necessary to bow the stem. A straight stem of reasonable diameter inserted into a bowed canal will inevitably perforate the anterior femoral cortex. Long straight stems may be used, but only if a femoral diaphyseal osteotomy has been carried out. This may result in some hyperextension of the knee, usually about 5° to 10°. Although this is probably not of great significance, it is preferable to use a bowed stem, especially if the knee tends to hyperextend in any case.

TABLE 1. *A comparison of head–neck and stem–sleeve junction zones in S-ROM retrievals*

	Head–neck (%)	Stem–sleeve (%)
Class A	47	37
Class B	40	41
Class C	13	24

From Bobyn JD, Dujovne AP, Krygier JJ, Young DC. Surface analysis of the taper junction of retrieval and in vitro tested modular hip systems. In: Morrey BF, ed. *Biological, material, and mechanical considerations of joint replacement.* New York: Raven Press, 1993;287–301.

POTENTIAL COMPLICATIONS OF STEM MODULARITY

Concerns exist about coupling dissociation. Most couplings are Morse tapers, and the taper must be locked by firm hammer blows. Care must be taken to avoid the presence of particulate debris, such as bone cement in the couplings. This debris may prevent the taper locking. Two cases of failure have been seen with the S-ROM. In one there was a coating of cement within the taper (1), and in the other, multiple wires were passed around the stem above the sleeve, thus preventing locking. In such a scenario, implant failure is inevitable. Other than these two cases, and a few cases reported in the literature of head–neck dissociation during reduction, the author is not aware of coupling failures to date with any modular system. In addition, no coupling fractures have been reported.

Fretting

All mechanically coupled metal–metal junctions must have some degree of micromotion under load. This micromotion results in one part moving on the other part, a process known as fretting. Fretting will result in a liberation of metallic debris. Wet testing in the laboratory has suggested that about 2 million particles per year will be liberated from the S-ROM junction. This pales into insignificance when compared with the 2 billion particles of polyethylene liberated per year from an apparently normal acetabular component.

Analysis of retrieved S-ROM specimens has shown less fretting than was predicted from laboratory studies. Bobyn et al. (1) divide fretting into class A, which shows no change, class B, which shows mild burnishing, and class C, which shows pitting and delamination. A comparison of the head–neck junction with the stem–sleeve junction showed little difference (Table 1). The only sleeve that demonstrated significant wear was the one in which bone cement had prevented the taper from locking.

With two decades of experience with modular heads and one decade with the S-ROM stem, fretting has not been found to be a clinical problem to date.

FURTHER DESIGN CONSIDERATIONS

Although it is not strictly germane to a discussion of hip modularity, any distally canal-filling prosthesis has the potential to produce end-of-stem pain. Any loose implant may, of course, produce end-of-stem pain, but stem pain in a nonloose implant was considered by the author to occur as a result of concentration of bending loads (7). Under load, all bones bend. The direction of bend is usually pretty obvious. They bend into or accentuate the bow. If a stiff metal implant fills the interior of the canal, the bone containing the implant cannot bend. Bending, therefore, is concentrated around the implant tip. If the bending stiffness of the implant is reduced sufficiently, the incidence of end-of-stem pain will almost be eliminated. The simplest way to do this is to split the implant like a clothes-pin in the plane of bending. End-of-stem pain is uncommon with cemented implants because they generally taper towards the tip, which reduces the bending stiffness. The cement also ensures that the bending is over an expanded area, which explains why cemented implants seldom produce end-of-stem pain.

It is theoretically possible to reduce bending stiffness by hollowing the implant. However, the wall thickness has to be reduced to 1.5 mm or so before a significant change in stiffness is noted. Manufacture of such an implant is technically difficult and to date it has not been done.

For the first 2 years after the introduction of the S-ROM, the author used a smooth-threaded socket (7). Although smooth-threaded sockets are still widely used in Europe, they are no longer used in North America because of their somewhat disappointing results. To avoid contamination of results, these cases have been excluded.

The author prefers to use the Paprosky classification (13) for revision hip surgery. The femur is classified after removal of the existing implant. A type 1 femur has a relatively normal metaphysis and diaphysis. A type 2 femur has a damaged metaphysis but a normal isthmus and diaphysis. A type 3 femur has a damaged metaphysis and isthmus.

With most systems, other than a very easy type 1, it is necessary to use specific revision stems because the geometry of the proximal femur has become distorted. However, in a proximally modular system such as the S-ROM, where a larger or oversized sleeve can be used, it is possible to use a primary stem in all type 1 cases and about 30% of type 2 cases. The criterion for use of a primary stem is that the cutting flutes must lock and provide rotational resistance when the implant is at least 2 cm away from final seating. If rotational stability is not achieved, then it is preferable to go to a longer stem.

In all type 3 cases, it is necessary to use a long-bowed stem. If there is significant bone loss in the region of the calcar, then a calcar replacement unit is required. The sleeve rests on host bone, and it can be left protruding at least 1 cm from the host bone. This 1 cm, coupled with a 46-mm neck length and a +12-mm head means that 68 mm of missing bone can be made up with metal. Because of this, it is very seldom necessary to use structural bone graft in an S-ROM revision case.

Revisions with S-ROM Primary Stem

The author's own series of S-ROM revisions have recently been updated. There were 54 cases with a 2- to 7-year follow-up. There were 20 men and 34 women, with an age range from 23 to 85. One patient died in under 2 years. There were no patients lost to follow-up and no stems were removed.

Prior operations consisted of 17 hip resurfacings, 12 press-fits, 18 short cemented stems, 3 proximal ingrowth implants, and 4 Girdlestone procedures. The prior operations consisted of 49 patients who had undergone one total hip replacement, 4 patients who had undergone two total hip replacements, and 1 patient who had undergone three total hip replacements. The original disease was osteoarthritis in 29 patients, rheumatoid arthritis in 2 patients, posttraumatic causes in 5 patients, congenital hip dislocation in 14 patients, Perthes disease in 2 patients, and other causes in 2 patients.

Additional preoperative problems consisted of trochanteric nonunion in four cases, a stem protruding from the femur in one case, absence of the tensor fascia lata in one case, and the leg too long in one case.

Intraoperative complications consisted of a crack of the greater trochanter in one case and a pelvic fracture during implant insertion. This was handled by using a cup with multiple screw holes to stabilize the ilium to the ischium. Concomitant procedures during the revision surgery consisted of a major structural acetabular grafting in seven cases, femoral strut grafts in two cases , a plate and screws in one case, and a calcar episiotomy in one case.

The Harris Hip Rating was excellent in 71.7%, good in 18.9%, fair in 7.5%, and poor in 1.8% of the cases. Fair and poor results included three trochanteric nonunions of previously un-united trochanters and one patient with significant co-morbidities.

Limp was absent in 73.6% of cases, mild in 9.4%, and moderate (i.e., Trendelenburg positive) in 17%. Pain was absent in 73.6%, insignificant (required no analgesics) in 22.6%, and significant (required analgesics) in 3.8% of the cases.

Further operations included one late dislocation treated with closed reduction, and one recurrent dislocation revised to a constrained socket. The hardware was removed from the greater trochanter in one case.

There are many ways of carrying out a radiographic analysis. One of the simplest systems rates the stem as types 1 (A and B), 2, and 3. A stem is rated as type 1A if there is no lucency at all between the stem and the bone. A type 1B stem shows incomplete lucency surrounding the stem, but not in the ingrowth zone. A stem is rated as type 2 if there is a continuous radiolucent line between the stem and the bone, the lines being parallel to the stem. If there is complete lucency with divergent lines, the stem is rated as type 3. A type 3 stem is radiologically loose, although it may not be clinically symptomatic. A type 1 stem is assumed to have bone ingrowth. A type 2 stem does not have bone ingrowth but is stable.

Radiographic analysis in the AP plane showed type 1A in 77.3% of cases, type 1B in 18.9%, and type 2 in 3.8% of cases. There were no type 3 cases. Using a zonal analysis, single-zone lucency (mostly zone 4) was present in 13.2% of cases, double-zone lucency in 3.8% of cases, and triple-zone lucency in 1.9% of cases. There was no high grade lucency other than the two cases of type 2 lucency.

In the lateral plane, 69.8% were type 1A, 26.4% were type 1B, 3.8% were type 2, and 0% were type 3. In the zonal lucency analysis, single-zone lucency (mainly zone 5) was present in 20.8% of cases. The reason for this relates to the entry of the implant into the bow. The anterior leg makes contact with the anterior femoral cortex. In those patients in whom the femur bows early, the posterior leg is left free in the medullary canal. Double-zone lucency was present in 3.8% of cases, and triple-zone lucency in 1.9%. The two stems that showed type 2 lucency were both significantly undersized.

Revision Results with a Long-Bowed Revision Stem

There were 88 cases in this series—45 men and 43 women, between 23 and 86 years of age. Three patients died before 2 years of follow-up and two patients were lost to follow-up. In addition, three stems were revised, leaving 80 cases for review with a 2- to 8-year follow-up. Original disease was osteoarthrits in 69 patients, rheumatoid arthritis in 1 patient, posttraumatic causes in 4 patients, congenital hip dislocation in 9 cases, tuberculosis in 2 cases, old sepsis in 2 cases, and ankylosing spondylitis in 1 case.

In this series, 71 cases had one hip replacement, 8 cases had two total hip replacements, 7 cases had three total hip replacements, and 2 cases had more than three total hip replacements. The prior operation was a short cemented stem in 43 cases, a long cemented stem in 7 cases, press-fit in 10 cases, proximal ingrowth in 8 cases, total ingrowth in 4 cases, Girdlestone in 12 cases, and other procedures in 4 cases.

In addition to aseptic loosening of the implant, the preoperative problems included six femurs that had fractured through zones of osteolysis. The stem had penetrated the side of the femur in five cases. In four cases, the femur had undergone bowing and developed a shepherd's crook deformity. This occurs as a result of serial microfractures in bone weakened by osteolysis. The proximal end of the femur develops a varus deformity (9). The proximal femur was absent in two cases.

Intraoperative complications included a crack fracture of the greater trochanter in four cases, usually fixed by lag screws. A crack of the calcar occurred in two cases, both of which were cerclage-wired. A longitudinal fracture of the femur occurred in three cases. The implant was withdrawn, cerclage wires inserted, and the stem re-inserted. A sciatic nerve injury occurred in two patients: one recovered completely and the other still suffers from dysesthesia. Early postoperative death occurred in one case as a result of cardiac complications.

Concomitant procedures included an extended trochanteric osteotomy in three cases, a transverse diaphyseal osteotomy in eight cases, a vertical osteotomy in four cases, dismantling in one case (2), a window in four cases, a calcar episiotomy in one case, a reduction osteotomy in one case, plate and screws in one case, internal

allograft in eight cases, strut allografts in 12 cases, structural femoral allografts in two cases, and major structural acetabular allografts in 18 cases (Fig. 8).

Further operations included four dislocations at 2, 3, 12, and 24 months. They were all treated with a closed reduction under anesthesia and have remained stable. Three stems were revised. One stem had been inserted into a femur that shattered at the time of initial prosthesis removal. The bone was inadequate to support the prosthesis and this was removed at 1 month. After fracture healing, a further revision was undertaken to reinforce the fractured femur with strut allografts. There was sepsis reactivation in one case at 3 years that necessitated implant removal. One stem, which was very long and ended just above the knee, was revised at 4 years because the patient complained of knee pain. The knee was arthroscoped and fairly minimal changes were found. It was felt possible that the stem was the source of the symptoms. The stem was, therefore, exchanged for a shorter stem that ended well above the knee. Unfortunately, the knee pain remained unchanged, suggesting that the stem was not, in fact, the source of this knee pain. Hardware was removed from the greater trochanter in one case. A supracondylar femoral osteotomy was carried out in three cases that had a significant valgus deformity at the knee, mainly as a result of longstanding CDH. Five acetabular revisions were required for aseptic loosening.

The Harris Hip Rating was excellent in 71.2% of the cases, good in 13.8%, fair in 6.2%, and poor in 15%. The fair and poor results included the sciatic nerve injury with residual dysesthesia, acetabular migration in four cases, an absent greater trochanter in three cases, knee pain in one case, and un-united strut allografts in one case. Limp was absent in 61.3% of the cases, mild in 17.5% of the cases, and moderate in 21.2% of the cases. Pain was absent in 75% of the cases, insignificant in 16.3%, and significant in 8.7%. The pain site was buttock and groin in 12 cases, greater trochanter two, femur in four, and knee in two. The pain related to the femur was significant in only two cases.

Stem lucency in the AP radiograph was type 1A, 63.8%; type 1B, 33.5%; type 2, 3.7%; and type 3, 0%. Using the zonal lucency system, excluding the type 2 cases, single-zone lucency (mainly zone 7) was present in 11.3%, two-zone lucency in 16.3%, three-zone lucency in 5%, and four-zone lucency in 0%. In the lateral radiograph, 62.5% were type 1A, 35% were type 1B, 2.5% were type 2, and 0% were type 3. Using the zonal lucency system, excluding the type 2 cases, single-zone lucency (mainly zone 7) was present in 17.5%; two-zone lucency, 12.5%, three-zone lucency, 3.7%; and four-zone lucency, 1.3%.

Further analysis of the three type 2 cases showed that one stem was too small because a cement ledge had been

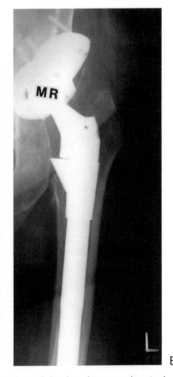

FIG. 8. This hip was infected and had a loose migrated acetabular component and significant calcar osteolysis. A resection arthroplasty was carried out **(A)**. Six months later, when there was no longer any sign of infection, a revision was performed using a bilobed ingrowth cup to restore the axis of rotation of the hip to normal. A calcar replacement stem was used to equalize leg lengths **(B)**.

left within the interior of the femur, one case had massive allograft struts that were probably un-united. The third case was a very large man with a fused ipsilateral knee. Interestingly, his most recent radiographs show a reduction in lucency. As this is difficult to believe and may be a radiologic artifact, he has been left with a type 2 grading for the time being.

SUMMARY

In summary, modularity has much to offer, greatly simplifying difficult hip surgery. The number of complications has been very low. To date, fretting, which is the main concern, has yet to show any significant effects with a follow-up of almost 10 years. The results in revision cases have shown that it is possible to use a proximal modular implant even in a severely damaged femur.

REFERENCES

1. Bobyn JD, Dujovne AP, Krygier JJ, Young DC. Surface analysis of the taper junction of retrieval and in vitro tested modular hip systems. In: Morrey BF, ed. *Biological, material, and mechanical considerations of joint replacement.* New York: Raven Press, 1993;287–301.
2. Cameron HU. Proximal femoral osteotomy in difficult revision hip surgery: how to revise the unrevisable. *Contemp Orthop* 1989;28:565–577.
3. Cameron HU. Use of a distally fluted long stem prosthesis in the correction of angular deformity of the femur. *Contemp Orthop* 1990;20:159–170.
4. Cameron HU. Use of a neck extension sleeve in total hip replacement. *Contemp Orthop* 1990;21:67–69.
5. Cameron HU. Ceramic head fractures in total hip replacement. *J Arthroplasty* 1991;6:185–188.
6. Cameron HU. Use of a distal trochanteric osteotomy in hip revisions. *Contemp Orthop* 1991;23:235–241.
7. Cameron HU, Bhimji S. Early clinical trials with a proximally fixed uncemented hip stem. *Contemp Orthop* 1988;17:31–46.
8. Cameron HU, Loehr J, Fornasier VL. Early clinical trials with a ceramic total hip prosthesis. *Orthop Rev* 1983;12:49–53.
9. Cameron HU, Paprosky WG. Shepherd's crook deformity of the proximal femur associated with aseptic loosening of cemented femoral components. *Contemp Orthop* 1992;25:593–596.
10. Dorr LD. Bone and total hip replacement. In: Cameron HU, ed. *Bone implant interface.* St. Louis, MO: Mosby Yearbook, 1994;49–73.
11. Hozack WJ, Mesa JJ, Rothman RH. Head/neck modularity for total hip arthroplasty: Is it necessary. *J Arthroplasty* 1996;11:397–400.
12. Lemons J. Morse taper modular connections. *Bull Am Acad Orthop Surg* 1996;44:9–10.
13. Paprosky WG, Lawrence J, Cameron HU. Femoral defect classification: clinical application. *Orthop Rev* 1990;19:9–15.
14. Pellicci PM, Haas B. Disassembly of a modular femoral component during closed reduction of the dislocated femoral component: a case report. *J Bone Joint Surg* 1990;72A:619–620.
15. Woolson ST, Pottorff GT. Disassembly of a modular femoral prosthesis after dislocation of the femoral component: a case report. *J Bone Joint Surg* 1990;72A:624–625.

The Adult Hip, edited by J. J. Callaghan,
A. G. Rosenberg, and H. E. Rubash.
Lippincott–Raven Publishers, Philadelphia © 1998.

CHAPTER 94

Revision of the Femoral Component: Bulk Allografts and Struts

Roger H. Emerson

As with many seemingly new orthopedic techniques, allografting is really an old idea that re-emerged in the early 1970s. Allografting is currently a topic of intense interest because it provides solutions to reconstructive problems involving significant bone loss, which are increasingly encountered in the hip after failure of a joint prosthesis. A positive correlation exists between the amount of bone loss and the number of prior total joint surgeries. Restoring the bone stock of the femur is an important part of revision surgery (9,14,46). Experience has shown that successful allograft surgery, like most orthopedic surgical techniques, requires special surgical knowledge and skills. The purpose of this chapter is to present the current status of bulk and strut allografts used for revision of the femoral component during revision total hip arthroplasty.

HISTORICAL OVERVIEW

Several key breakthroughs in orthopedic knowledge have permitted modern allografting techniques to develop. These include a better knowledge of bone healing and repair, as well as knowledge of allograft bone immunogenicity.

Lexer is generally given credit for publishing the first series on allograft transplantation in 1908, describing

the transplanting of 23 whole joints and 11 hemi-joints (30). He reviewed the results of his original series in 1925, reporting a 50% success rate (31).

It was not until after Chase and Herndon in 1955 (11), Bonfiglio et al. in 1955 (3), and Curtis et al. in 1959 (12) established the diminished immunogenicity of frozen bone that modern allografting could go forward. Two clinical series then appeared using hemi-joint fresh-frozen allografts to reconstruct defects left from *en bloc* excision of locally aggressive bone tumors: Parrish in 1966 (41) reported on 19 cases, and Ottolenghi in 1972 (40) reported on 62 cases. Both of these series reported good initial results.

The next significant contribution was the demonstration by Parrish in 1973 that these allografts subsequently were incorporated by the host and that the joints were preserved for many years (42). Parish studied his grafts roentgenographically and documented union in the majority of grafts by 6 to 8 months. He used radioisotope studies, with calcium-47 and strontium-85, to demonstrate incorporation of these grafts, noting higher isotope uptake at the 3- to 4-year mark compared to the 8 to 10-year mark.

The modern era of bone allografting began in the early 1970s, with the largest series done by Mankin et al. who utilized osteochrondral and intercalary whole bone allografts to treat locally aggressive orthopedic tumors (35). Spence et al. reported in 1976 on the use of crushed cortical allograft to pack bone cysts (45). With the appreciation that chemotherapy could treat metasta-

R.H. Emerson: Department of Orthopaedics, University of Texas Southwestern Medical School, Plano, Texas 75093-7916.

tic and microresidual tumor (13), even more aggressive tumors have been managed with allografting techniques, permitting the concept of limb preservation tumor surgery to move forward. The application of bone allografts to total hip revision began in the early 1980s (24).

BIOLOGY OF ALLOGRAFT HEALING ON THE FEMORAL SIDE

Successful allografting requires bone union at the host–graft junction. It is not known whether incorporation is also necessary for a satisfactory clinical outcome, although graft incorporation will not occur in the absence of union (5). Allograft healing and repair is part of the general biology of fracture repair and normal bone remodeling.

Normal Bone Union

Fracture healing is a series of processes: primary callus, bridging callus, late medullary callus, and bone remodeling. Each process is controlled in a different way by local environmental circumstances (37). The primary callus occurs in the first few days after fracture. It is a short-lived phenomenon. If contact with bone is not made, it will ultimately stop. It appears that the cells responsible for this primary callus are from the bony tissues. Most likely, complete bridging of the fracture site cannot be accomplished by the primary callus alone, but must rely on the bridging callus that arises from induction of cells in the surrounding soft tissues, is dependent on mechanical factors, and is suppressed by rigid immobilization. Bioelectric feedback and humoral mechanisms may be involved. This process will not continue indefinitely, and it will stop unless the fracture is bridged.

If bridging occurs between the fracture fragments and movement is arrested, late medullary callus forms. McKibbin (37) feels that this formation arises principally from the medullary cavity and is again dependent on mechanical influences, requiring rigid fracture stability. It can replace fibrous tissue with new bone, ultimately permitting the passage of osteons across gaps between fragments. Where gaps are large and external callus has failed, it may be capable of uniting the ends, although the process will be slow. Excessive motion will impede this process, so artificial stability may be necessary for late medullary callus to fully unite a fracture in the absence of immobilizing external callus. At this point, the remodeling process begins, removing unwanted bone, whether dead or alive, with osteons crossing the fracture site.

In the circumstances of extreme mechanical rigidity, the external callus is suppressed and healing is dependent on the activity of the medullary callus and direct osteonal penetration, as demonstrated by Schenk and Willenegger in 1967 (44). This is a slow process and does not appear to be accelerated by elimination of the external callus. It is diminished by the presence of dead bone, which must be removed. It requires absolute mechanical rigidity.

Allograft Union

Allograft union represents a special bone healing situation where new factors come into play, especially immune mechanisms. The immune inflammatory response appears to diminish the amount of osteoinduction (21). Burchardt et al. (5) compared autografting and allografting in the same canine fibular model. They found better bone union in the autograft situation. In this experiment, they removed a 4-cm section of proximal fibula, reversed it, and put it back into position, using local soft tissues and the adjacent tibia for stability of the bony segment. They documented three types of healing: type I, normal incorporation and fracture union; type II, abnormal healing with graft resorption, producing a substantial decrease in the diameter of the graft, with an increase in fatigue fractures and an increase in nonunions, or a combination of these; and type III, a complete lack of repair of the graft, resulting in resorption by 6 months. In their series of autograft controls, 86% exhibited type I repair. In contrast, using either fresh or freeze-dried allografts, 75% exhibited type II or III repair. Only 2 of 14 allografts had type I repair. Malinin et al. repeated similar allograft experiments with a dog radius, using dynamic compression plating of a freeze-dried segment of radius, and they found reliable bone union and incorporation (33).

This critical role of mechanical rigidity in allograft union was appreciated by the early allograft pioneers. Parrish (42) noted that internal fixation was required for graft union. More recently, Urbaniak and Black had more nonunions with nonrigid Rush pins compared to plating in their series of total elbow allografts (48). Makley (34) found rigid internal fixation necessary for optimal healing in his study of intercalary allografts. Mankin also advocates rigid internal fixation (35).

It is noteworthy that electrical stimulation (38), in the form of pulsed electromagnetic field stimulation, does not lead to any statistically significant change in the histology or biomechanical performances of canine fibular cortical autografts, suggesting that this repair process cannot be hastened and should not be used in the human allograft situation. Similarly, Makley (34) saw no difference in the incidence of union when allografts were supplemented with autografting at the junction. There was, however, improvement in the quality of the union in the grafted patients. Both Mankin (35) and Dick et al. (13) found autografting reliable treatment for allograft fractures and nonunions.

Allograft Immunogenicity

Modern studies have confirmed the decrease in immunogenicity of preserved bone and have shown that different preservation methods produce different amounts of immune response. The amount and type of immune response also depends on the assay method as well as the animal model used (20). Friedlaender et al. (18) compared deep freezing and freeze drying, using a microcytotoxicity assay for humoral and cell-mediated immunity in a rabbit model and found fresh cortical and corticocancellous allografts had significant levels of cell-mediated immunity. Deep-frozen corticocancellous allografts had decreased levels of immunity. Freeze-dried cortical allografts showed no immunity, while freeze-dried corticocancellous allografts produced some cell-mediated immunity in 2 of 5 cases. Therefore, freeze-dried cortex is the least antigenic of preserved grafts, but both deep freezing and freeze drying are associated with a significant reduction in graft antigenicity when compared to fresh bone.

Repeating the canine fibula allograft experiment with immunosuppression with azothioprine for either a short term of 6 weeks (6) or a long term of 12 weeks (4) revealed that more allografts in the immunosuppressed recipients healed with the pattern seen in the autograft controls. There was no increase in delayed unions and no difference in the strength properties or fatigue fractures in the immunosuppressed animals compared to the controls. They concluded that poor healing of bone allografts in the dog is an immunologic phenomenon. It appears that in this fibular allograft model, the superior osteoinduction potential of autograft bone produced sufficient callus to lead to initial bone stabilization to permit union. According to Goldberg et al., the inflammatory response to allograft bone, especially fresh, abrogates the osteoinduction phenomenon by destroying or displacing the progenitor cells (21), thereby preventing initial callus formation. Even with preserved grafts the low level of immunologic activity appears to diminish the quantity or quality of bone induction, thereby delaying the bone union.

Rigid internal fixation appears to lessen the osteoinduction requirements for successful union to take place. (It is well known that a rigidly fixed fracture can heal in the presence of an infection that would have prevented healing were there no internal fixation.) Mechanical rigidity may have other effects on immunologic events, possibly even favoring the creation of blocking antibodies, whose presence has been shown in animal models (11,29,39).

Human studies have not been as clear cut as animal studies. No correlation has been found between immune sensitization and clinical success in human studies. Friedlaender (20) has documented sensitization to anti-HLA (human leukocyte antigen) antibodies in 9 out of 43 human recipients of freeze-dried bone allografts. Follow-up of 8 of these 9 patients indicated no evidence for any detrimental effect on the clinical outcome. Mankin (35) has documented a high titer of anti-HLA antibodies in all but three of his first 83 frozen allograft patients. These titers also did not correlate with the end result. According to Friedlaender, it is premature at this time to ascribe all human allografts failures to immunologic causes (19). In fact, there is no consistent clinical or laboratory sign to suggest that preserved allograft implantation, whether by freezing or freeze drying, has any significant systemic effect on patients (20,34).

Clinical series to date are equally divided between use of freeze-dried and frozen allograft bone. Makley (34) found no difference in either the time to union or the time to incorporation with fresh-frozen or freeze-dried allograft. Pelker et al. (43) found, however, that freeze-dried bone is weaker in bending and torsion than frozen bone. There is no difference in compression. Head et al. preferentially used freeze-dried graft because of its diminished immunogenicity (24).

Allograft Repair

Bone junction healing initiates a process of incorporation of the allograft that arises from the healed junction and migrates down the medullary canal. It is the host's endosteal lining cells that are responsible for more than half of the new bone formation in the repair process; the remainder of the new bone is derived from the surrounding soft tissues (7).

In cortical autografts, the repair is initiated by osteoclasts rather than by osteoblasts. When the resorptive activity has sufficiently enlarged the haversian canals, osteoblasts appear and refill the area. Only 40% to 50% of the cortical graft cross section is repaired, about equal to the area of the haversian system repair. The allograft situation is similar, with the same sequence of events as seen with autograft use but occurring much more slowly. In fact, in rats at 8 months, the allograft is in the same histologic situation as the autograft at 1 month (7).

Whether or not revascularization of a cortical allograft is desirable is an unanswered question. In both the autograft and the allograft situations, such incorporation produces a porosity that profoundly decreases the strength of the graft (4–6,8,15,16). Bone necrosis does not alter the mechanical strength of bone. Therefore, cortical grafts are strongest initially, and then weakened by the revascularizing repair process by approximately 40% from 6 weeks to 6 months in dog cortical autografts. In the human autograft situation, porosity, mechanical strength, and radiographic density are not back to normal for 2 years (7). For example, in the series of Enneking and Burchardt (16) with human fibula autografts, there was a 45% incidence of stress fractures. Most healed without further treatment. There was an increased number of stress fractures with the longer grafts (those more than 12 cm). No stress fractures occurred if a nonunion was present. The stress fractures occurred between 6 and 39 months, with an average onset of 21 months. Berry et al. reported an increase in human allograft fractures at 2 to 3 years (2). Reconstructive techniques and patient management during the first 2 to 4 years after the allograft surgery should support the allograft segment during this predictable period of weakness.

Enneking et al. reported on a series of retrieved human allografts (17). The findings were consistent with the animal models. Bone union was on the periosteal side and derived from the host segment. Overall internal repair was slow, involving only 20% of the graft by 5 years. There was no evidence of any graft resorption around intramedullary stems or prostheses. Of note is that soft-tissue attachment occurred with deposition of a thin seam of new bone on the surface of the graft.

Strut Allografts

Struts, or cortical onlay allografts, are also an old technique that has found a new application. The original research and clinical applications were in fracture fixation. Kreutz et al. described the biology of these grafts in an animal model without stable graft fixation (28). Malinin et al. published a series of radius fractures in a dog model, comparing a metal plate to a "bone allograft plate," both fixed with screws. The allograft series healed more quickly with more strength (32). Allograft plates have been shown to revascularize and remodel into cancellous bone, becoming incorporated into the external callus (14).

Allograft struts follow the same biology as the whole bone segments. The very nature of these grafts, however, takes advantage of this biology. They can be rigidly fixed with ease and have an extensive surface area of contact with the host for union and incorporation. In a dog model, Malinin et al. showed that these grafts are very biologically active and incorporate rapidly (32). Although the grafts were distinguishable radiographically by 24 weeks, they were visually blended with the host, and had remodeled histologically to new bone. Not only were the grafts remodeled, but the host bone under the struts underwent similar remodeling. Radiographic study of human struts by Emerson et al. has shown the same sequence as in the dog model, and by 27 months, the grafts appeared to be incorporated. Some resorption of these struts was evident, usually a rounding-off that occurred all along the edge of the bone plate. There was also visible hypertrophy of some of the bone struts where new bone was laid down on top of the graft or at the proximal or distal ends (14). Further observation of these struts revealed that they ultimately took on the same appearance as the underlying host bone, apparently responding to the same local mechanical environment as the host bone.

USE OF ALLOGRAFTS FOR HIP RECONSTRUCTION

The use of allograft bone to restore femoral bone stock after a failed prosthesis began in the early 1980s. In 1987, Head et al. published a preliminary experience of the first 14 cases with 15 to 30 months' follow-up. Various fixation methods were used (24). This series has been followed and expanded, noting an increase in the complications with continued follow-up (25) but better clinical outcomes as a result of improved techniques. The most common serious complications are nonunion, dislocation, and deep infection. Comparing the first 50 cases from 1983 to 1986 to the next 70 cases from 1987 to 1989, the rate of union improved from 64% to 80% (the average time to union was 8 months), the dislocation rate improved from 28% to 16%, and the infection rate improved from 6% to 4%. The overall improvement in postoperative complications went from 67% to 53%. The average preoperative Harris Hip Score was 41 (range, 9 to 75) and the average postoperative score was 70 (range, 39 to 97). Defining excellent as an improvement in Harris Hip Score of 40 points, good as improvement of 20 points (with no complications), and fair as an improvement of 20 points (with one or more complications), 32 out of 70 patients (45%) were good to excellent, and 23 patients (32%) were fair (27).

Similar results have been reported by others. Zmolek and Dorr reported a nonunion rate of 18% and a dislocation rate of 54% in their series of 22 cases (49). Chandler et al. reported a nonunion rate of 7%, a dislocation rate of 16%, and an infection rate of 3% in their study that included 30 allograft revisions (10). Allan et al. (1) reported a nonunion rate of 19% and an infection rate of 6.8% in a series of 78 cases; 80% of the patients achieved a 20-point improvement in Harris Hip Score (Table 1).

TABLE 1. *Results with bulk allografts*

Authors (ref.)	Hips (N)	Follow-up (mo)	Nonunion (%)	Dislocations (%)	Infections (%)
Zmolek and Dorr (49)	22	48	18	54	na
Chandler et al. (10)	30	22	7	16	3
Allan et al. (1)	78	36	19	na	6.8
Head et al. (27)	120	30	20	16	4

Bone union remains the most difficult challenge of allograft femoral surgery, and it depends on two factors, the fixation of the prosthesis and the stability of the allograft–host bone junction. Generally, the more rigid the implant and junction is, the better the result. Head et al. demonstrated that cementing of the implant to the allograft correlated statistically with better union and fewer allograft fractures regardless of the junction type. Union varied from 50% with an all press-fit transverse graft junction secured to a host step-cut sleeve, to 100% with an allograft step-cut, long-side sleeve with the prosthesis cemented to the allograft and press-fit into the host (Fig. 1). Cementing into the allograft and into the host had a union rate of 75% (27). Although this is a very stable construct, some cement invariably migrates into the junction, which may explain the diminished union. Zmolek and Dorr have reported a better union rate with whole proximal femur than with femoral head, concluding that the latter did not provide enough structural support for a stable femoral component (49). Allan et al. also reported that small calcar grafts (average length, 2.4 cm) had a very low union rate of 17%, and, overall, 16 of 31 failed. Cement support of these small grafts improved the results (1).

The rate of infection in allograft surgery has been a concern, but Tomford et al. (47) have shown that infection is proportional to the complexity of the surgery rather than to the presence of allograft bone. Dick et al. found that two infections in a series of 36 allograft patients were both due to wound necrosis (13). Mankin et al. reported a 13.2% incidence of deep infections in allograft surgery in tumor patients, which were caused primarily by wound complications (35).

Graft fracture remains a late risk because of the increased porosity of the allograft bone as cortical repair progresses. Berry et al. showed that the risk of allograft fracture peaks at 2 to 3 years (2). Martin and Sutherland reported three allograft fractures out of four cases where a short-stemmed implant was cemented into the allograft with the graft junction below the tip of the stem. All fractures occurred at the tip of the implant despite a metal plate for juncture fixation (36). Head et al., however, found allograft fracture to be infrequent with long-stemmed components, with only four out of 70 cases. Each of these cases occurred when cement was not used to secure the allograft to the implant (27). Allan et al. reported two fractures out of 31 short calcar allografts (none in the larger segmental grafts). All stems were long and non-cemented into the allograft (1).

Cortical onlay struts have proven to be more reliable clinically than the whole-bone allografts. It should be noted, however, that the extent of the bone loss that can be reconstructed with a strut is much less than with whole-bone allografts, and it follows that strut cases are generally less complicated than those requiring bulk grafting. Allan et al. noted no nonunions, and an average improvement of 42 points with struts, compared to 35 points for the whole-bone grafts (1). Emerson et al. (14) have published a large series of femoral strut grafts,

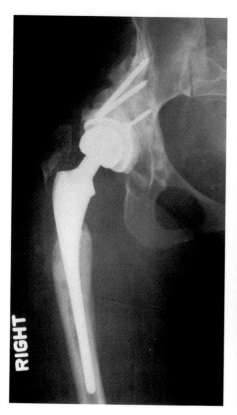
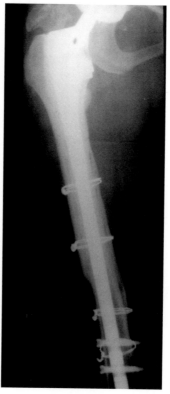

FIG. 1. A: Preoperative radiograph showing the deficiency of the proximal femur. **B:** Postoperative radiograph after proximal femoral allograft with a side-sleeve junction showing union all along the graft–host interface at 4 years. A strut graft has been placed on the medial host femur to strengthen the host femur to support the revision femoral component and bulk allograft. Note the interlocking screws used in the stem of the femoral component, since the junction is below the isthmus.

A

B

146 grafts in 115 patients with an average follow-up of 34 months. The union rate was 96.6%. The time to union for the struts was 8.4 months, compared to 8 months for the bulk grafts. The average Harris Hip Score for this group of strut revisions was 79, compared to 70 for the bulk-allograft patients. When bone struts were used to restore the deficient femur, the clinical outcome was independent of the original femoral bone deficiency, whereas historical controls have shown that the clinical outcome is best in those femurs with the best starting bone stock (23).

INDICATIONS AND PRINCIPLES

Bone allografting is indicated whenever there is not sufficient host bone to revise the femur or there is concern about the ability of the femur to support a revision component. In the young patient with early bone loss, augmentation of bone stock should be considered, even if available host bone is probably sufficient at the time, in anticipation of future revisions.

Struts have the advantage over bulk allografts of permitting a viable bone–implant interface with the possibility of bony ingrowth to the femoral component. Regional bone loss is ideal for strut reconstruction. The strut should be long enough to span the area of deficiency and provide significant mechanical support to the adjacent femur. The most common significant regional bone loss is in the medial femoral calcar (Fig. 2A), from osteolysis or stress shielding, complicated by varus collapse of the failed prosthesis (Fig. 3A). The combination of a calcar-deficient prosthesis and a strut makes a very strong construct for this bone loss pattern, because this implant design puts axial load on the top of the strut, enabling the strut to provide some rotational support to the implant (see Figs. 2,3). However, the strut cannot provide full axial support of the implant. Windows made for cement removal significantly weaken the femur, especially when located near the tip of the revision stem. A long strut over the window area will protect the femur from fracture. The ideal strut is freeze-dried to diminish the immunologic impact, and any loss of graft strength is not a problem in this setting. Simple circlage wires are sufficient fixation.

A bulk allograft is needed if the graft is providing full support of the implant or if the graft is providing segmental replacement of the femur. Short calcar bulk grafts are not reliable, rather a calcar deficient prosthesis should be used. Bulk grafts require complete internal splinting from the prosthesis. Therefore, only long stems should be used. No extraneous holes should be put in the graft, which will not heal and will only be a stress riser for graft fracture. Remnants of host bone should be preserved and are better wired around the graft than screwed or sewn into the allograft. These host segments will permit better

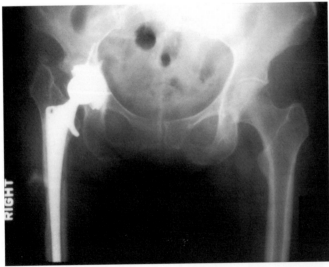
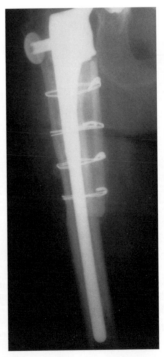
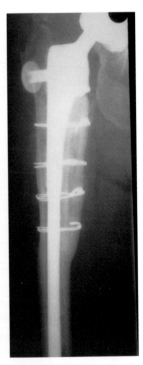

A–C

FIG. 2. A: Radiograph of failed cementless revision long-stem with marked compromise of medial bone stock and subsidence of the femoral component. **B:** Postoperative construct with a calcar-deficient implant and medial strut to augment the medial femoral shaft. **C:** Two-year follow-up of the medial strut demonstrating union to the shaft of the femur. Note the rounding-off of the graft edges.

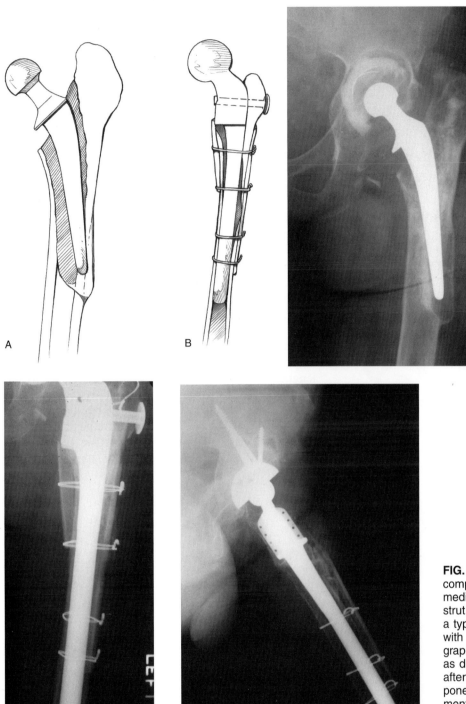

FIG. 3. **A:** Line drawing of a failed femoral component with varus shift and loss of medial calcar. **B:** Line drawing of a medial strut, calcar-deficient implant construct for a typical varus failure femoral component with medial osteolysis. **C:** The AP radiograph shows a femoral component failing as depicted in (A). **D:** The AP radiograph after revision shows the new femoral component and cortical allograft struts augmenting the deficient medial calcar and lateral cortex. **E:** Lateral radiograph showing the strut on the anterior cortex.

soft-tissue attachment to the allograft and will provide a vascularized autograft to aid in union with the host. The implant should be cemented to the allograft.

There is no clear consensus as to the best fixation method of the implant–allograft composite to the host, other than that the fixation must be rigid. Stronger and more rigid bone junctions will favor bone union. The best construct depends on the relative size of the host and the graft. With a larger graft and a smaller host, a long step-cut, side-sleeve junction has proved the most reliable. Alternatively, when the host and allograft are similar in diameter, a step-cut or oblique junction will increase contact and add stability (Figs. 1,4). Metal plates and wires can be used to further support the junction. A lateral tension band plate is especially important with a transverse junction to provide rotational stability (Fig. 5). Cable-

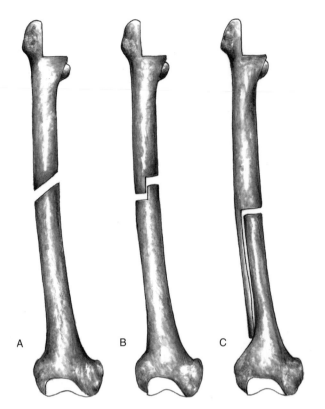

FIG. 4. Line drawing of the common junction constructs. The junction should provide stability as well as increased surface area. An oblique junction **(A)**, a step-cut junction **(B)**, and a lateral side-sleeve junction **(C)**.

plate devices have the advantage of avoiding screws through the graft.

The femoral prosthesis must be stable in the host bone, independent of the type of allograft–host junction used. In the case of a junction above the isthmus of the femur, a press-fit into the host is sufficient. However, below the isthmus, a press-fit cannot be achieved. In this latter circumstance, cement or interlocking screws in the prosthesis can achieve the needed stability. The use of such interlocking screws is on a custom basis (Fig. 6).

Re-attachment of the trochanter should be attempted only if the host trochanter is substantial. The main benefit is prevention of dislocation because of better soft-tissue support. Late trochanter fracture will be common. If the trochanter is deficient, re-attachment should not be attempted.

There is no one solution to prevent postoperative hip dislocation. The functional status of the periarticular soft-tissue envelope is difficult to assess in the operating room, but it can be presumed abnormal. The soft tissues at the end of the surgery must be left tighter than in the primary case, even at the expense of some leg lengthening, although in actual practice it is rare that the leg is lengthened significantly because most patients start out with considerable shortening. Postoperative bracing has a role in some patients. All patients must be educated about hip precautions. Bipolar cups or constrained cups should be considered if the soft-tissue envelope is obviously

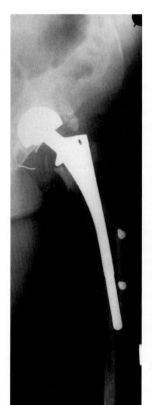

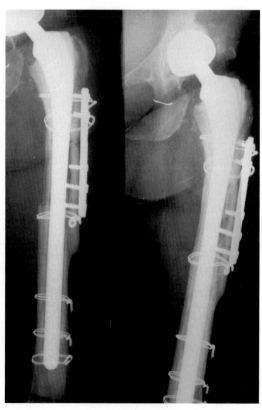

FIG. 5. A: Preoperative radiograph shows nonunion of a prior proximal femoral allograft, tipping into varus. **B:** Postoperative and 7-year follow-up radiograph of a proximal femoral bulk graft. The graft is united and remodeling is underway. A lateral plate is placed across the junction for rotational stability.

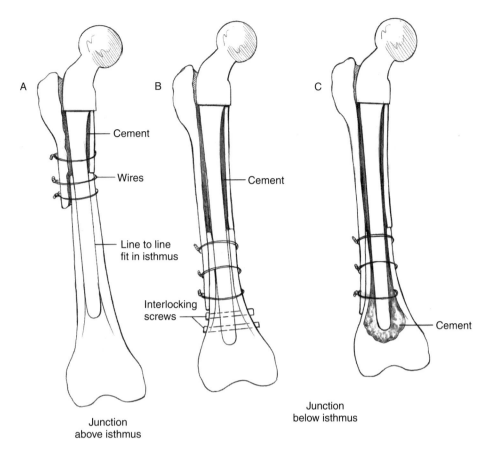

FIG. 6. Line drawing of different methods of achieving tip stability of the femoral prosthesis in host femur. **A:** Junction above the isthmus with press-fit of the stem. **B:** Junction below the isthmus with interlocking screws (custom implant). **C:** Junction below the isthmus with cement fixation.

deficient as with absence of the trochanter or previous dislocations.

Prevention of infection comes about primarily from avoidance of wound healing complications. Prophylactic antibiotics should be used; however, powdered antibiotics sprinkled in the wound should be avoided because of the documented deleterious effect on local osteoprogenitor cells (22). A reasonable practice is to continue the prophylactic antibiotics until all operative cultures are negative and the wound is dry. Bulk allografts in particular need an appropriate host environment for optimal union and repair. Such grafts are best covered with healthy muscle, as opposed to the scarred, relatively avascular subcutaneous tissue seen after radiation and occasionally after repeated surgeries. The surgical approach should facilitate muscle coverage of the allograft (26). If the local soft tissues at the allograft site are not sufficient, then healthy tissues must be brought into the site in the form of flaps or free tissue transfers as either an initial procedure or part of the bony reconstruction performed at a single stage. Strut allografts can irritate the iliotibial band if placed on the lateral shaft. Whenever feasible, these grafts should be placed medially on the femur.

With the fears of compromised wound healing, junctional stability, and hip instability, postoperative care must be carefully monitored. Range of motion, restricting adduction to neutral, and hip flexion to 60° should begin after the wound has stopped draining. Mobilization out of bed should wait until some muscular leg control has returned. Weight bearing should be protected, watching for clinical signs of junctional motion, usually increasing thigh pain. Substantial weight bearing should wait for radiographic evidence of union, usually at about 8 months. A cane may be required indefinitely for long walking, because of chronic abductor deficiency. Allograft patients need life-long orthopedic monitoring.

SUMMARY

Over the past decade, the need for femoral bone stock reconstruction has become evident, especially in the revision setting. Both bulk whole-bone allografts and cortical onlay strut allografts can successfully restore lost bone. In fact, the joint implant setting is ideally suited to these allografts that have certain liabilities inherent in their healing biology. The joint prosthesis needs the allograft for implant support and, likewise, the graft needs the implant to shield the allograft from excessive mechanical stresses during revascularization. The soft-tissue and bony aspects of these surgeries are equally important. Careful soft-tissue management will promote optimal wound healing and contribute to graft union, postoperative stability, and joint function. The best graft type, bulk or strut, freeze-dried or fresh-frozen, depends on the requirements of the particular case. The key principles to follow are rigid stability of the operative construct, at both the graft–host junction and the implant–bone interface.

REFERENCES

1. Allan DG, Lavoie GJ, McDonald S, Oakshott R, Gross AE. Proximal femoral allografts in revision hip arthroplasty. *J Bone Joint Surg* 1991; 73B:235–240.
2. Berry BH Jr, Lord CF, Gebhardt MC, Mankin HJ. Fracture of allografts. Frequency, treatment, and end-results. *J Bone Joint Surg* 1990;72A: 825–833.
3. Bonfiglio M, Jeter WS, Smith CL. The immune concept: its relation to bone transplantation. *Ann N Y Acad Sci* 1955;59:417–433.
4. Burchardt H, Glowczewskie F, Enneking WF. Allogeneic segmental fibular transplants in azothioprine-immunosuppressed dogs. *J Bone Joint Surg* 1977;59A:881–893.
5. Burchardt H, Jones H, Glowczewskie F, Rudner C, Enneking WF. Freeze-dried allogeneic segmental cortical-bone grafts in dogs. *J Bone Joint Surg* 1978;60A:1082–1090.
6. Burchardt H, Glowczewskie G, Enneking WF. Short-term immunosuppression with fresh segmental fibular allografts in dogs. *J Bone Joint Surg* 1981;63A:411–416.
7. Burchardt H. The biology of bone graft repair. *Clin Orthop* 1983; 174:28–42.
8. Burchardt H, Glowczewskie G, Enneking WF. The effect of adriamycin and methotrexate on the repair of segmental cortical autografts in dogs. *J Bone Joint Surg* 1983;65A:103–108.
9. Callaghan JJ, Salvati EA, Pellicci PM, Wilson PD, Ranawat CS. Result of revision for mechanical failure after cemented total hip replacement. *J Bone Joint Surg* 1985;67A:1074–1085.
10. Chandler H, Clark J, Murphy S, McCarthy J, Penenberg B, Danylchuk K, Roehr B. Reconstruction of major segmental loss of the proximal femur in revision total hip arthroplasty. *Clin Orthop* 1994;298:67–74.
11. Chase SW, Herndon CH. The fate of autogenous and homogenous bone grafts. *J Bone Joint Surg* 1955;37A:809–841.
12. Curtis PH Jr, Powell AE, Herndon CH. Immunological factors in homogenous-bone tranplantation. III. The inability of homogenous rabbit bone to induce circulating antibodies in rabbits. *J Bone Joint Surg* 1959;41A:1482–1488.
13. Dick H, Malinin T, Mnaymneh W. Massive allograft implantation following radical resection of high-grade tumors requiring adjuvant chemotherapy treatment. *Clin Orthop* 1985;197:88–95.
14. Emerson RH Jr, Malinin TI, Cuellar AD, Head WC, Peters PC. Cortical strut allografts in the reconstruction of the femur in revision total hip arthroplasty. A basic science and clinical study. *Clin Orthop* 1992; 285:35–44.
15. Enneking WF, Burchardt H, Puhl JJ, Piotrowski G. Physical and biological aspects of repair in dog cortical-bone transplants. *J Bone Joint Surg* 1975;57A:237–252.
16. Enneking WF, Burchardt H. Autogenous cortical bone grafts in the reconstruction of segmental skeletal defects. *J Bone Joint Surg* 1980; 62A:1039–1057.
17. Enneking WP, Mindell ER. Observations on massive retrieved human allografts. *J Bone Joint Surg* 1991;73A:1123–1142.
18. Friedlaender GE, Strong DM, Sells KW. Studies on the antigenicity of bone. *J Bone Joint Surg* 1976;58A:854–858.
19. Friedlaender GE. Editorial. *Clin Orthop* 1983;174:2–4.
20. Friedlaender GE. Immune responses to osteochondral allografts. *Clin Orthop* 1983;174:58–68.
21. Goldberg V, Bos G, Heiple K, Zika J, Powell A. Improved acceptance of frozen bone allografts in genetically mismatched dogs by immunosuppression. *J Bone Joint Surg* 1984;66A:937–950.
22. Gray J, Elves M. Osteogenesis in bone grafts after short-term storage and topical antibiotic treatment. *J Bone Joint Surg* 1981;63B:441–445.
23. Gustillo RB, Pasternak HS. Revision total hip arthroplasty with titanium ingrowth prosthesis and bone grafting for failed cemented component loosening. *Clin Orthop* 1988;235:111–119.
24. Head W, Malinin T, Berklacich F. Freeze-dried proximal femur allografts in revision total hip arthroplasty. *Clin Orthop* 1987;215:109–121.
25. Head WC, Berklacich FM, Malinin TI, Emerson RH Jr. Proximal femoral allografts in revision total hip arthroplasty. *Clin Orthop* 1987;225: 22–36.
26. Head W, Mallory T, Berklacich F, Dennis D, Emerson R, Watner K. Extensile exposure of the hip for revision surgery. *J Arthroplasty* 1987; 2:265–273.
27. Head WC, Hillyard JM, Emerson RH Jr, Peters PC. Proximal femoral allografts in revision total hip arthroplasty. *Semin Arthroplasty* 1993; 4:92–98.
28. Kreutz FP, Hyatt GW, Turner TC, Bassett AL. The preservation and clincial use of freeze-dried bone. *J Bone Joint Surg* 1951;33A: 863–872.
29. Langer F, Czitrom A, Pritzker KP, Gross AE. The immunogencity of bone. *J Bone Joint Surg* 1975;57A:216–220.
30. Lexer E. Substitution of whole or half joints from freshly amputated extremities by free plastic operation. *Surg Gynecol Obstet* 1908;6: 601–607.
31. Lexer E. Joint transplantations and arthroplasty. *Surg Gynecol Obstet* 1925;40:782–809.
32. Malinin T, Latta LL, Wagner JL, Brown MD. Healing of fractures with freeze-dried cortical bone plates. *Clin Orthop* 1984;190:281–286.
33. Malinin TI, Mnaymneh W, Wagner JL, Borja F. Healing of internally fixed intercalary canine allografts of freeze-dried bone. *Orthop Trans* 1985;9:339.
34. Makley J. The use of allografts to reconstruct intercalary defects in long bones. *Clin Orthop* 1985;197:58–75.
35. Mankin H, Doppelt S, Tomford W. Clinical experience with allograft implantation, the first ten years. *Clin Orthop* 1983;174:69–86.
36. Martin WR, Sutherland CJ. Complications of proximal femoral allografts in revision total hip arthroplasty. *Clin Orthop* 1993;295: 161–167.
37. McKibbin B. The biology of fracture healing in long bones. *J Bone Joint Surg* 1978;60B:150–162.
38. Miller G, Burchardt H, Enneking WF, Tylkowski C. Electromagnetic stimulation of canine bone grafts. *J Bone Joint Surg* 1984;66A: 693–698.
39. Muscolo D, Kawai S, Ray R. In vitro studies of transplantation antigens present on bone cells in the fat. *J Bone Joint Surg* 1977;59B:342–348.
40. Ottolenghi CE. Massive osteo and osteo-articular bone grafts. Technique and results of 62 cases. *Clin Orthop* 1972;87:156–164.
41. Parrish FF. Treatment of bone tumors by total excision and replacement with massive autologous and homologous grafts. *J Bone Joint Surg* 1966;48A:968–990.
42. Parrish FF. Allograft replacement of all or part of the end of a long bone following excision of a tumor. *J Bone Joint Surg* 1973;55A:1–22.
43. Pelker R, Friedlaender G, Markham T. Biomechanical properties of bone allografts. *Clin Orthop* 1983;174:54–57.
44. Schenk R, Willenegger H. Morphological findings in primary fracture healding. *Symp Biol Hungarical* 1967;8:75–86.
45. Spence KF, Bright RW, Fitzgerald SP, Sells KW. Solitary unicameral bone cyst: treatment with a freeze-dried crushed cortical-bone allograft. *J Bone Joint Surg* 1976;58A:636–641.
46. Stromberg CN, Herberts P. A multicenter 10-year study of cemented revision total hip arthroplasty in patients younger than 55 years old. A follow-up report. *J Arthroplasty* 1994;9:595–601.
47. Tomford W, Starkweather R, Goldman M. A study of the clinical incidence of infection in the use of banked allograft bone. *J Bone Joint Surg* 1981;63A:244–248.
48. Urbaniak J, Black L. Cadaveric elbow allografts. *Clin Orthop* 1985; 197:131–140.
49. Zmolek JC, Dorr LD. Revision total hip arthroplasty. The use of solid allograft. *J Arthroplasty* 1993;8:361–370.

The Adult Hip, edited by J. J. Callaghan,
A. G. Rosenberg, and H. E. Rubash.
Lippincott–Raven Publishers, Philadelphia © 1998.

CHAPTER 95

Revision of the Femoral Component: Proximal Porous Coating

David S. Hungerford and Michael A. Mont

The patient presenting with fixation failure of a cemented or cementless femoral stem (aseptic loosening) always has some loss of bone stock. This loss may range from minimal to catastrophic. For this reason, any approach to femoral revision must be individualized to address the bone loss. Although cementing into a femoral canal with minimal bone loss may have a high degree of success, this technique is not applicable to the situation of catastrophic bone loss after multiple failures. A review of the literature reveals five options for dealing with revision on the femoral side: (a) re-cement using modern cementing techniques (10,18,27,34,38,49,60, 62,65,66,67,70,75,79,80,85,92,93,95,97,104,105,111), (b) using a combination of bone graft and cement: compaction of cancellous bone graft followed by cementing of a smooth, tapered, polished prosthesis not designed to achieve cement–prosthesis bonding (37,39,86,101), (c) bone graft using an extensively coated prosthesis for cementless fixation (25,28–32,40,73,74,87,88), (d) bone graft using a proximally coated femoral prosthesis for cementless fixation (11,14,23,24,43,46,50,53,54,56–58,

61,71,83,91,106,107,109), and (e) massive structural bone allograft combined with any of the above (13,15, 44,45,51,52). The purpose of this chapter is to iterate the authors' rationale for, indications for, and experience with a proximally porous-coated femoral stem in the revision setting (8,9).

HISTORICAL PERSPECTIVES ON CEMENTLESS REVISION OF THE FEMORAL STEM

The main rationale for the use of porous-coated ingrowth stems for femoral-side revision include the generally poor reported results of cemented revision, and the generally favorable experience with cementless revision from multiple centers (11,14,23,43,54,56,72,76,78,83,98, 101,102,107). In the revision setting, it is difficult to achieve an optimal cement–bone interface, which is important in ensuring long-term survival at this interface. The femur usually presents as a sclerotic vascular tube in which cement interdigitation with host bone is difficult, if not impossible, to achieve. The truly catastrophic results of cemented revision total hip replacements reported in the 1970s and 1980s were the initial justifica-

D. S. Hungerford and M. A. Mont: Department of Orthopaedic Surgery, Johns Hopkins University at Good Samaritan Hospital, Baltimore, Maryland 21239.

tion for exploring the cementless option in the revision setting (2,7,12,19,20,26,33,42,59,68,69,84,89,90,94,108, 110). For first-generation cementing techniques, multiple studies report that actual revision rates plus radiographic failures approached or exceeded 60% in follow-ups of 5 to 10 years (59,68,89,90,110).

Although the modern cementing technique of distal canal plugging, pulsatile lavage, vacuum or centrifuge mixing of cement, retrograde filling, and pressurization has resulted in a dramatic reduction in aseptic loosening in the primary situation (49), the results in the revision setting are less convincing. Rubash and Harris (97) reported the results of a series of 43 revision femoral components in which modern cementing techniques were used with a minimum 5-year follow (average, 74 months). Although only 2% had been re-revised, an additional 9% were definitely loose radiographically. This same group was reported on by Estok and Harris (34): after an average duration of follow-up of 11.7 years, three additional femoral components had been revised because of aseptic loosening. Most recently, Mulroy and Harris (85) reported on this group at an average follow-up of 15.1 years (range, 14.2 to 17.5 years) and found a rate of loosening of 26% (9 of 35 hips). On the other hand, Callaghan and co-workers (10) reported only 66% good and excellent results for femoral component revisions with modern cementing techniques. With a mean follow-up of only 3.6 years, 20% of the stems were seen as radiographic or impending failures (10). In the case of re-revisions, the results are even worse. Retpen and co-workers (96) reported a failure rate of 18% within 5 years of first-time revisions, compared to a 33% failure rate after second revisions using cement.

The use of cement into impacted bone graft is an intriguing concept, as reported by Gie and co-authors (39) as an alternative to revision with cement alone. They reported good and excellent clinical results in 9 of 11 Charnley category A patients. However, at an average follow-up of 30 months (range, 18 to 49 months), 10 of 11 stems had subsided. Recently, Franzén and associates (37), utilizing stereophotogrammetric analysis to analyze for component migration, found a pattern almost identical to that observed in cemented revision arthroplasty (36). Therefore, the long-term outcome of this form of treatment is unknown.

In addition to the difficulties of achieving a good cement–bone interface in the revision setting, the problem of progressive bone loss is not addressed. Patients presenting for second or subsequent revisions have particularly poor results, even with modern cement technique (1,5).

CEMENTLESS REVISION

The options for use of cementless stems include ones that are proximally porous-coated and more fully coated (ranging from five-eights to fully coated). In both of these techniques, there is the possibility of the reestablishment of bone stock deficiencies with bone grafting.

Until recently, there were no long-term results of revisions performed with cementless components. Concerning extensively porous-coated long-stem revision components, Engh and Glassman and co-workers (29) reported a femoral-side re-revision incidence of 3.5% in a group of 127 hips at an average of 4.5 year follow-up. Of these patients, 30% had at least two previous cemented total hip arthroplasties. There were only 2.3% additional femoral components with definite radiographic loosening as indicated by circumferential radiolucent lines or subsidence. In a further follow-up study (9.2 years average, with range from 5 to 15 years), Glassman and Engh (40) have recently reported on an expanded group of 154 hips in 137 patients. Eighty-seven percent of the hips demonstrated radiographic signs of bone ingrowth, with implant stability in 93%. In no case was femoral fixation noted to deteriorate beyond the 2-year follow-up. Seven stems (4.5%) have been revised [one for infection, one for recurrent dislocation, and five (3.3%) for aseptic loosening]. There are five possible additional unstable stems (3.3%). The mechanical failure rate was 6.6% (10 of 152 hips). Survivorship probability was 91.8% using re-revision as the endpoint. Stress shielding was absent or mild in 78.6%, moderate in 14.3%, and severe in 7.1%.

Concerning proximally coated devices, Gustilo and Pasternak (46) reported a 2.8-year average follow-up (range, 2 to 6 years) in a group of 57 cementless femoral revisions using the Bias prosthesis (Zimmer, Warsaw, IN) with cancellous proximal bone grafting. They reported a 7% re-revision rate due to subsidence. An additional 3.5% had 5 to 11 mm of subsidence that did not progress after 1 year. In a series reported by Sotereanos and Rubash (103), 45 consecutive cementless femoral revision arthroplasties were performed utilizing a first-generation titanium femoral component with a long curved stem and a noncircumferential proximal fiber mesh (Bias, Zimmer, Warsaw, IN). At an average follow-up of 5.1 years, the overall mechanical loosening rate was 33%, with 11% of the patients re-revised and an additional 22% of the femoral components radiographically loose. In addition, in the entire series, only 24% of the 45 femoral components demonstrated stability from bone ingrowth into the proximal porous coating.

Hedley and co-workers (54) reported on the porous-coated anatomic (PCA) experience in 61 hips in 55 patients, with 90% good or excellent clinical results. They noted a 4% re-revision rate and a 9.5% symptomatic femoral loosening rate at an average follow-up period of less than 2 years (mean, 20.7 months; range, 12 to 50 months).

Thus, although these are mostly short-term reports, initial results of first-generation cementless technique for femoral component revision have improved upon older cemented results and are quite comparable or superior to most results with modern cementing techniques. Nonetheless, very recently, Woolson and Delaney (109) reported the results of cementless revision in 25 patients followed an average of 5.5 years (4 to 8 years) using the Harris-Galante proximally porous-coated femoral prosthesis. Five stems (20%) had been revised and a further nine (36%) had subsided 5 mm or more. The authors attributed the poor results to failure to achieve adequate apposition of host bone to the proximal fiber mesh pads.

INDICATIONS FOR PROXIMAL POROUS-COATED FEMORAL STEMS FOR REVISIONS

In 1988, we published the system we use for evaluating femoral bone stock at revision (58). Although other, more

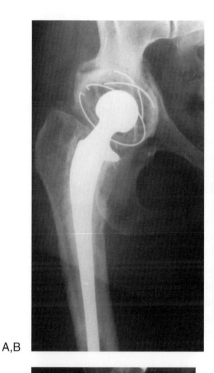
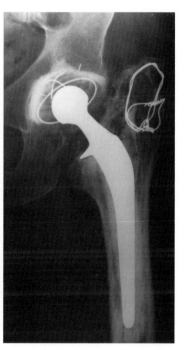

A,B

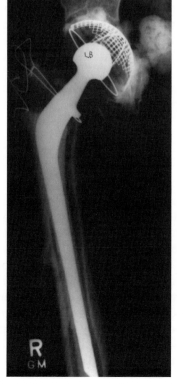
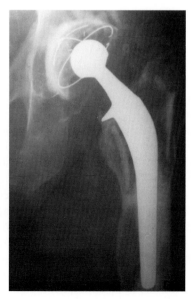

C,D

FIG. 1. Anteroposterior (AP) radiographs of cemented femoral stems needing revision, representing the four types of bone loss on our staging system. **A:** Minimal loss (type 1). **B:** Moderate bone loss, some bone graft required (type II). **C:** Severe bone loss and substantial bone graft required to ensure prosthetic stability (type III). **D:** Massive bone loss, whole allograft required (type IV).

TABLE 1. *Staging system for bone loss at revision arthroplasty*

Type	Degree of bone loss	Procedure(s) involved
Type I	Minimal loss, similar to primary total hip arthroplasties	Most hemi-arthroplasties; occasional total hip arthroplasties
Type II	Moderate loss requiring bone graft; revision prosthesis stabilized by host bone	Most total hip replacements
Type III	Severe bone loss; bone graft required to provide prosthetic stability	Most multiple revision cases
Type IV	Massive bone loss (with or without sepsis) requiring whole allograft	Rare; usually multiple revisions

complex systems are also in use (21,22), this simple system has been effective for us in deciding which patients are most appropriate for a proximally coated stem. This system is based on the degree of bone loss and the ability of the residual bone to support a prosthesis. Type I bone loss provides nearly complete support, whereas type IV bone loss provides virtually no proximal support without structural allograft (Fig. 1) (Table 1).

In our experience, all cases with type I and type II bone loss are satisfactory candidates for cementless revision with a proximally porous-coated device. Most type III cases have also performed well, but the surgeon must be prepared to go to a more extensively coated device if absolute stability cannot be achieved with the proximally coated stem. Proximally coated stems should not be used in type IV bone loss.

CONTRAINDICATIONS TO PROXIMAL POROUS-COATED DEVICES FOR REVISION ARTHROPLASTIES

If the patient has a limited life span as a result of age or medical condition (16), a cemented prostheses should be used. In the elderly, low-activity patient with marked femoral *and* acetabular bone loss, resection arthroplasty (3) should be considered. If the patient cannot participate in protected weight bearing, an extensively porous-coated device, cement, or cement-in-bone graft should be considered. If a proximally porous-coated device is considered, but stability cannot be achieved, an extensively porous-coated device or a cement-in-bone graft is a preferred alternative. In the case of active infection, a two-stage revision should be done. If a good bone–cement interface is possible, the second stage can be done with antibiotic-impregnated cement.

SURGICAL TECHNIQUE

Proximal Femoral Preservation

For proximally porous-coated devices in a revision setting, it is extremely important to preserve the integrity of the proximal femur. In fact, if the integrity of the proximal femur cannot be preserved, then in most instances, a proximally porous-coated device is inappropriate. For this reason, trochanteric osteotomy or trochanteric slide techniques for revision surgery are undesirable and, in our experience, not necessary (41,55). Both the posterior approach and the direct lateral transgluteal approach (47) are satisfactory. In cases when exposure is more difficult, the direct lateral approach can be extended to the removal of the posterior third of the gluteus medius muscle tendon, which is left attached to the tip of the trochanter in the standard direct lateral approach. This is taken off with a cutting cautery and reattached with a Krackow stitch (71) inserted through drill holes in the tip of the trochanter and tied over the metaphysis using No. 5 Ethibond nonabsorbable suture. This has proven to be a very satisfactory technique with excellent healing of this posterior third of the abductor mechanism noted in various cases at re-exploration for various reasons. By avoiding a trochanteric osteotomy, there is preservation of the integrity of the lateral cortex which is important for stability of the proximally porous-coated device and containment of the bone graft.

Once the proximal femur has been exposed, the proximal, accessible cement mantle must be removed before any attempt is made to disimpact the femoral stem from the cement bed. This is an important step, even if the prosthesis or the cement mantle is grossly loose in the femoral canal. Failure to create this proximal window runs the risk that cement attached to the prosthesis will blow out the greater trochanter during the extraction process (80). Again, preservation of the integrity of the proximal femur is a critical step in any femoral revision, but particularly important when using a proximally coated stem.

Cement Removal

Once the stem has been extracted, it is extremely important that all residual cement be removed by whatever technique the surgeon prefers. We use hand tools for the most part, although high-speed cutting tools under biplane fluoroscopic image intensification control occasionally may be necessary for removing distal cement. Once all of the cement has been removed, it is important to obtain anteroposterior and lateral hard-copy radiographs of the femur to definitively ascertain that all cement has been removed. Intensification does not offer sufficient detail to ensure that this has been carried out.

While the radiographs are being processed, the surgeon can turn his attention to removal of the acetabular component and preliminary acetabular preparation, thereby minimizing the delay.

Sizing the Femur

The first step in obtaining the proper fit of the femoral stem in the residual femoral bone stock is to gauge the diameter of the diaphysis with a flexible reamer. The size of the diaphysis determines the maximum size of the prosthesis that can be used, without enlarging the diaphysis. A wall chart is referred to, to determine the size of the prosthesis, corresponding to the diaphyseal size. The broach is initially inserted to see whether that particular size will achieve stability in the proximal femur. In the unlikely event that the proximal aspect of the broach is too large for the particular proximal femur, a smaller broach is chosen, and the broach is used to shape the proximal femur to receive the implant. The optimal goal is to achieve stability both proximally and distally; however, proximal stability is more important than distal stability for this type of device.

Proximal Preparation

Proximal preparation of the residual femur in a revision situation first requires visual inspection to note the presence of any dense cortical reactions to the previous implant. Gouges are used to approximate the lateral trochanteric bed to receive the broach. Because the revision stem is considerably larger than a primary stem, an

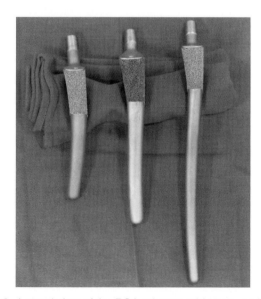

FIG. 2. Lateral view of the PCA primary, mid-stem, and long-stem prostheses showing the anterior distal and posterior proximal bowing.

adequate lateral window is essential to avoid fracture of the greater trochanter when using the broaches. Once the diaphyseal size has been determined, the mid-stem broach that corresponds to that size is inserted into the femur. Because the PCA mid-stem broaches and the long-stem trials have both an anterior distal bow and a proximal posterior bow (Fig. 2), the broach needs to be inserted in a severely anteverted position until the posterior portion of the proximal bow clears the posterior femoral neck. As insertion continues, the broach is progressively retroverted to the anatomic degree of anteversion (~10°). During this insertion in the broaching process, the surgeon needs to be sensitive to any severe hang-up or conflict with dense bony plates that might need to be preformed with a high-speed cutting tool prior to broaching for the final shape. The unique nature of this prosthesis makes this broaching process more complicated than canal preparation for a straight-stem prosthesis. However, once the broach is seated, much greater proximal canal filling is possible. Also, the curved shape of the prosthesis significantly contributes to rotational stability within the curved femoral canal. This works much the same way as a curved tapered cylinder passing into a curved, similarly shaped, tapered housing. Once the curved cylinder is fully seated in its bed, rotational stability is ensured as much by the curved shape of the cylinder and its bed as by friction between the two surfaces.

In the revision situation, because the bone loss is usually proximal, it is unlikely that proximal stability will be achieved before the diaphyseal cortex is embraced by the prosthesis. The more likely scenario is that the diaphysis will have to be expanded to arrive at a proximal size that is sufficient to fill. The diaphysis is then progressively reamed with flexible reamers to allow successively larger prostheses to be used until proximal stability is achieved. In the PCA revision system, there are two lengths with identical proximal geometries, the mid-stem prosthesis and the long-stem prosthesis. It is always preferable to use the mid-stem broach, but as each progressive size is used, the decision has to be made whether to go to the long-stem prosthesis in that size or to an increased size. It is undesirable to ream away any more diaphysis than is necessary because this creates an ever-increasing modulus mismatch of stiffer prostheses and more flexible bone. This has been implicated as a cause of enigmatic thigh pain (35). Therefore, if a mid-stem broach is close, but not quite stable, the long-stem trial should be used before going to the next size.

The additional diaphyseal purchase of the long stem will often provide rotational stability without the need to increase prosthetic size at the expense of diaphyseal bone. As necessary, progressive diaphyseal expansion is carried out until complete stability of the implant is ensured. To use a proximally porous-coated prosthesis without cement in the revision setting, stability must be achieved by host bone.

Leg-Length Equality

In the primary setting, preserving or reestablishing leg-length equality is important and achievable. In the revision setting, the index leg is usually short. Therefore, the risk of producing a leg longer than the other side is minimized. However, in the revision setting, the flexibility to adjust stem insertion level may be severely limited. To leave a stem more proud may compromise stability. To insert it more deeply into the femur risks a fracture. Therefore, in the revision setting, leg-length equality takes a decidedly secondary role.

Bone Grafting

We currently use exclusively fresh-frozen allograft bone for filling any residual defects in the femoral canal. Distal femur or distal femoral hemicondyle provides the best source of bone graft. The bone graft is prepared by using acetabular reamers to create a granular mix of cancellous and cortical bone to be mixed with bone morselated with a rongeur to produce 2- to 4-mm irregular morsels. The ground bone, combined with the morselated bone, produces a mix that can be packed into obvious cavitary defects. The canal is lightly packed and a central passageway created with a smooth medullary seeker. The long-stem trial is then used to pack this bone into place, starting with a trial that is two sizes smaller than the last broach used and ending with a trial one size smaller. The final compaction of the bone graft will take place with the final implant. As this progressive compaction takes place, it is usually necessary to remove some of the bone from the medullary canal using a curette to avoid fracturing the bone with the insertion of the prosthesis. With a proximally porous-coated device, primary stability rests with host bone. Bone grafting fills cavitary defects and provides some augmentation of stability. However, the interposition of bone graft between host bone that was in direct contact with the preparation broaches or trials and the prosthesis must be avoided.

POSTOPERATIVE MANAGEMENT

Because patients presenting for revision demonstrate a broad spectrum of bone stock and soft-tissue stability, the postoperative course varies considerably. Most revision patients require much greater soft-tissue dissection, so that in general we find they are more comfortable for the first 48 hours postoperatively in balanced suspension. Because of the extensive soft-tissue dissection, they are also more prone to dislocation, and therefore postoperatively we usually maintain the patient in a removable abduction brace. Because the cementless stem is considerably less resistant to force applied as an off-axis load (as with the hip in flexion) (63,64), we also limit hip flexion with the aforementioned brace to 45° for the first 6 weeks. Postoperative weight-bearing protection is a function of stem stability and bone loss. All patients have a minimum of 6 weeks of protective weight bearing using a walker or crutches, and with not more than 20 to 30 lb applied to the index extremity. For most patients with type I and type II bone loss, the initial 6 weeks are followed with protected weight bearing using a cane or a single crutch, with progression to full weight bearing at 3 months. For patients with more severe bone loss, the period of maximal-protection weight bearing is extended to 3 months and occasionally even 6 months, with full unprotected weight bearing not taking place for up to 1 year. We advise many patients with multiple failures, severe bone stock loss, and a severe compromise of the hip abductors, to use a cane or single crutch full time. Our current average hospitalization for a revision total hip replacement is 7 days.

OUR RESULTS

The senior author's experience with cementless revision of cemented failures began in October 1983. At that time, the primary PCA prosthesis was used, as well as the long-stem custom prosthesis that was the prototype for the PCA long-stem prosthesis. During this time, it also became apparent that there was a need for a shorter version of the long-stem prosthesis that preserved the metaphyseal/diaphyseal proportions of the long-stem prosthesis, and the PCA mid-stem prosthesis was developed. The complete system was available only in mid 1986. Prior to July 1986, 41 patients underwent cementless revision of a cemented failure, and of those, 13 have undergone re-revision. The incidence of osteolysis requiring revision is 24% (10 of 41). All patients were graded concerning bone stock loss into one of four types (see Fig. 1). The reasons for failure included failure to remove all the cement (one case), intraoperative fracture (three cases), undersized (and presumably unstable) prostheses (seven cases), and type 4 bone loss (two cases).

Between July 28, 1986, and December 31, 1989, 46 patients underwent cementless revision of a cemented failure. In all patients, the proximally circumferentially porous-coated cobalt femoral stem was used (PCA). This group included 23 men and 23 women who had an average age of 56 years (range, 26 to 89 years).

At an average follow-up of 5.5 years (range, 2 to 9 years), 41 hips (89%) had good and excellent outcomes measured by Harris Hip Score (48). Three stems (6%) have failed and been re-revised. Two of these re-revisions were in women at 6 and 7 years after surgery. They were both performed on stable stems surrounded by proximal femoral osteolysis. A 32-mm head had been used in the initial revision and marked polyethylene wear was noted at re-revision in both cases. The other re-revision was in a man who suffered an unrecognized intraoperative fracture (81). This patient was redone at 3 weeks and has had a successful result (Harris Hip Score of 92) at the 5-year follow-up. The other two poor results include a 42-year-old man with developmental dysplasia of the hip with six previous revisions. His revision of a stem in a femur with type III bone loss presently has an Engh fixation/stability score of –15 at 6 years follow-up. The patient has declined a revision procedure because he has no problem ambulating with one crutch. The other poor result is in a 78-year-old woman with previous catastrophic wear of the acetabulum requiring major structural allografting. At the 4-year follow-up, the acetabular component appears well-fixed but the femoral component has subsided 4 mm since surgery and may be impinging on the lateral cortex, which appears to be the source of her moderate-to-severe thigh pain. A cerclage allograft strut to strengthen the lateral cortex is being considered.

A radiographic analysis (82) revealed that 31 of the 46 hips (67%) had 2 mm of subsidence or less, 6 hips (13%) had 2 to 3 mm of subsidence, and 9 hips (20%), including the 5 poor results, had greater than 4 mm of subsidence. In the other four hips with greater than 4 mm of subsidence that were doing well, all had subsided in the first 6 months postoperatively and have been stable since

that time. Analyzing the hips by Engh fixation/stability scores (32), 38 hips (83%) had scores consistent with probable or suspected bone ingrowth (scores from 0 to +30). Four hips (9%) had scores consistent with fibrous stability (scores 0 to –10) and four hips (9%) had scores consistent with gross instability (less than –10 points) of which three have been revised as previously described.

Restoration of Bone Stock

A remarkable reconstitution of previously attenuated cortex is seen after removal of cement and membrane and the introduction of a bone graft with a noncemented stem (Figs. 3,4). Overall, there has been a positive response to cementless revisions on the femoral side. There has been excellent reconstitution of the cortex and apparent hypertrophy in areas of stress transfer in the metaphysis. Reconstitution of the thin cortical wall to increased thickness and density of bone at 12 to 24 months after surgery has been observed.

Ease of Re-Revision

Eight of the nine re-revisions in our series were done using a similar proximally coated porous prosthesis with

A–D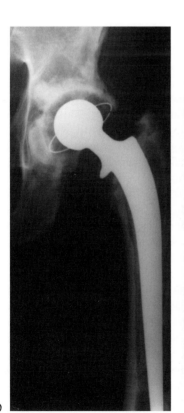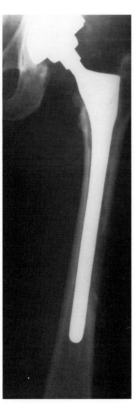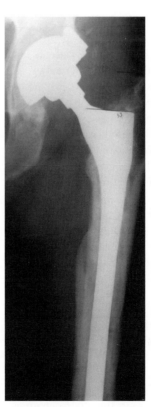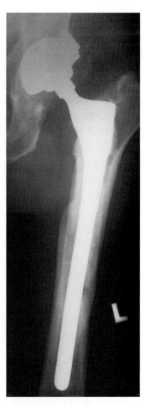

FIG. 3. Anteroposterior radiographs of a 52-year-old man with osteoarthritis with a loosened cemented femoral stem. **A:** Before revision. There is loosening of the femoral component and type II bone loss. **B:** Nine days after revision. **C:** Seven years after revision. **D:** Nine years after revision. The *arrow* indicates a lateral spot-weld that shows evidence of bone ingrowth and good fixation.

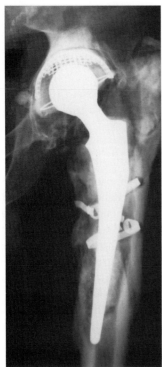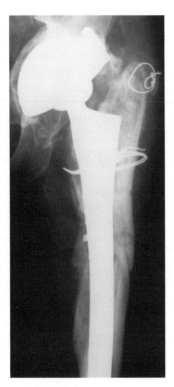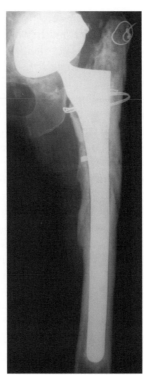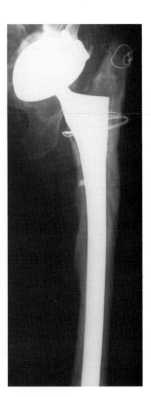

A–D

FIG. 4. Anteroposterior radiographs of a 62-year-old man with osteonecrosis and a grossly loosened cemented femoral stem. **A:** Before revision. There is massive osteolysis and type IV bone loss. **B:** Four months after revision. **C:** Three years after revision. **D:** Five years after revision. There is evidence of restoration of proximal bone stock. The series shows progressive calcar atrophy, and pedestal formation without radiolucencies, which are evidence of good fixation and stability.

re-bone-grafting of the femur. Four of these patients have an excellent clinical outcome (Harris Hip Scores greater than 90 points). Three have fair clinical outcomes and one has been re-revised secondary to loosening. The final revision was to a cemented stem that also loosened. The patient had a stroke 1 year after his last surgery and is currently wheelchair bound. These cases did not pose any inordinate difficulty as would have been found with revision of a cemented long-stem component or an extensively porous-coated stem.

Caveat emptor: It still is necessary to study the longer-term results to check for wear debris causing osteolysis, and to compare these results with other methods to determine the most viable options for particular situations.

COMPLETE CIRCUMFERENTIAL COATING VERSUS INCOMPLETE COATING

Incomplete coating of stems placed the porous coating proximally anteriorly, posteriorly, and medially in that surface area of the stem that contacts the intertrochanteric cancellous bone. This was believed to be the bone best suited for remodeling to permit proximal transfer of load. However, the incompleteness of the porous interface may

allow for distal migration of polyethylene or metal particles (99).

Woolson and Delaney (109) recently reported on the results of the Harris-Galante (Zimmer, Warsaw, IN) femoral prosthesis at a 5.5-year-average follow-up (range, 4 to 8 years). Five (20%) had undergone repeat femoral revision. An additional nine prostheses had subsided 5 mm or more. In total, there were 36% poor clinical results and 48% subsidence, thus making the use of this prosthesis not recommended. This prosthesis relied on diaphyseal fit but probably had both poor apposition of the pads to host bone and gaps between the pads to allow access of debris to the diaphysis (6).

Peters and co-workers (91) reported on the Bias prosthesis (curved, long-stemmed, titanium alloy, noncircumferentially porous-coated component) in 45 patients followed for 65 months (range, 45 to 87 months). Twenty-eight hips (57%) had at least 2 mm of subsidence during the first postoperative year. Using survivorship analysis, they found a 96% chance of component survival with revision as an end point, but only a 37% chance of survival with revision or progressive subsidence as an end point. They concluded that a noncircumferentially porous-coated, long-stem, titanium-alloy femoral component is not an appropriate implant for the revision of a hip with moderate or severe loss of metaphyseal bone.

The PCA prosthesis has a proximally one-third circumferential porous coating. Not only does this provide for a larger surface area, but it also helps to seal the diaphysis (6).

CONCLUSION

In using proximally porous-coated stems, it is clear from the literature that the coating must be completely circumferential. Any interruption in the coating provides a conduit for debris to access the diaphysis. It is also clear from our experience that not all patients presenting for revision are candidates for a proximally coated device or even a cementless revision. Our initial experience was compromised by not having all sizes or all lengths available. Also, until 1987, only PCA prostheses with 32-mm heads were available. Currently, eight sizes of mid-stem and eight sizes of long-stem prostheses are available in both right and left configuration. This allows stable fitting of most patients, except the few with catastrophic bone loss. Use of this device had achieved a high degree of stem stability with restoration of bone stock. In nearly all cases requiring re-revision, the condition of the bone was better than prior to the initial revision, and the re-revision proceeded without incident with additional bone grafting and insertion of the larger stem. Although modularity is a great temptation, particularly in the revision situation, it has not proven necessary in our experience, and it has the down-side of being another potential source of debris progression. In the few cases where proximal and distal relationships could not be accommodated with an off-the-shelf prosthesis, this was determined preoperatively by the templates, and a custom modification of the prosthesis was ordered (4,77).

REFERENCES

1. Amstutz HC, Luetzow WF, Moreland JR. Revision of femoral component: cemented and cementless. In: Amstutz HC, ed. *Hip arthroplasty.* New York: Churchill Livingstone, 1991;829–854.
2. Amstutz HC, Ma SM, Jinnah RH, Mai L. Revision of aseptic loose total hip arthroplasties. *Clin Orthop* 1982;170:21–33.
3. Ballard WT, Lowry DA, Brand RA. Resection arthroplasty of the hip. *J Arthroplasty* 1995;10:772–779.
4. Bargar WL, Murzic WJ, Taylor JK, Newman MA, Paul HA. Management of bone loss in revision total hip arthroplasty using custom cementless femoral components. *J Arthroplasty* 1993;8:245–352.
5. Barrack RL, Folgueras AJ. Revision total hip arthroplasty: the femoral component. *J Am Acad Orthop Surg* 1995;3:79–85.
6. Bobyn JD, Pilliar RM, Cameron HU, Weatherly GC. Osteogenic phenomena across endosteal bone-implant spaces with porous surfaced intramedullary implants. *Acta Orthop Scand* 1981;52:145.
7. Broughton NS, Rushton N. Revision hip arthroplasty. *Acta Orthop Scand* 1982;53:923.
8. Callaghan JJ. Current concepts review. The clinical results and basic science of total hip arthroplasty with porous-coated prostheses. *J Bone Joint Surg* 1993;75A:299–310.
9. Callaghan JJ. Total hip arthroplasty: clinical perspective. *Clin Orthop* 1992;276:33–40.
10. Callaghan JJ, Salvati EA, Pellici PM, Wilson PD Jr, Ranawat CS. Results of revision for mechanical failure after cemented total hip replacement, 1979 to 1982: a two to five-year follow-up. *J Bone Joint Surg* 1985;67A:1074–1085.
11. Cameron HU. The two- to six-year results with a proximally modular noncemented total hip replacement used in hip revisions. *Clin Orthop* 1994;298:47–53.
12. Carlsson ÅS, Gentz CF, Lindberg HO. Thirty-two non-infected total hip arthroplasties revised due to stem loosening. *Clin Orthop* 1983; 181:196.
13. Chandler H. Intramedullary grafting of the expanded femoral canal in total hip replacement. *Tech Orthop* 1993;7:33.
14. Chandler HP, Ayres DK, Tan RC, Anderson LC, Varma AK. Revision total hip replacement using the S-Rom femoral component. *Clin Orthop* 1995;319:130–140.
15. Chandler H, Clark J, Murphy S, et al. Reconstruction of major segmental loss of the proximal femur in revision total hip arthroplasty. *Clin Orthop* 1994;298:67–74.
16. Charnley J. Numerical grading of clinical results. In: Charnley J, ed. *Low friction arthroplasty of the hip: theory and practice.* New York: Springer-Verlag 1979;20–24.
17. Collier JP, Mayor MB, Jensen RE, et al. Mechanisms of failure of modular prostheses. *Clin Orthop* 1992;285:129–139.
18. Collis DK. Revision total hip replacement with cement. *Semin Arthroplasty* 1993;4:38–49.
19. Cook SD, Barrack RL, Thomas KA, Haddad RJ. Tissue ingrowth into porous primary and revision stems. *J Arthroplasty* 1991;6:S37–S46.
20. Dandy DJ, Theodorous BC. The management of local complications of total hip replacement by McKee-Farrar technique. *J Bone Joint Surg* 1975;57B:30.
21. D'Antonio J, McCarthy JC, Bargar WL, Borden LS, Capello WN, Collis DK, Steinberg ME, Wedge JH. Classification of femoral abnormalities in total hip arthroplasty. *Clin Orthop* 1993;296:133–139.
22. Dorr LD. Total hip replacement using APR system. *Tech Orthop* 1986; 1(3):22–34.
23. Dorr LD. Results of noncemented revision. *Semin Arthroplasty* 1993; 4:50–55.
24. Dorr LD, Diefendorf D, Carn RM. Principles of cementless total hip revision and use of APR revision hip. *Tech Orthop* 1987;2(1):20–33.
25. Egan KJ, Di Cesare PE. Intraoperative complications of revision hip arthroplasty using a fully porous-coated straight cobalt-chrome femoral stem. *J Arthroplasty* 1995;10:S45–S51.
26. Ejsted R, Olsen NJ. Revision of failed total hip arthroplasty. *J Bone Joint Surg* 1987;69B:57.
27. Engelbrecht DJ, Weber FA, Sweet MBE, Jakim I. Long-term results of revision total hip arthroplasty. *J Bone Joint Surg* 1990;72B:41–45.
28. Engh CA, Engh CA Jr, Cadambi A, Lauro G, Piston RW. Cementless revision of failed total hip arthroplasty: preoperative planning, surgical technique, and postoperative rehabilitation. *Tech Orthop* 1993; 7(4):9–26.
29. Engh CA, Glassman AH, Griffin WL, Mayer JG. Results of cementless revision for failed cemented total hip arthroplasty. *Clin Orthop* 1988;235:91–110.
30. Engh CA, Glassman AH, Suthers KE. The case for porous-coated hip implants. The femoral side. *Clin Orthop* 1988;235:63–81.
31. Engh CA, Massin P. Cementless total hip arthroplasty using the anatomic medullary locking stem: results using a survivorship analysis. *Clin Orthop* 1989;249:141–158.
32. Engh CA, Massin P, Suthers KE. Roentgenographic assessment of the biologic fixation of porous-surface femoral components. *Clin Orthop* 1990;257:107–128.
33. Esses S, Hastings D, Schatzker J. Revision of total hip arthroplasty. *Can J Surg* 1983;4:345.
34. Estok DM II, Harris WH. Long-term results of cemented revision surgery using second-generation techniques: an average 11.7 year follow-up evaluation. *Clin Orthop* 1994;299:190–202.
35. Franks E, Mont MA, Maar DC, Jones LC, Hungerford DS. Thigh pain as related to bending rigidity of the femoral prosthesis and bone. *Trans Orthop Res Soc* 1992;38:296.
36. Franzén H, Mjöberg B, Önnerfält R. Early loosening of femoral components after cemented revision: a roentgen stereophotogrammetric study. *J Bone Joint Surg* 1992;74B:721–721.
37. Franzén H, Toksvig-Larsen S, Lidgren L, Önnerfält R. Early migration of femoral components revised with impacted cancellous allografts and cement. *J Bone Joint Surg* 1995;77B:862–864.

38. Garcia-Cimbrelo E, Munuera L, Diez-Vazquez V. Long-term results of aseptic cemented Charnley revisions. *J Arthroplasty* 1995;10:121–131.

39. Gie GA, Linder L, Ling RSM, Simon J-P, Slooff TJJH, Timperley AJ. Impacted cancellous allografts and cement for revision total hip arthroplasty. *J Bone Joint Surg Br* 1993;75B:14–21.

40. Glassman AH, Engh CA. Cementless revision for femoral failure. *Orthopedics* 1995;18:851–853.

41. Glassman AH, Engh CA, Bobyn JD. Proximal femoral osteotomy as an adjunct in cementless revision total hip arthroplasty. *J Arthroplasty* 1987;2:47–63.

42. Goodman SB, Schatzker J. Revision hip surgery using the straight-stem Muller prosthesis. *J Arthroplasty* 1987;2:83.

43. Gorab RS, Covino BM, Borden LS. The rationale for cementless revision total hip replacement with contemporary technology. *Orthop Clin North Am* 1993;24:627–633.

44. Gross AE, Allen G, Lavoie G. Revision arthroplasty using allograft bone. *Inst Course Lect* 1993;42:363–380.

45. Gross AE, Lavoie MV, McDermott P, Marks P. The use of allograft bone in revision of total hip arthroplasty. *Clin Orthop* 1985;197:115–122.

46. Gustilo RB, Pasternak HS. Revision total hip arthroplasty with titanium ingrowth prosthesis and bone grafting for failed cemented femoral component loosening. *Clin Orthop* 1988;235:111–119.

47. Hardinge K. The direct lateral approach to the hip. *J Bone Joint Surg* 1982;64B:17–21.

48. Harris WH. Traumatic arthritis of the hip after dislocation and acetabular fractures: treatment by mold arthroplasty. An end-result study using a new method of result evaluation. *J Bone Joint Surg* 1969;51A:737–755.

49. Harris WH. Cemented revision for femoral failure. *Orthopedics* 1995;18:854–855.

50. Harris WH, Krushell RJ, Galante JO. Results of cementless revisions of total hip arthroplasties using the Harris-Galante prosthesis. *Clin Orthop* 1988;235:120–126.

51. Head WC, Berklacich FRM, Malinin TI, Emerson RH Jr. Proximal femoral allografts in revision total hip arthroplasty. *Clin Orthop* 1987;225:22.

52. Head WC, Emerson RH, Hillyard JM, Higgins LL. Management of the structurally deficient femur in revision total hip replacement. *Orthopedics* 1995;18:865–868.

53. Head WC, Wagner RA, Emerson RH Jr, et al. Revision total hip arthroplasty in the deficient femur with a proximal load-bearing prosthesis. *Clin Orthop* 1994;298:119–126.

54. Hedley AK, Gruen TA, Ruoff DP. Revision of failed total hip arthroplasties with uncemented porous-coated anatomic components. *Clin Orthop* 1988;235:75–90.

55. Holtgrewe JL, Hungerford DS. Primary and revision total hip replacement without cement and with associated femoral osteotomy. *J Bone Joint Surg* 1989;71A:487–495.

56. Hungerford DS. *Total Hip Arthroplasty: A Comprehensive Approach.* New York: Raven Press, 1994.

57. Hungerford DS, Jones LC. The rationale of cementless revision of cemented arthroplasty failures. *Clin Orthop* 1988;235:12–24.

58. Hungerford DS, Krackow KA, Lennox DW. The PCA Primary and Revision Hip Systems. In: Fitzgerald R, ed. *Non-cemented total hip arthroplasty.* New York: Raven Press, 1988;433–450.

59. Hunter GA, Welsh RP, Cameron HU, Bailey WH. The results of revision of total hip arthroplasty. *J Bone Joint Surg* 1979;61B:419–421.

60. Huo MH, Salvati EA. Revision total hip replacement using cement. *Tech Orthop* 1993;7(4):58–64.

61. Hussamy O, Lachiewicz PF. Revision total hip arthroplasty with the BIAS femoral component. Three to six year results. *J Bone Joint Surg* 1994;76A:1137–1148.

62. Izquierdo RJ, Northmore-Ball MD. Long-term results of revision hip arthroplasty. Survival analysis with special reference to the femoral component. *J Bone Joint Surg* 1994;76B:34–39.

63. Jasty M, Haire T, Tanzer M. Femoral osteolysis: a generic problem with cementless and cemented femoral components. *Orthop Trans* 1991;15:758–759.

64. Jasty M, Maloney WJ, Bragdon CR, O'Connor DO, Haire T, Harris WH. The initiation of failure in cemented femoral components of hip arthroplasties. *J Bone Joint Surg* 1991;73B(4):551–558.

65. Johnsson R, Thorngren K-G, Persson BM. Revision of total hip replacement for primary osteoarthritis. *J Bone Joint Surg* 1988;70B:56–62.

66. Katz RP, Callaghan JJ, Sullivan PM, Johnston RC. Cemented revision

total hip arthroplasty using contemporary techniques: a minimum ten year follow-up study *(abstr)*. *J Arthroplasty* 1994;9:103.

67. Kavanagh BF. Cemented revision of total hip arthroplasty. In: Callaghan JJ, Dennis DD, Paprosky WG, Rosenberg AG, eds. *Hip and knee reconstruction.* Rosemont, IL: American Academy of Orthopaedic Surgeons, 1995;207–213.

68. Kavanagh BF, Fitzgerald RH Jr. Multiple revisions for failed total hip replacement not associated with infection. *J Bone Joint Surg* 1987;69A:1144–1149.

69. Kavanagh BF, Ilstrup DM, Fitzgerald RH Jr. Revision total hip arthroplasty. *J Bone Joint Surg* 1985;67A:517–526.

70. Kershaw CJ, Atkins RM, Dodd CAF, Bulstrode CJK. Revision total hip arthroplasty for aseptic failure: a review of 276 cases. *J Bone Joint Surg* 1991;73B:564–568.

71. Krackow KA, Thomas SC, Jones LC. A new stitch for ligament-tendon fixation: brief note. *J Bone Joint Surg* 1986;68A:764–768.

72. Kyle RF, Gustilo RB. Revision total hip arthroplasty with the BIAS total hip system. *Tech Orthop* 1987;2(1):7–19.

73. Lawrence JM, Engh CA, Macalino GE. Revision total hip arthroplasty: long-term results without cement. *Orthop Clin North Am* 1993;24:635–644.

74. Lawrence JM, Engh CA, Macalino GE, Lauro GR. Outcome of revision hip arthroplasty done without cement. *J Bone Joint Surg* 1994;76A:965–973.

75. Lieberman JR, Moeckel BH, Evans BG, Salvati EA, Ranawat CS. Cement-within-cement revision hip arthroplasty. *J Bone Joint Surg* 1993;75B:869–871.

76. Lord G, Marotte J-H, Guillamon J-L, Blanchard J-P. Cementless revisions of failed aseptic cemented and cementless total hip arthroplasties: 284 cases. *Clin Orthop* 1988;235:67–74.

77. Malkani AL, Sim FH, Chao EYS. Custom-made segmental femoral replacement prosthesis in revision total hip arthroplasty. *Orthop Clin North Am* 1993;24:727–733.

78. Mallory TH. Preparation of the proximal femur in cementless total hip revision. *Clin Orthop* 1988;235:47–60.

79. Marti RK, Schuller HM, Besselaer PP, Haasnoot ELV. Results of revision of hip arthroplasty with cement: a five to fourteen year follow-up study. *J Bone Joint Surg* 1990;72A:346–354.

80. McLaughlin JR, Harris WH. Revision of the femoral component of a total hip arthroplasty with the calcar-replacement femoral component. Results after a mean of 10.8 years postoperatively. *J Bone Joint Surg* 1996;78A:331–339.

81. Mont MA, Maar DC. Fractures of the ipsilateral femur after hip arthroplasty. A statistical analysis of outcome based on 487 patients. *J Arthroplasty* 1994;9:511–519.

82. Mont MA, Maar DC, Krackow KA, Jacobs MA, Jones LC, Hungerford DS. Total hip replacement without cement for non-inflamatory osteoarthrosis in patients who are less than forty-five years old. *J Bone Joint Surg* 1993;75A:740–751.

83. Moreland JR, Bernstein ML. Femoral revision arthroplasty with uncemented porous-coated stems. *Clin Orthop* 1995;319:141–150.

84. Morrey BF, Kavanagh BF. Complications of revision of the femoral component of total hip arthroplasty. *J Arthroplasty* 1992;7:71–79.

85. Mulroy WJ, Harris WH. Revision total hip arthroplasty with use of so-called second-generation cementing techniques for aseptic loosening of the femoral component. A fifteen-year-average follow-up study. *J Bone Joint Surg* 1996;78A:325–330.

86. Nelissen RGHH, Bauer TW, Weidenhielm LRA, LeGolvan DP, Mikhail WEM. Revision hip arthroplasty with the use of cement and impaction grafting. Histological analysis of four cases. *J Bone Joint Surg* 1995;77A:412–422.

87. Paprosky WG, Bradford MS, Jablonsky WS. Cementless revision total hip arthroplasty. In: Callaghan JJ, Dennis DD, Paprosky WG, Rosenberg AG, eds. *Hip and knee reconstruction.* Rosemont, IL: American Academy of Orthopaedic Surgeons, 1995;215–225.

88. Paprosky WG, Jablonsky W, Magnus RE. Cementless femoral revision in the presence of severe proximal bone loss using diaphyseal fixation. *Orthop Trans* 1993;17:965–966.

89. Pellici PM, Wilson PD Jr, Sledge CB, Salvati EA, Ranawat CS, Poss R. Revision total hip arthroplasty. *Clin Orthop* 1982;170:34–41.

90. Pellici PM, Wilson PD Jr, Sledge CB, Salvati EA, Ranawat CS, Poss R. Long-term results of revision total hip replacement: a follow-up report. *J Bone Joint Surg* 1985;67A:513–516.

91. Peters CL, Rivero DP, Kull LR, Jacobs JJ, Rosenberg AG, Galante JO.

Revision total hip arthroplasty without cement: subsidence of proximally porous-coated femoral components. *J Bone Joint Surg* 1995; 77A:1217–1226.

92. Pierson JL, Harris WH. Cemented revision for femoral osteolysis in cemented arthroplasties. *J Bone Joint Surg* 1994;76B:40–44.

93. Pierson JL, Harris WH. Effect of improved cementing techniques on the longevity of fixation in revision cemented femoral arthroplasties. Average 8.8-year follow-up period. *J Arthroplasty* 1995;10:581–591.

94. Poss R, Walker P, Spector M, Reilly DT, Robertson DD, Sledge CB. Strategies for improving fixation of femoral components in total hip arthroplasty. *Clin Orthop* 1988;235:181–194.

95. Raut VV, Siney PD, Wroblewski BM. Revision for aseptic stem loosening revision using the cemented Charnley prosthesis. A review of 351 hips. *J Bone Joint Surg* 1995;77B:23–27.

96. Retpen JB, Varmarken JE, Röck ND, Steen Jensen J. Unsatisfactory results after repeated revision of hip arthroplasty. 61 cases followed for 5 (1–10) years. *Acta Orthop Scand* 1992;63:120–127.

97. Rubash HE, Harris WH. Revision of nonseptic, loose, cemented femoral components using modern cementing techniques. *J Arthroplasty* 1988;3:241–248.

98. Saker A, Cuckler JM. Results of cementless revision total hip arthroplasty. *Curr Opin Orthop* 1994;5(1):22–25.

99. Schmalzreid TP, Jasty M, Harris WH. Periprosthetic bone loss in total hip arthroplasty. Polyethylene wear debris and the concept of the effective joint space. *J Bone Joint Surg* 1992;74A:849–863.

100. Schüller HM, Marti RK, Besselaar PP. Aseptic failure in revision hip replacement. *Acta Orthop Scand* 1988;227:S34–S35.

101. Snorrason F, Kärrholm J. Early loosening of revision hip arthroplasty: a roentgen stereophotogrammetric analysis. *J Arthroplasty* 1990;5: 217–219.

102. Søballe K, Olsen NJ, Ejsted R, et al. Revision of the uncemented hip prosthesis. *Acta Orthop Scand* 1987;58:630.

103. Sotereanos N, Rubash HE. Personal communication, 1996.

104. Strömberg CN, Herberts P. A multicenter 10-year study of cemented revision total hip arthroplasty in patients younger than 55 years old: a follow-up report. *J Arthroplasty* 1994;9:595–601.

105. Strömberg CN, Herberts P, Ahnfelt L. Revision total hip arthroplasty in patients younger than 55 years old: clinical and radiological results after 4 years. *J Arthroplasty* 1988;3:47–59.

106. Turner RH, Mattingly DA, Scheller A. Femoral revision total hip arthroplasty using a long-stem femoral component: clinical and radiographic analysis. *J Arthroplasty* 1987;2:247–258.

107. Turner TM, Urban RM, Sumner DR, Galante JO. Revision, without cement, of aseptically loose, cemented total hip prostheses. *J Bone Joint Surg* 1993;75A:845–862.

108. Wilson PD Jr. Revision total hip arthroplasty: current role of polymethylmethacrylate. *Clin Orthop* 1987;225:218–228.

109. Woolson ST, Delaney TJ. Failure of a proximally porous-coated femoral prosthesis in revision total hip arthroplasty. *J Arthroplasty* 1995; 10:S22–S28.

110. Wroblewski BM. Revision surgery in total hip arthroplasty: surgical technique and results. *Clin Orthop* 1982;170:56.

111. Wroblewski BM. *Revision surgery in total hip arthroplasty*. London: Springer-Verlag, 1990.

The Adult Hip, edited by J. J. Callaghan,
A. G. Rosenberg, and H. E. Rubash.
Lippincott–Raven Publishers, Philadelphia © 1998.

CHAPTER 96

Revision of the Femoral Component: Cement

John J. Callaghan and Richard C. Johnston

HISTORICAL PERSPECTIVE

As experience with Sir John Charnley's total hip arthroplasty developed, various failure modes became apparent. In Charnley's initial experience with total hip arthroplasty, revision became necessary because of sepsis, which occurred relatively frequently. The need for acetabular revision was realized as acetabular component wear, osteolysis, and loosening occurred rapidly following the insertion of press-fit polytetrahydrofluoride acetabular components. The acetabular component loosening problem was addressed by changing from press-fit polytetrahydrofluoride to cemented polyethylene components, and sepsis was minimized by performing the total hip arthroplasty operation in clean air (15).

The next revision problem that Charnley faced was mechanical failure of the femoral component because of fracture, aseptic loosening, or osteolysis around fixed femoral components. Because polytetrahydrofluoride was never used for the acetabular component in the United States, and because prophylactic antibiotics *were* used in the the early total hip arthroplasties in the United States (thus limiting sepsis), mechanical failure of the femoral component, either because of component fracture or aseptic loosening, was a relatively early indication for performing revision surgery in this country (15).

As the initial total hip arthroplasty procedures were performed in relatively low-demand patients, the occurrence of clinically symptomatic mechanical failure was low during the first 15 years (late 1960s to early 1980s in

the United States) that the procedure was performed. Hence, no single surgeon or single institution had a large experience with revision surgery. At the Hospital for Special Surgery in New York City, the number of revision surgeries performed before 1983 was under 200 cases, and no surgeon had performed more than 75 (Fig. 1). Thus, experience was limited with this procedure that hip surgeons now appreciate requires a long learning experience for proficiency.

EARLY RESULTS

The studies of cemented revisions performed during the early evolution of revision hip surgery were not encouraging. According to Pellicci et al. (46), although the initial quality of an uncomplicated revision of a total hip replacement compares favorably with that of a primary total hip replacement, the durability of the result is substantially less. These authors demonstrated a 19% incidence of re-revision (18% on the femoral side), and a 29% incidence of loosening at an average follow-up of 8.1 years. Results were even worse if patients had had a previous revision, with Kavanagh and Fitzgerald (30) reporting a 50% clinical or radiographic failure at average 3-year follow-up. In addition to demonstrating a high incidence of aseptic re-revision, the early reports of revision surgery demonstrated a high incidence of complications when compared to primary cemented arthroplasty. Femoral fracture rates ranged from 2.1% to 8%, femoral canal perforation rates ranged from 4% to 13%, dislocation rates ranged from 8% to 10.6%, infection rates ranged from 1.2% to 3.4%, nerve palsy rates ranged from 0.5% to 7%, and trochanteric problems ranged from 6.2 to 12.7% (Table 1) (2,6,7,15–17, 26–28,31,33,37,40,41, 46–48,53–56,58–63, 65,66).

J. J. Callaghan and R. C. Johnston: Department of Orthopaedics, University of Iowa, Iowa City, Iowa 52242.

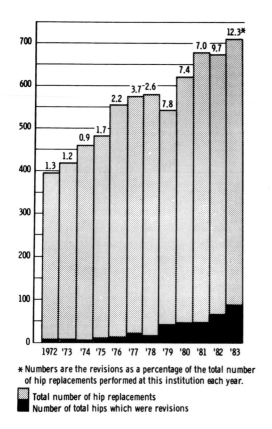

FIG. 1. Historical perspective of hip surgery. Few revisions were performed between 1970 and 1983 at a major institution (Hospital for Special Surgery) that performs revision hip surgery. (With permission from Callaghan et al. Results of revision for mechanical failure after cemented total hip replacement, 1979 to 1982. *J Bone Joint Surg* 1985; 67A: 1074–1085.)

CONTEMPORARY FEMORAL CEMENTING TECHNIQUE AND EXPERIENCE

In the initial experience with cemented revision total hip arthroplasty, the fibrous membrane between bone and loose cement, and the neocortex between the fibrous membrane and any residual cancellous bone were not ade-

quately removed. Cement delivery systems were not available, and, even when they did become available, the distal canal was not adequately restricted, especially when cement was to be injected distal to the isthmus of the femoral canal. (If cement is to be injected distal to the isthmus, a cement plug rather than a plastic plug is needed to ensure that cement will not extrude beyond the plug and prevent pressurization.) In addition, even after cement delivery systems became available, only two packs of cement would be mixed in many cases, and this would not provide adequate filling and pressurization of the canal with cement. Perforations of the femoral canal were not always appreciated and, even if recognized, were not always adequately bypassed. This led to inadequate pressurization of the cement with extrusion of cement outside the femoral canal. Because of the stress riser created by the perforations, femoral fractures could and did occur when the defects were not bypassed by the femoral stem.

In the late 1970s and early 1980s, surgeons in the United States began to recognize the need, in femoral canal preparation, to remove all femoral neocortex in areas where virgin cancellous bone could be obtained (Fig. 2A,B). In addition, in areas where there was only cortical bone, they began to appreciate the need to carefully burr or ream the bone to roughen the surface in the proximal femur and the femoral canal so as to provide interdigitation of cement into the bone. This is paramount if cement is to be used in the revision femur. Dohmae et al. (14) demonstrated (in a cadaveric human model) a 79% reduction in bone cement interface sheer strength in revision surgery when compared with primary replacement if such preparation is not performed.

After preparing the canal, the femur is carefully examined for any perforations by placing a cannulated guide wire (used for cannulated reaming) down the femoral canal and palpating distally to ensure that the wire abuts the distal femur at the knee and not the soft tissues. It is especially important to palpate anterolaterally in the femoral canal, as 90% of perforations occur at that location. In addition, this anterolateral aspect is the weakest area of the femur, as it is usually loaded in tension. If a

TABLE 1. *Early results of revision cemented total hip arthroplasty*

	HSS and Brigham Pellicci et al.	UCLA Amstutz et al.	MAYO Kavanagh et al.	HSS Callaghan et al.
Number of hips	110	66	166	139
Follow-up period (average)	3.4 yrs	2.1 yrs	4.5 yrs	3.6 yrs
Results (excellent/good)	60%	—	52%	66%
Loosening	13.6%	29%	20% to 40%	12%
Rerevision	5.4%	9.0%	6.0%	4.3%
Femoral fracture	—	6.0%	0.9%	2.1%
Femoral perforation	—	—	4%	13%
Dislocation	—	10.6%	9.0%	8.2%
Infection	1.8%	1.5%	1.2%	3.4%
Nerve palsy	—	7.0%	0.5%	0.7%
Trochanteric problems	12.7%	7.6%	6.6%	6.2%

perforation is noted, the femoral shaft is exposed by reflecting the posterior part of the vastus lateralis anteriorly. A rubber dam (a surgical glove is often convenient for this purpose) is placed over the perforation at the time of cementing, and if the bone in that area is thinned, a cortical strut graft is applied over the defect after removing all excess cement. As a trial femoral component is placed down the femoral canal, viewing it through the perforation can aid in determinating the desired prosthesis length, which should pass beyond the defect by 1.5 to 3 times the femoral shaft outer diameter (Fig. 3). However, if no distal defect is present, standard-length stems (120 to 140 mm) are used. Better cement pressurization occurs when a shorter rather than a longer column of cement needs to be filled.

Removing cortical femoral windows, especially when cement extends distal to the femoral isthmus, is preferable to multiple uncontrolled perforations (34,58). When making a window, it should be placed anteriorly to avoid the lateral tension surface, and the edges should be beveled to allow replacement of the window (before cementing) without much extrusion of the pressurized cement, and to avoid displacement of the fragment (Fig. 4). We perform more extended trochanteric osteotomies and cortical windows in the femur today than in the past to remove cement more easily and less traumatically, as maintenance of the femoral cortical tube and minimizing perforations allow for optimal cement pressurization. When cementing into a femur where an extended osteotomy has been performed, it is advisable to try to bevel the osteotomy bone edges, as is done for the cortical windows, to avoid cement extrusion. The femur is placed in the internally rotated position to take tension off the extended osteotomy, which has been reapproximated with cable prior to cement injection (Fig. 5). Cement is pressurized into the canal with direct vision of the osteotomy site, to remove any cement that interdigitates between the osteotomized piece of the greater trochanter and the femur. Supplemental cancellous bone graft may be applied over the osteotomy site to aid in union.

In preparing to cement the femur, the entire operating room staff should be prepared to help. Initially, a half pack of cement is mixed and placed in the Oh-Harris syringe (44). If the plug is to be placed distal to the isthmus, 6 to 8 cm of doughy cement is released from the syringe (see Fig. 2C). After this cement has cured, three to six packs of cement are mixed, depending on the size of the femoral canal (Fig. 6). In the revision situation especially, the surgeon should be sure that adequate cement is available for pressurization. Previous to mixing, 3.6 g tobramycin is introduced into each two packs of cement (1.8 g per pack). Studies have demonstrated minimal adverse effects on the mechanical properties of cement when under 2.0 g antibiotic powder (per pack) is introduced. Lynch et al. (36) demonstrated a reduction

in infection from 3.5% to 0.81% when antibiotics are added to cement in the revision situation. Porosity reduction of the cement by centrifugation or vacuum mixing is performed to strengthen it (5,10–13,68). Centrifugation is preferred because it is more predictable in removing bubbles. One to 2 minutes is the optimal centrifuge time. If there is a long, capacious canal to fill, chilling the monomer (with sterile ice) will allow longer setup time. Custom-designed twisting guns rather than caulking guns are useful to introduce the cement, and the distal end of the femur can be elevated so that the gravitational force will cause any blood to exit the femur proximally rather than to have it interdigitate with cement (see Fig. 2D). The canal is also dried with a sponge soaked in a 1:500,000 epinephrine solution prior to injecting cement into the femur. Pressurization can be applied with a proximal cement seal. The component is then placed down the femoral canal when the cement has cured to the doughy state. If a perforation has previously been noticed, it should be watched as the stem is introduced to avoid having the stem protrude through the defect in bone. Mechanical studies have demonstrated the need to bypass perforations with the femoral stem by two to three shaft diameters. This amount of bypass negates any stress-riser effect from the perforation (see Fig. 2E) (45). If an adequate amount of cement is utilized and inadequate pressurization is obtained in the canal, the surgeon should check by an intraoperative radiograph or by direct femoral shaft exposure to ensure that a perforation with cement extrusion or femoral component canal penetration has not inadvertently occurred (Fig. 7).

All cemented femoral components used today are made of chrome–cobalt and have wide, rounded medial surfaces to protect the cement mantle (8,9). In addition, higher-offset stems are available to help recreate the patient's natural femoral offset. This has become more important as surgeons attempt to perform revision surgery without removing the greater trochanter. In the past, offset adjustments were accomplished by distal and lateral advancement of the greater trochanter. In addition, calcar replacement prostheses should be available in cases with proximal femoral bone loss to allow adequate soft-tissue tensioning (Fig. 8). In the revision setting, even when offset and length have been adequately obtained, dislocation occurs in up to 10% of cases. We apply some form of bracing postoperatively after many revisions to protect the reconstruction during the first 6 to 8 weeks while the patient is gaining leg control and while the soft tissues and bony trochanteric attachment sites are healing. Adherence to these technical details have reduced the re-revision rate of cemented revision femoral components to 10% at 10 to 15 years, even in cases with extensive femoral osteolysis (Table 2) (3,4,18–20,24,25,29,39,42–44,49–52,57,64,67). Figures 2 through 10 demonstrate the principles outlined.

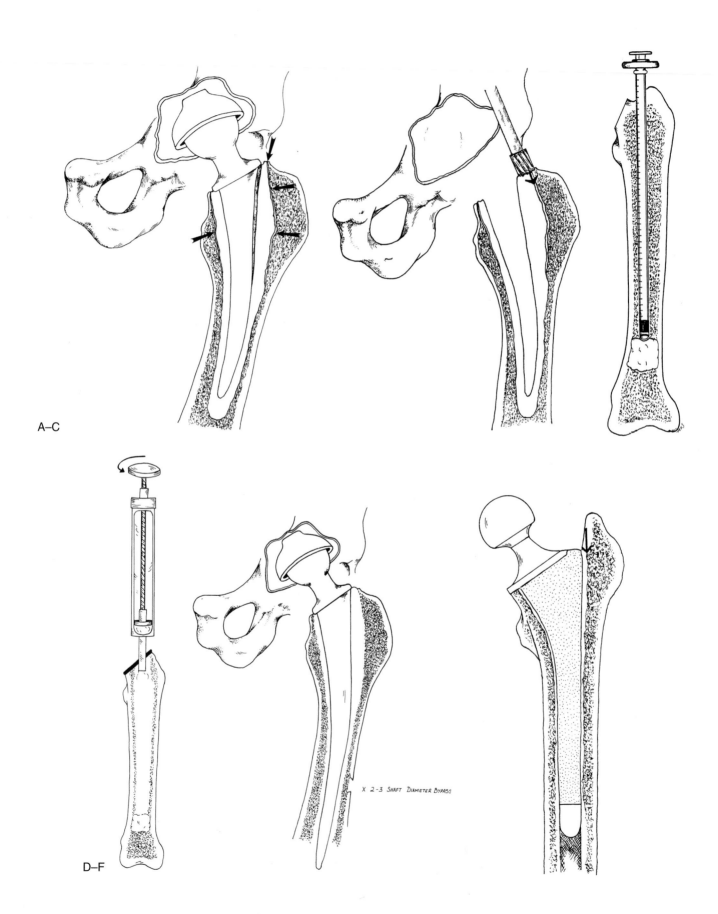

A–C

D–F

X 2-3 SHAFT DIAMETER BYPASS

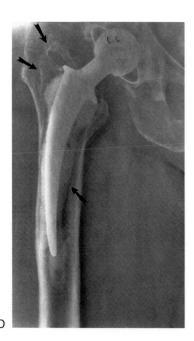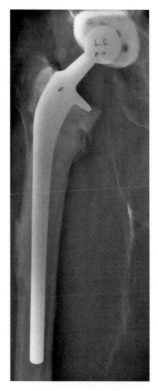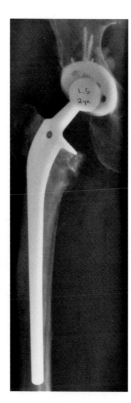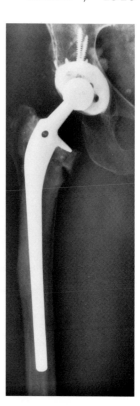

A–D

FIG. 3. This 82-year-old woman has a loose Müller prosthesis. Preoperative radiograph **(A)** demonstrates neocortex *(arrow)* around the loose femoral cement. Postoperative **(B)** and 2- **(C)** and 4-year **(D)** follow-up radiographs demonstrate the achievement of excellent cement penetration into bone with maintenance of the fixation. A long stem was used to bypass the thinned femoral cortex at the lateral aspect of the old femoral component.

SPECIAL TECHNICAL CONSIDERATIONS

Several situations warrant special technical considerations. If some or all of the cement mantle remains intact from the primary situation and if there are no signs of sepsis, the surgeon should consider hollowing out the cement column to slightly beyond the extent needed to introduce a new stem. After drying the hollowed canal (with previous cement intact) and introducing cement in a slightly liquid phase, a prosthesis can be inserted. Greenwald et al. (22) have demonstrated excellent bonding strength of cement in these situations, and McCallum and Hozack (38) and Lieberman et al. (35) have demonstrated excellent clinical results with recementing into an intact cement column. As suggested by the former group, ultrasonic cement-removing tools work well in tunneling out the secure cement shell (Fig. 9C). This technique is applicable in cases of cement–prosthesis failure (the case

FIG. 2. Contemporary cement technique in femoral revision. To optimize the interdigitation of cement into native cancellous bone in the revision situation, the surgeon must first address the neocortex that may form around the loose cement of a failed cemented or cementless implant. **A:** The *arrow* demonstrates the neocortex around the loose cement of a loose femoral component. **B:** The *arrow* demonstrates the path of a high speed burr that is removing neocortex after prosthesis removal. Although cement is still present, the burr is usually used in this manner after cement removal. **C:** A cement plug is made distal to the femoral canal isthmus to ensure an adequate seal to the distal canal. Six to 8 cm of cement is injected. **D:** Customized twisting cement gun is used to deliver the cement in the doughy stage (three to six packs of cement are used, requiring two delivery systems). The distal femur is lifted above the horizontal to allow blood to be expressed proximally so that it does not interdigitate with the cement. **E:** When the neocortex is removed, the same interdigitation of cement into bone can be obtained as in the primary situation. Note that the perforation is bypassed by two to three shaft diameters. A cortical cancellous graft is usually placed over such perforations. **F:** In the case of a loose uncemented component, a neocortex also forms *(arrow)*, and it must be removed to allow cement interdigitation into native cancellous bone to obtain optimal fixation.

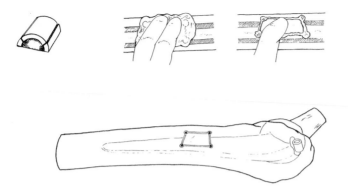

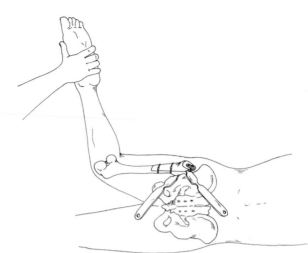

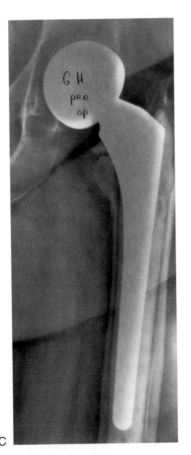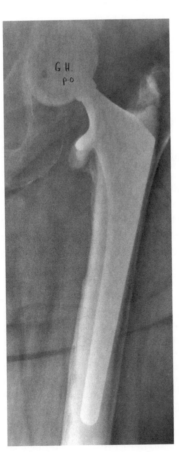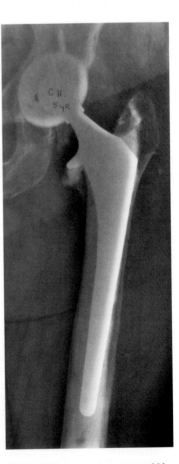

FIG. 4. Schematic of cortical window to remove cement. The edges are beveled *(top left)*. When replacing the window, a rubber dam is used to prevent cement extrusion *(top right)*. The remaining cement is curetted, and if the bone is thin, placement of a cortical cancellous strut graft is considered.

FIG. 5. A lower extremity where an extended greater trochanteric osteotomy had been performed to remove cement. The osteotomy has been reapproximated with cable fixation. The femur is internally rotated and the femoral canal is exposed as in a posterior approach. Observation at the osteotomy site with removal of any extruded cement during pressurization avoids interdigitation of cement between the osteotomy fragments.

A–C

FIG. 6. An active 69-year-old woman underwent a revision for loosening of a bipolar replacement **(A)**. Patient had thin cortical bone with a 20-mm diameter endosteal canal. Five packs of cement were needed to pressurize the femoral canal. Postoperative **(B)** and 5-year follow-up **(C)** radiographs demonstrate maintenance of a secure bone–cement interface.

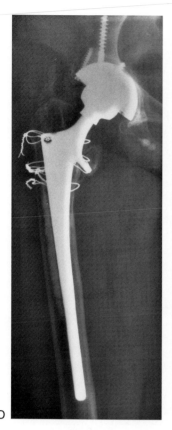
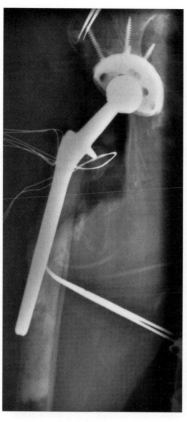
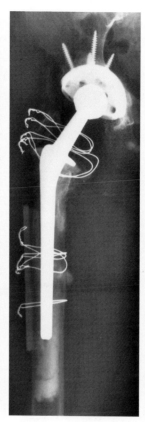
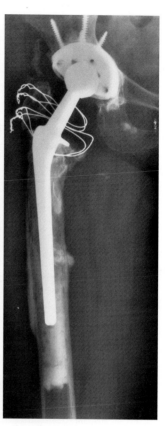

A–D

FIG. 7. This 68-year-old woman underwent a revision for loosening of a poorly performed uncemented femoral component; old cement was retained in the femoral canal **(A)**. Intraoperative radiograph **(B)**, obtained after placing the femoral stem because femoral canal cement pressurization was felt to be inadequate, demonstrated extraosseous penetration of the femoral component. The lateral femur was exposed, distal cement was removed, and a component was recemented under direct vision of the lateral femur, with a rubber dam placed over the perforation. A cortical cancellous graft was placed over the perforation **(C)**. A 5-year follow-up radiograph **(D)** demonstrated no change in the femoral cement–bone interface, and remodeling of the cortical cancellous graft.

with many Charnley prosthesis failures), femoral component fracture where the distal cement is intact (see Fig. 9), revision for instability or leg-length inequality, or in cases when the head size of an intact monolithic component needs to be changed (i.e., a 32-mm head in a young patient). An even more intriguing method has been employed by the New England Baptist group. If a femoral cement mantle is completely intact and the stem is not bonding to cement (not precoated or grit blasted), the stem is tapped out, acetabular revision is performed, and the stem is tapped back in.

When the femoral canal is very narrow, as in congenital hip dysplasia, a narrow nozzle is needed to introduce cement to the more distal aspect of the femur past the final distal position of the prosthesis stem. When placing the acetabular component in the high hip center position to avoid bone grafting, especially when using uncemented acetabular components, calcar and proximal femoral replacements are necessary (23) to preserve leg

length and to avoid the use of long-skirted head sizes that can hinder hip stability by early impingement (see Fig. 8) (32). In these high hip center cases, partial ischial resection may be necessary to prevent anterior instability in hip extension. This instability can be caused by posterior ischial impingement on the femur when the hip is in the high hip center position.

When revising failed uncemented femoral components to cemented femoral components (especially those that are not bone ingrown), a neocortex will have formed around the entire stem or parts of the stem (see Fig. 2F). High speed burrs and reamers can completely remove the neocortex, leaving a bed for bone cement interdigitation that is very much like the primary arthroplasty situation (Fig. 10).

Some final technical considerations concern the rare use of segmental allografts in the cemented femoral revision (1,69). If the surgeon is to cement the stem into the host bone, whether an oblique transverse or step cut is

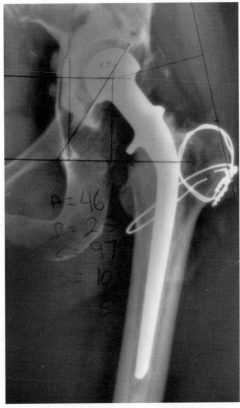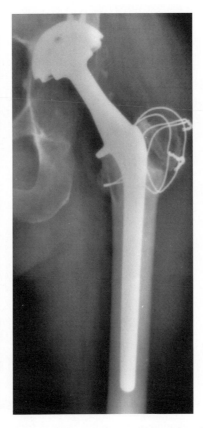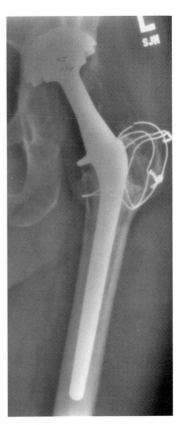

A–C

FIG. 8. This 60-year-old female patient developed loosening of a total hip arthroplasty initially performed for congenital hip dysplasia **(A)**. Hybrid revision was performed, placing the acetabular component in the high hip center position. This required the use of a long neck calcar-type femoral replacement **(B)**. The 5-year follow-up radiograph demonstrates a stable reconstruction **(C)**. Care must be taken to avoid anterior instability by providing adequate clearance of the ischium in extension.

created at the host–allograft junction makes little difference. However, to obtain adequate cement mantles in the allograft bone, the allograft should be sized to the endosteal surface of the proximal host femur (i.e., oversized to the outer shaft of the host femur) because the allograft usually has thick cortices (because of the young age of the donors). Reaming out the allograft should be avoided to maintain the strength of the allograft bone. The stem is first cemented into the allograft, and the distal stem is protected from cement adherence by covering it with the manufacturer's wrapping before it is skewered through the allograft, which has been previously pressur-

ized with very viscous cement. After cementing the allograft prosthesis composite into the host bone, cortical struts are placed at the host–allograft junction to add stability and to aid in the host–allograft junction healing (Fig. 11).

SUMMARY

Although the early reports of cemented revision total hip replacement were not encouraging, once newer techniques for cement delivery became available and once a

TABLE 2. *Results of cemented femoral revision total hip arthroplasty using contemporary cementing techniques*

Author (ref.)	Hips (N)	Age (avg.)	Follow-up (yr)	Re-revision incidence (%)	Radiographic loosening (%)
Raut et al. (51)	351	64	6	5.7	9.4
Weber et al. (64)	61	68	6.2	3	8
Katz et al. (29)	79	63.7	11.9	5.4	16.6
Mulroy et al. (42)	43	52.8	15.1	16	23
McLaughlin and Harris (39) (calcar replacements)	38	55	10.8	21	32

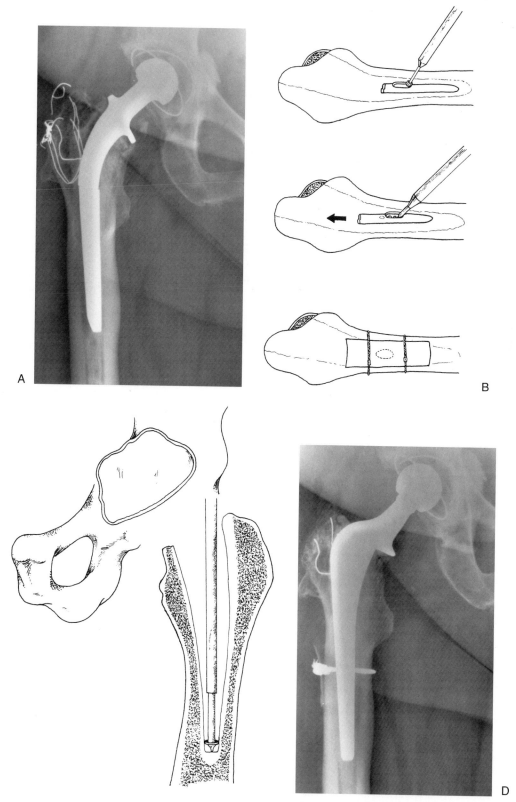

FIG. 9. This 70-year-old woman presented with a fracture of a T-28 femoral component **(A)**. The proximal component was easily excised, and the distal component was extracted by making an anterior femoral window 1 cm distal to the site of the fracture, using a carbide punch to knock the remaining stem out **(B)**. The distal cement canal was widened leaving the intact cement. This tunneling can be performed with the ultrasonic ski-pole burr **(C)**. The bone–cement interface was maintained and a short stemmed implant was able to bypass the window by two femoral shaft diameters. A supplemental cortical cancellous bone graft was applied **(D)**.

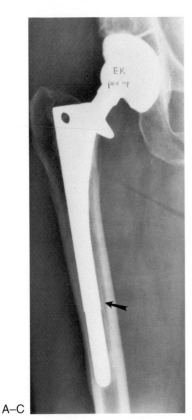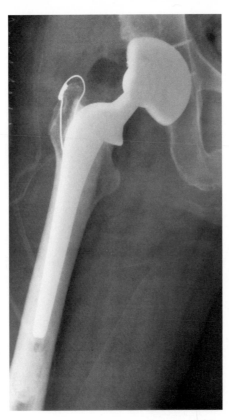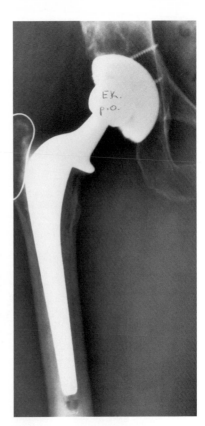

A–C

FIG. 10. Preoperative radiograph **(A)** of an uncemented femoral component that was loose at the time of revision. The neocortex around the device *(arrows)* was removed with a high speed burr and reamers. Excellent penetration into cancellous bone was obtained at revision surgery **(B)**. There was no need to use a long stem component and the distal pedestal of neocortex was used as the cement restrictor. The 2-year follow-up radiograph **(C)** demonstrates maintenance of the femoral bone–cement interface.

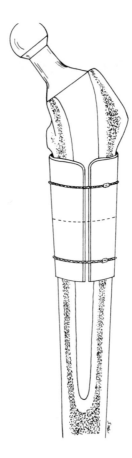

FIG. 11. Schematic of a proximal femoral allograft cemented stem composite positioned in the host bone. Cortical cancellous struts are used to aid in stabilization of the host–graft junction and to aid in host–graft union.

better understanding of the complexities of the operation were realized the results on the femoral side markedly improved. Nontraumatic cement removal and proper preparation of the femoral canal (removal of all neocortex that does not violate the femoral shaft cortical continuity) are essential. A chrome–cobalt femoral component with broad medial surfaces and no sharp corners, that bypasses any cortical defects, should be selected. A distal cement plug and adequate amounts of cement to pressurize the cement in the canal is paramount. Using these principles, cement can be used to provide durable femoral fixation in many cases. However, in cases with extensive osteolysis and in high-demand patients, it is wise to consider the use of other methods, such as impaction grafting with cement or the use of extensively coated porous stems (21).

REFERENCES

1. Allan DG, Lavoie G, McDonald S, et al. Proximal femoral allograft in revision hip arthroplasty. *J Bone Joint Surg* 1991;73B:235.
2. Amstutz HC, Mas SM, Jinnah RH, Mai L. Revision of aseptic loose total hip arthroplasties. *Clin Orthop* 1982;170:21–33.
3. Ballard W, Callaghan J, Johnston R. Revision of total hip arthroplasty in octogenarians. *J Bone Joint Surg* 1995;77A:585–589.
4. Barrack R, Mulroy R, Harris W. Improved cementing techniques and femoral component loosening in young patients with hip arthroplasty. A 12-year radiographic review. *J Bone Joint Surg* 1992;74B:385–389.
5. Burke DW, Gates EI, Harris WH. Centrifugation as a method of improving tensile and fatigue properties of acrylic bone cement. *J Bone Joint Surg* 1984;66A:1265–1273.
6. Callaghan JJ. Total hip arthroplasty. Clinical perspective. *Clin Orthop* 1992;276:33–40.
7. Callaghan JJ, Salvati, EA, Pellicci PM, Wilson, PDJ, Ranawat CS. Results of revision for mechanical failure after cemented total hip replacement, 1979 to 1982. A two to five-year follow-up. *J Bone Joint Surg* 1985;67A:1074–1085.
8. Crowninshield RD, Brand RA, Johnston RC, Milroy JC. An analysis of femoral component stem design in total hip arthroplasty. *J Bone Joint Surg* 1980;62A:68.
9. Crowninshield RD, Brand RA, Johnston RC, Milroy JC. The effect of femoral stem cross-sectional geometry on cement stresses in total hip reconstruction. *Clin Orthop* 1980;146:71.
10. Davies JP, Harris WH. Optimization and comparison of three vacuum mixing systems for porosity reduction of Simplex P cement. *Clin Orthop* 1990;254:261–269.
11. Davies JP, Burke DW, O'Connor DO, Harris WH. Comparison of the fatigue characteristics of centrifuged and uncentrifuged Simplex P bone cement. *J Orthop Res* 1987;5:366–271.
12. Davies JP, O'Connor DO, Burke DW, Jasty M, Harris WH. The effect of centrifugation on the fatigue life of bone cement in the presence of surface irregularities. *Clin Orthop* 1988;229:156–161.
13. Davies JP, Jasty M, O'Connor DO, Burke DW, Harrigan TP, Harris WH. The effect of centrifuging bone cement. *J Bone Joint Surg* 1989;71B(1):39–42.
14. Dohmae Y, Bechtold JE, Sherman RE, Puno RM, Gustilo RB. Reduction in cement-bone interface shear strength between primary and revision arthroplasty. *Clin Orthop* 1988;236:214.
15. Eftekhar NS, Smith DM, Henery JH, Stinchfield FE. Revision arthroplasty using Charnley low friction arthroplasty technique. With reference to specifics of technique and comparison of results with primary low friction arthroplasty. *Clin Orthop* 1973;95:48–59.
16. Ejsted R, Olsen NJ. Revision of failed total hip arthroplasty. *J Bone Joint Surg* 1987;69B:75.
17. Engelbrecht DJ, Weber FA, Sweet MB, Jakim I. Long-term results of revision total hip arthroplasty. *J Bone Joint Surg* 1990;72B:41–45.
18. Estok D, Harris W. Long-term results of cemented femoral revision

19. Fornasier VL, Cameron HU. The femoral stem/cement interface in total hip replacement. *Clin Orthop* 1976;116:248–252.
20. Garcia-Cimbrelo E, Munuera L, Diez-Vazquez V. Long term results of aseptic cemented Charnley revisions. *J Arthroplasty* 1995;10:121–131.
21. Gie G, Linder L, Ling R, Simon J, Slooff T, Timperley A. Impaction cancellous allografts and cement for revision total hip arthroplasty. *J Bone Joint Surg* 1993;75B:14–21.
22. Greenwald AS, Narten NC, Wilde AH. Points in the technique of rece-menting in the revision of an implant arthroplasty. *J Bone Joint Surg Br* 1978;60B:107–110.
23. Harris WH, Allen JR. The calcar replacement femoral component for total hip arthroplasty: design uses and surgical technique. *Clin Orthop* 1981;157:215–224.
24. Harris WH, McCarthy JC, O'Neill DA. Femoral component loosening using contemporary techniques of femoral cement fixation. *J Bone Joint Surg* 1982;64A:1063–1067.
25. Harris WH, McGann WA. Loosening of the femoral component after use of the medullary-plug cementing technique. Follow-up note with a minimum five-year follow-up. *J Bone Joint Surg* 1986;68A:1064–1066.
26. Hunter GA, Welsh RP, Cameron HU, Bailey WH. The results of revision of total hip arthroplasty. *J Bone Joint Surg* 1994;76B:419–422.
27. Iorio R, Eftekhar NS, et al. Cemented revision of failed total hip arthroplasty. Survivorship analysis. *Clin Orthop* 1995;316:121–130.
28. Izquierdo RJ, Northmore-Ball MD. Long-term results of revision hip arthroplasty-survival analysis with special reference to the femoral component. *J Bone Joint Surg* 1994;76B(1):34–39.
29. Katz R, Callaghan J, Sullivan P, Johnston R. Results of cemented femoral revision total hip arthroplasty using improved cementing techniques. *Clin Orthop* 1995;319:178–183.
30. Kavanagh BF, Fitzgerald RH Jr. Multiple revisions for failed total hip arthroplasty not associated with infection. *J Bone Joint Surg* 1987;69A:1144–1149.
31. Kavanagh BF, Ilstrup DM, Fitzgerald RH Jr. Revision total hip arthroplasty. *J Bone Joint Surg* 1985;67A:517–526.
32. Kelley SS. High hip center in revision arthroplasty. *J Arthroplasty* 1994;9(5):503–510.
33. Kershaw CI, Atkins RM, Dodd CAF, Bulstrods CJK. Revision total hip arthroplasty for aseptic failure: a review of 276 cases. *J Bone Joint Surg* 1991;73B:564.
34. Klein AH, Rubash HE. Femoral windows in revision total hip arthroplasty. *Clin Orthop* 1993;291:164–170.
35. Lieberman JR, Moeckel BH, Evans B, Salvati E, Ranawat C. Cement-within-cement revision hip arthroplasty. *J Bone Joint Surg* 1993;75B:869–871.
36. Lynch M, Esser MP, Shelley P, et al. Deep infection in Charnley low-friction arthroplasty: comparison of plain and gentamycin-loaded cement. *J Bone Joint Surg* 1987;69B:355–360.
37. Marti RK, Schuller HM, Besselaar PP, Vanfrank Haasnoot EL. Results of revision of hip arthroplasty with cement. A five to fourteen-year follow-up study. *J Bone Joint Surg* 1990;72A:346–354.
38. McCallum J, Hozack W. Recementing a femoral component into a stable cement mantle using ultrasonic tools. *Clin Orthop* 1995;319:232–237.
39. McLaughlin JR, Harris WH. Revision of the femoral component of a total hip arthroplasty with the calcar-replacement femoral component. Results after a mean of 10.8 years postoperatively. *J Bone Joint Surg* 1996;78A:331–339.
40. Michelson JD, Riley LH Jr. Considerations in the comparison of cemented and cementless total hip prosthesis. *J Arthroplasty* 1989;4(4):327–334.
41. Morrey BF, Kavanagh BF. Complications with revision of the femoral component of total hip arthroplasty. Comparison between cemented and uncemented techniques. *J Arthroplasty* 1992;7(1):71–79.
42. Mulroy WF, Harris WH. Revision total hip arthroplasty with use of so-called second generation cementing techniques for aseptic loosening of the femoral component. A fifteen-year-average follow-up study. *J Bone Joint Surg* 1996;78A:325–330.
43. Mulroy RD Jr, Harris WH. The effect of improved cementing techniques on component loosening in total hip replacement. An 11-year radiographic review. *J Bone Joint Surg* 1990;72B(5):757–760.
44. Oh I, Bourne RB, Harris WH. The femoral cement compactor. An

improvement in cementing technique in total hip replacement. *J Bone Joint Surg* 1983;65A:1335–1338.

45. Panjabi M, Trumble J, Hult E, Southwick W. Effect of femoral stem length on stress raisers associated with revision hip arthroplasty. *J Orthop Res* 1985;3:447–455.

46. Pellicci PM, Salvati EA, Robinson HJ. Mechanical failures in total hip replacement requiring reoperation. *J Bone Joint Surg* 1979;61A:28.

47. Pellicci PM, Wilson PD, Sledge CB, Salvati EA, Ranawat CS, Poss R. Revision total hip arthroplasty. *Clin Orthop* 1982;170:34.

48. Pellicci PM, Wilson PDJ, Sledge CB, Salvati EA, Ranawat CS, Poss R, Callaghan JJ. Long-term results of revision total hip replacement. A follow-up report. *J Bone Joint Surg* 1985;67A:513–516.

49. Pierson JL, Harris WH. The effect of second generation techniques on the longevity of fixation in revision cemented femoral arthroplasties. Average 8.8 year follow-up. *J Arthroplasty* 1995;10:581–591.

50. Raut VV, Siney PD, et al. Cemented revision Charnley low-friction arthroplasty in patients with rheumatoid arthritis. *J Bone Joint Surg* 1994;76B:909–911.

51. Raut VV, Siney PD, Wroblewski BM. Revision for aseptic stem loosening using the cemented Charnley prosthesis. *J Bone Joint Surg* 1995; 77B(1):23–27.

52. Raut VV, Wroblewski BM, Siney PD. Revision hip arthroplasty. Can the octogenarian take it? *J Arthroplasty* 1993;8:401–403.

53. Retpen JB, Varmarken JE, Jensen JS. Survivorship analysis of failure pattern after revision total hip arthroplasty. *J Arthroplasty* 1989;4:311–317.

54. Retpen JB, Varmarken JE, Sturup J, Olsen C, Solund K, Jensen JS. Clinical results after revision and primary total hip arthroplasty. *J Arthroplasty* 1989;4:297–302.

55. Retpen JB, Varmarken JE, Rock ND, Jensen JS. Unsatisfactory results after repeated revision of hip arthroplasty: 61 cases followed for 5 (1–10) years. *Acta Orthop Scand* 1992;63:120.

56. Retpen JB, Jensen JS. Risk factors for recurrent aseptic loosening of the femoral component after cemented revision. *J Arthroplasty* 1993;8:471.

57. Rubash HE, Harris WH. Revision of non-septic, loose, cemented femoral components using modern cementing techniques. *J Arthroplasty* 1988;3:241–248.

58. Shepherd BD, Turnbull A. The fate of femoral windows in revision joint arthroplasty. *J Bone Joint Surg* 1989;71A:716–718.

59. Snorrason F, Karrholm J. Early loosening of revision hip arthroplasty: a roentgen stereophotogrammetric analysis. *J Arthroplasty* 1990;5:217.

60. Stromberg CN, Herberts P, Ahnfelt L. Revision total hip arthroplasty in patients younger than 55 years old. Clinical and radiographic results after 4 years. *J Arthroplasty* 1988;3:47–59.

61. Stromberg CN, Herberts P. A multicenter 10-year study of cemented revision total hip arthroplasty in patients younger than 55 years old. A follow-up report. *J Arthroplasty* 1994;9(6):595–601.

62. Stromberg CN, Herberts P, Palmertz B. Cemented revision hip arthroplasty. A multi-center 5–9 year study for 204 first revisions for loosening. *Acta Orthop Scand* 1992;63:111–119.

63. Turner RH, Mattingly DA, et al. Femoral revision total hip arthroplasty using a long-stem femoral component. Clinical and radiographic analysis. *J Arthroplasty* 1987;2(3):247–258.

64. Weber K, Callaghan J, Goetz D, Johnston R. Revision of a failed cemented total hip prosthesis with insertion of an acetabular component without cement and a femoral component with cement—A five to eight-year follow-up study. *J Bone Joint Surg* 1996;78A:982–994.

65. Wilson PD. Revision total hip arthroplasty: current role of polymethylmethacrylate. *Clin Orthop* 1987;225:218.

66. Wirta J, Eskola A, et al. Revision of cemented hip arthroplasties. 101 hips followed for 5 (4–9) years. *Acta Orthop Scand* 1993;64(3): 263–267.

67. Wirta J, Eskola A, et al. Revision of aggressive granulomatous lesions in hip arthroplasty. *J Arthroplasty* 1990;5:S47–52.

68. Wixson RL, Lautenschlager EP, Novak M. Vacuum mixing of methylmethacrylate bone cement. *Trans Orthop Res Soc* 1985;10:327.

69. Zmollek JC, Dorr LD. Revision total hip arthroplasty: the use of solid allograft. *J Arthroplasty* 1993;8:361.

The Adult Hip, edited by J. J. Callaghan,
A. G. Rosenberg, and H. E. Rubash.
Lippincott–Raven Publishers, Philadelphia © 1998.

CHAPTER 97

Revision of the Femoral Component: Impaction Grafting

W. E. Michael Mikhail, Robin S. M. Ling, Lars R. A. Weidenhielm, and Graham A. Gie

HISTORICAL OVERVIEW OF IMPACTION GRAFTING FOR THE FEMORAL COMPONENT

Revision hip arthroplasty in the presence of proximal femoral bone loss poses a considerable challenge to surgical reconstruction. Impaction grafting and cement possess considerable potential to deal with this problem. In 1984, Slooff et al. (16) first reported their use of morselized allograft and cement for impaction in revision surgery on the acetabular side. After failure of impaction grafting *without* cement in a femoral revision performed at the Princess Elizabeth Orthopaedic Hospital (Exeter, United Kingdom) in 1985, the concept of impaction grafting and cement was adapted to femoral revisions and introduced into clinical practice in Exeter in the Spring of 1987 (5).

Initially, it proved difficult to achieve a neutral stem position in the center of the femoral canal when using this technique. To overcome this problem and make component alignment more predictable and repro-

ducible, dedicated instrumentation was developed (3,6,11,19). These instrumentation systems are based on the use of a collarless, double-tapered, polished stem that is cemented into a neomedullary canal formed by the tight impaction of morselized allograft in the proximal femur.

The results presented in this chapter were obtained with the use of this type of stem and may not apply to the use of other femoral component designs used with impaction grafting because of the high compressive element of load induced by this stem design (18). Time alone will tell.

BIOLOGY OF IMPACTION GRAFTING FOR THE FEMORAL COMPONENT

Animal Studies

In 1994, B. W. Schreurs published his thesis from Nijmegen (15). Together with Slooff and Huiskes, he carried out an experimental study of impaction grafting in goats. Histologic examination performed after 12 weeks showed revascularization and remodeling of the graft. Bone apposition and resorption of the graft resulted in a mixture of graft and new bone at 12 weeks.

W. E. M. Mikhail: Regency Orthopaedics, Toledo, Ohio 43623.
R. S. M. Ling and G. A. Gie: The Quadrant, Exeter EX2 4LE, Devon, England.
L. R. A. Weidenhielm: Department of Orthopaedics, St. Goran Hospital, S-11281 Stockholm, Sweden.

The authors concluded that the stability of the loaded, cemented stems in combination with impacted, morselized allograft permitted incorporation of the graft. The same *in vivo* goat model was used to study a noncemented titanium stem implanted in the impacted bone graft without cement. Histologic examination showed that graft lysis was evident in the mid-shaft region and distally around the prosthesis. Incorporation of graft occurred in the biomechanically stable implants, but in the majority of cases initial stability was not achieved.

Retrieval Study

Ling and co-workers (9) examined the proximal femur retrieved at autopsy from a patient 3.5 years after cemented revision with impaction grafting. A segment of femur in the region of a large lateral cortical defect in zone 2 had been dealt with by covering the cortical defect with wire mesh and cerclage and then carrying out an impaction grafting procedure in the usual way. The histology demonstrated three zones: regenerated cortical zone, interface zone, and deep layer zone. The layer closest to the implant contained necrotic bone entombed in cement. The intermediate zone showed direct contact between methylmethacrylate and osteoid, with scattered foreign-body-type giant cells, an appearance similar to that described by Charnley (2) in the femur after primary cemented hip arthroplasty. No direct contact between viable mineralized bone and cement was apparent. The outer zone contained histologically normal cortex and fatty bone marrow with a few islands of dead bone. Over 90% of the total surface area of the sections of new cortical bone contained filled osteocyte lacunae. There was no continuous fibrous membrane between cement and new bone.

Human Biopsies

Nelissen et al. (12) have published results on biopsies from the proximal femur in four patients 11 to 27 months after revision with impaction grafting. Recently, another biopsy consisting of a circumferential section of the femur at the level of the tip of the femoral stem has been obtained. These cases show features similar to those reported by Ling and co-workers (9). Three zones were also noted. The inner zone contained trabeculae of partially necrotic bone, fibrosis, occasional lymphocytes, and bone cement consistent with cemented bone graft undergoing remodeling. Several areas of viable mineralized bone were found directly adjacent to bone cement, although the significance of this is uncertain. The middle layer contained occasional particles of bone cement as well as viable trabecular bone in all cases. Review of the radiographs obtained at the time of revision arthroplasty suggests that some, if not all, of

this bone is the result of incorporated and remodeled allograft. In two of the cases, trabecular condensation was noted at the inner aspect of this zone, suggesting the formation of a neocortex similar to the circumferential rim of new bone surrounding stable, conventionally cemented implants as described by Jasty and co-workers (8). Although not specifically described in the histologic specimen, radiographs included in the autopsy retrieval report by Ling et al. (9) show a similar, if incomplete, neocortex around the bone cement.

The outer layer in the biopsies reported by Nelissen et al. (12) uniformly consisted of viable cortex, as noted by Ling et al. (9). Bone density is difficult to evaluate histologically without a contralateral control, but the porosity of the femoral cortex at this level appears to be increased. Although the viability of this bone suggests that it has been loaded, the increased cortical porosity also supports the presence of a component of proximal stress shielding even with this design.

It is important to emphasize that these biopsies of Nelissen et al. (12) were all from stable implants and that the study reported by Ling et al. (9) was from a patient who, during life, had a "forgotten" hip. Patients who met the standards of the former group were regarded by Charnley as essential to clarify the significance of the histologic findings between cement and bone in the femur, because this level of clinical function implied excellent stability of the device. Thus, the histology from human retrievals available so far in cases that have undergone impaction grafting is likely to represent the most optimistic end of an histologic spectrum, and it will almost certainly be less favorable when stability is compromised. Under those circumstances, extensive areas of fibrous tissue are to be expected. Much more remains to be learned about the biology of this technique and the factors that control bone regeneration.

INDICATIONS

This revision technique is indicated in patients with mechanical failure of cemented and cementless femoral stems, regardless of their length. In the presence of infection, the procedure is done in two stages. It is also indicated in cases with bone loss of the proximal femur with cortical defects and thinning from stress shielding and wear-induced osteolysis. The prerequisite for the procedure is that an intact femoral "tube" can be reconstructed and that the defects can be covered with strut grafts and/or wire mesh to allow for tight packing of the bone graft, and stable fixation of the femoral component in the impacted graft. Osteolytic lesions in the distal part of the femur or around long stems are not contraindications for this procedure. In these cases, however, reinforcement of the femur with cortical strut allografts, and a long stem option to bypass the lytic or defective areas, is sometimes advisable. Long stems of two different lengths, with a neck–shaft angle of 135° and the appropriate offset, are currently available. The lytic lesions usually disappear with time and a normalization of the distal femur occurs. For patients with an infected loose total hip arthroplasty (THA), a two-stage exchange is recommended. The infected THA is removed and the infection is treated. When the infection is under control, a prosthesis can be implanted with impaction grafting technique as will be described.

SURGICAL TECHNIQUE

In the preoperative planning of THA revision, a proper analysis of the femoral environment, including integrity of the bone–cement interface, the presence or absence of cortical defects, and the thickness of the femoral cortex both proximally and distally to the stem should be performed. Many classifications of bone-stock loss exist today. Assessment of bone-stock loss on a four-grade scale according to the Endo-Klinik classification (4) has worked well.

Exposure of the hip is performed according to the surgeon's preference. It is absolutely essential for the surgeon to recognize that this operation cannot be properly performed through an inadequate exposure. A free soft-tissue release is needed so that the upper end of the femur can be delivered into the wound, to allow the proximal end of the canal to be opened up into the greater trochanter at least 1 cm lateral to the midline axis of the canal. Only then can the new medullary canal

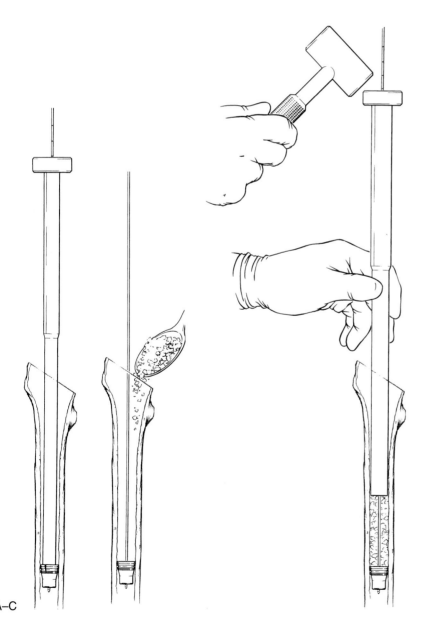

A–C

FIG. 1. A: Insertion of the distal plug. **B:** Grafting the femoral canal. **C:** Packing the distal one-third of the canal.

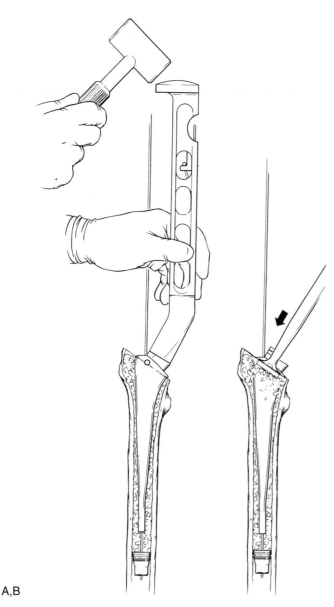

A,B

FIG. 2. A: Proximal packing with cannulated tamps. **B:** Final packing with proximal packers.

be correctly orientated, adequately impacted, and properly cemented. Trochanteric osteotomy is not favored because of possible loss of containment for the proximal and lateral parts of the graft.

The old femoral component is removed. Cement, fibrous membrane, particulate debris, and granulomatous material are cleaned from the femoral canal, which is then thoroughly lavaged. Defects in the cortex are patched with wire mesh and/or strut allograft secured with cerclage wires prior to packing. Prophylactic wiring of the femur before packing (or even before removal of the old implant) is recommended when cortical integrity is tenuous. A guide wire is threaded into a stiff medullary polymethylmethacrylate (PMMA) plug, and this is placed in the distal canal with the largest can-

nulated tamp that the femur can accommodate. The wire should be threaded completely through the plug with approximately 5 mm of pin protruding through the bottom of the plug. The plug is driven distal to areas of lytic bone, and a packer, smaller in size than the plug, is used to confirm seating (Fig. 1A). It is essential to ensure that the plug does not subside during the later packing/tamping process. Any tendency for the plug to subside during impaction can be controlled by driving a small Kirschner wire across the femur and either through the plug or just below it (13). This wire is removed once impaction has been completed. The guide wire should exit the proximal femur near the lateral endosteal cortex, which is in line with the axis of the center of the femur. The intramedullary plug will center the guide wire in the distal canal. The use of a cannulated system has greatly reduced the incidence of malposition of the stem. Three- to 5-mm diameter, fresh-frozen allograft chips are used (see Fig. 1B). It is a serious mistake to use chips that are too small, because stability is thereby compromised.

Cancellous allograft is obtained from femoral condyles, proximal tibiae, or femoral heads as appropriate. The allograft is inserted into the femur and packed vigorously into the canal with sharp hammer blows on a small-diameter cannulated packer. This step is repeated until the distal one third of the proximal femur has been filled (see Fig. 1C). Larger-diameter packers are used as the diameter of the canal increases more proximally. Packing *must* be vigorous. A cannulated tamp approximately one or two sizes smaller than the final component is introduced over the guide wire. More graft material is introduced and the tamp is vigorously impacted until fully seated (Fig. 2A). This process is repeated, progressing up in tamp size, until the planned size is firmly seated. The tamp of the planned size should allow for a uniform layer of bone graft, the optimal thickness of which is at present unknown. Graft thickness will be dictated to some extent by the geometry of the femoral canal. The driving handle is detached and final packing of the canal is completed with proximal packers around the tamp (see Fig. 2B). The tamp should be absolutely stable at the conclusion of impaction, to the extent that manual twisting or extraction without the use of a hammer is impossible. If it is not, it is best to extract the graft and repack the canal more tightly. It is important to note that any sudden reduction in the force needed to impact the tamp may mean that the femur has been fractured. Under such circumstances, the fracture should be stabilized by whatever means is appropriate, and the packing redone.

Pooled blood at the distal end of the stem is extracted by applying suction to the guide wire hole in the tamp. The tamp is left in place until immediately before cement insertion. The tamps are oversized compared to the corresponding stems to allow for a uniform 2- to 3-

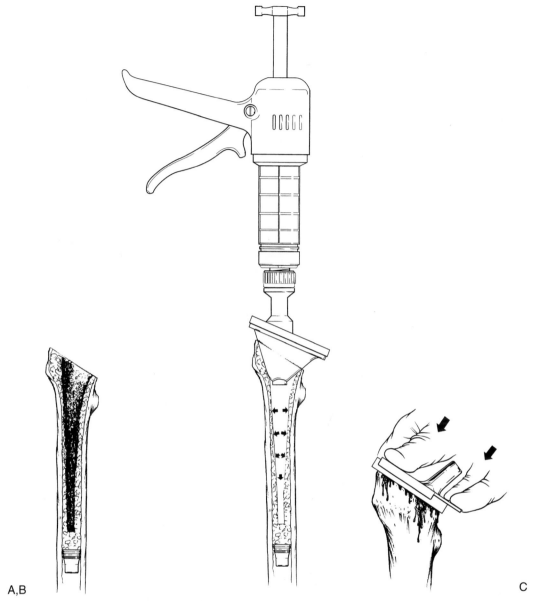

A,B   C

FIG. 3. A: The neomedullary canal. **B:** Pressurizing cement with proximal seal. **C:** Introducing the stem and final pressurization with plate.

mm-thick cement mantle. A complete "neomedullary" canal has been formed (Fig. 3A).

The same amount of cement as that used for primary THAs is impregnated with antibiotics and introduced into the neomedullary canal in a retrograde fashion. Conventional Simplex-type cement is used. It is important that the cement dough that is introduced into the canal be in a relatively low-viscosity state, otherwise the distal part of the neomedullary canal cannot be filled, and adequate penetration of the graft by cement cannot be achieved (1). A cement gun with a small tapered nozzle is used to inject cement into the narrow distal part of the neomedullary canal. A second, larger nozzle is used

to complete filling of the proximal femur. The femoral pressurizer seal and plate are then impacted into the opening at the upper end of the neomedullary canal while the cement continues to be injected, allowing the canal to be pressurized. Pressurization continues until the cement reaches a doughy consistency. The centralizer is applied to the distal end of the implant and the wings of the centralizer are cut off prior to insertion. The appropriate-sized, tapered, polished, collarless stem is inserted. Oversizing the stem is a major error and will be at the expense of the thickness of both the graft and the cement mantle. Prophylactic antibiotic treatment and prophylactic anticoagulation are routinely used.

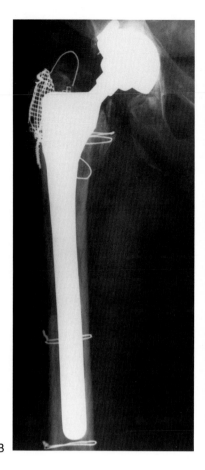 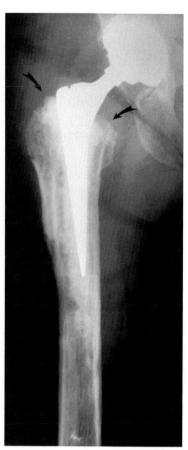

A,B

FIG. 4. A: At revision, Case 1 arthroplasty shows a non-cemented, long-stem PCA component and cerclage wires around the femur. **B:** At biopsy, there is a well-cemented femoral stem without radiolucent lines around the cement mantle. The stem has subsided 3 mm within the cement mantle. The bone in the proximal femur shows signs of trabecular remodeling, especially on the lateral side of the stem. The strut graft is radiologically incorporated.

CASE EXAMPLES

Case 1

A 61-year-old man received a cemented THA (Dual Lock, DePuy Corp., Warsaw, IN) for osteoarthritis in 1980. Revision arthroplasties were performed in 1984 [with a cemented porous-coated anatomic (PCA) stem, Howmedica Corp., East Rutherford, NJ] and in 1987 (with a noncemented long stem PCA, autogenous bone graft, and a PCA acetabular cup). In June of 1991, the uncemented PCA was revised because of aseptic loosening accompanied by gross proximal femoral bone loss (Fig. 4A). Most of the graft was resorbed and the remaining part was dead bone and fibrous tissue around the PCA stem. A cemented tapered, polished, collarless stem was inserted with impaction grafting technique, using two morselized femoral condyles and two ounces of cancellous allograft bone chips. Additional strut allografts were applied to reinforce the stress-shielding proximal femoral cortex. Cultures obtained at revision surgery were negative. A technetium single photon emmision computed tomography (SPECT) scan performed 12 months after revision surgery showed increased uptake in the proximal femur.

Postoperatively, the patient did well but developed lateral thigh pain caused by the cerclage wires. The wires were removed 27 months after revision arthroplasty, at which time biopsies of the proximal femur and the structural grafts were obtained. Radiographs at the time of biopsy showed a well-cemented femoral stem, without radiolucent lines at either interface. The bone in the proximal femur showed signs of trabecular remodeling, especially on the lateral side of the stem. The strut graft was radiologically incorporated (see Fig. 4B). The proximal femoral biopsy had a histologic appearance very similar to that of all the other biopsied cases. Three zones could be identified (Fig. 5A). An inner zone approximately 1 to 2 mm thick contained partially necrotic trabecular bone with evidence of ongoing bone remodeling ("creeping substitution") (see Fig. 5B). Fibrous tissue and bone cement were present between the remodeling bone chips. The second zone contained histologically viable trabecular bone with a few additional fragments of bone cement (see Fig. 5C). A suggestion of trabecular condensation could again be identified. The outer zone consisted of viable cortex. The biopsy of the structural bone graft showed necrotic bone with very little evidence of remodeling activity.

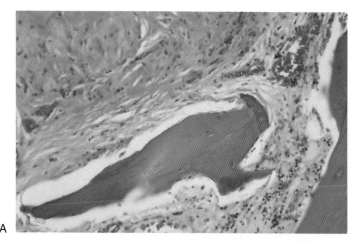

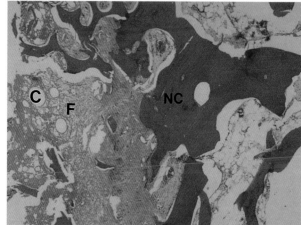

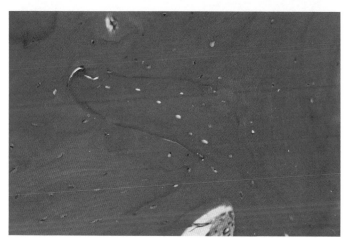

FIG. 5. Photomicrographs of the inner zone **(A)**, the middle zone **(B)**, and the outer zone **(C)** from Case 1.

Case 2

A 38-year-old woman sustained a subcapital fracture of the neck of her left femur at the age of 18. The fracture was treated by reduction and internal fixation. Union was achieved, but segmental collapse from avascular necrosis supervened. In 1978, she underwent a double cup replacement arthroplasty that failed after 4 years. Revision was carried out with the insertion of a banana-stemmed Müller prosthesis. Initially the result was good, but within 3 years pain recurred and eventually she was able to walk only with crutches. The Müller hip arthroplasty was removed and impaction grafting of both the socket and femur carried out. A satisfactory recovery ensued. Figure 6 shows the preoperative radiograph before revision with impaction grafting was performed. Note the loss of cortex in zones 2 and 3. Figure 7 shows the postoperative film, Figure 8 shows the appearances at 1 year, and Figure 9 shows the appearances at 4 years. The restitution of the cortex in 1 year in zones 2 and 3 is remarkable, and the trabecular remodeling evident in zones 2, 3, 6, and 7 is striking. The patient has been restored to full activities, including sports.

RESULTS

Mechanical Stability of the Implant

Schreurs et al. (15) studied the initial stability of both cemented and uncemented femoral stems implanted in goat femurs in a loading experiment. Displacement of the stems relative to bone was determined with roentgen-stereophotogrammetric analysis. The most important movements were axial rotations (cemented stems up to 2.1°, uncemented stems up to 6.8°) and subsidence (cemented stems up to 0.5 mm, uncemented stems up to 2.9 mm). Malkani et al. (10) presented a loading experiment in which the mechanical stability of a femoral prosthesis implanted in a cadaver femur with impaction-grafting technique was compared to a cemented THA in a cadaver femur simulating the primary situation. The mechanical stability for the prosthesis implanted with impaction–grafting technique was equal to the primary cemented THA.

Smith et al. (17) reported on *in vitro* studies of impaction grafting in which the loads were applied cyclically. They showed that when nonheparinized blood was

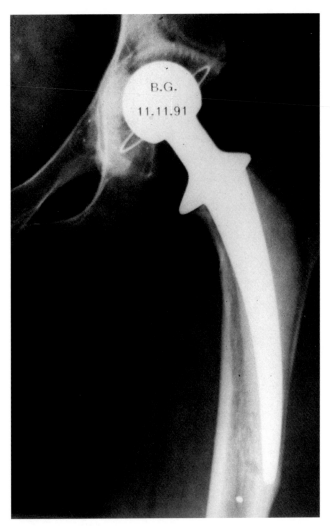

FIG. 6. Preoperative radiograph from Case 2 prior to impaction grafting. Note the loss of cortex in zones 2 and 3.

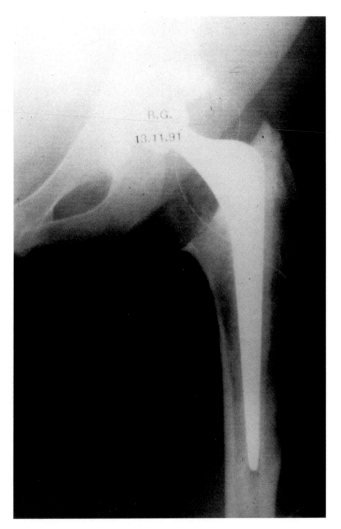

FIG. 7. The postoperative radiograph from Case 2.

mixed with the graft, substantially increased stability was obtained by comparison with the situation using dry graft or graft mixed with heparinized blood. This investigation has important implications for further *in vitro* experimental studies.

It is important to recognize that primary implant stability with this technique depends on the adequacy of containment and impaction of the graft, together with effective cementing.

Clinical and Radiographic Results

Gie et al. (7) reported a 44- to 78-month follow-up of 68 patients in whom impaction grafting and cementing had been combined with the use of a polished, double-tapered, collarless stem. The clinical results were comparable to primary surgery with incorporation of bone graft and, in a high proportion of the cases, trabecular remodeling and cortical healing. Radiolucent lines at the

graft–host and cement–graft interfaces were uncommon and complications few. Since the initial report, Gie et al. have performed another 310 cases, and, in the whole series of some 370 hips, only one had to be re-operated on for recurrent loosening of the stem. In this case, the technical performance of the impaction grafting operation left a great deal to be desired. The 2- to 6-year results of Mikhail and Timperly (11) with a stem of similar geometry in 132 patients are similarly favorable clinically and radiographically. There has been no failure to date, and none are impending. No re-revision has been performed to date. Fifteen patients with a minimum follow-up of 18 months, revised using the impaction grafting technique with appropriate instrumentation, have been reported by Mikhail and Timperley (11). The favorable clinical results in this series of patients support the findings of Gie et al. (7).

Elting and his colleagues (3) presented a preliminary report of impaction grafting for exchange femoral arthroplasty. Satisfactory results were reported for 67 patients, with a 2- to 5-year follow-up. The major complication in

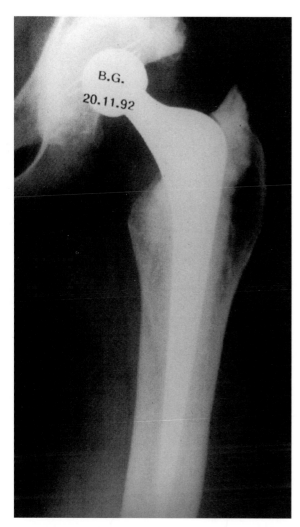

FIG. 8. The appearance at 1 year. The restitution of the cortex in 1 year in zones 2 and 3 is remarkable, and the trabecular remodeling evident in zones 2, 3, 6, and 7 is striking.

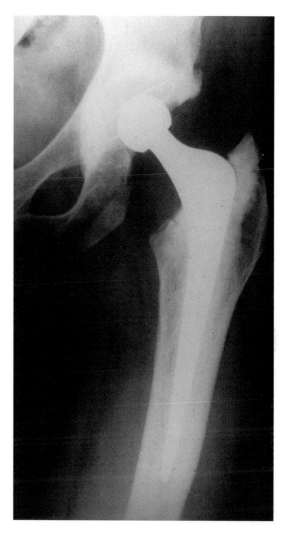

FIG. 9. The appearances at 4 years.

this series and in the overall series in Exeter has been late fracture of the femur.

PITFALLS

The availability of allograft is usually limited. There is a risk of transmitted disease resulting from contamination of the allograft, although none has been reported yet in over 1000 cases covering up to 7 years in multiple U.S. centers. Impaction grafting is not a forgiving procedure. It is important to use a precise technique and avoid short cuts. The need for a full and free exposure of the upper femur, together with all diaphyseal defects, cannot be overemphasized.

An intraoperative femoral fracture is most commonly produced by inadequate soft-tissue release. Modern instrumentation has made the technique reproducible and the outcome predictable. It helps to achieve a central position of the stem in the femoral canal. Oversizing the

stem is a mistake. At present, the optimal thickness of graft is not known, but a cement mantle not less than 2 mm in thickness and expanding to 4 mm proximally and medially is regarded as desirable. In cases with a substantial preoperative bone loss, particularly near the stem tip, there is an increased risk for postoperative femoral fracture. Prevention is probably best achieved using strut grafts with cerclage wire and/or a plate with a standard length stem. There may be a place for a longer stem in certain cases, but the authors are fundamentally opposed to the routine use of long stems in this procedure.

These patients should be instructed to limit their activities until healing of the osteolytic lesions has taken place. The results with this procedure are probably technique and design dependent. If possible, a trochanteric osteotomy should also be avoided, because it will disturb the proximal packing of the graft. However, Rosenberg (14) has shown in *in vitro* experiments that the stability of impaction grafting after fixation of an extended trochanteric osteotomy is virtually identical to impaction grafting in intact femora.

Impaction grafting is associated with increased costs compared to a cemented or uncemented revision, because of the costs of the allograft. The operative procedure can be time consuming, thus adding to costs.

The reported results to date from a number of centers lead to guarded optimism with regard to the long-term outcome in this procedure, and it is reasonable at this stage to conclude that it does have a definite place in the armamentarium of the revision surgeon. It is important to emphasize and reemphasize that although the operation is not technically difficult, the exposure, a vital prerequisite for adequate surgery, may sometimes be challenging. Thereafter, a successful result demands attention to the operative details and a commitment to take the time and energy to achieve adequate and vigorous packing of the femur with graft, followed by careful cementing and accurate femoral component insertion. It has to be remembered that the stability of the revision implant and its in-service life depends on the effectiveness of these operative details.

The extent to which the clinical results and bone remodeling are stem geometry dependent is at present unknown.

SUMMARY

1. This revision technique is indicated in the following cases:

   A. Mechanical failure of cemented and cementless femoral stems, regardless of their length.
   B. Cases with bone loss of the proximal femur, with cortical defects and thinning from stress shielding and wear-induced osteolysis.

2. The prerequisite for the procedure is that an intact tube can be reconstructed and the defects covered with strut grafts and/or wire mesh to allow for tight packing of the bone graft and stable fixation of the femoral component in the impacted graft.

3. Three- to 5-mm-diameter fresh-frozen allograft chips are used.

4. The prosthetic component should be well centered in the femoral canal, surrounded by a uniform layer of bone graft, the optimal thickness of which is at present uncertain, and a 2- to 3-mm-thick cement mantle.

5. Septic cases should never be tackled in one stage.

REFERENCES

1. Botha PJ, Snowdowne RB, Van Zyl AA. Allograft bone impaction grafting—what cement should be used and why? *South Afr Bone Joint Surg* 1995;5:25–28.
2. Charnley J. The reaction of bone to self-curing acrylic cement: a long-term histological study in man. *J Bone Joint Surg* 1970;52B:340–353.
3. Elting JJ, Mikhail WEM, Zicat BA, Hubbell JC, Lane LE, House B. Preliminary report of impaction grafting for exchange femoral arthroplasty. *Clin Orthop* 1995;319:159–167.
4. Engelbrecht E, Heinert K. *Klassifikation und Behandlungsrichtlinien von knockensubstansverlusten bei Revisionsoperationen am huftgelenk—mittelfristige Ergebnisse. Primare und revisionsalloartroplastik Hrgs—Endoklinik, Hamburg.* Berlin: Springer-Verlag, 1987; 189–201.
5. Gie GA, Linder L, Ling RSM, Simon J-P, Slooff TJJH, Timperley AJ. Impacted cancellous allografts and cement for revision total hip arthroplasty. *J Bone Joint Surg* 1993;75B:14–21.
6. Gie GA, Linder L, Ling RSM, Simon J-P, Sloof TJJH, Timperley AJ. Contained morsellized allograft in revision total hip arthroplasty. Surgical technique. *Orthop Clin North Am* 1993;24:717–725
7. Gie GA, Linder L, Ling RSM, Simon J-P, Slooff TJJH, Timperley AJ. Femoral reconstruction: cement with graft. In: Galante JO, Rosenberg AG, Callaghan JJ, eds. *Total hip revision surgery.* New York: Raven Press, 1995;367–373.
8. Jasty M, Maloney WJ, Bragdon CR, Haire T, Harris WH. Histomorphological studies of the long-term skeletal responses to well fixed cemented femoral components. *J Bone Joint Surg* 1990;72A: 1220–1229.
9. Ling RSM, Timperley AJ, Linder L. Histology of cancellous impaction grafting in the femur. *J Bone Joint Surg* 1993;75B: 693–696.
10. Malkani AL, Voor MJ, Fee KA, Bates CS. Femoral component revision with impaction morselized cancellous graft and cement: biomechanical evaluation of implant stability. *Trans Orthop Res Soc* 1995;20:729.
11. Mikhail WEM, Timperley AJ. Tight packing of morcellized allograft: new method for managing bone lysis. *Orthopedic Special Edition* 1994;3:21–22.
12. Nelissen RGGH, Bauer TW, Weidenhielm LRA, LeGolvan DP, Mikhail WEM. Revision hip arthroplasty with the use of cement and impaction grafting. *J Bone Joint Surg* 1995;77A:412–422.
13. Northmore-Ball MD, Narang ON, Vergroesen D. Distal femoral plug migration with cement pressurisation in revision surgery and a simple technique for its prevention. *J Arthroplasty* 1991;6:199–201.
14. Rosenberg AG. Personal communication, 1995.
15. Schreurs BW. *Reconstructive options in revision surgery of failed total hip arthroplasties.* Thesis, Nijmegen, The Netherlands, 1994.
16. Slooff TJ, Huiskes R, van Horn J, Lemmens A. Bone grafting in total hip replacement for acetabular protrusion. *Acta Orthop Scand* 1984; 55:593–596.
17. Smith EJ, Richardson JB, Learmonth ID, Nelson K, Lee RG, Dyson JR, Evans GP. In vitro impaction grafting. *Trans Eur Orthop Res Soc* 1995;5:48.
18. Verdonschot N, Huiskes R. Can polished stems reduce mechanical failures of the cement–bone interface in man? *Trans Eur Orthop Res Soc* 1995;5:42.
19. Weidenhielm LRA, Nelissen RGHH, Mikhail WEM, Bauer TW. Surgical technique and early results in revision THA with a cemented, tapered, collarless, polished stem and contained morselized allograft. *J Orthop Techniques* 1994;2(3):113–122.

The Adult Hip, edited by J. J. Callaghan,
A. G. Rosenberg, and H. E. Rubash.
Lippincott–Raven Publishers, Philadelphia © 1998.

CHAPTER 98

Revision of the Femoral Component: Hydroxyapatite Enhancement

Rudolph G. T. Geesink and Nicolette H. M. Hoefnagels

Revision hip surgery is an increasing challenge for the orthopedic surgeon, as a result of increasing numbers of primary total hip replacements and the expansion of indications to an ever younger population of patients. In contrast to the current excellent results of primary total hip replacements, revision hip surgery still has somewhat mediocre results.

Much of the controversy in the literature focuses on the use of cemented or cementless techniques in revision surgery. Published results of both cemented (6,10,18,22, 24–27) and cementless (3,8,19,20) revision arthroplasty are encouraging despite failure rates that remain generally higher than those of primary hip surgery. Successful results depend on several factors, including, but not limited to, cementing technique, implant design, bone–implant contact, quality of bone stock, implant stability, and age (10,16,17,20,23,24,31).

The cementless approach often is preferred because the sclerotic smooth endocortex of the femur does not allow for any trabecular interdigitation of a cemented stem, which is necessary for adequate cemented fixation. Several possibilities for cementless alternatives exist if used in conditions of poor bone stock. For instance, extensively porous-coated stems have been used with distal fixation, and the use of allografts has been advocated. Also, modular implants have been used to accommodate for the various types and locations of bone deficiencies.

Although the decision to use cemented or cementless fixation is important, the essential problem in hip revi-

sion surgery is loss of bone stock. If there is no balance between the amount of bone and the amount of implant, the implant will fail because the weak remaining bone cannot provide for long-term implant stability. This is true for both massively cemented stems and massive/ modular cementless implants if used in conditions of poor bone stock. Therefore, repair and augmentation of bone defects is mandatory at the time of hip revision surgery. One such technique as reported by Gie et al. (12) has gained considerable interest in recent years. This technique uses compressed trabecular bone graft in combination with cement on both the femoral and the acetabular side. Results (13,21), with a follow-up extending to 6 years, are promising.

The use of hydroxylapatite (HA) coatings in primary cementless hip surgery has resulted in significantly better results than obtained with previous generations of press-fit devices. In primary total hip replacements, excellent clinical results have been obtained, with survival rates of 100% for the femoral stem up to 6 years (11). Excellent persistence of bone stock has been documented using the dual energy x-ray absorptiometry (DEXA) technique as well (28). After 7 years of implantation, full bone stock is maintained in 6 out of 7 Gruen zones of the femur, versus only 30% loss of bone mineral density in the proximal medial part of the femur above the level of the lesser trochanter.

These properties of HA have led to the use of HA coatings in revision surgery as well as primary cementless hip surgery.

The use of bone graft in conjunction with HA coatings is necessary to improve the mechanical stability of the construct, as well as to provide an improvement in bone

R. G. T. Geesink and N. H. M. Hoefnagels: Department of Orthopaedic Surgery, University Hospital Maastricht, 6202 AZ Maastricht, The Netherlands.

stock. Bone ingrowth between HA coating and bone can occur only in the presence of well-vascularized native bone. HA coatings by themselves are known to be able to fill gaps of 1 to 2 mm wide, provided there is adequate mechanical stability of the implant (29,30). Initially, these conditions caused some reticence about the application of bone grafts in cases with minor bone deficiencies. Whether there will be any bone ingrowth between bone transplant and HA coating remains uncertain. If, however, long-term bone status is improved, any necessary future surgery will be easier. In addition, closure of any bone deficiencies in the proximal femur will improve the sealing effect between bone and stem, thereby limiting migration of polyethylene (PE) wear particles into the distal implant–bone interface.

Bone deficiencies are usually located in the proximal femur. If they are contained, trabecular chip grafts can be packed in the cavities and, with impaction of the stem, compressed between the stem and the surrounding femoral cortex. Bone ingrowth fixation will be obtained between the lower part of the HA coating and the metaphyseal or diaphyseal part of the femur. If bone deficiencies extend more distally, the use of longer stems becomes necessary, and a more distal HA coating will secure bone ingrowth fixation. If femoral bone deficiencies are segmentary and include significant parts of femoral cortex, then it is necessary to use additional structural grafts. The indications for bone grafting became more clear with longer experience. The first operations using HA coated devices in revision surgery were performed in 1987 and thus now allow a longest follow-up of 9 years.

Since 1987, 58 patients with 61 problem hips have undergone revision hip surgery as a result of mostly mechanical failure of cemented or cementless femoral components. This study is concerned only with femoral component revisions. Many patients had acetabular revisions as well, but they are not the issue of this study. Septic loosenings were excluded from this study. The average patient age was 58 years (range 34 to 75 years) with a female-to-male ratio of 1.3:1. The mean age of the male population was 54 years and the mean age of the female population 61 years.

There was no difference in the left-to-right ratio, and the average follow-up was 53 months (range, 7 to 102 months). With respect to the Charnley function classification, 49% of patients could be classified to class A, having unilateral hip disease and no other problems; 31% to class B, having bilateral hip disease and no other problems; and 20% to class C, having other orthopedic and/or medical problems that might reduce their scores regardless of the results of the hip replacement itself (4).

The relative obesity of patients was expressed in the Quetelet index, defined as weight in kilograms divided by the squared height in meters. The mean Quetelet index was 25.8 (range, 19 to 35), including 6% with obesity (index > 30).

Of the revised femoral components, 54% were revision of a failed cemented stems and 43% of a failed uncemented stems, and 3% consisted of conversion of an endoprosthesis to a THA. The reason for revision was mechanical loosening of both femoral and acetabular components in 57% of the cases, loosening of just the femoral stem only in 15% of the cases, and revision of mechanically well-fixed implants that had to be revised because of malposition, recurrent dislocation, or otherwise in the remaining 28% of the cases.

Many cases were multiply revised patients: 40% of the cases concerned a first implant revision, 35% of the cases a second revision, and 25% of the cases a third to fifth revision. The average time interval between current revision and previous hip implantation was 5 years (range, 0 to 19 years). Bone deficiencies were grouped according to Engh's classification of bone stock damage (7): 43% were rated as having minimal or no bone damage, 22% were rated as having proximal damage only (neck and intertrochanteric), and 35% were rated as having both proximal femur and femoral shaft damage.

The HA-Omnifit (Osteonics, Allendale, New Jersey) was used for revision of the femur in 88% of the cases. In the remaining 12% of the cases, longer stem length with a longer HA-coating was utilized.

The Osteonics stems with HA coating are manufactured from Ti-6Al-4V (90% titanium, 6% aluminum, 4% vanadium) alloy and have a macrotextured surface. Approximately 40% of the proximal stem length is HA coated. The HA coating has a 50-μm thickness with a porosity below 3%, an HA purity of 97%, and an approximately 65% crystallinity. The currently available revision stems have stem lengths of 160 to 300 mm with similarly textured surfaces but a longer length of HA coating extending to the diaphyseal part of the femur.

The surgical approach is usually a posterolateral one, but it may include a trochanteric slide or Wagner transfemoral osteotomy to remove distal well-fixed parts of cement or implant. These access osteotomies are usually repaired using cerclage wires or Dall-Miles cables. Bone graft augmentation (either heterologous or autologous) was used in 40% of the cases.

All patients received a 24-hour period of antibiotic prophylaxis, usually cephalosporins, and a 3-month period of anticoagulation. Depending on the mechanical stability of the surgical construct, most patients were kept on a regimen of restricted weight bearing for at least 6 weeks and usually up to 3 months after surgery. Then progressive weight bearing was allowed, with physiotherapy as needed. Use of crutches was left to the patient's comfort.

All patients were seen at least once at follow-up and were clinically reviewed with respect to the Harris Hip Score (HHS) (15) and the Pain–Motion–Activity rating

(PMA) (1). At the same time, anteroposterior and lateral radiographs of the pelvis were taken at each review to evaluate bone apposition, reactive line formation, cortical remodeling, osteolysis per Gruen zone (14), and bone resorption and heterotopic bone formation according to Brooker (2). Roentgenographic assessment of fixation and stability of the femoral component was performed using the radiographic score of Engh et al. (9). Additionally, polyethylene wear was measured using the method of Charnley and Halley (5). (See cases 3 and 4 for a discussion of clinical or radiographic failure.)

Statistical methods were applied, including the Student's *t*-test, to assess any variable differences (i.e., male/female, age, left/right, Charnley group A–B/Charnley group C, one or more previous surgeries, amount of bone damage, the use of bone graft or not) in regard to clinical (HHS and PMA) and radiographic scores (Enghscore, Brooker, and PE-wear). Statistical significance was assumed when $p < .05$. From 3 years on, no further statistical analysis could be executed because of the unequal sizes of the comparing groups.

COMPLICATIONS AND REOPERATIONS

No complications or reoperations were related to the HA coating. Dislocations were the most prominent feature (five cases) and all but one of these were successfully treated by closed reduction. Most patients with obvious soft-tissue instability at surgery were prophylactically treated in a flexion–abduction brace for 3 months after surgery.

There were four reoperations that were not related to implant fixation problems. One was for exchange of the cup insert because of recurrent dislocation. Two other reoperations concerned the removal of osteosynthesis including cerclage wires and trochanteric fixation devices, because of persistent pain and local osteolysis. The fourth reoperation involved repair of a symptomatic trochanteric nonunion.

One patient died of non-hip-related causes 6 months after revision arthroplasty. His autopsy retrieval histology is detailed in case 5.

There were three re-revisions of the femoral component for implant failure: two for mechanical loosening and one for septic failure without loosening. One example of mechanical loosening will be discussed in case 3. These patients were re-revised with satisfactory clinical results.

CLINICAL RESULTS

Clinical results are listed in Table 1. The early disappearance of pain is remarkable, although walking activi-

TABLE 1. *Mean Harris Hip Score (HHS) and Merle d'Aubigné classification score after revision THA with HA enhancement*

	Follow-up (mo)		
	3 (N=50)	6 (N=44)	12–72
HHS	78	84	88
Merle d'Aubigné score			
Pain	5.3	5.3	5.4
Motion	5.2	5.6	5.6
Walk	3.4	4.3	4.8

THA, total hip arthroplasty; HA, hydroxylapatite.

ties may remain restricted for quite a long period after surgery. The use of walking aids is necessary to compensate for limp or other gait disorders in the rehabilitation period.

Statistical analysis found differences in Charnley groups. Patient group Charnley C had significantly better pain rates up to 1 year after surgery as compared to Charnley groups A and B. Conversely, at 3 and 6 months the walking ability score was worse in Charnley group C as compared to Charnley groups A and B.

There was also a statistical difference in pain ratings at the 3-year follow-up between patients having more than one previous implant revision. In addition, first time revisions had a significantly better range of motion at 3 months, and a better ability to walk at 12 months than those with multiple previous surgeries.

Similar differences could be calculated in regard to the amount of bone deficiency and the use of autografts or allografts at surgery. Patients having both proximal femur and femoral shaft damage, which frequently necessitated the use of bone graft, had a significantly worse walking ability and range of motion at 3 and 6 months as compared to patients having minimal or no bone damage. These diminished abilities probably resulted in the significantly lower Harris Hip Score for this group at 3 months. After 6 months, no differences could be found between these groups. Regarding the difference between male and female patients, the pain and HHS scores for men were significantly better up to 3 years as compared to women.

RADIOLOGIC RESULTS

Radiologic parameters, such as bone apposition and formation of radiolucent lines, are listed in Tables 2 and 3. The general pattern is one of early bone ingrowth with bone apposition in Gruen zones 1, 2, 6, and 7, which are over the medial and lateral proximal parts of the stem. These patterns are fairly similar to those seen after primary total hip replacement using HA coatings (11). Most

TABLE 2. *Occurrences of bone apposition per Gruen zone after revision THA with HA enhancement*

Gruen zone	Follow-up (mo)			
	3 (N=50)	12 (N=42)	24 (N=44)	36–72
1	10	50	68	72
2	10	62	72	88
3	—	2	—	20
4	—	5	4	9
5	—	—	4	29
6	14	83	82	92
7	28	71	86	84
Stems showing apposition (%)	38	98	98	100
Mean peri-implant length of bone ongrowth area (mm)	19	79	105	148

TABLE 3. *Occurrence of reactive line formation per Gruen zone after revision THA with HA enhancement*

Gruen zone	Follow-up (mo)			
	3 (N=50)	12 (N=42)	36 (N=34)	48–72
1	2	5	9	11
2	2	9	21	21
3	2	33	76	68
4	—	62	82	82
5	2	40	59	52
6	—	14	34	31
7	—	—	6	5
Stems showing reactive line formation (%)	6	67	91	88
Mean peri-implant length of reactive lines (mm)	4	55	104	96

patients show clearly positive signs of bone ingrowth fixation in the proximal part of the femur in the first 1 to 2 years after implantation (Figs. 1,2). According to Engh's radiologic fixation and stability score (Table 4), 93% of patients have confirmed bone ingrowth fixation 2 years after implantation.

The number of cases with reactive line formation around the distal noncoated parts of the stem increases until the 3-year follow-up. From 3 years on, a decreasing tendency is visible. Similarly, the mean length of the reactive lines increases until the 3- to 5-year follow-up, then decreases in favor of bone apposition.

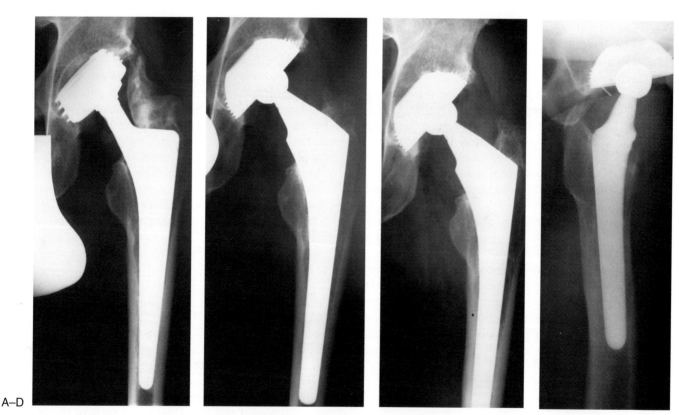

A–D

FIG. 1. A: Osteolysis around loose cementless stem in a 35-year-old man. **B:** Revision to an HA-coated stem without bone grafting. Postoperative condition: osteolytic areas still visible. **C:** At 5 years, there is stable bony fixation, good bone stock. Bony defects have spontaneously filled. **D:** Lateral view at 5-year follow-up.

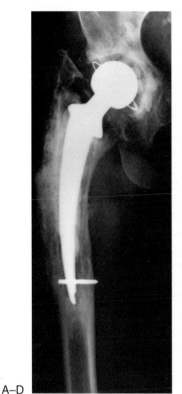 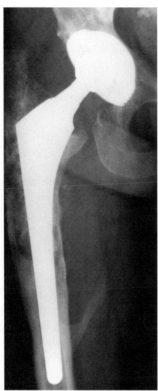 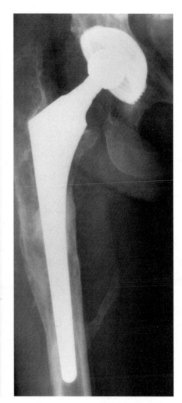 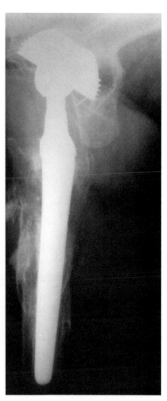

A–D

FIG. 2. A: Loosening of cemented stem and cup in a 57-year-old woman after multiple previous implant surgeries. Extensive bony defects. **B:** Postoperative radiograph shows revision to an HA femoral stem and cup. There is bone grafting at the lateral defect area of the stem. **C:** Five-year follow-up. Good bony integration of autograft area. Stable bony fixation of both stem and cup. Good bone stock. **D:** Lateral view of (C).

Cortical remodeling (Table 5), in the form of hypertrophy in mid or distal stem areas, was much less frequent than in primary hip implantation series. The incidence was 23% of cases at 5 years and usually was confined to Gruen zones 5 and 6. The incidence was still increasing thereafter. Heterotopic bone formation was not a major problem in this series (Table 6). At the 5-year follow-up, only 9% had Brooker grade III heterotopic ossification and there was no grade IV.

Calcar resorption, on the other hand, showed an increasing tendency as follow-up years increased. At the 5-year follow-up, 54% of cases showed mild to moderate signs of calcar atrophy. This tendency continued after 5 years.

TABLE 4. Average scores (by Engh's method of assessment) of radiologic fixation and stability after revision THA with HA enhancement

	Follow-up (mo)			
	3 (N=50)	12 (N=42)	24 (N=44)	36–72
Fixation	5.3	9.1	8.5	8.5
Stability	13.7	10.3	9.1	9.0
Total	19	19.4	17.6	17.6

TABLE 5. Occurrences of cortical remodeling per Gruen zone after revision THA with HA enhancement

	Follow-up (mo)		
Gruen zone	6 (N=44)	60 (N=22)	72 (N=11)
2	—	—	—
3	2	—	9
5	2	18	27
6	—	9	9
Stems showing cortical remodeling (%)	4	23	27
Mean peri-implant length of cortical remodeling (mm)	3	15	27

TABLE 6. Occurrence of heterotopic bone formation (in % of stems) per Brooker grade after revision THA with HA enhancement

	Follow-up (mo)	
Brooker grade	3 (N=50)	60 (N=22)
0	76	59
I	18	27
II	4	5
III	2	9
IV	—	—

In only a few cases (5%), small areas of osteolysis became visible in Gruen zone 7 at the 3-year follow-up and in Gruen zone 1 at the 5-year follow-up. The mean polyethylene wear was calculated as 0.5 mm (average) after 6 years, and it was detectable in 18% of cases.

There were two cases with radiographic failure of the femoral component (see case 4). These may be revised in the near future.

CASE DISCUSSIONS

Case 1

A young male patient developed corticosteroid-induced avascular necrosis of both hips after treatment for renal disease. At the age of 31, he received a bilateral Cementless Spotorno (CLS) (Protek, A. G. Bern) cementless total hip replacement. The left hip remained symptomatic and at radiologic follow-up 3 years later there was severe osteolysis in the mid as well as the distal stem region, with loosening and migration (see Fig. 1A). At the age of 35, a revision procedure was performed. The implant appeared loose and there was severe metallosis with black staining of all the tissues. Cultures were negative and all the granuloma tissue was cleared away. Because of the extensive metallosis, no bone transplantation was done. Early mechanical stability of the HA-coated stem was good (see Fig. 1B), and at longer-term follow-up all the osteolytic lesions had healed with restoration of the cortex. At 5 years follow-up, the patient is pain free on the left side. The implant shows confirmed bony fixation and the bone quality is excellent (see Fig. 1C,D).

The right hip also has been replaced with an HA stem because of progressive osteolysis. At 2 years, the right hip is excellent in both clinical and radiologic appearance.

Case 2

A female patient underwent bilateral cemented total hip replacement at the age of 50 after a previous osteotomy of the hip. Two years later, the right hip was replaced again with a cemented hip because of symptomatic loosening. Five years later she again presented with radiologic appearance of mechanical loosening. Ancillary studies did not suggest septic loosening, and reoperation was carried out in 1990. There was extensive osteolysis on the lateral side of the hip with "severe" bone stock damage (Engh's classification) and with perforation of the lateral cortex (see Fig. 2A). Extensive bone grafting was carried out over two thirds of the stem length on the proximal side laterally (see Fig. 2B). Mechanical stability of the construct was good and the clinical course was uneventful.

Radiologic examination showed revascularization of the bone graft area and, over the follow-up course of 5 years, the implant remained stable with confirmed bony fixation and no signs of migration (see Fig. 2C,D).

Case 3

The first reoperation for mechanical failure of an HA-coated stem was in a 62-year-old female patient. She underwent a fourth revision arthroplasty for loosening after three previous cemented femoral implantations (Fig. 3A). The femoral cortical wall was very thin, and there were multiple perforations of the shaft on the lateral side. On revision arthroplasty, bony defects were autografted on the lateral side, but not on the medial side. She received an HA-coated femoral stem and cup, and early postoperative recovery was uneventful (see Fig. 3B). There was apparent bone regeneration and the grafted areas improved in appearance. Two and a half years after surgery, she fell and the hip became symptomatic. The hip was painful and radiographs showed 1-cm subsidence of the stem (see Fig. 3C). Because the symptoms persisted, reoperation was performed and the femoral component was found to be loose. Overall bone quality was already better than at the previous revision. A next-bigger-size HA stem was implanted in combination with more extensive bone grafting of slits and spaces around the stem and a reduction osteotomy of the femur (Fig. 3D,E). Results at 3 years after the last revision are satisfactory.

The retrieved HA stem was analyzed for any remnants of HA coating. As usual with mechanically loose HA-coated stems, most of the HA coating had disappeared, although in some areas a 5- to 10-μm HA-coating remnant was found. The periprosthetic fibrous tissue did not show any HA particle remnants, although the usual giant cells and macrophages were visible.

Case 4

One of the two radiographic failures in this study involves a 35-year-old male patient with a history of two previous failures involving a cemented as well as a cementless implant (Fig. 4A). The femoral canal was very wide and the largest implant available at that time was not large enough to completely fill the canal (see Fig. 4B). The implant became loose with radiolucent lines in all Gruen zones and stem subsidence up to 0.5 cm at 5 years (see Fig. 4C). The patient's complaints have been minor, and there has been no progressive bone loss. It is possible, however, that the patient will be revised in the future.

Case 5

A 54-year-old male patient with a renal transplant was referred after a pathological fracture of the left

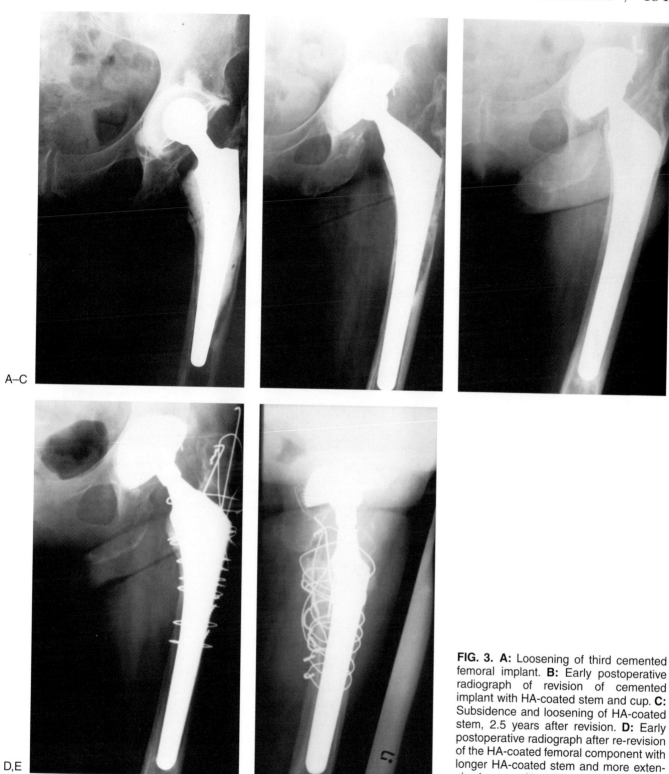

FIG. 3. A: Loosening of third cemented femoral implant. **B:** Early postoperative radiograph of revision of cemented implant with HA-coated stem and cup. **C:** Subsidence and loosening of HA-coated stem, 2.5 years after revision. **D:** Early postoperative radiograph after re-revision of the HA-coated femoral component with longer HA-coated stem and more extensive bone grafting. **E:** Lateral view of (D).

femur because of osteolysis around a loose cemented hip component. The cemented stem was removed, the fracture plated, and the acetabular component left in place (Fig. 5A). After fracture healing and plate removal, the hip was reimplanted using an HA-coated stem in combination with an HA-coated threaded cup because the present polyethylene component had surface damage (see Fig. 5B). The postoperative course was uneventful and the clinical performance at both the 3- and the 6-month follow-up was excellent. The patient

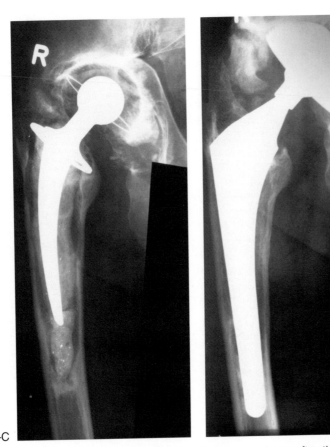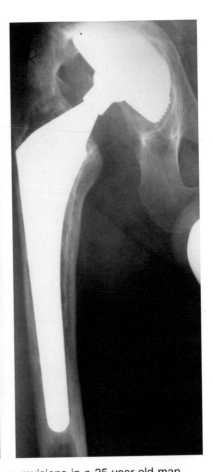

A–C

FIG. 4. A: Loosening of cemented stem and cup after three previous revisions in a 35-year-old man. Extensive bone loss of acetabulum and femur. **B:** Postoperative condition after revision to HA-coated stem and cup. **C:** At 5 years, there is migration of femoral stem with extensive line formation and pedestal formation at the tip. Radiologically loose implant. No complaints to justify revision.

was pain free and had good ambulating capacity, and the radiologic appearance at the last follow-up was good (see Fig. 5C). Six months after hip surgery, the patient was admitted into the hospital because of septic complications caused by a perforated intestine, probably masked by the immunosuppressive medication that he received in relation to the renal transplantation. Ultimately, the patient died because of septic complications and his left hip was retrieved at autopsy. The explant radiograph showed excellent bony apposition against the stem surface and no radiolucent line formation between bone and HA coating (see Fig. 5D). Microscopic sections (Thomas Bauer, pathologist, Cleveland, OH) confirmed this excellent bone apposition of the bone against the HA coating (see Fig. 5E). In addition, there was no fibrous tissue between the HA coating and the bone, and on quantification of the amount of bone ingrowth almost 40% of the available surface area with HA coating was found in contact with healthy bone. The average coating thickness was approximately 35 µm and more than 95% of the HA coating was still intact. Occasionally, there was localized osteoclastic remodeling of the coating, whereby the HA coating was replaced by bone, now being in direct contact with the titanium substrate of the stem.

CONCLUSIONS

Both the clinical and radiographic results have been very satisfying after the use of HA coatings in revision applications. Although the HHSs are not as high as those in primary hip implantation series, which acquire an HHS of 97 after 7 years and longer, an average HHS in revision surgery of 88 at between 1 and 7 years of follow-up is very satisfying. This is especially true because the pain rates are also excellent in the revision group. The scores are decreased primarily because of restrictions in walking ability. Many patients have had multiple previous surgeries, which have a deleterious effect on muscle quality and soft-tissue scarring, resulting in some restrictions in range of motion, in limping, and often in the need for a cane. The subjective rating by the patients, however, is usually very good because the pain levels are so low.

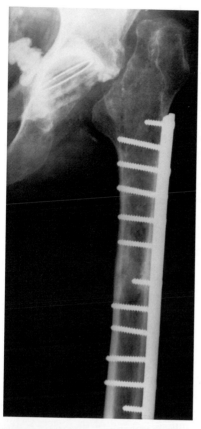
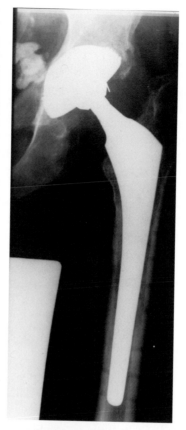
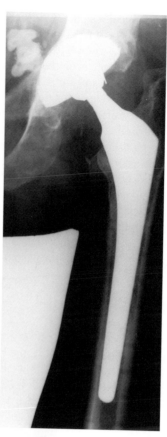

A–C

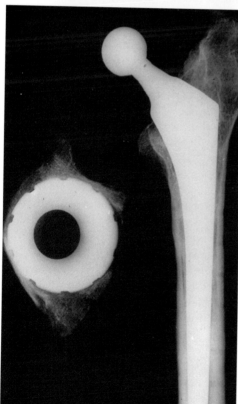

D

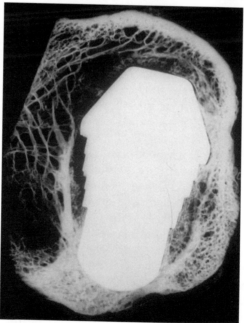

E

FIG. 5. A: Osteosynthesis for pathological fracture after loose cemented hip component. The acetabular component is left in place. **B:** After fracture healing and plate removal, the patient underwent revision to an HA-coated femoral and (threaded) acetabular component. Radiograph 7 weeks after surgery. **C:** Follow-up at almost 6 months. Good bony apposition against the stem surface and no radiolucent line formation between bone and HA coating. **D:** Radiograph of the hip after retrieval at autopsy. **E:** Transection of the proximal femur at autopsy. There is good bone apposition and gap filling of the HA coating over a significant area of the stem. There is no fibrous tissue between the HA coating and the bone.

The good clinical results are further supported by good radiologic results as far as bony fixation is concerned. Even with some restrictive use of bone graft, at 2 years almost 93% of patients acquired confirmed bony fixation by Engh's criteria. This result is substantiated by the ever-increasing area of bone apposition (which is still progressive after 6 to 7 years) and the regression in the amount of reactive lines around distal noncoated parts of the implant with increasing follow-up. After a peak incidence of distal reactive lines at 3 years, these rapidly regress in favor of bone apposition over the more distal parts of the stem, providing a strong secondary line of defense against implant loosening in areas where there is no HA coating. This phenomenon is similar to results found with primary implantations where increasing osseointegration of noncoated stem areas is observed after longer-term follow-up.

BONE STATUS

The statistical differences between the various Charnley groups is intriguing. Possibly, the healthy individuals from Charnley groups A and B have higher demands on their implants or higher activity levels at those follow-up intervals and, therefore, experience more pain than the patients in Charnley category C. The differences in clinical results between patients with and without bone graft, or between those with minor and those with extensive bone loss, are probably related to the treatment after surgery. For example, extensive bone loss is usually treated by bone transplantation, and these patients have a longer period of restricted weight bearing after surgery and, consequently, lower hip scores and PMA ratings. From 6 months on, there are no longer statistically significant differences in this respect. This leads to the conclusion that once bony fixation is obtained, clinical results are good. This is probably true irrespective of the bone status being good or compromised. Even cases with compromised bone stock appeared to be able to acquire bone ingrowth with HA coatings. Although bone graft may augment the ultimate bone stock, there are many examples of cases with initially compromised bone stock acquiring bony fixation and improving on their bone stock even without bone grafting. At the same time, the failures that have been observed in this study can clearly be attributed to lack of bone augmentation at the time of revision. These cases might have been better off with more extensive bone transplantation or the use of special revision implants with longer stems and HA coatings, custom designs, or other.

As a learning experience, it is of paramount importance that adequate mechanical stability be obtained at the time of surgery. The use of bone graft augmentation should be considered if the mechanical stability of the construct at the time of surgery is not adequate and/or bone stock is compromised in the form of segmentary or cavitary defects. Although bone graft may not contribute to the early implant fixation in biologic terms, it still provides mechanical stability for the surgical construct of bone and implant. Early bone ingrowth fixation is possible only between the HA coating and viable and vascularized bone. Sometimes, if there are extensive proximal bone deficiencies, this will require the use of longer stems with more extensive areas of HA coating.

The retrieval histology of well-fixed components is telling. There is excellent bony contact between the surrounding bone and the HA coating in contact with the stem. There are no signs of osteolysis on the microscopic level, and the HA coating is well accepted by the bone. There is neither foreign body response nor macrophage, giant cell, or other response. The great majority of the coating is still intact, with an average thickness of 35 to 40 μm, which is approximately 10 to 15 μm thinner than the implantation thickness of 50 μm. This thinning is caused by some physicochemical dissolution during the period of bone ingrowth. Once bony fixation of the HA coating is obtained, further dissolution will stop, which usually occurs around the 3rd month after surgery. After this time interval, only degradation by a cellular response is possible. Osteoclastic activity will remodel bone continually, and calcium phosphates, being physiologic material, are no exception to this osteoclastic degradation mechanism. Thus, very localized transformation of HA can be seen and, at the end of the osteoclastic cycle, an osteoblastic response fills the resorbed lacunae with new bone. Therefore, on specific areas around the stem, the HA can disappear, resulting in locations where the bone comes in direct contact with the titanium substrate of the implant. This process is linear with time and it is to be expected that with longer-term follow-up, more of the coating will be replaced by bone.

From animal work, where histologic follow-up of up to 10 years is available, it is evident that the amorphous portion of the HA coating is subject to degradation, whereas the crystalline portion is probably fully stable with time, although more prone to fatigue failure. It should be clear that there are no remnants of HA material left in the surrounding bone after degradation of the HA layer. The histologic acceptance is excellent, and if any parts of the HA coating are seen separate from the implant surface in the process of degradation, the histologic appearance is always benign and the fragments are surrounded by bone similar to the HA material used as bone graft substitute. There are no local osteolytic phenomena.

On the contrary, the loose stem observed in this study was macroscopically bare metal, although with accurate microscopic analysis, remnants of HA coating could be seen on the metal surface. The remaining coating was usually very thin, between 5 and 10 μm. If mechanical failure of an HA-coated stem occurs, it is usually because of lack of mechanical fixation, too much micromotion, and a lack of bone ingrowth. Because of persistent micromotion, the HA coating is rubbed away against the bone and therefore the disappearance of the HA coating is probably secondary to the loosening phenomenon. Also, in these cases, the HA-coating material will be degraded and hardly any remnants of calcium phosphate material will be found in the tissues around the hip. It should be noted that on all of an HA-coated stem, there is only 600 mg of HA material available. If this amount is released in a short time interval, some particle reaction with local osteolysis is theoretically conceivable. However, in the histology obtained thus far, none of these phenomena have been observed, probably just because degradation is so slow and thus the amount of HA material released in the periprosthetic area is minimal. The regular appearance of a well-fixed HA-coated stem is one of very healthy bone in contact with the HA coating. This human histologic evidence suggests that HA coatings provide a good substrate for bony fixation on the implant surface and that this can be a permanent situation.

This early series provides adequate proof for the good results possible with HA coatings in revision surgery, with follow-up of up to 9 years. The results in clinical terms, as well as the low total failure rate of 8%, are very promising. The results are at least comparable or similar to many published results on cementless or cemented applications with the same period of follow-up.

Because almost 93% of patients have confirmed bony ingrowth fixation at 2 years, continued good results can be expected for the next few years, despite the two cases pending for revision. In addition, our currently better understanding of implant biology, in combination with current availability of improved specific revision implants, will facilitate even better results for future patients. Of course, longer-term follow-up will be necessary to confirm whether the current good results will be maintained in the future. Data on primary HA-coated total hip replacement (which has currently between 9 and 10 years of follow-up) have demonstrated, however, that once implants have acquired bony stability, the prospect for long-term implant survival is very favorable.

ACKNOWLEDGMENT

The authors thank Angélique Janssen-Meertens for the secretarial assistance.

REFERENCES

1. Aubigné RM d', Postel M. Functional results of hip arthroplasty with acrylic prosthesis. *J Bone Joint Surg* 1954;36A:451–475.
2. Brooker AF, Bowerman JW, Robinson RA, Riley LH. Ectopic ossification following total hip replacement. *J Bone Joint Surg* 1973;55A:1629–1632.
3. Cameron HU. The two- to six-year results with a proximally modular noncemented total hip replacement used in hip revisions. *Clin Orthop* 1994;298:47–53.
4. Charnley J. The long-term results of low-friction arthroplasty of the hip performed as a primary intervention. *J Bone Joint Surg* 1972;54B:61–76.
5. Charnley J, Halley DK. Rate of wear in total hip replacement. *Clin Orthop* 1975;112:170–179.
6. Engelbrecht DJ, Weber FA, Sweet MBE, Jakim I. Long term results of revision total hip arthroplasty. *J Bone Joint Surg* 1990;72B:41–45.
7. Engh CA, Glassman AH, Griffin WL, Mayer JG. Results of cementless revision of failed cemented total hip arthroplasty. *Clin Orthop* 1988;235:91–110.
8. Engh CA, Glassman AH, Suthers KE. The case for porous-coated hip implants. *Clin Orthop* 1990;261:63–81.
9. Engh CA, Massin P, Suthers KE. Roentgenographic assessment of the biologic fixation of porous-surfaced femoral components. *Clin Orthop* 1990;257:107–127.
10. Estok DM, Harris WH. Long-term results of cemented femoral revision surgery using second-generation techniques. *Clin Orthop* 1994;299:190–202.
11. Geesink RGT, Hoefnagels NHM. Six-year results of hydroxyapatite-coated total hip replacement. *J Bone Joint Surg* 1995;77B:534–547.
12. Gie GA, Linder L, Ling RSM, Simon J-P, Slooff TJ, Timperley AJ. Contained morselized allograft in revision total hip arthroplasty. Surgical technique. *Orthop Clin North Am* 1993;24:717–725.
13. Gie GA, Linder L, Ling RSM, Simon J-P, Slooff TJJH, Timperley AJ. Impacted cancellous allografts and cement for revision total hip arthroplasty. *J Bone Joint Surg* 1993;75B:14–21.
14. Gruen TA, McNeice GM, Amstutz HC. "Modes of failure" of cemented stem-type femoral components. *Clin Orthop* 1979;141:17–27.
15. Harris WH. Traumatic arthritis of the hip after dislocation and acetabular fractures: treatment by mold arthroplasty. *J Bone Joint Surg* 1969;51A:737–755.
16. Havelin LI, Espehaug B, Vollset SE, Engesaeter LB. Early aseptic loosening of uncemented femoral components in primary total hip replacement. A review based on the Norwegian Arthroplasty Register. *J Bone Joint Surg* 1995;77B:11–17.
17. Head WC, Wagner RA, Emerson Jr RH, Malinin TI. Revision total hip arthroplasty in the deficient femur with a proximal load-bearing prosthesis. *Clin Orthop* 1994;298:119–126.
18. Izquierdo RJ, Northmore-Ball MD. Long-term results of revision hip arthroplasty. *J Bone Joint Surg* 1994;76B:34–39.
19. Kolstad K. Revision THR after periprosthetic femoral fractures. An analysis of 23 cases. *Acta Orthop Scand* 1994;65:505–508.
20. Lawrence JM, Engh CA, Macalino GE, Lauro GR. Outcome of revision hip arthroplasty done without cement. *J Bone Joint Surg* 1994;76A:965–973.
21. Ling RS. Femoral reconstruction with morselized bone graft and cemented stem. *Chir Organi Mov* 1994;79:305–311.
22. Marti RK, Schüller HM, Besselaar PP, Vanfrank Haasnoot EL. Results of revision of hip arthroplasty with cement. *J Bone Joint Surg* 1990;72A:346–354.
23. Önsten I, Sanzén L, Carlsson Å, Besjakov J. Migration of uncemented, long-stem femoral components in revision hip arthroplasty. A 2–8 year clinical follow-up of 45 cases and radiostereometric analysis of 13 cases. *Acta Orthop Scand* 1995;66:220–224.
24. Pierson JL, Harris WH. Cemented revision for femoral osteolysis in cemented arthroplasties. Results in 29 hips after a mean 8.5-year follow-up. *J Bone Joint Surg* 1994;76B:40–44.
25. Raut VV, Siney PD, Wroblewski BM. Long-term results of cemented Charnley revision arthroplasty for fractured stem. *Clin Orthop* 1994;303:165–169.
26. Raut VV, Siney PD, Wroblewski BM. Cemented Charnley revision arthroplasty for severe femoral osteolysis. *J Bone Joint Surg* 1995;77B:362–365.
27. Raut VV, Siney PD, Wroblewski BM. Revision for aseptic stem loosening using the cemented Charnley prosthesis. A review of 351 hips. *J Bone Joint Surg* 1995;77B:23–27.
28. Scott DF, Shubin Stein K, Geesink RGT, Yaffe WL. Seven-year radiographic and densitometric results of hydroxyapatite-coated femoral components. *Transactions of the Am Assoc Orthop Surgeons* 1995;1:1.
29. Soballe K, Hansen ES, Brockstedt-Rasmussen H, et al. Gap healing enhanced by hydroxyapatite coating in dogs. *Clin Orthop* 1991;272:300–307.
30. Stephenson PK, Freeman MAR, Revell PA, Germain J, Tuke M, Pirie CJ. The effect of a hydroxy apatite coating on ingrowth of bone into cavities in an implant. *J Arthroplasty* 1991;6:51–58.
31. Strömberg CN, Herberts P, Palmertz B. Cemented revision hip arthroplasty. A multicenter 5–9 year study of 204 first revisions for loosening. *Acta Orthop Scand* 1992;63:111–119.

The Adult Hip, edited by J. J. Callaghan,
A. G. Rosenberg, and H. E. Rubash.
Lippincott–Raven Publishers, Philadelphia © 1998.

CHAPTER 99

Surgical Treatment of Osteolysis

Raj K. Sinha, William J. Maloney, Wayne G. Paprosky, and Harry E. Rubash

Although the understanding of the pathophysiology of osteolysis has increased, its treatment and prevention remain challenging. This chapter provides a rational approach for the management and surgical treatment of osteolysis in total hip arthroplasty based on the current level of understanding.

When treating patients with periprosthetic osteolysis in total hip arthroplasty, the surgeon must adhere to some basic tenets (Fig. 1) (6,8,10,11). The finding must be discussed with patients, and the importance of close follow-up cannot be understated. Further, the reasons for the development of the lesions should be explored. The underlying cause of osteolysis is the generation of particulate debris in the articular space. Particle generation is influenced by several factors. These include the patient's age, activity level, and bone quality. The shape, type of porous coating, polyethylene thickness, and method of fixation of the implant also influence particle generation and its effects. Once the underlying mechanisms have been assessed, a decision for management can be made.

Important considerations in determining treatment include patient symptoms, location and the likelihood of progression of the lesions, the amount of bone loss, and the status of fixation of the components. After all avail-

able data are reviewed, surgical intervention may be the best form of treatment. The surgical procedure must address the osteolytic lesion and the particle generators (the sources of increased wear). Potential particle generators include worn or loose polyethylene liners, scored or burnished femoral heads, 32-mm heads, titanium (Ti) femoral heads, and fractured cement, among others. Therefore, surgery would address removal of granulomatous material when appropriate, filling the defects with a graft material, and the possible exchange of components, depending on the extent of damage (Fig. 2). Attention to normal anatomy and wide exposure help the surgeon restore the appropriate biomechanical relationships.

FEMORAL OSTEOLYSIS

Management Approach

Linear osteolysis around cemented stems is often circumferential, involving all Gruen femoral zones, and it is believed to progress to the point of loosening if left untreated. Radiographic examination at 3- to 6-month intervals is a reasonable approach until the patient becomes symptomatic, or until progressive lysis is observed. Although data are not available to indicate when observation should be abandoned in favor of surgery, sound surgical judgment would suggest that operative intervention be instituted when structural stability is threatened or when clinical symptoms are intolerable. Conditions that may threaten stability include loss of the proximal femoral cortical bone, including the calcar, and large osteolytic lesions that may lead to periprosthetic fracture, such as those at the tip of the stem.

　　W. J. Maloney: Department of Orthopaedic Surgery, Barnes-Jewish Hospital, Washington University School of Medicine, St. Louis, Missouri 63110.
　　W. G. Paprosky: Department of Orthopaedic Surgery, Rush-Presbyterian–St. Luke's Medical Center, Chicago, Illinois 60190.
　　H. E. Rubash and R. K. Sinha: Department of Orthopaedic Surgery, University of Pittsburgh Medical Center, Pittsburgh, Pennsylvania 15213-3221.

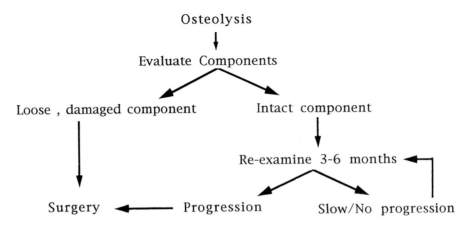

FIG. 1. Treatment algorithm for patients presenting with osteolysis.

When osteolysis already has resulted in symptomatic loosening, the decision to operate is determined principally by the patient's degree of pain. If the component is loose, it usually needs to be replaced, particularly to prevent further bone resorption. However, if the component is well fixed (as with cementless implants), then substantial bone loss can result from injudicious removal. Thus, curettage and grafting of the lytic lesion and retention of the stem, with exchange of the polyethylene liner, may be appropriate. Preliminary results indicate that this may be the appropriate approach, although long-term data are not yet available (6,8,10,11).

Rubash et al. (10) have recently proposed an algorithm for the management of femoral osteolysis (Fig. 3). They advocate revision of all loose stems. Cemented stems are considered to be definitely loose by evidence of migration or subsidence of the component, stem debonding, stem fracture or bending, or cement fracture (3). A circumferential radiolucency at the bone–cement interface suggests probable loosening (3). For cementless components, migration and subsidence are most indicative of a loose stem. Additional signs of likely instability include cortical or cancellous hypertrophy at the stem tip, distal pedestal formation, shedding of the porous coating, and radiolucent lines along the porous coating (1,2).

Surgery may be indicated for well-fixed stems when there is evidence of progression of osteolysis on serial radiographs. Other mitigating factors include the size and

location of the lesion, and patient age, activity, and medical status. For stems with focal and cavitary osteolysis in zones 1 and 7, the lytic lesions may be grafted, although this has not been regularly done. In addition, the particle generators should be removed. This may include changing the polyethylene liners for ingrown acetabular cups, downsizing modular femoral heads to 26 or 28 mm, and replacing titanium-aluminum-anadium (Ti6Al4V) with cobalt-chromium-molybdenum (Co-Cr-Mo) heads. For progressive diaphyseal osteolysis distal, the stem often requires revision. For small focal lesions or linear osteolysis, we recommend revision for physiologically young patients and observation for elderly and less active patients.

The location, extent, and type of porous coating also must be considered for uncemented stems. For proximal focal osteolysis, if the component is porous-coated circumferentially, the lesion can be packed with particulate graft and the particle generators exchanged. A noncircumferentially coated component may be retained in elderly, sedentary patients, with exchange of the particle generators and grafting of the lesions when appropriate. This approach may be applied to young, active patients if the stem is well fixed. However, if the stem is also a particle generator (e.g., monoblock titanium, extensive fretting of the modular taper), then it should be revised as well. For osteolysis distal to zones 1 and 7, the femoral stem and polyethylene liner should usually be changed.

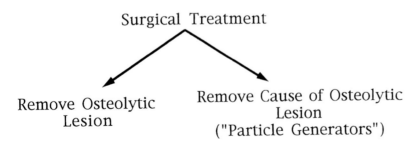

FIG. 2. Goals of surgical treatment for osteolysis.

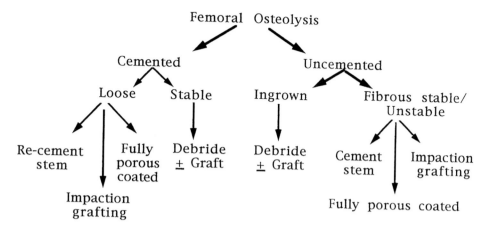

FIG. 3. Treatment algorithm for femoral osteolysis.

Because distal osteolysis is usually progressive with non-circumferentially coated stems, even if they are well fixed, revision of the stem should be strongly considered. Cavitary lesions distal to the stem tip present a high risk of periprosthetic fracture and also should be revised with a stem that bypasses the lesion. Distal osteolysis in extensively coated stems has not been reported; therefore, its appearance may imply loosening of the stem.

Surgical Treatment

Several surgical principles must be observed during revision of femoral components associated with osteolysis. Wide exposure is necessary for full and accurate visualization of defects of the femoral canal. Extensive subperiosteal elevation of the overlying musculature may be required to fully assess the lytic lesions. Likewise, an extended osteotomy of the femur may be necessary, particularly in cases of distally ingrown stems. During revision, the osteolytic membrane should be entirely removed, followed by curettage and reaming of the canal to remove neocortex, thus creating an appropriate bed of host bone for either a cemented or an uncemented stem. All structural defects should be reinforced with cortical femoral struts or intact distal femoral allografts. The graft should be contoured with a high-speed burr to allow close contact with host bone. Once cortical support has been reestablished, the endosteal cavities can be packed with particulate allograft. Then, the neutral axis of the femur must be identified so that the revision stem can be placed in the proper alignment. This is readily accomplished by passing a beaded guide wire into the cancellous bone proximal to the knee. This step also confirms the absence of cortical perforations. Finally, the particle generators must be addressed. Titanium heads, which are associated with higher rates of polyethylene wear, should be replaced with Co-Cr heads. Similarly, 32-mm heads should be replaced with 28-mm heads and new polyeth-ylene liners. Also, monoblock stems with extensive scoring of the head generally should be replaced, although advanced patient age, decreased activity, and poor medical status may be reasons to consider retaining otherwise well-fixed components.

ACETABULAR OSTEOLYSIS

Management Approach

The algorithm in Figure 4 provides a systematic approach to the treatment of acetabular osteolysis. For cemented cups, the first step is to evaluate stability. Linear or focal osteolysis in two or three acetabular zones has been associated with 71% and 94% incidences of loosening of the component, respectively (4). A loose cemented component must be revised, preferably with an ingrowth cup. Bone stock deficiencies must be treated with the appropriate graft. If the cup is not loose, the degree of wear should be evaluated. Worn cups with eccentricity of the femoral head should be replaced. Thirty-two-millimeter heads, which have been shown to have the highest degree of volumetric wear, and 22-mm heads have the highest degree of linear wear, should be replaced by 28-mm heads and liners.

Uncemented cups have been classified into three separate groups (Fig. 5). The type I cup is stable with discrete focal osteolysis, including zones 1 and 3, and it is occasionally adjacent to screws. The component usually can be retained, and particulate graft can be packed into the defect if readily accessible. In addition, the polyethylene liner in modular cups can be replaced as long as the locking mechanism is intact. For nonmodular metal-backed cups, periodic observation of the osteolysis may be appropriate, although early revision is recommended when progression of the osteolysis has been documented. Type II components are also stable by virtue of bone ingrowth, but the function of the cup is compromised. For example, the locking mechanism of a modular cup may

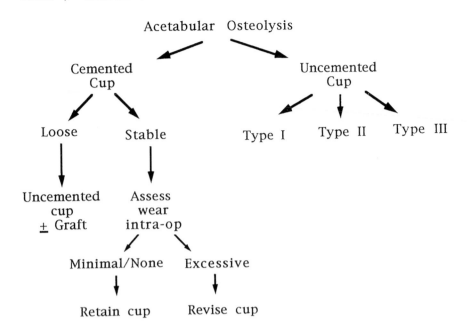

FIG. 4. Treatment algorithm for acetabular osteolysis.

be damaged, there may be extensive wear of the shell, or the shell may be malpositioned. In these cases, the entire component should be removed, defects filled with the appropriate graft, and a new cup re-implanted without cement. Rarely, an all-polyethylene cup can be cemented into a well-fixed metal shell, as long as the polyethylene is greater than 8 mm thick. Type III cups are unstable and have migrated into the osteolytic lesion, necessitating exchange. Cavitary acetabular defects with adequate rim integrity can be packed with particulate allograft. Structural rim deficiencies may require bulk allograft for support. Additionally, threaded screw-in design acetabular components are to be avoided for revisions because of the high rate of early loosening.

Surgical Treatment

Wide exposure allows complete visualization of the periphery of the cup to facilitate removal of modular polyethylene liners. The appropriate extraction device for each manufacturer's cup should be available to remove the polyethylene liner without damaging the locking mechanism. If it is not, a useful technique is to drill a hole in the polyethylene liner and then place a 4.5-mm cortical screw in the hole. As the screw contacts the metal shell, it disengages the liner from the shell. The locking mechanism must be examined to determine whether it is functional.

If the shell must be removed, then the entire acetabular rim must be accessible. The first step in removal is to separate the cup from the underlying cement mantle or bone bed. Specially shaped osteotomes or gouges are available to facilitate this step. Occasionally, the component must be broken into pieces for removal because the underlying bond with cement or bone cannot be broken. During component removal, care must be taken not to breach the medial wall, thereby compromising structural support and threatening the intrapelvic contents. Generally, the cup cannot be removed until it is released hemispherically past the widest diameter from underlying bone or cement (Fig. 6).

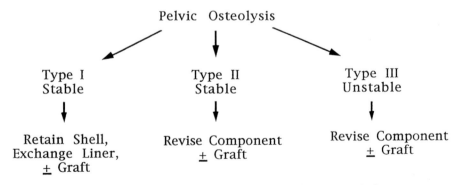

FIG. 5. Treatment algorithm for pelvic osteolysis in uncemented cups.

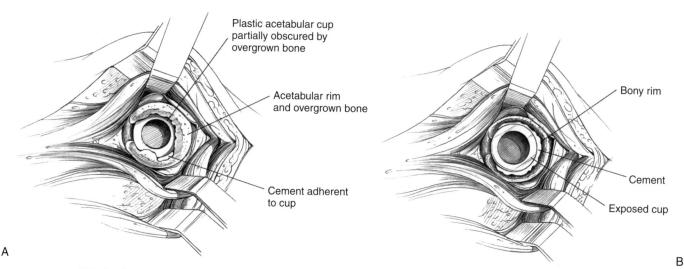

FIG. 6. A: Illustration of overhanging bone and soft tissue prevents complete visualization of an acetabular component that must be removed. **B:** Overhanging bone has been removed from the periphery of the cup, allowing access to the implant–cement interface. Disruption of the interface hemispherically past the widest diameter will be necessary before the implant can be removed.

The next step is to break the cement mantle to facilitate removal of the cement. In cases where there is a large amount of intrapelvic cement, forceful extraction could rupture underlying vessels. When of concern, a computed axial tomographic (CAT) scan and/or contrast venogram will identify the anatomic relationships between pelvic structures and components. If the cement is adherent to pelvic vessels, an intrapelvic surgical approach can be used to dissect the vessels from cement or implants (9). After removal of the cement, all osteolytic membrane must be curetted, especially within anchor or screw holes. The appropriate grafting technique is used to address the bony defects. Structural grafts should be oriented so the trabeculae are aligned to withstand axial compressive forces across the hip joint (7).

Next, the acetabulum is prepared for a porous-ingrowth cup. The acetabular bed is reamed hemispherically to preserve as much host bone as possible and to maximize the area of bone–component contact. Subchondral or sclerotic bone is the strongest bone for initial stability and should not be breached. The cup should be placed as near the anatomic position as possible. Screw fixation is often required to secure the cup. Once adequate stability of the component is achieved, a 28-mm polyethylene liner is recommended. In some situations, a polyethylene cup may need to be cemented, such as when allograft comprises greater than 60% of the contact area between component and structural bone (7), or when the pelvic bed has been previously irradiated (5).

CONCLUSIONS AND FUTURE DIRECTIONS

There are two keys to the effective treatment of femoral osteolysis. First, identify and remove the sources of the particles. Potential sources include worn polyethylene liners, modular junctions of metallic components, scored femoral heads, and fragmented cement. Third-body wear is the primary mechanism of wear *in vivo*, and the presence of any particulate matter predisposes to this modality. Second, treat the interfacial bone loss. Removal of loose components and the appropriate grafting of bony defects is often required. The issue of removing a well-fixed cementless stem with focal osteolysis should be addressed on an individual case basis using the guidelines described.

Future research should provide considerable insight into osteolysis and its treatment. Results of the management approaches proposed here, which are being employed at many centers, will be available. Improved models of osteolysis will enable more detailed study of particular treatment methods such as improved grafting materials and techniques, pharmacologic intervention, or immunologic modulation. In addition, the use of nonmodular femoral stems and the development of improved polyethylene, ceramic, or highly polished metal-on-metal articulations may reduce the production of particulate debris. Although much has been learned about osteolysis, the prospects for a higher level of understanding remain.

REFERENCES

1. Callaghan JJ, Salvati EA, Pellicci PM, et al. Results of revision for mechanical failure after cemented total hip replacement, 1979 to 1982. *J Bone and Joint Surg* 1985;67A:1074–1085.
2. Engh CA, Bobyn JD. The influence of stem size and extent of porous-coating on femoral bone resorption after primary cementless hip arthroplasty. *Clin Orthop* 1988;231:7–28.
3. Harris WH, Schiller AL, Scholler JM, et al. Extensive localized bone resorption in the femur following total hip replacement. *J Bone Joint Surg* 1976;58A:612–618.
4. Hodgkinson JP, Shelley P, Wroblewski BM. The correlation between

the rontgenographic appearance and operative findings at the bone-cement junction of the socket in Charnley low friction arthroplasties. *Clin Orthop* 1988;228:105–109.

5. Jacobs JJ, Kull LR, Frey GA, et al. Early failure of acetabular components inserted without cement after previous pelvic irradiation. *J Bone Joint Surg* 1995;77A:1829–1835.
6. Maloney WJ. Management of pelvic osteolysis. *The 26th annual Hip Course.* Boston 1996.
7. McGann W, Welch RB, Picetti GD. Acetabular preparation in cementless revision total hip arthroplasty. *Clin Orthop* 1988;235:35–46.

8. Paprosky WG, Kronick JL, Barba ML. When to operate on femoral osteolysis. *The 26th annual Hip Course.* Boston, 1996.
9. Petrera P, Trakru S, Mehta S, et al. Revision total hip arthroplasty with a retroperitoneal approach to the iliac vessels. *J Arthroplasty* 1996;11:704–708.
10. Rubash HE, et al. Osteolysis: clinical manifestations and management. *Symposium at the 63rd annual meeting of the American Academy of Orthopaedic Surgeons.* Atlanta, 1996.
11. Schmalzried TP. Management of pelvic osteolysis. *The 26th annual Hip Course.* Boston, 1996.

The Adult Hip, edited by J. J. Callaghan,
A. G. Rosenberg, and H. E. Rubash.
Lippincott–Raven Publishers, Philadelphia © 1998.

CHAPTER 100

Conversion Total Hip Replacement

Michael H. Huo and John J. Carbone

Total hip replacement has been applied principally to the treatment of degenerative and inflammatory arthropathies of the hip. It has also been used for a wide variety of other hip disorders, as well as to salvage failures of previous hip surgeries. Conversion total hip replacement is generally defined as a total hip replacement performed for failed previous hip surgeries other than an index total hip replacement. The various etiologies include the following:

1. Failure of internal fixation of previous hip fracture.
2. Failure of hemiarthroplasty.
3. Failure of surface replacement.
4. Failure of previous femoral osteotomy.
5. Failure of previous arthrodesis or ankylosis of the hip.

Different technical challenges, considerations for implant selection, clinical results, and complications are present for each one of these various situations.

M.H. Huo and J.J. Carbone: Department of Orthopaedic Surgery, Johns Hopkins Bayview Medical Center, Baltimore, Maryland 21224-2780.

TOTAL HIP REPLACEMENT AFTER FAILED INTERNAL FIXATION OF THE HIP

Indications

It is estimated that over 250,000 fractures of the hip occur each year in the United States (36). The mainstay of surgical treatment of femoral intertrochanteric and neck hip fractures remains anatomic reduction with internal fixation (36,37). This, unfortunately, has not been uniformly successful in every case. On average, the failure rate resulting from nonunion after internal fixation of femoral neck fractures has been reported to be approximately 33%, especially if the fracture was initially displaced (36,40). The incidence of femoral head osteonecrosis has been reported to be approximately 16% (40). Although the incidence of nonunion has been reduced to 4% (6) with improved surgical techniques, the incidence of osteonecrosis has remained at 25.7% for the same series of patients. The overall failure rate for intertrochanteric hip fractures treated by internal fixation has been reported to be in the range of 4% to 12% (37), with malrotation, nonunion, and loss of fixation being the primary modes of failure.

Total hip replacement has been utilized for the salvage of failed treatment of hip fractures with internal fixation in over two-thirds of such cases (40). Various technical difficulties may be encountered during conversion surgery. These technical challenges not only may predispose the patients to increased morbidity during the perioperative period, but they also may compromise the clinical results and durability of the hip replacement.

Technique

Conversion surgery for failed treatment of femoral neck and intertrochanteric hip fractures should be considered separately because there are different technical issues in each case. These issues primarily relate to the femoral reconstruction. Surgical exposure, acetabular preparation, and selection of cup designs are similar to routine primary total hip replacements. The subchondral bone of the acetabulum may be very soft as a result of disuse osteoporosis, and care should be taken while reaming so as not to violate the central acetabulum or the posterior wall.

Failure of Femoral Neck Fractures

In these situations, the most frequently encountered internal fixation devices are multiple screws or pins. They are usually easily removed, and femoral neck osteotomy can be performed at the appropriate level. On rare occasions, the screw heads may be buried below the lateral cortex. Moran (46) described a technique to remove these buried screws in a retrograde fashion in order to complete the total hip replacement. The remaining calcar is rarely deficient, and a standard femoral stem design can be used with or without cement, based on the principles used for primary total hip replacements. The screw or pin holes can be plugged by hand, or by the removed screws themselves as described by Patterson et al. (51) to facilitate pressurization of the cement (if cement fixation of the stem is selected). These small cortical defects can be either left alone, or grafted using bone from the femoral head.

Failure of Intertrochanteric Hip Fractures

Conversion surgery for failed internal fixation of intertrochanteric hip fractures is more difficult than conversion surgery for failed femoral neck fractures. There is often medial displacement of the shaft in relation to the femoral neck, thus making reaming and broaching with straight instruments a technical challenge (Fig. 1). In addition, there is often malrotation of fracture reduction during the index internal fixation surgery, which further distorts the proximal femoral geometry for femoral preparation (37). The calcar is often deficient to a level below the lesser trochanter. The greater trochanteric frag-

A–C

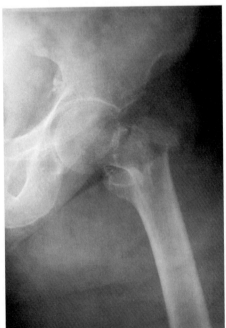 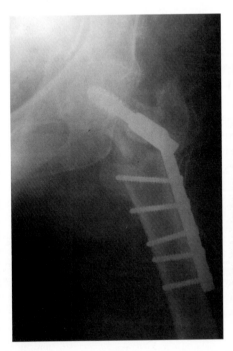 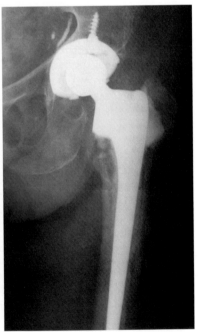

FIG. 1. A: Anteroposterior (AP) radiograph of a comminuted intertrochanteric hip fracture in a 72-year-old woman. **B:** Failure of fixation with sliding hip compression screw at 8 months after surgery. **C:** AP radiograph 2 years after conversion surgery performed with hybrid total hip replacement.

ment may not yet have healed, therefore necessitating supplemental fixation using multiple wires or cable system. (Fig. 2). The greater trochanter is often very thin, and care must be exercised in reattaching it so as not to cause further fragmentation.

Breakage of cortical screws of the side plate in hip compression screw/plate devices is occasionally a prob-

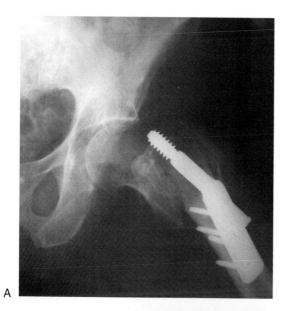

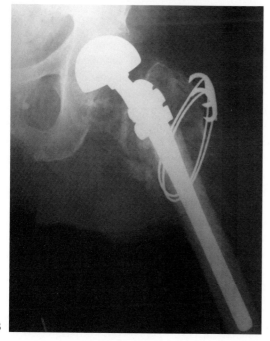

FIG. 2. A: Lateral radiograph demonstrating failure of fixation of an intertrochanteric hip fracture 3 months after surgery. **B:** Lateral radiograph 6 months after conversion surgery performed using a calcar-replacement stem inserted with cement, and a Dall-Miles cable/grip system to reattach the nonunited greater trochanter fragment.

lem. These broken screws may interfere with reaming and broaching of the femoral canal. These can be addressed either by overdrilling the lateral cortex and removing the screws, or by cutting the intramedullary portion of the screws using a high speed burr.

The distorted proximal femoral anatomy can usually be adequately addressed using stem designs inserted with cement. Selection of a stem of sufficient length to bypass the most distal cortical defect is recommended (50). Proximal bone deficiency can be addressed by using a calcar-replacement stem design. Leg length can be addressed using modular femoral head components. Restoration of soft-tissue tension and femoral offset can be addressed with the modular neck lengths of the prosthesis, and/or advancement of the trochanteric fragment. Patterson et al. (51) described a technique of plugging the cortical defects from the screws by using the screws themselves while pressurizing cement during insertion of the stem. This technique allows for plugging of the lateral cortex only. This will maximize the pressurization effect and minimize cement extrusion, which has been reported to result in stress fracture of the femur (22). The authors have generally found that the soft tissues on the medial side are not disturbed by surgical dissection, and they can most often keep cement extrusion to a minimum.

Occasionally, a stem design for insertion without cement may be desirable in a particular case. The distorted femoral geometry may compromise the surgeon's ability to achieve maximal fit-and-fill of the canal. Furthermore, there is the risk of perforations or fractures, because, in inserting stems without cement, the principal object is to obtain as much cortical contact as possible. The surgeon may consider using modular stem designs that allow fitting the proximal and distal femoral geometries separately. In addition, corrective osteotomy may be necessary if there is significant deformity. These issues will be further discussed in the section of conversion surgery for failed previous femoral osteotomies later in this chapter.

Results

The overall clinical results of conversion total hip replacements for failed internal fixation of previous hip fractures are generally satisfactory. The reported series, however, have indicated inferior results to routine primary total hip replacements. Turner and Wroblewski (66) reported satisfactory pain relief, joint motion, and walking ability in nearly 90% of the 205 patients who underwent conversion total hip replacements for late complications of femoral neck fractures. Internal fixation was the initial treatment in 146 of these patients. The major complications in this series were superficial wound infection (7.8%) and late deep sepsis (3.9%). The incidence of aseptic loosening was reported to be 3.4% at an unspecified follow-up interval. These cases were done with early cementing techniques and implant designs. The dislocation rate was only 0.5%, which could be attributed to the use of the transtrochanteric surgical approach.

Stambough et al. (61) reported on 27 cases of conversion surgery for failed internal fixation of hip fractures. The overall clinical results were mostly satisfactory. Complications with the trochanteric osteotomy and malpositioning of the stem each occurred in 26% of the hips. There was a 3.7% rate of revision for aseptic loosening, at a mean follow-up of 6.3 years. More important, the authors observed radiographic loosening in 33% of the cups and in 22.2% of the stems. Dislocation was again not a problem despite of the occurrence of nonunion or migration of the greater trochanter. There was no incidence of sepsis in this series.

Mehlhoff et al. (41) compared the results of conversion surgery for failed femoral neck and intertrochanteric hip fractures separately. The mean operating times were 143 minutes for the group with failed femoral neck fractures, and 170 minutes for those with failed intertrochanteric hip fractures. The mean estimated blood losses were 960 mL and 1216 mL, respectively. These were in contrast to a mean operating time of 125 minutes and an estimated blood loss of 730 mL in a group of patients undergoing routine primary total hip replacements at the same institution. The overall clinical results were generally satisfactory. There were more good and excellent results in the femoral neck fracture group. Dislocation occurred in none of the patients with a failed treatment of femoral neck fractures, but in 23% of those who underwent conversion surgery for failed intertrochanteric hip fractures. Franzen et al. (26) reported specifically on the incidence of mechanical failures of conversion total hip replacements for failed internal fixation of femoral neck fractures in 84 patients at 6 to 12 years of follow-up. Revision surgery was necessary in nine patients: four for recurrent dislocation, two each for infection and loosening, and one for fracture of the stem. There were 42 surviving hips at final follow-up; among these, six stems (14.3%) were radiographically loose, but none of the cups were loose. Survivorship analysis demonstrated an overall 2.5 times greater risk of failure of the conversion hip replacements than routine primary total hip replacements done at the same institution over the same time interval.

Conclusion

Conversion total hip replacements for patients with failed internal fixation of previous hip fractures provide excellent pain relief and improvement of overall function. The technical difficulties in reconstructing failure of femoral neck fractures are relatively few, and the perioperative complication rate is low. In contrast, reconstruction of failed intertrochanteric hip fractures can be tech-

nically demanding and there are more perioperative complications. The medium- to long-term survival of the conversion total hip replacements are inferior to that of routine primary total hip replacement. Some of the reported results could be partly due to older surgical techniques and selection of implants.

TOTAL HIP REPLACEMENT FOR FAILED HEMIARTHROPLASTY

Indications

Hemiarthroplasty reconstruction of the hip using endoprostheses has most frequently been applied to the treatment of acute femoral neck fractures. On occasion, they have been used as primary mode of treatment for young patients with osteoarthritis or femoral head osteonecrosis (8,9,44,52), with the hope of preserving acetabular bone stock for future reconstructions. Discussion in this section will be limited to conversion for failure of a primary hemiarthroplasty reconstruction, and it will not address the special situation of failure of a hemiarthroplasty used for revision of a previous total hip replacement (13).

The most common indication for conversion total hip replacement after previous hemiarthroplasty is pain. Pain can result from loosening of the femoral stem (48), erosion of the acetabulum (67,69), a combination of the two, and sepsis. More recently, two additional indications are disassembly (7) and wear (42) of modular hemiarthroplasty components (Fig. 3).

Workup for loosening and sepsis is similar to the workup for patients with conventional total hip replacements. Careful follow-up with serial radiographs should be done in patients with asymptomatic osteolysis caused by wear debris once it has been observed. If progression of the lesions is evident, early surgical intervention should be performed prior to significant compromise of the bone stock. A similar principle should be followed in cases of acetabular protrusion caused by the endoprosthesis.

One of the most commonly encountered clinical situations is the need for conversion surgery in patients who received reconstruction with an Austin-Moore-type prosthesis for displaced fractures of the femoral neck. Subsidence of the prosthesis is common, but many patients with such subsidence can remain clinically satisfied. Erosion of the acetabular cartilage, however, has been shown to be one of the primary mechanisms resulting in significant pain that necessitates conversion surgery to a total hip replacement. Whittaker et al. (68) reported a 64% incidence of loss of acetabular cartilage, with a 24% incidence of development of protrusio acetabuli at 15 years after hemiarthroplasty surgery. Kofoed and Kofod (35) reported a 37% incidence of conversion to total hip replacement within the first 2 years after hemiarthroplasty using the Austin-Moore prosthesis in 106 patients with femoral neck fractures. The incidences of subsidence and radiographic loosening of the stem were similar for those patients who went on to conversion surgery and for those who remained clinically satisfied. The most significant finding ($p < .001$) was that the presence of acetabular degeneration was 4 times greater in those patients who underwent conversion surgery. Another important finding in that study was that over two thirds of those patients needing conversion surgery were younger and more active.

Dalldorf et al. (18) recently reported evidence of acetabular cartilage degeneration using histology of biopsied specimens during conversion surgery in those patients who had previously undergone hemiarthroplasty surgery. They found a significant difference in the histology of the cartilage when compared to a group of control patients who were undergoing primary hip replacement surgery for femoral neck fractures. Moreover, the degree of cartilage degeneration was significantly related to the duration of articulation with the metallic implant. The fate of the acetabular cartilage that had articulated with a unipolar prosthesis was similar to that of the cartilage that had articulated with a bipolar prosthesis.

Technique

Technical challenges of conversion total hip replacement of a previous hemiarthroplasty are similar to those of revision surgery of a failed total hip replacement. Preoperative workup should determine whether only acetabular reconstruction is necessary, or if stem revision is also necessary. Selection of implant(s) should be based on templating and the same criteria as those used for routine revision total hip replacement. Surgical approach should be based on the individual surgeon's preference, previous surgical incisions, and the specific requirements of each case. The transtrochanteric approach may be more practical if only acetabular reconstruction is necessary in the case of a fixed-head stem. This will allow for more versatility in restoring soft-tissue tension with advancement of the trochanter. This particular limitation can be accommodated with various neck lengths that are available in the newer modular systems.

Removal of the stem with a unipolar component such as an Austin-Moore endoprosthesis is usually necessary because of stem loosening or acetabular erosion. Some newer designs have offered modular unipolar components. Exchange to a regular femoral head component with the appropriate taper and neck length will allow for retaining the original stem if only acetabular reconstruction is necessary. In cases with a bipolar component, the shell can be removed without removing the stem. In addition, the femoral head component in modular systems can be removed to better expose the acetabulum. The femoral stem must be carefully examined for stability and orientation. If the stem is to remain *in situ*, the neck–taper junction or the femoral head itself must be protected from abrasion during retraction.

Acetabular reconstruction is similar to primary total hip replacement. In some cases, subchondral bone of the acetabulum can be extremely weak, especially in elderly patients with previous femoral neck fractures. Careful reaming, therefore, is necessary, to avoid perforating the medial wall or compromising the posterior column. Acetabular cups inserted with cement may be best in these cases with porotic bone. In other cases, sclerosis of the subchondral bone is present, which presents as an obstacle to optimal cement–bone interface. Acetabular

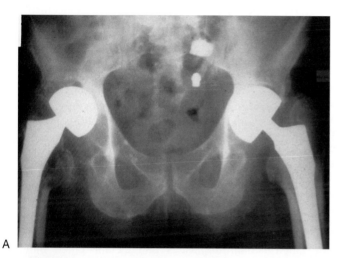

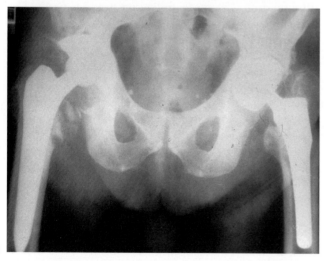

FIG. 3. A: AP radiograph demonstrating polyethylene wear of a bipolar prosthesis inserted without cement originally for osteonecrosis of the femoral head. There is significant protrusion of the neck of the stem into the bipolar cup, indicative of polyethylene wear. There is also extensive osteolysis in the acetabulum and the proximal femur. **B:** AP radiograph 6 months after conversion total hip replacement using a prostheses inserted without cement.

cups inserted without cement, with or without adjunct screw fixation, may be better. Bone grafting may be necessary if significant protrusion of the acetabulum is present. Deficiency of the acetabulum is generally mild, and major structural graft is usually not necessary.

If the femoral stem is to be removed, the same principles and techniques used when removing cemented or cementless stems in a previous total hip replacement should be followed. Femoral reconstruction is similar to routine femoral revision surgery. It is unnecessary to use a longer stem unless the femoral cortex is violated, either from stem removal or the loosening process itself. If the stem is to remain *in situ*, areas of osteolysis in the proximal femoral zones should be grafted using autograft or allograft.

Postoperative care is similar to routine revision total hip replacement, based on the surgical approach, implant selection, and other clinical issues.

Results

Conversion total hip replacement surgery for failed hemiarthroplasty resembles revision total hip replacement surgery. Sarmiento and Gerard (55) reported a mean operating time of 2.3 hours and nearly 2000 mL of blood loss during conversion surgery for failed hemiarthroplasties. Similarly, Stambough et al. (61) reported a mean operating time of 3.2 hours and blood loss of 824 mL in a group of conversion surgeries done for a variety of causes. Surgeries in the latter series were performed under hypotensive anesthesia.

Dupont and Charnley (20) were among the first to report the clinical results of conversion total hip replacement. They reported overall excellent success among 217 conversion surgeries. There were 121 femoral osteotomies, 51 endoprostheses, and 45 various other diagnoses including arthrodesis, pseudoarthrosis, and failed cup arthroplasties. Satisfactory pain relief was achieved in 96% of the 51 conversions for failed endoprostheses. Hip motion was good to excellent in 96% as well. Length of follow-up was not specified, but it was considered to be relatively short. The major complication was infection (3.7%) in the entire group. Most importantly, 23.6% had positive bacterial cultures from the hip joint at the time of conversion surgery. Similarly, Turner and Wroblewski (66) reported infection to be the major problem (3.9%) in their series of 205 conversion total hip replacements for late complications of femoral neck fractures. Forty-five of the procedures were done for previous hemiarthroplasties. Length of follow-up for the entire group was 2.8 years. Mechanical failure other than sepsis occurred in 3.9%.

Amstutz and Smith (2) reported the results of 41 conversion total hip replacements using early cementing techniques for failed hemiarthroplasties at a mean follow-up of 3 years. The mean interval between initial hemi-

arthroplasty and the conversion procedure was 5.5 years. Overall satisfactory clinical results were achieved in nearly all patients. They specifically focused on the discussion of femoral loosening. Radiographic evidence of suboptimal fixation of the stem was present in 13 (31.7%) cases, with six being progressive. They concluded that a previous femoral hemiarthroplasty, even without cement, could significantly compromise the quality of bone–cement interface at conversion surgery. Sarmiento and Gerard (55) reported on a series of 95 conversion hip replacements after failed hemiarthroplasties, also using early cementing techniques. Mean follow-up was 2.8 years. Satisfactory clinical results were achieved in over 95% of the patients. Loosening was evident in six (6.3%) stems and one cup. The major complication was dislocation, with a 5.5% rate that was similar to many early reported series of revision total hip replacements (15) (Fig. 4). Improved cementing techniques developed over the past two decades probably should offer better results today (23).

Stambough et al. (61) reported on a series of 140 conversion surgeries, with 32 having been done for failure of hemiarthroplasties. The length of follow-up was a minimum 4 years with a mean of nearly 8 years. Radiographic loosening of the stem was evident in 22%, with a 9.3% subsidence rate. Cup loosening was present in 34%. Revision surgery was necessary in two patients (6.3%) in this subgroup. In addition, trochanteric complications occurred in 28.5%. However, overall clinical improvement was consistently satisfactory. Llinas et al. (38) reported on a series of 120 conversion surgeries, with 99 for failed hemiarthroplasties and 21 for failed mold arthroplasties. The mean follow-up was 7.6 years. The incidences of radiographic loosening of the components were presented in survivorship analysis format and then compared to the results of patients after routine primary total hip replacements. The probability of cup survival was better in the group of conversion surgeries for failed hemiarthroplasties than for primary hip replacements. In contrast, the femoral stems in the conversion group were at significantly greater ($p < .001$) risk of cement fracture, cement–bone radiolucencies, and progressive loosening. The overall revision rate was 6%.

Conclusion

Conversion total hip replacement for a failed hemiarthroplasty can consistently offer improved clinical results. The perioperative morbidity approximates that of revision total hip replacements, rather than that of primary surgeries. Most important, femoral stem fixation using cement has been reported to be inferior to that of primary total hip replacement. Currently, avoidance of having to remove the stem in the more contemporary modular hemiarthroplasty systems, improved cementing techniques, and selected use of stem designs inserted

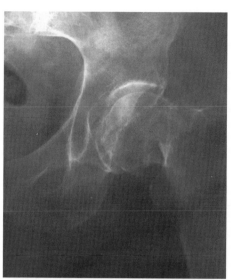

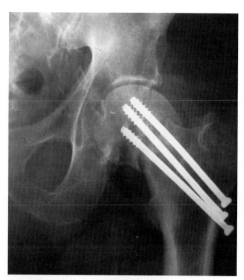

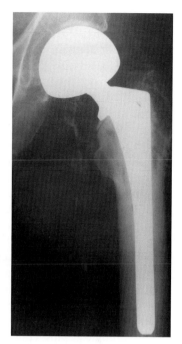

A–C

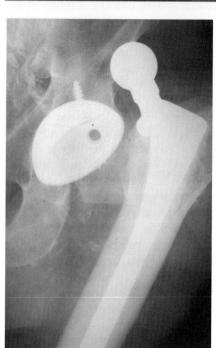

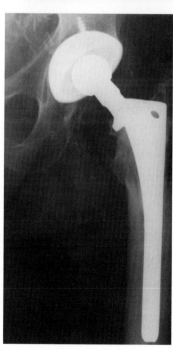

D,E

FIG. 4. A: AP radiograph of a displaced femoral neck fracture in a 65-year-old man. B: Nonunion of the fracture 8 months after initial surgery. C: AP radiograph of conversion surgery using a stem inserted with cement and a bipolar prosthesis. D: Dislocation after a second conversion surgery for pain, with an acetabular cup inserted without cement and exchange of the modular femoral head component to a longer neck length, 15 months after the bipolar replacement. This was complicated by perioperative dislocation. E: AP radiograph 2 years after the second conversion surgery. The patient's clinical result was successful, without any further dislocation.

without cement, may offer better durability of femoral reconstruction in conversion surgery for failed hemiarthroplasty.

TOTAL HIP REPLACEMENT AFTER FAILED SURFACE REPLACEMENT

Indications

Surface replacement arthroplasty of the hip was introduced in the 1970s as an alternative treatment option to conventional stem-type total hip replacement. The most important proposed advantage of surface replacement is preservation of femoral bone stock, thus facilitating further revision surgery should that become necessary. It has therefore been principally applied to younger patients in whom durability of any prosthetic replacement remains a significant problem.

The clinical results of surface replacements unfortunately have been disappointing. One of the largest clinical experiences with surface replacement has been at The University of California at Los Angeles (UCLA) using the THARIES design (2–4). Nearly 27.5% of the THARIES surface replacements have failed over the past 15 years. In addition to aseptic loosening of prosthetic fixation, osteolysis resulting from wear debris has become a major mode of failure (32,56). The proposed modes of failure (3) of a surface replacement include aseptic loosening, fracture of the femoral neck, osteolysis from wear debris, and sepsis.

The clinical presentation of failure of a surface replacement resulting from the various mechanisms is no different from failure of a conventional stem-type total hip replacement, with pain being the leading symptom. Two-thirds of the failures caused by aseptic loosening reported in the UCLA experience were on the acetabular side. Approximately 90% of the cup failures were a result of debonding at the bone–cement interface, and 10% were a result of debonding between the cup and cement. Newer prosthetic designs with porous-coated surfaces that would allow for bony-ingrowth and biologic stabilization were introduced in the 1980s. Loosening has not occurred in these cups. However, significant pelvic osteolysis has occurred in 17% of the hips at a mean follow-up of 5.3 years (56). Revision surgery has been necessary in some of these cases.

On the femoral side, loss of fixation has been primarily between cement and bone. Femoral neck fracture is another important mechanism of failure. The causes of the fracture include fatigue failure, osteonecrosis, trauma, and wear-debris-induced osteolysis. Osteolysis accounted for 50% of the failures on the femoral side with porous-coated surface replacements in the UCLA experience (4).

Radiographic criteria for the evaluation of cup loosening are similar to those proposed for conventional total hip replacement with or without cement. Radiographic evaluation of the femoral component is more challenging, because the prosthesis overshadows the bone–implant interface. Migration of the component is indicative of loss of fixation. Serial bone scans have been proposed to be efficacious in detecting femoral component loosening (16,64). In addition, contrast arthrography can be useful.

Technique

Conversion total hip replacement of a failed surface replacement is more difficult than routine primary total hip replacement. It is, however, easier than revision surgery of a failed total hip replacement. Acetabular reconstruction is similar to revision of a conventional hip replacement. There is generally adequate wall remaining on the anterior and posterior sides of the acetabulum. Reconstruction using a hemispherical cup with porous surface inserted without cement is often sufficient. Morselized bone graft may be necessary to fill cystic defects resulting from osteolysis and old cement anchor-

ing holes. The remaining femoral head and neck can serve as a source of the bone graft.

Reconstruction on the femoral side has most frequently been done with conversion to a stem-type prosthesis, with or without cement. Femoral preparation and implant selection are similar to routine primary total hip replacement. Current modular prosthetic systems should offer a sufficient selection of neck lengths to fulfill the requirements of equalization of leg lengths and maximizing femoral offset. In rare circumstances of significant bone loss resulting from osteolysis of the proximal femur, a transtrochanteric approach may be indicated to allow for the versatility of tightening the abductors to minimize dislocation.

Conversion of a failed surface replacement to another surface replacement is possible. This can be done only if the remaining femoral neck is without any significant erosion and shortening. In such situations, trochanteric osteotomy is necessary to provide wide access to the femoral neck. Care must be exercised while removing the original femoral component to preserve as much bone as possible.

McClelland et al. (43) reported conversion surgery for the femoral component using a stem-type bipolar prosthesis in three patients in whom the acetabular components were stable and without wear. They selected the bipolar prostheses to match the inner diameters of the cup of the surface replacement. The patients were all doing well at a mean of 2.5 years of follow-up. Failure of the femoral component has been the predominant problem in surface replacements done without cement. In situations of femoral reconstruction alone, exchange of the polyethylene cup liner to one that matches the diameter of the femoral head of the new stem without removing the cup can be easily done with modular cups.

In the presence of sepsis, removal of the components followed by a two-stage reimplantation protocol, similar to that used in the management of an infected routine total hip replacement, is recommended. The longer length of the remaining neck in a surface replacement theoretically offers better prognosis in a resection arthroplasty situation than a failed stem-type total hip replacement (29).

Results

There have been only a few earlier reported series of conversion hip replacement specifically for failure of a surface replacement (Table 1). A common finding in these three studies was that the mean time interval to failure of the index surface replacement was approximately 2 years. This relatively accelerated rate of failure probably resulted in only minimal loss of bone stock in both the acetabulum and femur, making conversion surgery less technically challenging than revision surgery of failed cemented total hip replacements.

TABLE 1. *Etiology of failed surface replacements*

Author (ref.)	Hips (N)	Time to failure of surface replacement (yr)	Reason for conversion surgery			
			Loosening	Fracture	Sepsis	Other
Bradley and Freeman (11)	28	1.8	21	5	1	1
Capello et al. (17)	24	2.5	17	4		3
Thomas and Amstutz (65)	17	1.8	15		1	1

Only Thomas and Amstutz (65) reported data on intra-operative parameters for conversion surgery. There were only four cases of conversion to stem-type total hip replacements; the other 13 cases were converted to another surface replacement. The mean operating time was 198 minutes with an estimated blood loss of 1439 mL. Postoperative complications were minimal in all three series, although none were specified. Stambough et al. (61) reported 12% trochanteric healing problems in 17 cases of conversion surgery for failed surface replacements.

The main problems in all reported series of conversion surgery for failed surface replacement are loosening and infection (Table 2). The rate of loosening has been especially a problem with the cup. Durability of the femoral stem has approximated that of primary total hip replacements. The relatively young age at conversion surgery is perhaps a major factor in the higher failure rates observed in these patients. Bradley and Freeman (11) reported three failures, one of which was for infection. Capello et al. (17) reported no failures for loosening, but there were two infections. In addition, they reported radiolucencies around the components in a majority of the 15 hips done using a stem-type prosthesis. Thomas and Amstutz (65) reported three failures resulting from loosening, all in patients who initially underwent cup revisions only using another surface replacement. More importantly, they reported radiolucencies greater than 2 mm around almost half of the cups.

In another study, Llinas et al. (38) reported on the results of conversion surgery for failed mold arthroplasties. They found a significantly higher incidence of complete radiolucencies around the cups than in the conventional primary total hip replacements that served as controls ($p < .008$). Radiographic evaluation of the femoral stems was not different from the primary cases. Recently, Ash et al. (5) reported the long-term follow-up results of 96 conversion surgeries using cemented stem-type prostheses for failed cup arthroplasties. Another revision surgery for cup failure resulting from aseptic loosening was necessary in 16% in those hips followed a minimum of 10 years. Survivorship analysis demonstrated an 84% probability of cup survival at 20 years. No femoral stem required further revision surgery to correct aseptic loosening. There was, however, an 8% incidence of infection. When radiographic loosenings were considered, cup loosening was found in 53%, which was significantly greater ($p < .005$) than a previous reported series of cemented total hip replacements performed by the same senior surgeon (and measured at long-term follow-up) (57). The cup revision rate was, however, not statistically higher in the conversion series ($p = .07$).

Amstutz and Navarro (4) have reported the results of a relatively large series of patients with failed surface replacements. They found a failure rate over 70% at a mean follow-up of 5.4 years in those cases revised with another surface replacement. In contrast, they found a 10.3% failure rate among the 58 patients who underwent conversion surgery to stem-type prostheses using cement. Survivorship analysis demonstrated 83% survival at 6 years. No data were given separately for the cups and the stems. In another 71 patients, conversion surgeries were done using prostheses inserted without cement. Overall failure rate was 17.6% at a mean follow-up of 3 years. Survivorship analysis demonstrated 93% survival of the stems, but only 82% survival of the cups. The main reason for the higher cup failure rate was the use of macro-threaded designs in some of the cases, according to the authors.

TABLE 2. *Results of conversion surgery for failed surface replacements*

Author (ref.)	Age at THR (yr)	F/U after THR (mo)	Success (%)	Revision (%)	Sepsis (%)	Radiographic loosening (%)	
						Cup	Stem
Ash et al. (5)	58	120 (minimum)	91.4	18	8	53	5
Bradley and Freeman (11)	66	34	89.3	7.1	3.6	*	*
Capello et al. (17)	43	25	87.5	0	83	85	43
Stambough et al. (61)	48	87	*	5.9	0	47	17.5
Thomas and Amstutz (65)	38	65	*	17.7	0	47	*

*Insufficient data given.

THR, total hip replacement; F/U, follow-up.

Conclusion

Technical challenges and complications of conversion hip replacement surgery of a failed surface replacement are generally few. The technique can be expected to provide good clinical results at least at short- to medium-term follow-up intervals. Some of the unsatisfactory results may be the result of multiple previous operations prior to conversion to a total hip replacement. Results of conversion to another surface replacement have been disappointing. When conversion is done with cement, durability of the cup has been predictably less satisfactory than primary surgery. Conversion surgery using current cup designs implanted without cement may improve the results. Durability of the femoral stem is expected to be the same as for primary surgery with or without cement.

TOTAL HIP REPLACEMENT AFTER FAILED FEMORAL OSTEOTOMY

Indications

Reconstructive osteotomies of the proximal femur have been widely applied to patients with hip disease, especially in Europe. The advancement of prosthetic arthroplasties over the past three decades has led to a significant decrease in the use of joint-sparing procedures such as proximal femoral osteotomy. The long-term success of well-performed proximal femoral osteotomies has been estimated to be approximately 50% at 10 years (45). Conversion total hip replacement is an accepted treatment option in patients whose clinical conditions have deteriorated further after proximal femoral osteotomies. The most common indication for conversion total hip replacement is progression of pain and loss of function from the underlying disease process. Nonunion of the osteotomy is another indication.

The technical challenges of total hip replacement in the presence of a previous proximal femoral osteotomy can be formidable because of the distorted anatomy. The complication rate has been reported to be greater than that of primary total hip replacements (24,63). Moreover, the clinical results and durability have been less predictable than those of primary total hip replacements (24,59,62).

Technique

Different technical issues require attention to implant selection and reconstructive goals when performing conversion total hip replacement surgery in patients with failed proximal femoral osteotomies. The surgical approach is generally according to the surgeon's preference for primary total hip replacement. If there is significant deformity from the osteotomy, a transtrochanteric approach would offer the best access to the proximal femur during the reaming and broaching process, therefore minimizing the risks of perforations and fractures.

Acetabular reconstruction is similar to routine primary total hip replacement. Many of these patients have undergone the proximal femoral osteotomies for hip dysplasia. Acetabular dysplasia therefore is frequently present. The principles and techniques used in such situations should be followed. The majority of the cases can be successfully reconstructed using porous-coated cups inserted without cement. On occasion, cups with smaller outer diameters are necessary because of acetabular dysplasia. It may be more appropriate to consider using femoral head components of smaller diameters (such as 22 mm or 26 mm), or using an all-polyethylene cup inserted with cement, to maximize the polyethylene thickness.

The major challenge is femoral reconstruction in the presence of deformed geometry and previous hardware. It has been suggested that removal of the hardware used for fixation of the osteotomy should be done as a separate procedure prior to conversion total hip replacement (24). This is to allow for healing of the cortical defects from the screws. It is probably not necessary if the principles outlined above in the section of conversion surgery for failed internal fixation devices are followed in terms of modification of cementing techniques and implant selection (50,51).

The deformed femoral geometry is often not a significant limitation if the stem is implanted with cement. It does, however, pose a problem if cementless stems are to be used. The majority of the cementless stem designs are straight and do not fit the distorted proximal femur. Furthermore, maximal cortical contact of the stem (fit-and-fill) is a critical factor in predicting the durability of the stem, so undersizing should be avoided. A corrective osteotomy may be necessary in some cases (19,28,31,33,49). Various techniques for corrective osteotomy have been described. The general principles are making the osteotomy at the level of the greatest deformity, correcting all components (axial and rotational) of the malalignment, removing as little bone as possible to minimize shortening, providing secure fixation of the osteotomy, and selecting a stem design that bypasses the osteotomy sufficiently to prevent periprosthetic fractures.

Custom-designed stems can be used in some cases, although they are not routinely necessary, especially if corrective osteotomy is performed as a part of the conversion total hip replacement. Another option is to use modular designs such as the S-ROM system (Johnson and Johnson, Raynham, Massachusetts), which offers the versatility of maximizing fit proximally and distally. This may allow for adequate femoral reconstruction without a corrective osteotomy. Regardless of what stem design is selected, attention must be given to restoring leg length, abductor offset, and soft-tissue tension.

Results

Conversion total hip replacement for failed proximal femoral osteotomy involves longer operating time and more blood loss than primary total hip replacement. Ferguson et al. (24) reported on the experience with a series of 215 conversion surgeries for failed femoral osteotomies. The mean operating time was 171 minutes, the mean estimated blood loss was 1340 mL, and the mean blood transfusion was 3.3 units. Moreover, the mean hospital stay was 17 days for that series. Similarly, Suominen et al. (63) reported a mean operating time of 142 minutes, and a mean estimated blood loss of 1680 mL in a series of 42 conversion total hip replacements.

Dupont and Charnley (20) first reported on 121 conversion total hip replacements for failed femoral osteotomies. Clinically satisfactory results were achieved in 87% of the patients at short-term follow-up. No information was given concerning mechanical failure, because of the short follow-up.

Benke et al. (10) reported on 105 conversion total hip replacements for failed femoral osteotomies. The mean follow-up was 4.7 years. Overall clinical success was 82%. There were, however, an infection rate of 8.6%, and a complication rate of 17% due to technical difficulties.

Soballe et al. (59) reported on 112 conversion total hip replacements for failed osteotomies and compared the results to a series of routine primary total hip replacements. Mean follow-up was 4.7 years. Satisfactory results were maintained in nearly 90% of the patients. There was no difference when compared to the routine hip replacement patients. In fact, there was less malpositioning of the stem, and less mechanical failures in the conversion group. There were six (5.4%) fractures in the conversion group, with four involving the greater trochanter and only two involving the femoral shaft. This rate could have been lower if the authors had used trochanteric osteotomy for the surgical approach. They reported no incidence of infection.

Nagi and Dhillon (47) reported 93% clinical success in 15 cases of conversion total hip replacements for failed McMurray femoral osteotomy. There was no deep infection, but superficial infection occurred in two cases (13.3%). Radiographic loosening of either component, however, occurred in 27% at a mean follow-up of 5.3 years. Although it was not specified, contemporary cementing techniques were not utilized in these patients.

The success and durability of conversion total hip replacements after femoral osteotomies are not confirmed by other studies, especially with longer follow-up. Ferguson et al. (24) reported on 215 such conversion hip replacements at a mean follow-up of 10 years. There were technical problems at surgery in 23%, with a total perioperative complication rate of 11.8%. Deep infection occurred in 2.3%, and trochanteric nonunion occurred in 6.7%, both of which were higher than the incidences for routine primary total hip replacements. More importantly, 18.1% of the hips required revision, with a rate of 14.9% for aseptic failures. Moreover, radiographic loosening was present in 30.9% of the stems and 19.8% of the cups. Survivorship analysis further demonstrated 20.6% probability of failure of the conversion total hip replacement at 10 years, and 33% failure probability at 15 years.

In another series, Suominen et al. (63) reported the results of 45 conversion surgeries done with cemented and cementless prostheses at a mean follow-up of 6 years. Revision rate was 6.7%, with another 35.7% of the hips showing signs of radiographic loosening. Echeverri et al. (21) reported on a series of 127 conversion total hip replacements at a mean follow-up of 10.4 years. Seventy-two of these cases were done for failed femoral osteotomies. No specific data were given for the osteotomy group. The overall revision rate for the entire group was 20%, and half of these were for infections. In addition, radiographic loosening was evident in 58% of the stems and 56% of the cups. One of the factors that could have potentially influenced the results in these three series was that the mean age at conversion surgery was approximately 60 years. Another important factor was that contemporary cementing techniques or current cementless prosthetic designs were not utilized in any of these patients.

Shinar and Harris (58) recently reported the long-term follow-up results of 19 cemented total hip replacements following proximal femoral osteotomies. The mean follow-up was 15.5 years. All stems were cemented using second-generation techniques. Revision rate for aseptic loosening was 10.5%, with an additional 10.5% rate of radiographic loosening. The overall mechanical failure rate for the stem was therefore 21.2%. The mechanical loosening rate for the cemented cups was, however, 47.4%. All four hips with mechanical failure of the stem had significant deformity of the proximal femur, making the surgical challenge considerable.

Conclusion

Conversion total hip replacement surgery for failed femoral osteotomies can be technically challenging. Selection of stem design should be carefully considered to meet the limitations of distorted femoral geometry. Short-term clinical and radiographic results have matched those of routine primary total hip replacements. Medium- to long-term results, however, have been less satisfactory. Two primary modes of failure reported in the literature are loosening and infection. Loosening may be improved with contemporary cementing techniques and prosthetic designs. Infection may be improved with careful preoperative work-up, intraoperative cultures and histologic examination of the periarticular tissues, and possibly approaching those cases with suspected sepsis using a two-stage protocol.

TOTAL HIP REPLACEMENT AFTER FAILED HIP ARTHRODESIS OR ANKYLOSIS

Indications

Hip arthrodesis remains an excellent alternative in the treatment of painful conditions of the hip joint. Arthrodesis is especially useful in young patients with unilateral disease. Sponseller et al. (60) reported the clinical results in 53 patients at an average of 38 years of follow-up. All patients were 35 years or younger at the time of arthrodesis. Satisfactory results were found in 78% of the patients. However, 57% had some low back pain, 45% had some ipsilateral knee pain, approximately 60% had some laxity of the collateral ligaments of the knee, and 17% complained of pain in the contralateral hip. In another study, Callaghan et al. (14) reported the results of 28 patients with hip arthrodesis at a mean follow-up of 35 years. Their findings paralleled those of Sponseller et al.: 60% had low back pain, 60% had ipsilateral knee pain, and 25% had contralateral hip pain.

Reconstructive surgeries of the painful joint(s) in patients with an arthrodesed or ankylosed hip have been done with relative success. Garvin et al. (27) reported the results of 13 total hip replacements of the contralateral hip, and eight total knee replacements of the ipsilateral knee in 20 patients with successful hip fusions. Overall results were satisfactory. Multiple revision surgeries were, however, necessary in three hips for mechanical loosening. Moreover, 7 of the 8 knees required a total of 15 manipulations for poor motion after surgery. Romness and Morrey (54) reported 16 total knee replacements in 13 patients with ipsilateral hip fusion. Conversion of the fusion to total hip replacement prior to the total knee replacement was done in 12 of the 16 cases. Only one knee required manipulation in that series. Authors of both studies cautioned against performing contralateral hip replacement or ipsilateral knee replacement without first converting the fusion to hip replacement, especially if the position of the fusion was suboptimal.

The major indications for converting a fused hip to total hip replacement are, therefore, the following:

1. Persistent low back pain.
2. Ipsilateral knee pain.
3. Painful pseudoarthrosis from the fusion attempt.
4. Poor position of the fusion.

Technique

Conversion of ankylosed hips to total hip replacements is technically far more demanding than conventional primary surgeries. Factors that necessitate consideration include distortion of anatomy, longstanding contractures of the soft tissues, loss of routine bony landmarks, leg-length discrepancy, and weakness of the abductors.

Preoperative templating using the contralateral normal hip is valuable in determining the hip rotation center and the abductor offset. In addition, this would aid in the selection of implants, especially if cementless designs are to be used. Occasionally, computerized tomography (CT) may be useful in assessing the bony geometry of both the pelvis and the femur. The CT scan can also be used to evaluate the presence and integrity of the hip abductors, extensors, and adductors; the location of the femoral neurovascular bundle anteriorly; and possibly the location of the sciatic nerve posteriorly (Fig. 5). Moreover, the degree of atrophy and fatty infiltration of the abductor muscles can be compared to the contralateral hip.

Many patients may have had multiple previous surgeries that would in part dictate the skin incision. The transtrochanteric approach is most frequently recommended because it offers the greatest versatility in addressing the anatomic variations that may be encountered during conversion surgery.

Integrity and strength of the abductor muscle is difficult to assess in patients with longstanding hip arthrodesis or ankylosis. Electromyographic evaluation and muscle biopsy have been attempted, but they have not proven to be valuable. Physical examination by palpation of abductor muscle contraction may be the best method of evaluation (1,25,34). Atrophy of the muscle is present in all cases. Care must be taken at the time of surgery to avoid devascularization and extensive dissection of the muscle off the ilium.

The femoral neck must be osteotomized *in situ* to allow mobilization of the femur. Care should be taken not to perform the osteotomy too close to the pelvis, so as to avoid creating a pelvic fracture or leaving insufficient acetabular bone stock. Releases of the soft tissues are necessary to correct longstanding contractures. If release of the adductors is necessary, it should be done after the completion of the hip replacement in those cases where adequate passive abduction under anesthesia cannot be achieved.

The principles of acetabular preparation are similar to those of routine total hip replacements. Identification of the inferior border of the acetabulum can be done by using the obturator foramen as a reference. Reaming should begin with smaller reamers to reach the depth of the new acetabular fossa. Limitation of the reaming is determined by the thickness of the posterior wall. The majority of the cups were cemented in published series of total hip replacements in ankylosed hips. In cases of spontaneous ankylosis, there is usually good cancellous bone with remodeled trabeculation, which allows for excellent cement interdigitation. In some cases of posttraumatic ankylosis, pseudoarthrosis of a fusion attempt, or multiple previous surgeries, a hard sclerotic bony bed may be present in the acetabulum. Porous-coated cups inserted without cement may be preferable because suboptimal cup cement–bone interface has been observed in these situations when cement was used. If a small cup is

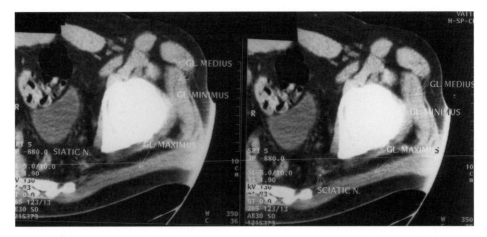

FIG. 5. Multiple CT scan images demonstrating the gluteus maximus, gluteus medius, hip adductors, femoral neurovascular bundle, and the sciatic nerve around a hip that has pseudoankylosis caused by advanced degenerative arthritis secondary to slipped femoral epiphysis.

necessary because of the size of the acetabulum, downsizing of the femoral head dimension should be considered to maximize polyethylene thickness, especially if a modular metal-backed component is selected.

Femoral canal preparation is generally routine. Selection of stem designs for cement or cementless application should be based on the same criteria used for routine primary cases, according to the surgeon's preference. If previous femoral osteotomy was done in conjunction with the ankylosis, realignment osteotomy may be necessary to accept the femoral stem without the risk of perforations or fractures. Consideration should be given to select a stem design that would offer maximal gain in femoral

offset to decrease impingement and to increase abductor biomechanics (Fig. 6).

Postoperative rehabilitation is critical to the clinical outcome of these patients. Partial weight bearing is recommended for the initial 6 to 8 weeks to allow for union of the trochanteric osteotomy. Walking support such as a cane is encouraged for a long time, because the atrophic abductor muscle will continue to improve over several years. Kilgus et al. (34) reported the average abductor strength to be 3.7 on a scale of 1 to 5, with 5 being the strongest, at final follow-up. One third of the patients continued to have a positive Trendelenburg test. The eventual muscle strength depends on several factors,

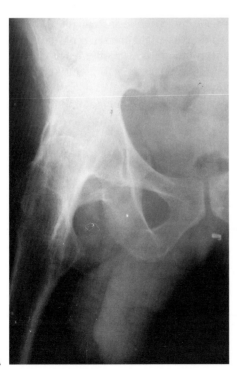

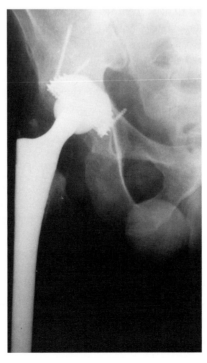

A

B

FIG. 6. A: Preoperative AP radiograph showing a fused right hip. **B:** Postoperative AP radiograph showing reconstruction using prostheses inserted without cement.

TABLE 3. *Results of conversion hip replacement for ankylosed hips*

Author (ref.)	Hips (#)	Mean F/U (yr)	Overall clinical success (%)	Relief of back pain (%)	Relief of knee pain (%)	Flexion arc of hip	Residual leg-length discrepancy (cm)
Brewster et al. (12)	33	1–3.5	91	94	94	76°	2.9
Hardinge et al. (30)	112	8.2	*	80	*	*	2.4
Kilgus et al. (34)	41	7.0	78	80	67	87°	2.5
Lubahn et al. (39)	18	*	59	92	100	70°	*
Reikeras et al. (53)	46	8.0	76	*	*	*	*
Strathy and Fitzgerald (62)	74	10.4	45	*	*	*	*

*Insufficient data given.
F/U, follow-up.

including quality of the muscle before surgery, adequacy of maximizing hip biomechanics, and postoperative rehabilitation.

Results

There have been only a few reports on the results of conversion of an ankylosed hip to total hip replacement (1,12,30,34,39,62) (Table 3). The initial experience was quite satisfactory. With longer follow-up, Strathy and Fitzgerald (62) reported only 45% good or excellent overall clinical results in 80 conversion total hip replacements for ankylosed hips at a mean follow-up of 10 years. Revision surgery was necessary for mechanical loosening in 11, for infection in 9, and for recurrent dislocation in 1, making an overall rate of 26.3%. They found 95% successful results among the 19 hips that were converted from a spontaneous ankylosis. In contrast, there was only a 45% success rate among those hips in which conversion was done after surgical ankylosis. Twenty of the 21 revisions in this series were also in this second subgroup. Moreover, the success rate for patients less than 50 years old at the time of conversion hip replacement was only 50% of the rate of success in those patients who were 50 years or older. In addition, failure occurred in two thirds of those hips with three or more previous operations. Similarly, Kilgus et al. (34) determined that age less than 45 years, and two or more previous surgeries, were the

most significant predictors in the failure of conversion total hip replacements in ankylosed hips. They observed that 50% of the failures were in patients whose ankylosis or arthrodesis began with traumatic injury, possibly because the more sclerotic bone bed (especially in the acetabulum) resulted in poor cement fixation of the cups.

The most frequently reported complications are infection and loosening (Table 4). The majority of the infections occurred in cases with multiple surgeries. Infection was rare in ankylosed hips that resulted from childhood sepsis or tuberculosis. The incidence of dislocation was relatively low. This could have been partially a result of routine use of the transtrochanteric approach, careful handling of the abductor muscles, proper selection of implant sizes, and having a majority of these reported cases being performed at tertiary centers of hip reconstruction.

Conclusion

Conversion of an ankylosed hip to total hip replacement can be extremely satisfying to the patient. Relief of back pain is more predictable than the relief of knee pain. Total mean arc of hip motion is generally less than 90°. Residual leg-length discrepancy of 1 to 2 cm is frequent (see Table 3). Abductor muscle strength and resolution of the Trendelenburg gait will continue to improve even years after surgery.

TABLE 4. *Complications after conversion hip replacement for ankylosed hips*

Author (ref.)	Hips (N)	Complications (N)	Radiographically loose (N)		Revisions[a] (N)	
			Cup	Stem	Cup	Stem
Brewster et al. (12)	33	2 inf, 1 disloc, 1 nerve	*	*	*	*
Hardinge et al. (30)	112	2 inf, 11 nerve, 32 HO	6	9	3	3
Kilgus et al. (34)	41	3 inf, 2 disloc, 1 nerve, 1 HO	2	21	3	2
Lubahn et al. (39)	18	1 inf, 1 disloc, 2 HO	*	*	0	1
Reikeras et al. (53)	46	*	0	2	7	7
Strathy and Fitzgerald (62)	74	9 inf, 1 disloc	*	*	21	21

*Insufficient data given.
[a]Includes aseptic and septic cases.
Inf, infection; disloc, dislocation; nerve, sciatic or femoral nerve palsy; HO, heterotopic bone.

If there is disabling contralateral hip disease, total hip replacement can be performed without converting the ankylosed hip first. However, loosening is a problem, especially if the ankylosed hip is in suboptimal position. Similarly, ipsilateral total knee replacement can be performed without converting the ankylosed hip first. Poor motion is often a problem. Clinical results of total knee replacement are generally superior in those patients in whom conversion total hip replacements have been done first.

The high incidence of failure of the total hip replacement after conversion surgery has been reported to be associated with young age, multiple previous surgeries, and posttraumatic injuries. Prosthetic fixation may be enhanced with cementless designs, especially on the acetabular side in cases of sclerotic bone bed. Improved cementing techniques and stem designs should offer improved fixation on the femoral side.

REFERENCES

1. Amstutz HC, Saikai DN. Total joint replacement for ankylosed hips. Indications, techniques and preliminary results. *J Bone Joint Surg* 1975;57A:619–625.
2. Amstutz HC, Smith RK. Total hip replacement following failed femoral hemiarthroplasty. *J Bone Joint Surg* 1979;61A:1161–1166.
3. Amstutz HC, Campbell P, Nasser S, Kossovsky N. Modes of failure of surface replacements. In: Amstutz HC, ed. *Hip arthroplasty*. New York: Churchill Livingston, 1991;507–534.
4. Amstutz HC, Navarro RA. Surface replacement revision. In: Amstutz HC, ed. *Hip arthroplasty*. New York: Churchill Livingston, 1991; 855–860.
5. Ash SA, Callaghan JJ, Johnston RC. Revision total hip arthroplasty with cement after cup arthroplasty. Long-term follow-up. *J Bone Joint Surg* 1996;78A:87–93.
6. Asnis SE, Wanek-Sgaglione L. Intracapsular fractrues of the femoral neck. Results of cannulated screw fixation. *J Bone Joint Surg* 1994; 76A:1793–1803.
7. Barmada R, Mess D. Bateman hemiarthroplasty component disassembly. A report of three cases of high-density polyethylene failure. *Clin Orthop* 1987;224:147–149.
8. Barnes CL, Berry DJ, Sledge CB. Dislocation after bipolar hemiarthroplasty of the hip. *J Arthroplasty* 1995;10:667–669.
9. Bateman JE, Berenji AR, Bayne O, Greyson ND. Long-term results of bipolar arthroplasty in osteoarthritis of the hip. *Clin Orthop* 1990;251: 54–66.
10. Benke GJ, Baker AS, Dounis E. Total hip replacement after upper femoral osteotomy. A clinical review. *J Bone Joint Surg* 1982;64B: 570–601.
11. Bradley GW, Freeman MAR. Revision of failed hip resurfacing. *Clin Orthop* 1983;178:236–240.
12. Brewster RC, Coventry MB, Johnson Jr EW. Conversion of the arthro-desed hip to a total hip arthroplasty. *J Bone Joint Surg* 1975;57A:27–30.
13. Brien WW, Bruce WJ, Salvati EA, et al. Acetabular reconstruction with a bipolar prosthesis and morseled bone grafts. *J Bone Joint Surg* 1990; 72A:1230–1235.
14. Callaghan JJ, Brand RA, Pedersen DR. Hip arthrodesis. A long-term follow-up. *J Bone Joint Surg* 1985;67A:1328–1335.
15. Callaghan JJ. Results and experiences with cemented revision total hip arthroplasty. *Instr Course Lect* 1991;40:185–187.
16. Capello WN, Wilson NM, Wellman HN. Bone imaging: a means of evaluating hip surface replacement arthroplasty. In: *The hip. Proceedings of the eighth open scientific meeting of The Hip Society*. St. Louis: CV Mosby, 1980;192.
17. Capello WN, Trancik TM, Misamore G, Eaton R. Analysis of revision surgery of resurfacing hip arthroplasty. *Clin Orthop* 1982;170:50–55.
18. Dalldorf PG, Banas MP, Hicks DG, Pellegrini Jr VD. Rate of degeneration of human acetabular cartilage after hemiarthroplasty. *J Bone Joint Surg* 1995;77A:877.
19. DeCoster TA, Incavo S, Frymoyer JW, Howe J. Hip arthroplasty after biplanar femoral osteotomy. *J Arthroplasty* 1989;4:79–86.
20. Dupont JA, Charnley J. Low-friction arthroplasty of the hip for the failures of previous operations. *J Bone Joint Surg* 1972;54B:77–87.
21. Echeverri A, Shelley P, Wroblewski BM. Long-term results of hip arthroplasty for failure of previous surgery. *J Bone Joint Surg* 1988; 70B:49–51.
22. Eschenroeder Jr HC, Krackow KA. Late onset femoral stress fracture associated with extruded cement following hip arthroplasty. *Clin Orthop* 1988;236:210–213.
23. Estok III DM, Harris WH. Long-term results of cemented femoral revision surgery using second generation techniques. An average 11.7-year follow-up evaluation. *Clin Orthop* 1994;299:190–202.
24. Ferguson GM, Cabanella ME, Ilstrup DM. Total hip arthroplasty after failed intertrochanteric osteotomy. *J Bone Joint Surg* 1994;76B:252–257.
25. Ferrari A, Charnley J. Conversion of hip joint pseudarthrosis to total hip replacement. *Clin Orthop* 1976;121:12–19.
26. Franzen H, Nilsson LT, Stromqvist B, et al. Secondary total hip replacement after fractures of the femoral neck. *J Bone Joint Surg* 1990;72B: 784–787.
27. Garvin KL, Pellicci PM, Windsor RE, et al. Contralateral total hip arthroplasty or ipsilateral total knee arthroplasty in patients who have a long-standing fusion of the hip. *J Bone Joint Surg* 1989;71A:1355–1362.
28. Glassman AH, Engh CA, Bobyn JD. Proximal femoral osteotomy as an adjunct in cementless revision total hip arthroplasty. *J Arthroplasty* 1987;2:47–64.
29. Grauer JD, Amstutz HC, O'Carroll PF, Dorey FJ. Resection arthroplasty of the hip. *J Bone Joint Surg* 1989;71A:669–678.
30. Hardinge K, Murphy JCM, Frenyo S. Conversion of hip fusion to Charnley low-friction arthroplasty. *Clin Orthop* 1986;211:173–179.
31. Holtgrewe JL, Hungerford DS. Primary and revision total hip replacement without cement and with associated femoral osteotomy. *J Bone Joint Surg* 1989;71A:1487–1495.
32. Howie DW, Cornish BL, Vernon-Roberts B. Resurfacing hip arthroplasty. Classification of loosening and the role of prosthesis wear particles. *Clin Orthop* 1990;255:144–159.
33. Huo MH, Zatorski LE, Keggi KJ. Oblique femoral osteotomy in cementless total hip arthroplasty. Prospective consecutive series with a 3-year minimum follow-up period. *J Arthroplasty* 1995;10:319–328.
34. Kilgus DJ, Amstutz HC, Wolgin MA, Dorey FJ. Joint replacement for ankylosed hips. *J Bone Joint Surg* 1990;72A:45–54.
35. Kofoed H, Kofod J. Moore prosthesis in the treatment of fresh femoral neck fractures. A critical review with special attention to secondary acetabular degeneration. *Injury* 1983;14:531–540.
36. Koval KJ, Zuckerman JD. Hip fractures: I. Overview and evaluation and treatment of femoral-neck fractures. *J Am Acad Orthop Surg* 1994; 2:141–150.
37. Koval KJ, Zuckerman JD. Hip fractures: II. Evaluation and treatment of intertrochanteric fractures. *J Am Acad Orthop Surg* 1994;2:151–156.
38. Llinas A, Sarmiento A, Ebramzadeh A, et al. Total hip replacement after failed hemiarthroplasty or mould arthroplasty. Comparison of results with those of primary replacements. *J Bone Joint Surg* 1991;73B: 902–907.
39. Lubahn JD, Evarts CM, Feltner JB. Conversion of ankylosed hips to total hip arthroplasty. *Clin Orthop* 1980;153:146–152.
40. Lu-Yao GL, Keller RB, Littenberg B, Wennberg JE. Outcomes after displaced fractures of the femoral neck. A meta-analysis of one hundred and six published reports. *J Bone Joint Surg* 1994;76A:15–23.
41. Mehlhoff T, Landon GC, Tullos HS. Total hip arthroplasty following failed internal fixation of hip fractures. *Clin Orthop* 1991;269:32–37.
42. Messieh M, Mattingly DA, Turner RH, et al. Wear debris from bipolar femoral neck-cup impingement. A cause of femoral stem loosening. *J Arthroplasty* 1994;9:89–93.
43. McClelland SJ, Godfrey JD, Benton PC, Slemmons BK. Revision of failed hip surface replacement arthroplasties with a bipolar prosthesis. Three case reports with two- to three-year follow-up observations. *Clin Orthop* 1986;208:243–248.
44. McConville OR, Bowman Jr AJ, Kilfoyle RM, et al. Bipolar hemiarthroplasty in degenerative arthritis of the hip: 100 consecutive cases. *Clin Orthop* 1990;251:67–75.
45. Miegel RE, Harris WH. Medial-displacement intertrochanteric osteo-

tomy in the treatment of osteoarthritis of the hip. *J Bone Joint Surg* 1984;66A:878–887.

46. Moran MC. A technique for removal of cannulated screws with buried heads from the femoral neck in the course of total hip replacement. *J Bone Joint Surg* 1992;74A:1245–1246.

47. Nagi ON, Dhillon MS. Total hip arthroplasty after McMurray's osteotomy. *J Arthroplasty* 1991;6:S17–S22.

48. Nilson LT, Stromqvist BN, Thorngren KG. Secondary arthroplasty for complications of femoral neck fracture. *J Bone Joint Surg* 1989; 71B:777–781.

49. Paavilainen T, Hoikka V, Solonen KA. Cementless total replacement for severely dysplastic or dislocated hips. *J Bone Joint Surg* 1990;72B: 205–211.

50. Panjabi MM, Trumble T, Hult JE, Southwick WO. Effect of femoral stem length on stress raisers associated with revision hip arthroplasty. *J Orthop Res* 1985;3:447–455.

51. Patterson BM, Salvati EA, Huo MH. Total hip arthroplasty for complications of intertrochanteric fracture. A technical note. *J Bone Joint Surg* 1990;72A:776–777.

52. Prieskorn D, Burton P, Page BJ, Swienckoski J. Bipolar hemiarthroplasty for primary osteoarthritis of the hip. *Orthopaedics* 1994;17: 1105–1111.

53. Reikeras O, Bjerkreim I, Gundersson R. Total hip arthroplasty for arthrodesed hips. 5- to 13-year results. *J Arthroplasty* 1995;10: 529–531.

54. Romness DW, Morrey BF. Total knee arthroplasty in patients with prior ipsilateral hip fusion. *J Arthroplasty* 1992;7:63–70.

55. Sarmiento A, Gerard FM. Total hip arthroplasty for failed endoprostheses. *Clin Orthop* 1978;137:112–117.

56. Schmalzried TP, Guttmann D, Grecula M, Amstutz HC. The relationship between the design, position, and articular wear of acetabular components inserted without cement and the development of pelvic osteolysis. *J Bone Joint Surg* 1994;76A:677–688.

57. Schulte KR, Callaghan JJ, Kelley SS, Johnston RC. The outcome of Charnley total hip arthroplasty with cement after a minimum twenty-year follow-up. The results of one surgeon. *J Bone Joint Surg* 1993; 75A:961–975.

58. Shinar AA, Harris WH. Total hip arthroplasty following previous femoral osteotomy. An average fifteen year follow-up study. *(Personal communication, 1996.)*

59. Soballe K, Boll KL, Kofod S, et al. Total hip replacement after medial-displacement osteotomy of the proximal part of the femur. *J Bone Joint Surg* 1989;71A:692–697.

60. Sponseller PD, McBeath AA, Perpich M. Hip arthrodesis in young patients. A long-term follow-up study. *J Bone Joint Surg* 1984;66A: 853–859.

61. Stambough JL, Balderston RA, Booth Jr RE, et al. Conversion total hip replacement. Review of 140 hips with greater than 6-year follow-up study. *J Arthroplasty* 1986;1:261–268.

62. Strathy GM, Fitzgerald RH. Total hip arthroplasty in the ankylosed hip. *J Bone Joint Surg* 1988;70A:963–966.

63. Suominen S, Antti-Poika I, Santavirta S, et al. Total hip replacement after intertrochanteric osteotomy. *Orthopaedics* 1991;14:253–257.

64. Thomas BJ, Amstutz HC, Mai LL, Webber MM. Identification of hip surface replacement failures with TcSC/TcmDP radionuclide imaging. *Clin Orthop* 1982;167:106–112.

65. Thomas BJ, Amstutz HC. Revision surgery for failed surface arthroplasty of the hip. *Clin Orthop* 1982;170:42–49.

66. Turner A, Wroblewski BM. Charnley low-friction arthroplasty for the treatment of hips with late complications of femoral neck fractures. *Clin Orthop* 1984;185:126–130.

67. Vazquez-Vela E, Vazquez-Vela G. Acetabular reaction to the Bateman bipolar prosthesis. *Clin Orthop* 1990;251:87–91.

68. Whittaker RP, Abeshaus MM, Scholl HW, Chung SM. Fifteen years' experience with metallic endoprosthetic replacement of the femoral head for femoral neck fractures. *J Trauma* 1972;12:799–805.

69. Yamagata M, Chao EY, Ilstrup DM, et al. Fixed-head and bipolar hip endoprostheses. A retrospective clinical and roentgenographic study. *J Arthroplasty* 1987;2:327–341.

The Adult Hip, edited by J. J. Callaghan,
A. G. Rosenberg, and H. E. Rubash.
Lippincott–Raven Publishers, Philadelphia © 1998.

CHAPTER 101

Rehabilitation

Michael C. Munin, Peggy S. Hockenberry, Patrick G. Flynn, and Wendy Toplak

The ultimate goal of rehabilitation after total hip arthroplasty (THA) is to maximize functional performance and improve an individual's ability to perform daily activities. Common physical impairments that must be overcome include pain, limited range of motion at the hip, and muscular weakness. These impairments lead to disability that, if not corrected, can negate the beneficial effects of surgery (5).

Successful treatment after THA is dependent on the efforts of the interdisciplinary team comprising rehabilitation physicians, physical therapists, occupational therapists, and other allied health disciplines (2,5,17). With an estimated 80,000 to 130,000 hip arthroplasties performed each year in the United States, this group accounts for a large percentage of referrals (25). Joint replacement surgery and subsequent rehabilitation have resulted in high measures of success in the categories of pain relief, increased function, and return to normal activity (2,5,29). Most benefits of rehabilitation are achieved by 3 to 6 months after surgery (17). However, patients can continue to make gains within a period of 2 years. Many biomedical factors may affect rehabilitation outcome, including the method of fixation, surgical approach and difficulty of the procedure, complications and comorbidities, strength, coordination, weight, and cognition. Among the latter

points, cognitive deficits may account for slow progress early after surgery, because 11% of patients in one study had postoperative delirium regardless of whether general or epidural anesthesia was used (57).

COMPONENTS OF REHABILITATION

Education, exercise, and functional mobility training are the three main components of rehabilitation after hip arthroplasty. Rehabilitation programs must include education against dislocation of the endoprosthesis during functional mobility and self-care activities. After a posterior surgical approach, dislocations tend to occur when the operated limb is adducted past midline, internally rotated, and flexed more than 90°. After an anterior approach, extreme external rotation, adduction, and extension should be avoided. To prevent dislocation, a small triangular abductor cushion may be worn between the thighs when the patient is sitting, and a thick pillow between the knees may be worn when in bed. A knee immobilizer when in bed is also effective, and for some it is less cumbersome (43). Precautions are maintained at least 12 weeks after surgery, and some surgeons continue precautions for an even more extended period (5). Dislocations can occur for reasons other than failure to observe hip precautions. Other causes include a malpositioned prosthesis, profound soft tissue weakness, trauma, and falls (5).

It may be necessary for the revision patient to wear a hip abduction orthosis with an adjustable hinge for 6 to 12 weeks. The hip abduction orthosis should seat evenly over the pelvis and allow free hip flexion up to 60° to 70° (31). Although some authors (31) suggest abducting the

M. C. Munin: Division of Physical Medicine and Rehabilitation, Department of Orthopaedic Surgery, University of Pittsburgh Medical Center, Pittsburgh, Pennsylvania 15213-3221.

P. S. Hockenberry and P. G. Flynn: Department of Physical Therapy, University of Pittsburgh Medical Center, Pittsburgh, Pennsylvania 15213-3221.

W. Toplak: Department of Occupational Therapy, University of Pittsburgh Medical Center, Pittsburgh, Pennsylvania 15213-3221.

limb 15° to 20°, it is very difficult for patients to ambulate if abduction is set more than 5° to 10°. Moreover, it is most critical to properly don the orthosis with the prosthetic hip joint positioned over the greater trochanter rather than in an internally rotated position in relation to the anatomic hip joint. Occupational therapy is important for proper donning and doffing of the orthosis without violating hip precautions.

There is a wide variation in the type of exercise that is initiated in the postoperative phase. Strickland et al. (52) observed that rehabilitation procedures appear to be largely based on local custom. Enloe et al. (14) reported that some facilities utilize only walking programs, whereas other postoperative protocols include instruction in specific exercises and functional training. A THA exercise protocol by consensus has been developed that includes quadriceps sets, gluteal sets, ankle pumps, and active hip flexion (heel slides) (14).

Several authors have advocated direct strengthening of the hip abductor muscles (3,6,14,28,44). The hip abductors maintain a level pelvis during stance phase by preventing the contralateral hip from tilting laterally during swing phase (49). Ipsilateral hip strengthening is achieved by active concentric hip abduction in a supine position (14). However, abduction exercises such as isometric hip abduction against resistance should not be included initially, especially when a trochanteric osteotomy has been performed (16,36). Resisted strengthening of the distal leg muscles can be undertaken with proper isolation. Strengthening of the contralateral hip and lower trunk stabilizers can be useful to realign forces through the joint and enhance stability (9,32,47). Vaz and colleagues (54) demonstrated a moderate correlation between hip abductor torque and distance walked during a 6-minute test. Strength of the hip abductors tended to be greater for individuals with better functional performance in the immediate postoperative period (38).

Progression to short-arc quads and straight-leg raising should occur at a later stage when partial or full weight bearing is permitted. This recommendation, based on data from a three-axis load-cell implanted in the femoral head of a single subject, showed that straight-leg raising applied a force of 1.5 to 1.8 times body weight at 16 and 31 days postoperatively (9). Placement of a bolster under the knee can minimize hip stress during terminal quadriceps extension. If pain persists with the straight-leg raise, it may be beneficial to exercise the component's hip flexion and knee extension separately (9,48).

All muscle groups, including hip flexors, extensors, and abductors, continue to show increases in strength from 6 months through 1 year postoperatively in both the operated and non-operated limbs (47,48). In one study, weakness in the hip abductors on the operated side was observed 2 years after surgery (33). In another, even the non-operated hip produced 20% less energy than a group of able-body controls (32). Although these data support

the need for a carefully monitored follow-up exercise program, clinical studies documenting the functional benefits of prolonged exercise are lacking (39).

Functional tasks encompass activities such as transfers, gait training on level and uneven surfaces, stair climbing, and lower extremity dressing. Patients are first instructed to transfer to the uninvolved side by leading with the non-operated limb both into and out of bed. Transferring is then progressed to either side of the bed because patients may be required to do this at home. With stair climbing, patients should lead with the uninvolved leg. Descending stairs, the operated limb should lead to optimize control of body weight through the uninvolved leg. When initiating transfers and other activities early after surgery, contact forces are significantly reduced by the use of upper extremity support or elevated seating surfaces (16,52).

Studies by Zavadak and colleagues (59) have shown a progression in the attainment of functional milestones after surgery. For example, transfers from a sitting to standing position, performed independently by the patient, required a mean of 5.5 physical therapy sessions. Supine-to-sit transfers and ambulation to 100 feet needed a mean of 8.1 sessions, whereas independent stair climbing was the most difficult activity, requiring a mean of 9.5 physical therapy sessions. Davy et al. (9) demonstrated that stair climbing yielded a force equivalent to 2.6 times body weight, with a significant force component out of the plane of the prosthesis, creating a torsional force on the femoral stem. With poor technique, functional activities can produce as much contact pressure as vigorous exercises (9,52).

As length of stay after surgery is decreased, patients may not be independent in functional tasks by discharge. Munin et al. (38) observed that less than 40% of total joint replacement patients were independent for basic functional tasks before discharge to home. However, more than 80% attained a supervision functional level, meaning that they could complete the maneuvers if provided with standby assistance or verbal cueing from another person. This exemplifies the need for education and family training with functional activities prior to discharge home.

CONSIDERATIONS ABOUT WEIGHT BEARING AND ASSISTIVE DEVICES

Weight-bearing restrictions prescribed by the surgeon directly impact the level of functional independence attained by discharge. In general, when a cemented femoral stem has been utilized, patients are instructed to perform partial weight bearing (PWB) for 6 weeks before advancement to full weight bearing, although some surgeons allow weight bearing as tolerated with a walker immediately. Clinically, 30% to 50% of body weight is intended by the professional recommending PWB, but studies have shown that patients have difficulty estimating percentage of body weight and sustain forces closer to 65% to 85% (1,9). For PWB, we have found that patients best understand the instruction not to exceed one half of body weight, rather than learning a specific figure such as 30% body weight. Uncemented porous ingrowth femoral stems or complicated revisions require more limited touchdown weight bearing (TDWB) for 6 to 12 weeks (20,43). TDWB should apply no more than 10% body weight and is described as walking on eggshells. TDWB is preferred over non-weight bearing (NWB), because the latter may actually create greater pressures as a result of muscle forces acting across the hip to maintain correct positioning (9,16). This is especially true in cases where the knee is maintained in extension, lengthening the lever arm (9).

There are no outcome studies supporting empiric weight-bearing restrictions that are used in common clinical practice. Weight-bearing restrictions can negatively affect the rehabilitation program. Elderly patients with impairments such as muscle weakness, balance deficits, peripheral neuropathy, and hand joint deformities may not be able to perform strict NWB or TDWB ambulation. Moreover, because gait training with restricted weight bearing is more difficult, length of stay may be prolonged. From a rehabilitation standpoint, surgical implants that permit early partial (50%) weight bearing, or weight bearing as tolerated, are preferred and surgeons should consider the functional implications in their decisions for implant selection.

Joint unloading is provided by assistive devices such as walkers, crutches, and canes. When choosing the appropriate assistive device, weight-bearing status, energy costs, strength, and other joint impairments should be considered (23,52). Walkers are usually the first choice for many THA patients, because they provide the greatest stability, increase the patient's base of support, and unload the affected leg (41). The use of a walker reduced contact forces at the hip to 1.0 times body weight during ambulation and 0.5 times body weight during double-limb stance (9,52). Rolling walkers produced higher self-selected walking speeds (13.5 m/min versus 7.5 m/min) when compared to standard walkers, although they were more difficult to manipulate over carpeted surfaces (22). The peak risks for tipping a standard walker occur in the initial loading phases and just before lift off. In the case of upper extremity pain or severe hand joint involvement from rheumatoid arthritis, platform attachments may be added to relocate damaging forces from the carpal and interphalangeal joints to the forearms. Because walkers require the use of both hands, patients may feel restricted when carrying objects and performing self-care activities. Walkers occasionally do not fit through doorways and are not recommended for use on stairs (42).

Axillary crutches allow the fastest gait and, consequently, the least stability, utilizing four-point or three-point step-to-gait patterns. Axillary crutches are appropriate for younger, more agile patients. They are inexpensive and can be used on stairs (42). Holder et al. (23) demonstrated that axillary crutches yielded better energy efficiency in NWB healthy subjects, as measured by oxygen consumption. Crutches tend to exert pressure on the axilla, which could potentially lead to nerve compression injuries if used incorrectly (41). Users of crutches also require better control of the lower leg, the ability to understand gait sequence, and better overall balance than users of walkers.

A cane functions to widen the base of support and to provide stability. Canes are not indicated when patients are limited to PWB, TDWB, or NWB conditions. Several studies have shown that individuals can load between 10% and 20% body weight onto a cane placed on the contralateral side after total hip replacement (10,13,40). This amount of force through the cane decreases ipsilateral vertical hip contact forces to 2 times body weight (4). Contralateral cane use also improves stride length, cadence, and velocity, although one study showed that ipsilateral positioning caused less mean hip joint motion (13). Canes are inexpensive, can be used on stairs, and allow a reciprocal walking pattern (42). Canes should be sized to the patient so that the crook of the handle is even with the radial styloid process, and so that the elbow is flexed to 15° to 30° (41).

Progression from one assistive device to another is dependent on numerous factors. Most patients transition easily from gait training in the parallel bars to ambulating with a walker. From that point, transition to crutches, one crutch, or a cane is dependent on the ability of the patient to maintain prescribed weight-bearing restrictions, to control the operated limb, and to be comfortable with the chosen gait aid. The physical therapist weighs these factors along with the amount of assistance required for sit-to-stand transfers and other functional tasks. Individuals with advanced age, less family support, and multiple comorbid conditions tend to progress slowly because of an increased risk of falling.

ACUTE CARE REHABILITATION

At the University of Pittsburgh Medical Center (UPMC), patients are introduced to the interdisciplinary team through preoperative teaching sessions that occur approximately 1 to 2 weeks prior to the surgical procedure. Patients meet with nurses, physical and occupational therapists, social workers, and, if necessary, nutritional consultants. They learn about the rehabilitation process, including expectations of length of stay in the hospital. At this time, patients who live alone or have several comorbid conditions are identified as high risk for requiring prolonged rehabilitation services (38). In conjunction with clinical pathways that standardize daily treatment regimens, mean length of stay at our institution and elsewhere for hip arthroplasty has been 5 days, with greater than two thirds of individuals going directly home (15).

Physical therapy is begun in the afternoon of postoperative day 1 (Table 1). Approximately 50% are able to go to the gym for strength assessments, sit-to-stand transfers, and gait training in the parallel bars. The nursing staff also place the patient in a chair twice a day for one-half hour at a time.

From postoperative day 2, the patient is scheduled in the physical therapy gym twice a day during weekdays and once a day on weekends. Several recent studies have cited the benefits of 7-day therapy in reducing length of stay; this differs from older literature (5,24,30). Transfers and gait training are advanced with respect to the patient's weight-bearing status, and strengthening exercises are continued. Ambulation progresses from simple walking on level surfaces to attempting curbs, ramps, and steps as dictated by the patient's needs. Moreover, car transfers may be started on postoperative day 4 or 5. Patients often go home in a car and need to practice this transfer while observing hip precautions. Because of the low seating level found in bucket seats, patients are advised to use cars with bench-type seating (7). Additional recommendations include sitting on a pillow to prevent hip flexion past 90° while entering the vehicle.

Patients are assessed in occupational therapy on the second postoperative day for lower-extremity dressing, bathing, and toilet transfers utilizing adaptive equipment to maintain hip precautions. Patients may be issued a raised toilet seat, extended handle reacher, leg lifter, long-handled bath sponge, hand-held shower extension, stocking cone, long-handled shoe horn, elastic shoelaces, and a device that attaches to a walker or crutches to assist in carrying items. A patient survey showed the raised toilet seat and reachers to be the most useful pieces of adaptive equipment (46). All patients receive adaptive equipment to maintain hip precautions unless they indicate that a family member will complete self-care activities for them.

GOALS UPON DISCHARGE FROM ACUTE CARE

Generalized goals for discharge home include independence with the home exercise program, adherence to hip precautions, the ability to ambulate farther than 100 feet on level indoor surfaces, and attainment of at least a supervision functional level for bed transfers, toilet transfers, and activities of daily living using adaptive equipment (5,15,24,37,38). Discharge is facilitated by the presence of strong family support and hampered if the patient lives alone and has no such resources (15,24,38).

Given the increasing pressure to discharge patients more quickly after surgery, it is important to predict whether a patient can be safely discharged home. Guide-

lines have been developed to assist surgeons in discharge decision-making (38,56). Weingarten et al. (56) developed a set of medical criteria that, if satisfied, permitted safe discharge home after the 5th postoperative day. Munin and colleagues (38) studied 162 patients prospectively to determine factors that predicted the need for inpatient rehabilitation after surgery. They found that patients transferred to an inpatient rehabilitation unit tended to live alone (51% versus 17%), were significantly older (mean age, 71.4 years versus 65.1 years), had increased comorbid conditions, and reported significantly greater pain levels as measured by daily visual analog recordings. The relationship between increased coexistent medical conditions and decreased functional outcome after hip replacement has been identified in another study (19). A two-factor logistic regression model predicted 76% of the discharges to the rehabilitation unit early after surgery, depending on whether the patient lived alone and whether the patient failed to achieve a supervision level for sit-to-stand transfers after three physical therapy sessions (38).

COMPREHENSIVE INPATIENT REHABILITATION

Comprehensive inpatient rehabilitation has been the primary setting for patients who require more than a few days of postoperative rehabilitation. Significant functional improvement, as documented by improved Functional Independence Measure scores (a validated benchmark for rehabilitation outcome), has been shown after THA (18,51). For admission into an inpatient rehabilitation unit, patients must demonstrate the need for continued skilled care, should be able to physically tolerate at least 3 hours of therapy per day, and should have a good chance of returning home within a reasonable time frame. Patients who are likely to return to a long-term-care facility are usually excluded from inpatient rehabilitation.

Comprehensive inpatient rehabilitation differs from the acute hospital by providing significantly more total therapy time, while maximizing function of the entire patient rather than solely addressing the impairments from the operated hip. In the inpatient rehabilitation unit, patients are treated twice a day in both physical and occupational therapy with 45 to 60 minutes allocated for each session. Recreational therapy is also employed to facilitate community re-entry. The inpatient rehabilitation setting provides a greater opportunity for interdisciplinary treatment in combination with intensive family training. Weekly interdisciplinary patient care conferences are held to update progress, set short-term goals, and plan all follow-up services upon discharge. Some centers foster group exercise classes or aquatic therapy programs.

Medical management is similar to the acute care setting and includes aggressive pain control, bowel and

TABLE 1. Clinical pathway for acute care after total hip arthroplasty[a]

	Day of surgery	Postop day 1	Postop day 2	Postop day 3	Postop day 4	Postop day 5
1. Assessment/evaluation: (a) Immediately postop; (b) Continued assessment	Check following systems: skin, respiration, cardiovascular, GI/GU, mental/emotional, NVS	Same	Same	Same	Same	Same
2. Activity: positioning, hip precautions, strengthening, gait, ADLs	Explain use of abduction pillow; turn every 2 hr; instruct in hip precautions	Same; OOB chair × 2 for 0.5 hr each; PT evaluation at bedside; instruct isometric exercises q 4 hr; note weight bearing status assistive devices	Same; OOB chair × 3 for 1 hr each; PT in department; OT consult	Same; independent hip precautions; OOB all meals; begin hallway ambulation; PT begins stair training; OT for ADL and assistive devices	Same; hallway ambulation with minimal assist; stair training with minimal assist; bathe in chair at sink with minimal assist	Same; independent ambulation and stairs utilizing assistive device
3. Treatments: O$_2$, incentive spirometry, SCDs, stockings, drains	Instruct/reinforce O$_2$ as needed, I.S. q 4 hr while awake, SCD/TED hose; monitor drainage	Same; check dressing q 4 hr; D/C O$_2$	Same; D/C drain; wound check	Same	Same; change dressing q day	Same
4. Pain management	Assess pain level q 4 hr; assess effectiveness of epidural, PCA, IM injection	Same	Same	Same; wean to PO analgesics	Same	Same
5. Medications: anticoagulant (coumadin); antibiotics	Give coumadin as ordered at 6 PM, qd PT/INR draw 7 AM; IV antibiotics and fluids as ordered	Same	Same	Same	Same	Same
6. Tests	AP hip x-ray in PACU	Hb & Hct	Hb & Hct	Hb & Hct	Venous Doppler scan done in late afternoon	AP pelvis/lateral oblique hip
7. Bladder function	I&O q 8 hr; Foley catheter	Same; D/C Foley	Same; straight catheterize q 8 hr. prn if no void	Same	Same	Same
8. Bowel elimination	Check status; offer bedpan q 4 hr	Same	Same; offer laxative prn; bedside commode; bathroom privileges	Same	Same; if no BM, Dulcolax or Fleets Enema	Same
9. Consults: preop clearance, Physical Medicine and Rehabilitation	Note consultant's assessment, ensure timeliness of consult; review recommendations	Same	Same	Same	Same	Same
10. Discharge plan: Social Service consult	Review preop assessment	Discuss rehab choice, home care needs	Plan home care program	Instruct patient about wound care, symptoms of infection, medications	Same	Discharge instructions reviewed; written instructions given to patient and family

[a]Used at the University of Pittsburgh Medical Center.

Postop, postoperative; preop, preoperative; GI, gastrointestinal; GU, genitourinary; NVS, nervous system; ADL, activities of daily living; OOB, out of bed; OT, occupational therapy; PT, physical therapy; SCD, Sequential Compression Device; TED, thromboembolic disease; I.S. incentive spirometry; PCA, patient-controlled analgesia; PACU, Post Anesthesia Care Unit; D/C, discontinue; PT/INR, prothrombin time/international normalized ratio; IM, intramuscular; IV, intravenous; PO, by mouth; I&O, intake and output; BM, bowel movement; Hb, hemoglobin; Hct, hematocrit; qd, every; q, every; qd, every day; prn, as needed.

bladder management, deep vein thrombosis prophylaxis, and monitoring of overall health status, especially comorbid illnesses such as neurologic disorders or cardiopulmonary disease. Nursing is very important to carry over tasks learned in therapy and to prevent secondary disability from decubitus ulcers, which can occur over the calcanei by prolonged supine lying. Most individuals receive a psychology assessment to help with adjustment after surgery, they are provided relaxation training in cases of extreme pain or anxiety, and they are screened for psychiatric disease such as depression or dementia. At times, a home visit may be necessary to problem-solve environmental barriers such as a narrowly positioned toilet or bathroom doorway. A typical clinical pathway is listed in Table 2.

REHABILITATION ALTERNATIVES AND COST-EFFECTIVENESS

Managed care networks and other health-care initiatives have caused significant changes in the delivery of health-care services based on cost considerations. Subacute or nursing home rehabilitation has grown as an alternative to comprehensive inpatient rehabilitation, because it offers a less expensive daily charge by utilizing 1 hour of therapy per day (21). Patients who are placed in subacute rehabilitation generally can not withstand the 3 hours per day therapy requirements of an inpatient rehabilitation program and are at a low risk for medical instability. Subacute rehabilitation was developed as a complement to inpatient rehabilitation; however, it is now being used more as a substitute in certain regions (45).

Outcome studies are needed to determine the most cost-effective approach for patients who can not go home after surgery. To date, there have been very few studies attempting to compare comprehensive inpatient rehabilitation and subacute rehabilitation (26). We have prospectively examined whether high-risk patients unable to go home after surgery can tolerate comprehensive inpatient rehabilitation early after surgery. Our preliminary data demonstrated that high-risk patients had improved short-term functional outcome and reduced total cost when inpatient rehabilitation was begun on postoperative day 3 as compared to patients transferred to inpatient rehabilitation on postoperative day 7 (MC Munin, personal correspondence, 1997). The area of cost-effectiveness and functional outcomes requires much more intensive research to develop appropriate clinical pathways after hip arthroplasty.

REHABILITATION AT HOME

The continuation of therapy from the hospital to the home environment can be important to ensure safety and carryover of learned information. Strategies for maneuvering specific barriers in the home setting, such as a bed located on the second floor or a staircase without handrails, can be developed. General goals for home therapy include (a) decreased pain, (b) increased range of motion of the involved hip, (c) increased strength, (d) progression to a cane or independent ambulation as appropriate, and (e) increased access to the community. For more agile and active patients, an outpatient therapy program may be more appropriate to attain rehabilitation goals.

Resumption of recreational activities after THA is important to an individual's self-worth. Conventional wisdom dictates that patients who have undergone THA should avoid high-impact activities such as running, water-skiing, football, basketball, handball, karate, soccer, and racquetball (8,12,55). Several studies have noted that high-impact activities have contributed to decreased longevity of the hip endoprosthesis (8,11). Kilgus et al. (27) observed that patients who participated in sporting activities or heavy labor were at twice the risk of revision than less active patients.

A survey of 28 orthopedic surgeons at the Mayo Clinic regarding appropriate sporting activities after THA revealed that sailing, swimming, scuba diving, cycling, and golf were most recommended (35). Visuri and Honkanen (55) found similar results with an increased percentage participating in walking, swimming, cycling, and cross-country skiing. Tennis was not one of the recommended sports, but doubles tennis was favored over singles tennis (35). One patient was noted to play tennis with bilateral hip arthroplasties over 14 years on sand or clay surfaces, which absorb friction better than hard court surfaces (12). Social dancing is permitted if hip precautions are observed and if vigorous dancing is avoided (7).

Driving ability, as measured by right foot brake reaction tests, is affected to a greater extent after right THA than after left (34). Some patients with right THA may not recover sufficient hip function to return to driving at 2 months after surgery, even though other aspects of rehabilitation appear normal (34). For certain patients, driving reactions should be formally tested in occupational therapy and, in most cases, patients may resume driving when they are comfortable in the seated position at approximately 8 weeks after the procedure (5,34).

Difficulties with sexual intercourse have been reported in 75% of patients preoperatively and in 40% postoperatively (53). After THA, sexual activity can safely resume between 1 and 2 months after an uncomplicated arthroplasty (50). Women report supine positioning or side-lying on the uninvolved side to be more comfortable, whereas men find the supine position most comfortable (50). Patients should be advised to play a more passive role in the first few weeks. Men can assume the more traditional prone orientation 2 to 3 months after surgery. Pillows can be used to position the operated leg to maintain hip precautions by preventing excessive hip internal rota-

TABLE 2. *Clinical pathway for inpatient rehabilitation after total hip arthroplasty[a]*

	Preadmission	Day 1 (admission)	Day 2	Day 3	Day 4	Day 5	Day 6	Day 7
1. Consults	Physical Medicine and Rehabilitation, Utilization Review	PT, OT, Social Service, home care; notify orthopedic surgeon	Recreational Therapy and Neuropsychology evaluations	—	—	—	—	—
2. Tests	—	CBC, PT/INR if on coumadin, EKG (copy prior tracing), urinalysis (if not recently obtained)	—	PT/INR if indicated	—	—	PT/INR if indicated	—
3. Treatments	—	Thigh-high TED stockings, dry dressing; ice applied to hip pm pain; SCDs while patient <5 days postop	Same; PT and OT therapies, each 2× per day	Same; recreational therapy 1× per day; Neuropsychology if indicated	Same	Same; community living skills group	Same	Same; wear elastic stockings until 4 wk postop
4. Medications	—	Current medications; oral analgesics 0.5 hr prior to AM and PM therapies; anticoagulant; bowel program	Same	Same	Same	Same	Same	Same
5. Nutrition		Diet as indicated	Same	Same	Same	Same	Same	Same
6. Activity and safety	Review performance in acute care therapies; assess potential for rehabilitation	Hip precautions; weight bearing as ordered; pillow between legs in bed; ambulation and transfers in room with assistance per PT evaluation; bathroom privileges	Same	Same; ambulate 20 ft to bathroom and hallway with supervision prn; self-care and dressing with adaptive equipment	Same; ambulate to 1 meal to dining room	Same; ambulate to 2 meals to dining room	Same; ambulate all meals to dining room	Same; modified independent level with ambulation, transfers, and self-care
7. Assessment	Review performance in acute care therapies; assess potential for rehabilitation	Decubiti risk assessment; vitals per routine; wound check assess pain management; document last BM	Same	Same	Same	Same	Same; understand PT/OT instructions; complete car transfer	Same
8. Discharge planning	—	Assess and review of discharge destination	Review home environment, caregivers, and equipment needs	Schedule family training if indicated	Plan discharge transportation	Identify home equipment needs, arrange home care including nursing, PT, and O.T. as indicated	Same; order home equipment; arrange physician follow-up; inform patient/family of details	Same; confirm discharge plans; answer patient questions; discharge to home if goals met
9. Psychol/social	—	Family support; coping skills	Same	Same; observe readiness for discharge	Same	Same	Evaluate readiness for discharge	—
10. Patient education	Introduction to Rehab Unit routines and philosophy by admissions coordinator	Orient to unit; review safety and hip precautions	Review treatment rationale, rehab goals, pain management, hip precautions, wound infection	Same	Same; teach home exercise program, review hip precautions	Family training if indicated; review medications, drug interactions, home exercises, hip precautions	Same	Same

[a]Used at the Inpatient Rehabilitation Unit at the University of Pittsburgh Medical Center.
See Table 1 for abbreviations; CBC, complete blood cell count; PT/INR, prothrombin time/international normalized ratio; EKG, electrocardiogram.

tion and adduction. Kneeling should be avoided for any activity for 3 to 4 months following surgery (58). It should also be noted that most patients wished to be provided with more information on this topic but were too uncomfortable to request additional information from their surgeon (50).

REFERENCES

1. Baxter ML, Allington BA, Koepke GH. Weight-distribution variables in the use of crutches and canes. *Phys Ther* 1969;49:360–365.
2. Bayley KB, London MR, Grunkemeier GL, et al. Measuring the success of treatment in patient terms. *Med Care* 1995;33:AS226–235.
3. Beber CA, Convery FR. Management of patients with total hip replacement. *Phys Ther* 1972;52:823–828.
4. Brand RA, Crowninshield RD. The effect of cane use on hip contact force. *Clin Orthop* 1980;147:181–184.
5. Brander VA, Stulberg SD, Chang RW. Rehabilitation following hip and knee arthroplasty. *Phys Med Rehabil Clin North Am* 1994;5:815–836.
6. Burton DS, Imrie SH. Total hip arthroplasty and postoperative rehabilitation. *Phys Ther* 1973;53:132–140.
7. Carpenter ES. *Information for our patients: total hip joint replacement.* rev. ed. Professional Staff Association, Rancho Los Amigos Hospital, Downey, CA; 1979.
8. Chandler HP, Reineck FT, Wixson RL, et al. Total hip replacement in patients younger than thirty years old. *J Bone Joint Surg* 1981;63A: 1426–1444.
9. Davy DT, Kotzar GM, Brown RH, et al. Telemetric force measurements across the hip and after total arthroplasty. *J Bone Joint Surg* 1988;70A: 45–50.
10. Deathe AB, Hayes KC, Winter DA. The biomechanics of canes, crutches, and walkers. *Crit Rev Phys Rehabil Med* 1993;5:15–29.
11. Dorr LD, Takei GK, Conaty JP. Total hip arthroplasties in patients less than forty-five years old. *J Bone Joint Surg* 1983;65A;474–479.
12. Dubs L, Geschwind N, Munzinger U. Sport after total hip arthroplasty. *Arch Orthop Trauma Surg* 1983;101:161–169.
13. Edwards BG. Contralateral and ipsilateral cane usage by patients with total knee or hip replacement. *Arch Phys Med Rehabil* 1986;67:734–740.
14. Enloe LJ, Shields RK, Smith K, et al. Total hip and knee replacement treatment programs: a report using consensus. *J Orthop Sports Phys Ther* 1996;23:3–11.
15. Erickson B, Perkins M. Interdisciplinary team approach in the rehabilitation of hip and knee arthroplasties. *Am J Occup Ther* 1994;48:439–445.
16. Givens-Heiss DL, Krebs DE, Riley PO, et al. In vivo acetabular contact pressures during rehabilitation, part II: postacute phase. *Phys Ther* 199272:700–705.
17. Gogia PP, Christensen CM, Schmidt C. Total hip replacement in patients with osteoarthritis of the hip: improvement in pain and functional status. *Orthopedics* 1994;17:145–150.
18. Granger CV, Ottenbacher KJ, Fiedler RC. The uniform data system for medical rehabilitation. *Am J Phys Med Rehabil* 1995;74:62–66.
19. Greenfield S, Apolone G, McNeil BJ, et al. The importance of co-existent disease in the occurrence of postoperative complications and one-year recovery in patients undergoing total hip replacement: comorbidity and outcomes after hip replacement. *Med Care* 1993;31:141–154.
20. Haddad RJ, Look SD, Thomas KA. Biological fixation of porous-coated implants. *J Bone Joint Surg* 1987;69A:1459–1466.
21. Haffey WJ, Welsh JH. Subacute care: evolution in search of value. *Arch Phys Med Rehabil* 1995;76:SC2–4.
22. Hamzeh MA, Bowkar P, Sayegh A. The energy costs of ambulation using two types of walking frame. *Clin Rehabil* 1988;2:119–123.
23. Holder CG, Haskvitz EM, Weltman A. The effects of assistive devices on the oxygen cost, cardiovascular stress, and perception of nonweight-bearing ambulation. *J Orthop Sports Phys Ther* 1993;18:537–542.
24. Hughes K, Kuffner L, Dean B. Effect of weekend physical therapy on postoperative length of stay following total hip and total knee arthroplasty. *Physiother Canada* 1993;45:245–249.
25. Katz JN, Wright EA, Guadagnoli E, et al. Differences between men and women undergoing major orthopedic surgery for degenerative arthritis. *Arthritis Rheum* 1994;37:687–694.
26. Keith RA, Wilson DB, Gutierrez P. Acute and subacute rehabilitation for stroke: a comparison. *Arch Phys Med Rehabil* 1995; 76:495–500.
27. Kilgus DJ, Dorey FJ, Finerman GAM, et al. Patient activity, sports participation, and impact loading on the durability of cemented total hip replacements. *Clin Orthop* 1991;269:25–31.
28. Kisner C, Colby LA. *Therapeutic exercise: foundations and techniques.* Philadelphia: FA Davis, 1985;343–347.
29. Liang MH, Cullen KE, Larson MG, et al. Cost-effectiveness of total joint arthroplasty in osteoarthritis. *Arthritis Rheum* 1986;29:937–943.
30. Liang MH, Cullen KE, Larson MG, et al. Effects of reducing physical therapy services on outcomes in total joint arthroplasty. *Med Care* 1987;25:276–285.
31. Lima D, Magnus R, Paprosky WG. Team management of hip revision patients using a post-op hip orthosis. *J Prosthet Orthop* 1994;6:20–24.
32. Loizeau J, Allard P, Duhaime M, et al. Bilateral gait patterns in subjects fitted with a total hip prosthesis. *Arch Phys Med Rehabil* 1995;76: 552–557.
33. Long WT, Dorr LD, Healy B, et al. Functional recovery of noncemented total hip arthroplasty. *Clin Orthop* 1993;288:73–77.
34. Macdonald W, Owen JW. The effect of total hip replacement on driving reactions. *J Bone Joint Surg* 1988;70B:202–205.
35. McGrorey BJ, Stuart MJ, Sim FH. Participation in sports after hip and knee arthroplasty: review of literature and survey of surgeon preferences. *Mayo Clin Proc* 1995;70:342–348.
36. Minns RJ, Crawford RJ, Porter ML, et al. Muscle strength following total hip arthroplasty: a comparison of trochanteric osteotomy and the direct lateral approach. *J Arthroplasty* 1993;8:625–627.
37. Möller G, Goldie I, Jonsson E. Hospital care versus home care for rehabilitation after hip replacement. *Int J Technol Assess Health Care* 1992; 8:93–101.
38. Munin MC, Kwoh CK, Glynn NW, et al. Predicting discharge outcome after elective hip and knee arthroplasty. *Am J Phys Med Rehabil* 1995;74:294–301.
39. National Institutes of Health. Total hip replacement. *NIH Consens Statement* Sep 12–14, 1994;12:1–31.
40. Opila KA, Nicol AC, Paul JP. Forces and impulses during aided gait. *Arch Phys Med Rehabil* 1987;68:715–722.
41. O Sullivan SB, Schmitz TJ. *Physical rehabilitation: asessment and treatment,* 2nd ed. Philadelphia: FA Davis, 1988;293–300.
42. Palmer ML, Toms JE. *Manual for functional training,* 3rd ed. Philadelphia: FA Davis, 1992;119–128.
43. Rao JP, Bronstein R. Dislocations following arthroplasties of the hip: incidence, prevention, and treatment. *Orthop Rev* 1991;20:261–264.
44. Richardson RW. Physical therapy management of patients undergoing total hip replacement. *Phys Ther* 1975;55:984–990.
45. Salcido R, Moore RW. Acute and subacute rehabilitation (letter). *Arch Phys Med Rehabil* 1996;77:100–101.
46. Seeger M, Fisher L. Adaptive equipment used in the rehabilitation of hip arthroplasty patients. *Am J Occup Ther* 1982;36:503–508.
47. Shih CH, Du YK, Lin YH, et al. Muscular recovery around the hip joint after total hip arthroplasty. *Clin Orthop* 1994;302:115–120.
48. Smidt WR, Clark C, Smidt GL, et al. Short-term strength and pain changes in total hip arthroplasty patients. *J Orthoped Sports Phys Ther* 1990;12:16–23.
49. Soderberg GL. *Kinesiology: applications to pathological motion.* Baltimore: Williams & Wilkins, 1986;183–185.
50. Stern SH, Fuchs MD, Ganz SB, et al. Sexual function after total hip arthroplasty. *Clin Orthop* 1991;269:228–235.
51. Stineman MG, Hamilton BB, Goin JE, et al. Functional gain and length of stay for major rehabilitation impairment categories. *Am J Phys Med Rehabil* 1996;75:68–78.
52. Strickland EM, Fares M, Krebs DE, et al. In vivo acetabular contact pressures during rehabilitation, part I: acute phase. *Phys Ther* 1992;72: 691–699.
53. Todd RC, Lightowler CDR, Harris J. Low friction arthroplasty of the hip joint and sexual activity. *Acta Orthop Scand* 1973;44:690–693.
54. Vaz MD, Kramer JF, Rorabeck CH, et al. Isometric hip abductor strength following total hip replacement and its relationship to functional assessments. *J Orthop Sports Phys Ther* 1993;18:526–531.
55. Visuri T, Honkanen R. Total hip replacement: its influence on spontaneous recreation exercise habits. *Arch Phys Med Rehabil* 1980;61: 325–328.
56. Weingarten S, Riedinger M, Conner L, et al. Hip replacement and hip

hemiarthroplasty surgery: potential opportunities to shorten lengths of hospital stay. *Am J Med* 1994;97:208–213.

57. Williams-Russo P, Sharrock NE, Mattis S, et al. Cognitive effects after epidural versus general anesthesia in older adults. *J Am Med Assoc* 1995;274:44–50.

58. Yoslow W, Simeone J, Huestis D. Hip replacement rehabilitation. *Arch Phys Med Rehabil* 1976;57:275–278.

59. Zavadak KH, Gibson KR, Whitley DM, et al. Variability in the obtainment of functional milestones during the acute care admission after total joint replacement. *J Rheumatol* 1995;22:482–487.

Subject Index

Subject Index

Note: Page numbers followed by f indicate figures; those followed by t indicate tables.